Fundamentals of

SURGERY

Fundamentals of
SURGERY

First Edition

Edited by

John E. Niederhuber, MD
Professor of Surgery and Oncology
   and Director, University of Wisconsin
   Comprehensive Cancer Center
University of Wisconsin Medical School
Madison, Wisconsin

Formerly
Chair, Department of Surgery
Stanford University School of Medicine
Stanford, California

With the Assistance of

Shireen L. Dunwoody
Senior Editorial Coordinator
Department of Surgery
Stanford University School of Medicine
Stanford, California

APPLETON & LANGE
Stamford, Connecticut

Notice: The authors and the publisher of this volume have taken care to make certain that the doses of drugs and schedules of treatment are correct and compatible with the standards generally accepted at the time of publication. Nevertheless, as new information becomes available, changes in treatment and in the use of drugs become necessary. The reader is advised to carefully consult the instruction and information material included in the package insert of each drug or therapeutic agent before administration. This advice is especially important when using, administering, or recommending new or infrequently used drugs. The authors and publisher disclaim all responsibility for any liability, loss, injury, or damage incurred as a consequence, directly or indirectly, of the use and application of any of the contents of this volume.

Copyright © 1998 by Appleton & Lange
A Simon & Schuster Company

All rights reserved. This book, or any parts thereof, may not be used or reproduced in any manner without written permission. For information, address Appleton & Lange, Four Stamford Plaza, PO Box 120041, Stamford, Connecticut 06912–0041

98 99 00 00 01 02 / 10 9 8 7 6 5 4 3 2 1

Prentice Hall International (UK) Limited, *London*
Prentice Hall of Australia Pty. Limited, *Sydney*
Prentice Hall Canada, Inc., *Toronto*
Prentice Hall Hispanoamericana, S.A., *Mexico*
Prentice Hall of India Private Limited, *New Delhi*
Prentice Hall of Japan, Inc., *Tokyo*
Simon & Schuster Asia Pte. Ltd., *Singapore*
Editora Prentice Hall do Brasil Ltda., *Rio de Janeiro*
Prentice Hall, *Upper Saddle River, New Jersey*

ISBN 0–8385–0509–0
ISSN 1096

Acquisitions Editor: Shelley Reinhardt
Development Editor: Cara Lyn Coffey
Production Editor: Sondra Greenfield
Senior Art Manager: Eve Siegel
Designer: Mary Skudlarek
Cover illustration: *Improvisation: The Deluge* by Wassily Kandinsky

PRINTED IN THE UNITED STATES OF AMERICA

ISBN 0-8385-0509-0

90000

9 780838 505090

Contents

Authors

Edward J. Alfrey, MD
Assistant Professor of Surgery, Department of Surgery, Stanford University School of Medicine, Stanford, California
Internet: ealfrey@leland.stanford.edu
Transplant Immunology; Transplant Immunopharmacology

Kayvan Ariani, MD
Fellow in Pain Management, Stanford University Medical Center, Stanford, California
The Management of Perioperative Pain & Anxiety

J. Augusto Bastidas, MD
Department of Surgery, Stanford University School of Medicine, Stanford, California
The Stomach, Small Intestine, & Appendix; The Pancreas

Ramin E. Beygui, MD
Fellow, Vascular Surgery, Stanford University Medical Center, Stanford, California
Cerebrovascular Occlusive Disease; Peripheral Vascular Occlusive Disease

Robyn L. Birdwell, MD
Assistant Professor of Radiology, Stanford University School of Medicine, Stanford, California
Internet: robyn. birdwell@forsythe.stanford.edu
The Breast

Henry Brem, MD
Professor of Neurosurgery and Oncology; Director, Neurosurgical Oncology, Johns Hopkins University School of Medicine, Baltimore, Maryland
Neurosurgery

Jay B. Brodsky, MD
Professor of Anesthesiology; Medical Director of Postanesthesia Care Unit, Stanford University Medical Center, Stanford, California
Internet: jbrodsky@leland.standord.edu
Recovery Room Care

Jimmy J. Brown, DDS, MD
Assistant Professor, Drew University of Medicine and Science, Los Angeles, California
Internet: jibrown@crewu.edu
Emergency Airway Management; The Head & Neck

Thomas A. Burdon, MD
Assistant Professor of Cardiothoracic Surgery, Stanford University School of Medicine; Chief, Surgical Services, Veteran's Administration Health Care System, Palo Alto, California
Internet: sfwv46a@prodigy.com
Acquired Disease of the Heart

Sharon Butler, RN, BSN, MSN
Staff Nurse, Stanford University Hospital, Stanford, California
Internet: butler_s.@hosp.stanford.edu
Operating Room Setup & Basics of Sterile Technique

Helen Collins, MD
Acting Assistant Professor, Stanford University School of Medicine, Stanford, California
Internet: hlcollins@aol.com
Principles of Chemotherapy

Waldo Concepcion, MD
Assistant Professor of Surgery, Stanford University School of Medicine, Stanford, California
Internet: concepcion_w@hosp.stanford.edu
Liver Transplantation

Donald C. Dafoe, MD
Associate Professor, Department of Surgery, Chief, Division of Transplant Surgery, Stanford University School of Medicine, Stanford, California
Historical Perspectives; Pancreas Transplantation; Intestinal Transplantation

Ronald L. Dalman, MD
Assistant Professor, Division of Vascular Surgery, Department of Surgery, Stanford University School of Medicine, Stanford; Chief, Vascular Surgery, Surgical Service, Veterans Affairs Palo Alto Health Care System, Palo Alto, California
Internet: mu.rad@forsythe.stanford.edu
Evaluation of Patients With Vascular Disease; Peripheral Vascular Occlusive Disease

John M. Daly, MD, FACS
Lewis Atterbury Stimson Professor and Chairman, Department of Surgery, The New York Hospital-Cornell Medical Center, New York, New York
Internet: jmdaly@mail.med.cornell.edu
Nutritional Support

Carlos O. Esquivel, MD, PhD
Professor of Surgery; Director of Liver Transplant Program, Stanford University School of Medicine, Stanford, California
Internet: esquivel_c@hosp.stanford.edu
Liver Transplantation

C. Garrison Fathman, MD
Professor of Medicine and Chair, Department of Immunology and Rheumatology, Stanford University School of Medicine, Stanford; Director for the Center for Clinical Immunology at Stanford (CCIS), Stanford, California
Transplant Immunology

Willard E. Fee, Jr, MD
Edward G. & Amy H. Sewall Professor and Chairman, Stanford University School of Medicine, Stanford, California
Internet: wfee@leland.stanford.edu
Emergency Airway Management; The Head & Neck

Stephen P. Fischer, MD
Assistant Professor of Anesthesia; Medical Director, Anesthesia Preoperative Evaluation Program, Department of Anesthesia, Stanford University School of Medicine, Stanford, California
Medical Assessment of the Surgical Patient

Raymond R. Gaeta, MD
Assistant Professor of Anesthesia; Director, Pain Management Center, Stanford University School of Medicine, Stanford, California
Internet: gaeta@leland.stanford.edu
The Management of Perioperative Pain & Anxiety

Susan Galel, MD
Assistant Professor of Pathology, Stanford University School of Medicine, Stanford, California
Internet: galel_s@hosp.stanford.edu
Transfusions & Blood Component Therapy

Maritza Gonzalez, MD
Staff Physician and Clinical Assistant; Professor of Pathology, Stanford University School of Medicine, Stanford, California
Internet: mx.mxg@forsythe.stanford.edu
Transfusions & Blood Component Therapy

F. Carl Grumet, MD
Professor of Pathology, Stanford University School of Medicine, Stanford, California
Internet: mm.fcg@forsythe.stanford.edu
Transfusions & Blood Component Therapy

E. John Harris, Jr, MD
Assistant Professor of Surgery, Stanford University School of Medicine, Stanford, California
Internet: mu.ejh@forsythe.stanford.edu
Venous Disorders

Edmund J. Harris, Sr, MD
Clinical Professor of Surgery, Stanford Health Services, Department of Surgery, Division of Vascular Surgery, Stanford, California
Venous Disorders

Richard F. Heitmiller, MD
Associate Professor of Surgery and Oncology; Chief, Division of Thoracic Surgery, Johns Hopkins Hospital, Baltimore, Maryland
Pulmonary Diseases; Chest Wall & Pleural Disease; Lung Cancer

Danny O. Jacobs, MD
Associate Professor of Surgery, Harvard Medical School; Associate Surgeon, Department of Surgery, Brigham & Women's Hospital, Boston, Massachusetts
Internet: dojacobs@bics.bwh.harvard.edu
The Esophagus

R. Brooke Jeffrey, Jr, MD
Professor of Radiology, Stanford University School of Medicine, Stanford; Chief of Abdominal Imaging, Department of Radiology, Stanford University Medical Center, Stanford, California
Internet: ma.rbj@forsythe.stanford.edu
Imaging the Surgical Patient

Stefanie S. Jeffrey, MD
Assistant Professor of Surgery; Chief of Breast Surgery, Division of Surgical Oncology, Stanford University School of Medicine, Stanford, California
Internet: ah.ssj@forsythe.stanford.edu
The Breast

Nancy Krieger, MD
Resident in General Surgery, Stanford University Medical Center, Stanford, California
Internet: nrk@leland.stanford.edu
Transplant Immunology

Dainis K. Krievins, MD
Research Fellow, Stanford University School of Medicine, Stanford, California
Internet: cdm@com.latnet.lv
Aneurysms

Michael D. Lieberman, MD
Assistant Professor of Surgery, Cornell University Medical College, New York, New York
Nutritional Support

Yuan-Chi Lin, MD, MPH
Assistant Professor of Anesthesia and Pediatrics, Stanford University School of Medicine, Stanford, California
Internet: yclin@leland.stanford.edu
Anesthesia Principles

Jeffrey R. Lukish, MD
Chief Surgery Resident, National Naval Medical Center, Bethesda, Maryland
Pediatric Surgery

Paul N. Manson, MD
Professor and Chief, Plastic Reconstructive and Maxillofacial Surgery, Johns Hopkins School of Medicine, Baltimore, Maryland
Internet: pmans@welchlink,welch.jhu.edu
Plastic Surgery

Lori J. Morgan, MD
Assistant Professor, University of Iowa Hospitals and Clinics, Iowa City, Iowa
Internet: ljmorgan@worldnet.att.com
Fluids, Electrolytes & Acid-Base Balance

Randall E. Morris, MD
Research Professor and Director, Transplantation Immunology, Department of Cardiothoracic Surgery; Stanford University School of Medicine, Stanford, California
Transplant in Immunopharmacology

David W. Mozingo, MD
Associate Professor of Surgery and Anesthesiology, University of Florida College of Medicine, Gainesville; Director, Shands Burn Center at the University of Florida, Gainesville, Florida
Internet: mozingo@surgery.ufl.edu
Burn Trauma & Surgery

Kurt D. Newman, MD
Professor of Surgery and Pediatrics, George Washington University Medical School, Washington, DC; Vice Chairman, Department of Pediatric Surgery, Children's Hospital, Washington, DC
Pediatric Surgery

Camran R. Nezhat, MD
Clinical Professor of Surgery, Clinical Professor of Obstetrics and Gynecology, Stanford University School of Medicine, Stanford; Director, Stanford Endoscopy Center for Training and Technology, Stanford, California; Clinical Professor of Obstetrics and Gynecology, Mercer University School of Medicine, Macon, Georgia; Director, Center for Special Pelvic Surgery, Atlanta, Georgia
Internet: cnezhat@leland.stanford.edu
Laparoscopic Surgery

Ceana H. Nezhat, MD
Clinical Assistant Professor of Obstetrics and Gynecology, Stanford University School of Medicine, Stanford; Co-Director, Stanford Endoscopy Center for Training and Technology, Stanford, California; Clinical Associate Professor of Obstetrics and Gynecology, Mercer University School of Medicine, Macon, Georgia; Director, Center for Special Pelvic Surgery, Atlanta, Georgia
Internet: yjqs41a@prodigy.com
Laparoscopic Surgery

Farr R. Nezhat, MD
Clinical Professor of Obstetrics and Gynecology, Mercer University, Macon, Georgia ; Clinical Professor of OB/GYN, Stanford University Medical Center, Stanford; Co-Director, Stanford Endoscopy Center, Stanford, California
Internet: cnezhat@lelend.stanford.edu
Laparoscopic Surgery

Ronald Lee Nichols, MD, MS, FACS
William Henderson Professor of Surgery; Professor of Microbiology and Immunology, Tulane University School of Medicine, New Orleans, Louisiana
Internet: rnichol1host.tcs.tulane.edu
Surgical Infections and Antibiotics

John E. Niederhuber, MD
Professor of Surgery and Oncology, and Director, University of Wisconsin Comprehensive Cancer Center, University of Wisconsin Medical School, Madison. Formerly: Chair, Department of Surgery, Stanford University School of Medicine, Stanford, California
Internet: niederhu@biostat.wisc.edu
The Surgery Service & Surgery Training; Incisions, Wound Closures, & the Healing Process; Basic Technical Procedures; Fluids, Electrolytes & Acid Base Balance; Chronic Vascular Access; The Liver; The Biliary System; The Pancreas; Soft Tissue Sarcomas

David Oakes, MD
Associate Professor of Surgery, Stanford University School of Medicine, Stanford, California
Hernias

Harry A. Oberhelman, Jr, MD
Professor and Chief of Gastrointestinal Surgery, Stanford University School of Medicine, Stanford, California
Internet: hf.jmh@forsythe.stanford.edu
The Stomach, Small Intestine, and Appendix

Cornelius Olcott IV, MD
Professor of Surgery, Stanford University Medical Center, Stanford, California
Internet: hf.wgw@forsythe.stanford.edu
Renovascular Hypertension & Mesenteric Ischemia (Visceral Artery Disease)

Glen S. O'Sullivan, MD
Assistant Professor, Functional Restoration (Orthopaedics), Stanford University Medical Center, Stanford, California
Internet: ml.gso@forsythe.stanford.edu
Orthopedic Surgery

Hee Wan Park, MD, PhD
Postdoctoral Scholar, Division of Otolaryngology, Head and Neck Surgery, Stanford University School of Medicine, Stanford, California; Chief of Head and Neck Surgery, Kwang Ju Christial Hospital, Kwang Ju, Korea
The Head & Neck

Joseph C. Poen, MD
Assistant Professor, Department of Radiation Oncology, Stanford University Medical Center, Stanford, California
Principles of Radiotherapy

Basil A. Pruitt, Jr, MD
Professor of Surgery, Department of Surgery, University of Texas Health Science Center at San Antonio, San Antonio, Texas
Internet: jtrauma@uthscs.edu
Burn Trauma & Surgery

Bruce A. Reitz, MD
The Norman E. Shumway Professor and Chairman, Department of Cardiothoracic Surgery, Stanford University School of Medicine, Stanford, California
Internet: breitz@leland.stanford.edu
Congenital Disease of the Heart; Cardiac Transplantation; Lung & Combined Heart-Lung Transplantation

Robert C. Robbins, MD
Assistant Professor, Department of Cardiothoracic Surgery, Stanford University School of Medicine, Stanford, California
Internet: robbins@leland.stanford.edu
Congenital Disease of the Heart

John A. Rock, MD
James Robert McCord Professor and Chairman, Department of Gynecology and Obstetrics, Emory University School of Medicine, Atlanta, Georgia
Gynecologic Surgery

Myer Rosenthal, MD
Professor of Anesthesia, Medicine and Surgery Program Director of Critical Care Anesthesiology, Stanford University School of Medicine, Stanford, California
Internet: mhr@leland.stanford.edu
Emergency Airway Management

Jeffrey P. Salomone, MD
Assistant Professor of Surgery, Emory University School of Medicine, Atlanta, Georgia
Surgical Infections and Antibiotics

Oscar Salvatierra, Jr, MD
Professor of Surgery and Pediatrics and Director, Pediatric Renal Transplantation, Stanford University Medical Center, Stanford, California
Kidney Transplantation

Daniel S. Seidman, MD
Department of Obstetrics and Gynecology, Sheba Medical Center, Tel-Hashomer and Sackler School of Medicine, Tel-Aviv University, Israel
Internet: dannys@leland.stanford.edu
Laparoscopic Surgery

Adam Seiver, MD
Acting Chief, Surgical Medical Care, Stanford University School of Medicine, Stanford, California
Basic Considerations in Critical Care; Shock & Resuscitation; Multiple Organ Dysfunction Syndrome

Samuel K. S. So, MD
Associate Professor of Surgery; Associate Director, Liver Transplant Program, Stanford University School of Medicine, Stanford, California
Liver Transplantation

Donald R. Stanski, MD
Professor and Chairman, Department of Anesthesia, Stanford University School of Medicine, Stanford, California
Internet: dstanski@leland.Stanford.edu
Anesthesia Principles

Gary D. Steinberg, MD
Assistant Professor of Surgery/Urology, Pritzker School of Medicine, The University of Chicago, Chicago, Illinois
Internet: gsteinbe@surgery.bsd.uchicago.edu
Urologic Surgery

Frank E. Stockdale, MD, PhD
Maureen Lyles D'Ambrogio Professor of Medicine; Chief, Comprehensive Breast Clinic, Stanford University School of Medicine, Stanford, California
Internet: ml.fes@forsythe.stanford.edu
The Breast

James M. Stone, MD
Private Practice, Northern California Surgical Group, Redding, California
Internet: jmstone@e_zone.net
Surgical Endoscopy; The Colon, Rectum, & Anus

Alan Ting, PhD
Associate Professor of Pathology; Co-Director of Stanford Histocompatibility Laboratory, Stanford University School of Medicine, Stanford, California
Internet: alan.ting@forsythe.stanford.edu
HLA & Histocompatibility Testing

Chris Traver, MD
Attending Trauma Surgeon, San Jose Medical Center, San Jose, California
Basic Technical Procedures

Mark Vierra, MD
Assistant Professor of Surgery, Department of Surgery, Stanford University Medical Center, Stanford, California
Internet: mu.mav@forsythe.stanford.edu
Laparoscopic Surgery; The Biliary System; The Spleen & Lymphatics

Jeffrey Warshaw, MD
Assistant Professor, Department of Obstetrics and Gynecology, Emory University School of Medicine, Atlanta, Georgia
Internet: jwarsha@emory.edu
Gynecologic Surgery

Mark C. Watts, MD
Instructor, Department of Neurosurgery, Johns Hopkins Hospital, Baltimore, Maryland
Internet: mcw@welchlink.welch.jhu.edu
Neurosurgery

Phyllis G. Weber, RN
Executive Director, California Transplant Donor Network, San Francisco, California
Internet: pweber@ctdn.org
Organ Donation

Ronald J. Weigel, MD, PhD
Associate Professor of Surgery, Stanford University School of Medicine, Stanford, California
Cancer Biology; The Endocrine System

Stephen C. Yang, MD
Assistant Professor of Surgery and Oncology; Staff Surgeon, Division of Thoracic Surgery, Johns Hopkins University School of Medicine, Baltimore, Maryland
Internet: syang@welchlink.welch.jhu.edu
Pulmonary Diseases; Chest Wall & Pleural Disease; Lung Cancer

David D. Yuh, MD
Postdoctoral Fellow, Department of Cardiothoracic Surgery, Stanford University School of Medicine, Stanford; Chief Resident in General Surgery, Department of Surgery, Stanford University School of Medicine, Stanford, California
Internet: davidyuh@leland.Stanford.edu
Congenital Disease of the Heart; Cardiac Transplantation; Lung & Combined Heart-Lung Transplantation

Kwok L. Yun, MD
Assistant Professor, Division of Thoracic and Cardiovascular Surgery, Ohio State University, Columbus, Ohio
Acquired Disease of the Heart

Gregory P. Zagaja, MD
Resident, University of Chicago, Chicago, Illinois
Urologic Surgery

Christopher K. Zarins, MD
Chidester Professor of Surgery, Stanford University School of Medicine, Stanford; Chief of Vascular Surgery, Stanford University Medical Center, Stanford, California
Internet: ma.ckz@forsythe.stanford.edu
Cerebrovascular Occlusive Disease; Aneurysms

Preface

Fundamentals of Surgery is the first edition of a text in general surgery designed to introduce the discipline of surgery to the third-year surgery clerkship students and to the beginning postgraduate trainees in surgery. This book is intended to provide a broad base of information concerning surgical diseases to be used by medical students and residents in surgery training. The book aims to help the student make the transition from the lecture hall and laboratory to the practice of surgery in the operating room, intensive care unit, and clinic and at the bedside. To accomplish this, efforts were made to introduce the structure of the surgical service in a teaching hospital, the concepts of graduated responsibility in surgical training, and the details of procedures commonly performed in the day-to-day running of a busy surgical service.

When possible, in the disease-based chapters, key terms and ideas have been summarized (in a Key Facts box feature at the beginning of the chapter) and highlighted (in boldface type throughout the text) for emphasis. Algorithms, figures, and tables have been liberally used. Although the desire has been to provide quick access to the most important information, every effort has been made to make each chapter comprehensive regarding significant clinical features of surgical diseases. References have been selected primarily for their ability to provide additional review of a subject. Finally, an attempt has been made throughout the text to introduce some of the important aspects of the history of surgery. The selection of individuals to be featured in the Historical Facts boxes was often quite obvious. Of course, some selection decisions were arbitrary, and other equally deserving individuals could easily have been chosen to highlight notable contributions.

The efforts of all of the authors are greatly appreciated. Each was extremely cooperative and responded enthusiastically to endeavors to make the format of the text as uniform in its presentation as possible. Each of the authors brings to this work a considerable experience in both surgery and surgical education. In addition, it is personally extremely pleasing to see this text take its place among the other outstanding books of the Lange student series.

Dedication

Next to my family, it is the students and surgery residents who have brought the most joy, reward, excitement, and learning to each day of my academic life. They have been and are the stimulus behind this first edition. The students and residents at Michigan, Johns Hopkins, and Stanford have experienced the influence of my mentors—most notably Doctors R. M. Zollinger, G. C. Child, and W. Fry—in the operating room and on teaching rounds. They have patiently tolerated my stories of past experiences and have accepted gracefully the direction I have offered. It is hoped that the students and residents who use this book will also share in that heritage. It is to these individuals—mentors, students, and residents—that I dedicate this book as a small thank you for all they have given me during my career as a surgeon.

Acknowledgments

Everyone who participated in the writing and production of *Fundamentals of Surgery* shares in the claim that Ms. Shireen Dunwoody is deserving of saintly designation. Ms. Dunwoody worked with unusual energy, enthusiasm, and dedication on this project. She contributed an enormous number of hours, editing chapters, procuring graphic materials, and working directly with all of the authors to ensure cohesive presentation of the chapters. She is in large part responsible for helping all of us develop the Historical Facts boxes as a unique feature of the book. Ms. Dunwoody is expert at the art of gentle persuasion, and without her daily assistance this book would not have been possible.

I owe a great deal of thanks, as always, to my assistant,

Joan Witsel. She not only managed my full and busy schedule to provide the time for me to be involved in this rewarding project but also patiently typed and retyped my chapters.

A special thank you goes to Diane Abeloff, who provided the wonderful original art used throughout the text. Ms. Abeloff is well known for her outstanding contributions in medical illustration, and it was a special honor to have her work with us on this book.

Shelley Reinhardt, Senior Editor at Appleton & Lange, and the staff, specifically Cara Coffey and Eve Siegel, have been a great group to work with. I personally want to thank Ms. Reinhardt for her confidence in me and for being a good friend.

As always in academic life, it is one's wife and children who make the necessary sacrifices so that these projects can be completed at night and on weekends. I owe my wife, Tracey, my children, Matt and Beth, and my niece, Lindsey, much for the gracious way in which they tolerate my absences and for our many late dinners. My mother, Helen, at age 90 remains an active member of our household. Although she would deny it, she brings much wisdom and common sense to our dinner discussions and to my work in academic medicine.

John E. Niederhuber, MD
December 1997
Madison, Wisconsin

Section I

Introduction to Surgical Care

1

The Surgery Service & Surgery Training

John E. Niederhuber, MD

To study the phenomenon of disease without books is to sail an uncharted sea, while to study books without patients is not to go to sea at all.

—Sir William Osler, 1849–1919,
Professor of Medicine, Oxford, England

For the medical student, the first days of a third-year clerkship in general surgery can be overwhelming. Almost immediately, however, the initial fears and apprehension give way to the excitement and enthusiasm that comes with being an integral part of a well-managed team. Every medical student will tell you that the key to an outstanding experience on a surgery rotation is the surgery residents, and the most important member of this team is the service's chief resident. Even though as professors we are many years removed from our student days, you will find that each of us has amazingly clear recollections of the chief residents with whom we worked so intensely during our student and resident years.

ORGANIZATION OF THE SURGERY SERVICE

As a student beginning a surgery clerkship, it is important to understand the organization of the service to which you are assigned. In most medical schools and university-based surgery training programs, there will be a chief resident, a more junior resident (in the third or fourth year of clinical training), and one or more residents in their first or second years of the residency program. These individuals form the team, and you as a student are integrated into this team and expected to be an effective contributor. Surgery services tend to be very busy and this is not a place for idle observers.

The residents on the surgery service have different re-sponsibilities, depending upon their level of experience. This is often referred to as "graded responsibility." The chief resident is the individual responsible for the welfare of the patients and for running the daily activities of the service in an efficient and effective manner. Thus, every member of the team must keep the "chief" maximally in-formed—even regarding the smallest detail.

Each service will generally have a group of attending staff surgeons who admit their patients to the service for in-hospital care and surgery. Obviously, as the attending surgeon for a given patient, the admitting surgeon is the one with ultimate responsibility and authority for the care of the patient and the conducting of any surgical or inter-ventional procedures. The admitting surgeon may dele-gate certain of these activities as appropriate. On some services, especially in academic medical centers, one of the "attendings" may serve as the service chief or division chief.

Thus, the team has many members and each member has responsibilities appropriate to his or her level of expe-rience and training. As a student member of the team, you will be learning by doing as well as by listening, reading, and asking. The central feature of a well-run service is communication between all the members of the team. As you will see, a great deal of information must be gathered each day, much of which must be easily accessible for safe and effective patient care. At times, you may feel your role is to be a large data bank. What you need to re-member throughout this experience is that the more infor-mation you have firmly fixed in your mind about each of your patients, the more effectively you can contribute to the activities of the whole team; and most important of all, the more you will understand and learn from the manage-ment of your patient.

The very best surgical care is directly dependent upon the skills and devotion of the residents and students. Being a student or resident on a surgery service involves many responsibilities, including standing in for the at-tending, representing the attending, and communicating between patient and attending. The importance of this role cannot be overemphasized. It requires the student and resident to be totally supportive of the attending and of the institution. The patient and the patient's family need to have the utmost confidence in both—often, this is greatly assisted by the students and resident staff.

The "Why?" and "What if?" questions are extremely important to your training, and, more importantly, are welcomed by any attending or chief resident. The rule to remember is that such discussions always need to take place out of ear-shot of the patient and patient's family. While this may be a simple rule, it is too frequently forgotten during the pressure of patient rounds. A rule to remember at all times has to do with our attitude toward our patients; simply stated, it is: Strive to treat each patient with courtesy, respect, sensitivity, and reverence.

BASIC CONSIDERATIONS IN CARING FOR THE SURGICAL PATIENT

There is a wonderful prayer that we all would do well to recite each day as we begin our work. I can think of no better introduction to the paragraphs that follow regarding the care of the surgical patient.

> Medical Litany of Sir Robert Hutchison, 1871–1960, Consulting Physician to the London Hospital, London, England:
>
> From inability to leave well alone;
> From too much zeal for what is new and contempt for what is old;
> From putting knowledge before wisdom, science before art, cleverness before common sense;
> From treating patients as cases; and
> From making the cure of a disease more grievous than the endurance,
> Good Lord, deliver us.

Surgery is the oldest method of dealing with human disease. It originated not as a science but as an art, long before there existed an understanding of pathology, physiology, and the principles of diagnosis. Today, surgery no longer stands alone but is an integral and integrated aspect of the diagnosis and treatment of human disease. Surgery's achievement of this status is based on years of participating in, and often leading, the creation of new knowledge and the development of the scientific foundation of modern medicine. Even so, "the art" of surgery is what sets it apart from the other fields of medicine. This art of surgery remains essential, even in our era of rapidly advancing knowledge, such as in the avantgarde fields of molecular genetics and protein structure/function analysis.

The modern surgeon who has developed an outstanding clinical reputation is very much the complete physician, with a broad knowledge of medicine and diagnosis. This background and broad knowledge base helps the surgeon evaluate the complaints of the patient, determine what tests and procedures will establish a diagnosis or probable cause for the patient's symptoms, and remain constantly vigilant for comorbid diseases that could endanger a safe operation. In carrying out these preoperative responsibilities on behalf of the patient, the modern surgeon is much more integrated with other physician specialists than were surgeons of prior generations. To be optimally effective in this role requires great breadth and depth of knowledge.

It is only on the basis of a careful and thorough preoperative evaluation that the surgeon can make proper decisions regarding the indications for operation and the appropriate timing of surgery. Careful and thorough preoperative preparation positions the surgeon to institute essential safeguards to manage effectively any associated diseases, such as previously unsuspected heart disease. All of this effort prepares the surgeon to make decisions during the operation itself—decisions that ensure surgical success and a recovery free of complications. A sample format for a history and physical examination as well as operative and postoperative notes are shown in Figure 1–1.

The surgeon who is equally as intense in providing postoperative care as in operating is the one who will consistently achieve the best results. Certainly, most patients recover uneventfully, but not all do, and often when we least expect a problem is when it occurs. The postoperative period is not the time to relinquish the patient's care to another physician, for many aspects of patient management, both intraoperatively and postoperatively, are directly related to experience. The good surgeon develops a consistent routine for close observation during the critical early phase of recovery. Rigorous and repeated observation is time well spent and is the only way to detect, at their earliest stage, impending events—such as an early calf thrombophlebitis—that could have a disastrous outcome.

You will learn that the relationship between a patient and his or her surgeon is unique in medicine—a very personal affair. Often, of course, the act of operating on a patient will ultimately determine whether the patient lives or dies. In discussing this unique relationship with my residents, I have often stated that no matter how specialized the surgery and the surgeon, the surgeon often becomes the patient's primary caregiver. I tell the residents that they will always know when they have been at their best, if their patients call them for advice and counsel on even their nonsurgical medical problems.

Finally, patients and their families need to appreciate and draw strength from this close personal relationship. They need to feel and sense the confidence of their surgeon. The thoroughness and availability of their surgeon adds to this confidence. For the patient, a major surgery is

<table>
<tr><td>

History and Physical Format

Identification of Patient and Reason for Referral:
  A. Source of history
  B. Referring physicians (include address and
     phone numbers)

Current Medications:

Gynecologic History (for female patients):

Past Medical History:
  A. Infant and childhood illnesses
  B. Medical illnesses
  C. Surgeries
  D. Injuries
  E. Allergies
  F. Blood transfusions/coagulation problems

Family History:
  A. Mother
  B. Father
  C. Siblings
  D. Inherited diseases

Social History:

Review of Systems:

History of Present Illness:

Physical Examination:

Review of X-rays, Scans, Labs, and Outside Pathology:

Impression:

Recommendations/Plan:

A
</td><td>

Brief Operative Note Format

Date:
Start Time: _____   Completion: _____
Preoperative Diagnosis:
Postoperative Diagnosis:
Operation:
Findings:
Complications:
Specimens:
Drains:
Estimated Blood Loss:
Blood Replacement:
Total Fluids:
Anesthesia:
Status:

B

Postoperative Note Format

Postoperative Day No. 1   Time: _____
Vital Signs:
Maximum Temperature:
Mental Status:
Medications:
I&O: (ie, drains, avg. hourly urine output)
Examination:
Status:
Plan:

C
</td></tr>
</table>

Figure 1–1. Sample format. **A:** Standard history and physical examination form. **B:** Brief operative note for chart. **C:** Daily postoperative note for chart.

the maximum of physical and mental stress. The postoperative patient needs more than ever to draw on the presence of his or her surgeon during those initial hours and days of recovery.

THE TYPICAL STUDENT DAY

While a typical student day on the surgery service may differ from institution to institution, one thing is certain: the day usually begins well before dawn and ends late at night. For the student, this means being in the hospital a few minutes ahead of everyone else in the morning to quickly check charts and have a word with the night nurse regarding any events that occurred during the few hours you were absent. The team convenes to make morning rounds, usually at 6:00 AM. Each service carries "The Book," which contains important information on each patient. On morning rounds, progress for each patient is noted, preoperative patients are given a final check, and plans are established for work that needs to be accomplished during the day. By the end of rounds (usually around 7:00), everyone knows his or her assignment for the day.

Shortly after 7:00 AM, it is off to the operating room for the first case of the morning. As a student, you may not have a patient in the operating room on a particular day, but whenever possible, plan to stop by to observe the critical aspects of interesting cases.

During the day, participate as much as possible in hands-on patient care: dressing changes, wound care, line placements, and so forth. One learns best by repeatedly performing procedures. One or more days each week should include time in the ambulatory setting where new patients are evaluated and others are followed postoperatively.

Most services expect the student to write a daily note on the patient's chart. Do this early in the day. In the late afternoon, there are didactic lectures interspersed with clinical conferences. Some of the most interesting and informative for you will be the multidisciplinary clinical care conferences.

Well after 5:00 PM, your team will reconvene again to begin afternoon rounds. This set of rounds is at a slower pace, with more time for discussion, questions, and teaching. Often, teaching takes the form of questions directed at the student and junior housestaff. Be prepared on these rounds to present your patient to the team. Presentations should be concise and well-organized for pertinent facts. Evening rounds often start in the x-ray suite to review films and then progress to the floor, concluding in the surgical intensive care unit (SICU).

Yes, it is a long day and you will feel the exhaustion, but you will also feel the exhilaration of caring for your patients and making a difference in their lives. In writing this, I am reminded of my surgery clerkship and a fellow student that shared the rotation with me. Charles Montgomery is now an ophthalmologist in Florida; back then, he was committed to a career in neurosurgery. Charles was as fanatic about surgery as I was. Frequently, it would be close to midnight as we collected our belongings to leave the floor. But before we left the hospital, Charles would always want to make one last stop by the operating room to see if an interesting case was going on. There usually was, and another pair of hands to retract was almost always welcomed. We seldom slept, but we saw a lot of surgery!

THE STUDENT IN THE OPERATING ROOM

The medical student experiences both the excitement of the opportunity to scrub for an operative procedure as well as a certain fear of what is to come. The student knows that all too often the operative field will not be easily seen and, frozen to the handle of a retractor, muscles will ache. Fatigue, in such circumstances, can be overwhelming, or at least sufficient enough to significantly impair one's thinking. The student knows all too well that this is likely to be the setting during which he or she will be asked a variety of what seem to be unrelated questions regarding diagnosis, pathophysiology, anatomy, organ function, risks of surgery, and disease prognosis.

To minimize this fear and to ensure an enjoyable experience, it is essential that you come prepared. The knowledge that you have prepared goes a long way in shifting the balance of emotions toward elation rather than trepidation. Obviously, the better prepared you are the more you will learn from the experience. Most attendings very much enjoy having students present at the operating table and are kind and sensitive to them. When a student is obviously well prepared, the surgeon shares in a sense of pride—is honored that the student was sufficiently interested and committed to be so. You will quickly learn that this also usually enhances the performance of the surgeon as a teacher, again to your ultimate benefit (Table 1–1).

In the operating room, your assistance to the operating room staff and residents is important. You should plan to be present when the patient arrives. As you assist with the proper positioning of the patient, you will learn how the patient is protected from injury while the surgical team is provided the appropriate exposure. You should become familiar with the basic equipment, surgical instruments, and supplies used in the operating room. A number of

Table 1–1. Student preparation for surgery.

1. Review patient's hospital chart thoroughly.
2. Commit key facts to memory.
3. Review a surgical atlas description of planned operation.
4. Review specific anatomy and organ physiology.
5. Review facts about results of treatment, potential complications, and future needs of the patient.
6. Discuss the patient and review the case thoroughly with the senior resident.

principles are followed by the operating room staff. These include:

- maintaining and protecting the airway at all times
- establishing appropriate vascular access
- ensuring adequate exposure of vascular access sites and monitoring sites for anesthesia staff
- protecting patient's peripheral nerves, circulation, and skin
- safety—safety—safety

It is important to remember that conversation in the operating room should be limited and essential to the task at hand. The patient, while awake, needs to sense the seriousness with which all are proceeding. Today, many surgical procedures are performed with the patient awake and lightly sedated. Conduct by everyone during such procedures must be entirely appropriate and sensitive to the patient's presence.

You will learn that there is an order to which the surgical technician (scrub technician) has arranged all instruments and sutures on the Mayo stand and the back table. This is the private territory of the scrub technician, and there are two rules to remember. First, never reach for anything on the Mayo stand, or put your hands on the Mayo stand and back table—these are sacred territory. Second, even when you feel you know what is needed next, avoid either repeating what the surgeon has asked for or asking for what you think is needed. Silence is a virtue in the operating room. Much of what transpires between surgeon and scrub tech is by subtle sign language.

Be attentive and ready to assist at all times. Usually you will be helping by cutting suture, assisting with exposure, and occasionally manning the suction to keep the field dry. Remember to always move carefully and purposefully and, as much as possible, without obstructing the surgeon's view of the field.

At the completion of the case you will often be asked to assist with moving the patient from the operating table to the bed and to accompany the patient to the recovery area or the intensive care unit. Again, protecting vital vascular lines and monitoring lines, airway, and patient status are essential. Learn to write the postoperative orders and the brief operative note for the patient's chart.

Through all of the activities within the operating room, it is easy to see the importance of maintaining an absolutely sterile environment. Your role toward this end is no less than that of the operating surgeon. Everyone in the room is responsible at all times for maintaining sterility, and everyone shares the responsibility of immediately calling attention to any break or suspected break in sterile technique—even you.

The operating room is the "home" of the surgeon and the surgical service you have joined. You will always remember your days in the OR, even if you choose another discipline in medicine. The OR is where you will learn much about surgical disease and many things that you will use throughout your career in medicine.

TRAINING IN SURGERY

> We need a system, and we shall surely have it, which will produce not only surgeons but surgeons of the highest type, men who will stimulate the youths of our country to study surgery and devote their energies and their lives to raising the standard of surgical science.
>
> William S. Halsted, 1852–1922.
> Address delivered at Yale University, 1904.

Frequently, I am asked by students how they should proceed in selecting a surgery training program. The guidelines are fairly simple. First of all, select a good university and medical school with a strong department of surgery—a surgery department with an excellent history of training and a strong commitment to research as well as teaching. Be aware that university teaching hospitals vary in size; generally, you should select the larger hospitals with full-time faculties and more than 750 beds. Such institutions are more likely to provide the full range of outstanding residency programs and a high volume of interesting and complex cases upon which to build experience.

Learn as much as you can regarding any affiliated hospital used in the training program. How are the faculty at these affiliates selected? What is their relationship to the parent department? Avoid selecting places where there is tension between full-time faculty and private attendings. A divided house is never a good place to spend 5 or more years of one's life.

Finally, spend time reviewing the current surgical literature. How often do you find publications originating from the faculty of the department you are considering? This will tell you a great deal about the vibrancy and intellectual energy within this setting, and about the potential for your involvement with the faculty. No matter what your ultimate career goals, it is always wisest to train at the best possible program for which you qualify.

The first years of residency place heavy emphasis on learning the basics of surgical diseases—their diagnoses, their physiologic sequelae, and their histopathology. The first- and second-year surgical residents begin to learn about the importance of surgical decision-making and to develop a sense of timing vis-à-vis surgical intervention. It is often said that in surgery, timing is everything. During these first years of training, the resident begins to learn how important good judgment is to outcome. It is also a time to learn how to work with and manage critically ill patients—patients whose recovery will depend, not on finely honed operative skills, but rather on the diligently practiced skills developed by long hours of work in the surgical intensive care unit.

One of the most difficult concepts to communicate to the first-year trainee in surgery is the notion that learning to operate is only part of the training, and, for that matter, perhaps the smaller part. Although significant time is spent in the operating room, the greater emphasis at this stage must be placed on learning about surgical disease. The overused cliché that the best surgeon is, in reality, the consummate internist with additional technical skills is even more true today. The first-year trainee, with all the desired impatience of a race horse in the starting gate, has a difficult time waiting his or her turn in the operating theater. The responsibility of being the operating surgeon is one that must be earned; hence, it is a late occurrence in the spectrum of surgical training.

Lord Berkeley Moynihan (1865–1936), the well-known surgeon scholar and for many years the chair of clinical surgery at London University in England, stated it perhaps as well as anyone: "Surgery is not only a question of operating. . . . The operation itself is but one incident, no doubt the most dramatic, yet still only one in the long series of events which must stretch between illness and recovery."

The first 2 years of training are also a time to develop organizational skills. The life of a surgeon is a busy one, and one that is almost always accompanied by an element of fatigue. It is a life that demands discipline, character, and high moral and ethical standards. It is not a career for everyone, and it is only possible with highly developed time management and leadership skills.

In addition, the first 2 years are the time for gaining an appreciation of the other surgical disciplines. The pressures of today's specialty training programs, unfortunately, too often restrict the time allotted to gain experience in the diagnosis and management of diseases seen exclusively in neurosurgery, urology, orthopedic surgery, reconstructive surgery, and pediatric surgery.

The remaining clinical training is accomplished over the next 3 years, for a total of 5 years of clinical training. This, plus a certain volume of operative experience, qualifies the resident to sit for the written part of the examination of the American Board of Surgery. One must pass the written component to be eligible to take the oral examination. The various surgical subspecialties have specific requirements for training. Some, such as cardiothoracic and pediatric surgery, require full training in general surgery followed by an additional 2–3 years of subspecialty training to qualify for their board exams. Specialties such as neurosurgery, orthopedic surgery, and urology require a preliminary year of general surgery experience prior to entry into these respective training programs.

If one's goal is to become a professor of surgery, the training must include a significant period devoted to acquiring the skills of a scientist. Thus, many trainees in university-based residencies will devote 2–4 years to expanding their experience as a laboratory or clinical investigator.

During the final 3-year segment of the residency, greater emphasis is placed on developing technical skills and leadership. The latter is extremely important. Nowhere else in medicine is the term "captain of the ship" more appropriate, for the surgeon is required to be this captain for the patient. To accomplish this within the complexities of today's highly subspecialized environment requires all the leadership and communication skills commonly ascribed to a corporate executive of a major company.

Today, more time is spent during training in the ambulatory setting. This is one of the most significant changes in surgery education and is the result of changes in health care reimbursement that have moved so much of diagnostic evaluation and postoperative care to the outpatient setting. In addition, the disappearance in recent years of "ward services" where patient care is under the sole direction of surgical residents has placed all patients in the surgery program into a private care mode. The result is a closer association between the trainee and the faculty, more of a preceptorship, and has significantly increased time spent in an ambulatory setting. Gone are the days of admitting a patient for a lengthy diagnostic workup in preparation for surgery.

Proficiency in the performance of surgery comes only with experience and with considerable practice. As in sports, practice and more practice are the essentials to success. Becoming an outstanding surgeon evolves over time and requires, not only knowledge, but sound decision-making. The latter is extremely difficult to teach. Perhaps the skills of sound decision-making are best acquired through the close relationship you will have with your preceptors, which is unique and so vital to surgery training.

In addition to the required solid foundation of knowledge regarding surgical disease, skills in decision-making, and leadership, the truly outstanding surgeon has an intense interest in and a complete knowledge of the anatomy in the operations he or she performs. I recall my days as an intern on Dr. Robert Zollinger's service. The intern was required to prepare a new anatomy sketch of each case and tape it to the operating room wall. One day, time was short and I quickly taped up an old sketch of the anatomy of the colon. When Dr. Zollinger entered the operating room he took one look at my drawing and promptly sent me off to make a new one. To this day I cannot figure out how he knew it was an old sketch. The lesson, however, has never left me.

The training program, although long in years, is really only the beginning. The surgeon who completes these years is poised to begin clinical practice—gaining experience and building on the foundation of the residency years. It is an ongoing process, and as for the young artist, the greatest years lie ahead—years devoted to becoming the "master surgeon."

> Surgery is not learned easily. The training is arduous and protracted; indeed, it lasts a man's lifetime. It must begin under a master's eye and be influenced by his criticism, and not less by his spiritual encouragement. It must not be light-heartedly or recklessly undertaken, nor can it ever be a matter of display. . . . In surgical work, craftsmanship is much and knowledge is much and wisdom, which is the timely and rightful application of knowledge, is more, but as we establish our place in the world it is chiefly character that counts. . . .
>
> Lord B. Moynihan, 1865–1936,
> Chair of Clinical Surgery,
> London University, London, England

THE ART OF FIRST ASSISTING

There is an art to being the very best surgical resident, and the operating room is where the truly superb are most evident. To be an outstanding resident requires focus and dedication, as well as an understanding of the role and of the tremendous educational benefits that befall those who excel at being a dedicated apprentice. Surgery continues to be a discipline that is handed down from one generation to the next, and the bonds formed between mentor and student last a lifetime.

The resident who understands the value of this tradition will derive the most in terms of experience and exposure. The tradition of apprenticeship begins with learning to be a superb first assistant and progresses to the point at which the senior surgeon begins to relinquish more and more of the procedure to his or her resident trainee. The resident must remember that such participation is not a right, but a reward to be earned by demonstrated competence.

As the first assistant for a specific case, the resident should always be present when the patient enters the operating room. The resident assists in positioning the patient and, therefore, must be thoroughly familiar with the planned procedure, the likes and dislikes of the senior surgeon, and the safe methods of securing appropriate positioning. While the patient is undergoing anesthetic induction, the resident is observant of all activities and ready to assist or manage any emergent situation. It is also a time during which the resident determines whether the instruments selected by the operating room staff are appropriate, including retractors and the individual preferences of the senior surgeon. The resident should also review the selection of suture to be used during the operation with the circulating nurse and the scrub technician.

When the patient is anesthetized and turned over to the operating team by the anesthetist, the resident prepares the operating site, checks the position of the operating room lights, and checks all ancillary equipment, including monitors, footpedals, and so forth. The placement of a Foley catheter, if needed, is supervised or performed by the resident. The resident should also review with the anesthesia team the choice of vascular access, both for intraoperative volume replacement as well as monitoring of cardiovascular parameters. Both the anesthesia team and surgical team must be comfortable that they are optimally prepared according to the potential risks of the planned procedure.

To function as an outstanding assistant and to be ready to learn both by observing and by actually performing some aspects of the operation, the resident must obviously have a thorough knowledge of the surgical condition and of the planned operation. There are two key points to remember when striving to be a good first assistant: to be gentle in all actions that involve the handling of tissue, and to be alert toward maintaining a clear field of vision for the surgeon. The saying, "exposure, exposure, exposure," is a maxim of good surgery. In all that you do as an assistant, exercise gentleness—sponge, don't wipe; clamp with precision small amounts of tissue; guard against placing undo tension on clamps, sutures, and retractors. Be atraumatic as much as possible in all that you do. Make your movements purposeful and work hard to maintain focus and to anticipate the next move in the procedure.

Along with maintaining exposure, the first assistant has the responsibility to ensure that the lights remain focused appropriately in the operating field at all times. Don't make sudden movements or movements that disrupt the surgeon's line of vision. The operating room is an environment that demands and deserves complete focus. As part of the team you must stay cool and calm, even under the most stressful situations. Moments of great peril to the patient must be met with equanimity and clearness of mind to maximize judgment and improvisation.

As you progress to the point in your training where you and the senior surgeon become interchangeable—a smooth working team—you will then, and only then, feel the exhilaration of an artfully accomplished procedure. You will gradually learn to use all your senses, and you will marvel to yourself on how much information flows from the tips of your fingers to your brain and your eyes.

Over the years, I have frequently emphasized to my residents the importance of keeping a journal that documents what they have encountered during each operation and what they have learned. A good surgical atlas is the perfect place to make these notes and to easily find them years later when reviewing for tomorrow's cases. Over the years, as new insights have emerged from the repetition of procedures learned long ago, they have found their way onto pages alongside the notes from years past. These pages of notes, I promise you, will become a treasure.

Finally, remember that you can never watch too much surgery. Each time I observe a surgeon perform an operation, I always learn. Learning surgery is a continuous process, even for the most seasoned surgeon—a lifetime of effort and a lifetime of reward.

SUGGESTED READING

Alkinson LJ, Kohn ML: *Berry and Kohns's Introduction to Operating Room Technique*. McGraw Hill, 1978.

Bunch WH et al: The stresses of the surgical residency. J Surg Res 1992;53:268.

Cooley DA: Acquiring and improving surgical skills. Curr Surg 1995;52:327.

Moynihan B: *Addresses on Surgical Subjects*. Saunders, 1928.

Moynihan B: *Essays on Surgical Subjects*. Saunders, 1921.

Rhoads JE et al: Surgical philosophy. In: Harkins HN et al (editors): *Surgery Principles and Practice*, 2nd ed. Lippincott, 1961.

2

Operating Room Setup & Basics of Sterile Technique

Sharon Butler, RN, BSN, MSN

▶ Key Facts

- ▶ Students must quickly and thoroughly learn operating room (OR) protocol in order to be an effective member of the surgical team.

- ▶ OR traffic must be kept to a minimum in order to prevent cross-contamination of patients. Only persons directly involved with the case should be in restricted areas.

- ▶ Proper OR attire includes clean scrub suits, caps, or hoods that confine hair, and masks that properly cover the nose and mouth.

- ▶ Personal protective equipment is provided for all members of the OR staff and includes scrub clothes, gloves, masks, face shields, and sterile gowns.

- ▶ The sterile field is created to isolate the surgical incision site from the unsterile environment. Scrubbed persons should stay as close to the in-

cision site as possible, while unscrubbed persons should remain several feet away while observing in order to prevent contamination.

- ▶ Contamination of the supplies or personnel within the sterile field should be taken care of immediately.

- ▶ Surgical instruments fall into four basic categories: (1) dissectors; (2) retractors; (3) graspers; (4) clamps.

- ▶ Sutures are divided into two categories, absorbable and nonabsorbable. Needles vary greatly in shape, size, and point design. Choice of needle depends on the tissue to be penetrated.

- ▶ Surgical counts are an essential safety measure, and each member of the OR team must understand what is counted. Counted items must not leave the room or be thrown into the trash.

The operating room, often referred to simply as the "OR," is a demanding and intense environment, and it can sometimes be quite daunting to the surgical student. There are strict protocols that must be followed in order to insure the safety of the patient and operating room personnel. It is of vital importance to be familiar with the operating room environment and the meticulous practice of asepsis and sterile technique. Principles of asepsis are utilized to provide a suitable environment for surgical intervention. Most students soon recognize that the code of conduct is straightforward and designed to be easily learned.

Operating room personnel include both scrubbed and unscrubbed persons. The scrubbed surgical team consists of the operating surgeon, the surgical assistants, and the scrub nurse or operating room technician. The unscrubbed team members include the anesthesiologist, the circulating nurse, and others, such as x-ray or radiation therapy technicians.

The operating surgeon is responsible for the preoperative and postoperative care as well as the selection of the operation to be performed. Although the surgeon assumes full responsibility for the management of the patient, the concept of a team effort should be utmost in the minds of everyone within the operating room environment.

SCHEDULING

Preparation of the surgical suite and monitoring of sterile technique are most often the function of the nursing staff. However, the surgeon schedules the procedure and should indicate during scheduling any special equipment that may be required. From this information the perioperative nurse assembles equipment, sterile supplies, and instrumentation to complete the surgical procedure.

In most institutions, the perioperative nurse makes liberal use of computerized surgeon preference lists for specific cases. The surgeon must request all specialty items that will be needed for the procedure. Many surgical procedures now require special rooms and equipment that may have limited availability. Due to the cost of some of the new technology, such as lasers, microscopes, video cameras, and red blood cell savers, only a limited amount of the equipment can be purchased. Therefore, it is usually reserved on a first-come/first-served basis. Some procedures may require a particular operating room with special facilities, such as intraoperative radiation capabilities or ceiling-mounted microscopes. If the surgeon is not specific in the scheduling of the procedure, equipment may not be available resulting in surgery delays, angry patients, cancellations, institutional financial loss, and loss of the surgeon's time.

OPERATING ROOM SETUP

Setting up the OR by the staff may require only a few minutes or an hour or more. The increased use of high-technology equipment within the OR has escalated the preparation time for the OR staff and also the amount of technical knowledge necessary for staff members. Each piece of equipment must be obtained and tested prior to the beginning of the procedure. It is important for all operating room caregivers to understand how such equipment works and the safety measures applicable to each piece. This requires that the operating room director maintain ongoing programs for in-service training, not only for operating room staff, but also for the surgeons using such equipment.

Additionally, all sterile supplies, instruments, and sutures must be gathered and prepared by the scrub nurse and the circulating nurse. After it has been determined that all necessary equipment and supplies are present and working, the circulating nurse and the anesthesiologist will bring the patient into the operating room. It is important that a member of the surgical team be present. This assignment often falls to the more junior member of the team. One can readily see that this puts a significant burden on the junior resident to quickly learn as much as possible about the specific tasks assigned to each member of the operating room staff.

TRAFFIC PATTERNS

Traffic patterns within the operating room are developed to enhance the flow of patient supplies, equipment, and personnel in order to reduce cross-contamination of the surgical patient. The operating room consists of three areas: (1) unrestricted; (2) semirestricted; and (3) restricted. Each of these areas have different apparel requirements. Unrestricted areas allow both scrub clothes and street clothes. The unrestricted areas include locker rooms, lounges, and, in most hospitals, the OR main desk (the main desk is very much like a control tower at a busy airport).

Semirestricted areas allow only persons in scrub clothes, which includes some type of head covering that confines the person's hair. Semirestricted areas include storage areas for sterile supplies and the area directly adjacent to the individual operating rooms. The pre- and postanesthesia care units (PACU) may also be semirestricted areas.

Restricted areas require scrub clothes, hair covering, and a mask (see following section). Restricted areas are the individual operating rooms where the surgical procedures are performed. Most operating rooms have a window that allows observation without entering. Only persons directly involved with patient care should be in the restricted areas. The more persons in and out of each OR, the greater the chance of cross-contamination of patients. It is good practice to observe before entering to determine if a mask is needed. A mask is required if sterile supplies are open for a surgical procedure.

SURGICAL ATTIRE & SCRUBBING

Personnel as well as patients are the major sources of contamination in the operating room. All personnel entering the surgical suite must be in proper OR attire. This includes clean scrub suits, caps or hoods that confine hair, and masks that properly cover the nose and mouth. Scrub suits should be changed between cases, and every effort should be made to restrict their use to the surgery suite and other interventional units in the hospital. It is good patient care to change to a clean set of scrubs upon returning to the OR if you have been outside the operating suite.

Shoe covers are required in some hospitals and are available in others for personnel to use to maintain clean, dry footwear. Footwear utilized for the OR should be easy to clean. It is preferable that such footwear be restricted to use in the surgical suite. Protective eyewear and gloves must be used for any procedure involving contact with the patient's body and bodily fluids.

Prior to donning sterile gown and gloves, the surgical team must do a surgical hand scrub. It is not possible to sterilize the skin, however, it is possible to reduce the amount of bacteria contained on the skin in order to prevent patient contamination. Scrubbing procedures are fairly standard and absolutely necessary for all persons within the sterile field. Preparations for surgical scrubbing include keeping fingernails short and unpolished, as well as removing all jewelry. Some institutions also recommend a pre-scrub of the hands and arms.

There are two methods for surgical scrubbing: the so-called "timed method" and the "counted stroke method." For the timed method, a 5-minute total scrub is recommended with either povidone-iodine or chlorhexidine gluconate. Both are rapid-acting broad-spectrum antimicrobials that are effective against gram-positive and gram-negative microorganisms. Other products may require longer scrub time.

The counted stroke method includes a prescribed number of bristle brush strokes for the fingers, hands, and arms. The standard is 30 strokes for nails, 20 strokes to each area of the fingers, hands, and arms. Each side of the forearm is scrubbed with a circular motion up to the elbow. Both methods follow a prescribed anatomic pattern of scrubbing that includes the fingernails, four surfaces of each finger, the dorsal and palmar surface of the hand, and the area over the wrists and extending up the arm to 2 inches below the elbow (Figure 2–1). After the scrub, the hands and forearms are held higher than the elbows in order to keep contaminated water away from the hands (Figure 2–2). The hands should always be kept above the waist.

Hand washing before and after exposure to a patient is mandatory to prevent cross-contamination of the patient as well as to protect yourself from infections. This practice should become habitual, both in the operating room as well as in other patient care areas.

After the hand scrub, the surgeon enters the operating room, receives a towel from the scrub nurse to dry his or her hands, and is then assisted into a sterile gown by the circulating nurse, who also assists in this process by pulling the gown over the shoulders, fastening snaps, or tying the back of the gown. The gown can be made of a reusable densely woven cotton or a disposable water-repellant material. The sterile gown is only considered sterile from the nipples to the waist and up to the elbows of the arm.

The scrub nurse or operating room technician assists with gloving the surgeon and assistants. When the surgical gown is put on, hands should not be advanced beyond the

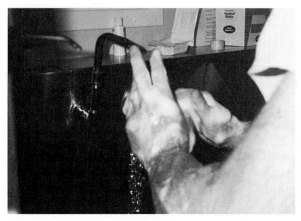

A

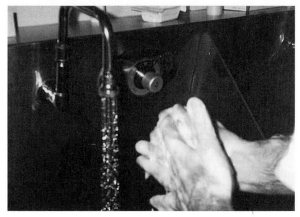

B

Figure 2–1. Techniques for surgical scrubbing. **A:** Scrubbing of individual. **B:** Thorough scrubbing of the palmar surface of the hand.

cuffs until gloves are placed. The hands are pushed through the cuffs as the gloves are placed by the scrub nurse or operating room technician (Figure 2–3). When away from the operating table it is a good habit to keep the hands folded on the chest in order to avoid contamination. At the operating table, always find a safe place to rest the hands when not actively assisting. To remove the gown and gloves properly, the gown should be pulled off at the shoulders, turning the sleeves inside out while the arms are removed. The hand should not touch the outer portion of the glove, which is soiled.

STERILIZATION

All OR personnel (especially the scrub nurse or operating room technician) must understand the principles of sterilization to provide the surgeon with sterile instru-

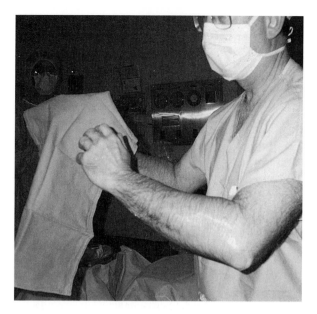

Figure 2–2. When hands are dried, arms should be held away from body so contaminated water falls away from hands and forearms.

tion can be used on almost any product but it is currently only available in industrial settings. The three most frequently used forms of sterilization within hospitals are steam, ethylene oxide, and hydrogen peroxide.

Steam is the cheapest and most reliable form of sterilization, but it also has limitations with some equipment, such as the cameras and lenses used in endoscopic surgical procedures. Steam is also the quickest method, requiring as little as 3 minutes of exposure for a few instruments to 20 minutes for an entire set of instruments.

Ethylene oxide has been utilized for many years for delicate and heat-sensitive supplies, but it is hazardous to the employees and to the environment. The sterilization process is quite lengthy, ranging from 3–4 hours, and all materials must go to the aeration chamber for 12–14 hours to remove the gas from the packaging and the supplies. Failure to remove the gas can result in burns and tissue damage to patients and to the surgical team. Ethylene oxide sterilization is rapidly being replaced by ionization techniques. Several companies are now marketing low-temperature sterilizers that utilize hydrogen peroxide, or acetic acid in ionized form to sterilize delicate instruments and equipment.

ments and supplies for the surgical procedure. **Sterilization** is the process that renders items free of microorganisms and spores. Several methods are available for the numerous items needed for each procedure. Most of the paper and disposable supplies are purchased from companies who use gamma radiation to sterilize. Gamma radia-

ASEPTIC TECHNIQUE

Asepsis is briefly defined as a condition that is free from germs and infection—sterile. The goal of aseptic technique is to provide an environment for the surgical pa-

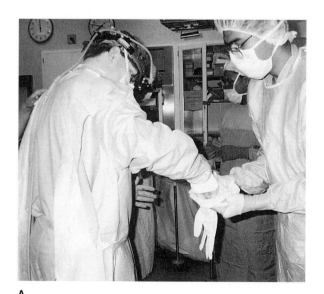

A

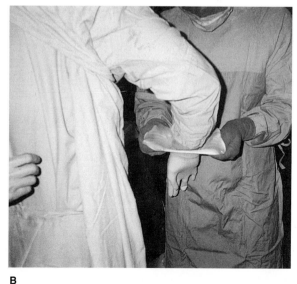

B

Figure 2–3. Gowning and gloving techniques. Gown is fastened by circulating nurse. **A:** Hands should not be extended through the gown until scrub nurse or operating room technician assists the surgeon into the sterile glove. **B:** Glove is placed over gown wristlet.

tient that will promote healing, prevent surgical infections, and minimize the length of recovery from surgery.

Universal precautions assume all patients are infectious and that all patients should be treated in the same manner. Personal protective equipment (PPE) is provided for all members of the operating room staff and include scrub clothes, gloves, masks, face shields, and sterile gowns (Figure 2–4). Utilization of protective barriers protects operating room personnel as well as the patient.

Aseptic technique is the foundation of practice within the operating room. Principles of aseptic technique include the staff's use of sterile surgical attire the establishment of a sterile operating field. A sterile operating field is created by the draping of sterile sheets and towels in a prescribed way based on the procedure and the surgeon's preference. However, before the sterile drapes are placed, the patient's skin at the operating site must be cleaned as thoroughly as possible.

Trays for prepping the skin are commercially available and usually include gauze sponges, antiseptic soap, disposable razors, and towels. Razors are used to remove hair

from the incision site. If large areas are involved, hair should be removed prior to bringing the patient to the OR. The skin is scrubbed with antiseptic solution, beginning at the incision site and working outward in a circular motion toward the periphery of the field. Cleansing should be vigorous and involve chemical as well as mechanical action. The most common antiseptic skin scrubs are iodine-based soaps and solutions. After the skin has been prepared, the patient is ready for draping.

Draping

Draping is the process of covering the patient and surrounding areas with a sterile barrier in order to maintain a field of sterility. Drapes are fluid-resistant, antistatic, abrasive-free, lint-free, and made to fit contours. They are usually blue, green, or gray in order to reduce glare and eye fatigue. There are a number of different types of drapes, including towels, stockinettes for extremities, fenestrated sheets, split sheets, single sheets, and plastic incise drapes. Each drape has a specific use, for example, fenestrated sheets have a fenestration that exposes the op-

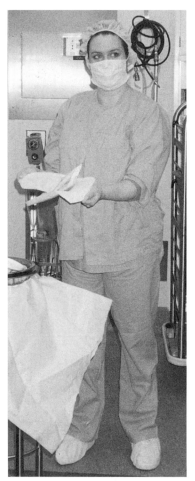

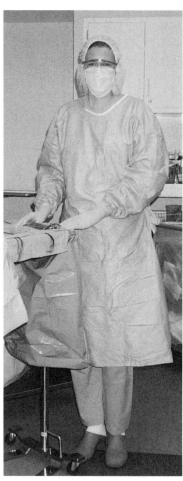

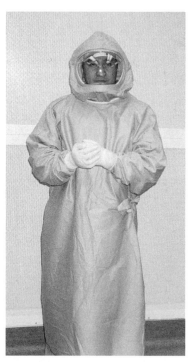

C

Figure 2–4. Scrub attire. ***A:*** Standard scrub attire for a circulating nurse. ***B:*** Standard scrub attire for a scrub nurse or operating room technician. ***C:*** Scrub attire (including hood and oxygen) for specialized procedures where rigorous asepsis is essential (ie, orthopedic procedures taking place within an operating room equipped with laminar air flow).

A   **B**

erating site (Figure 2–5), while single sheets are used for draping nonspecific areas, such as the area between the surgical team and the anesthesiologist (Figure 2–5). Drapes should be handled as little as possible, as the air current can contain contaminants. Drapes should not be adjusted, once placed. If a drape is placed improperly it should be discarded. If a hole is found after a drape is placed, it should be covered with another barrier or discarded.

STERILE FIELD

A sterile field is created to isolate the surgical incision site from the unsterile environment. Sterile drapes are used to create the sterile field. Only the top surface is considered sterile. All items within the sterile field must be sterile. The circulating personnel will provide additional sterile supplies and instruments throughout the procedure. Scrubbed persons should stay as close to the sterile field as possible while the nonscrubbed persons remain at a distance (usually several feet, while observing) that will prevent contamination of the sterile field.

The sterile field includes the draped patient, surgeon, surgeon's assistants, and the scrub nurse. The scrub nurse maintains the sterile instruments and supplies on two surfaces, called the **back table** and the **Mayo stand** (Figure 2–6). The Mayo stand holds the supplies and instruments that the surgeon will need to have most accessible during the procedure. The back table holds supplies and instruments that may be needed at various times throughout the

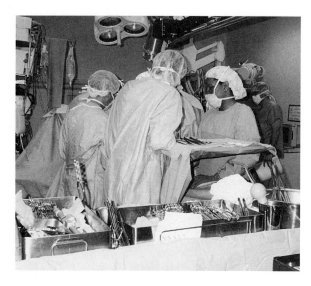

Figure 2–6. Figure shows back table in foreground and Mayo stand centered between scrub nurse and medical student.

procedure. The scrub nurse will move items back and forth as called for by various stages in the operation.

Contamination of supplies or personnel within the sterile field should be handled immediately. This includes changing gowns and gloves and removing from the field any instrument or supply that has become contaminated. Good judgment by the scrub team dictates how the sterile field is maintained. Everyone must have a strong surgical

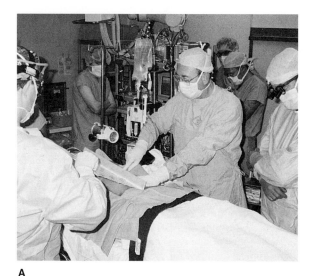

A

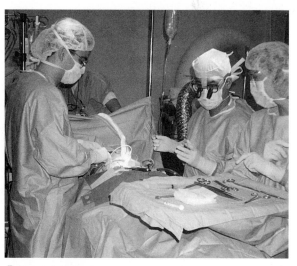

B

Figure 2–5. Patient being draped for a surgical procedure. **A:** Incision site is exposed but isolated. The surgeons place a loban steri-drape over the incision site in order to prevent contamination from the skin. **B:** Patient is draped for the operation, including placement of a single sheet drape between the patient and the anesthesiologist.

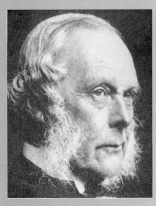

Jospeh Lister (1827–1912).

J oseph Lister (1827–1912) is considered the father of asepsis. In fact, the practice of asepsis is still often said to be based on "Listerian principles." Lister was a technically adept surgeon, but he was disappointed in the high mortality rate (~50%) associated with the amputations and excisions he performed.

When Lister learned of the work of Louis Pasteur (1822–1895) in bacteria and infection, he immediately began to consider methods of antisepsis in surgery. It is interesting to note that Lister's father had an avid interest in microscopy and optics. Lister's early education and familiarity with the microscope most likely enabled him to accept the work of Pasteur without question. The extreme heat that Pasteur had proposed to destroy bacteria was impractical in the surgical setting, so Lister began to consider methods of chemical antisepsis. He first began experimenting with the use of carbolic acid in 1865.

In 1867 Lister published two large papers describing his two-year experience of using carbolic acid in the practice of surgery. Lister not only used carbolic acid to sterilize wounds, he sterilized his own hands with this solution and also sprayed the operating field and table with it. Although Lister's methods were not met with unanimous approval during his lifetime, they were eventually incorporated into hospitals worldwide. His career was marked by other great achievements, including the development of absorbable sutures and the drainage tube. Despite early objections to his antiseptic techniques, he was widely respected and received a baronetcy in 1883.

conscience to protect the patient. It is everyone's individual responsibility to immediately call attention to the surgeon any observed breaks in sterile technique and, for that matter, any suspected possible break. It is always best to err on the side of caution. The patient's life depends on the team's focus and intensity. There is no room for error.

INSTRUMENTATION

Instrumentation for each surgical procedure is chosen based on the procedure, size of the patient, anatomical approach, and surgeon preferences. Instruments fall into four major categories: (1) dissectors; (2) retractors; (3) graspers; and (4) clamps. A combination of these instru-

ments makes up each instrument set. Each surgical specialty has instruments from these four categories designed to meet its special operating needs.

Instruments used for dissection include scissors and scalpels. Scissors used for tissue dissection should not be used to cut suture. Suture material will rapidly dull the scissors that are designed for tissue. Many of the scissors used are very delicate, with easily damaged tips. It is an expectation of the surgeon that the scrub nurse has examined all the instruments prior to handing them to the surgical team to make sure they are functioning properly.

Instruments utilized for grasping and holding tissue include forceps, sponge forceps, stone forceps, and needle holders. Tissue forceps are available with and without teeth. Forceps with teeth will be used on tissue such as muscle, skin, and fascia where little damage to this tissue will occur. Forceps without teeth are used on delicate structures and vessels. The size of a needle and the suture ligature will determine the size and shape of the needle holder.

Clamping instruments are primarily used for hemostasis. Clamps may be very delicate for small vessels or very large with special surfaces for clamping the aorta. Nursing staff will select appropriate clamps by the scheduled procedure.

Instruments used for retraction are self-retaining or hand-held. Retractors provide the necessary visibility to assist the surgeon in performing the surgery. Visualization is critical. Without proper exposure, procedure time may be prolonged and technical errors can occur.

Although minimally invasive (endoscopic, laparoscopic) surgical techniques once were utilized primarily by specialty groups, they are now common for almost all surgical specialties (see Chapters 11 and 12). Endoscopic equipment is easily damaged and costly to repair. When equipment is out of service for repair, surgeons may have to delay or cancel procedures. Great care must be taken to

NEEDLE SHAPE	APPLICATIONS	
Straight	Gastrointestinal tract Nasal cavity Nerve Oral cavity	Pharynx Skin Tendon Vessels
Half-curved	Skin (rarely used)	
1/4 Circle	Eye (primary application) Microsurgery	
3/8 Circle	Aponeurosis Biliary tract Dura Eye Fascia Gastrointestinal tract Muscle Myocardium	Nerve Perichondrium Periosteum Peritoneum Pleura Tendon Urogenital tract Vessels
1/2 Circle	Biliary tract Eye Gastrointestinal tract Muscle Nasal cavity Oral cavity Pelvis Peritoneum	Pharynx Pleura Respiratory tract Skin Subcutaneous fat Urogenital tract
5/8 Circle	Anal (hemorrhoidectomy) Cardiovascular system Nasal cavity Oral cavity Pelvis Urogenital tract (primary application)	
Compound curved	Eye (anterior segment)	

Figure 2–8. Choice of needle depends upon tissue to be penetrated. (Reprinted, with permission, from Ethicon, Inc, New Jersey.)

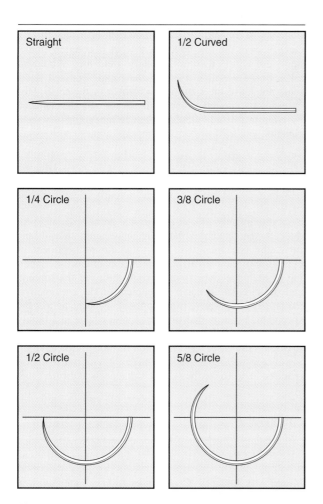

Figure 2–7. Different types of needles used in surgical procedures. (Reprinted, with permission, from Ethicon, Inc.)

avoid dropping a lens or bending a fiberoptic light cord. Camera, lens, or light cord damage will severely affect the visualization of the surgeon and require costly repair.

Careful handling of sharps is mandatory for all health care providers. Many operating rooms have established procedures for the handling of sharps during surgery. Even if formal procedures do not exist, most surgeons and scrub nurses will determine prior to the first incision how sharps will be handled during the case. Most of the sharps will be passed by the scrub nurse to the surgeon and the assistant. Other persons should try to stay clear of this area.

Students need to be especially aware of the location of sharps and avoid getting their hands inadvertently in the path of the transfer process. The knowledgeable student avoids over-reaching for an instrument on the Mayo stand. Even though the student is often stationed in close proximity to the Mayo stand, it is the scrub nurse or operating room technician who is responsible for instruments in this area.

SUTURES

Sutures are divided into two categories: absorbable and nonabsorbable. Types of absorbable sutures include plain, chromic, collagen, and glycolic acid polymers. Plain chromic and collagen are natural products obtained from animal intestines. Glycolic acid polymers are synthetic absorbable sutures.

Nonabsorbable sutures fall into three classes: class I—silk or synthetic fibers; class II—cotton or linen fibers, or coated natural or synthetic fibers; class III—wire. Types of nonabsorbable sutures include silk, cotton, nylon, polyester fiber, polypropylene, and stainless steel wire.

Along with determining the suture type and size, the nurses must determine what needle types and sizes the surgeon will require. Needles vary greatly in shape, size, and point design (Figure 2–7). Choice of needle depends on the tissue to be penetrated (Figure 2–8). Tissue such as bowel and kidney require a taper or blunt point, whereas skin that is dense requires a cutting point. The suture may be attached to the needle, or the scrub nurse may thread free strands of the ligature on needles during the procedure. The latter technique is rare today, as most sutures come attached. Some of the attached sutures are "pop-off" in design. This means that after placement, the needle can be removed by a gentle tug. Other attached sutures require the needle to be removed by cutting the suture material. It is always preferable, when possible, to remove the needle prior to tying the knot to minimize glove punctures and skin injury.

Sutures are used to provide hemostasis during the procedure, to maintain a surgical anastomosis, and to close the surgical wound. They are also sometimes used to mark surgical specimens for pathological purposes. Selection of sutures is based on the tissue to be sutured and the surgeon's preference.

SURGICAL COUNTS

Retained sponges, instruments, needles, and any other foreign object left by the surgical team can be costly in terms of patient injury, extended hospitalization, added operative procedures, and litigation. The nursing staff assumes responsibility for tracking all these items and will notify the surgeon before the incision is closed that all items are accounted for and removed. It is critical that all caregivers in the OR understand what is counted, and if items are removed from the sterile field they should always be in a visible place in the room. Counted items must not leave the room or be thrown in the trash. Discrepancies in counts occasionally occur and are managed by appropriate radiographs of the patient prior to wound closure.

SPECIMENS

Approximately 80% of all surgical procedures will produce a specimen for pathological examination. Many times the specimen will determine future treatment or even cure of the patient. Careful documentation and labeling of each specimen is the responsibility of the surgeon and the circulating nurse. Placement of the specimen in the proper preservative is also critical, as is seeing that the specimen is transported to the pathology suite in a timely manner. Frequently, the pathologist will come to the OR to discuss the case, the orientation of the specimen, labeling of margins, and any additional information that will be required to optimize the patient's diagnosis and care.

SUGGESTED READING

Bell RM, Bell PM: The—OR-home of the surgeon. In: Lawrence PF (editor): *Essentials of General Surgery*. Williams & Wilkins, 1992.

Meeker MH, Rothrock JC: *Alexander's Care of the Patient in Surgery*, 10th ed. Mosby, 1995.

3

Medical Assessment of the Surgical Patient

Stephen P. Fischer, MD

▶ Key Facts

▶ The preoperative evaluation should be performed in exactly the same manner each time so that no step is omitted. A preoperative medical questionnaire facilitates efficiency and focuses the evaluator to specific concerns.

▶ Cardiovascular diseases most frequently associated with surgical complications are ischemic heart disease with a history of myocardial infarction or angina, congestive heart failure, hypertension, and major arrhythmias or heart block.

▶ Acute and chronic pulmonary disorders, such as asthma and chronic obstructive pulmonary disease, are common and can be a significant source of postoperative morbidity and mortality.

▶ In general, most surgical procedures can be performed safely in patients with chronic renal disease, however, an understanding of fluid management and intraoperative electrolyte and

acid-base therapies are important to prevent acute renal dysfunction.

▶ Acute hepatitis is a relative contraindication to elective surgery and anesthesia.

▶ Diabetes mellitus is the most common endocrine disorder in surgical patients. Diabetic patients may be more prone to hyperglycemia, wound and urinary tract infections, and cardiovascular disorders.

▶ A thorough preoperative neurological assessment involves evaluation of both peripheral and central nervous system function.

▶ The preoperative patient may be considered compromised if his or her capacity to physiologically respond is impaired because of malnutrition, immune system compromise, advanced age, obesity, or the use of illicit or addictive drugs.

The preoperative evaluation of the surgical patient enhances the practitioner's awareness of a patient's medical condition and facilitates the plan of intra- and postoperative care. The purpose of the preoperative evaluation is to: (1) obtain pertinent information regarding the patient's current and past medical history; (2) perform a complete physical examination; (3) develop a plan of surgical intervention; (4) obtain the patient's informed consent; (5) reduce the patient's anxiety and fears through education about the proposed surgery, perioperative care, and options for postoperative pain control; (6) determine the appropriate laboratory tests and diagnostic studies; (7) answer any questions from the patient or family.

The preoperative evaluation of the patient should be performed in exactly the same manner each time so that no step is omitted. The time and level of detail of the evaluation will depend upon the patient's medical history and the proposed surgical procedure in terms of complexity and potential blood loss. The use of a preoperative medical questionnaire completed by the patient prior to the evaluation may facilitate efficiency and serve as a foundation for focusing the evaluator into pertinent areas of concern.

The practice of preoperative evaluation has changed during the past decade. Fewer patients are admitted prior to surgery unless their medical condition is unstable or requires optimization. Currently, 70–80% of surgeries in the United States are performed on an outpatient or same-day admission basis. This includes major cardiac and neurosurgical procedures. This change in the manner of preoperative evaluation requires the surgeon to achieve a high level of efficiency and accuracy in the history assessment and the physical examination with less time.

RISKS OF SURGERY & ANESTHESIA

Advances in surgical and anesthetic techniques have significantly reduced perioperative morbidity and mortality in the past 20 years. Approximately 26 million patients undergo a surgical procedure each year in the United States. Most patients have few complications as a result of the surgical or anesthetic procedure. Perioperative deaths occur in approximately 0.3% of all surgical patients. Post-

operative morbidity is often related to the patient's underlying medical condition, preoperative stability, and associated risk factors for each organ system. Patients 70 years of age or older, compared with younger patients, have an increased morbidity and mortality secondary to coexisting medical disorders. Elderly patients also have more emergency and cancer-related surgeries.

The American Society of Anesthesiologists developed a physical status classification for patients requiring surgery and anesthesia (Table 3–1). The concept was to classify and standardize physical categories of a patient's medical condition preoperatively in terms of his or her surgical risk and potential predisposition toward morbidity or mortality. The classification serves as a means of alerting the practitioner to a patient's physical condition and facilitates the plan of intra- and postoperative care.

SURGERY IN THE MEDICALLY COMPROMISED PATIENT

CARDIOVASCULAR SYSTEM

The preoperative cardiovascular evaluation is directed toward the severity, progression, and functional limitations of a patient's cardiovascular disease. Cardiovascular diseases most frequently associated with increased surgical morbidity and mortality include ischemic heart disease with a history of a myocardial infarction or angina, congestive heart failure, hypertension associated with either cardiac or renal failure, and major arrhythmias or heart block.

Cardiovascular complications account for 25–50% of deaths following noncardiac surgeries. Perioperative risk factors, such as myocardial infarction within 6 months and congestive heart failure, have been associated with an increase in surgical morbidity and mortality. The preoperative evaluation of a patient with cardiovascular disease requires attention to risk factors (Table 3–2), evaluation of the patient's medical history (Table 3–3), and a detailed physical examination. Diagnostic testing to determine the patient's stability and appropriateness for surgery is based on the severity of the disease, degree of impairment, and coexisting major organ dysfunction, such as of the pulmonary, hepatic, or renal system. The patient's physiologic compensatory mechanisms, as well as current drug therapy, should be thoroughly reviewed and evaluated.

HYPERTENSION

Hypertension is a common preoperative abnormality in the surgical patient, which appears more commonly with advancing age. Hypertension is a major risk factor for

Table 3–1. American Society of Anesthesiologists classification of physical status.

Class	Physical Status
1	The patient with no organic, physiologic, biochemical, or psychiatric disturbance (eg, is normally a healthy individual).
2	The patient with mild to moderate systemic disease that may or may not be related to the proposed surgical disorder (eg, mild diabetes, essential hypertension, nonlimiting organic heart disease).
3	The patient with severe systemic disease from a cause that is not incapacitating (eg, uncontrolled diabetes mellitus, systemic heart disease that limits activity, poorly controlled hypertension, angina, moderate to severe pulmonary insufficiency).
4	The patient with incapacitating systemic disease that is life-threatening with or without surgery (eg, unstable angina, congestive heart failure, and advanced renal, hepatic, pulmonary, endocrine, or cardiac failure).
5	The moribund patient who is not expected to survive with or without the operation. Surgery is performed in a desperate attempt for survival (eg, abdominal aneurysm rupture with profound shock, major cerebral trauma, massive pulmonary embolus).
E	Added to any patient's classification who undergoes emergency surgery (eg, appendectomy, incarcerated hernia with nausea and emesis, trauma).

Table 3–2. Preoperative cardiovascular risk factors.

Non-Clinical Criteria	Male gender Increasing age Obesity Cigarette smoking Lack of exercise (sedentary lifestyle) Family history of early cardiac disease Menopause Use of oral contraceptives (by women who smoke)

Clinical Criteria	Coronary artery disease
	Previous myocardial infarction
	Angina pectoris
	Significant aortic stenosis
	Dysrhythmias
	Congestive heart failure
	(S_3 gallop with increase jugular venous
	   pressure on examination)
	Arterial hypertension
	Hypercholesterolemia
	Diabetes mellitus
	History of cerebrovascular or vascular
	   disease
	Major emergency surgeries

cerebral, renal, and cardiac diseases. Complications of hypertension include congestive heart failure, cerebrovascular hemorrhage (eg, stroke), myocardial infarction, renal failure, and aortic and other vascular aneurysms with dissection or rupture. When hypertension is severe with systolic pressures greater than 195 mm Hg or diastolic blood pressure greater than 110 mm Hg, the patient should be treated medically prior to an elective surgery.

The preoperative evaluation of the patient with hypertension should assess the duration and severity of the disease, current and past drug therapy (as well as compliance with the current prescribed regimen), a history of chest pain, paroxysmal nocturnal dyspnea, symptoms of myocardial ischemia, impaired peripheral vascular profusion, ventricular failure, dependent edema, postural light-headedness, and symptoms of transient ischemic attacks or cerebrovascular impairment.

Table 3–3. Symptoms and signs of cardiac disease.

Symptoms	Signs
Chest pain	Cyanosis
Dizziness	Diaphoresis
Syncope or presyncope	Bradycardia/tachycardia
Visual blurring	Hypotension/hypertension
Shortness of breath	Diminished peripheral pulses
Dyspnea on exertion	Delayed cardiac upstroke
Paroxysmal nocturnal dyspnea	Jugular venous elevation Hepatojugular reflux
Unexplained fatigue	Rales or bibasilar dullness on pul-
Palpations	monary examination (think pleural
Leg/ankle edema	effusion and congestive heart
Ascites	failure)

Cough (think congestive
  heart failure)
	Abnormal heart sounds and
	  murmurs

ISCHEMIC HEART DISEASE

The most common cause of ischemic heart disease is atherosclerosis of the coronary arteries. The patient's medical history, physical examination, electrocardiogram, and chest x-ray are the foundation of the cardiac evaluation of the patient with known or suspected ischemic heart disease. The common clinical manifestations of coronary artery disease are ischemia (usually described as angina), arrhythmias, myocardial infarction, or ventricular dysfunction as manifested by congestive heart failure.

The surgical risk for a myocardial infarction and the potential for reinfarction during the perioperative period are listed in Table 3–4. Approximately one third of patients with significant coronary artery disease who have not sustained a myocardial infarction will have a normal baseline electrocardiogram. Patients experiencing angina may demonstrate electrocardiogram evidence of ischemia only during episodes of chest pain. Specialized studies such as exercise electrocardiography, thallium scintigraphy, two-dimensional echocardiography, and coronary angiography are diagnostic studies utilized in patients with suspected coronary artery disease, but have a low predictability in normal patients or when used as screening tests for preoperative patients.

VALVULAR HEART DISEASE

The preoperative assessment of patients with valvular heart disease focuses on the degree of impairment of myocardial function and the presence of associated major organ complications. The hemodynamic significance of a valvular lesion can be a precipitating factor for myocardial ischemia in some patients (eg, in severe aortic stenosis or regurgitation).

The most common cardiac murmur is the "innocent" flow murmur or a generally benign murmur of aortic sclerosis or mitral valve prolapse. Severe aortic stenosis increases the operative risk, especially in patients with aortic valve orifice areas less than 1 cm^2 (normal: 2.5–4 cm^2) and transvalvular pressure gradients greater than 50 mm Hg. The characteristic triad of associated symptoms with severe aortic stenosis include angina pectoris, dyspnea on exertion, and a syncopal history. Patients with aortic stenosis have an increased incidence of sudden death.

Table 3–4. Risk of perioperative myocardial infarction in patients undergoing non-cardiac surgery.

Patient Category	Infarction Incidence (%)
Patients without history of MI	0.13
Prior MI > 6 months	4.2
Prior MI 4–6 months	7.3
Prior MI < 3 months	18.6
Previous coronary artery bypass	1.2

MI = myocardial infarction.

Aortic stenosis should be clinically suspected in patients with the presence of a harsh murmur in the second intercostal space to the right of the sternum with radiation to the carotid arteries. Additionally, these patients often have diminished carotid pulsations and electrocardiographic evidence of left ventricular hypertrophy. In elderly patients whose activities are reduced, aortic stenosis may progress even to a severe stage without overt clinical symptoms.

Mitral regurgitation is another valvular disorder for which surgery carries increased morbidity and mortality. Mitral regurgitation is often secondary to rheumatic fever and is usually associated with some degree of mitral stenosis. Regurgitation flow results in left atrial volume overload with a decrease in left ventricular stroke volume and left ventricular dysfunction. Preoperative and intraoperative treatment of patients with mitral regurgitation is directed toward reducing systemic vascular resistance. The purpose is to increase forward stroke volume and decrease the retrograde flow. Mitral regurgitation is best auscultated at the cardiac apex and is characterized as a pansystolic murmur radiating to the axilla.

RESPIRATORY SYSTEM

The adverse impact of preexisting pulmonary disease on surgery and anesthesia can be significant. Acute and chronic pulmonary disorders are common and can be a significant source of postoperative morbidity and mortality.

Preoperative pulmonary risk factors include (1) a history of preexisting pulmonary dysfunction; (2) smoking history; (3) obesity; (4) surgeries involving the upper abdomen or thorax; and (5) age greater than 70 years. There is also a relationship between a prolonged surgical procedure under general anesthesia (> 4 hours) and the potential for postoperative pulmonary compromise, especially in patients with known risk factors.

The preoperative evaluation should determine the type, severity, functional limitations, and duration of any preexisting pulmonary disease, along with the current therapy. Physical activity limitations secondary to dyspnea often reflect the severity of the underlying pulmonary disease and the potential for perioperative respiratory compromise.

ASTHMA

Asthma is a common disease that affects 3–5% of adults in the United States. Preoperative evaluation of the asthmatic patient is directed toward the frequency and severity of asthmatic attacks and the adequacy of current treatment. Symptoms and signs of asthma include: (1) wheezing; (2) cough; (3) dyspnea; (4) tachypnea.

Asthma is considered a disorder of reversible airway inflammation and bronchoconstriction. The physical and emotional stress of surgery and the intubation of a patient's airway during anesthesia can trigger an acute asthmatic attack.

Severity of airflow obstruction can be measured preoperatively by spirometry and is especially useful when compared to the patient's previous baseline determinations. The patient taking oral bronchodilators should continue treatment as prescribed, including the day of the surgery.

CHRONIC OBSTRUCTIVE LUNG DISEASE

Chronic obstructive lung disease afflicts approximately 10 million people in the United States and is primarily due to smoking of tobacco. Chronic obstructive lung disease includes pulmonary emphysema and chronic bronchitis, with many patients having features of both disorders.

Chronic Bronchitis

Chronic bronchitis is clinically characterized by the presence of a productive cough with frequent pulmonary infections. Bronchial mucous and edema cause airflow obstruction, which can lead to chronic hypoxemia, pulmonary hypertension, and potentially right heart failure (cor pulmonale). Arterial blood gases can help delineate patients who have chronic hypoxemia and CO_2 retention. A $PaCO_2$ that is greater than 50 suggests an increased risk of postoperative respiratory compromise or failure. Preoperative assessment is directed towards treatment of any underlying acute bacterial infection, optimization of bronchodilator therapy, use of an incentive spirometer to minimize atelectasis, nuritional support, and cessation of smoking, which is often the most difficult aspect of the patient's preoperative treatment.

Emphysema

Pulmonary emphysema is a pathologic process based on destruction of the alveolar walls. This results in an irreversible alveoli enlargement and loss of elastic recoil. The etiology of emphysema is almost always related to cigarette smoking. Patients can develop bullae or large cystic areas in the lung; patients with severe emphysema often present with significant dyspnea. Characteristics of chronic bronchitis and pulmonary emphysema are presented in Table 3–5.

RENAL SYSTEM

The kidneys play an important role in regulating intravascular volume, eliminating metabolic toxins, and producing hormones, such as erythropoietin and renin. The possibility of impaired renal function during surgery

Table 3–5. Characteristics of chronic obstructive lung disease.

Characteristic	Emphysema	Chronic Bronchitis
Dyspnea	Progressive and severe	Intermittent and moderate
Cough	Infrequent	Persistent
Sputum	Little or no sputum	Excessive sputum production
Elastic recoil	Decreased	Normal
Airway resistance	Normal	Increased
Auscultation	Decreased breath sounds	Rhonchi, wheezing
PaO_2 mm Hg	Mild to moderately decreased ("pink puffer")	Markedly decreased (< 60) ("blue bloater")
$PaCO_2$ mm Hg	Normal to decreased	Increased
Chest x-ray	Hyperinflation with flat diaphragm Increased anteroposterior diameter Bullae, blebs	Increased lung markings
Heart	Normal, vertical	Large, horizontal
Cor pulmonale	Mild and late in disease	Marked and early in disease
Hemoglobin	Normal	Increased

$PaCO_2$ = partial pressure of carbon dioxide in arterial gas; PaO_2 = partial pressure of arterial oxygen.

should be considered in patients with renal disease and also in healthy patients undergoing major surgical procedures. In general, most surgical procedures can be performed safely in patients with chronic renal disease. An understanding of fluid management and intraoperative elec-trolyte and acid-base therapies are important to prevent intraoperative acute renal dysfunction (see Chapter 19). Table 3–6 contrasts acute from chronic renal failure.

The surgeon should be familiar with the various types of diuretics that are frequently employed in the periopera-

Table 3–6. Signs and symptoms of acute and chronic renal failure.

System	Signs and Symptoms Acute Renal Failure	Signs and Symptoms Chronic Renal Failure
Cardiac		Increased cardiac output Systemic hypertension Congestive heart failure Peripheral edema and ascites Dysrhythmia Pericarditis
Respiratory		Shortness of breath Dyspnea on exertion Rales, pleural effusion
Gastrointestinal	Nausea and emesis Anorexia	Gastrointestinal bleeding

Renal	Polyuria, nocturia
	Oliguria, anuria
	Sudden increase in creatinine and
	  blood urea nitrogen
		Progressive increase in creatinine and blood
		  urea nitrogen

Neuromuscular		Neuromuscular irritability Leg cramps Paresthesias Asterixis
Hematopoietic		Coagulopathy Platelet dysfunction Easy bruisability, ecchymosis Anemia
Metabolic	Metabolic acidosis Hypocalcemia Hyperphosphatemia	Metabolic acidosis Hypocalcemia Hyperkalemia Hypermagnesemia Hyperphosphatemia
Mental status	Fatigue, weakness	Fatigue, weakness Mental status changes Stupor
Other findings		Increased susceptibility to infections Pruritus Skin is yellow–brown.

tive period to correct common problems such as hypertension and intravascular fluid overload associated with cardiac, hepatic, and renal impairment. Additionally, renal disease can contribute to increased bleeding secondary to platelet dysfunction with uremia. Renal impairment can lead to anemia, peripheral neuropathies, and drug, metabolic, and excretion abnormalities.

The operative complications of patients with kidney disease are primarily dependent on the severity of the renal dysfunction rather than the type of disease. The preoperative evaluation of these patients includes the appropriate use of tests to assess renal function. The trends of testing results are more useful than isolated measurements. Tests for assessment of glomerular filtration rate are creatinine clearance, plasma creatinine, and blood urea nitrogen. Diagnostic tests for evaluation of renal tubular function determine proteinuria, hematuria, sodium excretion, urine concentrating ability and volume, and urine sediment by miscroscopic evaluation.

Anesthetic drugs used during the surgical procedure can have both a direct nephrotoxic effect as well as an indirect effect on renal function. Both drug metabolism and excretion are influenced by glomerular filtration rate and renal blood flow. Perioperative adjustments in drug dosage and frequency must be considered in patients with renal failure.

HEPATIC & GASTROINTESTINAL SYSTEM

The adult liver weighs approximately 1500 g and has a normal hepatic blood flow of approximately 25% of total body volume per minute (30 mL/min per kg body weight). The liver has a large functional reserve, and clinically significant liver dysfunction following surgery is uncommon. The four major physiologic functions of the liver include: (1) drug, hormone, protein, and fat metabolism; (2) glucose homeostasis; (3) protein synthesis; (4) bilirubin formation and excretion. Disorders of hepatic function have important implications for the surgeon. Many of the drugs given perioperatively, including the anesthetic drugs, are metabolized through the hepatic system. Diminished liver function may prolong drug effect and increase toxicity to the patient.

Liver function tests (LFTs) are utilized to determine the presence of liver disease preoperatively and to distinguish the differential diagnosis of hepatic dysfunction. However, LFTs are neither very sensitive nor very specific. Considerable liver dysfunction or damage must be present before any LFT abnormalities are evident, secondary to the liver's large functional reserves. A detailed medical history and physical examination is important and can provide the clinical "clues" of a patient's potential hepatic dysfunction.

Acute hepatitis is a relative contraindication to elective

Table 3–7. Preoperative differential diagnosis of upper abdominal pain.

Cholecystitis
Pancreatitis
Appendicitis
Acute viral or alcoholic hepatitis
Cardiac (myocardial infarction or angina pectoris)
Peptic ulcer disease
Gastritis
Enlarging abdominal aortic aneurysm
Acute pyelonephritis
Pneumonia
Hepatitic idiosyncratic drug reaction

surgery and anesthesia. Signs and symptoms of acute viral hepatitis include fatigue, anorexia, nausea and vomiting, dark urine, fever, pruritus, abdominal pain, and lighter-colored stools. Both morbidity and mortality increase approximately 10% during surgeries in patients with acute viral hepatitis. The patient with chronic hepatitis may appear without signs or symptoms characteristic of hepatitis except for a mild increase in LFTs. These patients can usually undergo surgery safely by avoiding potentially hepatotoxic drugs and maintaining hepatic vascular pressure through blood pressure control.

Patients with liver cirrhosis often manifest evidence of portal hypertension. Intraoperative hypotension from any cause (eg, blood loss, vasodilation, cardiac failure) can result in a decrease in hepatic blood flow and oxygenation to the liver. Hepatic ischemia can lead to tissue injury, necrosis, and hepatic failure. Prolonged hypotension in patients with cirrhosis must be avoided.

Patients with gallbladder or biliary tract disease often present with severe mid-gastric pain and progressive jaundice if biliary tract obstruction has occurred. Cholecystitis must be differentiated from other causes of upper abdominal pain (Table 3–7).

Patients with gastrointestinal disorders may indicate history of gastric reflux, suggesting the presence of an esophageal hiatal hernia. These patients have an increased risk of pulmonary aspiration during the anesthesia induction and in the postoperative period. Patients with a history of gastrointestinal bleeding may present with associated signs and symptoms of nausea and vomiting, weakness and fatigue, dehydration, and associated organ system dysfunction (eg, tachycardia, high-output cardiac failure, acute renal failure, altered mental status).

ENDOCRINE & METABOLIC SYSTEM

Endocrine gland disorders of overproduction and underproduction of hormones can have significant physiologic effects in surgical patients. Dysfunctions of the pancreas, thyroid, parathyroid, and the adrenal gland can increase perioperative morbidity and mortality.

PANCREAS

Diabetes mellitus is the most common endocrine disorder in the surgical patient. It is characterized by an impairment of carbohydrate metabolism secondary to a deficiency of insulin production. Diabetic patients are prone to hyperglycemia, increased wound and urinary tract infections, and cardiovascular disorders, such as congestive heart failure and myocardial infarction. Diabetes mellitus affects approximately 6 million patients in the United States, of which only 10% are insulin-dependent diabetics. These patients are more susceptible to metabolic abnormalities and end-organ dysfunction (Table 3–8).

Diabetes is diagnosed when the patient's fasting blood glucose is greater than 140 mg/dL, when a 2-hour postprandial plasma glucose is greater than 200 mg/dL, and when either ketonemia, ketouria, or glycosuria is evident. The preoperative evaluation of the diabetic patient is directed toward whether the diabetes and the end-organ complications of the disease have been optimally controlled. Patients with diabetes mellitus can have autonomic dysfunction, which may cause a decrease in gastric emptying and the potential for pulmonary aspiration. Patients with diabetic autonomic neuropathy may demonstrate signs of orthostatic hypotension, a resting tachycardia, a neurogenic bladder, and painless myocardial ischemia. Diabetic renal dysfunction is first indicated by proteinuria, followed by an elevation in serum creatinine.

THYROID

Hyperthyroidism can be caused by Graves' disease, multinodular toxic goiter, thryoiditis, thyroid-secreting tumor of the pituitary, a functional thyroid adenoma, or an over-dosing of thyroid replacement therapy. Hypothyroidism may be caused by Hashimoto's thyroiditis (eg, autoimmune disease), thyroidectomy, iodine deficiencies, failure of the pituitary hypothalamic axis, anti-thyroid medications, or the exposure to radioactive iodine. Preop-

erative patients presenting for thyroid surgery may have received a course of medical therapy preoperatively.

Elective surgical procedures for patients with clinically evident hyperthyroidism, including subtotal thyroidectomy, should be postponed until the patient is euthyroid with medical therapy. Patients with thyrotoxicosis undergoing operative procedures can manifest cardiovascular dysfunction, including congestive heart failure, high-output cardiac failure, and shock.

Hypothyroidism in the adult patient is often insidious and may present with few clinical symptoms. Patients with overt signs of clinical hypothyroidism may show adverse (hypometabolic) responses associated with perioperative management. Patients may demonstrate increased sensitivity to depressant drugs, slow metabolism, hypodynamic cardiovascular responses in heart rate and cardiac output, decreased baroreceptor reflexes, delayed gastric emptying, hypothermia, and hypovolemia. Elective cases in patients with severe clinical hypothyroidism should be postponed until the patient is euthyroid. Signs and symptoms of hyperthyroidism and hypothyroidism are presented in Table 3–9.

PARATHYROID

Parathyroid hormone is the primary regulator of calcium hemostasis. Hyperparathyroidism causes excessive release of parathyroid hormone, which stimulates bone reabsorption and the decreased renal excretion of calcium. The preoperative clinical manifestations of hyperparathyroidism are due to hypercalcemia and are often insidious in onset and nonspecific. Therefore, the diagnosis is often dependent on obtaining an elevated serum calcium with an associated increased parathyroid hormone level. Etiologies of primary hyperparathyroidism include carcinoma, adenoma, and parathyroid gland hyperplasia. Secondary hyperparathyroidism is a response to hypocalcemia from intestinal malabsorption disorders or renal failure.

The preoperative evaluation of a patient with hypoparathyroidism is directed toward the clinical signs and symptoms of hypocalcemia. Hypoparathyroidism can occur secondary to a deficiency of parathyroid hormone following parathyroidectomy. Occasionally, the parathyroid glands are accidentally removed during a thyroidectomy procedure because of their proximity to the thyroid gland. In addition to hypoparathyroidism, other causes of hypocalcemia include renal failure, acute pancreatitis, hypomagnesemia, and vitamin D deficiency.

Patients with hypoparathyroidism and hypocalcemia often manifest two clinical signs of neuromuscular irritability. **Chvostek's sign** is elicited by tapping over the facial nerve, which causes a painful twitching of the facial musculature. **Trousseau's sign** is the occurrence of carpopedal spasm following inflation of a tourniquet above systolic blood pressure for 3 minutes. It should be noted that on occasion both of these signs are present in normal individuals. Table 3–10 reviews the signs and symptoms

Table 3–8. Preoperative concerns and complications of diabetes mellitus.

Acute	Chronic
Hyperglycemia	Cardiomyopathy
Ketoacidosis	Coronary artery disease
Dehydration, hypovolemia	Silent myocardial ischemia
Osmotic diuresis	Cerebrovascular disease
Electrolyte imbalance	Peripheral vascular disease
Hyperkalemia	Retinopathy
Hypophosphatemia	Sensory neuropathy
Nausea and vomiting	Autonomic neuropathy
Abdominal pains	Gastroparesis
Tachypnea	Tachycardia, dysrhythmias
Weakness, fatigue	Orthostatic hypotension
Mental status changes	Prone to dermopathies and pressure ulcers
	Increased susceptibility to infections
	Delayed wound healing

Table 3–9. Signs and symptoms of hyper- and hypothyroidism.

System	Signs and Symptoms	Signs and Symptoms
	Hyperthyroidism	**Hypothyroidism**
Cardiac	Tachycardia Atrial fibrillation Congestive heart failure	Bradycardia Decreased cardiac output
Gastrointestinal	Diarrhea Weight loss	Constipation Weight gain Delayed gastric emptying
Neuromuscular	Hyperactive muscle reflexes Tremor Skeletal muscle weakness	Hyperactive muscle reflexes Skeletal muscle weakness
Skeletal	Bone resorption	
Hematopoietic	Anemia Thrombocytopenia	Anemia
Ocular	Exophthalmos	
Metabolic	Heat intolerance Warm and moist skin Menstrual irregularity	Cold intolerance Dry skin Peripheral vasoconstriction Menorrhagia
Mental status	Nervousness Anxiety	Dull facial expression Lethargy, depression
Other findings	Goiter	Hyponatremia Excessively large tongue Possible pleural, pericardial, or abdominal effusions Hoarseness

Table 3–10. Signs and symptoms of hyper- and hypoparathyroidism.

System	Signs and Symptoms	Signs and Symptoms
	Hyperparathyroidism with Hypercalcemia	**Hypoparathyroidism with Hypocalcemia**
Cardiac	Shortened QT interval Prolonged PR interval Hypertension Heart block	Prolonged QT interval Hypotension Congestive heart failure
Respiratory		Inspiratory stridor
Gastrointestinal	Weight loss Anorexia Polydipsia Nausea and emesis Epigastric pain Constipation	
Renal	Polyuria Hematuria Decreased glomerular filtration rate Renal stones	
Neuromuscular	Skeletal muscle weakness Headache	Skeletal muscle weakness Neuromuscular irritability (positive Chvostek or Trousseau sign) Tetany, muscle cramps Carpopedal spasms Seizures
Skeletal	Bone pain Cystic lesions Pathologic fractures	
Hematopoietic	Anemia	
Ocular	Conjunctivitis	Cataracts
Mental status	Lethargy, somnolence Insomnia Apathy, depression Psychosis	Restlessness Depression, dementia Psychosis
Other findings		Laryngospasm Tingling of lips, hands, & feet Thin, brittle nails Skin dry and scaly

of hypo- and hyperparathyroidism and the associated surgical concerns.

ADRENAL GLAND

Preoperative evaluation of patients with adrenal gland dysfunction depends on the anatomy of the disturbance and the resulting physiologic effects. Chronic or primary adrenocortical insufficiency (hypoadrenocorticism) is referred to as **Addison's disease** and is secondary to a destruction of the adrenal cortex, resulting in glucocorticoid and mineralocorticoid deficiency. A principal concern in patients with Addison's disease is the increased risk of circulatory collapse secondary to their inability to respond to stress. This acute adrenal crisis is caused by insufficient cortisol. Intraoperatively, severe hypotension can occur with decreased systemic vascular resistance and left ventricular stroke index. Postoperative instability may be greater than during the operative procedure. Etiologies of primary adrenocortical insufficiency include autoimmune destruction of the adrenal cortex (80% of cases), adrenal hemorrhage (use of anticoagulants), sepsis, tuberculosis, Hashimoto's disease, and congenital adrenal hyperplasia.

Hyperadrenocorticism is referred to as **Cushing's syndrome**, and its common clinical presentation is secondary to an excess of glucocorticoids. Etiologies include adrenal hyperplasia, adenoma, carcinoma, and iatrogenic causes. Clinical manifestations of hypo- and hyperadrenocorticism are listed in Table 3–11.

Pheochromocytomas are tumors of rare occurrence that account for fewer than 0.1% of all patients with hypertension. The clinical manifestations of a pheochromocytoma are secondary to its secretion of catecholamines. The hallmark of a pheochromocytoma is paroxysmal hypertension with associated tachycardia, headache, and diaphoresis. Patients with pheochromocytoma are a significant perioperative management concern with a high risk for morbidity.

Carcinoid syndrome is another rare endocrine disorder

Table 3–11. Clinical manifestations of adrenal cortical dysfunctions.

Hyperadrenocorticism (Cushing's Syndrome)	Hypoadrenocorticism (Addison's Disease)
Diastolic hypertension	Weight loss, anorexia
Hypokalemia	Nausea and vomiting
Hyperglycemia	Diarrhea
Leukocytosis	Amenorrhea
Skeletal muscle wasting	Abdominal pains
Osteoporosis, osteopenia with pathologic fractures	Sparse axillary hair
Weakness, fatigue	Skeletal muscle weakness
Truncal obesity	Hypotension
Hirsutism	Cardiopenia
Mental status changes	Arrhythmias if hyperkalemia
Amenorrhea, oligomenorrhea	Neutropenia, lymphocytosis
Impaired wound healing	Severe dental caries
Susceptibility to infection	Hyperkalemia
"Moon faces"	Hyponatremia
"Buffalo hump" (supraclavicular fat pad)	Hypoglycemia
Thin skin with striations	Hyperpigmentation over palmar surfaces & pressure points
Easy bruisability	
Headaches	

Table 3–12. Signs and symptoms of intracerebral hemorrhage.

Nausea and emesis
Depressed level of consciousness
Triad of meningeal irritation:
  Photophobia
  Headaches
  Meningismus
Focal neurological signs
Cranial nerve palsies
Hypothermia
Seizures
Increased intracranial pressure (see Table 3–14)

that appears as a slow-growing tumor, often in the gastrointestinal tract. The release of various vasoactive substances into the circulation results in a variety of preoperative clinical manifestations, including abdominal pain and cramping, diarrhea, dehydration, bronchospasm, hypertension with paroxysmal hypotension, and cutaneous skin flushing.

CENTRAL NERVOUS SYSTEM

Preoperative neurological assessment involves evaluation of both peripheral and central nervous system function. Evaluation is based upon a detailed history and a focused physical examination. The purpose of the preoperative neurological examination is: (1) to determine the general extent and location of the neurological lesion; (2) to document in the surgical record the absence or presence of nervous system malfunction for perioperative comparison; (3) to record and determine the patient's preoperative stability or instability; (4) to develop an appropriate surgical perioperative management plan. Patients with nervous system disorders present with a variety of symptoms dependent on the location of the neurological disease or injury.

CEREBROVASCULAR DISEASE

The four major neurological disorders of a patient with neurological cerebrovascular disease include intracranial aneurysms, arteriovenous malformations, hypertensive intracerebral disease, and carotid artery disease. The patient with cerebrovascular disease may demonstrate preoperative signs and symptoms of a nonspecific nature. Patients may indicate dizziness, headaches, orbital pain, and mild motor or sensory abnormalities. With the rupture of a intracranial lesion, the signs and symptoms are more specific (Table 3–12). An intracerebral hemorrhage with increased intracranial pressure may also affect the electrocardiogram, causing ST segment elevation or depression, and the presence of U-waves, a prolonged QT interval, and T-wave inversion or flattening. A primary focus preoperatively should be directed towards controlling any systemic hypertension.

Patients presenting with carotid artery or vertebrobasilar artery disease usually have manifested signs or symptoms of either a transient ischemic attack (TIA) or a completed stroke. There is an associated higher incidence of hypertension, coronary artery disease, and valvular heart disease in patients presenting with carotid artery disease. Cerebral and lacunar infarction occurs with the thrombotic or embolic occlusion of a cerebral vessel. The preoperative neurological deficits are related to the particular vessel(s) involved and the extent of any collateral circulation.

TIAs are characterized by focal ischemic deficits that can last anywhere from minutes up to 2 hours. Approximately 30% of patients with a history of stroke have TIAs. Table 3–13 reviews the clinical findings of a patient with TIAs. Since TIAs are transient, patients may have a normal examination at the time of their preoperative assessment.

INTRACEREBRAL TUMORS & INCREASED INTRACRANIAL PRESSURE

Intracranial tumors present preoperatively according to size, location, and intracranial pressure. Slow-growing tumors may present with minimal symptoms. A rapidly expanding mass often evokes acute neurological compromise and symptoms. The preoperative assessment of a patient presenting with an intracranial tumor is directed towards determining if increased intracranial pressure (ICP) is present. Table 3–14 lists the signs and symptoms of increased ICP. If ICP is significant, there may be evidence of brain herniation manifested by: (1) apnea; (2) pupil(s)

Table 3–13. Signs and symptoms of transient ischemic attacks.

Carotid Territory	Vertebrobasilar Area
Contralateral arm, leg, or face weakness, paresthesias, or numbness	Extremity weakness, paresthesias, or numbness (either uni- or bilateral)
Dysphagia	Dysarthria
Visual monocular loss (contralateral to the affected limb)	Diplopia, visual dimness or blurring
Hyperreflexia	Ataxia
External plantar response on the affected side	Drop attacks or falling to floor from leg weakness

dilated and unreactive pupil(s); (3) contralateral hemiplegia; (4) bradycardia; and (5) altered mental consciousness.

HEAD TRAUMA

The preoperative evaluation of a patient presenting with a head trauma is often influenced by the extent of the injury and whether it has precipitated an open or closed skull fracture. Associated trauma, such as abdominal injuries and long bone fractures, may be present. Patency of the airway, ventilation, and treatment of shock are the initial focus of the surgeon. The preoperative evaluation is then directed toward the absence or presence of increased ICP.

In patients with acute head trauma, the preoperative evaluation must proceed concomitantly with management of unstable or urgent conditions. Seizures may accompany cerebral trauma and suggest the expansion of an intracranial hematoma. Both hypertension and hypotension are manifestations of head injuries and require immediate preoperative treatment. Comatose patients with decerebrate or decorticate posturing have severe hemispheric dysfunction, deterioration, and probable intubation requirements.

The preoperative assessment in any trauma patient may be limited by the extreme urgency to proceed to the operating room. In addition to laboratory and diagnostic tests, a drug screen should be performed in all trauma patients, since illegal and prescription drugs may influence intra- and postoperative surgical management.

Table 3–14. Signs and symptoms of increased intracranial pressure.

Headache (often worsened by cough)
Nausea and emesis
Altered mental status
Hypertension
Bradycardia
Visual disturbances
Papilledema
Unilateral pupillary dilatation
Abducens (cranial nerve VI) or oculomotor (cranial nerve III) palsy
Neck rigidity
Seizures
Decreased alertness
Stupor or coma

ADDITIONAL FACTORS AFFECTING SURGICAL RISK

The preoperative patient may be considered compromised if their capacity to respond in a normal physiologic fashion to trauma or infection is significantly impaired. Recognition of factors that may delay wound healing and recovery and increase susceptibility to infection are essential to evaluate and, if possible, optimize preoperatively.

NUTRITIONAL ASSESSMENT

Metabolic and nutritional disorders can cause patient malnutrition, weight loss, and an overall deterioration in general health (see Chapter 20). Patients with malnutrition have an increased rate of perioperative morbidity and mortality as well as postoperative infections Acute weight loss in excess of 10% of body weight may indicate the need for preoperative nutritional support prior to elective surgery. Additionally, patients with moderate to severe dehydration should be treated preoperatively, with close regard to avoiding fluid overload and pulmonary edema.

IMMUNE SYSTEM ASSESSMENT

Preoperative patients with immune system disorders are susceptible to increased infections and have a higher incidence of perioperative morbidity and mortality. Several immune deficiency disorders are linked to severe malnutrition states, such as the acquired immune deficiency syndrome (AIDS).

Certain drugs may increase the patient's susceptibility to infection in the perioperative period, such as corticosteroids and cytotoxic or immunosuppressive drugs. Additionally, prolonged antibiotic therapy may reduce the surgical patient's resistance to infection. Certain hematologic diseases as well as diabetes mellitus, for example, are known to decrease the immune competence of the preoperative patient, thus increasing operative risk.

THE ELDERLY PATIENT

The elderly surgical patient has an increased risk of morbidity and mortality when concurrent cardiovascular, pulmonary, renal, or other significant systemic disease is present. Age is not usually considered a contraindication for most major operative procedures. However, it is often difficult to delineate the physiologic process of increasing age from that of coexisting disease.

The preoperative evaluation of the elderly patient should be detailed and comprehensive in a judgment of his or her medical condition and stability. An absence of overt signs and symptoms may not indicate an absence of significant disease. The clinical manifestations of coronary artery disease, which is often present in patients over 65 years, may not be obvious in elderly patients who have a generally sedentary lifestyle. However, the physiologic stress of surgery and anesthesia may unexpectedly demonstrate the underlying cardiovascular or other systemic disorder. There is a general decline of organ function with increasing age, and occult diseases such as cancer are not infrequent.

Elderly patients generally require smaller doses of anesthetics, narcotics, and preoperative medications. These patients have an increased susceptibility to the adverse and toxic effects of certain drugs. Enhanced sensitivity to sedatives and depressant drugs may cause mental confusion or increased somnolence.

In addition to the medical history and physical examination, information on the elderly patient's activity levels and exercise tolerance are useful in estimating their cardiopulmonary status and physiologic reserve. Surgical risk of the elderly patient should be judged on the basis of physiological status and stability rather than on chronological age alone.

THE OBESE PATIENT

There is no precise definition between patients who are considered overweight and obese. Morbid obesity has been clinically defined to be as little as 20% above ideal body weight to 100% or greater above ideal body weight. In either case, the adverse effects of morbid obesity, both intra- and postoperatively, are well documented. Table 3–15 reviews the perioperative concerns and adverse effects of the morbidly obese patient for surgery.

PRESCRIPTION & ILLICIT DRUGS

The patient's current medications should be reviewed as to their preoperative continuation or discontinuation and any adjustment in frequency or dosage. The physiologic effects of a patient's drug regimen may be altered during the intra- and postoperative periods from the surgical intervention, metabolic changes, or concomitant new drug use. Patients using diuretics, for example, may present preoperatively mildly to moderately dehydrated and may have hypokalemia. Patients taking aspirin or nonsteroidal anti-inflammatory drugs may benefit from discontinuation of these drugs preoperatively in surgical cases where a large blood loss is expected. Certain drugs,

Table 3–15. Adverse physiologic effects of morbid obesity.

Systemic and pulmonary hypertension
Increased blood volume
Increased cardiac output
Ischemic cardiac disease
Cardiac arrythmia and conduction defects
Cardiomegaly
Congestive heart failure
Restrictive lung disease
Obesity-hypoventilation syndrome
Arterial hypoxemia
Hiatal hernia and reflux
Delayed gastric emptying
Hyperacidic gastric fluid
Diabetes mellitus
Obstructive sleep apnea
Fatty liver infiltration and insufficiency
Hypercholesterolemia and hypertriglyceridemia
Osteoarthritis

such as monoamine oxidase inhibitors, can have significant adverse effects on a patient's cardiovascular stability during anesthesia, surgery, and the postoperative period. The surgeon must be familiar with the potential adverse and toxic effects of the patient's drugs. Any drug that is unfamiliar to the practitioner should not be simply listed under the "medication" history without personal knowledge of the drug's effects and potential adverse reactions.

Patients taking illicit and addictive drugs are often reluctant to indicate their substance abuse disorder. This is of concern, since the use of cocaine and amphetamines can cause a reduction or depletion of catecholamine receptor store. Intraoperatively, these patients may have a blunted response to hypotension and an associated decrease in cardiac output. This can result in shock and cardiovascular collapse.

A careful history should be obtained from any patient who indicates illicit or addictive drug use. Patients utilizing cocaine or amphetamines should have elective surgeries postponed and may benefit from referral to a substance abuse rehabilitation program.

COST-EFFECTIVE PREOPERATIVE LABORATORY & DIAGNOSTIC TESTING

The value and utility of preoperative diagnostic studies have become a central issue in evaluating cost-effective health care in the surgical patient. It is estimated that up to $3 billion is spent in the United States annually in preoperative laboratory and diagnostic studies.

Unnecessary testing is inefficient, expensive, and requires additional technical resources. Inappropriate studies may lead to evaluation of "borderline" or false-positive laboratory abnormalities. This may result in unnecessary operating room delays, cancellations, and potential patient risk through additional testing and follow-up. The surgical patient requires preoperative laboratory and diagnostic studies, which should be consistent with his or her medical history, the proposed operative procedure, and the potential for blood loss. Preoperative laboratory and diagnostic testing should be ordered for specific clinical indications, rather than simply because the patient is about to undergo a surgical procedure.

SUMMARY

The preoperative evaluation of the surgical patient is a comprehensive, systematic assessment of a patient's medical history and current status. The ultimate goal is to reduce the potential for perioperative morbidity through enhanced practitioner awareness and patient management.

The preoperative evaluation is defined by the nature of the proposed surgical procedure in view of the patient's underlying medical disorder, and alerts all team members to potential difficulties.

Each individual patient for surgery requires the highest level of comprehensive preoperative evaluation and presents the surgeon with significant clinical challenges in providing the most appropriate care and the best outcome possible.

SUGGESTED READING

Celli BR: What is the value of preoperative pulmonary function testing? Med Clin N Am 1993;77:309.

Elliot DL et al: Medical evaluation before operations. West J Med 1982;37:351.

Friedman LS, Maddrey WC: Surgery in patients with liver disease. Med Clin N Am 1987;71:453.

Gluck R et al: Preoperative and postoperative medical evaluation of surgical patients. Am J Surg 1988;155:730.

Goldman L, Mangano DT: Preoperative assessment of the patient with known or suspected coronary artery disease. N Engl J Med 1995;333:1750.

Kaufman BS, Contreras J: Preanesthetic assessment of the patient with renal disease. Anesth Analg 1994;78:143.

Kroenke K: Preoperative evaluation: the assessment and management of surgical risk. J Gen Int Med 1987;2:257.

Ladenson PW et al: Complications of surgery in hypothyroid patients. Am J Med 1984;77:261.

MacPherson D: Preoperative laboratory testing: should any tests be "routine" before surgery? Med Clin N Am 1993;77:289.

Martin DE, Kammerer WS: The hypertensive surgical patient. Surg Clin N Am 1983;63:1017.

Merli GJ, Bell RD: Preoperative management of the surgical patient with neurologic disease. Med Clin N Am 1987;71:511.

Mohr DN, Jett JR: Preoperative evaluation of pulmonary risk factors. J Gen Int Med 1988;3:277.

Pasulka PS et al: The risks of surgery in obese patients. Ann Intern Med 1986;106:540.

Schiff RL, Emanuele MA: The surgical patient with diabetes mellitus: guidelines for management. J Gen Int Med 1995; 10:154.

Wyatt WJ et al: Pitfalls in the role of standardized pre-admission laboratory screening for ambulatory surgery. Am J Surg 1989; 55:343.

Anesthesia Principles

Yuan-Chi Lin, MD, MPH, & Donald R. Stanski, MD

► Key Facts

- ► Premedications are often given to surgical patients prior to anesthesia and include sedatives, opioids, tranquilizers, and anticholinergics.

- ► The goals of general anesthesia are to provide amnesia, analgesia, reflex suppression, and muscle relaxation for surgical procedures.

- ► The four phases of general anesthesia are induction, maintenance, emergence, and recovery.

- ► Endotracheal intubation is the most common technique for maintaining the airway in general anesthesia.

- ► The four major methods for the maintenance of general anesthesia are pure inhalation agents, nitrous oxide-opiate-relaxant technique, total intravenous anesthesia, and combination.

- ► Common regional anesthesia techniques include spinal anesthesia, epidural anesthesia, peripheral nerve block anesthesia, and intravenous regional anesthesia.

- ► Local anesthetics are administered intradermally or subcutaneously for infiltration anesthesia by blocking impulse conduction nerve fibers.

The primary responsibility of the anesthesiologist is to facilitate surgical procedures by providing analgesia and amnesia for patients in a safe manner. The practice of anesthesia is no longer confined to the operating room. Anesthesiologists provide care for invasive and noninvasive procedures outside the operating room, including magnetic resonance imaging, lithotripsy, computed tomography, electroconvulsive therapy, cardiac catheterization, and interventional radiologic procedures. Anesthesiologists are members of the cardiopulmonary resuscitation team. The American Board of Anesthesiology now provides certification examinations for special qualification in critical care medicine and in pain management.

The practice of anesthesia has changed significantly over the past few decades because of new drugs, monitoring techniques, and advances in surgical techniques. Surgeons and anesthesiologists comprise an integrated team dedicated to optimal patient care. This chapter describes the following fundamental aspects of anesthesia practice: preanesthesia assessment, intraoperative monitoring, general anesthesia, regional anesthesia, monitored anesthesia care, and local anesthesia.

PREANESTHESIA ASSESSMENT

Prior to a surgical procedure, the anesthesiologist evaluates the patient's medical, surgical, and psychological status. The anesthesiologist formulates a therapeutic plan that utilizes knowledge of the patient's medical condition

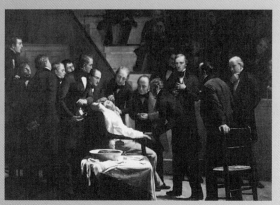

Ether Day by Robert Hinckley (1853–1941). Artist's depiction of the first public demonstration of chemical anesthesia at Massachusetts General Hospital on October 16, 1846. (Courtesy of Boston Medical Library.)

In the mid-1800s, as surgical techniques improved, the need for safe and effective methods of pain prevention became a priority. Prior to the discovery of ether, nitrous oxide, and chloroform, numerous agents—including narcotics, alcohol, and hypnotic trances—had been used to relieve patients of their pain and discomfort during surgical procedures.

The first published account of the use of anesthesia during a surgical procedure appeared on November 18, 1846, in the *Boston Medical and Surgical Journal* (vol. 35, pp. 309–317 and 379–382). This paper described operations performed by John Collins Warren and George Hayward with ether anesthesia administered by William Morton, a practicing dentist who had used his preparation on his patients for tooth extractions. News of this phenomenon spread rapidly, and a new age in the history of medicine was begun.

It is interesting to note that the first "clinical trials" of ether anesthesia took place in the parlor of the American surgeon, Dr. Crawford Long. In the early 1840s, he took note of the reactions of his friends during fashionable "ether parties," and it was not lost on him that they were "feeling no pain." He was using ether anesthesia in his practice as early as 1842, but did not publish his findings until 1849.

and the planned operative procedure. Ideally, the patient arrives in the operating room apprehension-free, lightly sedated, and fully cooperative. The preoperative visit is important in reducing patient anxiety. For outpatients, the preoperative interview can be conducted via the telephone. Chapter 3 provides a detailed description of the preoperative assessment.

Prior to delivering anesthesia, the anesthesiologist checks the safety and the function of the equipment for anesthetic delivery and monitoring (Figure 4–1), tests the laryngoscope, prepares the proper sized endotracheal tube, prepares the intravenous (IV) fluids, and examines the function of the suction tubing and connectors. The necessary medications and blood products are prepared or made readily available.

In addition, premedications are commonly given to surgical patients to reduce anxiety. Most premedications are administered orally, intravenously, or intramuscularly; rectal suppositories and intranasal approaches are also utilized (especially in children). For outpatient surgery, intravenous premedications are usually administered in the preoperative holding area since most patients are not hospitalized prior to the surgical procedures. Premedications are individualized to specific needs and include sedatives, opioids, tranquilizers, and anticholinergics. Common premedications are listed in Table 4–1.

Patient positioning during induction and during surgery is important. During induction, most patients are positioned supine with extremities in a neutral anatomic position. The anesthesiologist ensures that the legs are uncrossed, that the head and arms are comfortably positioned, that the restraining devices do not create pressure points, and that the restraining belt is properly positioned above the knees. After induction, the positioning may be

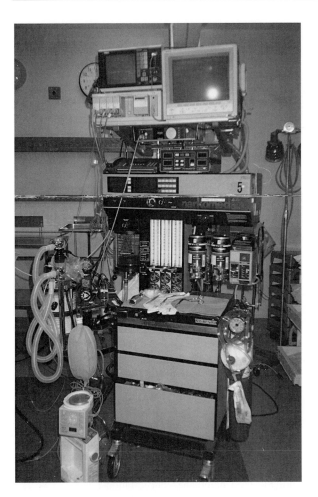

Figure 4–1. Anesthetic machine and monitors.

modified to facilitate surgical exposure. In addition, the optimal position depends on other factors, including the cardiac venous return, the pulmonary ventilation-to-perfusion relationship, and the prevention of peripheral nerve injuries. For patients in the supine position, arm extension beyond 80 degrees is avoided, and the eyes are protected.

Table 4–1. Common premedications, routes, and dosages.

Medications	Route and Dosage	Time Prior to Induction
Diazepam (Valium)	PO 5–10 mg	1 h
Lorazepam (Ativan)	PO 1–2 mg	1 h
Morphine sulfate	IM 5–10 mg	1 h
Scopolamine	IM 0.2–0.4 mg	1 h
Midazolam (Versed)	PO 0.5–0.75 mg/kg	1/2 h
Midazolam (Versed)	IV 1–2 mg	Immediately preinduction
Fentanyl (Sublimaze)	IV 25–100 μg	Immediately preinduction

Most complications related to positioning (eg, nerve injury, pressure sore, corneal ablation) can be prevented by careful patient positioning and proper equipment usage.

INTRAOPERATIVE MONITORING

Monitoring devices enable the rapid detection of physiologic abnormalities or trends that may endanger patient safety. The American Society of Anesthesiologists has published standards for basic intraoperative monitoring. However, in emergency situations, appropriate life support measures take precedence. One standard states the following: "Qualified anesthesia personnel shall be present in the room throughout the conduct of all general anesthetics, regional anesthetics, and monitored anesthesia care." Another standard states the following: "During all anesthetics, the patient's oxygenation, ventilation, circulation, and temperature shall be continuously evaluated."

Sufficient illumination and patient exposure are necessary to evaluate skin color, adequacy of ventilation, and adequacy of circulatory function. Standard noninvasive intraoperative monitors include oxygen analyzer with a low concentration limit alarm, pulse oximetry, capnography or mass spectrometry, esophageal or precordial stethoscope, continuous electrocardiography, arterial blood pressure, and body temperature electrocardiography. The standard noninvasive monitors and invasive monitors are listed in Table 4–2.

Table 4–2. Noninvasive monitors and invasive monitors.

Noninvasive	
Monitors	**Measured Functions**
Pulse oximetry	Arterial oxygen saturation, heart rate
Automatic blood pressure (Dinamap)	Mean, systolic diastolic arterial pressure, heart rate
Precordial/esophageal stethoscope	Heart sounds, breath sounds
Electrocardiography	Heart rate, rhythm
Capnography	Inspired/expired CO_2 concentration
Oxygen analyzer	Inspired oxygen concentration
Mass spectrometry	Inspired/expired CO_2 concentration, inhalation Anesthetic concentration
Temperature probe	Oral, rectal, esophageal, or tympanic temperature
Peripheral nerve stimulator	Neuromuscular blockade status

Invasive	
Monitors	**Measured Functions**
Intra-arterial catheter	Intra-arterial blood pressure
Central venous catheter	Central venous pressure
Pulmonary arterial catheter	Pulmonary arterial pressure, wedge pressure
Intraventricular catheter	Intracranial pressure
Foley catheter	Urine output

GENERAL ANESTHESIA

The goals of general anesthesia are to provide amnesia, analgesia, areflexia, and muscle relaxation for surgical procedures. The choice of the general anesthetic agent depends on several factors, including patient medical and surgical status, planned surgical procedure, availability of anesthetic and monitoring equipment, and clinical experience of both the anesthesiologist and the surgeon. General anesthesia is achieved by several different anesthetic agents: inhalation anesthetics, intravenous anesthetics, opioid analgesics, and muscle relaxants. Inhalation anesthetics are administered by temperature-compensated vaporizer, which is calibrated to deliver a specific volume percent of inhalation anesthetic. The dosages of inhalation anesthetics are expressed as the **minimal alveolar concentration** (MAC), the concentration at one atmosphere at which 50% of patients do not move in response to surgical stimulus (Table 4–3). Intravenous anesthetics are popular because of their rapid redistribution and systemic effects. The intravenous anesthetics include barbiturates, benzodiazepines, ketamine, and propofol. Opioid analgesics both relieve pain during surgery and provide adequate postoperative analgesia. The opiates act by binding to both central and peripheral receptors. Morphine, fentanyl (Sublimaze), alfentanil (Alfenta), sufentanil (Sufenta), meperidine (Demerol), and hydromorphone (Dilaudid) are commonly used opiates. Muscle relaxants reduce muscle tension by interfering with acetylcholine transmission at neuromuscular junctions. They facilitate endotracheal intubation (Table 4–4) and provide muscular relaxation during surgery. High-dose potent inhalation agents also produce muscle relaxation.

The four phases of general anesthesia are induction, maintenance, emergence, and recovery. The **induction phase** begins when the anesthetic is first given and ends when the surgical level of anesthesia is achieved. Possible complications during induction include upper airway obstruction, gastric content regurgitation, laryngospasm, hypotension, hypertension, arrhythmia, and oxygen desaturation. Induction may be achieved by the following methods: intravenous induction, inhalation induction, and rapid sequence induction.

Table 4–3. MAC of inhalation anesthetics.

Inhalation Anesthetics	MAC (% atmosphere; with oxygen only)
Halothane (Fluothane)	0.7
Enflurane (Ethrane)	1.7
Isoflurane (Forane)	1.2
Desflurane (Suprane)	6.0
Sevoflurane	2.0
Nitrous oxide	104

MAC = minimal alveolar concentration.

Table 4–4. Muscle relaxants for intubation.

Drug	Dosage (mg/kg)	Onset (min)	Duration (min)
Depolarizing muscle relaxant			
Succinylcholine (Anectine)	1	1/2–1	4–6
Nondepolarizing muscle relaxant			
Mivacurium (Mivacron)	0.1–0.2	1–2	6–10
Rocuronium (Zemuron)	0.6–1.0	1–2	45–75
Vecuronium (Norcuron)	0.1	2–3	25–30
Atracurium (Tracrium)	0.6	2–3	25–30
d-Tubocurarine (Curare)	0.6	3–5	60–100
Pancuronium (Pavulon)	0.1	3–4	60–120

INDUCTION OF ANESTHESIA

Intravenous induction requires the establishment of a functioning catheter. Common hypnotic agents for induction include thiopental (3–5 mg/kg IV), methohexital (1–2 mg/kg IV), and propofol (2–2.5 mg/kg IV). Thiopental and methohexital are potent ultrashort-acting barbiturates; the dosages are reduced for elderly or hypovolemic patients. When propofol is given, patients often experience pain during injection secondary to venous irritation. To decrease this effect, most anesthesiologists use a large catheter (16 gauge) or mix lidocaine (0.01%) with propofol.

Inhalation induction is used when cannulation is difficult (eg, pediatric patients) or when major airway obstruction exists (eg, upper airway tumor). At the beginning of inhalation induction, only oxygen or nitrous oxide-oxygen mixture is given through the mask. Once the patient tolerates the mask, halothane is then added in 0.5% increments until the total halothane concentration reaches 3%. The patient takes three to four breaths between each incremental increase, since too rapid an increase induces coughing and laryngospasm. Enflurane, isoflurane, and desflurane are not commonly used for inhalation induction secondary to their pungency and airway irritative effects. Sevoflurane, which is less irritable to the airway, can be used for inhalation induction.

AIRWAY ISSUES

For patients with risk factors for aspiration pneumonitis (eg, recent meal, gastroesophageal reflux, pregnancy, morbid obesity, bowel obstruction, or symptomatic vomiting), rapid sequence induction and endotracheal intubation are usually employed. The patient is preoxygenated with high-flow 100% oxygen via mask for at least 3 minutes. Then, an induction agent (eg, thiopental, propofol, ketamine, or etomidate) and a muscle relaxant (succinylcholine) are given intravenously. Simultaneously, an assistant applies cricoid pressure by compressing the cricoid cartilage, effectively occluding the esophagus. Cricoid pressure is maintained until successful endotracheal intubation is confirmed.

After induction, the airway is maintained by three methods: mask, laryngeal mask airway, and endotracheal intubation (Figure 4–2). The mask airway can provide inhalation anesthesia for patients not at risk for gastric regurgitation and aspiration pneumonitis or for short-duration surgical procedures. The laryngeal mask airway is inserted posterior to the larynx, seals the glottic opening, and

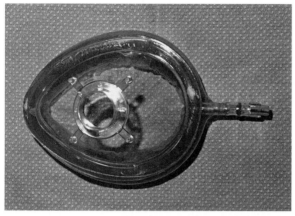

A

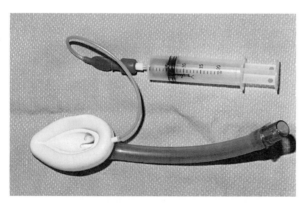

B

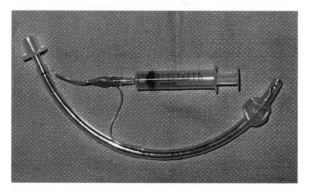

C

Figure 4–2. Airway equipment. **A:** mask; **B:** laryngeal mask airway; **C:** endotracheal tube.

maintains a patent airway (Figure 4–2). This device comes in six different sizes; most adults require size three or size four. Its placement requires topical or general anesthesia. It does not prevent gastric regurgitation or aspiration pneumonitis. Endotracheal intubation is a common technique for maintaining the airway in general anesthesia. It is essential when aspiration pneumonitis is a concern, when airway maintenance by mask is difficult, or when prolonged controlled ventilation is necessary. The appropriate endotracheal tube size depends on the patient's age, the body habitus, and the surgical procedure. A 7.0-mm endotracheal tube is utilized for most women, and an 8.0-mm endotracheal tube is utilized for most men. In general, the appropriate endotracheal tube size (mm) is calculated using the following formula: 4 + [age (years) ÷ 4]. Prior to endotracheal intubation, a muscle relaxant is usually given after confirming adequate ventilation via the mask airway.

Because endotracheal intubation may be difficult, the equipment necessary for alternative techniques must be readily available. If a difficult intubation is anticipated, flexible fiberoptic orotracheal or nasotracheal intubation is performed with the patient awake ("awake intubation"). To facilitate awake intubation, several techniques have been employed, including (1) aerosolized local anesthetic (4% lidocaine) applied to the nasopharynx, oropharynx, and pharynx; (2) superior laryngeal nerve and recurrent laryngeal nerve block; (3) sedative-narcotics, including midazolam, fentanyl, meperidine, propofol, or ketamine; (4) spontaneous ventilation using an inhalation agent; and (5) a combination of the above. If intubation attempts and airway maintenance by mask or laryngeal mask are unsuccessful, emergency airway techniques, including percutaneous needle cricothyroidotomy, surgical cricothyroidotomy, and tracheostomy, may be performed.

MAINTENANCE OF ANESTHESIA

After induction, an adequate depth of general anesthesia is maintained for the duration of the procedure. **Maintenance** refers to the period that begins with surgical anesthesia and ends with emergence. There are four major methods for the maintenance of general anesthesia: pure inhalation agents, nitrous oxide-narcotic-relaxant technique, total anesthesia, and combination.

When pure inhalation agents are used, the anesthetic dosage is titrated to the patient's somatic and autonomic responses to surgical stimulation. These responses include body movement, blood pressure, heart rate, and changes in respiratory rates and tidal volume. Nitrous oxide can be added to other potent inhalation agents, however, adequate oxygenation must be ensured. If the surgical procedure requires minimal muscle relaxation, spontaneous ventilation is usually allowed. In the nitrous oxide-narcotics-relaxant technique, nitrous oxide 60–70% is combined with narcotics given early in the operation. Because muscle relaxants are given, the ventilation is controlled via endotracheal intubation. Total anesthesia utilizes continuous infusion or repeated boluses of short-acting anesthetics, narcotics, or hypnotics, with or without a muscle relaxant. Lastly, combinations of inhalation agents with nitrous oxide-narcotics-relaxant technique are often employed.

Most surgical cases require fluid therapy for preoperative fluid deficit, maintenance fluid requirement, third space fluid loss, and blood loss. The preoperative fluid deficit is calculated by multiplying the number of NPO (nothing by mouth) hours by the hourly maintenance requirement. Half the deficit is replaced during the first hour of the surgery; a quarter of the deficit is replaced both during the second hour of surgery and during the third hour of surgery. The purpose of preoperative NPO is to minimize gastric contents and to prevent aspiration pneumonitis. Current recommendations are for the patient to have no solid food for 6–8 hours preoperatively and no clear liquids for 2–3 hours preoperatively.

The maintenance fluid requirement is calculated by the following: 4 mL/kg/h for the first 10 kg of body weight, 2 mL/kg/h for the second 10 kg of body weight, and 1 mL/kg/h for the additional body weight greater than 20 kg. The amount of third space fluid loss depends on the operative procedure and is replaced accordingly, ranging from 0 to 10 mL/kg/h (Table 4–5). The optimal solution is a relatively isotonic, balanced salt solution. Blood loss is usually replaced with 3:1 volume of balanced salt solution or 1:1 volume of colloid solutions (eg, packed red blood cells, 5% albumin, or 6% hydroxyethyl starch).

EMERGENCE FROM ANESTHESIA

At the conclusion of the operation, the patient is allowed to emerge from surgical anesthesia. The **emergence phase** of general anesthesia refers to the progression from an unconsciousness state to an awake state, with spontaneous ventilation and ability to protect the airway. If a nondepolarizing muscle relaxant was given during the case, reversal is usually achieved with neostigmine 3 mg IV and glycopyrrolate 0.4 mg IV. Extubation is performed either while the patient is still significantly anesthetized (**deep extubation**) or after the protective laryngeal gag reflex has returned (**awake extubation**). After deep extubation, the patient may require assistance to maintain a

Table 4–5. Third space fluid replacement.

Fluid Translocation	Example	Replacement (mL/kg/h)
Little or none	Craniotomy	0
Mild	Inguinal herniorrhaphy	2–3
Moderate	Thoracotomy	4–5
Severe	Colon transposition	7–8

patent airway. If aspiration pneumonitis is a concern, awake extubation is necessary.

Laryngospasm during extubation is treated with head extension, anterior displacement of the mandible, and gentle positive pressure ventilation via a mask delivering pure oxygen. During emergence from nitrous oxide anesthesia, diffusion hypoxia may occur; this is prevented by having the patient breath 100% oxygen before breathing room air.

At the end of the surgical procedure, the anesthesiologist and the surgeon are responsible for patient transportation from the operating room to the postanesthesia care unit (PACU). The PACU provides close monitoring for patients after anesthesia care. The anesthesiologist ensures that the patients maintain patent airway, adequate ventilation, and stable cardiovascular function during transportation. Some patients require a portable pulse oximeter, electrocardiogram, blood pressure monitoring, and oxygen E cylinder with ventilatory circuit during transport. Many complications can occur during the immediate postoperative period. For a detailed discussion of patient care in the PACU, refer to Chapter 7.

REGIONAL ANESTHESIA

Regional anesthesia involves the injection of local anesthetics adjacent to the spinal cord or the peripheral nerves to provide adequate analgesia during and after surgery. Regional anesthesia can be utilized as the sole anesthetic or combined with general anesthesia. If regional anesthesia is combined with general anesthesia, the need for anesthetic agents is decreased, and emergence from general anesthesia is more rapid. The advantages of regional anesthesia include minimal physiologic alteration, less risk of aspiration pneumonitis, and provision of postoperative analgesia. The absolute contraindications for regional anesthesia include patient refusal, infection of the potential injection site, systemic blood-borne bacteremia, and uncorrected coagulopathy.

Common regional anesthesia techniques include spinal anesthesia, epidural anesthesia, peripheral nerve block, and regional anesthesia. Spinal anesthesia involves the administration of local anesthetics into the subarachnoid space (Figure 4–3) via 22-gauge, 25-gauge, or 27-gauge Quincke needles. Sprotte and Whitacre needles, featuring a pencil point design with a side opening, are also commonly used. Smaller needles decrease the incidence of postdural puncture headache. The patient can be in a sitting, prone, or lateral decubitus position for the dural puncture. A common anatomic landmark is that the line defined by the bilateral iliac crests crosses the L4 spinal process. Dural puncture is usually performed at the L2-L3, L3-L4, or L4-L5 interspace via midline or paramedian approach. The spinal anesthesia level depends on the local anesthetic dosage (Table 4–6), volume, and baricity. Hy-

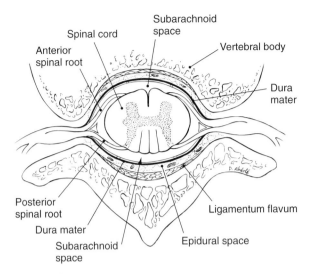

Anterior spinal root
Spinal cord
Subarachnoid space
Vertebral body
Dura mater
Posterior spinal root
Dura mater
Subarachnoid space
Ligamentum flavum
Epidural space

Figure 4–3. Cross-sectional diagram of the vertebral column, indicating the epidural space and the subarachnoid space.

perbaric solutions (Table 4–6), prepared by adding dextrose to local anesthetics, flow to the dependent portion of the cerebrospinal fluid (CSF) column by gravity. Adding epinephrine 0.2 mg to spinal anesthetics prolongs the duration of tetracaine anesthesia.

Common side effects of spinal anesthesia include hypotension, dyspnea, and headache. Hypotension often occurs immediately after spinal anesthesia is induced. The incidence of hypotension is decreased by pretreatment with 500–1000 mL of isotonic solution prior to the administration of the spinal anesthesia. Intravenous ephedrine (5–10 mg IV) or phenylephrine (50–100 μg IV) may be necessary for some patients.

Dyspnea is a common complaint with high spinal anesthesia and is related to loss of chest wall sensation. The patient can be reassured by performing a forceful exhalation with a hand near the mouth.

Postdural puncture headache is usually a postural severe headache with onset 24–48 hours after the initial dural puncture. The headache may be related to continuous CSF leak through the puncture hole, resulting in low CSF pressure and traction on the meningeal nerves and CNS blood vessels. The incidence is higher in younger patients. The treatment consists of bed rest, analgesics, and intravenous fluids. If the headache is prolonged and

severe, an **epidural blood patch** may be performed, which is the injection of 10–15 mL of sterile autologous blood into the epidural space at the prior dural puncture site. Neurological impairment after spinal anesthesia is very rare. Cauda equina syndrome has been reported after small-bore catheter continuous spinal anesthesia.

Epidural anesthesia can be performed by the single-shot technique or continuous catheter technique. Most commonly, the 17-gauge Tuohy needle is used to identify the epidural space via loss of resistance technique or hanging drop technique. The lumbar epidural space, which has the widest epidural space, is most commonly utilized. Thoracic epidural anesthesia provides upper abdominal and thoracic anesthesia with a smaller dose of local anesthetic. After placement of the epidural catheter, a test dose of 3 mL of 1–2% lidocaine with 1:200,000 epinephrine is injected. The response to the test dose determines whether the catheter tip is located in the subarachnoid space, the epidural venous plexus, or the targeted epidural space. Epidural anesthesia is used for both intraoperative anesthesia and postoperative analgesia. Accidental dural puncture can occur in 1% of patients. The management of postdural puncture headache is as previously described.

Peripheral nerve block is used for anesthesia, postoperative analgesia, and chronic pain syndrome diagnosis and treatment. Peripheral nerve block requires identification of the appropriate nerve and adjacent injection of local anesthetics. Additional sedation may be administered to some patients. Cervical plexus block is commonly used for head and neck regional anesthesia. Brachial plexus block can be performed through the interscalen, supraclavicular, or axillary approach. For upper extremity peripheral nerve blockade, the median nerve, ulnar nerve, or radial nerve may be targeted. Multiple intercostal nerve blocks may be performed to provide postoperative analgesia after thoracic or abdominal surgery or to relieve pain related to rib fractures.

The lower extremity is supplied by widely separated nerves (eg, sciatic nerve, femoral nerve, lateral femoral cutaneous nerve, and obturator nerve). Therefore, lower extremity blockade is more easily achieved by epidural or spinal block than by attempting to block all the involved nerves. For certain surgical procedures involving the foot, an ankle block can provide anesthesia if a tourniquet is not required. The major nerves approachable at the ankle level include the saphenous, superficial peroneal, deep peroneal, sural, and posterior tibial nerves.

Intravenous regional anesthesia (Bier block) pro-

Table 4–6. Common local anesthetics for spinal anesthesia in 70-kg adult male of average height.

Local Anesthetic	Dosage for Level T10 (umbilicus) (mg)	Dosage for Level T6 (xiphoid process) (mg)	Duration (min)
Lidocaine (5% in 7.5% dextrose)	50	75	30–90
Tetracaine (0.5% in 5% dextrose)	8	10	90–120
Bupivacaine (0.75% in 8.5% dextrose)	7.5	10.5	90–120

Table 4–7. Parenteral sedatives and analgesics used during monitored anesthesia care.

Drug	Usual Intravenous Dosage
Opioids	
Alfentanil (Alfenta)	20–120 µg/kg/min
Fentanyl (Sublimaze)	1–2 µg/kg
Sufentanil (Sufenta)	0.1–0.2 µg/kg
Meperidine (Demerol)	1–2 mg/kg
Morphine sulfate	0.1–0.2 mg/kg
Sedative-anxiolytics	
Midazolam (Versed)	0.02–0.03 mg/kg
Propofol (Diprivan)	2–3 mg/kg
Thiopental (Pentothal)	3–5 mg/kg
Non-opioid–analgesics	
Ketamine (Ketalar)	0.25–0.5 mg/kg

duces anesthesia for the upper or lower extremity by the injection of large-volume local anesthetics while the circulation to that extremity is occluded by a double tourniquet. The onset of anesthesia is rapid, and the degree of muscle relaxation is profound. The anesthesia duration depends on the total time that the tourniquet is inflated. The major risk of regional block anesthesia is the potential for anesthetic systemic toxicity if the tourniquet is deflated prematurely.

MONITORED ANESTHESIA CARE

Monitored anesthesia care provides patient comfort and safety during procedures performed both within the operating room and remote from the operating suite. Many diagnostic or therapeutic procedures, such as cataract extraction, herniorrhaphy, lithotripsy, vascular access placement, interventional cardiovascular procedures, cosmetic surgery, breast biopsy, and cystoscopy, are performed under monitored anesthesia care. The preoperative preparation and standards for basic intraoperative monitoring are identical to that for general anesthesia.

The medications used during monitored anesthesia care include opioids, sedative-anxiolytics, and non-opioid–analgesics (Table 4–7). Nitrous oxide and low-dose volatile anesthetics are also used. The ideal medication for sedation has a rapid onset of action, predictable amnesia and anxiolytic effect, and rapid recovery. Midazolam, a

water-soluble benzodiazepine, is a popular drug for anxiolysis and sedation. Flumazenil, a benzodiazepine antagonist, rapidly reverses the central nervous system effects of midazolam and diazepam. Opioids are often added to benzodiazepines. Compared to benzodiazepines, opioids produce more profound sedation and analgesia but with the disadvantage of potential respiratory depression. Ketamine causes dissociative mental status, amnesia, and sedation without respiratory depression. Propofol has a short onset of action, rapid elimination, and prompt recovery. Low-dose propofol infusion (25–100 µg/kg/min IV) is commonly used for sedation.

LOCAL ANESTHESIA

Local anesthetics (Table 4–8) may be administered intradermally or subcutaneously for infiltration anesthesia by blocking impulse conduction in nerve fibers. The choice of local anesthetics depends on pharmacological properties of various anesthetic agents, planned anesthetic or surgical procedures, and patient status. There are two basic groups of local anesthetics: amino-ester and amino-amide. The amino-ester group includes cocaine, procaine, tetracaine, and chloroprocaine. The amino-amide group includes lidocaine, prilocaine, etidocaine, mepivacaine, and bupivacaine. Both ester and amide groups have similar pharmacological properties.

The anesthetic activity of local anesthetics depends on physical-chemical properties, such as pKa (the pH at which the amount of ionized and nonionized drug is equal), lipid solubility, and protein binding ability. The pKa is responsible for the onset of action. The relative potency of local anesthetics varies according to lipid solubility. The anesthesia duration is determined by protein binding ability. Adding a vasoconstrictor, usually epinephrine 1:200,000, retards the systemic absorption and prolongs the duration of infiltration anesthesia. Epinephrine is not used in areas with poor circulation.

Several topical anesthetics are now available. Topical EMLA (eutectic mixture of 2.5% lidocaine and 2.5% prilocaine) decreases the pain associated with percutaneous insertion of needles and cannulas. Topical EMLA produces cutaneous anesthesia in skin-grafting procedures. This preparation must be applied under an occlu-

Table 4–8. Local infiltration anesthesia.

Drug (Concentration %)	Plain Solution			Epinephrine-Containing Solution		
	Max dose (mg)	(mg/kg)	Duration (min)	Max dose (mg)	(mg/kg)	Duration (min)
Chloroprocaine (1–2%)	800	15	15–30	1000	20	30–90
Lidocaine (0.5–1%)	300	5	30–60	500	7	120–360
Mepivacaine (0.5–1%)	300	5	45–90	500	7	120–360
Bupivacaine (0.25–0.5%)	175	3	120–240	225	3	180–420

sive bandage for 45–60 minutes to obtain effective cutaneous analgesia.

Most local anesthetics are free of localized or systemic toxic effects if appropriately utilized. Local anesthetic agents rarely produce localized nerve damage. The amino-ester type of local aesthetics, such as procaine, may cause allergic reactions as a consequence of the metabolite p-aminobenzoic acid. To avoid intravascular injection, negative pressure aspiration is performed prior to injecting the local anesthetic. Inadvertent intravascular injection and overdose result in central nervous or cardiovascular toxicity.

Central nervous system toxicity occurs only when the plasma concentration exceeds the toxic level. Initial symptoms include light-headedness, metallic taste, disorientation, visual disturbance, and auditory disturbance. Objective signs include shivering, tremors, and generalized tonic-clonic convulsions. Initial treatment of seizures includes ventilatory support with oxygen. If seizure activity persists, treatment with benzodiazepines (midazolam 1–2 mg IV) or barbiturates (thiopental 50–200 mg IV) is indicated.

The cardiovascular system is less susceptible to systemic side effects. However, cardiovascular side effects are more resistant to therapy. The treatment includes ventilatory support with oxygen, cardioversion, bretylium, and cardiopulmonary bypass therapy until drug redistribution. Bupivacaine 0.75% is no longer recommended for obstetric anesthesia because of cardiotoxic effects in pregnant women.

SUGGESTED READING

Barash PG et al (editors): *Clinical Anesthesia*, 3rd ed. Lippincott, 1996.

Jaffe RS, Samuels SI: *Anesthesiologist's Manual of Surgical Procedures*, Raven Press, 1994.

Miller RD: *Anesthesia*, 4th ed. Churchill Livingston, 1994.

Morgan GE Jr, Mikhail MS: *Clinical Anesthesiology*, 2nd ed. Appleton & Lange, 1996.

5

The Management of Perioperative Pain & Anxiety

Kayvan Ariani, MD, & Raymond R. Gaeta, MD

► Key Facts

► Nociception is the transmission of the pain stimulus from the periphery to the brain.

► Untreated pain leads to an alteration in the patient's physiologic homeostasis and predisposes the patient to perioperative morbidity.

► Systemic opiates are the most commonly used tool for postoperative pain management.

► Patient-controlled analgesia allows the patient to self-administer analgesic therapy using a programmed pump with adjustable parameters.

► Opiates or local anesthetic administered via an epidural catheter can provide effective postoperative analgesia after chest, abdominal, pelvic, and lower extremity surgical procedures.

► Benzodiazepines are currently the most effective class of medications for anxiolysis.

Effective management of perioperative pain and anxiety is an essential component in the care of the surgical patient. Patient satisfaction, positive surgical outcome, and speedy return to preoperative functional state are enhanced when the individual needs of the patient with regard to analgesia and anxiolysis are met. Regimens that are effective for the majority of patients may fail if applied universally without consideration of each patient's unique physiology and psychology. This chapter outlines current concepts regarding perioperative analgesia and anxiolysis and summarizes the tools at the disposal of the physician to provide effective therapeutic interventions.

PAIN: DEFINITION & ANATOMIC CONSIDERATIONS

Pain is defined by the International Association for the Study of Pain as "an unpleasant sensory and emotional experience associated with actual or potential tissue damage or described in terms of such damage." This definition implies that both patient- and stimulus-related factors coalesce to create the pain experience. While undoubtedly primitive, the current anatomic and biochemical model of pain transmission is consistent with this definition (Figure 5–1).

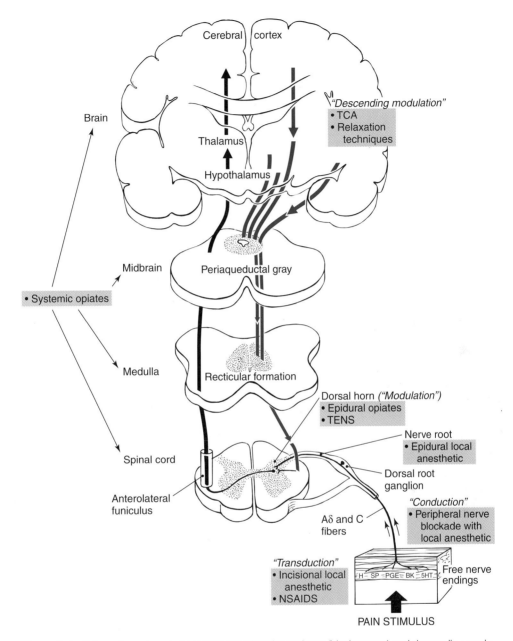

Figure 5–1. Schematic portrayal of ascending nociceptive pathway (black arrows) and descending modulation of nociception (blue arrows). Boxed items indicate analgesic interventions and their sites of action. Serotonin (5-HT), bradykinin (BK), substance P (sP), prostaglandins (PGE), histamine (H), transcutaneous electrical nerve stimulation (TENS), tricyclic antidepressants (TCAs), nonsteroidal anti-inflammatory drugs (NSAIDs).

Nociception is the transmission of the pain stimulus from the periphery to the brain. This begins with **transduction** of the physical stimulus to an electrical signal by free nerve endings in somatic and visceral tissues. Tissue damage releases chemical substances locally that stimulate these nerve endings. The small-diameter **Aδ** and **C**

fibers, whose cell bodies are contained in the dorsal root ganglion, carry these signals from the periphery to the spinal cord and synapse in the dorsal horn with the cell bodies of second-order neurons. This process is called **conduction**. The second-order neurons cross the spinal cord and the axons ascend to the brain via the **anterolat-**

eral **funiculus**, a collection of nerve tracts located in the anterolateral white matter of the spinal cord. The anterolateral funiculus transmits nociceptive information to the brainstem and thalamus. Synaptic transmission occurs in these areas, and fibers ascend to the limbic system, parietal cortex (postcentral gyrus), and frontal cortex for final processing of nociceptive information with regard to location, intensity, and emotional response.

Modulation of nociceptive information occurs in the dorsal horn of the spinal cord. Descending pathways travel from the cortex, limbic system, and brainstem down the spinal cord to inhibit second-order neuron firing in the dorsal horn via release of enkephalins, endogenous opiates. Central states, such as environmental and psychological factors, are represented by these descending pathways.

Modulation can also occur with stimulation of peripheral nerve fibers that mediate vibration or touch. Stimulation of these fibers inhibit firing of second-order neurons in the dorsal horn involved in nociception; hence, the phenomenon of rubbing a painful site to decrease the pain. The tools of pain management act at differing sites along the pain pathway to modulate nociception (Figure 5–1).

PHYSIOLOGIC EFFECTS OF PAIN IN THE SURGICAL PATIENT

Surgical intervention with consequent tissue disruption results in a barrage of nociceptive input to the central nervous system. Untreated, this leads to an alteration in the patient's physiologic homeostasis and predisposes the patient to perioperative morbidity (Figure 5–2). Spinal cord reflexes result in a variety of deleterious effects, including reflex muscle spasms, which can reduce pulmonary compliance when the chest and upper abdomen are involved. Coupled with decreased respiratory excursion by the patient in an effort to minimize pain, atelectasis with increased ventilation/perfusion mismatching, hypoxemia, pneumonia, and respiratory failure can result. Other spinal cord reflexes can result in impaired gastrointestinal motility, urinary retention, and increased peripheral vascular resistance. Further physiologic perturbation is mediated by release of a variety of sympathetic and catabolic mediators and hormones. Among other responses, elevated heart rate and blood pressure, increased metabolic rate and oxygen consumption, impaired tissue repair and immune response, sodium and water retention, negative nitrogen balance, and hypercoagulability with possible deep venous thrombosis can occur. This **surgical stress response** can also be exacerbated by cortical factors, such as fear and anxiety. In addition to providing comfort for the patient, perioperative pain management can minimize the impact of surgery on the patient's homeostatic state and facilitate postoperative recovery.

PERIOPERATIVE PAIN MANAGEMENT

Preoperative preparation is essential for successful management of postoperative pain. This involves obtaining a pain history from the patient, educating the patient about postoperative pain and intervention options, and developing a preliminary management plan.

The pain history should contain information regarding prior surgical and pain experiences in order to avoid repeating medications or management strategies that have failed previously. It is essential to determine if opiate or anxiolytic use is ongoing preoperatively. The chronic pain patient on opiate medications develops some degree of tolerance to these medications, and postoperative opiate requirements in these patients may be far in excess of what would normally be expected. In addition, the chronic pain patient's response to nociception and expectations regarding analgesia are often higher than usual, making these patients especially difficult to manage.

Preoperative determination of a method by which the patient is to report his pain is important to facilitate postoperative communication between the patient and physicians or nurses. Numeric scales, visual analog scales, or descriptive adjective scales are introduced to the patient preoperatively (Figure 5–3).

The patient's attitude with regard to pain should be sought; patients may perceive pain medication as addictive and attempt to avoid these at all costs. Education with regard to these issues can preempt postoperative confusion and unnecessary suffering and morbidity.

PAIN MANAGEMENT MODALITIES

Knowledge of and familiarity with the tools of pain management increase the likelihood that postoperative pain will be managed successfully, in even the most difficult cases (Table 5–1). Reliance on standard regimens for all patients will likely lead to unsatisfactory results in exactly those patients for whom effective pain management is most essential.

OPIATES

Systemic opiates are the most commonly used tool for postoperative pain management. Opiates act at specific receptors in the spinal cord and brain to produce analgesia. There are a variety of subtypes of opiate receptors, with each particular receptor mediating a constellation of opiate effects (eg, analgesia, sedation, miosis, nausea). Opiate **agonists** bind to these receptors and activate them. Opiate **antagonists**, on the other hand, bind to the receptors but do not activate them; these agents actually reverse the effects of opiate agonists. **Mixed agonist-antagonists**

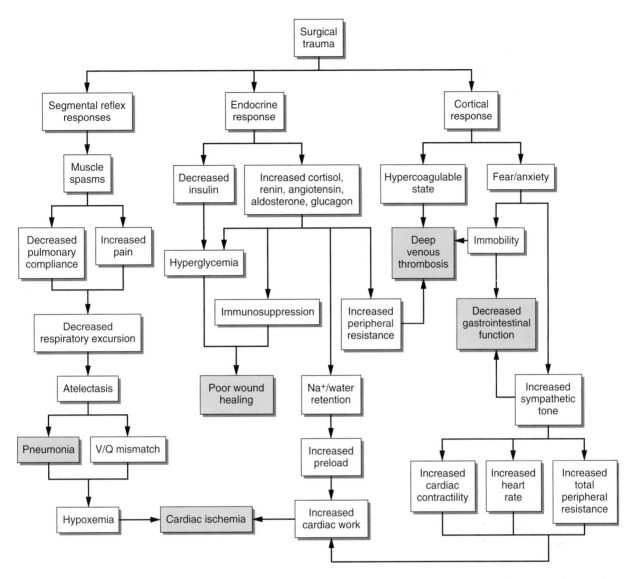

Figure 5–2. Pathophysiologic response to surgical trauma. Untreated, morbidity (blue shading) and prolonged postoperative convalescence can result.

act as agonists at some opiate receptors and antagonists at others. They can be useful in providing analgesia while minimizing side effects, such as respiratory depression.

To effectively use opiates, the physician must be knowledgeable about potency, pharmacokinetics, and special characteristics of the various commonly used opiates. Table 5–2 summarizes the more commomly used opiates. **Equianalgesia** refers to an equal amount of pain relief achieved with different opiates. For example, 0.1 mg of intravenous (IV) fentanyl is equianalgesic to 10 mg of IV morphine or 75 mg of IV meperidine, since each of these

doses of opiate provides the same amount of pain relief. **Potency**, in contrast, refers to the inherent strength of an opiate. Thus, using the above example, fentanyl is more potent than morphine, which is more potent than meperidine. Consideration of equianalgesia and potency avoids improper dosing when alternating between opiates or changing dosing route.

Route of administration is an often overlooked factor in providing effective opiate therapy. In fact, one could argue that route of administration of opiate is a more important factor in achieving effective analgesia than the

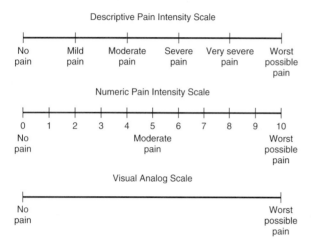

Figure 5–3. Descriptive scales, numeric scales, and visual analog scales are useful tools for communicating pain intensity between patient and health care providers. The visual analog scale is used by measuring the distance along the scale.

particular opiate used. While **intramuscular** administration remains a popular mode of delivering opiates, it is fraught with inconsistent uptake from the depot site and delay in achieving analgesic effect. The advantage of **intravenous** administration is fast onset, consistent absorption, and lack of need for a functioning gastrointestinal system for effectiveness. **Oral** administration is not appropriate in the patient with impaired gastrointestinal function, such as patients who have just undergone gastrointestinal surgery. In addition, with oral dosing, the issues of first-pass metabolism and bioavailability must be considered. Those with poor intravenous access are candidates for **subcutaneous** delivery of opiate, however, the previously discussed limitations of intramuscular (IM) delivery apply. **Rectal** preparations, which do not require a functioning gastrointestinal tract, are available for selected opiates. Transdermal fentanyl uses a **skin patch system** to deliver a constant hourly dose of fentanyl that is proportional to patch size.

Patient-controlled analgesia (or PCA) is a concept that allows the patient to self-administer analgesic therapy. A programmed pump that has adjustable parameters in terms of dose and dosing interval is employed to allow safe self-administration of opiate by the patient. The ad-

Table 5–1. Tools for postoperative pain management.

Systemic opiates and nonsteroidal anti-inflammatory drugs
Patient-controlled analgesia
Epidural administration of opiates and local anesthetics
Intermittent peripheral nerve blocks with local anesthetics
Transcutaneous electrical nerve stimulation (TENS)
Cognitive/behavioral techniques, such as relaxation, self-hypnosis, visualization

vantage of PCA pumps are immediate access to drug when the patient feels pain, which avoids the inherent delays that occur when a nurse must respond to a request for medication. In addition, smaller doses of opiate can be given more frequently with a PCA pump, resulting in a more constant plasma level of opiate, less total opiate used, and improved pain management (Figure 5–4). When used properly, PCA pumps minimize the risk of overdosage and respiratory arrest. For guidelines regarding initial PCA dosing recommendations, see Table 5–3.

While standard dosing regimens exist, each patient may respond differently to a dose of opiate. Particularly, those chronically taking opiates will have developed tolerance to the drug and will require more than the usual dose. On the other hand, reduced dosing may be required in the elderly and those with coexisting respiratory, hepatic, or renal disease. Table 5–4 summarizes conditions that warrant caution in the use of opiates with perhaps more conservative dosing schedules.

The most effective way to determine the appropriate dose of opiate for a patient is to titrate the drug intravenously at the bedside while asking the patient to rate his pain using a pain scale. Because of the relatively fast onset of intravenous dosing, the physician can quickly determine the optimal analgesic dose of opiate that minimizes side effects (eg, respiratory depression); a rational dosing schedule can then be developed using knowledge of the drug's pharmacokinetic parameters.

Side effects of opiate therapy include sedation and respiratory depression, decreased bowel function, pruritus, urinary retention, and nausea and vomiting. Physical dependence to opiates may develop with prolonged, continuous usage, and withdrawal symptoms (rhinorrhea, sweating, mydriasis, insomnia, abdominal cramps, diarrhea, nausea, vomiting, hypertension, tachycardia) may occur with abrupt discontinuation of the drug.

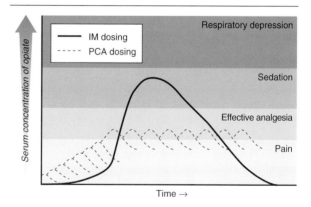

Figure 5–4. Comparison between intermittent intramuscular (IM) administration of opiate and patient-controlled analgesia (PCA). IM dosing produces peak serum drug levels resulting in sedation and trough serum drug levels resulting in inadequate analgesia. PCA dosing results in serum drug levels within the therapeutic range for analgesia for a greater period of time.

Table 5–2. Characteristics of commonly used opiates.

Drug (Trade Name)	Equianalgesic Dose[1] (mg)		Peak (min)	Duration (h)	Standard Dosage[2] (adults > 50 kg)	Comments
Agonist						
Propoxyphene (Darvon)	Oral	400	60–90	4–6	65 mg Q 4h	Weak analgesic; overdose may lead to convulsions.
Codeine (Tylenol #3)	Oral Parenteral	200 120	45–90	4–6 4–6	15–60 mg Q 4–6h 15–60 mg Q 4–6h	
Meperidine (Demerol)	Oral Parenteral	300 75	60–120 30–60	3–6 2–4	Not recommended 50–100 mg Q 3–4h	1) Limit dose to less than 600 mg/24 hr, as metabolite normeperidine can accumulate (esp. in those with renal failure) and lead to CNS excitation (seizures). 2) Combination with MAO inhibitors has caused fatalities. Avoid this combination. 3) Has atropine-like effect and can induce tachycardia. 4) Small dose can control postop shivering (12–25 mg IV).
Hydrocodone (Vicodin, Lortab)	Oral	40	30–60	4–5	5–10 mg Q 3–4h	Available in combination with acetaminophen, which limits dosing to maximal 4 gm acetaminophen per day (adults > 50 kg).
Oxycodone (Percocet, Tylox)	Oral	30	60	4–5	5–10 mg Q 3–4h	See comment for hydrocodone.
Morphine (Roxanol, MS Contin)	Oral Parenteral	30 10	90–120 30–60	4 3–5	5–30 mg Q 2–4h 5–15 mg Q 4h	Oral slow release formulation MS Contin useful for long-acting therapy (eg, in cancer patients). This formulation is dosed Q 8–12 hr.
Methadone (Dolophine)	Oral Parenteral	10 10	90–120 30–60	4–12 4–8	2.5–20 mg Q 12h 2.5–20 mg Q 8h	1) Long and variable half-life (12–48 hr) render this agent good for long-acting treatment. Effect may persist for days after drug is discontinued. 2) Oral bioavailability essentially equal to parenteral.
Hydromorphone (Dilaudid)	Oral Parenteral	4 2	90–120 30–60	4–6 3–4	2–4 mg Q 4–6h 1–2 mg Q 4–6h	Available in suppository form.
Fentanyl (Sublimaze, Duragesic)	Parenteral	0.1	3–20	0.5–1	0.05–0.1 mg Q 1–2h	1) Available in skin patch for transdermal administration. Achieving therapeutic level is delayed for 12 hours as drug passes through skin initially. In addition, removal of patch still leaves drug in skin, thus delaying actual end of dosing. 2) Excellent agent to titrate intravenously, as high lipid solubility allows for rapid onset of action (within 5 min). 3) Associated with less hemodynamic instability than morphine or meperidine secondary to less histamine release and no vagolytic effect.
Sufentanil (Sufenta)	Parenteral	0.02	3–20	0.5–1	0.005–0.02 mg Q 1–2h	Similar to fentanyl except more potent and less accumulation of drug with infusion.
Mixed Agonist-Antagonist						
Butorphanol (Stadol)	Parenteral	2	30–60	2–4	1–2 mg Q 3–4h	1) Nasal preparation available (10 mg/mL; one spray in one nostril is equal to 1 mg). 2) See pentazocine.
Nalbuphine (Nubain)	Parenteral	10	30–60	3–6	10 mg Q 3–6h	1) Similar to pentazocine, except fewer hallucinations.
Pentazocine (Talwin)	Oral Parenteral	150 30	90–120 30–60	2–4 2–4	50 mg Q 3–4h 30 mg Q 3–4h	1) When given to patient chronically on pure opiate agonist, may precipitate withdrawal symptoms. 2) May cause hallucinations.

[1]Note: "Equianalgesic dose" refers to the dose of opiate that would produce the same amount of analgesia as 10 mg of parenterally administered morphine. It does not represent dose recommendations.

[2]"Standard dosage" may be excessive in patients with conditions outlined in Table 5–4.

Table 5–3. Intravenous patient-controlled analgesia dosing regimens.

Drug	Initial Bolus	Basal Rate	Lockout Dose	Lockout Interval (min)
Morphine	0.1 mg/kg	0–2 mg/h	1–4 mg	10–20
Fentanyl[1]	0.5–2.0 µg/kg	0–25 µg/h	10–25 µg	6–15
Hydromorphone	0.5–2 mg	0–0.4 mg/h	0.2–0.6 mg	10–20

[1]Note fentanyl dosing is in micrograms. Analgesic requirements may vary among patients; see Tables 5–2 and 5–4.

Naloxone (Narcan), an opiate antagonist, reverses the effects of opiate agonists and is used clinically to reverse respiratory depression and excessive sedation that results from opiate overdosage. Initial dose is 0.1–0.4 mg IV. Because of its short half-life, naloxone needs to be continued in the form of a drip (0.05–0.2 mg/hr) when opiate overdose is due to the effect of a long-acting opiate. Note that as well as reversing the respiratory depressant effects of opiate agonists, naloxone will reverse the analgesic effects and may produce withdrawal symptoms in those chronically taking opiates.

NONSTEROIDAL ANTI-INFLAMMATORY DRUGS

Prostaglandins are potent mediators of inflammation and are released locally in response to tissue damage. They act by facilitating transduction at free nerve endings to augment nociception. There is also evidence for a central effect. **Nonsteroidal anti-inflammatory drugs** (NSAIDs) act by inhibiting the enzyme cyclooxygenase, thus preventing the synthesis of prostaglandins. A diverse array of compounds are classified as NSAIDs, including salicylic acid derivatives (aspirin), para-aminophenol derivatives (acetaminophen), proprionic acid derivatives (ibuprofen, naproxen), indole derivatives (indomethacin, ketorolac), and others.

Interest in the use of these NSAIDs in the postoperative setting has increased with the recent development of **ketorolac** (Toradol). Ketorolac is approved by the FDA for parenteral use and has potent analgesic effects. Its use, along with opiates, in the immediate postoperative period can significantly reduce opiate requirements while providing effective analgesia. Ketorolac is dosed 15 mg IM or IV every 6 hours. Parenteral dosing should be limited to 5 days.

NSAIDs can produce significant morbidity, including gastrointestinal bleeding resulting from peptic ulcer formation, renal dysfunction, and impaired platelet aggregation predisposing to coagulopathy and bleeding. They should not be used in at-risk groups (Table 5–5). An exception is **acetaminophen** (Tylenol), which does not produce the above-mentioned side effects. Instead, acetaminophen can cause hepatotoxicity, especially in those with hepatic dysfunction or when dosed greater than 4000 mg per day. In addition, acetaminophen is unique in that it does not have a peripheral anti-inflammatory effect and appears to provide analgesia via a central effect.

In the patient who is tolerating oral intake, popular opiate/NSAID combined formulations are available (eg, Vicodin, Percocet). The physician must be knowledgeable as to the contents of these formulations to prevent use of these medications in excessive doses or when contraindicated. For example, Vicodin contains 5 mg of hydrocodone and 500 mg of acetaminophen. Because of the acetaminophen content, dosing of Vicodin should be limited to eight or fewer tablets per day (less than 4000 mg of acetaminophen per day). In addition, caution should be used in prescribing Vicodin in the patient with preexisting hepatic dysfunction.

EPIDURAL ANALGESIA

The **epidural space** surrounds the spinal cord just outside the dura mater. The space contains fat, an epidural venous plexus, and nerve roots. Placement of an epidural catheter involves identifying the space with a needle attached to a syringe filled with saline or air (Figure 5–5). Constant pressure is applied to the plunger as the needle is slowly advanced through the interspinous ligament that connects the spinous processes of vertebrae. As the needle

Table 5–4. Conditions requiring caution when using opiates.

Chronic lung disease
Impending airway obstruction
Advanced liver disease
Renal failure
Head injury
Increased intracranial pressure
Use of MAO inhibitors
Concomitant central nervous system depressants
Elderly patients

MAO = monoamine oxidase.

Table 5–5. Conditions requiring caution when using NSAIDs.[1]

Concomitant anticoagulant therapy
Renal dysfunction
History of peptic ulcer disease/gastritis
Aspirin allergy
Intracranial hemmorhage risk

[1]Note: The risk of nephrotoxicity, coagulopathy, and gastrointestinal bleed is minimal with acetaminophen; acetaminophen is, however, associated with hepatotoxicity when provided in dosages of greater than 4 g/d or given to persons with preexisting hepatic disease.

NSAIDs = nonsteroidal anti-inflammatory drugs.

is advanced through the ligamentum flavum, sudden "loss of resistance" with advancement of the plunger and injection of the saline/air identifies the epidural space. A catheter is passed through the needle into the epidural space and the needle is removed.

The use of epidural analgesia for postoperative pain management requires coordination between the surgical team and the anesthesia team. Optimally, the epidural catheter is placed preoperatively by the anesthesia team. The catheter can be used during surgery as the sole anesthetic, to supplement a general anesthetic, or only for postoperative pain management, depending on the preference of the anesthesiologist. Medications given via an epidural catheter consist of opiates and local anesthetics.

When opiates are injected into the epidural space, a portion of the drug diffuses across the dura and arachnoid mater into the cerebrospinal fluid where it reaches its site of action, opioid receptors in the dorsal horn of the spinal cord. Here, opiates act to modulate nociceptive input to the spinal cord. Hydrophilic opiates such as morphine or hydromorphone (Dilaudid) have a slow onset and long du-

ration of action such that a single dose of drug lasts 12–24 hours. Usually, a dose of hydrophilic opiate is given intraoperatively. Postoperatively, dosing can be continued with either bolus dosing or an infusion of low-dose opiate via the epidural catheter. Side effects from epidurally administered opiates are the same as with opiates given by other routes, and include sedation, respiratory depression, urinary retention, pruritus, and nausea and vomiting.

Local anesthetics, such as lidocaine (Xylocaine) and bupivacaine (Marcaine), injected into the epidural space diffuse through the dura and act at the spinal nerve roots. Here, they block sodium channels and block conduction of the pain signal. Depending on the concentration used, local anesthetics can block sensory fibers only (low concentration) or both sensory and motor fibers (high concentration). In general, for postoperative pain management, a continuous infusion of low-concentration local anesthetic is used. Common side effects from epidural administration of local anesthetics include lower extremity numbness with inability to ambulate and hypotension resulting from blockage of sympathetic input to the vasculature. Rarely, local anesthetic toxicity resulting in seizures or cardiac arrest may occur but is unlikely, given the low doses of local anesthetics used for epidural postoperative analgesia. Total spinal anesthesia may also occur, secondary to inadvertent placement of the epidural catheter into the subarachnoid space with injection of local anesthetic directly into the subarachnoid space.

Ideally, the anesthesiologist managing the epidural catheter for postoperative analgesia uses a combination of opiates and local anesthetics, leaning more heavily towards one or the other, depending on the patient and situation. In the overly sedated patient, local anesthetics would probably be a better choice, as the sedative and respiratory depressant effects of opiates would be avoided. In the hemodynamically unstable patient, opiates would probably be preferable, as the sympatholytic effects of local anesthetics with resulting hypotension would be avoided. Of note, the use of epidural local anesthetic is more effective than epidural opiate or systemic opiate in blocking the spinal cord reflexes and release of sympathomimetic/catabolic mediators associated with the surgical stress response (see above).

PERIPHERAL NERVE BLOCKADE

Local anesthetic in the epidural space blocks afferent pain fibers at the spinal cord level. More distally, application of local anesthetic along peripheral nerves can provide postoperative analgesia limited to the duration of action of the local anesthetic. In the case of chest or abdominal surgery, blockade of intercostal nerves with 3–5 mL of 0.25% bupivacaine containing epinephrine at a concentration of 1:200,000 can provide 6–12 hours of analgesia.

This is carried out by identifying the involved dermatomes and the corresponding ribs. The posterior angle of the rib is identified, and a 22-gauge needle is walked

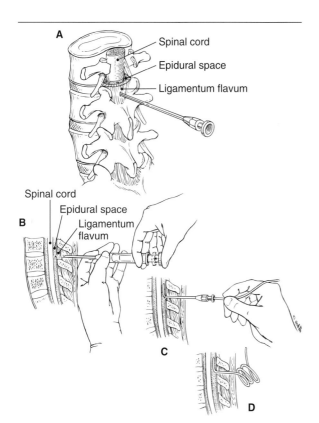

Figure 5–5. A: Anatomy and illustration of "loss of resistance" technique for identification of epidural space. **B:** Once the epidural space is identified, **C:** a catheter is passed through a needle into the epidural space **D:** and the needle is removed. Continuous epidural anesthesia or analgesia may then be provided.

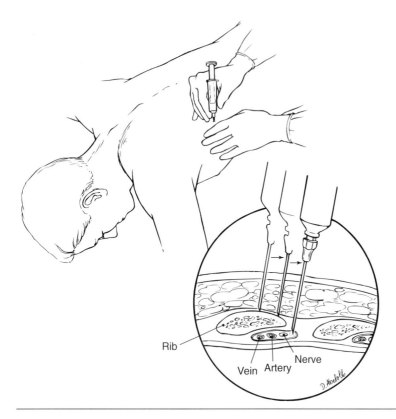

Figure 5–6. Technique for intercostal nerve blockade. (See text for details.)

off the inferior aspect of the rib into the intercostal space, where the local anesthetic is injected (Figure 5–6). Care is taken not to advance too deeply, as pneumothorax can result. Visceral pain is not affected; this is a disadvantage of this technique as compared to epidural analgesia. In addition, this technique requires a number of needle sticks to block the involved intercostal nerves, and the blocks must be repeated after the effect of the local anesthetic has waned. Placement of an intrapleural catheter with continuous local anesthetic infusion or injection of local anesthetic into an indwelling chest tube can provide a similar effect to intercostal nerve blocks without the need for multiple needle sticks.

Intraoperative infiltration of local anesthetic into the incision site prior to closure can have a limited analgesic effect as well. A comprehensive review of peripheral nerve blocks for postoperative analgesia is beyond the scope of this chapter (see Cousins or Katz references for comprehensive review).

NONPHARMACOLOGIC ANALGESIC INTERVENTIONS

Transcutaneous electrical nerve stimulation (TENS) is the application of low-intensity electrical stimulation to the skin surface via electrode pads. The analgesic effect of TENS is due to its stimulation of large-diameter sensory fibers that inhibit nociceptive input at the dorsal horn of the spinal cord via interneuron interactions. Peri-incisional application of TENS has been shown to be useful in reducing pain scores and improving objective physiologic parameters in postoperative patients.

Relaxation, self-hypnosis, and **visualization** are techniques that can have a significant impact on postoperative pain in patients susceptible to these modalities. Preoperative teaching of these techniques enhances success.

ANXIETY & THE SURGICAL PATIENT

For most patients, the surgical experience is a significant life event and a source of anxiety preoperatively. In the postoperative period, anxiety over surgical outcome and recovery can augment the pain experience and the surgical stress response. Anxiety can be a source of physiologic perturbation and instability, especially in the patient with coexisting disease states. For example, anxiety-induced tachycardia and hypertension in the patient with coronary artery disease or cardiac dysfunction can lead to cardiac ischemia or heart failure. The surgeon must be prepared to effectively provide anxiolysis in the perioperative patient without causing significant side effects from the intervention. Thus, in selecting the best techniques or medications to reduce anxiety, the surgeon must consider their **therapeutic index**.

NONPHARMACOLOGIC ANXIOLYSIS

Clinical data support the use of nonpharmacologic methods to reduce preoperative anxiety in the surgical patient. In fact, several studies suggest that these techniques are more effective anxiolytics than are medications, and produce far fewer side effects.

The surgeon's preoperative visit, during which the surgery and postoperative course are clearly explained and the patient's questions are answered, can have a significant anxiolytic effect. The same can be said of the anesthesiologist's visit; in fact, studies have shown it to be more effective than pharmacologic therapy in easing the patient's anxiety. While not a replacement for the preoperative visit by the surgeon, pamphlets or videos can inform the patient of what to expect and can be an effective means of reducing anxiety. Relaxation techniques, such as visualization or deep breathing, can also help reduce anxiety. These methods must be developed prior to the immediate preoperative period.

PHARMACOLOGIC ANXIOLYSIS

While many combinations of medications have been used in the past for anxiolysis, **benzodiazepines** are currently the most effective class of medications for anxiolysis. This class of drugs acts via the GABA/benzodiazepine receptor complex to produce anxiolysis, sedation, and amnesia. In general, benzodiazepines have a high therapeutic index, but must be used with caution in the elderly or with concomitant use of opiates or other sedatives, as respiratory arrest has been reported. In addition, benzodiazepines are probably not indicated in situations of altered mental status (oversedation can lead to obtundation and aspiration of gastric contents), hypovolemia (may lead to further hypotension), increased intracranial pressure (respiratory depression can lead to futher increases in intracranial pressure), or respiratory distress/airway obstruction. While many different benzodiazepines are on the market, diazepam, lorazepam, and midazolam are most frequently used in the perioperative period (Table 5–6).

Diazepam (Valium) is the classic benzodiazepene; it has anxiolytic and sedative properties, but is not a very effective amnestic. It is most useful in oral form, as the parenteral form is water-insoluble and can cause thrombophlebitis when given intravenously or muscle discomfort when given intramuscularly. Pharmacokinetically, it is characterized by slow onset and a long half-life, making it a more appropriate agent for treatment of anxiety the night before or the morning of a surgical procedure. Dosage is 5–20 mg.

Lorazepam (Ativan) is similar to diazepam, but is associated with less thrombophlebitis and muscular discomfort with parenteral use. Although it is eliminated more rapidly than diazepam, its sedative effect may last longer than diazepam's, secondary to slower dissociation from the benzodiazepine receptor. In addition, lorazepam is associated with more amnesia, as compared to diazepam. Dosage is 0.5–2.0 mg.

Midazolam (Versed) differs from diazepam and lorazepam in many ways. First, its amnestic properties are superior to both diazepam and lorazepam. Secondly, while it is water-soluble at acidic pH and is ideal for parenteral use, at physiologic pH it undergoes a structural change that renders it lipid-soluble. This lipid solubility allows midazolam to cross the blood-brain barrier rapidly and allows for a rapid onset. In addition, it is relatively rapidly eliminated from the body. Midazolam is not approved for oral use, but has been used orally for preoperative sedation in children. Midazolams's rapid onset makes it an ideal agent for intravenous titration in the operating room holding area prior to the patient's entering the operating room.

Table 5–6. Characteristics of commonly used benzodiazepines.

Drug	Trade Name	Routes	Dosage (mg) (adults > 50 kg)	Peak (min)	Elimination Half-life	Amnestic	Comments
Diazepam	Valium	PO, IV	5–20	PO: 60–120 IV: < 20	30 h	+	Water-insoluble; can lead to pain with IM or IV injection. Active metabolite can lead to prolonged effect.
Lorazepam	Ativan	PO, IV, IM	0.5–2.0	PO: 60–120 IM: 30–90	15 h	++	High receptor affinity may prolong activity.
Midazolam	Versed	IV, IM	0.5–4.0	IM: 30–90 IV: < 6	2 h	+++	Rapid onset and short half-life make it ideal agent for preoperative sedation in operating room holding area. Used orally for sedation in children, but not FDA-approved for this.

In addition, the short elimination half-life makes midazolam an ideal agent for outpatient use, in that it minimizes residual sedation.

Flumazenil (Romazicon) is a benzodiazepine antagonist that acts at the GABA/benzodiazepine receptor complex to reverse the sedative effects of benzodiazepines. Titration of 0.2 mg IV every 1–2 minutes up to 1 mg total dose should produce a clinical effect if sedation is due to benzodiazepine. In those chronically dependent on benzodiazepines or alcohol, withdrawal seizures can be precipitated with flumazenil. Because of the short half-life of flumazenil (1 hour), resedation is possible.

SUGGESTED READING

Acute Pain Management Guideline Panel, Agency for Health Care Policy and Research, Public Health Service: *Acute Pain Management: Operative or Medical Procedures and Trauma. Clinical Practice Guideline.* AHCPR Pub. No. 92-0032. US Department of Health and Human Services, Rockville, MD, February 1992.

Bonica JJ: *The Management of Pain,* 2nd ed. Lea & Febiger, 1990.

Cousins MJ, Bridenbaugh PO: *Neural Blockade in Clinical Anesthesia and Management of Pain,* 2nd ed. Lippincott, 1988.

Gilman AG et al: *The Pharmacological Basis of Therapeutics,* 8th ed. Macmillan, 1990.

Katz J: *Atlas of Regional Anesthesia.* Appleton-Century-Crofts, 1985.

Kehlet H: Surgical stress, the role of pain and analgesia. Br J Anaesth 1989;63:189.

Sinatra RS et al: *Acute Pain: Mechanisms and Management.* Mosby–Year Book, 1992.

6

Transfusion & Blood Component Therapy

Susan Galel, MD, Maritza Gonzalez, MD, & F. Carl Grumet, MD

► Key Facts

- ► Timely identification of specific blood deficit(s) and proper replacement levels is essential.

- ► Intravascular volume loss is the first deficit that must be identified, followed by degree of anemia, platelet count, and coagulation factor deficits.

- ► A working knowledge of the elementary rules of immunohematology as well as the characteristics of blood products is vital for the proper selection of appropriate transfusions.

- ► Clinically, it is important to be familiar with the hematological concepts behind the ABO, Rh, and HLA antigen systems in order to assess the need for compatibility.

- ► Routine compatibility testing is necessary for transfusion of red blood cell products unless the harm of transfusion delay outweighs the hazard of a possible transfusion reaction.

- ► The "unit" concept used in transfusion therapy is based on the standard 500 mL (1 unit) of whole blood from one donor; each of the components (red blood cells, plasma, or platelets) separated from that donation is then called a "unit" of that component.

- ► Autologous blood transfusion is the collection of a patient's own blood or blood components for later reinfusion.

- ► Complications of transfusion must be clearly understood and evaluated; these include hemolytic reactions, allergic reactions, and transmission of infectious agents.

Several simple and basic principles provide general guidance for effective and safe blood transfusion of surgical patients. First, there is no substitute for clear and timely identification of the specific blood deficit(s) and definition of proper replacement levels. Second, selection of the most appropriate transfusions demands a working knowledge of the elementary rules of compatibility and the characteristics of available blood products. Third, the risks and complications of transfusion must be understood and given due consideration in the process of deciding what, when, and how much to transfuse. Fourth, the guidelines presented below are not rigid formulas, but are reasonable starting points for therapeutic decisions.

The clinical impact of specific deficits is often complicated by concomitant other deficits, drugs, or underlying disease. Therapeutic responses to each identifiable deficit must therefore always be considered in the context of the complete clinical presentation. Finally, transfusion related problems should be addressed by early and open communication with knowledgeable laboratory personnel and physicians trained in transfusion medicine.

BASIS & RATIONALE FOR BLOOD REPLACEMENT

BLOOD VOLUME

Intravascular blood volume loss is the first deficit that must be identified and distinguished from the depletion of specific blood components. Normal blood volume is approximately 70 mL/kg, or 3500 mL in an adult female and 5000 mL in an adult male. Loss of intravascular volume decreases cardiac output by decreasing preload to the heart. This effect is offset by a vasoconstriction mediated by the sympathetic reflex, which, in otherwise normal patients, is sufficient to maintain normal blood pressure in the face of volume losses of up to 10–15% (500–750 mL in an adult male). Volume losses greater than 20–25% (1000–1250 mL) require volume replacement to avoid hypotension. Volume replacement therapy is generally initiated with electrolyte and/or colloid solutions, and then blood components are added only if the components themselves are also indicated, as described below. In general, components containing red blood cells (RBC) are the first to be considered.

RED BLOOD CELLS

The red cell transfusion trigger is determined by the degree of anemia. Red blood cells can be thought of as packages of hemoglobin whose function it is to deliver oxygen to the tissues, as described by the following equation:

$$O_2 \text{ delivery} = \text{cardiac output} \times \text{arterial } O_2 \text{ content}$$

Arterial O_2 content, in turn, is a function of the concentration of hemoglobin and the degree to which this hemoglobin is saturated with oxygen. In a patient with healthy heart and lungs, oxygen saturation is near 100%, so the major determinant of arterial O_2 content is the blood hemoglobin concentration. With decreased hemoglobin concentration, the body can maintain O_2 delivery by increasing cardiac output. As long as intravascular volume is sufficient to provide adequate preload for the heart, cardiac output may increase enough to maintain adequate oxygen delivery despite hemoglobin concentrations as low as 3 g/dL (corresponding to a loss of three quarters of the body's red blood cells).

The adequacy of O_2 delivery at a given hemoglobin level is affected by clinical factors, such as myocardial disease, which limits the ability to increase cardiac output; pulmonary disease, which causes decreased hemoglobin O_2 saturation; vascular disease, which limits blood flow to critical tissues; or fever, which causes increased O_2 consumption. In the presence of any of these factors, O_2 delivery will become inadequate at hemoglobin levels well above 3 g/dL.

Currently, no single laboratory test is accepted as an indicator of the adequacy of O_2 delivery. In the absence of a specific test, the following general guidelines for red blood cell replacement therapy may be used for otherwise healthy children or adults.

With maintenance of intravascular volume, hemoglobin concentrations down to 7 g/dL are well tolerated, compensated for by an increase in cardiac output. Oxygen delivery to the myocardium will become inadequate and heart failure will occur at a hemoglobin level between 3 and 6 g/dL. Transfusion of red cell products is usually indicated in patients with a hemoglobin less than 6 g/dL (representing less than one half of the blood's normal red cell mass). For patients with anemia near this level or with massive bleeding, the decision to infuse red cell products is made on a case-by-case basis as determined by the presence of ongoing blood loss, signs or symptoms of impaired oxygen delivery, or signs of impending cardiac failure. For patients with known systemic vascular or coronary artery disease, there may be increased risk of myocardial ischemia at a hemoglobin level below 9 g/dL; it is reasonable to maintain such patients at hemoglobins above this value.

In summary, current guidelines suggest that red cell transfusion is usually indicated in patients with a hemoglobin less than 6 g/dL and is usually not necessary in patients with a hemoglobin greater than 10 g/dL. Between these values, the need for red cell transfusion must be assessed individually, as described above, with packed RBC used for normovolemic anemia, and either packed RBC or whole blood for hypovolemic anemia.

The hemoglobin triggers discussed above presume a normovolemic state. Hemoglobin levels, expressed as a concentration (g/dL), will appear artifactually lower in overhydrated patients and elevated in dehydrated patients. The physician should adjust reported hemoglobin levels for the patient's state of hydration before deciding whether to transfuse.

PLATELETS

The **platelet transfusion trigger** relates to the physiologic role of platelets in ameliorating *microvascular* hemorrhage (ie, "oozing" rather than bleeding from severed larger vessels). General guidelines are based on the following principles: In patients with normal platelet function, hemostasis is not affected until the platelet count is below 100,000/μL. Platelet transfusion is appropriate in patients whose platelet counts are between 50 and 100,000/μL with significant microvascular hemorrhage or with procedures involving sites where the consequences of bleeding may be devastating. In other surgical patients or in traumatically bleeding patients with counts below 50,000/μL, platelet transfusion is appropriate. Significant *spontaneous* bleeding generally does not occur until the platelet count is less than 10–20,000/μL.

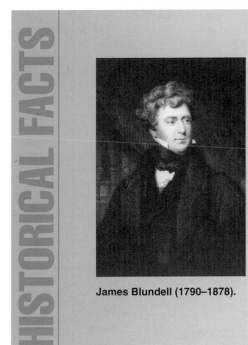

James Blundell (1790–1878).

The first human-to-human transfusion was performed in 1818 by James Blundell (1790–1878), who was a professor of physiology and obstetrics at St. Thomas' and Guy's Hospitals in England. Unfortunately, the patient died 56 hours after the transfusion. It was not until 1828 that Blundell performed the first transfusion in a human that did not result in the death of the patient. Blundell is responsible for establishing the fundamentals of transfusion, including the incompatibility of transfusions between different species and the method of indirect transfusion.

In the treatment of massive bleeding (discussed in detail later), dilutional thrombocytopenia is the most common cause (other than severed vessels) of impaired hemostasis. The patient's platelets become diluted by the infusion of large volumes of fluids and blood products that do not contain platelets. The effect of dilution is blunted, however, by mobilization of platelets from bone marrow and spleen, and platelet counts generally do not fall to levels requiring replenishment until *two blood volumes* have been replaced. On the other hand, tissue damage and fever may increase platelet consumption and cause a more rapid fall in platelet count. Therefore, in a massive transfusion situation, the need for platelet transfusion is best guided by clinical assessment of bleeding and platelet count (if quickly available), rather than by a precise formula related to volume of blood loss.

Platelet dysfunction secondary to mechanical (eg, cardiopulmonary bypass), genetic, drug (eg, aspirin and other salicylates), or other effects (eg, uremia) can impair hemostasis even if the platelet count is normal. Hematology consultation is strongly advised in such patients because appropriate therapy may require steps other than platelet transfusion. Therapy should be guided by the presence of diffuse microvascular bleeding or the risk of clinically significant bleeding from an invasive procedure. Unfortunately, the template bleeding time does not appear useful as a predictor of clinical bleeding or as a guide to the usefulness of platelet transfusion.

OTHER COMPONENTS

Plasma (fresh frozen), cryoprecipitate, and coagulation factor triggers vary substantially according to the therapeutic goal. Plasma serves many functions, including maintenance of intravascular volume and oncotic pressure, and carriage of specific proteins. Many commercially available plasma protein derivatives, such as albumin, gamma globulin, or concentrated coagulation factors, have been physically or chemically treated to reduce viral disease transmission, however, virus-inactivated whole plasma is not yet licensed in the United States. Therefore, infusion of plasma (stored in the fresh frozen state to optimally preserve coagulant factors) is indicated only if the patient is in need of multiple coagulation factors or a specific factor (eg, factor V) for which no virus-inactivated or recombinant product is available.

Regarding coagulation factor levels, in general, as little as 30% of normal is adequate for hemostasis. In massive bleeding, coagulation factors do not fall below these levels until after replacement of a complete blood volume. Prothrombin time (PT) and partial thromboplastin time (PTT) measurements are helpful in assessing the need to transfuse plasma. Bleeding patients with PT or PTT more than 1.5 times normal should benefit from the infusion of fresh frozen plasma. Fresh frozen plasma may also be used to reverse warfarin therapy if urgent correction is needed. For patients with acquired or inherited deficiencies of specific coagulation factors, virus-inactivated or recombinant-DNA–derived factor concentrates are the treatment of choice. Hematology consultation is recommended for proper use of these pharmaceutical agents.

Cryoprecipitate is a plasma component enriched for high-molecular-weight proteins, such as fibrinogen, factor VIII, factor XIII, and von Willebrand's factor. Because it is not virus-inactivated, it is no longer the treatment of choice for hemophilia but is most frequently used for fibrinogen replacement (indicated for bleeding patients with fibrinogen levels less than 100 mg/dL) or topically in fibrin sealant. It may also be considered as an adjunct to improve hemostasis in patients with uremia.

CONCEPTS & APPLICATION OF COMPATIBILITY

Understanding the basic rules of immunohematology permits an understanding and the efficient use of clinical transfusion compatibility testing. The ABO, Rh, and HLA antigen systems are by far the most important clinically.

THE ABO SYSTEM

The **ABO antigens** (Table 6–1) are carbohydrate (CHO) chains on large, membrane-bound glycosphingolipid molecules that differ only in their terminal sugar. The genes responsible for these differences are alleles at the ABO locus on chromosome 9 that encode specific transferases. The A gene transferase appends an N-acetylgalactosamine onto the common precursor chain whereas the B gene transferase appends a galactose instead; these effects are genetically codominant. The O gene does not produce a functional transferase, and its effect is genetically recessive.

ABO antigens are expressed early in gestation and at high density on almost all human cells. ABO antibodies do not arise spontaneously but are normally induced during the first year of life by exposure to ABO-like CHOs common to flora that colonize the normal gut. Infants then develop antibodies to the A antigen or B antigen, or both, absent from their own cells. CHO antigens induce strong and persistent IgM antibody responses, and this class of immunoglobulin is an effective hemolysin and activator of serum complement.

The clinical impact of the ABO system follows from its immunologic characteristics. After infancy and independent of any prior transfusions, each patient will have "naturally occurring," pre-formed antibodies to foreign ABO antigens. Because these antibodies are usually IgM, they will very rapidly lyse transfused ABO-incompatible RBC (eg, A RBC into an O recipient), causing intravascular hemolysis, complement activation and release of cytokines, and hemoglobinemia and hemoglobinuria (ie, an **acute hemolytic transfusion reaction**). Likewise, transfusion of ABO-incompatible plasma (eg, O plasma into an A recipient) can result in hemolysis of recipient RBC. Small amounts (< 500 mL in an adult) of transfused incompatible plasma are well tolerated because donor antibodies will be greatly diluted into the recipient's blood volume and will also be "mopped up" by ABO antigens on recipient endothelium. ABO incompatibility plays a minor role in platelet transfusions because the lower antigen density on those cells results only in limited target cell damage without clinical symptoms.

THE Rh SYSTEM

Rh antigens are proteins that appear early in gestation, are found only on the membranes of red blood cells and their precursors, and are expressed at relatively low density. Encoded by a multilocus complex on chromosome 1, the Rh system functionally behaves as three tightly linked genes, each having two major alleles: D and d; C and c; E and e. The D antigen is by far the most immunogenic. Its allele, d, is immunologically silent, apparently as a result of the deletion of several codons. Common usage of the term **Rh typing** refers to D antigen testing; ie, D(+) people are called Rh-positive, and D(–) are called Rh-negative, regardless of the other (C,c, E,e) antigens of the Rh system. Rh-like antigens are not encountered naturally in the environment, therefore, anti-Rh antibodies are produced only by patients exposed to these proteins through transfusions or pregnancies.

As expected for an immune response to protein antigen, anti-Rh antibodies are initially IgM but rapidly switch to IgG with persistence and immune memory (ie, rapid recall with increased titers following rechallenge). IgG are less effective than IgM antibodies in activating complement, particularly with a low density of antigen on the target

Table 6–1. The ABO system.

Patient ABO Characteristics				Compatible Blood Products	
Blood Type	Genotype	Antigens on RBC	Antibodies in Plasma	RBC	Plasma
A	A/A or A/O	A	Anti-B	A or O	A or AB
B	B/B or B/O	B	Anti-A	B or O	B or AB
O	O/O	None	Anti-A, anti-B	O	O, A, B, or AB
AB	A/B	AB	None	AB, A, B, or O	AB

RBC. Therefore, immune destruction of RBC due to Rh alloimmunity is primarily by IgG-mediated extravascular phagocytosis rather than intravascular lysis. Of special note is the problem of Rh alloimmunity in pregnancy because maternal IgG crosses the placenta and can cause clinically significant hemolytic destruction of Rh-incompatible fetal RBC. This problem of hemolytic disease of the newborn primarily affects D(–) women carrying a D(+) fetus.

The clinical impact of the Rh system also is explained by its immunologic characteristics. The strong immunogenicity of the D antigen dictates that donors and recipients should be typed for D compatibility in order to avoid anti-D sensitization. D(–) recipients should (except for emergencies) receive only D(–) RBC, but D(+) recipients can accept either D(+) or D(–) RBC. In the event that a nonsensitized D(–) patient is inadvertently exposed to D(+) RBC, prompt administration of hyperimmune anti-D immunoglobulin preparation should be considered to block the induction of an active anti-D immune response. This is particularly important in women of childbearing age in order to prevent hemolytic disease of the newborn in future pregnancies. The anti-D immunoglobulin will cause removal of the D(+) cells. If more than 1 unit of D(+) cells has been transfused, consideration should first be given to performing an exchange transfusion to minimize the volume of RBC to be destroyed.

Rh transfusion reactions are less severe than ABO for several reasons. Patients without prior transfusions or pregnancies will not have pre-formed anti-Rh antibodies that could cause acute transfusion reactions. The antibodies induced by Rh sensitization will be primarily IgG, therefore, RBC destruction will be extravascular and relatively slow, occurring over hours or days (ie, a **delayed hemolytic transfusion reaction**), usually without overt clinical symptoms. Further, if incompatible RBC are given to an already Rh-sensitized patient (eg, D(+) RBC to a patient with anti-D), the RBC destruction will still be primarily extravascular and, thus, more a delayed than an acute reaction. Because Rh expression is limited to RBC, and because anti-Rh antibodies do not occur naturally, platelet and plasma transfusions and solid organ transplants are not affected by Rh incompatibility.

Typing for the other, less immunogenic, Rh antigens is not routinely performed unless there has been a positive antibody screen or crossmatch, or the patient has a history of sensitization against one of those antigens.

Other RBC alloantigen systems produce relatively infrequent transfusion complications in the surgical setting. The most common (eg, Kell, Kidd and Duffy systems) mechanistically resemble Rh, particularly in their absence of naturally occurring antibody and induction of mostly IgG immune response. Other plasma and cellular allosensitization, such as anti-IgA, anti-platelet, anti-granulocyte and anti-drug antibodies, are of a range and complexity beyond the scope of this text and warrant consultation with a specialist trained in transfusion medicine.

COMPATIBILITY TESTING

Clinical compatibility testing is routine for transfusion of RBC products (ie, whole blood and packed RBC). Donor and recipient RBC are typed for ABO and D to assure compatibility for those antigens. Recipient serum is tested against selected cell panels (**antibody screen**) and against donor RBC (**serologic crossmatch**) to identify any "irregular" antibodies to other RBC antigens that may have been induced by prior transfusion or pregnancy. (If the antibody screen is negative, some laboratories now forgo the serological crossmatch.) Donor units incompatible by any of these tests are then avoided.

In emergencies, some compatibility testing for whole blood or RBC may be bypassed if the potential harm of a transfusion delay outweighs the hazard of a possible transfusion reaction. For example, a patient of unknown ABO type who is in shock could be given uncrossmatched type O RBC immediately, and uncrossmatched but ABO- and Rh-type-specific RBC or whole blood would be available within 5–10 minutes. Failure to complete an antibody screen or crossmatch (ie, full compatibility testing) exposes the patient to increased risk of a hemolytic transfusion reaction. The decision to eliminate these normal safeguards should never be made lightly.

THE HLA SYSTEM

The basics of the HLA system are covered in detail elsewhere in this text. Here, the most relevant features are the protein nature of these antigens; their very low to absent expression on RBC but strong expression on white blood cells, platelets and almost all other tissue; and the absence of naturally occurring antibodies.

Patients may become sensitized to HLA proteins through pregnancies, transfusions, or transplants. HLA antibodies do not diminish the efficacy of RBC transfusions, but may cause febrile transfusion reactions due to reactivity with donor leukocytes in the blood product (see below). Because HLA antigens are expressed on platelets, sensitized patients may require platelets selected for HLA compatibility to attain a therapeutic effect.

TRANSFUSION OPTIONS

Once a clinical objective is defined, prompt initiation of appropriate transfusion therapy requires knowledge of the range, impact, and limitations of useful blood products.

Transfusable blood components are generally referred to as **units**. The standard amount of whole blood (1 unit) given by a donor is ~500 mL, including citrate anticoagulant. Each of the components derived from that original volume are then also referred to as a unit (of that specific component). A pheresis "unit" is somewhat different because the pheresis procedure consists of the combined yield of a specific component (eg, platelets) obtained from several sequential whole blood unit equivalents, with almost all of the other components returned to the donor. Table 6–2 summarizes the important characteristics of the standard blood products available.

AUTOLOGOUS BLOOD TRANSFUSION

Autologous blood transfusion is the collection for later reinfusion of a patient's own blood or blood components. In general, this is the safest transfusion option, eliminating the potential for transmitted infection and immune transfusion reactions. Several autologous collection strategies are available, and each should be judged by the degree to which it reduces the need for allogeneic (see below) blood transfusion.

Preoperative blood donation refers to the collection of one or more units of blood in advance of anticipated surgery. This option is most effective in reducing the need for allogeneic blood when adequate time (ideally, 1 week or more) is allowed after collection for the patient to regenerate red cells prior to surgery. **Intraoperative** and **postoperative blood salvage** refer, respectively, to the collection and reinfusion of blood lost during surgery or through postoperative drainage. Only red cells are salvageable, and salvage procedures are most useful when the red cell content of the salvaged fluids is high. Salvaged fluids should be washed to remove free hemoglobin and activated clotting factors or other unwanted materials, although infusion of small unwashed volumes is generally well tolerated.

Acute normovolemic hemodilution refers to the collection of autologous blood in the operating room immediately prior to surgery, and immediate replacement with adequate colloid/crystalloid to maintain intravascular volume. Mathematical models suggest that acute normovolemic hemodilution does not reduce the need for allogeneic blood transfusion unless the patient is dramatically hemodiluted and the anticipated surgical blood loss is large.

Several significant factors limit the benefit of autologous blood collection strategies. These include the possibility that the patient will not require any transfusion, the low risk of transfusion-related infection from allogeneic blood, and the consideration that high-risk or elderly patients will expire from other causes well before developing morbidity from transfusion-related infections. In some cases the use of autologous blood may pose *increased* risks, such as in the collection of autologous units from patients with unstable cardiovascular disease or with occult bacteremia. The risks and benefits of autologous transfusion must always be carefully assessed for each patient.

Allogeneic (formerly called homologous) blood refers to blood collected from a person other than the patient. The great majority of the blood supply in the United States is allogeneic blood obtained from volunteer community donors. All donors are extensively questioned regarding potential exposure to infectious diseases, and donated blood is subjected to multiple infectious disease tests.

Table 6–2. Standard blood components.

Component	Unit Volume (mL)	Therapeutic Indication	Therapeutic Impact/Unit[1]	Approximate Emergency Dose[2]	Preparation, Compatibility Testing Time, or Both
Whole blood	500	Acute hypovolemia with anemia	↑Hgb ~1 g/dL ↑blood vol ~10%	Determined by estimated volume deficit	Type and cross-match[3] (30–60 min)
Red blood cells[4]	250[5]	Anemia	↑Hgb ~1 g/dL ↑blood vol ~5%	Determined by degree of anemia	Type and cross-match[3] (30–60 min)
Fresh frozen plasma	200	Acute replacement of coagulation factors pending definitive diagnosis of deficit, Warfarin reversal, Factor V deficit	↑coagulation factors ~8% ↑blood vol ~4%	4 U (10–15 mL/kg)	Thawing (15–30 min)
Platelet concentrate[4] a) Single unit b) Pheresis unit	a) 50 b) 250	Thrombocytopenia	↑platelet count by a) 5–10,000/μL b) 30–50,000/μL	a) 6 U b) 1 pheresis U	None
Cryoprecipitate	25	Hypofibrinogenemia	↑fibrinogen ~3% (also includes factors VIII, XIII, von Willebrand factor)	15 U (1 U/5 kg)	Thawing and dilution (15–30 min)

[1]Anticipated response expressed either as a directly measurable increment or as a percent of normal replacement in an adult.
[2]Initial dose for an adult when therapy must be started before laboratory test results are available.
[3]See text for modifications in emergencies.
[4]May be leukodepleted or washed to avoid nonhemolytic transfusion reactions; preparation times may, thus, become longer.
[5]Volume may be increased by addition of red cell nutrient solutions.

Blood centers actively recruit donors in their communities in order to have blood components of all types readily available. Some patients may request transfusion of blood components from allogeneic donors that they choose (**directed** or **designated** donors). Directed donors are subjected to the same infectious disease screening as volunteer community donors and have been shown to be *no safer*.

RISKS & COMPLICATIONS OF TRANSFUSIONS

IMMUNE-MEDIATED REACTIONS

Immune-mediated reactions can result from sensitization to red cells, white cells, or plasma proteins.

Hemolytic reactions involve red cells and may be acute or delayed. Acute hemolysis is the result of immediate intravascular destruction, usually of ABO-incompatible RBC, and may be followed by hypotension, renal failure and disseminated intravascular coagulation, with a high risk of mortality. When an acute reaction is suspected, the infusion must be stopped immediately, the identification of the unit and recipient must be confirmed, and the remainder of the unit returned to the laboratory. The patient should receive blood pressure support with aggressive fluid resuscitation and with diuresis to maintain renal blood flow. Most ABO reactions are caused by errors in patient identification, either at the time the blood sample for typing is drawn or when the blood is administered. This type of "clerical" complication is preventable by simple diligence and careful attention to identification procedures at the bedside!

Delayed hemolysis is extravascular and is usually not life threatening. It is caused by antibody formation to incompatible red cell antigens other than ABO. Such sensitization can arise within 1–3 weeks of a first transfusion, or even sooner if the recipient has been immunized by prior transfusions or pregnancy. Signs of this type of red cell destruction include hyperbilirubinemia and failure of an expected posttransfusion rise in hemoglobin concentration. An unexplained fall in hematocrit accompanied by jaundice within days or weeks of transfusion should alert physicians to the possibility of a delayed hemolytic reaction.

Because not all hemolysis is immune-mediated, other causes must be considered in evaluating any hemolytic reaction, for example, lysis of blood induced by osmosis (mixing nonisotonic solutions with RBC in the patient's intravenous line), mechanical means (forced transfusion through a small-bore needle), and heat (overheated blood warmers).

Febrile nonhemolytic reactions may also occur, caused by the interaction between recipient antibodies, usually anti-HLA, and passenger leukocytes in the transfused blood. Cytokine release from leukocytes in stored blood components has also been recently implicated as the cause of some febrile, nonhemolytic reactions. Rarely, donor antibodies in the transfused blood may interact with recipient white cells and cause similar reaction symptoms.

Symptoms may include chills, nausea, vomiting, hypertension, and dyspnea, with pulmonary edema seen in the most severe and rare cases. Treatment consists of discontinuing the transfusion, administering antipyretics, and appropriately treating the other symptoms. Leukocyte reduction of cellular blood products (currently most efficiently achieved by filtration) is an effective way to prevent febrile reactions.

Allergic reactions, most often consisting of mild urticaria, are caused by antibodies primarily to plasma proteins and are treated and prevented by administering antihistamines. True anaphylactic reactions (eg, anti-IgA in IgA-absent individuals) are very rare; such patients present with flushing, hypotension, and respiratory distress or wheezing. For life-threatening reactions, treatment includes discontinuation of the transfusion, aggressive fluid resuscitation, and administration of epinephrine. To prevent future reactions after the occurrence of a severe allergic reaction, cellular products should be washed in order to remove offending substances in the plasma.

INFECTIOUS TRANSMISSION

Transmission of infectious agents is the other major type of transfusion complication. The most important infections are described here briefly. Hepatitis and human immunodeficiency virus (HIV) can be transmitted by any of the blood products listed in Table 6–2; human T-cell lymphotropic virus (HTLV) and cytomegalovirus (CMV) are transmitted only by blood products containing leukocytes, ie, whole blood, RBC, and platelet concentrates. Because blood is a biological product, a "zero risk" blood supply is impossible to achieve because no test procedures are perfect. Many measures are in place, however, to lower the risks as much as possible. Table 6–3 shows current estimates of risk.

Hepatitis B Virus (HBV). The hepatitis B virus infects about 300,000 persons in the United States each year and is transmitted parenterally and percutaneously. Intravenous drug use and sexual contact are the most important modes of transmission. A highly effective vaccine is available and should be used to immunize at-risk individuals (eg, health care workers and household contacts of HBV-infected persons). Blood donated in the United States has been tested for HBV surface antigen since 1972 and, more recently, for antibodies to HBV core antigen. In addition, prospective blood donors with history of IV drug use or hepatitis are not allowed to donate.

Hepatitis C Virus (HCV). Hepatitis C was discovered in 1989 and is the etiologic agent responsible for the majority of the cases of non-A, non-B hepatitis. Sexual transmission appears to be very inefficient, while parenteral inoculation accounts for at least 50% of the total HCV cases, with a high prevalence of infection among intra-

Table 6–3. Risks of transfusion complications.

Complication	Estimated Risk Per Unit Transfused[1]
Acute hemolytic reaction	~1/20,000
Delayed hemolytic reaction	1/500 – 1/1000
Allergic (urticarial) reaction	~1/100
Febrile, nonhemolytic reaction	~1/100
HCV	1/3000 – 1/6000
HIV	1/400,000 – 1/600,000
HBV	1/50,000 – 1/200,000
HTLV I/II	1/50,000 – 1/200,000
Bacterial contamination	1/10,000 – 1/30,000

[1]Unfortunately, transfusion complication rates may be underreported (eg, failure to recognize or failure to report) or overreported (eg, hepatitis from source other than transfusion). Therefore, estimates of risk must be understood to be projections based on limited data. Current rates for infectious complications are so low that they are difficult to measure with precision.

HBV = hepatitis B virus; HCV = hepatitis C virus; HIV = human immunodeficiency virus; HTLV I/II = human T-cell lymphotropic virus I and II.

Table 6–4. Noninfectious complications of transfusion.

Cause	→	Result
Acute Reactions		
ABO incompatibility	→	shock, hemolysis, renal failure
Bacterial contamination	→	septic shock
Anti-IgA	→	anaphylaxis
Plasma proteins alloimmunity	→	urticarial rash
Leukocytes, cytokines	→	fever/chills, without hemolysis
Volume overload	→	dyspnea, heart failure
Delayed Reactions		
Recipient antibodies to:		
RBC antigens (other than ABO)	→	shortened RBC survival, crossmatch difficulties, need for compatible donors, hemolytic disease of newborn
Platelet antigens	→	posttransfusion purpura
HLA antigens	→	platelet transfusion refractoriness, need for HLA-compatible platelets
Leukocytes in transfused blood	→	graft vs host disease in immunosuppressed patients
Iron overload	→	hemochromatosis in chronically transfused patients
Immunomodulation?	→	suspected ↑ postoperative infection or cancer recurrence

RBC = red blood cells.

venous drug users and hemophiliacs. The transfusion risk decreased markedly in 1990 when the first HCV antibody test for blood donors was implemented and has continued to decrease with more sensitive tests.

Additional viruses that may cause hepatitis have been recently identified and are under study to determine potential transmissibility and rates of infection.

Human Immunodeficiency Virus (HIV). Despite its low risk of transfusion-associated infection, HIV is probably the most feared complication of transfusion. Almost all HIV infection will result in the development (median time, 7–10 years) of acquired immunodeficiency syndrome (AIDS). Once it was recognized that a blood-borne agent was causative, measures were implemented to exclude from donation individuals with symptoms of, or risk factors for, AIDS. Since 1985 all blood donations have been tested for HIV antibody. Antibody testing cannot prevent all infections because of the several-week "window" delay between infection with the virus and development of detectable levels of antibody. Efforts to further decrease risk to patients have included more sensitive antibody tests and screening donated blood for the early appearance of HIV antigen.

Cytomegalovirus Virus (CMV). A herpesvirus that produces a self-limited, mostly asymptomatic disease in immunocompetent hosts, CMV is found in almost half of the adult population. In immunosuppressed or immunoincompetent hosts, however, CMV can produce significant morbidity and mortality. Like other herpesviruses, CMV remains latent in tissues following acute infection, with the potential for re-activation at later times. Blood products obtained from uninfected donors (ie, donors negative for anti-CMV antibody) are the product of choice for patients at risk for severe CMV disease, such as uninfected transplantation recipients and pregnant women, and premature infants born to CMV-antibody-negative mothers. Recently, leukocyte reduction of cellular blood products

has also been shown to effectively reduce transfusion-transmitted CMV.

Human T-Cell Lymphotropic Virus I and II (HTLV-I/HTLV-II). HTLV-I retrovirus is the causative agent of adult T-cell lymphoma/leukemia and an HTLV-associated myelopathy (tropical spastic paraparesis). HTLV-II is closely related to HTLV-I, sharing many antigenic specificities, but disease associations for HTLV-II presently are not clear. Donated blood is tested for antibody to HTLV-I/II, and positive units are discarded.

Parasites. A number of parasites can be transmitted by blood transfusion. In the United States, all donors are deferred if they have a history of babesiosis or Chagas' disease and are temporarily deferred after travel to areas endemic for malaria. Questioning does not exclude all potentially infectious donors, however, because these infections may be chronic and asymptomatic. We and others are investigating improved donor screening strategies, such as selective serologic testing of blood from donors immigrating from Chagas' endemic areas. Currently, no serologic tests for parasitic infection are licensed for routine blood donor screening in the United States.

Other Complications. A number of other complications have been associated with transfusion (Table 6–4). Additional complications may occur as a result of rapid and massive transfusion. Hypothermia from massive infusion of refrigerator-stored blood may be avoided by use of well-controlled blood warmers. Hypocalcemia due to the citrate anticoagulant in blood units may occur with rapid (1 U/5 min) infusion and in settings of impaired hepatic clearance of citrate (eg, hypothermia or severe liver dysfunction). In such situations, electrocardiographic (ECG) or ionized calcium monitoring would be appropriate; calcium should not be administered according to fixed schedules, since this could result in life-threatening hypercalcemia. Because stored whole blood or RBC contain elevated levels of plasma potassium, transient hyperkalemia has been reported in infants but is rarely seen in adult patients. ECG monitoring may be appropriate with extremely rapid (2 U/5 min) whole blood or RBC infusions and in patients with preexisting hyperkalemia or acidemia.

SUGGESTED READING

Anderson N: *Scientific Basis of Transfusion Medicine. Implications for Clinical Practice*. Saunders, 1980.

Fresh-Frozen Plasma, Cryoprecipitate, and Platelets Administration Practice Guidelines Development Task Force of the College of American Pathologists (CAP): Practice parameters for the use of fresh-frozen plasma, cryoprecipitate, and platelets. JAMA 1994;271:777.

Mollison PL, Engelfriet CP, Contreras M: *Blood Transfusion in Clinical Medicine*, 9th ed. Blackwell, 1993.

Rossi EC et al (editors): *Principles of Transfusion Medicine*, 2nd ed. Williams & Wilkins, 1996.

7

Recovery Room Care

Jay B. Brodsky, MD

▶ Key Facts

▶ Every patient undergoing anesthesia should be cared for postoperatively in a properly equipped and staffed postanesthesia care unit (PACU).

▶ All patients undergoing anesthesia should be given oxygen while being transferred from the operating room to the PACU to prevent hypoxemia.

▶ As many as 24% of all patients undergoing anesthesia will experience some complication in the PACU.

▶ Recovery from inhalational and fixed anesthetic agents is a function of many variables; recovery time will differ for each patient.

▶ The most common cause of airway obstruction is pharyngeal obstruction from a sagging tongue in an unconscious patient.

▶ For problems involving the respiratory system, initial therapy begins with administration of 100% oxygen.

▶ Central respiratory depression can follow both inhalation and intravenous anesthesia.

▶ Nausea and vomiting are the most common complications of anesthesia and surgery.

▶ Many patients arrive in the PACU hypothermic after major procedures, as they become poikilothermic during general anesthesia and cannot control their body temperature.

POSTANESTHESIA CARE UNIT

Every patient having general, regional, or monitored anesthesia should be cared for postoperatively in a properly equipped and staffed recovery room (postanesthesia care unit, or PACU). A member of the intraoperative anesthesia care team (physician anesthesiologist or certified nurse anesthetist) must always accompany the patient during transfer to the PACU. The PACU should be located close to the operating suite to keep transit time short and to allow for subsequent quick return of the anesthesia

and surgical team, if necessary. Open wards are preferred for patient observation, but at least one isolation room should be available for severely immunosuppressed patients or for patients with contaminated wounds. A ratio of one nurse for every three patients is recommended, but more critically ill patients will require more intensive nursing care.

Each PACU bed space should have piped-in oxygen, air, and vacuum capable of both intermittent pressure for gastric suction and high pressure for airway and chest suction. Each station should have routine monitoring equipment (electrocardiogram [ECG], pulse oximetry, blood pressure). Emergency equipment must be readily available and should include an "airway cart" containing laryngoscopes, bronchoscopes, endotracheal tubes, oral and nasal airways, and a manual-ventilation device. A "crash cart" containing cardiopulmonary resuscitation equipment and emergency drugs must be close by at all times and fully stocked with chest tubes, cut-down trays, and tracheostomy and cricothyrotomy trays. There should also be access to equipment for pulmonary artery catheterization, a synchronized defibrillator, a 12-lead ECG, a pacemaker and pacing wires, appropriate transducers, and a cardiac output monitor. Radiographic, blood bank, blood gas, and other clinical services must be readily available.

ROUTINE RECOVERY FROM ANESTHESIA

Although recovery from anesthesia and surgery begins in the operating room as soon as the anesthetic is discontinued, actual time to full recovery from general or intravenous anesthesia will differ with each patient.

All patients undergoing general anesthesia or intravenous sedation should be given oxygen while being transferred from the operating room to the PACU, since as many as one in three patients monitored during transport experience hypoxemia ($SaO_2 < 90\%$) if allowed to breathe air.

Upon the patient's arrival in the PACU, the anesthesiologist gives the PACU nurse a full verbal report (Table 7–1). The anesthesiologist reevaluates the patient and remains physically present and available until the nurse accepts responsibility for the care of the patient. The anesthesiologist should never leave an unstable patient. A physician capable of managing postanesthetic complications and cardiopulmonary resuscitation (CPR) must always be available to the PACU.

Routine postoperative PACU orders (including analgesic, antiemetic, and other medication; fluid replacement; monitoring; and special discharge criteria) are written by the surgeon or anesthesiologist.

Oxygen by mask or nasal prongs, and monitoring of blood pressure, cardiac rate and rhythm, oxygen saturation, and temperature are begun. The patient's vital signs are recorded upon admission and then periodically on a flow sheet while the patient is in the PACU.

POSTOPERATIVE COMPLICATIONS IN THE PACU

For most patients, recovery from anesthesia and surgery is routine and uneventful, but for others it can be a life-threatening experience. As many as 24% of all patients undergoing general, regional, or local anesthetic care experience some complication in the PACU. Most problems are minor and easily treated, but very serious complications can follow even the simplest and most straightforward surgical or anesthesia procedure.

DELAYED AWAKENING FROM ANESTHESIA

Most patients usually begin to respond to verbal or physical stimuli following general anesthesia while still in the operating room. For patients slow to awaken, usually patience and occasionally ventilatory support are all that is needed. Recovery from inhalational and fixed anesthetic agents is a function of many variables, and recovery time will differ for each patient (Table 7–2).

Antagonist drugs can be given in the postoperative period to reverse the unwanted persistent sedative effects of intraoperative medications. Naloxone in 40-μg increments

Table 7–1. PACU admission assessment report.

Patient's name, sex, age, and native language
Surgical procedure(s) (including surgeon's name and any surgical complications)
Anesthetic technique(s) (anesthetic and reversal agents)
Intraoperative course (vital signs—stable or unstable; fluid balance, including blood loss; urinary output and fluid and blood replacement; and any anesthetic complications)
Previous medical history (including medications, allergies, smoking, use of recreational drug(s), and alcohol)
Pending laboratory and radiologic studies

PACU = postanesthesia care unit.

Table 7–2. Factors causing delayed awakening from anesthesia.

Prolonged drug action (depends on many factors, incuding patient's age and physical status, dose of anesthetic, hepatic and renal clearance, and ventilatory status)

Metabolic
  Hypothermia
  Hypoglycemia
  Hyperosmolar nonketotic hyperglycemia
  Hepatic encephalopathy
  Uremia
  Adrenal insufficiency
  Thyroid disturbance (hypothyroidism and hyperthyroidism)

Electrolyte
  Hyponatremia (inappropriate ADH secretion, water intoxication—following laparoscopy or transurethral resection of the prostate)
  Hypo- or hyperkalemia

Neurologic injury
  Cerebral edema from head injury (preoperative or intraoperative)
  Cerebrovascular accident (embolism, hemorrhage, anoxia due to intraoperative hypotension or hypoxemia)
  Paradoxical air embolism (patent foramen ovale)

ADH = antidiuretic hormone.

Table 7–3. Common respiratory complications in the PACU.

Airway obstruction
Hypoxemia
Alveolar hypoventilation (hypercapnia)
Aspiration

PACU = postanesthesia care unit.

intravenously (IV) will reverse opioid-induced sedation. Flumazenil (up to 1.0 mg IV) reverses the effects of benzodiazepines, such as midazolam. Physostigmine (1.0–2.0 mg IV) will reverse the central effects of anticholinergics, such as scopolamine or atropine.

If the patient fails to awaken within a reasonable time, or if a documented intraoperative event suggests cerebral injury, a diagnostic workup with neurology consultation is indicated.

RESPIRATORY COMPLICATIONS

Most problems involving the respiratory system in the PACU can be detected by pulse oximetry before organ damage occurs (Table 7–3). Whatever the cause, initial therapy begins with administration of 100% oxygen. If air movement is occuring, it is important to determine the nature of the breath sounds (wheezing, rales, rhonchi) and whether the breath sounds are equal bilaterally or unequal. If unequal, the physician must determine if one side is dull or hyperresonant to percussion. If no air movement is occuring, a patent airway must be established. The need for reintubation of the trachea in the PACU is uncommon, occuring in fewer than 0.2% of patients. The usual reasons for reintubation include anesthetic or sedative overdose, excessive fluid administration, persistent muscle relaxation or upper airway obstruction.

Airway Obstruction

The most common cause of airway obstruction (Figure 7–1) is pharyngeal obstruction from a sagging tongue in an unconscious patient. This is managed by combining a backward tilt of the head with anterior displacement of the mandible. A nasal or oral airway may be helpful. A nasal airway is better tolerated, since it will not stimulate gagging or vomiting. If the airway cannot be opened by physical means, positive-pressure ventilation with a bag, mask, and 100% oxygen is indicated. If this maneuver fails, a small amount of succinylcholine (10–20 mg IV) should allow successful manual-assisted mask ventilation. If succinylcholine is used, assisted ventilation should be continued for at least 5 minutes after the obstruction is relieved.

Laryngeal obstruction can also occur from laryngeal spasm, which is treated by manual mask ventilation and IV succinylcholine. Orotracheal intubation by direct laryngoscopy is indicated only when the previous steps are unsuccessful. In very rare cases, emergency cricothyrotomy or tracheostomy may be necessary.

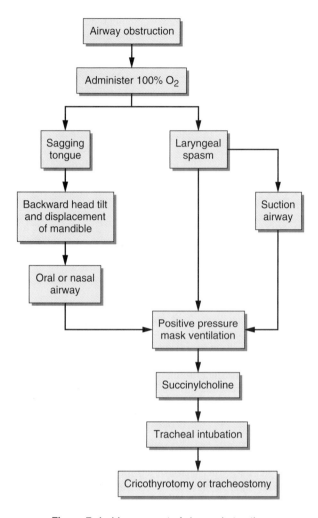

Figure 7–1. Management of airway obstruction.

Airway trauma or anaphylactic reaction can cause laryngeal edema. Initial treatment consists of supplemental oxygen, steroids (dexamethasone 4–8 mg IV), and inhalation of racemic epinephrine. Tracheal intubation, cricothyrotomy, or tracheostomy may be needed to secure a patent airway.

Hypoxemia

Hypoxemia following anesthesia and surgery can be due to many factors (Table 7–4). If hypoxemia (SaO_2 <90%, PaO_2 <60 mm Hg) persists despite the administration of 100% oxygen by face mask, tracheal intubation and mechanical ventilation are indicated. Continuous positive airway pressure by face mask (mask-CPAP) can be considered in a hypoxemic patient who demonstrates adequate carbon dioxide elimination. A chest radiograph and an arterial blood gas sample should be obtained.

A 10–20% pneumothorax in a spontaneously breathing patient can be observed with frequent upright chest x-ray

Table 7–4. Causes of hypoxemia in the PACU.

Low inspired concentration of oxygen (FiO$_2$)
Failure to administer oxygen, patient breathes room air
Diffusion hypoxia—can occur when nitrous oxide is replaced with air following a general anesthetic if no supplemental oxygen is administered
Crossed gas pipelines (rare)

Hypoventilation
Central respiratory depression
Inadequate respiratory muscle function
Increased carbon dioxide production

Low ventilation/perfusion relationship

Intrapulmonary right-to-left shunt
Atelectasis
Bronchial obstruction (secretion, blood)
Endobronchial intubation
Pneumothorax

Hypotension

Increased oxygen demand
Sepsis
Shivering
Malignant hyperthermia (rare)

PACU = postanesthesia care unit; FiO$_2$ = forced inspiratory oxygen.

Table 7–5. Respiratory insufficiency in the PACU.

Factors that depress the respiratory center
Drugs (volatile anesthetics, opioids, barbiturates, elevated carbon dioxide)
CNS injury (neurosurgery, trauma)

Factors that impair chest-wall mechanics
Incomplete reversal of neuromuscular blocking agents
Mechanical (tight dressing, body casts, suboptimal positioning of obese patients)
Neuromuscular disorders (Eaton-Lambert syndrome, myasthenia gravis, Guillain-Barré syndrome, hypocalcemic tetany following parathyroidectomy)

Factors that increase airway resistance
Upper airway obstruction (sagging tongue, uvular edema, sublingual hematoma, bilateral hypoglossal nerve injury, recurrent laryngeal nerve injury)
Laryngeal spasm, laryngeal edema secondary to trauma or anaphylactic reaction
Lower airway obstruction (tracheal compression: extrinsic—neck hematoma, intrinsic—mediastinal mass, tracheomalacia)
Pulmonary aspiration of gastric contents
Increased airway resistance (bronchospasm [asthma, reactive airways in COPD, anaphylactic reaction]; pneumothorax, hemothorax, or hydrothorax; pulmonary embolism [thrombus, fat, air])

Conditions affecting lung compliance or ventilation/perfusion relationship
Pulmonary edema (cardiac and noncardiac)
Pneumonia
Atelectasis
Aspiration of gastric contents

CNS = central nervous system; COPD = chronic obstructive pulmonary disease; PACU = postanesthesia care unit.

films. A pneumothorax >20% in a spontaneously breathing patient, or any pneumothorax in a mechanically ventilated patient, should be treated by insertion of a chest tube. A tension pneumothorax occurs when the pleural cavity fills with air and compresses the lung and mediastinum, leading to circulatory collapse. If a tension pneumothorax is suspected, immediate insertion of a 14-gauge needle in the second intercostal space can be life-saving.

Pulmonary edema, which usually occurs within the first 60 minutes following surgery, is often preceded by hypertension. Treatment consists of lowering hydrostatic pressure in the lungs while maintaining adequate systemic organ perfusion. Diuretics (furosemide, 20 mg IV), fluid restriction, and vasodilators (nitroprusside IV infusion) are used. Positive-pressure ventilation may be needed if there is severe hypoxemia and hypercapnia. A central venous pressure (CVP) or pulmonary artery catheter should be inserted to monitor these patients.

The diagnosis of pulmonary embolism is suspected in the patient with sudden pleuritic chest pain, shortness of breath, pleural effusion, or tachypnea. The ECG may reveal evidence of acute right-heart strain. Massive emboli result in hypotension, pulmonary hypertension, and elevated central venous pressure. Diagnosis is made by pulmonary angiography.

Hypercapnia

Reduced alveolar ventilation results in an increase in arterial carbon dioxide tension (PaCO$_2$). Hypoventilation usually occurs as a result of poor respiratory drive, poor respiratory muscle function, or a high rate of carbon dioxide production, or as a direct result of acute and chronic lung disease (Table 7–5).

Hypertension and tachycardia are two common signs of carbon dioxide retention that may not be seen in postsurgical patients, especially elderly patients with an attenuated response to elevated carbon dioxide levels. Direct measurement of PaCO$_2$ from an arterial blood sample is the best method to diagnose hypoventilation. Capnography is only useful if the patient's trachea is intubated.

Central respiratory depression can follow both inhalation and intravenous anesthesia. Opioid-induced respiratory depression can be reversed with naloxone. Naloxone should be administered in small increments (40 µg IV), since larger doses will reverse opioid analgesic effects, resulting in sudden pain. Sudden, severe pain can increase heart rate and blood pressure and result in myocardial ischemia in patients with coronary artery disease.

Failure to adequately reverse neuromuscular blocking agents will result in poor postoperative respiratory muscle function. Persistent neuromuscular blockade can be due to inadequate excretion of the drug as a result of poor renal function, or the presence of other drugs that attenuate neuromuscular blockade (eg, gentamicin, neomycin, clindamycin, or furosemide). Respiratory acidosis and hypokalemia inhibit reversal of neuromuscular blockade, while hypermagnesemia and hypothermia potentiate neuromuscular blockade. Obesity, gastric dilation, tight dressings, and body casts also inhibit normal respiratory muscle function.

Increased carbon dioxide production from sepsis or shivering can result in an elevated $PaCO_2$, especially in sedated patients who cannot increase minute ventilation.

CIRCULATORY COMPLICATIONS

Hypotension

Since prolonged hypotension will reduce tissue perfusion and cause ischemic organ damage, prompt diagnosis and treatment is essential. Before instituting treatment, one should assess whether the hypotension is real or an artifact. Inaccurate blood pressure readings can be due to an improperly placed or improper-sized blood pressure cuff, unequal pressures in the upper extremities (eg, cervical rib, aortic coarctation), or an inaccurately calibrated or positioned pressure monitor transducer.

In the PACU, hypotension is usually due to either decreased ventricular preload, reduced or ineffective myocardial contractility, or profound reduction in systemic vascular resistance (Table 7–6). Whatever the cause, the patient should be given 100% oxygen immediately.

Decreased ventricular preload is usually due to intravascular volume depletion from blood loss, inadequate replacement of third-space fluid and urinary losses, or septicemia that is associated with vasodilation and capillary fluid leak. Other causes to consider include acute massive pulmonary embolism (thrombus, air, fat), a pneumothorax, cardiac tamponade, inadvertent administration or incorrect dosage of drugs that dilate the systemic vasculature, and the occurence of an anaphylactic reaction to blood or medications. Hypovolemia may be acutely unmasked by sudden position changes in patients with blunted autonomic nervous system reflexes. This can occur following spinal or epidural blocks, in patients with autonomic neuropathy secondary to diabetes, and in patients receiving antihypertensive medications.

Ventricular preload can be increased by elevating the legs to promote venous return to the heart and by administering IV fluids. The surgical wound should be examined for evidence of blood loss, and a hematocrit ordered. Occult bleeding can present with recurrent episodes of hypotension that may transiently respond to fluid challenges.

If, despite fluid resuscitation, hypotension perists, ventricular preload must be quantitated and the specific etiology treated. In patients with normal left ventricular function, a CVP is adequate. For patients with left ventricular dysfunction, a pulmonary artery catheter is necessary to

Table 7–6. Causes of hypotension in the PACU.

Decreased ventricular preload
Reduced or ineffective myocardial contractility
Reduced systemic vascular resistance

PACU = postanesthesia care unit.

Table 7–7. Diagnosis of shock.

Hypovolemic shock
Low PAOP (<5–10 mm Hg)
Normal or low cardiac index (2.5–4.0 L/min/m²)
Normal or elevated SVR[1]
Cardiogenic shock
Increased PAOP (>15 mm Hg)
Low cardiac index
Elevated SVR
Septic shock
Low PAOP
High cardiac output
Low SVR

[1]SVR = MAP – CVP/CO × 80 (CO = cardiac output; CVP = central venous pressure; MAP = mean arterial pressure; SVR = systemic vascular resistance).
PAOP = pulmonary artery occlusion pressure.

measure pulmonary artery occlusion pressure (PAOP) (Table 7–7).

Hypovolemia is treated with intravenous crystalloid fluid and blood. Starch solutions can also be used for colloid replacement. Albumin is expensive and offers no additional benefits to crystalloid or starch.

Continued depressant effects of anesthetic drugs, preexisting ventricular dysfunction, or the development of perioperative myocardial infarction can all reduce myocardial contractility. Patients with suspected left ventricular failure should have an ECG and chemical analysis of fractionated creatinine phosphokinase (CPK). Elevated CPK-MB in the first 24 hours after surgery is specific for myocardial muscle damage. Total CPK is nonspecific and useless, since it will be elevated because of skeletal muscle damage during surgery.

Cardiogenic shock is managed first by optimizing ventricular preload. Fluid and blood are given to increase PAOP to 15–20 mm Hg, and inotropic support with dopamine (3–10 μg/kg/min IV) is begun. If a low cardiac output with high systemic vascular resistance still persists despite optimal preload and inotropic support, a peripheral vasodilator, such as sodium nitroprusside, should be instituted to lower outflow impedance to ventricular ejection, thereby improving myocardial function.

Profound reductions in systemic vascular resistance usually occur with septicemia, but can also be seen in anaphylactic reactions, in chronic hepatic failure, and with adrenal insufficiency. Septic shock is managed by replacing fluid lost to capillary endothelial leak. Crystalloid salt solutions are preferred. Albumin may be dangerous since it can leak out into the interstitium, further reducing intravascular fluid. An inotropic agent (dopamine) is necessary to increase cardiac output and raise arterial blood pressure. Alpha-adrenergic agonists, such as norepinephrine or phenylephrine, may be needed in severe sepsis with lowered vascular resistance if the patient is unresponsive to fluids and inotropes.

Concurrent with starting appropriate therapy, arrange-

Table 7–8. Complications secondary to hypertension.

Left ventricular failure
Myocardial ischemia
Arrhythmia
Pulmonary edema
Cerebral hemorrhage

Table 7–9. Causes of agitation in the PACU.

Pain
Fear
Drugs (scopolamine, atropine, ketamine, phenothiazines, and bar-
   biturates)
Respiratory problems (hypoxemia, hypercapnia)
Gastric and urinary bladder distention
Toxic delirium (hyperthermia, thyroid storm)
Metabolic disturbances (hypoglycemia, hyperosmolar hyper-
   glycemia, hyponatremia, uremia, hepatic encephalopathy)
Withdrawal syndromes associated with chronic chemical sub-
   stance dependency (alcohol, drugs)

PACU = postanesthesia care unit.

ments should be made to transfer the patient from the PACU to the ICU.

Hypertension

Severe hypertension can lead to serious complications (Table 7–8). More than half the patients who develop hypertension in the PACU have a history of preexisting hypertension. Postoperative hypertension may be made worse if antihypertensive medications are withheld prior to surgery. Management of hypertension first involves treating the cause, which in the PACU is usually pain, hypercapnia, hypoxemia, or fluid overload.

If hypertension persists, a short-acting antihypertensive agent, such as hydralazine (5 mg IV in increments) is indicated. Beta-blocking drugs are also effective. Incremental boluses of labetalol (5 mg IV) or an intravenous infusion of esmolol (25–300 µg/kg/min) are used. Propranolol (0.5–1.0 mg IV) is effective, especially if the patient is on beta-adrenergic blocking medication.

Arrhythmias

Ventricular ectopy, if present preoperatively, usually requires no treatment other than observation postoperatively in the PACU. If ectopy becomes more frequent or multifocal, intervention may be necessary. Correction of the underlying etiology usually is the only treatment needed. Arrhythmias first appearing in the PACU are usually due to hypertension from a variety of causes, including pain, electrolyte imbalance (usually hypokalemia or hypocalcemia), hypoxemia, hypercapnia, acid-base disturbances, or preexisting heart disease. Factors such as hypothermia or drugs that increase vagal tone (eg, excessive acetylcholinesterase inhibitor used to reverse muscle relaxants) can lead to bradycardia with ventricular escape beats.

POSTOPERATIVE AGITATION

Postoperative agitation, or "emergence delirium," can be due to many factors but the usual causes are pain or fear, especially in pediatric patients (Table 7–9).

Scopolamine and atropine can cause a "central anticholinergic syndrome." Symptoms may present as delirium, restlessness, confusion, or obtundation. The patient may have a dry mouth, hot and dry skin, blurred vision, photophobia, and fever. The effects are reversed with physostigmine (1.0–2.0 mg IV). Pulse rate must be closely monitored, since physostigmine may cause marked bradycardia.

PAIN

Pain is not a complication, but if inadequately treated pain can result in serious complications. The goal is to achieve optimal pain relief with minimal side effects. Opioids (intramuscular, IV [continuous or patient-controlled], epidural) remain the mainstay of analgesic therapy in the PACU (see Chapter 5).

Preoperative analgesic dependency influences postoperative needs. These patients often require extraordinarily large amounts of analgesic drugs.

Opioids can cause respiratory depression (decreased respiratory rate, decreased tidal volume), nausea and vomiting, pruritus, and urinary retention. A nonsteroidal antiinflamatory agent (NSAID) like ketorolac (30 mg IV) does not depress ventilation and is an excellent supplement to opioid analgesia. NSAIDs should be avoided in patients with a history of bleeding or gastric ulcers.

NAUSEA & VOMITING

Nausea and vomiting are probably the most common complications of anesthesia and surgery. Antiemetics, such as droperidol (75 µg/kg IV) or metoclopromide (10 mg IV), can be given. Odansetron (4 mg IV) is most effective in preventing or treating nausea and vomiting, but, because of its expense, it is seldom used as prophylaxis unless the patient has a history of severe postoperative nausea and vomiting. Odansetron is indicated for nausea and vomiting refractory to other treatments.

A stomach distended by air should be decompressed with an oral or nasal gastric tube.

HYPOTHERMIA & SHIVERING

Patients become poikilothermic during general anesthesia and cannot control their body temperature. Many patients arrive in the PACU hypothermic after major procedures, especially when a body cavity has been open for a long time. A cold patient is uncomfortable and will shiver. Shivering causes a marked increase in oxygen consumption (up to 500%) with an increase in metabolic rate, resulting in increased cardiac output and minute ventilation. The prevention and treatment of hypothermia in the PACU includes supplemental oxygen, warming IV fluids and blood, and external warming with heating blankets and lights.

Following inhalational anesthetics, many normothermic patients shiver. Meperidine (10–20 mg IV) is effective in this setting to stop shivering and decrease oxygen consumption.

VISUAL DISTURBANCES

Petroleum-based eye lubricants, used to protect the eyes, may cause decreased or blurred vision in the PACU.

A more serious complication, corneal abrasion, may be due to direct trauma, irritation from liquids or prep solution, and decreased tear production after failure to protect the eyes during surgery. The patient complains of a foreign body sensation, has marked tearing and photophobia, and has pain that is aggravated by blinking and with eye movement. The diagnosis of corneal abrasion is made by fluorescein staining of the eye and subsequent ophthalmic examination. Corneal abrasions are treated by patching the injured eye and applying a topical antibiotic solution.

Acute glaucoma is characterized by a painful eye and decreased visual acuity, often associated with severe headaches and nausea and vomiting. These attacks usually occur in patients with narrow-angle glaucoma and are precipitated by the administration of mydriatics (eg, atropine) or corneal edema. The incidence of glaucoma attacks is reduced if the patient uses his topical medications on the morning of surgery. When an attack occurs, it is treated with parenteral acetazolamide, osmotic diuretics, and topical instillation of miotics and timolol.

Following surgery, blindness resulting from central retinal artery or vein occlusion can occur from extrinsic pressure on the globe in patients put in the prone position for extended periods, or from hypotension in patients with increased intraocular pressure. Visual loss can also occur from retinal vessel hemorrhage secondary to malignant hypertension. Transient bilateral visual loss has been associated with ketamine anesthesia and with water intoxication following transurethral prostate resection.

HEARING COMPLICATIONS

Hearing impairment following anesthesia is usually the result of tympanic membrane rupture. The patient complains of decreased or total hearing loss and tinnitus and has blood in the ear canal. Displacement of a tympanic membrane graft, disruption of ossicular reconstruction, or direct injury to the middle ear can result from high middle ear pressures during a nitrous oxide anesthetic or from negative ear pressures following cessation of nitrous oxide.

The tympanic membrane can be ruptured intraopera-

tively or postoperatively by a tympanic membrane temperature probe.

RENAL COMPLICATIONS

The most common cause of what appears to be anuria in the PACU is actually a kinked or blocked urinary catheter. Always check the patency of the catheter in the anuric patient.

Urinary retention is not uncommon, especially after spinal or epidural anesthesia in elderly male patients. A full bladder should be considered in a patient with marked blood pressure swings and a distended abdomen.

Postoperative oliguria (urine output <15 ml/hr) is usually prerenal, due to poor renal perfusion from hypovolemia or circulatory failure. Administration of 250–500 ml of crystalloid solution is often adequate treatment. If oliguria is not due to hypovolemia, then cardiac failure should be considered. Inotropic support (dopamine 2–10 μg/kg/min) increases cardiac output and renal blood flow. Diuretics (furosemide, 5–10 mg IV) will restore urine

Table 7–10. Guidelines for discharge from the PACU.

General	Oriented to time and place
	Responds to verbal instructions
	Stable vital signs
	Available destination appropriate for patient
Cardiovascular	Systolic blood pressure ± 20% of resting preoperative level
	Stable heart rate and rhythm
Airway	No need for artificial airway support
	Protective gag reflexes intact
	SpO$_2$ >92% (room air); SpO$_2$ >96% supplemental oxygen
	Oxygen available for transport (if needed)
Pain control	Adequate analgesia
	At least 30 min since last parenteral opioid injection
	Appropriate orders for analgesics after PACU discharge
Renal function	Urine output >30 ml/hr (with catheter)
	Spontaneous voiding has occurred in PACU
Laboratory	Acceptable laboratory, ECG, and chest x-ray (if ordered)
Ambulatory patients	Ability to ambulate without dizziness, hypotension, or support
	Adequate control of nausea and vomiting
	Adult present to accompany and care for patient
Regional anesthesia	Evidence that the block is receding or has worn off

ECG = electrocardiogram; PACU = postanesthesia care unit; SpO$_2$ = percent oxyhemoglobin saturation as measured by pulse oximetry.

flow in patients with oliguria stemming from circulatory failure, but diuretic therapy is dangerous in a hypovolemic patient. A central venous pressure catheter or pulmonary artery catheter should be used to monitor volume status prior to administering diuretics.

Postrenal oliguria, a less common cause of oliguria in the PACU, may be due to obstruction of the urinary collecting system. This condition is treated with nephrostomy tubes or ureteral catheters. Acute tubular necrosis in the PACU is very rare. In this situation, fluid intake is minimized and the patient is treated with dialysis.

BLEEDING COMPLICATIONS

Postoperative bleeding may be occult or may present as hypotension. One should examine the patient for a distended abdomen. Following head and neck surgery, bleeding into the neck may cause acute upper airway obstruction.

PERIPHERAL NERVE INJURIES

Proper patient positioning during surgery is extremely important, since nerve injuries can occur from stretching or direct compression or from trauma. Prolonged periods of hypotension, hypothermia, improperly functioning automatic blood pressure devices, or the use of tourniquets can all injure peripheral nerves.

A complete preoperative medical history is important, since coexisting factors, such as cervical rib, can contribute to the injury. Chronic medical problems, such as preexisting neuropathy (for example, due to alcoholism, diabetes, or pernicious anemia) can be exacerbated by anesthesia and surgery. A neurologic consultation should be obtained.

DISCHARGE FROM THE PACU

Immediately prior to leaving the PACU, the patient must meet the hospital's criteria for discharge (Table 7–10). Every patient should be arousable and oriented and have stable vital signs.

For "same-day" ambulatory surgical patients, a responsible adult must be present to accompany the patient home and care for any patient who has undergone general anesthesia or IV sedation.

SUGGESTED READING

Feeley TW: The postanesthesia care unit. In: Miller RD (editor): *Anesthesia.* Churchill-Livingstone, 1986.

Hines R et al: Complications occurring in the postanesthesia care unit: A survey. Anesth Analg 1992;74:503.

Mathew JP et al: Emergency tracheal intubation in the postanesthesia care unit: Physician error or patient disease? Anesth Analg 1990;71:691.

Mecca RS: Postoperative recovery. In: Barash PG, Cullen BF, Stoelting RK (editors): *Clinical Anesthesia.* Lippincott, 1989.

Van der Walt JH et al.: The Australian Incident Monitoring Study. Recovery room incidents in the first 2000 incident reports. Anaesth Intensive Care 1993: 21:650.

8

Imaging the Surgical Patient

R. Brooke Jeffrey, Jr, MD

▶ Key Facts

- ▶ X-rays are a form of radiant energy with a short wavelength, which gives them the ability to penetrate substances that are opaque to light.

- ▶ A radiographic image distinguishes between air, fat, tissues of differing water density, and metallic densities.

- ▶ In order to distinguish structures of similar densities on a radiographic image more definitively, chemical compounds known as "contrast media" may be injected or swallowed.

- ▶ Ultrasonographic imaging makes use of ultrasonic waves (high-frequency sound waves) rather than ionizing waves and presents no significant hazard to the patient.

- ▶ Ultrasonography is widely available and is the least expensive of the radiological techniques.

- ▶ Recent advances in imaging have greatly facilitated the early diagnosis of many acute surgical disorders.

- ▶ The use of exploratory laparotomy merely for diagnosis has greatly diminished with the development of high resolution CT and ultrasonography.

- ▶ CT, ultrasonography, and MRI are increasingly important diagnostic techniques in the detection and staging of abdominal and thoracic malignancies.

It is very important that every surgeon possess an understanding of the techniques of diagnostic imaging as well as basic skills in ordering and interpreting radiological images. Amazing advances in diagnostic radiological imaging over the last decade made the acquisition of this skill increasingly difficult. However, the responsible surgeon knows that initially ordering the proper radiological studies and accurately interpreting results are essential parts of modern-day practice. It is not sufficient to be satisfied with merely reading a radiological report. The surgeon must also be able to intelligently discuss the films with the consulting radiologist.

IMAGING MODALITIES

CONVENTIONAL RADIOGRAPHY

Conventional radiography is based on the principle of differential absorption of x-ray photons by different types of body substances. X-rays are a form of radiant energy with a short wavelength; this gives them the ability to penetrate substances that are opaque to light and produce an image or shadow that can be recorded on photographic film. A radiographic image distinguishes between air, fat, tissues of differing water density, and metallic densities.

This seemingly simple concept has obviously proved enormously valuable and is still the basis for the most commonly used imaging modality.

Contrast Media

The efficiency of radiography largely depends on the density of different structures, which determines their ability to produce shadows of varying intensity on an x-ray. It is obvious that many structures do not differ strongly in density and will, therefore, be difficult to discern. In order to distinguish between these structures, chemical compounds known as "contrast media" may be injected or swallowed. A very common contrast medium is barium. It is used in "barium meals" and "barium enemas" to obtain images of gastrointestinal structures. Organic iodine is another compound widely used for imaging everything from the kidney (intravenous pyelogram, or IVP) to various vascular structures (angiograms).

Unfortunately, some patients experience moderate-to-severe allergic reactions to iodinated contrast material. The protocol used by the author for pretreating patients with a history of allergy is outlined in Table 8–1.

Table 8–1. Protocol for premedication of patients with allergic history receiving iodinated contrast.

Although there is no one "correct" approach for the pretreatment of patients receiving iodinated contrast with a prior history of allergy, the following protocol is documented as extremely safe and efficacious. It consists of:
1. 50 mg of prednisone orally 13 hours prior to the examination.
2. 50 mg of prednisone orally 7 hours prior to the examination.
3. Both 50 mg of prednisone and 50 mg of diphenhydramine hydrochloride (Benadryl®) orally 1 hour prior to the examination.

ULTRASONOGRAPHY

Ultrasonography is widely available and is the least expensive of the radiologic techniques. Ultrasonic diagnosis is not an x-ray examination, since it makes use of ultrasonic rather than ionizing waves. This technique has an advantage over the use of x-rays in that there are no significant hazards to the patient from the waves themselves at the levels used in diagnostic examinations. Ultrasonographic waves are high-frequency vibrations (sound waves) generated by electrical stimulation of a piezoelec-

HISTORICAL FACTS

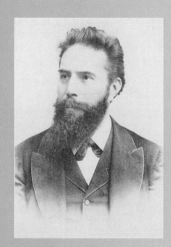
Wilhelm Roentgen (1845–1923).

In 1901, Wilhelm Roentgen (1845–1923) was awarded the Nobel Prize for physics for his discovery of x-rays in November of 1895. As is the case with many landmark scientific discoveries, it was quite by accident. Roentgen was very interested in the phosphorescence from metallic salts exposed to light. He was passing electrical current through a vacuum tube when he noticed a glow radiating from a screen painted with a phosphorescent substance (barium platinocyanide). As he experimented further with this phenomenon, he found that these invisible rays were able to pass through wood, metal, and, most notably, the soft tissues of the body. He set up a photographic plate to capture his findings on film, and history was made.

Roentgen's discoveries were accepted and put into practice in the medical community very quickly. Numerous applications were developed to aid surgeons in the diagnosis of fractures, dislocations, and the locations of foreign bodies. Unfortunately, the dangers of x-rays were not immediately appreciated and there were a number of injuries related to its use.

tric crystal. These vibrations pass through the body and are reflected or attenuated to varying degrees, depending upon the density of the underlying tissue. Ultrasonographic transducers first emit the sound waves, then subsequently detect the reflected sound wave. These findings are electronically amplified and displayed, and a photograph of the image can be taken and used as a permanent record, if necessary.

Ultrasonic Doppler is a technique that utilizes the Doppler effect arising when continuous ultrasonic waves reflect off a moving object, indicating the rate of movement of the object. This technique is now used extensively for intraoperative ultrasonography.

CT

Computed axial tomography (CT) first became available for examination of the cranium in 1972 and has continued to revolutionize radiography since that time. It is the technique of obtaining an image of a transverse slice of a person's body. A fan beam of x-rays is passed through the patient in an axial direction as the x-ray source rotates about the patient. Instead of photographic film, opposite the x-ray source is an array of detectors that measure the amount of x-ray absorption. A computer uses complex mathematical calculations to process and store the data. Photographic films may be produced from the information for a permanent record.

"Contrast enhanced" CT images may be produced when contrast media is injected intravenously. If the patient is scanned within a specified period of time, normal and abnormal structures and tissues show a higher density due to the selective increase in chemical (usually iodine) concentration within them.

MRI

Magnetic resonance imaging, or MRI, is not as readily available as ultrasonography or CT because of its expense. For example, the cost of an MRI to assess a liver tumor is six to eight times that of ultrasonography and twice that of CT. Like ultrasonography, MRI does not involve the use of x-rays and is noninvasive. The principle of this imaging system is that the presence of a magnetic field can influence the resonance (behavior) of protons in the nuclei of atoms (usually the hydrogen atom). In a strong magnetic field the protons will spin. By varying the strength of the magnetic field, changes in cell biochemistry and the composition of tissue can be demonstrated. At the heart of the system is a huge cylindrical magnet (metallic objects such as scissors should not be taken into the scanning room). The patient is placed in the center of this magnet. The information is fed to a computer and 3-D pictures are produced and stored.

IMAGING FOR ACUTE SURGICAL DISORDERS

The development of high-resolution CT and ultrasonography, and other advances in imaging, have greatly facilitated the early diagnosis of many acute surgical disorders and diminished the need for exploratory laparotomy. These cross-sectional techniques have made a major contribution to the diagnosis of blunt trauma, abdominal abscesses, acute inflammatory disorders, and bowel ischemia.

BLUNT TRAUMA

Contrast-enhanced CT is the imaging method of choice to evaluate hemodynamically stable patients with blunt abdominal trauma. Unstable patients require diagnostic peritoneal lavage and/or urgent laparotomy. CT is highly accurate in detecting lacerations of the liver, spleen, and kidney, and in determining the extent of hemoperitoneum (Figure 8–1). Contrast enhancement is essential for a diagnosis of visceral lacerations. Normal parenchymal tissues will enhance significantly following intravenous contrast. Avascular hematomas will not enhance, thus, lacerations appear as low-attenuation lesions.

Because of the high protein content, CT attenuation values can be used to diagnose hemoperitoneum (typically 30–60 HU) and distinguish it from other fluid collections, such as bile, urine, or ascites (typically 0–10 HU). In selected patients, active arterial extravasation can be demonstrated with bolus administration of contrast.

CT is not as accurate for early diagnosis of pancreatic lacerations and luminal injuries to the gastrointestinal (GI)

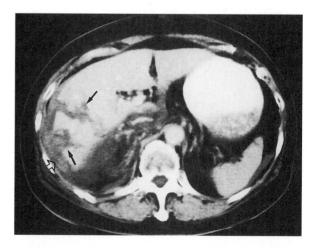

Figure 8–1. CT diagnosis of hepatic laceration. Contrast-enhanced CT demonstrates multiple linear low-attenuation lacerations from blunt trauma **(arrows)**. Note adjacent high-attenuation hemoperitoneum **(open arrow)**.

tract. A small percentage of patients with bowel and mesenteric injuries may have very subtle abnormalities on initial CT scans. The CT findings may include pneumoperitoneum, mesenteric hematoma, extravasated oral contrast, or free fluid between the reflections of the mesentery.

Pancreatic lacerations may also be difficult to diagnose on scans obtained within a few hours of injury. Follow-up scans may demonstrate posttraumatic pancreatitis and peripancreatic fluid collections that may not be evident in the immediate posttrauma period.

ABDOMINAL ABSCESSES

In patients with suspected hepatic or pelvic abscesses, ultrasonography is the imaging method of choice (Figure 8–2). For all other patients, contrast-enhanced CT is the most useful technique for diagnosis of intra-abdominal abscesses. The hallmark of an abscess on imaging studies is a complex fluid collection with mass effect. With contrast enhancement, inflamed tissues adjacent to an abscess demonstrate a significant increase in attenuation. However, liquefied pus will not enhance because it is avascular.

One of the main values of cross-sectional imaging is to provide guidance for percutaneous catheter drainage of abdominal abscesses (Figure 8–3). The majority of localized abdominal abscesses can be successfully treated with percutaneous techniques. In patients with infected pancreatic necrosis, however, catheter drainage is less effective, as necrotic tissue in the pancreatic bed requires surgical debridement.

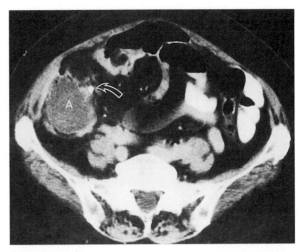

A

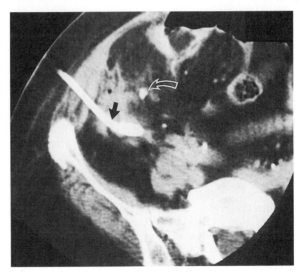

B

Figure 8–3. CT-guided percutaneous drainage of periappendiceal abscess. **A:** Note low-density fluid collection representing abscess **(A)** adjacent to calcified appendicolith **(curved arrow)**. **B:** After insertion of a catheter into the abscess **(black arrow),** the fluid collection completely resolves. The appendicolith is still evident **(curved arrow)**. (Reprinted, with permission, from Jeffrey RB J.: *CT and Sonography of the Acute Abdomen.* Raven Press, 1989.)

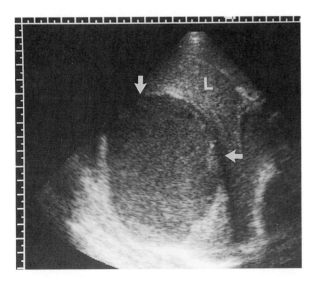

Figure 8–2. Amoebic abscess diagnosed by ultrasonography. Sagittal scan of the liver demonstrates a large hypoechoic amoebic abscess **(arrows)** near the dome of the liver **(L)**. (Reprinted, with permission, from Jeffrey RB Jr: *CT and Sonography of the Acute Abdomen.* Raven Press, 1989.)

ACUTE CHOLECYSTITIS

Ultrasonography and biliary scintigraphy are the primary diagnostic methods to evaluate patients with suspected biliary colic or acute cholecystitis. Ultrasonography has the advantage of demonstrating gallstones and gallbladder wall thickening. When the gallbladder is normal, the rest of the abdomen can be imaged to make alter-

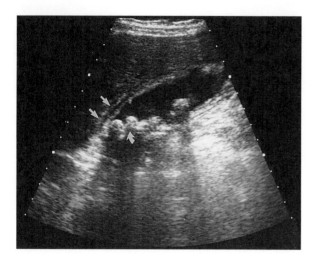

Figure 8–4. Acute cholecystitis. Note multiple gallstones *(curved arrow)* as well as edema of the gallbladder wall *(arrows)*. Patient had a positive sonographic Murphy's sign, and acute cholecystitis was confirmed surgically. (Reprinted, with permission, from Freeney PC, Stevenson GW: *Margulis and Burhenne's Alimentary Tract Radiology*, 5th ed. Mosby, 1994.)

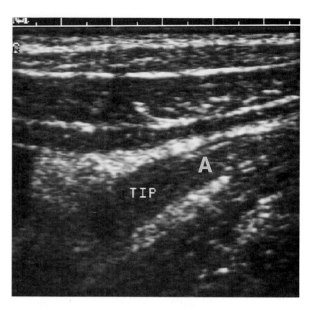

Figure 8–5. Ultrasonographic diagnosis of acute appendicitis. Graded-compression sonography of the right low quadrant demonstrates a noncompressible thickened appendix *(A)*. The tip of the appendix is indistinct due to focal gangrenous change *(Tip)*. (Reprinted, with permission, from Jeffrey RB Jr: Acute appendicitis confined to the appendiceal tip: evaluation with graded compression sonography. J Ultr Med 1992;11:205.)

nate diagnoses. The primary sonographic findings in acute cholecystitis are gallstones and a positive sonographic Murphy's sign (focal tenderness elicited directly over the gallbladder) (Figure 8–4). Secondary findings include gallbladder wall thickening, pericholecystic fluid, and intraluminal membranes (representing fibrinous strands or hemorrhage). When ultrasonography is indeterminate, biliary scintigraphy is indicated to confirm the diagnosis. In patients with calculous cholecystitis, isotope will not enter the gallbladder as a result of cystic duct obstruction.

APPENDICITIS

The clinical assessment of acute right lower quadrant pain is often challenging, due to the broad spectrum of diagnostic possibilities. This is particularly true of women of child-bearing age, as there is significant overlap between acute gynecologic abnormalities and the clinical presentation of acute appendicitis. Ultrasonography relies on the graded-compression technique with direct visualization of a noncompressible appendix greater than 6 mm in maximal diameter (Figure 8–5).

Identification of an appendicolith also indicates a positive study. Obese patients are often best evaluated with CT, as graded compression of the abdominal wall may be difficult in these patients. Inflammatory changes in the pericecal fat may be an important clue to appendicitis on CT, although they are nonspecific and may be the result of cecal diverticulitis, inflammation of the terminal ileum, or a tubo-ovarian abscess.

DIVERTICULITIS

CT and contrast enemas are the primary methods used to evaluate patients with suspected diverticulitis. CT is generally performed in patients with high fever and leukocytosis and suspected abscesses (Figure 8–6). A discreet, well-defined paracolonic abscess may be draining percu-

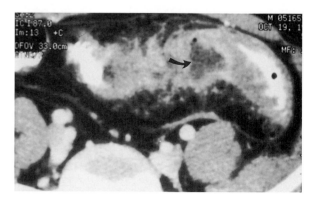

Figure 8–6. CT diagnosis of diverticulitis with adjacent abscess formation. On contrast-enhanced CT, a well-defined, low-attenuation abscess *(arrows)* is noted adjacent to a thickened segment of sigmoid colon from diverticulitis.

taneously, thus eliminating the need for a diverting colostomy. In selected patients, a single-stage surgical resection may then be performed following successful percutaneous drainage of the abscess.

CROHN'S DISEASE

Barium studies and CT are used most often to evaluate the extent of involvement of the GI tract in patients with Crohn's disease. The main value of CT is in demonstrating mesenteric or intraperitoneal abscesses. Small-bowel contrast studies, including enteroclysis, are quite valuable in assessing mucosal involvement in Crohn's disease and determining the discrete segments of involvement. Often, there are "skip areas" of involvement that can only be determined with barium studies.

PANCREATITIS

Contrast-enhanced CT is the imaging method of choice to evaluate patients with suspected pancreatitis. The CT findings may include pancreatic enlargement, peripancreatic fluid, and inflammatory masses (Figure 8–7). Ultrasonography is useful in evaluating for gallstones as a potential cause for pancreatitis. Complications of pancreatitis, such as necrosis, pseudocyst, or pseudoaneurysm formation, are best imaged with contrast-enhanced CT.

BOWEL ISCHEMIA & INFARCTION

Early intestinal ischemia may be very difficult to diagnose with current imaging studies. The initial screening study should be a contrast-enhanced CT because a variety of acute abdominal disorders (pancreatitis, bowel obstruction, perforated duodenal ulcer) may mimic intestinal ischemia. The CT findings of bowel ischemia include identification of a thrombus within the superior mesenteric artery or vein, thickening of the bowel wall, pneumatosis, portal venous gas, and mesenteric hematoma or fluid (Figure 8–8). Bowel wall thickening is nonspecific and may be caused by a variety of infections or inflammatory disorders. When CT is equivocal, mesenteric angiography may be performed to diagnose major vaso-occlusive disease of the superior mesenteric artery or vein.

TUMOR IMAGING

CT, ultrasonography, and MRI are increasingly important diagnostic techniques in the detection and staging of abdominal and thoracic malignancies. Percutaneous biopsy guided by cross-sectional imaging techniques has largely replaced open surgical biopsy for confirmation of most neoplasms. A combination of techniques can be used to follow the patient's response to chemotherapy and radiation therapy.

GASTROINTESTINAL TRACT TUMORS

Endoscopy and barium studies remain the primary techniques for diagnosing tumors of the GI tract. The depth of mural invasion of gastrointestinal tumors is best evaluated with endoscopic ultrasonography, since discrete layers of the bowel wall, including the submucosa and muscularis

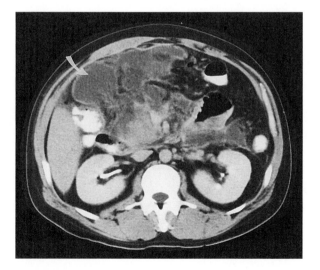

Figure 8–7. Peripancreatic fluid from acute pancreatitis. Contrast-enhanced CT demonstrates extensive fluid extending into the transverse mesocolon secondary to acute pancreatitis **(arrow)**.

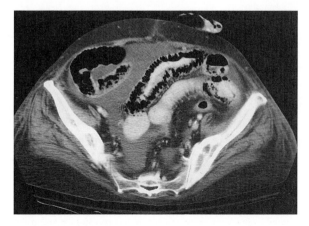

Figure 8–8. CT diagnosis of bowel infarction. Extensive pneumatosis is demonstrated from infarction of the distal small bowel.

propria, can be directly imaged with high-frequency ultrasonography. Identification of deep mural invasion is critically important information for the treatment of esophageal and rectal tumors.

Preoperative radiation and chemotherapy may be performed in these patients prior to definitive surgical resection. Distant metastasis to the liver and lungs is generally evaluated with CT, although hepatic metastasis may also be readily imaged by MRI. Intraoperative ultrasonography is a highly accurate technique to detect many small, nonpalpable hepatic metastases from colorectal tumors.

PANCREATIC NEOPLASMS

Contrast-enhanced CT and MRI are the current modalities of choice for evaluating patients with suspected pancreatic neoplasms (Figure 8–9). Ultrasonography is an excellent technique to evaluate for biliary tract obstruction. Once an obstructing mass is noted within the head of the pancreas, however, further imaging studies are required with CT or MRI to accurately stage the tumor. CT can accurately determine the presence of arterial encasement, venous occlusion, and hepatic metastasis, which generally preclude radical surgical resection.

HEPATIC NEOPLASMS

Contrast-enhanced CT and MRI are the primary imaging techniques to diagnose hepatic metastases. The recent development of spiral (helical) CT allows rapid scan acquisition during both the arterial phase (25–55 s after intravenous contrast injection) and portal venous phase

(70–100 s). This enables imaging of hypervascular tumors during the arterial phase (Figure 8–10). Because of its lower cost, ultrasonography is often utilized as a screening modality for hepatocellular carcinoma in patients with known hepatitis.

For the preoperative assessment of liver turmos, CT arterial portography is a highly sensitive technique that utilizes intra-arterial injection through a catheter placed in either the superior mesenteric artery or the splenic artery. The liver is then imaged 30 s after this injection, during the portal venous phase.

Intraoperative ultrasonography is an increasingly important technique to guide surgical planning for liver resection. Intraoperative ultrasonography can detect small, nonpalpable lesions that often cannot be adequately imaged preoperatively.

RENAL NEOPLASMS

CT and MRI are the imaging techniques of choice to evaluate patients with known or suspected renal tumors detected by either intravenous urography or ultrasonography. Both techniques can determine invasion of the renal vein, regional lymphadenopathy, and extension of tumor through Gerota's fascia.

THORACIC NEOPLASMS

CT and MRI are routinely used to preoperatively stage carcinoma of the lung. These techniques can greatly aid in the diagnosis of mediastinal and vascular invasion, lymphadenopathy, and chest wall involvement. Pancoast tu-

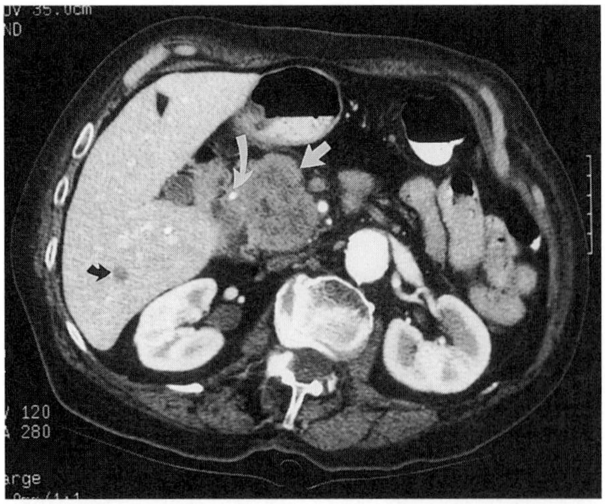

Figure 8–9. CT diagnosis of nonresectable pancreatic carcinoma. A large pancreatic mass is noted *(arrow)*, encasing the gastroduodenal artery *(curved white arrow)*. Note the low-density liver metastasis *(curved black arrow)*.

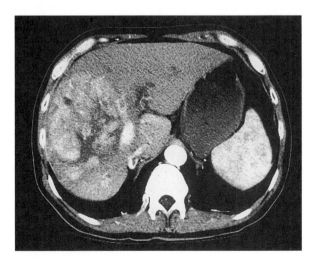

Figure 8–10. Arterial-phase spiral CT images of hepatocellular carcinoma. Arterial-phase images from a spiral CT scan of the liver demonstrate a hypervascular tumor mass consistent with hepatocellular carcinoma.

mors at the lung apex are often best imaged with MRI, as coronal images readily demonstrate supraclavicular invasion, bone destruction, and involvement of the brachial plexus. Pulmonary parenchymal metastases are best imaged with CT. Thin sections (high-resolution CT) may also demonstrate lymphatic metastases.

SUGGESTED READING

Brown JJ, Wippold FJ: *Practical MRI: A Teaching File*. Lippincott-Raven Publishers, 1996.

Fishman EK, Jeffrey RB Jr: *Spiral CT: Principles, Techniques, and Clinical Applications*. Raven Press, 1995.

Jeffrey RB Jr, Ralls PW: *Sonography of the Abdomen*. Raven Press, 1995.

Jeffrey RB Jr, Ralls PW: *CT and Sonography of the Acute Abdomen*, 2nd ed. Lippincott–Raven Publishers, 1996.

Putnam CE, Ravin CR: *Textbook of Diagnostic Imaging*, 2nd ed. Saunders, 1994.

Ros PR, Bidgood WD Jr: *Abdominal Magnetic Resonance Imaging*. Mosby–Year Book, 1993.

Section II

Basic & Special Procedures

9

Incisions, Wound Closure, & the Healing Process

John E. Niederhuber, MD

▶ Key Facts

▶ Incisions must be carefully planned, for they are the key to a successful operation. The incision must be long enough to allow for adequate exposure, but appropriately placed and of a size that will optimize the patient's rapid recovery.

▶ When possible, incisions should be designed to follow the normal "wrinkle lines" of the skin. This is especially true of the face, neck, and other exposed areas of the body.

▶ An incision cannot heal properly with minimal scarring unless it is carefully made with a sharp blade and with careful attention to "drawing" the incision in a manner exactly perpendicular to the flattened skin.

▶ During the operation, wound edges must be kept moist with wet sponges to protect the soft tissues of the chest wall, abdominal wall, and so forth from pressure damage from retractors and from drying during exposure.

▶ The placing of a knot actually creates a weak point in the suture. The goal is to set the knot as a square rather than a series of loops.

▶ Before putting a needle into an area to be sutured, the free end is carefully passed to the assistant's side with care. Thus, the suture can be easily grasped for prompt tying to prevent it from becoming tangled with other sutures or with instruments in the field.

▶ The healing of a tissue wound, whether made by the surgeon's scalpel or by a traumatic injury, occurs via a series of overlapping phases: coagulation, inflammation, granulation with angiogenesis, and scar formation.

▶ The healing process of a wound may be negatively affected by a number of conditions, including, but not limited to, malnutrition, diabetes mellitus, peripheral vascular disease, immunodeficiency states, and irradiation.

The making of wounds by incising normal tissues as well as wounds that result from traumatic injury, and the repair or treatment of such wounds, is central to the science of surgery. By its very nature, surgery is the process of wound repair and healing. Thus, for the beginning trainee and student, certain fundamental principles are important to understand.

As would be expected, much of the early science of surgery had to do with advances in the management of traumatic injury, infection, and wound healing. The great army surgeon, Ambröise Paré (1510–1590), was initially distraught when in the midst of battle he ran out of boiling oil, which was routinely used to treat battle wounds. Later, impressed with the results of healing he observed in

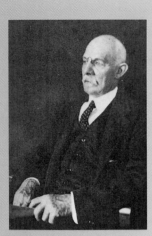

William Steward Halsted (1852–1922).

William S. Halsted (1852–1922) is certainly one of the greatest and most renowned figures in American surgical history. Although he is best known for his unprecedented educational philosophy, which set the tone for modern American surgical training, his insistence on fastidious tissue handling and wound care were, and continue to be, an important part of his influence on the practice of surgery. The Halsted stitch, which is placed through the subcuticular fascia for exact skin approximation, is still widely used today. He introduced silver as a suture material and as a covering for wounds because of its bactericidal qualities. He also introduced gutta-percha (purified latex from trees) in the form of a protective dressing for open wounds. He showed how silk could be safely buried in tissue and designed delicate pointed forceps for hemostasis. In order to decrease wound infection, he also introduced rubber gloves into surgery in the early 1890s and is credited with their widespread use throughout the United States. His innovative clinical procedures included a technique for the treatment of inguinal hernia, the radical mastectomy for the treatment of breast cancer, and the introduction of a metal band in place of a ligature for the occlusion of arteries.

the wounds that were not subjected to boiling oil, he began to advocate a new approach to managing battle wounds that avoided harmful interference in the body's ability to heal itself. An inscription on his statue reads, "Je le pansay, Dieu le guarit" ("I treated him, God healed him"), should serve as our guide in facilitating the ability of the patient to recover and heal the required incisions made in an effort to treat a surgical disease or repair an injury.

INCISIONS & TECHNIQUE

The student of surgery has been taught anatomy and histopathology on tough, fixed tissues. As a result, the transition to working with living tissues requires a change in approach and the adoption of a view that gentleness is essential in the performance of any invasive or surgical procedure. The basis of modern surgery and the principles of gentleness and careful technique emanate from the teachings of William Stewart Halsted (1852–1922). Halsted is credited with first demonstrating that careful hemo-

stasis and avoidance of tissue injury were the difference in whether recovery was smooth and complication-free or protracted and complicated.

While the following comments have often been stated and frequently written, they are certainly worth repeating here. First of all, students and junior surgical trainees should not be impressed by the speed of the operation and by those more interested in accomplishing the day's work as rapidly as possible. For surgeons concerned only with speed, there is little time for considering careful technique, the avoidance of unnecessary tissue injury, the avoidance of unnecessary blood loss, and the careful, meticulous repair of tissue. As you progress through years of training and are exposed to many surgeons, you will observe that those concerned only with the speed of an operation have more complications and more patients with serious septic problems. You will also observe that such individuals rarely question the reason for a complication and are quick to lay blame on the patient.

Incisions must be carefully planned, for they are the key to a successful operation. As such, an incision becomes a balance between a wound that will heal rapidly with minimal scarring and disfigurement and a wound that

In 1889, Halsted was appointed surgeon-in-chief to the outpatient dispensary and acting surgeon to the hospital at The Johns Hopkins University School of Medicine in Baltimore. He gained a full professorship in 1892. From early on in his career, Halsted had a vision of surgery that was entirely unique for his time. Many feel this is due to the two years he spent studying surgery in Europe in the late 1870s. During his travels through the German-speaking countries, he was invited to view the work of Billroth, von Bergmann, and Volkmann. He could not help but appreciate the incredible contrast between the surgical training programs in Germany with those in America. These impressions would be translated into a new order of surgical training inaugurated by Halsted at The Johns Hopkins Hospital.

Halsted insisted on a professionalism that moved surgery from the operating "theater" to the sterile, organized operating "room" and the privacy of the research laboratory. He insisted on the highest professional standards and attributes. Halsted's influence was indeed astounding, as his aim to train the best possible surgical teachers as well as clinician/scientists was certainly realized in his own lifetime. During his 33 years as director of surgical training he guided the careers of the most influential names in American surgery, including Harvey Cushing, Stephen Watts, George Heuer, Mont Reid, John Churchman, Robert Miller, Emile Holman, Roy McClure, James Mitchell, Joseph Bloodgood, Walter Dandy, and Hugh Young. In a moving tribute to him after his death, Harvey Cushing wrote, "Halsted was a man who taught by example rather than precept. He was a safe, fastidious, and finished surgeon . . ."

offers ample access to the task at hand. I recall well the admonitions of Dr. Robert Zollinger, who repeatedly reminded us that incisions heal "side-to-side," not "end-to-end." An incision must be long enough to allow for the operating surgeon and the assistant to perform the procedure without struggling to maintain exposure of the field, but appropriately placed and of a size that will optimize the patient's rapid recovery.

There are a few simple rules to follow. In general, incisions should be planned to follow the normal "wrinkle lines" of the skin (Figure 9–1). This is especially true of the face, neck, and other exposed areas of the body. The wrinkle lines are not always the lines of "Langer." Langer's lines are often misunderstood, as they resulted from a study of skin distraction forces acting on puncture wounds created in cadaver skin. Wrinkles in living skin, on the other hand, result from the persistent action of underlying muscles and occur over time.

The *first rule* is to remember that the scar of the skin incision will become adherent to the deep tissue and, thus, move with the action of deep structures. For this reason, avoid placing scars across joints or in the line of long muscles where they may form a restricting band. Rather, the incision should be placed transversely across muscles and joints so that the healed scar simply moves normally with the deep structures rather than against them (Figure 9–2).

The *second rule* involves the chest. Here, incisions follow the line of the ribs. The deep aspect of the chest incision is made along the superior surface of the rib to avoid injury to the neurovascular bundle located along the inferior border of each rib (Figure 9–3A).

The *third rule* has to do with abdominal incisions. Abdominal incisions need to be planned so that they do the least amount of damage to the nerves, vessels, and muscles of the abdominal wall. In addition, they should be planned to allow for easy extension in case the intra-abdominal findings dictate a change in plans or require greater exposure to other structures. In some circumstances, it may be prudent to close one incision and make a second incision. For example, a McBurney incision (Figure 9–3B) for acute appendicitis is usually best closed when the findings dictate a different pathology and require exposure to the stomach, duodenum, gallbladder, or left colon.

My preference is short, transverse incisions (Figure 9–3C) or, more often, the vertical midline incision (Figure 9–3D). The latter, especially for cancer operations, does

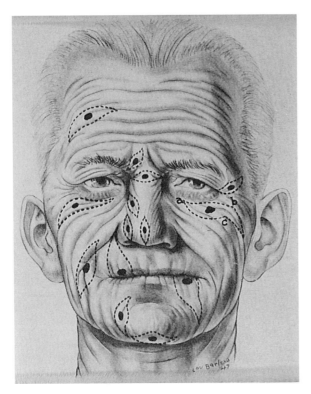

Figure 9–1. Diagram of suggested lines of excision on the face to allow the ultimate scar to fall in normal wrinkles. (Reproduced, with permission, from Kraisl CJ, Conway H: Excision of small tumors of the skin and face with special reference to the wrinkle lines. Surgery 1949;25:529–600, p. 598.)

the least damage to nerves and muscles and can be easily extended for greater access to all intra-abdominal organs or, for that matter, into the mediastinum or chest. Cancer patients often require repeated surgeries of the abdominal cavity; this is another reason for choosing the midline approach at the time of the initial operation—it facilitates repeated surgeries at different locations within the abdominal cavity.

The *fourth rule* is perhaps as important as the other three. It is the scar of the incision that the patient lives with and sees each day. It is also the discomfort, should that unfortunate circumstance arise, that will be a burden to the patient. The patient has little knowledge or awareness of all that the surgeon accomplished deep within the chest or abdomen. The incision cannot heal properly with minimal scarring unless it is carefully made with a sharp blade, with careful attention to "drawing" the incision in a manner exactly perpendicular to the flattened skin (Figure 9–4). Often, it is helpful to make several scratch marks with a sharp needle perpendicular to the line of incision. These marks facilitate exact reapproximation of skin edges. The correct placement and making of the incision are, thus, the first steps in an often complex operation, with meticulous closure at the conclusion of surgery being equally important.

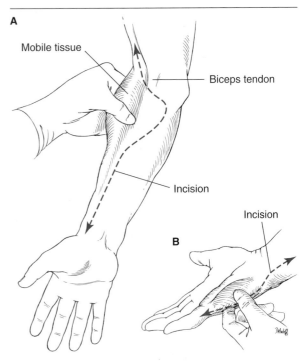

Figure 9–2. **A:** Incision for anterior exposure of the radius. **B:** Incision for exposure of the deep ulnar branch. Incision for the skin and fascia follow the dorsal edge and then go up the forearm—ulnar to flexor carpi tendon.

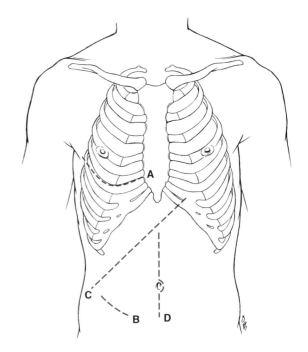

Figure 9–3. **A:** Chest incision along the line of the ribs. **B:** McBurney incision. **C:** Transverse incision. **D:** Vertical midline incision.

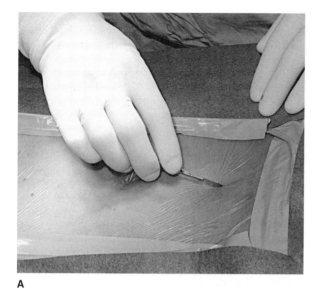

A

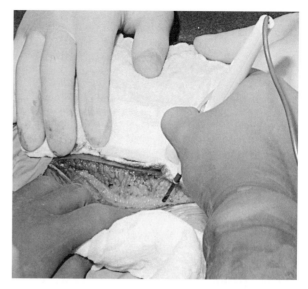

Figure 9–5. Incision through the subcutaneous fat, muscle, fascia, and so forth is carried out with electrocautery.

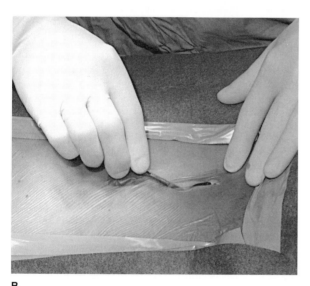

B

Figure 9–4. *A:* Scalpel grip for drawing of skin incision. *B:* To complete incision, the scalpel is held exactly perpendicular to the skin.

SKIN PREPARATION & WOUND CARE

The preparation of skin prior to making the incision has become quite standardized in our clinical and operating facilities. While there may be some variations from institution to institution, these procedures are designed to minimize contamination from skin flora and to provide a sterile field. I prefer to utilize a plastic adherent skin drape whenever possible, especially in the abdomen and chest. This provides a large, completely sterile field through which to place the incision, rather than a surgically clean field.

During the operation wound edges must be kept moist with wet sponges to protect the structures of the chest wall, abdominal wall, and so forth from pressure damage caused by retractors. Often the procedures we perform in the abdomen or chest are lengthy and involve potential contamination or shedding of viable cancer cells. Placing a wound protector (plastic drape), which inserts inside the wound and isolates it from the operative field, adds additional protection of the wound. Such drapes also help to protect the other drapes from soaking.

While the incision through the epidermis and dermis is made sharply, once this is accomplished the rest of the deeper incision through the subcutaneous fat, muscle, fascia, and so forth is best made by electrocautery (Figure 9–5). This technique provides excellent hemostasis with minimal tissue trauma, and does so without the placement of many sutures. Hemostasis of the wound is just as important as it is throughout the operation. The reasons for meticulous hemostasis in surgery are simple: (1) to prevent unnecessary blood loss, which may lead to shock, and to minimize the requirement for blood replacement; (2) careful, accurate dissection requires a relatively bloodless field; (3) careful hemostasis limits clot formation and hematomas that may become seeded with the patient's bacteria during recovery.

Incisions that are cleanly made with minimal tissue damage, and where blood supply is preserved and careful hemostasis is undertaken, have the least chance of becoming infected and provide the greatest opportunity to heal promptly.

SUTURE MATERIALS, KNOT-TYING, & SKIN STAPLING

SUTURE MATERIALS

The first use of thread for the closure of a wound and ligation of blood vessels appears in the Edwin Smith papyrus, 1500 BC. As would be expected, prior to the introduction of methods to sterilize these materials, they were always associated with infection and posed a great problem to surgeons. The predominant suture materials were catgut, silk, cotton, and linen until the 1930s, when steel wire was introduced. Synthetic absorbable suture materials are actually quite new, with sutures of polyglycolic acid first being introduced in 1970.

We tend to group suture materials as absorbable and nonabsorbable and as monofilament or multifilament. Their origin is also important. For example, catgut is absorbable monofilament suture of organic material. Catgut is made from the submucosa of sheep intestines or serosa of bovine intestine and is 90% collagen. The raw catgut is "tanned" to crosslink the collagen fibers by exposure to chrome or aldehyde. The more "tanning," the longer the suture will maintain its strength.

With the advent of synthetic materials that are absorbable, the production and use of catgut has decreased significantly. The newer synthetic materials are much easier to produce in a uniform, standardized fashion. They have been improved tremendously for ease of handling and strength and cause very minimal tissue reaction. The rate at which they lose their strength in tissue is not altered by the presence of infection or by exposure to digestive enzymes.

These sutures, marketed under trade names of Dexon, Vicryl, Maxon, and PDS, lose significant strength during the first 7 days. Dexon and Vicryl require about 3 months for absorption, with strength decreasing essentially as a straight line over 4 weeks. Maxon and PDS maintain strength for an additional 1–2 weeks.

The mainstream of nonabsorbable sutures are stainless steel, silk, synthetic materials made from polyester (Dacron), polyamide (nylon), and polyolefines (Surgilene, Prolene). While silk is considered nonabsorbable, it is, in fact, a protein made by a special silk worm. The silk fiber is braided by a technique termed "braided cordage" originally developed for making venetian blind cords. Silk loses its strength over about 6 months and causes a fair tissue reaction in the process.

Silk has maintained its place in surgery largely because of its handling properties. I use silk often because I am working with young surgeons. It is easier for them to set the first knot and not have it slip when the tension is released. A square knot can then be laid down to secure the ligature and the suture cut close to the knot. In general, you will find that all other materials are always compared to silk for handling and knot-tying ability.

Standards for suture are described in the United States Pharmacopoeia (USP). Since 1976, sutures have been classified as medical devices under the supervision and control of the Federal Food and Drug Administration. The USP sets standards for dimensions according to a numerical scale of 1, 0, 1–0, 2–0, 3–0 to the most fine suture 9–0 and 10–0, and for strength based on the force required to break the suture when being knotted. Examples of the USP standards are given in Tables 9–1 and 9–2.

Today, virtually all suture needles are disposable and of the atraumatic type (eyeless) with pre-packaged suture material attached. Some needles with suture attached allow for expedient separation of the needle from the suture with a gentle tug after the stitch is placed. These are commonly known as "pop-off" sutures. They are especially useful when multiple interrupted stitches are required, as in an intestinal anastomosis.

Figure 9–6 illustrates the various needle curvatures and needle points. The tissue to be sutured determines which needle will be used. For skin, fascia, and tough tissues, a needle with a cutting point is required (also see Chapter 2).

KNOT-TYING

Tying suture correctly with efficiency requires hours of practice. The placing of a knot actually creates a weakness point in the suture. The goal is to set the knot as a square rather than a series of loops. Tumbled, half hitches give poor knots with only about 20% of the security of square knots. Modern suture materials that are braided and coated require an extra throw on each knot to make them secure.

The three most common methods of tying sutures are shown in Figure 9–7, including the instrument tie. Over the years it has been my pleasure to observe a number of surgeons considered by their peers to be the very best. What has impressed me is always how careful and meticulous they are in setting their suture knots—almost without exception using a two-hand tie.

SKIN STAPLING

Disposable skin and fascia staplers employing stainless steel staples have gained widespread popularity because of their ease of use and the significantly reduced amount of time required for wound closure. The cosmetic result is certainly acceptable, and staple removal (which requires a special device) is often less painful for the patient than the removal of conventional suture material, as the skin does not adhere to it as readily (Figure 9–8).

Table 9–1. USP specifications for collagen suture.

USP Size	Metric Size (Gauge No.)	Limits on Diameter (mm)		Limits on Knot-Pull Tensile Strength (kg)
		Min.	Max.	
	0.01	0.001	0.009	
	0.1	0.010	0.019	
	0.2	0.020	0.029	
9–0	0.3	0.030	0.039	0.023
	0.4	0.040	0.049	0.034
8–0	0.5	0.050	0.069	0.045
7–0	0.7	0.070	0.099	0.07
6–0	1	0.10	0.149	0.18
5–0	1.5	0.15	0.199	0.38
4–0	2	0.20	0.249	0.77
3–0	3	0.30	0.339	1.25
2–0	3.5	0.35	0.399	2.00
1–0	4	0.40	0.499	2.77
1	5	0.50	0.599	3.80
2	6	0.60	0.699	4.51
3	7	0.70	0.799	5.90
4	8	0.80	0.899	7.00

Reprinted, with permission, from Anderson RM, Romfh RF: *Technique in the Use of Surgical Tools.* Appleton-Century-Crofts, 1980, p. 185.

Table 9–2. USP specifications for synthetic absorbable suture.

USP Size	Metric Size (Gauge No.)	Limits on Diameter (mm)		Limits on Knot-Pull Tensile Strength (kg)
		Min.	Max.	
12–0	0.01	0.001	0.009	
11–0	0.1	0.010	0.019	
10–0	0.2	0.020	0.029	
9–0	0.3	0.030	0.039	0.045
8–0	0.4	0.040	0.049	0.07
7–0	0.5	0.050	0.069	0.14
6–0	0.7	0.070	0.099	0.25
5–0	1	0.10	0.149	0.68
4–0	1.5	0.15	0.199	0.95
3–0	2	0.20	0.249	1.77
2–0	3	0.30	0.339	2.68
1–0	3.5	0.35	0.399	3.90
1	4	0.40	0.499	5.08
2	5	0.50	0.599	6.35
3 and 4	6	0.60	0.699	
5	7	0.70	0.799	

Reprinted, with permission, from Anderson RM, Romfh RF: *Technique in the Use of Surgical Tools.* Appleton-Century-Crofts, 1980, p. 185.

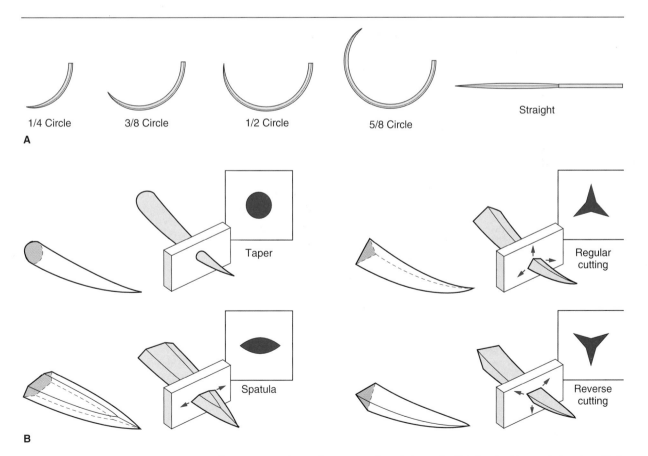

Figure 9–6. **A:** Various needle curvatures. **B:** Various needles and corresponding stitch canals. (Reprinted, with permission, from Zederfeldt BH, Hunt TK: *Wound Closure: Materials and Techniques*. Davis & Geck, 1990, p. 37.)

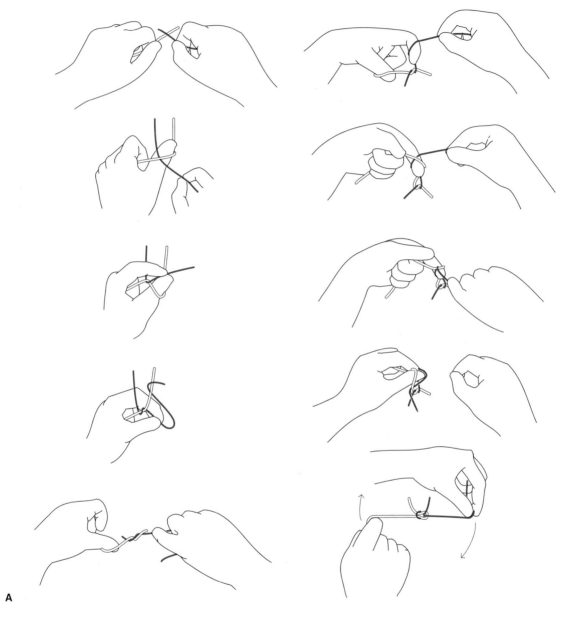

Figure 9–7. **A:** Two-hand knot. **B:** One-hand knot. **C:** Tying with needle holder. (Reprinted, with permission, from Zederfeldt BH, Hunt TK: *Wound Closure: Materials and Techniques*. Davis & Geck, 1990, pp. 56–61.) (figure continues)

SUTURE TECHNIQUE

The most important step in placing a suture is the one most often omitted by students and residents. Before putting the needle into the area to be sutured, the free end should be carefully passed to the assistant's side, where it can be easily grasped for prompt tying (Figure 9–9), preventing it from becoming tangled with other sutures or with instruments in the field.

The second step is to place the needle point at the proper site to penetrate the tissue, but also insure that it is directly perpendicular to the tissue. It is important to avoid "stuttering." Be resolved in your mind, keep your eye focused, and place the needle point in exactly the correct place with the first pass. Correctly position yourself to optimize your ability to sew with an easy forehand motion (Figure 9–10). If your elbow is touching your side, then you are not in an optimal position to place your stitches.

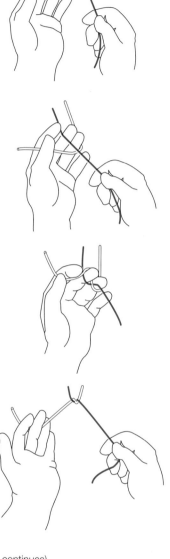

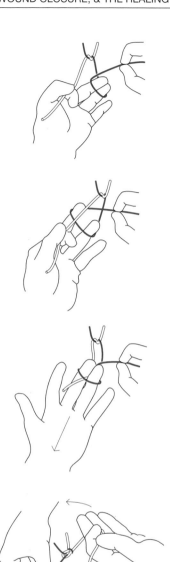

B

Figure 9–7. (figure continues)

The actual passage of the needle is all wrist. The hand begins slightly angled outward at the wrist and in full pronation. The rotation of the hand gently passes the needle through the tissue in a very atraumatic arc. Always follow the curve of the needle. Often, it may be necessary to reset the needle holder on the back of the needle for further passage. When it is possible to extract the needle, grasp the needle toward the point end, being careful not to damage the point (Figure 9–11). Make every effort to grasp the needle perpendicular to the needle holder

with the hand pronated so that you can continue the 180-degree rotation along the curve of the needle as it is extracted from the tissue. Attention to these details avoids unnecessary tearing and trauma to the tissue being sutured.

When continuous suture is being used, the needle is reset during extraction or by hand before pulling the suture through. This saves unnecessary maneuvers and, therefore, time. As an assistant, you are often called upon to keep sutures in order and to assist by following a con-

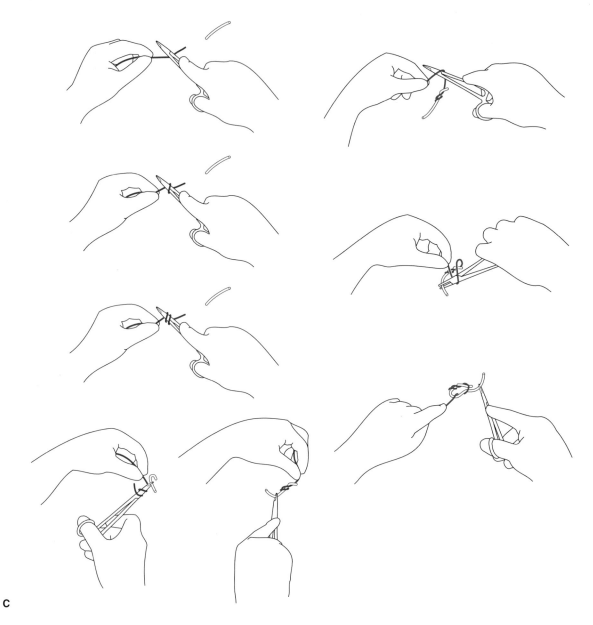

C

Figure 9–7. (continued)

tinuous suture. In following a continuous suture, you maintain appropriate tension (not too much) on the suture and you keep the suture out of the way of the surgeon as the next stitch is placed. Keep the stitches loose to avoid strangulating the tissue and producing ischemia. Injured tissue responds with edema; remember that the suture will tighten automatically within 12–24 hours. Examples of various types of stitches used in tissue repair are shown in Figure 9–12.

CLASSIFICATION OF WOUNDS

Clean wounds comprise approximately 75% of all wounds and usually occur during elective surgery. These incisions are made under sterile conditions and are not predisposed toward infection. It is also implied that no break in aseptic technique occurs in the operative setting during the procedure. The surgeon does not enter the

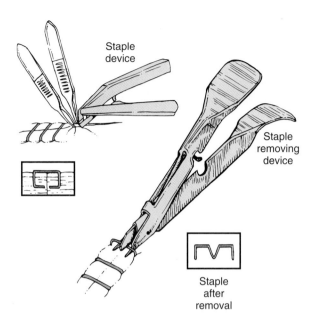

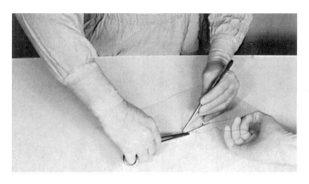

Figure 9–10. Optimal method for a forehand stitch is to start with a prone hand and sew toward oneself, according to full 180 scope to rotate the needle through the tissue. (Reprinted, with permission, from Anderson RM, Romfh RF: *Technique in the Use of Surgical Tools*. Appleton-Century Crofts, 1980, p. 53.)

Figure 9–8. The skin is closed with a stapling device using stainless steel staples. A special staple remover is used to extract the staple from the skin. (Reprinted with permission, from Lawrence PF: *Essentials of General Surgery*, 2nd ed. Williams & Wilkins, 1992.)

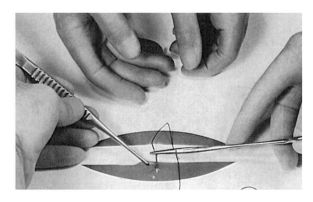

Figure 9–9. To insure against tangling and to allow for prompt knot tying, pass the free suture end to the assistant's side before stitching. (Reprinted, with permission, from Anderson RM, Romfh RF: *Technique in the Use of Surgical Tools*. Appleton-Century-Crofts, 1980, p. 51.)

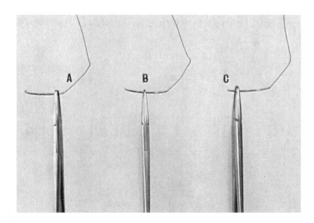

Figure 9–11. ***A:*** Grasping the needle near the eye works best for soft tissue. It allows maximum needle length to be inserted through tissue, least risk of needle slippage, and maximum exposure of point for regrasping. ***B:*** When the needle is grasped near midpoint, rather than near the eye, greater force is available to advance the needle through tissue, with less risk of breakage. ***C:*** For tough tissue, the needle is grasped near the point, for greatest driving force. As the needle is advanced, the holder is repositioned nearer to the eye. (Reprinted, with permission, from Anderson RM, Romfh RF: *Technique in the Use of Surgical Tools*. Appleton-Century-Crofts, 1980, p. 45.)

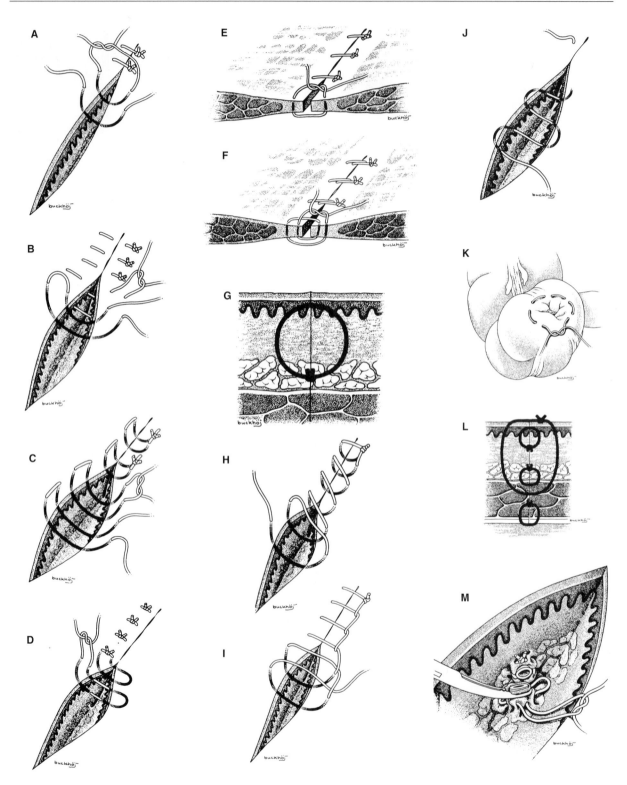

Figure 9–12. **A:** Simple interrupted skin suture. **B:** Interrupted vertical mattress suture. **C:** Interrupted horizontal mattress suture. **D:** Semi-mattress suture, Allgöwer suture. **E:** Single-loop fascial suture. **F:** Double-loop far and near "Snead Jones" suture. **G:** Interrupted inverted intracutaneous suture. **H:** Continuous over-and-over suture. **I:** Continuous interlocking suture. **J:** Continous intracutaneous suture. **K:** Purse string suture. **L:** Retention suture. **M:** Suture ligature. (Reproduced, with permission, from Zederfeldt BH, Hunt TK: *Wound Closure: Materials and Techniques*. Davis & Geck, 1990, pp. 41–50.)

oropharyngeal cavity or the respiratory, alimentary, or genitourinary tracts.

Clean-contaminated wounds include appendectomies and vaginal operations, as well as clean wounds that become contaminated by minimal (not significant) spillage of viscus contents. If the genitourinary or biliary tracts are entered, there is no contamination from infected urine or bile.

Contaminated wounds include traumatic injuries, such as open fractures, soft tissue lacerations, and penetrating wounds. Operative wounds in which there is significant spillage from the gastrointestinal, genitourinary, or biliary tract, and any procedure in which there is a major break in aseptic technique, also fall into this category. Microorganisms multiply so rapidly that these wounds can become infected within 6 hours.

Dirty and infected wounds are those that have been heavily contaminated or are infected prior to the operation. These are wounds that contain infected foreign material or necrotic tissue, perforated viscera, abscesses, and so on. Infection present at the time of surgery can increase the infection rate of any wound fourfold.

WOUND HEALING

The healing of a tissue wound, whether made by the surgeon's scalpel or by a traumatic injury, occurs via a series of overlapping phases: coagulation, inflammation, granulation with angiogenesis, and finally by scar formation. This process may be negatively affected by a number of conditions, including malnutrition, diabetes mellitus, peripheral vascular disease, immunodeficiency states, and irradiation.

The initial phase involves the extravasation from the severed or injured vessels of plasma and platelets. This initial response is followed rapidly by the attraction of neutrophils, monocytes, and lymphocytes. Junctions between endothelial cells are opened and the complement cascade is initiated. The sticky platelets are critical to the plugging of small vessel openings but are also responsible for releasing substances such as platelet-derived growth factor (PDGF), cyclic adenosine monophosphate (cAMP), and transforming growth factor-β (TGF-)β, which are chemotactic. The presence of neutrophils, macrophages, and lymphocytes creates the inflammatory phase of wound healing.

The great influx of activated macrophages is essential for the degradation of damaged tissue and the phagocytosis of debris and decaying neutrophils. Various soluble factors produced by the cells responsible for the inflammation are involved in the generation of the granulation tissue phase of the healing process.

The granulation phase lasts from day 4 through day 21 and is the time when the healing wound begins to have a degree of tensile strength. There exists within the wound a loose matrix of fibrin, fibronectin, collagen, hyaluronic acid, and fibroblasts. During this phase fibroblasts are activated to proliferate and to synthesize components of the extracellular matrix. Endothelial migration and new vessel growth into the wound begins a few days after injury and originates from capillary loops in the wound margins. Angiogenesis is usually complete by the seventh day.

The final phase of scar formation and wound contracture begins between the eighth and tenth day of injury and is the result of the fibroblasts in the wound applying tension to the surrounding extracellular tissue matrix. Recent studies have shown that the fibroblasts of the granulation phase undergo a phenotypic change, probably as a direct result of specific cytokine stimulation. The fibroblasts develop cytoskeletal features similar to those of smooth muscle cells and as myofibroblasts are key to the contractile phase of scar formation.

When the wound is fully epithelialized and contracture ceases, myofibroblasts containing α-sm actin disappear, probably via apoptosis, the scar becomes much less cellular, and the myofibroblasts return to the classic fibroblast phenotype.

One of the most important components of the granulation phase of wound healing and the final phase of scar formation is the production of collagen. Actually, the production of the various types of collagen (Table 9–3) is a factor in wound healing for several weeks after the initial wound closure and reaches its peak synthesis between 14 and 21 days. The amount of collagen and collagen density within the wound returns to a normal rate of synthesis at approximately 3 weeks but the tensile strength of the wound continues to increase for up to 60 days. The tensile strength of the wound reflects the degree of intermolecular cross-linking of the collagen. The scar of the wound is a dynamic structure and continues to undergo remodeling for 2 or more years.

The future of the field of wound healing is focusing now on the pharmacologic modulation of soft tissue repair. The identification of growth factors and other cellular cytokines as mediators of tissue repair processes has opened a very promising area of investigation, and work in animal models has been very promising. Table 9–4 summarizes the various factors and their mode of action, suggesting the possible ways in which these agents may

Table 9–3. Collagen types.

Collagen Type	Tissue Distribution
I	Ubiquitous in most connective tissues, including skin, bones, tendons, ligaments, etc.
III	Skin, blood vessels, predominant in fetal tissues and in early wounds
IV	Basement membranes, anchoring plaques
V	Ubiquitous
VI	Extracellular microfibrils
VII	Skin, fetal membranes

Reprinted and modified, with permission, from Uitto J, Olsen PR, Fazio MJ: Extracellular matrix of the skin: 50 years of progress. J Invest Dermatol 1989;92:61s–71s.

Table 9–4. Growth factors and cytokines in clinical development.

Growth Factor/Cytokine	Preclinical Effect	Clinical Trial Results
PDGF-BB	↑Neovessels ↑Reepithelialization ↑Granulation tissue	↑Healing in pressure and diabetic ulcers: Phase III trials in progress

TGF-β2	↑Collagen-containing
	    granulation tissue
		↑Healing in venous stasis ulcers;
		    repair of macular holes not successful

TGF-β3	↑Healing ↓Scarring	Chronic ulcers, in progress

Basic FGF	↑Neovessels in a provisional matrix,
	    ↑reepithelialization
		Pressure ulcers—biological effect;
		    diabetic and venous stasis ulcers no effect

IL-1β	↑Healing in infected open wounds	Pressure ulcers, Phase I study in progress
GM-CSF	↑Healing in incisions	Chronic ulcers, in progress

Acidic FGF	↑Neovessels,
	    ↑matrix
		Diabetic and venous stasis ulcers,
		    in progress

EGF	↑Reepithelialization	Donor graft sites, chronic ulcers, minimal effects

EGF = epidermal growth factor; PDGF-BB = platelet-derived growth factor; TGF = transforming growth factor; FGF = fibroblast growth factor; IL = interleukin; GM-CSF = granulocyte-macrophage colony-stimulating factor.
Reprinted, with permission, from Pierce GF, Mustoe TA: Pharmacologic enhancement of wound healing. Annu Rev Med 1995;46:467.

be applied, either individually or in combination, to correct conditions of impaired healing and to enhance normal healing.

Of course, the advances to come in pharmacologic manipulation and perhaps even the introduction of genes producing specific growth factors and cytokines directly into the healing wound will not be substitutes for the key basic principles responsible for optimizing the healing process. These principles are: (1) minimizing tissue damage when introducing a wound and preventing further tissue damage in the case of traumatic injury; (2) eliminating from the wound any nonviable tissue or foreign body;

(3) maximizing vascular perfusion of the damaged tissue and, therefore, oxygenation; (4) optimizing nutritional status; (5) correcting metabolic abnormalities, such as hyperglycemia; and (6) maintaining a moist, clean, wound-healing environment.

The principles outlined in this chapter should provide the beginning student of surgery with important insights into the placement of incisions, the basics of closing the incision and traumatic wounds, a good background in suture materials, and the basics of the biology behind the healing process. These are important to the proper care of patients and, as such, cannot be reviewed too often.

SUGGESTED READINGS

American College of Surgeons et al: *Manual on Control of Infection in Surgical Patients.* Lippincott, 1976.

Anderson RM, Romfh RF: *Technique in the Use of Surgical Tools.* Appleton-Century-Crofts, 1980.

McCulloch JM, Kloth LC, Feedar JA: *Wound Healing: Alternatives in Management.* FA Davis, 1995.

Pierce GF, Mustoe TA: Pharmacologic enhancement of wound healing. Annu Rev Med 1995;46:467.

Zollinger RM Jr, Zollinger RM: *Atlas of Surgical Operations,* 7th ed. McGraw-Hill, 1993.

10

Emergency Airway Management

Myer Rosenthal, MD, Willard E. Fee, Jr, MD, & Jimmy J. Brown, DDS, MD

▶ Key Facts

▶ Therapeutic procedures that may require emergent intubation and ventilatory support include radiologic studies in an uncooperative patient requiring sedation, gastric lavage in a patient lethargic from drug ingestion, bronchoscopy, and esophagogastroscopy.

▶ The presence of significant facial and/or laryngeal trauma may mitigate against more common nasotracheal or orotracheal intubation and require immediate cricothyroidotomy or tracheostomy.

▶ A difficult intubation can be expected in patients with severe arthritis, obesity, a large tongue, small receding mandible, small mouth with full dentures, thick muscular neck, and long thyromental distance.

▶ After placing an endotracheal tube, auscultation of both sides of the chest laterally should be carried out to verify ventilation and positioning above the carina.

▶ The most common reason to emergently change the endotracheal tube is a dysfunctional cuff that prevents adequate ventilation.

▶ The two most common complications of cricothyroidotomy are bleeding from the cricothyroid artery and the development of cricoiditis.

▶ The main indications for tracheostomy are to relieve obstruction and to facilitate cleansing of the tracheobronchial tree.

▶ The placement of a permanent tracheostomy may be indicated for posttraumatic or postirradiation fibrosis of the larynx, chronic obstructive pulmonary disease, and obstructive sleep apnea.

▶ Always consider gaining assistance from more experienced practitioners when contemplating less familiar intubation techniques.

OVERVIEW

The principal factors most essential for successful management of the airway include clinical experience, proper preparation and equipment, an understanding of the implications of the process requiring airway manipulation, awareness of coexisting related factors in the patient's medical condition, appreciation of the pharmacology of agents selected to facilitate access to the airway, a willingness to accept the limitations of one's ability, and a willingness to seek assistance.

The first objective is to assess the patient to determine the need for endotracheal intubation. Does the patient have the ability to maintain a patent, protected airway, thus avoiding the risks of aspiration and inadequate gas exchange? This must be considered in patients with central nervous system compromise as in head trauma, metabolic encephalopathy, cerebral hemorrhage, stroke, seizures, pharmacologic depression, neuromuscular disease, cervical cord injury, Guillain-Barré, and airway trauma and hemorrhage, as well as any other process resulting in severe mental obtundation. Therapeutic procedures that may require emergent intubation and ventilatory support include radiologic studies in an uncooperative patient requiring sedation, gastric lavage in a patient lethargic from drug ingestion, bronchoscopy, and esophagogastroscopy. Rapid emergent access to the airway may also be required to provide ventilatory support in a wide variety of disease states resulting in hypoxemia or inadequate alveolar ventilation with respiratory acidosis.

Once it is determined that airway access is necessary, the clinician responsible for the patient should determine the rapidity needed and the availability of individuals with sufficient expertise to perform the necessary procedure. Furthermore, the most appropriate route to access the airway, including nasotracheal, orotracheal, or transtracheal approaches, must be considered. The presence of significant facial or laryngeal trauma may mitigate against more common nasotracheal or orotracheal intubation and require immediate cricothyroidotomy or tracheostomy.

With selection of the preferred technique should come assessment of the clinician's ability, assessment and recognition of coexisting disease or injury, attainment of necessary equipment, and, if possible, oxygenation and ventilation by bag and mask application. When determining the best route for intubation one should consider patient cooperation to allow oral access, facial characteristics that might indicate a difficult orotracheal intubation (particularly if sedation and neuromuscular blockade is contemplated), and the presence of coagulopathy, facial fractures, or suspected basal skull fractures that may preclude nasotracheal intubation.

There are a number of clinical situations where immediate placement of an artificial airway is necessary, however, available time may allow for a more optimal setting for the procedure and the ability to gain support of those with more expertise. A common situation warranting such consideration is that of partial airway obstruction due to edema, epiglottitis, tumor, neck hemorrhage, or foreign body. In such situations, anesthetizing the patient while maintaining spontaneous ventilation using inhalation anesthetics in an operating room prepared for transtracheal and fiberoptic approaches is advisable.

Coexisting processes might also influence approach to the airway. Suspected or proven cervical fracture requires immobilization of the neck and, thus, increases the difficulty in optimally positioning the patient. An assistant may need to steady the head to insure lack of neck movement during intubation or tracheostomy. Both neck trauma and head trauma with suspected increase in intracranial pressure (ICP) should raise concern for vigorous coughing with intubation, which may increase neck movement or ICP. Coughing may be minimized by intravenous lidocaine (1 mg/kg) given 1–2 minutes prior to intubation or the use of sedatives and paralytics.

The clinician is often faced with the dilemma of whether to sedate and paralyze a patient for emergent intubation. The temptation to alleviate discomfort and anxiety, as well as create a desirable environment, often results in the selection of pharmacologic agents to quiet and relax the patient. Major concerns must be recognized in determining the advisability of administering drugs and selection of the best agents. First is the likelihood of success and an estimation of the time to accomplish the procedure. A quick, yet thorough, evaluation of the patient's facial and neck characteristics will provide evidence to suggest the ease of successful laryngoscopy and intubation. The Mallampati classification is shown in Table 10–1, but may not be possible in the uncooperative patient who is unwilling or unable to open the mouth wide enough to perform the evaluation. Alternatively, difficulty can be anticipated in patients with severe arthritis, obesity, a large tongue, small receding mandible, small mouth with full dentures, thick muscular neck, and long (>6.5 cm) thyromental distance (thyroid cartilage to mandible).

It should also be recognized that, once sedatives and paralytics are administered, ventilation will decrease if not disappear. This eliminates the ability for the patient to continue to self-oxygenate which, in the presence of low functional residual capacity (FRC), leaves little time before significant hypoxemia may develop. Furthermore, as many patients requiring emergent intubation have liquid and particulate gastric contents, sedation and paralysis leading to the inability of the patient to protect the airway from passive aspiration requires a rapid intubation sequence, applying cricoid pressure so as to minimize the risk of regurgitation.

The decision to use sedatives and paralytics must include an awareness of the pharmacologic properties and side effects of the multitude of agents available. Time to onset and peak effect, cardiovascular depression, and effect on intracranial pressure are some of the considerations that must be evaluated in selecting preferred agents for an individual patient. Tables 10–2 and 10–3 outline the important pharmacologic characteristics of the commonly used sedatives and paralytics, respectively. Of particular concern is the release of potassium following

Table 10–1. Mallampati classification (sitting position, mouth open, tongue protruded).

Class I	Finding
1	Visualize faucial pillars
	Visualize soft palate
	Visualize uvula
2	Uvula obscured by
	base of tongue
3	Visualize only soft palate

Table 10–2. Pharmacologic characteristics of commonly used intravenous sedatives.

Drug	Dose (mg/kg)	Onset	Duration (min)	Sequelae
Thiopental	3–5	30 sec	5–20	Hypotension Apnea
Propofol	1.5–3	30–60 sec	4–8	Hypotension Pain at injection site Apnea Hypertonus
Etomidate	0.3	30–45 sec	3–12	Myoclonus Pain at injection site Adrenocortical depression
Ketamine	1–2	30–60 sec	10–15	Hypertension Tachycardia Increased intracranial pressure Hallucinations
Midazolam	.15–0.4	1–2 min	6–15	Unpredictable

muscle depolarization with succinylcholine. This complication is of major consequence in patients with neuromuscular diseases (muscular dystrophies), spinal cord lesions (syringomyelia), burns, paralysis (quadriplegia, paraplegia), and patients with preexisting hyperkalemia (renal failure, rhabdomyolysis), and contraindicates the use of succinylcholine.

Once the individual patient evaluation has been completed and the route for accessing the airway determined, necessary equipment must be collected. An abbreviated description of the techniques and equipment necessary to secure the airway are included in this chapter, however, for a more in-depth discussion of these options, a suggested reading list is provided at the end of the chapter. Table 10–4 provides a list of basic equipment that should be readily available at the bedside at the time of intubation. Table 10–5 lists additional equipment that should be accessible promptly, should more routine techniques not be successful.

Selection and functionality of equipment prior to the administration of medications and initiation of the procedure are paramount to avoiding untoward events. This should include testing for the proper functioning of the laryngoscope, testing the integrity of the endotracheal tube cuff, selecting the proper size laryngoscope blade (2 or 3 Miller, 3 MacIntosh for the average adult) and endotracheal tube (7–8 mm or 30–34 French for the average adult), and ensuring satisfactory intravenous access.

OROTRACHEAL INTUBATION

Provided cervical injury has been ruled out, the patient should be positioned supine in the sniffing position, facilitated by elevating the head on one or two folded towels with the nose pointed straight up towards the ceiling. The mouth is opened using the crossed fingers technique (index finger pushing on upper teeth and thumb on the

Table 10–3. Pharmacologic characteristics of neuromuscular blocking agents (relaxants).

Drug	Intravenous Dose (mg/kg)	Onset[1]	Duration[2] (min)	Sequelae
Succinylcholine	1	45–60 sec	10–12	Muscle pains Potassium release Vagotonic response Increased: Intraocular pressure Intragastric pressure Intracranial pressure Malignant hyperthermia
Vecuronium	0.1	2–3 min	60–80	Blocks histamine metabolism
Mivacurium	0.3	90–120 sec	30–40	Histamine release Hypotension
Atracurium	0.5–0.6	2 min	60–90	Hypotension Tachycardia Histamine release
Cis-Atracurium	0.4–0.6	45–90 sec	60–90	Minimal
Pancuronium	0.1	2–3 min	120–150	Tachycardia
Rocuronium	0.6	60 sec	20–60	Minimal

[1]Time to suitable conditions for intubation.
[2]Time to 95% return of muscle function.

Table 10–4. Equipment for routine intubation.

Suction apparatus	Laryngoscope handle
Large suction catheter	MacIntosh blades
Lidocaine ointment	Miller blades
Bag/mask/oxygen	Endotracheal tubes
Tincture of benzoin	10 cc syringe for cuff
Tape	Oral airways
Functioning IV	Stylette
Sedatives, Relaxants	Phenylephrine nasal spray
Liquid cocaine swabs	Magill forceps

lower) of the right hand to avoid being bitten by the patient. Depending on experience and preference, a proper size of Miller or Macintosh blade (Figure 10–1) is selected. The laryngoscope is grasped with the left hand and the blade is then placed into the mouth on the right side of the midline, advancing and moving toward the midline, sweeping the tongue towards the left. As the blade is advanced, structures should be identified, including the hard palate, uvula, and epiglottis. While advancing the laryngoscope, the handle should be lifted up at an angle of 60–75 degrees from the horizontal to avoid putting pressure on the upper teeth. Once the epiglottis is in view, exposure of the larynx and vocal cords differs, depending on the laryngoscope blade selected. When the curved Macintosh is used, the blade is placed in the vallecula. Lifting of the handle upwards without prying on the teeth will elevate the epiglottis and allow exposure of the larynx. If the straight Miller blade is chosen, the tip of the blade is advanced over the epiglottis and then lifted to provide similar exposure. Once the vocal cords are in view, an appropriately sized endotracheal tube is introduced on the right side of the mouth and advanced towards the larynx, with care to avoid obscuring the view of the cords. A stilette is often placed in the tube to its tip, but not beyond. The tube tip is bent to create a hockey stick appearance in order to facilitate direction toward the anterior larynx. Once the tip of the endotracheal tube has passed through the vocal cords, the stilette should be removed to prevent tracheal trauma prior to further advancement. The tube is then advanced under direct vision until the deflated cuff is beyond the vocal cords. The laryngoscope is then removed, the endotracheal tube cuff inflated, and the location verified.

Immediate verification of the endotracheal tube position is essential. Unfortunately, it is not uncommon for a

Table 10–5. Equipment recommended for difficult intubation.

14- and 16-gauge angiocaths
Cricothyroidotomy set
Tracheostomy set with tubes
Fiberoptic laryngoscope
Retrograde wire set
Airway tube exchanger
Jet ventilation apparatus
Light wand
Laryngeal Mask Airway

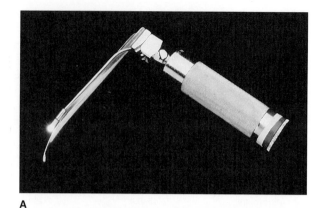

A

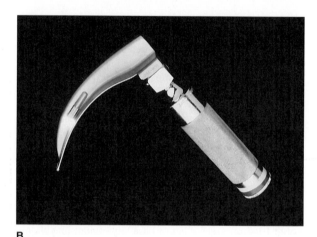

B

Figure 10–1. A: Miller blade. **B:** MacIntosh blade.

patient to suffer irreversible hypoxia as a consequence of the failure to recognize esophageal intubation. Failure to provide adequate oxygenation in the presence of successful tracheal intubation may be due to endobronchial intubation and unilateral ventilation, thus inducing a significant pulmonary shunt. If available, a qualitative end-tidal carbon dioxide indicator or quantitative capnograph is the preferable means of verifying endotracheal intubation. Also, a pulse oximeter is of value in assessing oxygenation. Auscultation of both sides of the chest laterally should be done to verify both ventilation and positioning of the endotracheal tube above the carina. Auscultation over the stomach is also of benefit in assessing for esophageal intubation. Once correct positioning is determined, the centimeter marking on the endotracheal tube at the teeth should be noted and the tube secured with tape.

Anticipating difficulty with oral intubation and preparing options is a responsibility of the individual performing the procedure. Failure to visualize the larynx should initially be approached with external tracheal manipulation, either using the operator's right hand or by a directed assistant. If this maneuver is unsuccessful, then repositioning the patient with less or more neck flexion and changing laryngoscope blades are further maneuvers.

During this period, oxygenation may require manual bag/mask ventilation, particularly if the patient has been given respiratory depressant drugs. If emergent intubation is required as a result of hypoxemia or extreme airway dysfunction, the early recognition of difficulty should be accompanied with plans for possible transtracheal approach.

Once it is determined that the usual orotracheal approach is not likely to succeed, there are other options. However, most require preexisting familiarity and experience to be successful and avoid catastrophic complications. As has been stressed several times already in this chapter, more experienced practioners can be of great benefit when less familiar options are contemplated. Figures 10–2, 10–3, 10–4, and 10–5 show the equipment used when routine intubation techniques are unsuccessful.

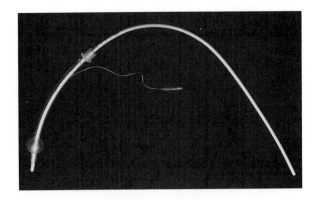

Figure 10–3. Tube changer.

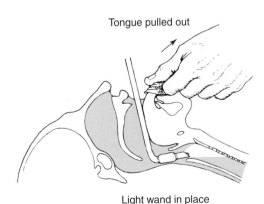

A

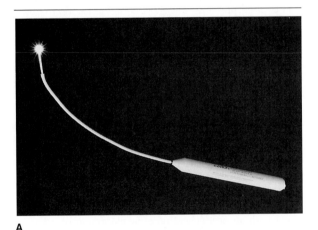

Tongue pulled out

Light wand in place

B

Figure 10–2. **A:** Light wand. **B:** Light wand in place. (Reprinted, with permission, from Benumof JL: *Clinical Procedures in Anesthesia and Intensive Care.* Lippincott, 1992, p. 174.)

NASOTRACHEAL INTUBATION

A blind nasotracheal intubation is an alternative to orotracheal intubation that may be preferable in patients unable to cooperate with an oral approach, and where sedation and paralysis is undesirable. Contraindications to this approach have been discussed earlier in this chapter. Since nasal hemorrhage is a common sequela, if time allows, a vasoconstrictive agent (phenylephrine nasal spray or cocaine swabs) should be placed in the nose. Also, to decrease gagging and improve patient tolerance, a local anesthetic spray can be applied to the mouth and throat. Superior laryngeal nerve blocks and transtracheal local anesthetic injection can also be used. However, it should be understood that anesthetizing the airway with local anesthesia may decrease airway protective reflexes.

The more patent nares should be selected for the procedure. In the average adult a 6- or 7-mm uncut endotracheal tube should be passed through the nares into the nasopharynx. The operator should not use excessive force

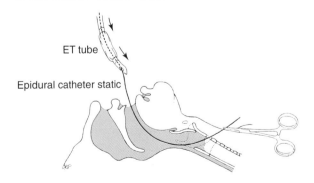

ET tube

Epidural catheter static

Figure 10–4. Epidural catheter fed into endotracheal tube central lumen via "Murphy Eye" in endotracheal tube. (Reprinted, with permission, from Benumof JL: *Clinical Procedures in Anesthesia and Intensive Care.* Lippincott, 1992, p. 164.)

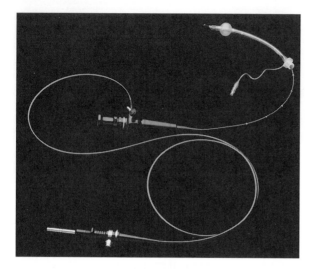

Figure 10–5. Fiberoptic scope with endotracheal tube and oral airway.

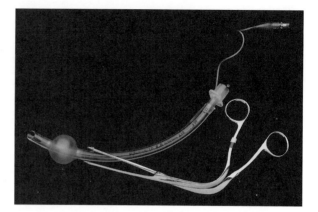

Figure 10–6. Magill forceps grasping endotracheal tube.

against an obstruction, as this may lead to submucosal canalization and extensive hemorrhage. The preferred patient position is 30–60 degrees sitting, with the tongue sticking out, if possible. With the endotracheal tube in the nasopharynx and the patient breathing spontaneously, the tube should be advanced during inspiration while listening to breath sounds at the distal end of the tube. If initial passage is unsuccessful, changing the patient's head position and twisting the tube 90 degrees may provide success. Finally, if the blind approach is failing, alternatives include placing a fiberoptic laryngoscope through the tube to visualize and access the larynx or using a laryngoscope to attempt direct visualization of the vocal cords. If necessary, a pair of Magill forceps (Figure 10–6) to direct the tube into the trachea may be used. Once it is determined that the tube is in the trachea, proper positioning should be verified in a similar manner, as discussed previously.

In recent years, many centers have been less enthusiastic with the use of nasotracheal tubes. Although better tolerated than orotracheal tubes, they are often more difficult to suction and require a smaller diameter than orally placed endotracheal tubes. Additionally, and of greater concern, is the incidence of bacterial sinusitis with prolonged placement of nasal catheters. Fever, leukocytosis, and other signs of sepsis should always raise suspicion for sinusitis in patients with nasotracheal and even nasogastric tubes.

CHANGING ENDOTRACHEAL TUBES

A procedure that often causes the greatest concern, even among the most experienced practitioners, is the emergent changing of an endotracheal tube, particularly in patients with neck traction devices (halo-traction) who are immobilized, or those in respiratory failure requiring full ventilatory support with high inspired oxygen and positive end-expired pressure. The most common reason to emergently change the endotracheal tube is a dysfunctional cuff that prevents adequate ventilation. Fortunately, if the tube is still within the trachea, enough ventilation can be delivered to allow time to assess the patient and acquire the necessary equipment. Often, a suspected ruptured endotracheal tube cuff may, in fact, be a result of outward migration of the tube with cuff herniation above the cords, precluding an adequate seal. Removal of cuff air, advancement of the tube, and re-inflation of the cuff may be all that is required. Adequate sedation and even paralysis can often be safely administered to optimize changing of the tube, if warranted.

Other reasons to change an endotracheal tube include obstruction of the existing tube, replacement of a nasotracheal with an orotracheal tube, or placement of a larger-diameter tube to allow better suctioning and to facilitate fiberoptic bronchoscopy. Similar equipment as outlined in Table 10–4 should be available, with assistance as required. Dependent upon the clinical status of the patient, a number of techniques may be employed, including direct vision with a laryngoscope, a fiberoptic laryngoscope placed alongside the existing tube, or the use of a tube changer (Figures 10–3 and 10–7). A tube changer has several advantages, including minimal invasiveness and the ability to ventilate through its own lumen using a jet ventilation device as shown in Figure 10–8.

With each of these techniques, proper preparation minimizes the risk and allows the procedure to be performed in minimal time. Removal of the existing tube, by either direct laryngoscopy or a fiberoptic approach, should not take place until visualization of the larynx or trachea is accomplished. The amount of time the patient will not be able to ventilate should then only be several seconds. Following replacement of the tube, the position should be verified, as previously described.

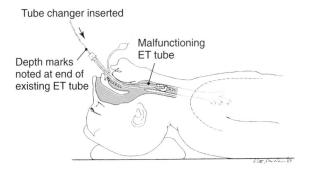

Figure 10–7. Passage of tube changer into endotracheal tube (Reprinted, with permission, from Benumof JL: *Clinical Procedures in Anesthesia and Intensive Care.* Lippincott, 1992, p. 180.)

TRANSTRACHEAL INTUBATION

Patient anatomy, airway trauma or disease, or limited practitioner skill may lead to inability to oxygenate or ventilate a patient using a bag-mask assist or a naso/orotracheal approach to secure the airway. In such conditions, the placement of a large-bore intravenous catheter into the trachea at the neck, with the application of a jet ventilation device, may be most advantageous, if not life-saving. Although such an approach may have existed as early as the 17th century, studies demonstrating its effectiveness appeared only 25 years ago. The percutaneous placement of a 12- to 14-gauge intravenous catheter through the cricothyroid membrane is accomplished by placing the needle at a 30- to 45-degree angle caudad. Localization of the needle/catheter assembly within the tracheal lumen, verified by syringe aspiration of air, is critical to avoid

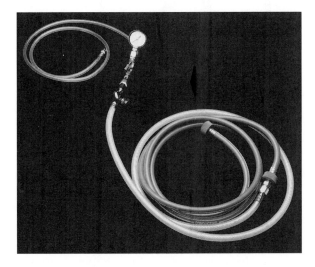

Figure 10–8. Jet ventilation device.

subcutaneous and mediastinal emphysema that will rapidly accumulate with jet ventilation.

Once the catheter is in place, ventilation is best accomplished using a transtracheal jet ventilation (TTJV) device powered by a regulated wall or tank oxygen source. Although with appropriate connections a manual resuscitation bag may be used, its effectiveness is far less than the TTJV. The clinician/practitioner employing this system must ensure that the natural airway remains patent to allow exhalation for the avoidance of barotrauma secondary to air trapping. Although potentially life-saving, the availability of proper equipment and expertise is essential for cricothyroidotomy.

CRICOTHYROIDOTOMY

Cricothyroidotomy, also known as cricothyrotomy, is an excellent way to establish an emergency airway in a patient who has airway obstruction at or above the vocal cords. If a patient has tracheal stenosis, intratracheal tumor, or a foreign body below the level of the cords, a cricothyrotomy will be ineffective; however, in some cases, a number 4 endotracheal tube can be passed through the obstruction and a satisfactory airway obtained until a tracheostomy can be performed below the level of the obstruction.

Two major and relatively frequent complications make cricothyroidotomy problematic. The first is that the cricothyroid artery, which is a branch of the superior thyroid artery, is approximately 1.5–2 mm in diameter and can result in considerable bleeding when violated as it crosses the cricothyroid membrane. The easiest way to handle this problem is to simply place an endotracheal tube through the cricothyroidotomy, inflate the cuff, and then place Vaseline gauze packing into the wound to achieve hemostasis. If one is lucky enough to have sutures or an electrocautery machine available, these can be used to effectively achieve hemostasis.

The second problem is development of cricoiditis due to the presence of a foreign body and an open wound. The longer the foreign body is left in place, the more likely the patient will develop this complication, which will eventually result in subglottic stenosis. Although several journal articles have been published to the contrary, most otolaryngologists have seen several cases of subglottic stenosis due to prolonged placement of a tube through the cricothyroid membrane. Therefore, we recommend conversion of a cricothyroidotomy to an elective tracheostomy as soon as the patient has stabilized.

The technique of cricothyroidotomy is relatively simple and can be performed by any surgeon with or without prior training. Since it is a life-saving maneuver with very few complications other then those mentioned above, it is something that every surgeon should practice. Before beginning the procedure, obtain a number 6 cuffed tracheostomy tube or endotracheal tube. There is nothing more distressing than to have successfully obtained an emergency airway, only to have it compromised by bleeding into the tracheobronchial tree. In the hospital setting, obtaining a tube is not usually a difficult problem, but out in the field this is another matter. Next, palpate the cricothyroid membrane, and, if time permits, prep and drape the area and instill 1% Xylocaine with 1:100,000 epinephrine into the area of the cricothyroid membrane; obviously, in a crash emergency, this step is not performed. Next, palpate the cricothyroid membrane *again* and ensure that it is the cricothyroid membrane. "Cricothyroidotomy" performed through the thyrohyoid membrane produces extensive destruction of the epiglot-

tis and supraglottic larynx. Using a number 10 or number 15 Bard-Parker blade in the middle of the cricothyroid membrane, make a cut through the skin, subcutaneous tissue, cricothyroid membrane, and subglottic mucosa (Figure 10–9); this can be done layer by layer. Once through the skin, use the cutting Bovie if you have time; but, since this is often not the case, the authors prefer to make a plunge into the airway with the knife, and then widen the incision to approximately 1.5 cm, cutting all layers at the same time. It is faster to simply place a number 6 endotracheal tube through the wound, blow up the cuff, and tamponade the bleeding with a half-inch Vaseline gauze, if available, or to use an unfolded 4 × 4

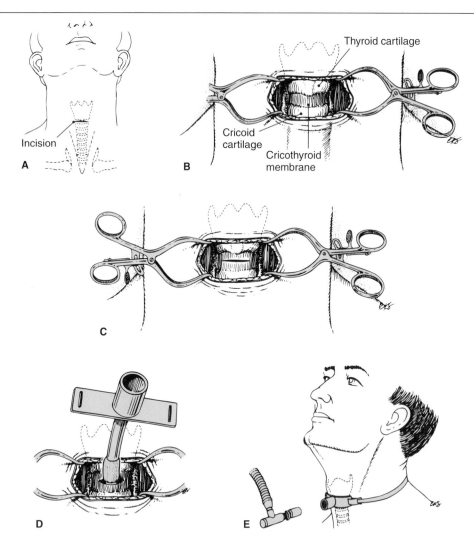

Figure 10–9. A: .Incision for cricothyroidotomy. **B:** Retraction of incision. **C:** Transverse incision in circothyroid membrane. **D:** Insertion of tracheostomy tube into incised cricothyroid membrane. **E:** Crichothyroidotomy tube in place. (Reprinted, with permission, from Benumof JL: *Clinical Procedures in Anesthesia and Intensive Care.* Lippincott, 1992, p. 222.)

sponge. The endotracheal tube is suctioned and the patient stabilized.

As soon as possible (preferably within the first 24 hours), the cricothyroidotomy should be converted to a tracheostomy. If the procedure was performed under unsterile conditions, the patient should receive prophylactic antibiotics until conversion to a tracheostomy. After conversion to tracheostomy, the cricothyroidotomy skin and subcutaneous tissues are closed with simple nylon sutures.

TRACHEOSTOMY

The main indications for tracheostomy are to relieve obstruction (or potential obstruction) and to facilitate cleansing of the tracheobronchial tree (pulmonary toilet). While the controversy of prolonged endotracheal tube intubation versus tracheostomy will not be settled in this chapter, some rather simple observations should be made. The first is that it is far more comfortable for the patient to have a tracheostomy tube than an endotracheal tube, and it is far easier for nursing care and suctioning of the patient. The second is that death from the tracheostomy procedure itself is exceedingly uncommon. There probably is nothing more distressing than a dislodged tracheostomy tube within the first 24 hours after performing the procedure; the potential calamity is great, but probably no greater than that of a dislodged endotracheal tube required for supraglottic narrowing of the airway and the calamities that follow emergency reintubation. Excellent results, as well as disasters, can occur by either method.

Many different techniques of tracheostomy have been advocated and, depending upon the situation, are clinically efficacious. Two different techniques will be described: temporary tracheostomy, where one anticipates that the tracheostomy tube will be required less than 6 months, and **permanent tracheostomy**, where it is assumed that the procedure is likely to be required for life, such as for severe sleep apnea.

TEMPORARY TRACHEOSTOMY

A temporary tracheostomy can be performed under local or general anesthesia, with or without an endotracheal tube in place. For those who have not mastered the skill or in those patients who, for whatever reason, cannot readily cooperate, general anesthesia with an endotracheal tube in place is the preferred methodology. The type and placement of the tracheostomy incision is important, and predicated upon what type of opening will be made in the trachea. The general idea is that on a horizontal plane, the skin incision should be at the same level as the tracheal incision. The safest tracheostomies are performed in between the second and third tracheal rings. A tracheal incision placed higher than that runs the risk of producing subglottic stenosis due to infection of the cricoid and sub-

glottic area. A tracheal incision placed below that runs the risk of the tracheostomy tube tip eroding through the anterior wall of the trachea into the innominate artery, producing a tracheal-innominate fistula. Because patients present with different anatomy, the decision of where to make the incision for tracheostomy can be difficult. The incision should fall in between the cricoid ring and the suprasternal notch; those with short necks may have only 1 cm between these two structures, resulting in a very difficult tracheostomy. A safe rule of thumb is that the incision should be placed two finger breaths (3 cm) above the suprasternal notch or slightly less than one finger breath (1 cm) beneath the cricoid cartilage (Figure 10–10).

PERMANENT TRACHEOSTOMY

Permanent tracheostomy may be indicated for posttraumatic or postradiation fibrosis of the larynx, chronic obstructive pulmonary diseases, and for obstructive sleep apnea. A permanent tracheostomy eliminates the need for a tracheostomy appliance.

The technique involves placement of skin incisions with dimensions of 2–3 cm horizontally and 1.5 cm vertically. The incisions are placed as inferiorly as practical and are undermined widely to elevate cervical skin flaps pedicled laterally. Excess fatty subcutaneous tissue is removed from the cervical skin flaps created.

The trachea and thyroid are approached in a similar fashion as a temporary tracheostomy. An inverted, rectangular-shaped flap pedicled inferiorly is created in the anterior tracheal wall incorporating tracheal rings 2–4. This tracheal flap is sewn to the cervical skin incision inferiorly. The superior skin incision and bilateral cervical skin flaps are also sewn to the trachea, creating a widely opened stoma.

TRACHEOSTOMY INCISIONS

Horizontal incisions in the neck are generally placed in relaxed skin tension lines and will, thus, result in the best overall cosmetic appearance. This incision is also easily revised if the cosmetic appearance is not satisfactory. A vertical incision placed precisely in the midline makes the procedure slightly easier, as the wound retracts laterally; some vertical incision tracheostomies heal very satisfactorily, especially when the tracheostomy tube is only required for a short period of time (3 days or less). However, should the vertical incision not heal satisfactorily, it is much more difficult to repair and produces a poor cosmetic outcome. In either event, those with less experience, with no assistant available, or who are faced with a procedure that is truly emergent are advised to use a vertical incision.

No matter what the incision, it is seldom necessary to make the incision longer than 2.5 cm. The incision is carried through the platysma muscle aponeurosis and the

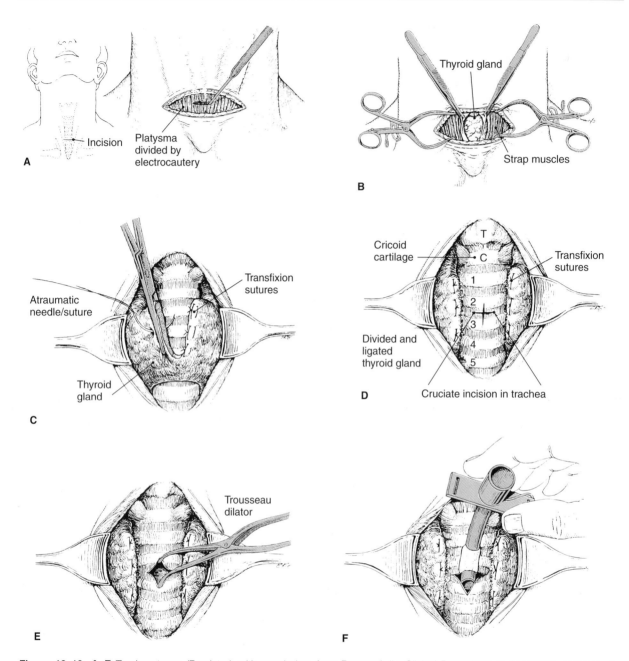

Figure 10–10. A–F: Tracheostomy. (Reprinted, with permission, from Benumof JL: *Clinical Procedures in Anesthesia and Intensive Care*. Lippincott, 1992, p. 220.)

platysma muscle fibers close to the midline. Next, a vertical incision is made precisely in the midline through the fascia surrounding the sternohyoid muscles. This vertical incision is generally 1–1.5 cm superior and 1–1.5 cm inferior to the midpoint of the incision. Rarely are the sternothyroid muscles encountered because they generally lie lateral to the midline. Once this fascia is incised, the isthmus of the thyroid gland is usually encountered and must

be lifted superiorly or inferiorly, or, better yet, divided in the midline and tied. Along the way to the thyroid gland are generally sizable veins, such as the anterior jugular vein, which must be divided and tied. The pretracheal fascia is dissected off the anterior tracheal wall, exposing the second, third, and fourth tracheal rings. At this point in the procedure, hemostasis is obtained and should be absolute.

Should the patient have a blood dyscrasia and generalized oozing cannot be controlled, this wound can be packed with Vaseline gauze and the patient kept intubated overnight until hemostasis is obtained and entry made into the trachea the following day. Once entry is made into the trachea itself, one is obligated to place a tracheostomy tube to prevent bleeding into the trachea. The tracheostomy balloon can be inflated below the tracheostomy wound, preventing aspiration of blood into the lungs, but blood continuing to exude from the wound after placement of the tube can present difficulty for the nursing staff. It is acceptable to place the tracheostomy tube and pack the tracheostomy wound with Vaseline gauze for 24 or 48 hours, postoperatively, to achieve hemostasis.

There are advantages and disadvantages with every type of incision made in the trachea, but that associated with the lowest incidence of tracheomalacia/tracheal stenosis is an inferiorly based, small, U-shaped incision incorporating the third and fourth ring. While there is much to be said for the U-shaped flap, it is the slowest to close upon extubation. A vertical incision through the second, third, and fourth tracheal ring with sacrifice of 5 mm of the third tracheal ring cartilage on either side of the midline, or the removal of 1 cm of the third tracheal ring, also produce excellent results. Simply making a horizontal incision between the second and third tracheal ring is likely to produce tracheomalacia of the second tracheal ring by virtue of pressure necrosis from the superior bend of the tracheostomy tube.

TRACHEOSTOMY TUBES

Many types of tracheostomy tubes are available, each with its own advantages and disadvantages. It is seldom necessary to use larger than a size 6 or 7 tracheostomy, regardless of the manufacturer. Because all of the tubes have low pressure cuffs, it is preferable to use a cuffed tracheostomy tube at the initial procedure, in case hemostasis is not satisfactory. The cuff should be inflated to the point where there remains a minimum leak with inspiratory pressure of 20 cm of water, so as to cause the least possible damage to the tracheal mucosa. Almost all ventilators can overcome any small inspiratory leak, and utilizing this technique will result in the lowest possible complication rate.

Having made the incision, a tracheal dilator is placed into the incision, separated, and the tracheostomy tube placed under direct vision. Without proper lighting and experience, creating a false passage anterior to the trachea and placing the tube into the tissues anterior to the trachea is much easier than one would expect. The best way to prevent this complication is to visualize the tracheostomy tube going into the trachea. A sterile dressing is then applied and the tracheostomy tube secured in the neck firmly, with an assistant placing two fingers beneath the tracheostomy ties and the ties secured snugly with square knots. Like any other clean contaminated open surgical wound, the tracheostomy wound itself should be cleansed with soap and water daily and a sterile dressing applied.

CHANGING OF THE TRACHEOSTOMY TUBE

If a different size or type of tracheostomy tube is required, this change can be safely made after 48 or 72 hours. Proper lighting and suction are required, and if the wound is fresh, a tracheal hook and tracheal dilator are sometimes needed. If the tracheostomy track is not firmly established, once again, care must be exercised to prevent placing the tube anterior to the trachea in a false passage. The first tracheostomy tube change is best done by the physician who did the procedure and not by the nursing staff or another team who are unfamiliar with the patient's anatomy.

SPECIALIZED APPROACHES

As a final comment regarding airway access, it is worthy to recognize two specific clinical states that may require a specialized approach. Tracheal obstruction secondary to tumor or scarring may prevent the advancement of the usually selected endotracheal tube after the tube has passed through the larynx. In such cases, vigorous pressure may further injure the trachea, resulting in perforation into the mediastinum. Alternatives include the placement of small tubes (as small as 4 mm or 18 French) without cuffs and the use of jet ventilation or, alternatively, ventilation with a mixture of helium and oxygen (Heliox). The addition of helium to oxygen significantly decreases the density of the gas mixture, producing less turbulence and, thus, less resistance to passage of the gas mixture. The typical concentration is 30–40% oxygen in helium. Heliox is, thus, limited by its low oxygen concentration and is most commonly used in children with croup in an effort to avoid intubation. The practitioner should be prepared to perform transtracheal ventilation when obstruction is suspected or recognized, if intubation attempts are unsuccessful, or if complete obstruction occurs.

The second clinical state that may require a specialized approach is bronchial hemorrhage. In such a situation, in-

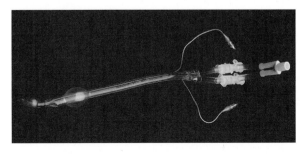

Figure 10–11. Double-lumen endotracheal tube.

tubation may be the only means to provide oxygenation. The goal of intubation is to isolate the origin of hemorrhage, provided it is unilateral. Several options exist, including placement of a double-lumen endotracheal tube (Figure 10–11), fiberoptic localization of an orotracheal tube in the nonbleeding bronchus, or the use of a bronchial blocker and endotracheal tube. In each of these situations, it is best to have experienced practitioners performing these procedures. A final alternative for the less experienced individual is to advance a small cuffed orotracheal tube into one of the bronchi. If the hemorrhage is originating from the other side, the patient will be able to be ventilated through the tube. If bleeding is coming through the endotracheal tube, a second small tube may be placed alongside the first into the trachea, allowing ventilation to the unaffected lung. Use of any of the above approaches will, hopefully, permit ventilation and oxygenation while definitive therapy is being sought.

Maintenance of an effectively protected airway is critical to the successful management of all patients. The need to emergently instrument the airway is one of the most challenging and worrisome procedures, even in the most experienced hands. Proper preparations, evaluation, familiarization, and experience are the best qualities to maximize success and avoid complications.

SUGGESTED READING

Benumof J: *Clinical Procedures in Anesthesia and Intensive Care.* Lippincott, 1992.

Cummings CW: *Atlas of Laryngeal Surgery.* Mosby, 1984.

Fee WE, Ward PH: Permanent tracheostomy: A new surgical technique. Ann Otol Rhinol Laryngol 1977;86:635.

11

Surgical Endoscopy

James M. Stone, MD

► Key Facts

► Endoscopy offers several advantages over radiologic examinations such as magnified, direct visualization of the mucosal surface as well as the ability to take directed biopsies and perform therapeutic maneuvers.

► The working length of an endoscope is dictated by its intended use.

► The majority of complications associated with endoscopic procedures are related to sedation.

► Most commonly, endoscopic sedation consists of benzodiazepines alone or in combination with an opiate.

► Although endoscopic procedures are increasingly being performed, documented cases of infectious complications are rare.

► Esophagogastroduodenoscopy is performed for upper gastrointestinal complaints, including dyspepsia, dysphagia, gastrointestinal bleeding or obstruction, removal of foreign bodies, or investigation of a mass.

► Flexible sigmoidoscopy is the most commonly used investigation for colorectal diseases.

► The ultimate investigation of the colon is achieved via colonoscopy, as the entire length of the colon, and sometimes even a portion of the distal ileum, may be visualized.

Flexible gastrointestinal endoscopy has dramatically altered the diagnosis and treatment of gastrointestinal disease. It offers several advantages over radiologic examinations, such as magnified, direct visualization of the mucosal surface, as well as the ability to take directed biopsies, remove lesions with snare-loop cautery, and perform such therapeutic maneuvers as coagulation of bleeding vessels, insertion of feeding tubes, dilation of strictures, removal of foreign bodies, and stenting of luminal obstructions. Radiographic studies, however, are still preferred in the initial evaluation of dysphagia or suspected

Zenker's diverticulum, identification of fistula tracts, elucidation of postoperative anatomy, evaluation of motility disorders, and demonstration of extrinsic masses.

INSTRUMENTATION

Flexible endoscopes may be categorized by their means of transmitting an image (fiberoptic or video) and the direction of view from the scope (forward, oblique, or side-viewing). The working length of the endoscope is dictated by the intended use. Shorter endoscopes are, in general, easier to use and manipulate, but longer endoscopes offer more versatility. The working length of a flexible sigmoidoscope ranges from 25–60 cm, upper endoscopes are 100 cm, and colonoscopes range from 140–180 cm. Endoscopes also vary in diameter. Narrower or "pediatric" endoscopes are more easily passed into the esophagus (require less sedation) and are useful for passing through pathologically narrowed areas at the expense of smaller biopsy/suction channels and less ease of advancing within the gastrointestinal tract.

Although design specifics are unique to each manufacturer, flexible endoscopes share certain common features. The portion of the endoscope from the handle to the area where the image is generated or viewed is called the **insertion tube**, the portion from the handle to the light source or image processor is called the **umbilical**. On the handle there are two buttons. The lower button, when covered lightly, causes the endoscope to insufflate air. When the lower button is pressed fully down, a jet of water is directed across the viewing objective. A hollow channel running the length of the endoscope may be used for suction by pressing the top button. This channel is also used for passing instruments, or injecting fluid for irrigation. On the right side of the handle are two spoked wheels. The inner, larger wheel controls movement in the up/down direction. The outer wheel controls movement in the left/right direction (Figure 11–1).

There are two general techniques for controlling endo-

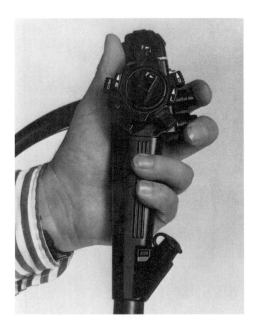

Figure 11–1. Correct "grip" for the standard endoscope; the index and middle fingers are left free to activate suction and air/water buttons, respectively.

scope movement. In the two-person technique, the endoscopist uses the left hand to control up-down motion and the right hand to control right-left movement while instructing an assistant to insert or withdraw the endoscope. In the one-person technique, the endoscopist controls both tip deflection and tube insertion. The left hand is used for up-down deflection while the left-to-right movement is accomplished by torquing the insertion tube with the right hand.

SEDATION & INFECTION CONTROL

SEDATION

The majority of complications associated with endoscopic procedures are related to sedation. Hypoventilation, hypotension, vasovagal episodes, aspiration, and airway obstruction are the most common problems. The risk of an adverse event is more likely in patients who are elderly, have concurrent significant medical problems, have more complex endoscopic procedures, or in patients who take sedatives or anxiolytic medications. An evaluation prior to the endoscopic procedure looking for cardiovascular, pulmonary, renal, and hepatic disorders, as well as allergies, is worthwhile. Measurement of level of consciousness, vital signs, and oximetry should be performed before, during, and after sedation.

Most commonly, endoscopic sedation consists of benzodiazepines alone or in combination with an opiate. Topical anesthesia is used prior to esophageal intubation. Medications should be administered slowly and in small increments, with adequate time for the sedative effect of the injected dose to be apparent before additional medications are given.

Benzodiazepines

Benzodiazepines act within the central nervous system at specific benzodiazepine receptor sites. They are capable of producing a dose-dependent effect ranging from mild sedation through general anesthesia. Midazolam (Versed) is currently the benzodiazepine of choice for conscious sedation. Midazolam is superior to diazepam (Valium) because its pharmacologic effects are more rapid ($\approx$ 3 minutes). There is a shorter elimination half-life (less than 12 hours), and its ability to induce amnesia is superior to diazepam.

Midazolam is metabolized in the liver and excreted by the kidneys. Its elimination half-life is prolonged two to three times the normal in patients with congestive heart failure, renal failure, and severe hepatic dysfunction. Caution should be used in patients with these problems and a longer period of observation after sedation is indicated. Discretion should also be exercised when giving a benzodiazepine to patients with chronic obstructive pulmonary disease because all benzodiazepines decrease minute ventilation.

Flumazenil competitively inhibits the benzodiazepine receptor in the central nervous system and, therefore, acts as a reversal agent for benzodiazepines. Flumazenil has an elimination half-life ($\approx$ 1 hour) that is much shorter than that of midazolam. The occurrence of oversedation and respiratory depression after elimination of flumazenil is, therefore, possible. It is important to recognize that flumazenil may precipitate acute benzodiazepine withdrawal when given to patients who chronically use benzodiazepines.

Narcotics

Narcotics bind to an opioid receptor within the central nervous system to cause analgesia, euphoria, and respiratory depression. Because respiratory depression can occur at doses lower than needed to achieve altered consciousness, use of opiates alone for conscious sedation has largely been abandoned. Opiates are, however, useful when combined with benzodiazepines because they potentiate the sedative effects of the benzodiazepines and add analgesic properties to the mix.

Elimination of narcotics is slow in patients with severe hepatic or renal dysfunction. Opioids should not be given to patients taking monoamine oxidase inhibitors and should be used with increased caution with other central nervous system depressants, including alcohol.

Meperidine (Demerol) has an onset of action approximately 5 minutes after intravenous administration and a half-life of approximately 2–3 hours. Its main side effects are respiratory depression and gastrointestinal upset. Fentanyl (Sublimaze) is preferred by some endoscopists because of its shorter duration of action (30–60 minutes versus 2–3 hours for Demerol). All narcotics are given in small, incremental doses. A dose of 10 mg of morphine is approximately equivalent to 0.1 mg of fentanyl or 75 mg of Demerol.

Naloxone (Narcan) competes for the opioid receptor without causing an opioid effect. Naloxone can, therefore, reverse the opioid-induced respiratory depression. Naloxone is rapidly eliminated via hepatic conjugation. Since naloxone elimination is more rapid than that of the narcotic effect, repeat sedation and respiratory depression may occur.

INFECTION CONTROL

Equipment Maintenance

Although an increasing number of endoscopic procedures are being performed, documented cases of infectious complications remain a rare occurrence. It should be clearly understood that organisms may be spread by contaminated equipment. Immediately after a procedure, the endoscope should be thoroughly mechanically cleaned with detergents and brushes before mucus, blood, or stool are allowed to dry. After mechanical cleaning, those parts of the endoscope that are immersible should be thoroughly rinsed with water. The handles, and other nonim-

mersible elements, should be cleaned with alcohol-dampened cloths and dried using forced air. The endoscope should then by disinfected by submersion into a 2% glutaraldehyde solution and dried using forced air. The scope should be hung in a well-ventilated area. Automated washing machines are available and range from simple to very elaborate computer-controlled systems.

Prophylactic Antibiotics

Although the risk of bacteremia with subsequent bacterial infection with endocarditis or infection of prosthetic material was once believed to be quite high, it is now understood to be quite uncommon. Antibiotic prophylaxis is now limited to high-risk procedures, such as endoscopic retrograde cholangiopancreatography (ERCP) with an obstructed biliary system, dilation of strictures, or esophageal sclerotherapy in high-risk patients, such as those with prosthetic heart valves, a history of endocarditis, systemic-pulmonary shunts, or recent synthetic vascular grafts. An acceptable prophylactic regimen consists of 2 g of ampicillin intravenously and 1.5 mg/kg of gentamycin given 30 minutes prior to endoscopy, followed by amoxicillin 1.5 g orally 6 hours after the procedure. Vancomycin (1 g) intravenously may be substituted for ampicillin in patients allergic to penicillin.

ROUTINE EXAMINATIONS

ESOPHAGOGASTRODUODENOSCOPY (EGD)

Indications & Contraindications

Indications for esophagogastroduodenoscopy (EGD) include dyspepsia without response to empiric therapy, duodenal ulcer without response to medical therapy, chronic dysphagia or odynophagia, upper gastrointestinal bleeding, gastric or duodenal obstruction, dilation of esophageal stricture, surveillance of premalignant conditions, and removal of foreign bodies; EGD is also indicated after a barium upper gastrointestinal study shows gastric ulcer or mass or esophageal stricture or mass (Table 11–1). Most of the contraindications to the performance of an EGD are relative and include an unstable medical condition or airway, suspected mechanical obstruction of the gastrointestinal tract, or diverticulum of the upper esophagus. An absolute contraindication includes any known or suspected perforation of the gastrointestinal tract.

Preparation & Technique

The patient should be instructed not to eat or drink for 4 hours prior to the endoscopy examination. In disease states associated with poor emptying of the stomach, longer periods of fasting or even gastric lavage may be necessary. If possible, the examination is performed with the patient in the left lateral decubitus position. Patients

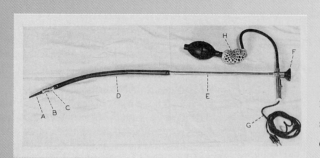

Schindler flexible gastroscope. *A:* rubber finger; *B:* electric lamp; *C:* objective; *D:* flexible portion; *E:* rigid portion; *F:* eyepiece; *G:* electric cable; *H:* air balloon. (Reprinted, with permission, from Schindler R: *Gastroscopy: The Endoscopic Study of Gastric Pathology.* University of Chicago Press, 2nd ed. 1954, p. 34.)

It is interesting to note that some of the first attempts at gastroscopy were inspired by sword-swallowers who were commonly seen in the late eighteenth and early nineteenth century at fairs throughout Europe. Accordingly, some of the first experiments using early gastroscopes were performed on sword-swallowers. However, it soon became apparent that the distance to the stomach from the mouth was so great that it was impossible to obtain adequate illumination.

The modern era of gastroscopy really began in 1932 when Rudolf Schindler (1888–1968) approached a talented instrument manufacturer, Georg Wolf (1873–1938), and asked for his assistance in developing a semiflexible gastroscope with a lens, lamp, and an air outlet to clear the lens. Schindler and Wolf achieved flexibility by making the lower half of the gastroscope tube out of a spiral of bronze with a protective outer covering of rubber (Figure).

Schindler became widely known as a promoter of gastroscopy and soon began instructing other physicians who traveled from Europe and North America to learn the proper techniques under his tutelage in Munich. Many of these individuals returned home to perform gastroscopy and promote the instrument themselves.

Unfortunately, not long after Schindler's instrument and techniques were introduced he was captured by the Nazis and placed in detention for 6 months. Fortunately, his American colleagues at the University of Chicago were able to secure his release. Schindler's presence in Chicago made it a mecca of gastroscopy for the next decade. Thus, the era between 1932 and 1957 (when fiberoptic scopes were introduced) is referred to as the "Schindler era."

may be repositioned to facilitate better exposure of surfaces covered with intraluminal content.

Flexion of the neck precedes initial insertion of the endoscope, which may be accomplished via a blind technique, using finger guidance, or under direct visualization. In the blind technique, the endoscope is held with the right hand 25 cm from the tip, and a gentle curve is placed in the endoscope to facilitate passage over the tongue and into the midline of the pharynx. When the tip is approximately 18 cm from the incisors, resistance from the cricopharyngeus will be felt. Very light pressure is held against the cricopharyngeus and the patient is instructed to swallow. The endoscope is advanced when a decrease in resistance is appreciated.

Finger guidance may be helpful when it is difficult to keep the endoscope in the midline, when patients cannot cooperate, or when patients have an endotracheal tube in place. In this technique, a mouth guard is threaded over the proximal endoscope but cannot be placed in the mouth until the examiner's fingers are removed. The second and third fingers of the examiner's left hand are placed over the tongue and used to hold the endoscope in the midline.

Table 11–1. Indications and contraindications for esophagogastroduodenoscopy (EGD).

Indications

Dyspepsia without response to empiric therapy

Duodenal ulcer on empiric therapy without response to medical therapy

Chronic dysphagia or odynophagia

Upper gastrointestinal bleeding

Gastric or duodenal obstruction

Dilation of esophageal stricture

Surveillance of premalignant conditions

Removal of foreign bodies

As further evaluation to barium upper gastrointestinal study showing:

    Gastric ulcer or mass

    Esophageal stricture or mass

Contraindications

Known or suspected perforation of the gastrointestinal tract

Unstable cardiac conditions

Food intake within 4 hours of procedure

Patient's lack of consent after the procedure is explained

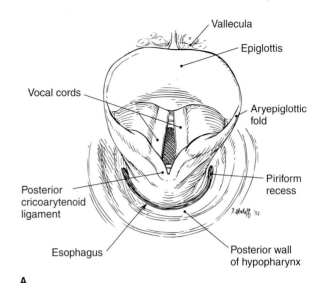

Figure 11–2. *A:* Hypopharyngeal endoscopic anatomy. ***B:*** Endoscopic view of the same structures.

The endoscope is then passed blindly through the cricopharyngeus.

Passage under direct vision is the preferred technique, although it requires the most skill. The endoscope is placed over the tongue in the midline and gently advanced until the epiglottis and then the cricoarytenoid cartilage is seen (Figure 11–2). The vocal cords may be seen in the anterior field of view. The endoscope is deflected down (away from the vocal cords) and is advanced beyond the cricoarytenoid cartilage where the field of view will be lost. The cricopharyngeal sphincter is passed by a combination of air insufflation, gentle pressure, and asking the patient to swallow. The area within the cricopharyngeal sphincter is poorly visualized with a flexible endoscope. Modern flexible endoscopes, by virtue of their wide field of view and flexibility, allow inspection of nearly all mucosa, from the esophagus to the second portion of the duodenum. Visualization is limited within areas with sphincteric function (ie, cricopharyngeus, lower esophageal sphincter, pylorus).

The endoscope is always advanced under direct vision. Inspection during insertion is worthwhile because mucosal trauma may easily be confused for subtle lesions, however, the best view is usually obtained on withdrawal of the endoscope.

Inspection of the esophageal body reveals indentation and pulsation from the left atrium. Ulceration of the mucosa at sites of physiologic narrowing may occur in patients who take certain medications when the pills lodge at these sites ("pill ulcers").

The esophagogastric junction is usually seen as an irregular line (Z–line) (Figure 11–3) where the grey-pink esophageal squamous mucosa meets the salmon-colored columnar gastric mucosa. The distal esophagus is inspected for signs of inflammation. The impression of the diaphragm on the stomach or esophagus is seen by having

the patient sniff through his or her nose. If the Z–line is located more than 2 cm above the diaphragmatic impression, a hiatal hernia is said to exist (Table 11–2).

With the endoscope buttons pointing upward, when the endoscope passes through the lower esophageal sphincter, the view is of the smooth lesser curve to the right and the parallel folds of the greater curve to the left; the posterior gastric wall is inferior and the anterior wall is superior. A pool of gastric juice marks the posterior wall of the greater curve.

In order to view the pylorus (Figure 11–4), the endoscope must be advanced over the spine and around the "J-shaped" curve of the stomach. This is accomplished by a combination of clockwise rotations of the endoscope and deflections of the tip upwards. The antrum and the pylorus may then be inspected. The pylorus is entered by ad-

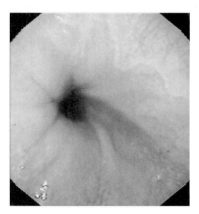

Figure 11–3. Endoscopic view of the esophagogastric junction or "Z" line.

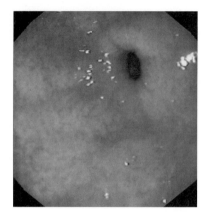

Figure 11–4. Endoscopic view of the pylorus.

vancing the endoscope until the pylorus fills the field of view. Gentle pressure is held against the pylorus until the endoscope pops into the duodenal bulb. The tip of the endoscope will usually impact against the duodenal wall, and it will be necessary to withdraw the endoscope to obtain a view.

The second portion of the duodenum is entered by placing the endoscope tip at the apex of the duodenal bulb and deflecting the tip while rotating the endoscope to the right (Figure 11–5).

All mucosal surfaces are inspected upon withdrawal of the endoscope. It may be necessary to advance and withdraw through an area several times to obtain a complete view. It may be necessary to pull back through the pyloric channel repeatedly, each time pressing on a different wall of the pyloric channel by deflecting the tip in a different direction. On pulling back into the stomach, air should be insufflated if the stomach is not well distended. The tip is deflected up approximately 90 degrees and the endoscope is gently rocked back until the incisura comes into view. All surfaces of the incisura can be seen by holding the endoscope stationary while an antral peristaltic wave comes through. The tip is then deflected a full 180 degrees upward to obtain a complete view of the lesser curve. Close-up views of the fundus, gastric cardia, and gastroesophageal junction are obtained by pulling the endoscope back and rotating to the left and right. The endoscope is then straightened and placed in view of the pylorus. The gastric mucosa is systematically visualized by deflecting the tip

in circles as the endoscope is withdrawn. Prior to reentering the esophagus, the endoscopist removes the insufflated air with suction. The esophagus is inspected and, after being pulled back through the cricopharyngeus, the vocal cords are easily seen and may be inspected for inflammation, tumors, and movement (Figure 11–6). Selected applications of EGD are listed in Table 11–3.

FLEXIBLE SIGMOIDOSCOPY & COLONOSCOPY

As mentioned earlier, the only difference between the endoscopes used for flexible sigmoidoscopy and colonoscopy is their length. However, it is important to understand that the degree of difficulty is increased as the length of the endoscope increases. Flexible sigmoidoscopy was performed using a 35-cm scope for a number

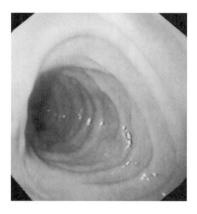

Figure 11–5. Endoscopic view of the second portion of the duodenum.

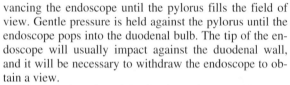

Table 11–2. Esophageal anatomic markers.

Structure	Approximate Distance (cm) from Incisors
Cricopharyngeus	18
Aortic arch impression	23
Left mainstem bronchus	26
Gastroesophageal junction	40

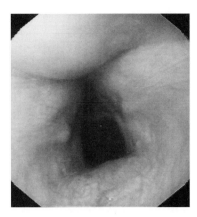

Figure 11–6. Endoscopic view of the vocal cords.

of years. Because of the proliferation of endoscopic training programs, this smaller endoscope has been largely abandoned in favor of the increased viewing area provided by the 60-cm size. The flexible sigmoidoscope is the most commonly used tool for investigation of colorectal diseases. Flexible sigmoidoscopy can usually be performed with minimal discomfort to the patient and a negligible risk of complications.

The ultimate examination of the colon is achieved via colonoscopy. The entire length of the colon, and sometimes even a portion of the distal ileum, may be visualized during this examination. There is a long-standing argument about the benefits of using contrast radiology (barium enema) rather than colonoscopy. While a barium enema is less expensive and may provide anatomic information difficult to visualize during colonoscopy, it is the latter that offers the single procedure for both diagnosis and treatment. In the best case scenario, barium enema and colonoscopy should be considered complementary investigations.

Indications & Contraindications

Indications for flexible sigmoidoscopy include screening of normal-risk patients for carcinoma, evaluation of

bright red rectal bleeding, or evaluation of other anorectal symptoms such as pruritus, pain, or perianal fistula. Flexible sigmoidoscopy is also indicated in the follow-up of patients with distal inflammatory bowel disease or neoplasms at high risk for local recurrence. It may, on occasion, be useful in the evaluation of chronic diarrhea or bowel evacuation disorders. Contraindications to this procedure include acute diverticulitis, peritonitis, toxic colitis, hemodynamic instability, or lack of consent after the procedure has been thoroughly explained to the patient (Table 11–4).

As mentioned earlier, colonoscopy is a more extensive procedure than flexible sigmoidoscopy. While colonoscopy is the ultimate examination for investigation of diseases involving the large bowel, it also requires more extensive bowel preparation, sedation and monitoring, and training for the endoscopist. Indications for this procedure include screening of high-risk patients for carcinoma, investigation and treatment of polyps, and evaluation of occult blood, colorectal hemorrhage, and vague colorectal symptoms, such as chronic constipation, diarrhea, and abdominal pain. It may also be used to determine the extent of colitis and Crohn's disease and to investigate abnormalities visualized during a barium enema. Contraindications to colonoscopy include toxic colitis, hemodynamic instability, peritonitis, acute diverticulitis, improperly prepared bowel, or lack of consent after the procedure has been thoroughly explained to the patient (Table 11–5).

Bowel Preparation

Bowel preparation for a flexible sigmoidoscopy consists of two fleet enemas given consecutively. A liquid diet for the 2 days preceding the procedure may help, but it is not necessary. The enemas can be self-administered by the patient (within 1 hour of the procedure) or given at the office.

Bowel preparation for colonoscopy is more extensive because the entire colon will be examined by the endoscope. It is essential that bowel preparation be thorough in

Table 11–3. Selected applications of esophagogastroduodenoscopy (EGD).

Application	Benefit
Upper gastrointestinal hemorrhage (UGI)	Early therapy can reduce transfusion requirements, shorten hospital stay, and diminish the need for emergency surgery
Percutaneous endoscopic gastrostomy (PEG)	Provides secure route for enteral feeding or gastric decompression
Dilation of strictures	Relieves obstructive symptoms
Removal of foreign bodies	Prevents perforation or obstruction

Table 11–4. Indications and contraindications for flexible sigmoidoscopy.

Indications
Screening for carcinoma
Bright red rectal bleeding
Chronic diarrhea
Distal inflammatory bowel disease
Perianal fistula
Anorectal symptoms:
  Pruritus
  Pain

Contraindications
Acute diverticulitis
Peritonitis
Toxic colitis
Hemodynamic instability
Improperly prepared bowel
Patient's lack of consent after the procedure is explained

Table 11–5. Indications and contraindications for colonoscopy.

Indications
    Screening for carcinoma in high-risk patients
    Investigation and/or treatment of:
        Polyps
        Suspicious bleeding
        Colorectal hemorrhage
        Vague colorectal symptoms:
            Constipation
            Diarrhea
            Abdominal pain
    Determine the extent of:
        Colitis
        Crohn's disease
    Investigate abnormalities visualized during barium enema

Contraindications
    Toxic colitis
    Hemodynamic instability
    Peritonitis
    Acute diverticulitis
    Improperly prepared bowel
    Patient's lack of consent after the procedure is explained

Table 11–6. Typical bowel preparation regimens.

Evening before examination:
5:00 PM: 1. Start clean liquid diet
           2. Take metoclopramide, 10 mg, orally
           3. May repeat × 1 for nausea
5:30 PM: 4. Four liters of balanced electrolyte polyethylene glycol (PEG) solution ingested over 3–4 hours

OR

Day before examination:
10:00 AM: 1. Begin clear liquid diet
           2. 45-cm³ dose of sodium phosphate preparation (Fleet, CB Fleet Co., Inc., Lynchburg, Virginia)
2:00 PM: 3. 3.8 oz clear liquid, 8 oz water
6:00 PM: 4. 30-cm³ dose of sodium phosphate preparation (Fleet)
10:00 PM: 5. 8 oz clear liquid, 8 oz water

order to accurately visualize the colon. Some individualization of the preparation for colonoscopy is rational because of the great variability in bowel habits. Patients with severe constipation may require longer periods of clear liquid diet and the addition of cathartics or enemas to their regime. Table 11–6 lists typical bowel preparation regimens for colonoscopy for patients with normal gut function.

Technique

The goal of the flexible sigmoidoscopy is to examine the rectum and the sigmoid colon. It is possible to obtain the appropriate information in approximately 90% of cases. In some flexible sigmoidoscopy examinations the splenic flexure can be reached, and in a limited number the transverse colon can be visualized. Colonoscopy is intended to inspect the entire colon and a portion of the distal ileum in some cases (Figure 11–7).

Before beginning the procedure, it is important to put the patient at ease with an explanation of what they will experience. They should be told that pain is a useful warning sign and to alert the operator when pain is felt during

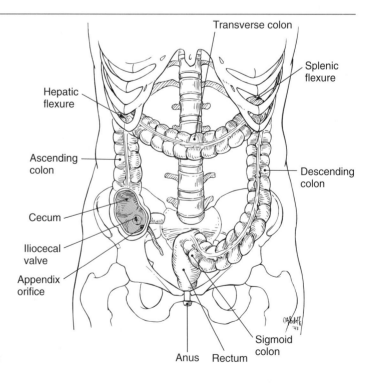

Figure 11–7. Colon anatomy.

the procedure. The two most common patient positions for both procedures are the knee-chest and left lateral positions. However, the left lateral position is less desirable for patients with anal complaints, as the anus is more easily inspected in the knee-chest position.

A digital examination is helpful to relax the anus and for a preliminary inspection. However, the most important reason for inserting a finger prior to the endoscopy is to digitally examine the posterior quadrant of the distal rectum. This area is not well visualized with standard straight-viewing endoscopes and is often the site of missed neoplasms. Examination of the prostate at this time is simply good medical care. If anal disease is extensive, the procedure may have to be postponed or the patient sedated in order to proceed. For both flexible sigmoidoscopy and for colonoscopy, the tip of the instrument is more easily inserted side-on than end-on. Patients are often very apprehensive about flexible sigmoidoscopy. However, they tolerate it very well if a gentle technique is used, adequate warning is given (ie, "I'm about to insert my finger/scope . . . inflate with air . . . go around a sharp turn," etc), and abundant reassurance is offered.

Proper techniques of push, pull, tip deflection, and torque (twist) are key components of a successful endoscopic examination. A rapid, thorough, and comfortable endoscopic examination can be performed when the endoscope is kept straight. Loop formation is uncomfortable for the patient and prevents adequate visualization of structures. The tip of the scope should be kept in the center of the lumen. This may be a difficult maneuver, especially when negotiating turns.

The first structure encountered after insertion of the endoscope is the rectum. Air insufflation is used to open the rectum. The scope will usually pass easily through this structure. The next structure, the rectosigmoid colon, is often the most difficult structure to negotiate. The sigmoid colon may either be in a loose position over the rectum or fixed over the rectum by pelvic adhesions or previous pelvic surgery (ie, hysterectomy). This creates an acute angle that may be difficult to negotiate and may cause discomfort for the patient. In order to proceed, it is important to keep the scope as straight as possible as it exits the rectum. It is beneficial to insufflate a minimal amount of air. Additional sedation may be required in unusually difficult cases. Under no circumstances should the endoscope be forced. Once this difficult turn is negotiated, the tip should be straightened.

The sigmoid colon is often highly mobile and may contain diverticula that are large enough to be mistaken for the true lumen. Passing the sigmoid colon without creating a loop greatly facilitates the remainder of the examination. A technique of clockwise torque and intermittent partial withdrawal of the scope is usually successful.

Spasms and cramps within this region may cause patient discomfort and inability to advance for the endoscopist. When spasm is encountered, it is usually best to resist the temptation to insufflate air. A common reason endoscopists fail to reach the cecum during colonoscopy

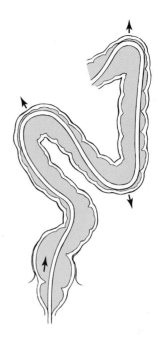

Figure 11–8. "N" loop formation within the colon.

is overinsufflation. A distended bowel is very uncomfortable for the patient, and it is impossible to shorten and straighten an overdistended colon. In areas where the lumen is relatively straight, it is usually possible to aspirate some air without losing the current view. In areas such as the hepatic flexure and ascending colon, aspirating air may move the colon over the stationary colonoscope and bring the more proximal lumen into view.

The descending colon is fixed to the retroperitoneum. The angle at the junction of the sigmoid and descending colon is determined by how effectively the endoscopist has shortened and straightened the sigmoid colon. When a

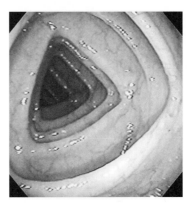

Figure 11–9. Endoscopic view of triangular folds of transverse colon.

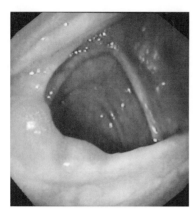

Figure 11–10. Endoscopic view of the ileocecal valve.

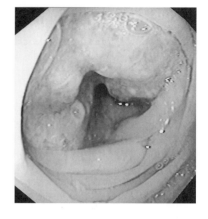

Figure 11–12. Typical appearance of colon carcinoma.

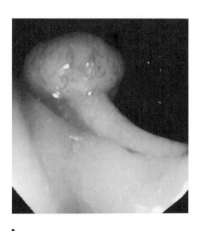

A

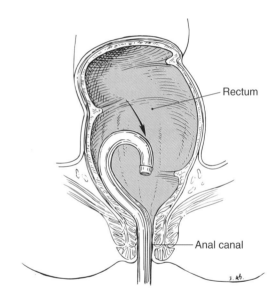

Figure 11–13. Retroflexion of the endoscope within the rectum.

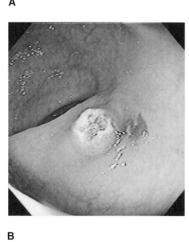

B

Figure 11–11. *A:* Pedunculated polyp. *B:* Polyp stalk after removal.

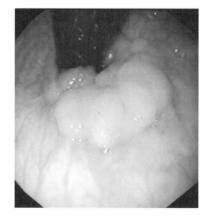

Figure 11–14. Sessile polyp in distal rectum (retroflex view of distal rectum).

Table 11–7. Selected applications of colonoscopy.

Application	Benefit
Endoscopic polypectomy	Decreases incidence of colorectal carcinoma
Surveillance of inflammatory bowel disease	Identifies premalignant mucosal changes
Surveillance and follow-up of colon cancer	Identifies metachronous polyps or tumors

sigmoid loop forms at the site of fixation of the descending colon, the endoscope is forced into three curves (up to the apex of the sigmoid loop, down to the sigmoid-descending junction, up to pass the descending colon). This so-called "N" loop (Figure 11–8) is identified by an inability to advance the endoscope tip and is remedied by withdrawing the endoscope while externally pushing the sigmoid colon into the left lower quadrant.

The next structure encountered is the splenic flexure. A purplish shadow may be visualized (the spleen) and a strong cardiac pulsation is present. It may be difficult or relatively easy to negotiate this structure, depending on patient anatomy. If a loop begins to form in the sigmoid colon, it may become impossible to negotiate the splenic flexure, as any force inserted on the scope only increases the loop.

Once reached, the transverse colon has a triangular appearance (Figure 11–9). If there is no loop in the sigmoid colon, the scope should advance easily through this structure. When the transverse colon is redundant, external splinting or a change in patient position may be necessary to allow the scope to pass.

The hepatic flexure is easily recognized by the prominent blue liver shadow. In the same manner as all other turns, a straight scope will pass easily. It is impossible to pass a looped scope at this point. If the scope can be passed, it will easily pass through the ascending colon. It may sometimes be difficult to determine if the cecum has been reached. The appendiceal orifice and the ileocecal valve are the most dependable landmarks. The ileocecal valve lies proximal to the base of the cecum and is often seen as a bulbous fold (Figure 11–10). It often has a yellowish tinge due to fatty infiltration. In order to visualize the distal ileum, patience is required to advance through the ileocecal valve. This maneuver should routinely be attempted in order gain skill for the instances in which it is necessary.

In general, the colon is better visualized and evaluated upon withdrawal of the scope. This is the time to generously insufflate air. However, forward pressure must be maintained in order to prevent rapid ejection. The patient may pass air upon withdrawal, causing collapse of the lumen wall. In this case, air insufflation may be necessary to properly visualize structures.

In general, polyps should be removed during withdrawal of the endoscope, although small lesions and polyps that may be difficult to find again can be removed or biopsied during insertion (Figure 11–11). When an obvious colon carcinoma is visualized (Figure 11–12), surgical excision is required and should be scheduled as soon as possible (Table 11–7). Polyps that would be removed in the standard surgical resection need not be removed at this time. The surgeon should be notified that adjacent polyps are present so that removal is assured. All polyps outside the surgical field should be removed endoscopically.

Upon withdrawal, the rectum may best be visualized by "retroflexing" the endoscope (Figure 11–13). This consists of distending the rectum by insufflating air, bringing the scope back into the lower third of the rectum, and then advancing it with maximum tip deflection. As the bent end of the scope comes in contact with the bowel wall, it should be further inserted so that the scope doubles back on itself. This provides an excellent view of the rectum, and it may be possible to visualize areas that may have been missed upon insertion (Figure 11–14). The retroflexed view of the rectum has been associated with rectal perforation, therefore, caution is indicated.

SUGGESTED READING

Baillie J: *Gastrointestinal Endoscopy: Basic Principles and Practice.* Butterworth-Heinemann, 1992.

Church JM: *Endoscopy of the Colon, Rectum, and Anus.* Igaku-Shoin, 1995.

Dent L et al: *Surgical Endoscopy.* Year Book Medical Publishers, 1985.

Tytgat GNJ, Classen M: *Practice of Therapeutic Endoscopy.* Churchill Livingstone, 1994.

12

Laparoscopic Surgery

Camran R. Nezhat, MD, Farr R. Nezhat, MD, Ceana H. Nezhat, MD,
Mark Vierra, MD, & Daniel S. Seidman, MD

▶ Key Facts

▶ The benefits of laparoscopic surgery include less postoperative pain, lower risk of wound dehiscence, early mobilization, as well as decreased adhesion formation and infection rates.

▶ Disadvantages of the laparoscopic approach include limited two-dimensional depth perception, lack of tactile feedback, and a steep learning curve.

▶ Practically all intra-abdominal procedures and many gynecologic and urologic procedures can be performed laparoscopically. Exceptions include the debulking of large tumors and organ transplants.

▶ Contraindications to laparoscopy include diffuse fecal peritonitis, severe cardiovascular compromise, acute inflammatory bowel disease, liver cirrhosis, large abdominal aortic aneurysm, and any condition which limits patient positioning and anesthesia tolerance (ie, massive obesity).

▶ Laparoscopic surgery for cancer is a technically demanding operation and should be performed only at centers where experienced oncologic and laparoscopic surgeons collaborate.

▶ Essential instruments for performing laparoscopic procedures include the laparoscope, an insufflator, camera equipment, suction irrigator probes, and a hydrodissection pump, as well as various tools designed to fit through the trocar sleeves, such as forceps, scissors, and CO_2 lasers.

▶ Extracorporeal knot tying simplifies laparoscopic suturing. Instruments to facilitate this process include a needle-holder, needle-driver, suture introducer, and scissors.

▶ The most effective use of CO_2 laser beam is through the operative channel of the laparoscope as a "long knife"; the beam does not ostruct the view and works well for delicate dissection.

ADVANTAGES

Most benefits of laparoscopic surgery are derived from the minimal access used and include less postoperative pain, lower risk of wound dehiscence, early mobilization, and generally more rapid convalescence (Table 12–1). Other recognized advantages of laparoscopy are decreased adhesion formation and reduced rates of infection. The reason for these superior outcomes is not completely understood. They have been attributed to lack of exposure of the abdominal organs to air and to less im-

Inspection of the abdominal cavity was first attempted by Philip Bozzinin of Italy in 1805 using a tube and a candle. Laparoscopy was developed during the early 20th century as a means to diagnose liver and spleen disease. Kelling, a surgeon from Dresden, was first to report in 1901 the use of a cystoscope to examine a canine abdominal cavity. He was also the first to perform this procedure by filling the abdominal cavity with filtered air, thus creating a pneumoperitoneum. Kelling's professional rival, Jacobaeus (Sweden, 1910), was the first to use laparoscopy with a pneumoperitoneum in humans. Laparoscopy was first performed in the United States in 1911 by Bernheim at Johns Hopkins.

Kalk, often regarded as the father of modern diagnostic laparoscopy, introduced improved obligue-viewing optics in 1929. In 1934, Ruddock was the first to use biopsy forceps equipped with monopolar electrocautery during laparoscopy. In the same year, Hope was the first to diagnose an ectopic pregnancy laparoscopically.

Despite initial good results, laparoscopy was far from being accepted in the first half of this century. However, the introduction of a new laparoscope that utilized fiberoptic (cold) light transmitted along a quartz rod in 1952 by Fourestier, Gladu, and Valmier renewed interest in the technique. Other major advancements included the development by Hopkins in 1966 of a rod lens system that doubled the transmission of light through the endoscope.

The prominent French gynecologist, Raoul Palmer, who began promoting the technique in the 1940s, is considered by many to be the father of modern operative laparoscopy. He was among the first to show the benefits of general anesthesia during laparoscopy and the need to monitor intra-abdominal pressure. In 1962, he reported the first human tubal fulguration.

Another pioneer of this technique is Kurt Semm of Kiel. His revolutionary contributions include the multiple-puncture laparoscopic approach using a straight laparoscope and multiple-accessory operating instruments. In addition, his group developed an automatic insufflating device that maintains a constant abdominal pressure. Semm introduced many of the instruments currently used in operative laparoscopy, including hook scissors, needle holders, clip applicators, and atraumatic forceps. Many advanced operations were first developed in Kiel, including laparoscopic appendectomy.

During the 1970s, other gynecologists, including Gomel and Bruhat, significantly contributed to the development of operative laparoscopy. Nevertheless, this new technique was confined to a limited group of surgeons and was not widely accepted.

In the late 1970s, Nezhat experimented with a video camera, attached to the eyepiece of the scope in animal laboratories and humans. The camera magnified the image and projected it onto video monitors in the operating room. The benefits of this approach include not only eliminating the back strain of the surgeon, but more importantly allowing synchronization of the surgical team, who were previously blinded to the entire procedure.

HISTORICAL FACTS *continued*

The first videolaparoscopic surgeries in humans were difficult because early cameras were cumbersome, weighing over 2 pounds, and the resolution and light sources were inadequate. In the early 1980s, miniature video cameras became available, and as manufacturers recognized the potential market, they produced lighter versions with higher resolution and better light sources.

Bruhat (1979) and Tadir (1982) were among the first to utilize the CO_2 laser in laparoscopy using a second puncture. In 1983, Nezhat introduced a new arrangement using a fixed coupler to secure the CO_2 laser in the operating channel of the laparoscope. The CO_2 laser has since been used extensively to treat endometriosis. The laparoscopic management of infiltrating endometriotic lesions was extended by Nezhat to include complex procedures, such as resection and reanastomosis of the rectosigmoid colon or the ureter.

In 1987, Mouret of France performed the first cholecystectomy using standard laparoscopic equipment. This new procedure was introduced to the USA by Reddick and Berci 1 year later. The remarkable rapid and wide acceptance of laparoscopic cholecystectomy was an important stimulus to the development of other laparoscopic techniques. In 1989, Dubois completed highly selective vagotomy laparoscopically, and Nathonson undertook suture toilet of a perforated duodenal ulcer. Laparoscopic inguinal hernia repair was first performed by Ger, and in the same year Kakhouda and Mouiel completed a truncal vagotomy and seromyotomy.

Gynecologists further expanded the scope of laparoscopy with techniques for hysterectomy and myomectomy. Similar advances have been made by urologists. Vancaillie and Schuessler were the first to report a laparoscopic Marshall-Marcehetti-Krantz (MK) bladder neck suspension in 1991. A year later, Nezhat described a laparoscopic Burch procedure.

One of the most fascinating developments in operative laparoscopy is the extension of the use of this technique to cancer surgery. Although still controversial, D'argent in 1989 and Querleu in 1991 reported on the performance of laparoscopic pelvic lymphadenectomy for cancer staging. In 1991, Nezhat was the first to perform a radical hysterectomy and report the extension of lymph node dissection to the para-aortic area.

It has been stated that laparoscopic surgery has more of a future than a past. The recent successful completion at Stanford of coronary bypass vascular surgery using laparoscopic techniques attests to the approach's expanding role. This revolutionary procedure, which avoids the need to split the sternum, was reported by Nezhat, using a porcine model, in 1992.

munosuppression owing to decreased physical stress. With this approach, there is less bleeding, resulting from increased intraperitoneal pressure created by pneumoperitoneum, and better hemostasis aided by the magnification. Indirect benefits include reduced use of analgesics and enhanced mobilization, resulting in more rapid return of bowel function and a lower rate of thromboembolic complications.

DISADVANTAGES

Basic surgical principles must always be adhered to, regardless of the approach. These include maximal exposure of the operative field, meticulous hemostasis, avoidance of spillage of the enteric or tumor contents in the peritoneal cavity, retrieval of the specimen intact for complete

Table 12–1. Advantages of laparoscopic surgery.

Elimination of large abdominal incision
- Less wound infection and dehiscence

Less bleeding
- High intra-abdominal pressure; limits bleeding from small blood vessels
- Meticulous hemostasis possible under magnified operative field

Better inspection of upper abdomen
- Excellent light source and magnification
- Allows visualization and biopsy of diaphragm, paracolic gutter, peritoneum, omentum

Improved laparoscopic access to rectovaginal space

Fewer adhesions
- Due to less manipulation of tissues, less bleeding, lowered pH in CO_2-rich Ringer's lactate, decreased infection rate

Decreased postoperative pain
- Less need for analgesia and related bowel paralysis
- Fully ambulatory earlier
- Reduced risk of thromboembolic complications
- Shorter hospitalization

More rapid recovery
- Easier postoperative care
- Earlier initiation of postoperative treatment (chemotherapy or radiotherapy)

---

pathologic analysis, and the performance of well-vascularized, tension-free anastomoses. Compensating for the inherent limitations of laparoscopy requires a high degree of skill and experience (Table 12–2). The surgeon's depth perception is reduced by the two-dimensional image on

Table 12–2. Disadvantages of laparoscopic surgery.

Two-dimensional vision
- Depth perception may be challenging

Direct palpation not possible
- Poor tactile feedback

Demands more skill and experience
- Prolonged operating time

Requires specialized equipment
- Higher costs

Optimal retraction difficult to achieve
- Limited exposure of the operative field

No protection possible for upper abdomen
- No intra-abdominal packing

More tumor manipulation, trauma
- Possibility of tumor spillage

High intra-abdominal pressure
- Adverse effect on lung ventilation
- Possible increased risk of tumor dissemination
- Excessive carbon dioxide absorption from pneumoperitoneum

Difficult to extract large tumors
- Not suitable for large bulky tumors

the video screen. Tactile feedback is also poor since direct palpation is not possible. In addition, it is difficult to achieve optimal retraction of abdominal organs, which occasionally may limit exposure of the operative field. Laparoscopy may be unsuitable for some patients because of the Trendelenburg positioning and the need for abdominal distention. Removing large tumors from the abdomen through trocars requires extensive morcellation, which is very time-consuming. Last but not least, the use of highly specialized equipment increases costs, a significant concern in the money-conscious health system. These extra expenses can be largely overcome by decreased use of costly and disposable instruments by more experienced laparoscopic surgeons. Further, in centers with a major interest in this approach, a higher patient load reduces the cost per use of "high-ticket" instruments, such as lasers. Additional cost savings is achieved through shorter hospital stays and early return to work.

INDICATIONS

The scope of surgical procedures that can be performed laparoscopically has expanded over the last decade. Practically all intra-abdominal procedures have been shown not only to be feasible, but to provide the patient with many of the advantages described above. The only types of surgery not suited for laparoscopy are debulking of large tumors and organ transplants. It seems that the acceptability of laparoscopic operations is mainly determined by the skill and experience of the surgeon.

The major role of laparoscopy as a diagnostic tool in both acute and chronic conditions has long been recognized. Subsequently, treatment of conditions causing acute pain, including appendicitis, torsion of ovarian cysts, and ectopic pregnancy, can often be best performed by laparoscopy.

Cholecystectomy is currently performed, in most cases, laparoscopically. In fact, the availability of this technique has, to a large extent, triggered the current interest of general surgeons in laparoscopic operations. Additional laparoscopic procedures, the roles of which are still under evaluation, include repair of inguinal hernias, Nissen fundoplication, and small bowel and colon resection. Practically all known abdominal operations have been completed laparoscopically; an exhaustive list is beyond the scope of this chapter.

Other surgical disciplines have also enthusiastically adopted the laparoscopic approach. In fact, for well over two decades, gynecologists frequently performed laparoscopic procedures, including tubal ligation, removal of ovarian cysts, adhesiolysis, and ablation of endometriosis. Recently, advanced gynecologic operations such as hysterectomy have become routine. Urologists have incorporated laparoscopy only over the last few years for procedures such as removal of an undescended testis, partial nephrectomy, and adrenalectomy. Ureteroureterostomy has been done successfully by laparoscopy. Genuine stress urinary incontinence is managed laparoscopically using the Burch and Marshall-Marchetti-Krantz procedures by both gynecologists and urologists. Minimal-access techniques similar to those used in laparoscopy are being adopted by thoracic surgeons, vascular surgeons, and even neurosurgeons. Endoscopy has long been used by ear, nose, and throat specialists and orthopedic surgeons (see Chapter 11).

CONTRAINDICATIONS

As the indications for laparoscopic surgery constantly evolve, so do the definitions of contraindications (Table 12–3). For example, acute inflammation in appendicitis and salpingitis, previously considered a contraindication, is now accepted as a common indication for laparoscopic diagnosis and management. The importance of careful patient selection for laparoscopic surgery must be emphasized. Accepted contraindications include diffuse fecal peritonitis, severe cardiovascular compromise, and inability to withstand the necessary positioning and anesthesia. Less common contraindications include the presence of large phlegmons, acute inflammatory bowel disease, liver cirrhosis, and large abdominal aortic aneurysm.

Relative contraindications include massive obesity, extensive multiple adhesions, unprepared bowel, diaphragmatic hernia, large tumors, and prior abdominal radiation therapy. The "relativity" of these contraindications depends on the experience of the surgeon, the anesthesiologist, and the entire operating room team.

CANCER SURGERY

For many years, cancer was considered a contraindication to laparoscopic surgery. Much effort was invested in preoperative patient screening to avoid an unexpected finding of malignancy. Although laparoscopy was used for some time in second-look explorations, it has only recently been attempted for tumor removal and staging. Experienced laparoscopists today can remove adequate tumor specimens and a number of lymph nodes comparable to that achieved at conventional open surgery.

Laparoscopic surgery has included bowel resection for colon cancer and radical hysterectomy for uterine malignancy. These and other cancer operations have been successfully combined with aggressive lymphadenectomy of the para-aortic, obturator, and iliac nodes.

The advantages of laparoscopic surgery are especially appealing for cancer patients. The minimal access reduces the rate of complications more common among these patients, including surgical scar dehiscence, infection, and thromboembolism. Further, the early ambulation and rapid recovery allow more immediate initiation of postoperative irradiation or chemotherapy.

The major concern regarding laparoscopic surgery in patients with malignant tumors is the absence of long-term survival data, since these techniques have only recently been introduced. Additional concerns include the risk of tumor dissemination caused by increased intra-abdominal pressure, inability to protect the upper abdomen with packing, and the difficulty of tumor removal through the trocar. Special retrieval bags are currently used to avoid spillage. Tumor implantation affecting the abdominal wall at the site of the trocar incision has been attributed to the aggressive nature of the cancer in these patients.

Laparoscopic surgery for cancer is a technically demanding operation and should be performed only at centers where experienced oncologic and laparoscopic surgeons collaborate.

TECHNIQUE

Laparoscopic operations begin with the placement of trocar ports through which a scope, coupled with a video camera, and various surgical tools are inserted. To create an operating field, the abdomen is distended by insufflating carbon dioxide (CO_2) gas, creating a pneumoperitoneum. Some surgeons first insert a needle and insufflate the abdomen before inserting the trocars, while others prefer to directly insert the trocars. When the latter approach is used, it is crucial to manually (with towel clips—see Figure 12–1) lift the abdominal wall to avoid injury to the abdominal organs. A number of mechanical devices have been recently introduced to elevate the abdominal wall, distending the abdomen. However, these "gasless" techniques are still under study.

The exact location of trocar insertion depends upon the procedure to be performed (Figure 12–1). The surgical team observes the operating field on video screens (Figure 12–2). Specially devised instruments are used. For example, laparoscopic appendectomy can be performed using bipolar electrodesiccation (Figure 12–3), CO_2 laser

Table 12–3. Contraindications to laparoscopy.

Absolute	Relative
Shock	Large tumors
Ileus or obstruction	Prior abdominal irradiation
Inability to withstand Trendelenburg positioning	Massive obesity
Inability to withstand local or general anesthesia	Known multiple adhesions
Diffuse fecal peritonitis	Diaphragmatic hernia

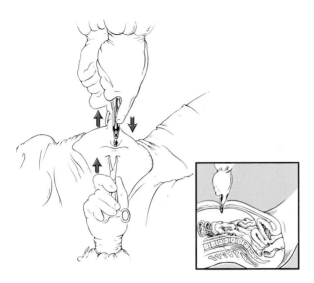

Figure 12–1. Insertion of trocar. Countertraction is applied by grasping the lower abdomen; the surgeon inserts the trocar into the abdomen by palming it and using the index finger as a guard against sudden entry into the abdomen. (Reproduced, with permission, from Nezhat CR et al: *Operative Gynecologic Laparoscopy.* McGraw-Hill, 1995.)

for cutting (Figure 12–4), Endoloops (Ethicon, Inc, Somerville, NJ) for suturing (Figure 12–5), or stapling devices for fast clip-and-remove procedures (Figure 12–6).

EQUIPMENT

The development of specialized instruments enabled surgeons to increase the diversity of laparoscopic procedures. The instruments are designed to fit through trocar sleeves 3–30 mm in diameter.

Successful operative laparoscopy requires proper instruments. Specialized instruments can make difficult procedures technically possible and safer. Most procedures can be performed with two or three forceps, a suction-irrigator probe, a bipolar electrocoagulator, a pair of scissors, and a CO_2 laser. Disposable, semireusable, and reusable instruments are available. Many ancillary instruments have a unipolar electrosurgical capability. Instruments should be carefully selected on the basis of cost and effectiveness; too many instruments clutter the field and increase operative time.

The CO_2 laser is placed through the operative channel of the laparoscope for cutting and hemostasis of small blood vessels. Electrocoagulation with a bipolar forceps is used to control bleeding from larger blood vessels. The CO_2 laser can be replaced by another cutting instrument.

DISPOSABLE OR REUSABLE INSTRUMENTS

When choosing instruments, several factors must be considered, including initial cost, cost per use, ease of use, and reliability. Reusable instruments involve initial and maintenance expenses, such as handling, sterilizing, sorting, and storing. For some reusable instruments, such as scissors, performance declines with use and they must be replaced periodically. However, most reusable instruments perform reliably, and their construction and materials allow a certain level of indelicate handling.

Disposable instruments cost the patient as much as $100 to $200 per instrument. The use of a stapler may add $1,000 to $3,000 to the operation, thus offsetting the cost savings achieved by laparoscopy. In addition, there remains the expense of handling and storing disposable instruments. The materials are not durable, and are not reliable with repeated use. Their main advantage, therefore, is high performance, including brand new sharp-edged blades and a theoretically reduced risk of disease transmission. Once discarded, however, environmental concerns are raised about disposal and biodegradability. The combination of disposable and reusable instruments helps maintain high performance standards.

ESSENTIAL INSTRUMENTS

Laparoscope

The endoscope must be in optimal condition for the procedure. Although the diameters of laparoscopes vary from 1–12 mm and the angle of view from 0–90 degrees, the most commonly used laparoscopes are the straight, diagnostic, and right angle operative laparoscopes. A direct 10-mm, 0-degree diagnostic laparoscope, and an 11-mm, 0-degree operative laparoscope for operative laparoscopy with the CO_2 laser, are preferable. The image transmitted by the diagnostic scope is superior because of the absence of an operative channel; its presence requires a reduction in the size of the lens system and number of fiberoptic bundles. The endoscope provides the access to the abdominal and pelvic cavity and is, thus, the most important piece of equipment.

Insufflator

To adequately observe the contents of the abdominal and pelvic cavity, the abdomen must be insufflated. CO_2 is most commonly used for operative laparoscopy. Advanced procedures require an automatic, electric insufflator that can deliver up to 15 L of gas per minute, or two insufflators, each delivering 9–10 L of gas per minute. The insufflator will compensate for any change when the intra-abdominal pressure is preset. Intra-abdominal pressure should not exceed 16 mm Hg to avoid complications, such as subcutaneous emphysema. Although a mechanical abdominal wall lifter can replace the establishment of a pneumoperitoneum, exposure is poor and complications,

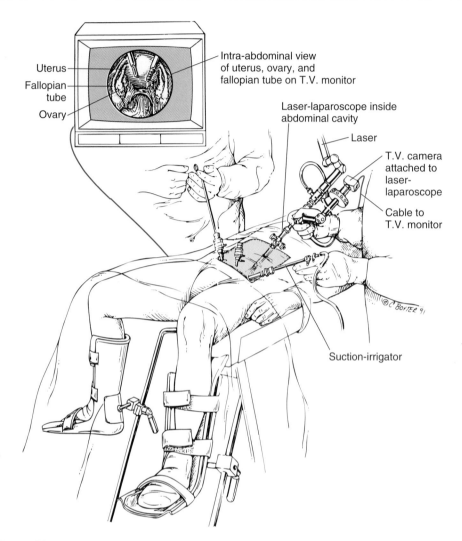

Uterus

Fallopian tube

Ovary

Intra-abdominal view of uterus, ovary, and fallopian tube on T.V. monitor

Laser-laparoscope inside abdominal cavity

Laser

T.V. camera attached to laser-laparoscope

Cable to T.V. monitor

Suction-irrigator

Figure 12–2. Suprapubic punctures are made to introduce the suction irrigator probe and grasping forceps. (Reproduced, with permission, from Nezhat CR et al: *Operative Gynecologic Laparoscopy.* McGraw-Hill, 1995.)

including femoral nerve injury, have been reported with these new devices.

Camera Equipment

In early endoscopic surgery, no medical video cameras were available, and endoscopists adopted cameras from the television trade. Camera tubes and single- and three-chip cameras followed the introduction of similar advancements in commercial cameras. That trend began to change, however, with the introduction of equipment specific for endoscopy, including the breakthrough of digital processing and chip-on-a-stick, three-dimensional, and virtual reality technologies.

The camera includes two components: the camera head with its cable and the CCU, or camera controller unit. The cable is plugged into the camera controller. The lens on

the medical camera is referred to as a "coupler." The coupler screws onto the camera head and is available in several sizes that magnify the image.

Suction-Irrigator Probe & Hydrodissection Pump

A suction-irrigation probe can be a versatile instrument. Controlled suction and irrigation enhances observation and improves the operative technique. This device serves as an extension of the surgeon's fingers and a backstop for the CO_2 laser. It facilitates hydrodissection, division of tissue planes and spaces, lavage, blunt dissection, and smoke and fluid evacuation.

Laparoscopic Tools

Many conventional instruments have been adapted for insertion through the trocar ports and use in the abdominal

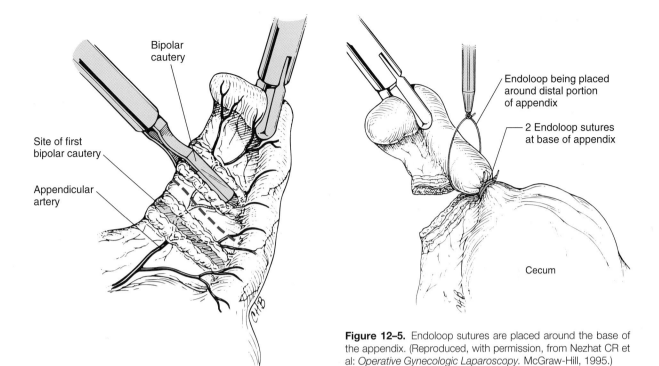

Figure 12–3. The mesoappendix is coagulated with bipolar forceps. (Reproduced, with permission, from Nezhat CR et al: *Operative Gynecologic Laparoscopy.* McGraw-Hill, 1995.)

Figure 12–5. Endoloop sutures are placed around the base of the appendix. (Reproduced, with permission, from Nezhat CR et al: *Operative Gynecologic Laparoscopy.* McGraw-Hill, 1995.)

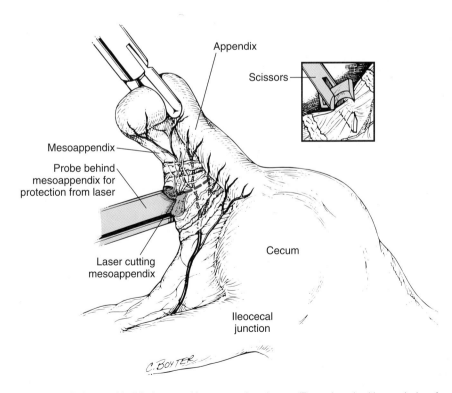

Figure 12–4. The mesoappendix is cut with CO$_2$ laser and laparoscopic scissors. (Reproduced, with permission, from Nezhat CR et al: *Operative Gynecologic Laparoscopy.* McGraw-Hill, 1995.)

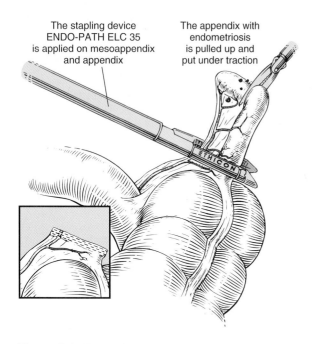

The stapling device ENDO-PATH ELC 35 is applied on mesoappendix and appendix

The appendix with endometriosis is pulled up and put under traction

Figure 12–6. The stapling device is applied directly across the mesoappendix and appendix. ***Inset:*** The appendix and meso-salpinx are clipped and cut. (Reproduced, with permission, from Nezhat CR et al: *Operative Gynecologic Laparoscopy.* McGraw-Hill, 1995.)

cavity. These include atraumatic, claw-toothed, and spoon graspers; curved, straight, and hooked scissors; biopsy forceps; and aspiration-injection needles.

Electrogenerator & Bipolar Forceps. One of the most important instruments widely adopted for laparoscopic surgery is the bipolar electrocoagulator. It is used effectively for hemostasis and to coagulate small and large blood vessels.

Clips. The laparoscopic clip applicators are used for reapproximation of peritoneal surfaces or hemostasis of medium-sized vessels. Disposable loaded applicators and reusable single-clip applicators are available.

Linear Stapler. The available staplers are disposable and can be reloaded with cartridges. The stapler is introduced through a 12-mm port. Each cartridge contains titanium staples arranged in two sets of triple-staggered rows. The instrument also contains a push bar knife assembly, which cuts between the two sets of triple rows, ligating both ends of the incised tissue. The cut line usually is shorter than the staple line. For example, the laparoscopic linear cutter 35 (Ethicon) cut line is approximately 33 mm with a stapler line of 37 mm.

The tissue to be clipped is held and stretched with grasping forceps, and the Endoclip applicator's jaws are placed at the desired incision site. When fired, it simultaneously places six rows of small titanium clips and cuts along the center, leaving three rows of clips on the edge of

each pedicle. This instrument can be used to seal blood vessels and cut pedicles.

Suture. The ability to suture laparoscopically increases the surgeon's versatility. Suturing can be used for hemostasis and to oppose tissues during reconstructive procedures. Different types of suture are available for endoscopic use. The Endoloop (Ethicon) suture, a preformed skipknot attached to a rigid, disposable 5-mm applicator, is available in 0 chromic, polyglactin, polydioxanone, and polypropylene. The loop is positioned around the pedicle by grasping the structure to be removed and pulling it through the loop. The loop is tightened against the applicator and cut above the knot.

Suture material is available with a straight or slightly curved needle, specifically designed for laparoscopic use. It is available in 0 chromic catgut, 4-0 polydioxanone with a swaged ST-4 needle, and polyglactin. The suture is grasped with forceps several centimeters from the needle. The grasper with suture is inserted intra-abdominally through the 5-mm accessory trocar sleeve with a 3-mm suture introducer.

Surgeons also can use any suture with a swaged needle of any size. To place the needle intra-abdominally, the grasper or needle driver is revolved along the trocar sleeve, which remains around the grasper's shaft. The suture is grasped about 5 cm from the needle and the grasper is reintroduced with the trocar sleeve, into the suprapubic incision site. The needle follows the grasper into the abdominal cavity. Once the suture is placed, several techniques can secure the knot.

An instrument tying method within the abdomen uses two forceps and suture material. Intracorporeal knotting is difficult and requires practice. The suture can get caught in the articulation point of the forceps and break. However, variations of the Fisherman's clinch knot, originally described in 1972, may prevent some difficulties. The principles of this instrument do not differ from those of tying suture deep in the pelvis, where the surgeon uses a finger to push and secure the knot.

Extracorporeal Knot Tying. Extracorporeal knot tying simplifies laparoscopic suturing. Instruments to facilitate this process include a needle-holder, needle-driver, suture introducer, and scissors. The surgeon first loads suture into the needle-holder, holding the suture below the swage point so the needle will collapse into the introducer. Next, the needle-holder is inserted into the introducer (Figure 12–7). The introducer is placed into a 5-mm sleeve and the needle-driver into a contralateral sleeve. The needle is advanced into the abdominal cavity and passed from the holder to the driver. While steadying the needle with the driver, the surgeon repositions the holder to the desired location. The needle is tapped with the driver to lock it into a right angle position, then rearmed with the driver. The driver is used to pass the needle through the tissue, then the tip is grasped and the needle is passed to the holder (Figure 12–8). To reduce the risk of pulling the suture out of the tissue, tension on the suture line is kept to a minimum.

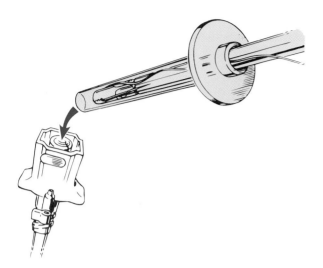

Figure 12–7. The needle-holder is inserted into the introducer. (Reproduced, with permission, from Nezhat CR et al: *Operative Gynecologic Laparoscopy.* McGraw-Hill, 1995.)

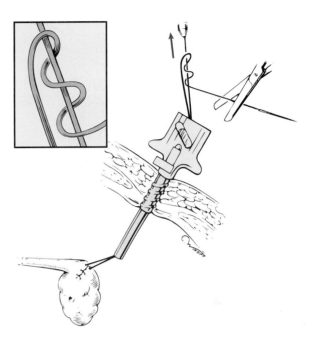

Figure 12–9. The surgeon makes a double-throw knot. (Reproduced, with permission, from Nezhat CR et al: *Operative Gynecologic Laparoscopy.* McGraw-Hill, 1995.)

The needle-holder and excess suture line are withdrawn from the abdominal cavity through the introducer. An assistant covers the introducer channel to maintain pneumoperitoneum. The surgeon cuts the suture below the swage point and makes a double-throw knot with the two suture ends (Figure 12–9). The knot is held securely with the thumb and third finger while three revolutions are made around both suture strands with the free end of the suture. The tail of the suture is inserted through the first loop directly above the surgeon's thumb. After the tail is passed through the loop, the operator pulls up on the tail to form the knot and cuts the tail approximately 0.6 cm

above the knot (Figure 12–10). The end of the Endoknot (Ethicon) shaft is snapped off at the colored band, allowing the shaft to slide the knot downward (Figure 12–10, inset). Placing the shaft perpendicular to the knot minimizes suture breakage and ensures knot security.

The Endoknot cannula is then placed in the introducer. By pulling back on the small end piece of the Endoknot shaft while sliding the plastic shaft forward, the surgeon allows the knot to move forward as the loop decreases in size. The Endoknot cannula acts as an integral knot pusher for placement of the formed knot (Figure 12–11). Scissors inserted through the contralateral trocar are used to cut the excess suture (Figure 12–12).

Extracorporeal Pre-tied Knot. An endoscopic pre-tied suture knot device can be used for extracorporeal knot tying. The pre-tied Endoknot consists of a synthetic absorbable suture material with a hollow plastic tube that is narrowed at one end and scored at the other. The center of the plastic tube has a 4-0 stainless steel suture that is looped at the narrow end and swaged at the surgical needle. The scored end of the device serves as the handle. The primary advantage of these devices is that the knot is made already and does not have to be manually tied by the surgeon (Figure 12–11).

Intracorporeal Knot Tying. Intracorporeal knot tying, which is used during microsurgery and fine sutur-

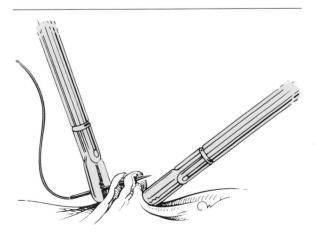

Figure 12–8. The suture is passed through the tissue. (Reproduced, with permission, from Nezhat CR et al: *Operative Gynecologic Laparoscopy.* McGraw-Hill, 1995.)

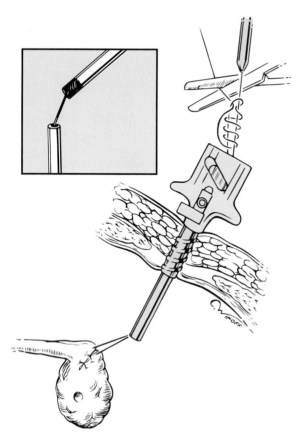

Figure 12–10. The suture tail is cut approximately 0.6 cm above the knot. The end of the Endoknot shaft is snapped off at the colored band, allowing the shaft to slide the knot downward. (Reproduced, with permission, from Nezhat CR et al: *Operative Gynecologic Laparoscopy.* McGraw-Hill, 1995.)

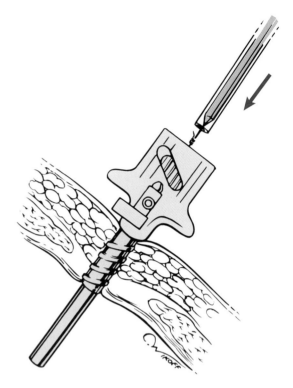

Figure 12–11. The Endoknot cannula acts as a knot pusher to place the formed knot. (Reproduced, with permission, from Nezhat CR et al: *Operative Gynecologic Laparoscopy.* McGraw-Hill, 1995.)

ing, is more difficult and time-consuming than extracorporeal knot tying. The instructions for introducing the needle and suture to the abdomen are the same as for extracorporeal knot tying. The needle and entire suture are placed in the abdominal cavity. After the needle is positioned, it is grasped with the needle-holder. While the grasping forceps apply pressure or hold the tissue being sutured, the suture is inserted through the tissue. The graspers hold the needle, and the needle-holder applies counterpressure to the tissue. The needle is removed from the tissue. Enough suture to form a knot is pulled through, leaving a sufficient tail. The needle is grasped with a grasping forceps and two or three loops are made around the needle-holder and brought inside the formed loops. Using both grasping forceps and the needle-holder, the surgeon ties the suture over the tissue, applying additional knots over the suture and reversing the direction of the sutures with each successive knot.

Lasers. Laser is an acronym for "light amplification by stimulated emission of radiation." The device produces

and amplifies light energy to create intense, coherent electromagnetic radiation. However, unlike the ionizing radiation of x-rays and gamma rays, which result from nuclear destruction, the energy emitted by laser results from the release of photons that occur when stimulated electrons circling their nuclei return from their "excited" (E2) to their "resting" (E1) states (E2 – E1 = photon). These intermediate energy photons induce molecular vibration and create heat when they interact with tissue. Therefore, although laser light is powerful and penetrating, it is neither mutagenic nor carcinogenic.

Because each lasing substance has a unique atomic and molecular structure with its characteristic electron orbit, the wavelength and frequency of emitted photons will be unique and uniform for each particular substance (CO_2, potassium titanyl phosphate, argon). Laser light is monochromatic, consisting of a single wavelength that cannot be separated into any other components, unlike regular light, which can be separated into the colors of the spectrum when passed through a prism. When all the light waves are exactly in phase with each other, the light is said to be coherent; when all waves are parallel, the light is collimated. Because light waves of lasers have exactly the same length (monochromatic), are in phase with each

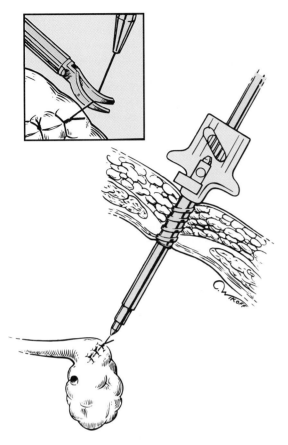

Figure 12–12. The knot is placed over the tissue, and the suture above the knot is cut. (Reproduced, with permission, from Nezhat CR et al: *Operative Gynecologic Laparoscopy.* McGraw-Hill, 1995.)

other (coherent), and always run parallel (collimated), the laser can be focused precisely by lenses into a very small spot, which can develop an extremely high power density.

Lasers have several unique characteristics that differentiate them from other medical instruments. The primary difference is that, with some exceptions, the tissue is not touched by surgical instruments but only by the laser beam. Thus, the depth of the incision is not controlled by the pressure exerted on the tissue, but by the power density and the time that the laser is focused on any one spot. This "action at a distance" allows for greater accessibility to the target tissue and, perhaps, less tissue trauma.

When used at laparotomy, the CO_2 laser is delivered with a hand-held probe or attached to the operating microscope. The former has the advantage of a shorter focal distance and, therefore, a smaller spot size, resulting in greater power density. The greater power density yields much higher penetrating power and significantly less thermal damage to the contiguous normal tissue. The hand-held probe is subject to hand tremor and less accurate beam delivery. Attaching the laser to the scope increases

precision because of the magnification and the absence of hand tremor; however, because of the longer focal length, the spot size is larger. With more precise lasers, very high power density is achievable through the laparoscope.

Although each laser has unique properties and tissue effects determined by wavelength and tissue absorption, by varying the power density or mode of delivery (sapphire tips, fiber diameter), the surgeon can achieve the desired tissue effects—such as ablation, coagulation, or vaporization—with most lasers.

The most effective use of the CO_2 laser beam is through the operative channel of the laparoscope as a "long knife"; the beam does not obstruct the view and works well for delicate dissection. The CO_2 laser is stopped easily by a water backstop. This characteristic of the CO_2 laser allows precise dissection in sensitive areas, such as bowel, bladder, ureter, and blood vessels.

THE FUTURE

Laparoscopic surgery successfully combines many technologic innovations, however, surgeons performing laparoscopic operations still face technical limitations. Fortunately, bioengineering advances may help convert this "patient friendly" procedure to a "surgeon friendly" technique. The most apparent limitations of laparoscopic compared to conventional surgery are the two-dimensional view with the former and the inability to palpate the tissues manipulated during surgery.

The laparoscopic surgeon must operate in a three-dimensional field while watching a two-dimensional television monitor. Most surgeons can operate by subconsciously comparing the size of instruments with body structures, using their prior knowledge of anatomical relationships to obtain an idea of depth. It may take some time for the inexperienced surgeon to become accustomed to operating in this way, while some surgeons never do.

To solve this lack of depth perception, the video camera must imitate human stereo vision. Devices are being developed using two video cameras or special computer programs that present a separate image to each of the surgeon's eyes. This is done utilizing special goggles that, through various techniques such as high-frequency shutters and polarized or color filters, exhibit on a single television screen separate images to each eye. Most available three-dimensional systems do not provide the resolution or picture quality available with standard laparoscopic cameras. Gradual improvements are likely to produce compatible devices within a few years. Another concern is the high cost of such systems and the inconvenience of wearing special goggles.

Automated instruments are being developed to transfer tactile sensation and force feedback to the operator's hand from the operating field. Other methods that allow the laparoscopic surgeon to see beyond the surface of the various organs include ultrasonographic probes that can be inserted through the trocars. Laparoscopic ultrasonography can provide accurate imaging of the organ's internal anatomy. It may help locate gallstones in the liver ducts or tumors in the bowel. These laparoscopic probes can also measure blood flow and help the surgeon differentiate between a vein and an artery. In the future, more sophisticated sensor probes will provide information on the actual functional properties of the abdominal structures.

Other technical advances include the development of remote control surgery, also called **telepresence**. In this procedure, the patient is connected to the instruments at one location, while the surgeon watches a video picture transmitted from a distance. The surgeon performs the operation using an instrument panel that simultaneously transmits the sensation of the tissues of the patient on whom surgery is being performed, and precisely interprets the surgeon's instrument use. When adapted for laparoscopic surgery and combined with three-dimensional images, this approach may provide sensation of the tissues and allow the surgeon to manipulate the instruments in a familiar way, more resembling conventional open surgery.

Virtual reality, a computer-generated three-dimensional image that responds to the viewer's signals, may prove to be the optimal training device for surgeons, preparing them to deal with surgical emergencies and complications.

Many surgeons resent the idea that they could be replaced someday by more precise and reliable robotic machines. The theoretical notion that robots could discriminately remove diseased tissue, however, is becoming a reality. Robots can drill a cavity in the thigh bone to perfectly match a hip prosthesis. Other automated systems have successfully facilitated the removal of the prostate gland. Robotics are used at laparoscopy as the surgeon's assistant and to allow tracking of the video camera according to the movements of the operator's head or eyes.

Progress in surgery is likely to decrease the technical difficulty associated with many laparoscopic operations. It is likely that as laparoscopic surgery becomes easier and safer, its role will expand.

SUGGESTED READING

American College of Surgeons: Statement on new laparoscopic and thoracoscopic procedures. Bull Am Coll Surg, September 1993.

Hatlie MJ: Climbing "the learning curve." New technologies, emerging obligations. JAMA 1993;270:1364.

Nezhat C et al (editors): *Operative Gynecologic Laparoscopy: Principles and Techniques*. McGraw-Hill, 1995.

Nezhat C, Nezhat F, Green B, Gonzalez G: Laparoscopic ureteroureterostomy. *J of Endourology* 1992;6:143.

Nezhat C, Nezhat F, Nezhat C: Operative laparoscopy (minimally invasive surgery): State of the art. J Gynecol Surgery 1992;8:111.

See WA, Cooper CS, Fisher RJ: Predictors of laparoscopic complications after formal training in laparoscopic surgery. JAMA 1993;270:2689.

Soper NJ, Brunt CM, Kerbil K: Laparoscopic general surgery. N Engl J Med 1994;330:409.

13

Basic Technical Procedures

Chris Traver, MD, & John E. Niederhuber, MD

► Key Facts

- ► There is no substitute for good patient communication and reassurance in the performance of bedside procedures.

- ► During venipuncture, the skin should be punctured rapidly in order to decrease the patient's discomfort, but once through the skin the needle should be advanced slowly through the subcutaneous tissue into the vein.

- ► Tapping or flicking the veins sharply, thus paralyzing the intrinsic vascular tone, may make them stand up more prominently.

- ► For long-term catheters, a subcutaneous tunnel is developed once the guide-wire has been placed. This increases the distance between the vein entrance site and the skin exit site, which decreases the incidence of catheter-borne septicemia.

- ► Chest tube placement is indicated for pneumothorax, hemothorax, pleural effusion, and empyema. Hemothorax or empyema require larger chest tubes (32–36 French), while pneumothorax or malignant effusion can be managed with smaller tubes (20–28 French).

- ► Thoracentesis is indicated for the evacuation of air or fluid in the lungs. For pleural effusion, it should only be used to evaluate the initial fluid collection, as repeated procedures may lead to hypoproteinemia and a decrease in osmotic pressure, leading to recurrence.

- ► Although urethral catheterization is often suspected of being the cause of serious urinary tract infections, allowing the bladder to become overly distended may cause prolonged dysfunction and infection.

The responsibilities of students and house officers vary widely from hospital to hospital. This chapter is meant to provide a brief overview of some of the procedures that a house officer, or a student with close house staff supervision, may be required to perform. Keep in mind that, in the performance of bedside procedures, there is no substitute for good patient communication. If a patient is properly prepared, and trusts that they are in good hands, the procedure will be much easier to perform. It is also important to understand that supervision is essential when any unfamiliar procedure is performed.

VENOUS ACCESS

PERIPHERAL VENIPUNCTURE

Peripheral venipuncture is indicated for the sampling of venous blood for laboratory analysis and is one of the most frequently performed procedures. It is likely to be one of the first tasks assigned to the medical student. There is a tremendous variation in venous accessibility from patient to patient and it is not uncommon for the beginner to miss the first few attempts at venipunctures. Of course, a failed attempt or attempts to obtain venous access may lead to anxiety and anger on the part of the patient. Even in the presence of an anxious or even angry patient, it is imperative that the physician avoid becoming distraught. Obviously, the chances of success are much higher when the physician is relaxed and endeavors, via conversation and demeanor, to maintain a calm, understanding patient.

In order to perform a venipuncture, you will need skin cleaning supplies, a syringe, a vacutainer syringe hub, a needle for the syringe, a tourniquet, appropriate venipuncture vacuum tubes for blood, gauze and tape, or Band-Aid dressing.

Procedure

The positioning of the patient for peripheral venipuncture is shown in Figure 13–1. It is difficult to determine the reaction of a patient to venipuncture, so the procedure should be carefully explained and the patient asked to look away, if necessary. Rest the upper extremity on a firm surface. Antecubital veins are the easiest site for phlebotomy, which is why they are used 95% of the time. The cephalic and basilic veins lie on the lateral and medial aspects of the antecubital fossa.

Apply the tourniquet above the antecubital fossa, remembering to talk to your patient as you proceed in order to give an indication of each step as you proceed. Remember, always be gentle and sensitive to your patient's feelings. Locate the vein and apply an alcohol wipe to the overlying skin. Inspect the antecubital space using the pads of the second and third fingers. The skin over the vessels should be gently pressed inward. The vein will feel much like an elastic cord, but understanding the exact tactile character of a patent vein comes with experience. Apply gentle traction to the vein distal to the planned puncture site. Puncture the skin, with the bevel of the needle pointed upward, directly over the vessel and guide the needle inward through the skin in the direction of the vein's long axis. The skin should be punctured rapidly in order to decrease the patient's discomfort, but once through the skin the needle should be advanced slowly through the subcutaneous tissue into the vein. When a flash of blood return is seen, aspirate blood into a syringe or attach specific venipuncture vacuum tubes to the vacutainer. Vacuum tubes are color-coded, depending on the presence of specific anticoagulants or other chemicals to provide the correct specimen for the requested blood tests.

Before withdrawing the needle, release the tourniquet and apply pressure to the venipuncture site with your thumb over a gauze pad. Have the patient apply pressure for approximately 1 minute and tape the gauze in place to absorb any additional oozing from the site.

PERIPHERAL VENOUS CATHETERIZATION

Peripheral venous catheterization is performed for venous access in both the outpatient and inpatient settings. The preferred sites for access are the veins of the forearm and the small veins on the dorsum of the hand. Blood products must be given through an 18-gauge or larger intravenous catheter. For the hypovolemic or trauma patient, a large-bore, 14- to 16-gauge intravenous catheter should be placed in the antecubital veins. The necessary supplies include those required for skin sterilization, a tourniquet, catheter-over-needle or scalp vein needles, intravenous (IV) fluid, appropriate connection tubing flushed with IV solution and fully assembled, tape, and a sterile dressing.

Procedure

The arm should be placed in a resting position and the tourniquet positioned above the antecubital fossa. Dangling the arm over the side of the bed for 1–2 minutes should make veins more visible. If possible, the patient should be asked to pump the fist in order to bring blood to the superficial veins. Tapping or flicking the veins sharply, thus paralyzing the intrinsic vascular tone, may make them stand up more prominently. Sterilize the skin after identifying the target vein, apply traction to the vein distal to the puncture site, puncture skin with the bevel of the needle pointed upward, and advance the needle slowly into the lumen of the vein. When a flash of blood is seen, advance only 1 mm more and watch for continued blood return. Then, slowly advance the catheter over the needle, gently leaving the catheter in the vein. Release the tourniquet, withdraw the needle, and attach IV tubing. Tape the

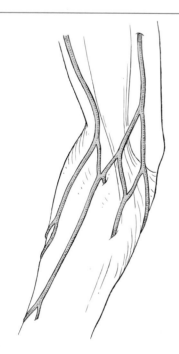

Figure 13–1. Positioning for peripheral venipuncture.

IV catheter securely to the skin and cover with a sterile dressing. Occasionally, the fluid will run more smoothly if the hub of the needle is slightly elevated by a small portion of folded tape or gauze, thereby depressing the tip into the lumen. It may be necessary to immobilize the hand when using a vein in the hand or wrist.

Possible complications of this procedure include hematoma, cellulitis, thrombosis, and extravasation. Local pain during infusion should cause suspicion of infiltration of the fluid being administered outside the vein into the surrounding tissue. The infusion should be stopped immediately and the intravenous catheter removed.

CENTRAL VENOUS ACCESS

1. SUBCLAVIAN VENIPUNCTURE: INFRACLAVICULAR APPROACH

The indications for a subclavian vein venipuncture utilizing the infraclavicular approach include inadequate peripheral venous access, the need to provide rapid infusion of fluids or blood products, the need for total parenteral nutrition, and the need to provide access for central venous or pulmonary artery pressure monitoring. A careful history and physical examination for evidence of previous catheters, trauma, clavicular fractures, radiation, and surgery should be carried out. The skin should be inspected for collateral veins or edema, which suggest that the subclavian vein is occluded. Findings from careful examination will help determine the best site for catheter placement.

Catheters can be single-, double-, or triple-lumen. Catheters to be used for long periods of time have a Dacron felt cuff to act as a barrier and are made of silicone rubber. These long-term catheters are designed to be placed through a subcutaneous tunnel between the venipuncture site and the skin exit site. Catheters designed for hemodialysis have a separation of 1–2 cm between the tip of the two lumens and are usually at least 12 French. Pre-assembled catheter insertion kits are available and have the following necessary items: the catheter, a guide-wire, a dilator with a tear-away sheath, local anesthetic (10 mL of 1% lidocaine), an insertion needle and syringe, sutures, a scalpel, gauze, tape, and a sterile dressing.

Procedure

The patient should be placed in a supine position, 15 degrees Trendelenburg or greater, to distend the veins and prevent air embolism (Figure 13–2). The head should be turned away from the venipuncture site.

After the patient is positioned, use sterile techniques to prep and drape the infraclavicular area. Continue the infusion of the local anesthetic medially; inject lidocaine into the skin at the venipuncture site 2 cm (approximately 2 finger-breadths) below the clavicle and at the junction of the middle and lateral thirds of the clavicle. Medially, inject the clavicular periosteum as well as the soft tissues

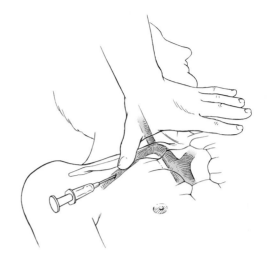

Figure 13–2. Positioning for subclavian venipuncture: infraclavicular approach.

along the anticipated tract toward the subclavian vein puncture site.

A large-caliber needle attached to a 6-mL syringe is used to puncture the skin at an angle. The needle and the syringe should then be lowered to a plane parallel to the frontal plane. The fingers of the opposite hand are placed in the suprasternal notch. While gently aspirating the syringe, advance the needle medially, posterior to the clavicle and toward the suprasternal notch. When a free flow of blood appears in the syringe, remove the syringe from the needle, carefully holding the needle in position and occluding the needle hub with a finger. Quickly insert the guide-wire into the needle hub and advance it (Seldinger technique) through the needle into the vein. If resistance is encountered, do not continue to advance the wire. Never forcefully withdraw the wire or use a "to and fro" motion, as such actions have resulted in shearing the wire, which may then embolize. If necessary, withdraw the wire and reposition the needle and syringe until a free flow of blood is again visible.

After the wire is advanced easily and smoothly into the vein, withdraw the needle, leaving the wire in place. Make a small nick in the skin at the wire insertion site. Pass the dilator over the wire, advance it into the insertion site, and withdraw, creating a tunnel. Advance the catheter over the wire by withdrawing the wire through the catheter. Grasp the wire as it exits the other end of the catheter, then advance the catheter into the vein. While holding the catheter in place, withdraw the rest of the wire. The tip of the catheter should be right above the atrium. Aspirate the lumen of the catheter to clear air and flush with heparinized saline. Suture the catheter to the skin, apply antibacterial ointment, and secure a sterile dressing to the skin exit site. It is advisable to obtain a portable upright chest radiograph to check for line placement and possible pneumothorax.

For long-term catheters, a subcutaneous tunnel is developed once the guide-wire has been placed. Inject skin and subcutaneous tissue with 1% lidocaine along the subcutaneous tract from the wire to a convenient exit site on the anterior chest. By creating a subcutaneous tract, and therefore increasing the distance between the vein and the skin exit site, infections of the vein are reduced significantly.

Direct a thin alligator clamp or tunneling device from the venipuncture site to the selected skin exit site through the anesthetized subcutaneous tissue. Make a small nick at the exit site and bring the tip of the clamp or tunneling device through it. Grasp the tip of the catheter with the clamp or secure the catheter to the tunneling device with a suture. Pull the catheter through the tunnel, leaving the catheter barrier cuff within the subcutaneous tissue approximately one half of the way between the two sites. After the dilator is used, a peel or tear-away sheath is placed over the dilator and both are passed again over the wire into the subclavian vein. The wire and dilator are removed and the catheter is quickly passed through the sheath. While holding the catheter in place, the tear-away sheath is removed, leaving the catheter in the vein. A good way to estimate the length of the catheter to be used is to lay the catheter in a gentle curve over the skin along the imagined route to a point four finger-breadths below the sternal notch on the midline of the sternum.

2. INTERNAL JUGULAR VENIPUNCTURE

The indications for this procedure are similar to those of the subclavian venipuncture, as is the equipment used for this procedure, except a 20-gauge "finder" needle is first used to identify the vein.

Procedure

For this procedure, the patient is positioned supine, in at least 15 degrees Trendelenburg with the head down and turned slightly away from the insertion site (Figure 13–3). The mastoid process and sternal notch should be palpated, and an imaginary line should be projected between them. Landmarks for this procedure are the triangle formed by the lower two heads of the sternocleidomastoid and the clavicle. The edge will stand out distinctly when the patient's head is turned away from the side selected for insertion of the catheter.

After positioning the patient, inject the skin with lidocaine at the apex of the triangle defined by the two heads of the sternocleidomastoid. With the finder needle attached to a 3-mL syringe, puncture the skin at the apex of the triangle defined by the two heads of the sternocleidomastoid, and advance the needle while gently aspirating the syringe in a direction parallel to the sagittal plane and 30 degrees posterior to the frontal plane.

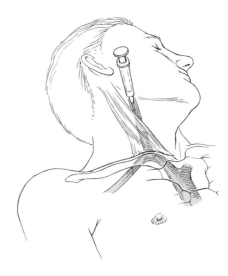

Figure 13–3. Positioning for subclavian jugular venipuncture.

When blood is aspirated make note of the trajectory of the needle and insert the larger introducer needle in the same direction. The finder needle may then be withdrawn. After blood is aspirated and freely flows into the syringe, carefully hold the position of the needle hub and remove the syringe. Immediately cover the needle hub with a finger, then advance the guide-wire through the needle. Withdraw the needle slowly and make a small nick in the skin at the wire entry point with a scalpel. Advance and withdraw the dilator over the guide-wire, then advance the catheter over the wire, slowly withdrawing the wire through the catheter, until it exits the hub end of the catheter. Then, continue to slowly insert the catheter while withdrawing the wire. Hold the catheter in place and, when the proper length of catheter has been inserted, withdraw the wire. Aspirate and flush the lumen of the catheter. Suture the catheter to the skin, apply antibiotic ointment to the skin exit site, and cover the exit site with a sterile dressing.

It is advisable to obtain an upright portable chest radiograph to check for line placement and possible pneumothorax. Possible complications for this procedure include hematoma, cellulitis, thrombosis, phlebitis, arterial puncture, pneumothorax, nerve injury, chylothorax, arteriovenous fistula, and bacteremia.

3. FEMORAL VENIPUNCTURE

Femoral venipuncture is indicated to obtain central venous access in a bed-bound patient or if subclavian or jugular access is not available. The equipment used for this procedure is similar to that used for the subclavian venipuncture.

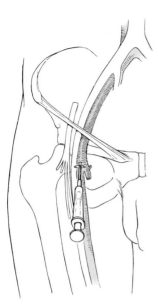

Figure 13–4. Positioning for femoral venipuncture.

Procedure

The patient should be placed in a supine position (Figure 13–4). The patient's proximal thigh should be prepped and draped in a sterile manner. Inject lidocaine into the skin 1 cm medial to the femoral pulse and several centimeters distal to the inguinal ligament. Palpate the femoral artery with the fingers of the left hand as a method of localizing the femoral vein, which lies medial to the artery. At a 30-degree angle to the frontal plane, advance the needle bevel up, cephalad, 1 cm medial to the arterial pulse. When venous blood freely flows into the syringe, lower the angle slightly and advance 1 cm more, ensure good blood return, then detach the syringe and partially advance the wire through the needle. Remove the needle, and make a small nick in the skin at the wire insertion site. Advance and then withdraw the dilator over the guide-wire. Advance the catheter over the wire by withdrawing the wire through the catheter. Grasp the wire as it exits the catheter hub, then place the catheter into the vein and remove the wire. Secure the catheter to the skin with a suture, apply antibacterial ointment, and secure a sterile dressing to the skin. Aspirate and flush the catheter lumen.

Possible complications from this procedure include arterial puncture, pseudoaneurysm, arteriovenous fistula, hematoma, cellulitis, phlebitis, and bacteremia.

VENOUS CUTDOWNS

There are many indications for venous cutdowns, including access for administration of fluids during shock and resuscitation, monitoring of central venous pressure,

and rapid or massive blood transfusions; venous cutdowns are also indicated when peripheral veins are unsuitable for standard venipuncture and venous infusions. The necessary equipment for this procedure includes a scalpel, 2-0 silk ties, a curved hemostat, nylon sutures, IV cannula, tubing, and sterile dressing.

Procedure

The preferred site for this procedure is the greater saphenous vein at the ankle (Figure 13–5). Alternate sites include the cephalic vein at the wrist, the basilic vein in the antecubital space, the cephalic vein at the shoulder, and the external jugular vein. The saphenous vein at the ankle is certainly the vein of choice when time is essential. It is identified approximately 2 cm anterior and superior to the medial malleolus. Prep and drape the skin in as sterile a manner as possible, given the situation or emergent circumstances. Inject lidocaine into the skin. Make a full-thickness, 3-cm transverse skin incision. Using a curved hemostat, bluntly dissect to identify the vein and dissect it free from the surrounding tissue. Approximately 2 cm of the vein should be exposed. Ligate the distal mobilized vein, leaving the suture intact for traction. Pass a tie around the proximal vein. Make a small transverse venotomy and gently dilate the vein with the closed tips of the hemostat. While holding traction on the distal tie, advance the cannula into the vein and secure the upper tie around the vein with the cannula in place. Attach IV tubing, close the incision with sutures, and apply a sterile dressing.

Possible complications include cellulitis, thrombophlebitis, and hematoma.

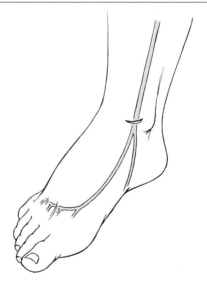

Figure 13–5. Positioning for a venous cutdown at the greater saphenous vein at the ankle.

ARTERIAL ACCESS

Indications for arterial access include continuous blood pressure monitoring and the necessity for frequent arterial blood sampling. The catheters for this procedure are usually single-lumen silastic IV cannulas, 18–22 gauge. Pre-assembled catheters come with a blood chamber and guide-wire already in place. A local anesthetic (10 mL of 1% lidocaine), sutures (for patients in the intensive care unit), and a sterile dressing are also necessary for this procedure.

Procedure

The most common site for arterial access is the radial artery. Radial arterial lines are placed in the distal radial artery at or just proximal to the wrist (Figure 13–6). The patient's history should be reviewed thoroughly, with particular note taken of any previous vascular surgery or access procedure, or symptoms or signs of any peripheral vascular disease. Check pulses and the condition of the extremity. If possible, the Allen test should be performed to assess the existence of adequate flow from the ulnar artery.

The procedure is performed by exposing the volar wrist and forearm. The area should be prepped and draped in a sterile manner. Inject lidocaine into the skin. Insert the catheter over the needle at an angle of 30–45 degrees. When arterial blood flashes, lower the angle and advance the needle slightly. With continued blood return, thread the catheter into the artery. If using a guide-wire system, advance the wire when blood returns, then advance the catheter over the wire. Alternatively, one can transfix the artery by passing through it, then slowly withdrawing the needle until blood returns. Attach pressure monitoring equipment as necessary and apply a sterile dressing to the skin. For long-term use in the intensive care unit, the catheter should be secured with sutures.

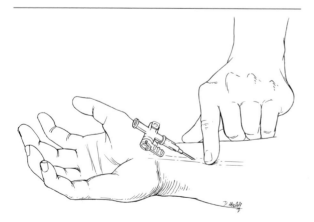

Figure 13–6. Positioning for arterial access at the distal radial artery.

Possible complications from this procedure include hematoma, pseudoaneurysm, arteriovenous fistula, thrombosis, hand ischemia, infections, and bacteremia.

CHEST TUBE PLACEMENT & REMOVAL

Indications for a tube thoracostomy, or chest tube placement, include pneumothorax, hemothorax, effusion, installation of intrapleural sclerosing agents, and empyema.

Hemothorax or empyema require larger chest tubes (32–36 French). Pneumothorax or malignant effusion can be managed with smaller tubes (20–28 French). The necessary equipment for this procedure also includes a drainage apparatus based on a three-bottle system with a trap, an underwater seal, a suction control, scalpel, Kelly clamp, local anesthetic (10 mL of 1% lidocaine), sutures (0 silk), and an occlusive dressing. Most centers have compartmentalized plastic chest drainage units, combining all the necessary elements.

Procedure

Positioning for this procedure is shown in Figure 13–7. The insertion site should be at or above the nipple level at the fifth intercostal space and in the anterior axillary line. The procedure begins with the patient in the supine position with the arm abducted and the hand placed behind the head, if possible. Parenteral sedation and analgesia should be provided if the patient's condition permits. The skin and subcutaneous tissue over the fifth rib in the anterior axillary line should be infiltrated with 1% lidocaine. Advance the needle through the intercostal space superior to the fifth rib until entering the pleural space as confirmed by aspirating air or fluid. Pull back the needle until just out of the pleural space and inject more lidocaine. Make a 2-cm transverse incision through the skin and subcutaneous tissue overlying the fifth intercostal space. With a Kelly clamp, tunnel over the fifth rib into the fourth intercostal space then spread the intercostal muscles to the level of the pleura. Close the clamp and puncture the pleura, entering the pleural space. Spread the clamp widely to enlarge the hole and pass a gloved finger into the pleural space to palpate for adhesions. Grasp the tip of the chest tube within the Kelly clamp and guide it into the pleural space. The radio-opaque marker line indicates the last hole which must be placed within the pleural cavity. The tube should be secured to the skin with large sutures (0 silk), and the tube should be connected to the suction drainage system. It should be noted that condensation in the tubing during respiration is a sign of intrapleural placement.

An occlusive dressing should be applied and all tubing connections should be checked and secured with tape. If possible, obtain a portable chest film to confirm proper

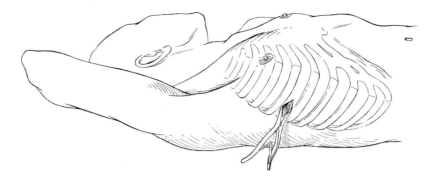

Figure 13–7. Positioning for insertion site of chest tube.

positioning and check for adequate drainage or lung re-expansion.

Possible complications include injury to intercostal vessels, nerves, great vessels, pulmonary structures, or abdominal organs as well as tube malposition and dislodgement, infection, and empyema.

The chest tube is removed when it is no longer indicated, typically for a pneumothorax if an air leak is not detectable for 24 hours, or for a drainage tube if the drainage has decreased to an acceptable amount (60–100 mL/24 h).

The equipment used to remove a chest tube includes a scalpel and occlusive dressing. Administer parenteral sedation, remove the old dressings, cut the sutures, and clean the skin. Keep pressure on the skin around the tube while removing it quickly when the patient is exhaling or performing the Valsalva maneuver. Apply an occlusive dressing for 24–48 hours.

THORACENTESIS

The primary indications for thoracentesis are the evacuation of air or fluid in the pleural space and the diagnosis of these conditions. The necessary equipment for this procedure includes materials for skin preparation, a local anesthetic (10 mL of 1% lidocaine), a 50-mL Luer-Lok syringe, 5-mL Luer-Lok, 18-gauge (2-inch) needle or 15-gauge (2-inch) needle, three-way stopcock, two Kelly clamps, tubing, specimen bowl, and a sterile dressing.

Procedure

Before beginning this procedure, it is vital to review the most current erect chest x-ray in order to verify the diagnosis, location, and approximate amount of pleural air or liquid. For removal of air, the patient should be in the supine position, the head slightly elevated, and the arm held over the head for a right-sided lateral approach. The entry site is the second or third intercostal space, midclavicular line (with care to avoid the internal mammary artery). For removal of liquid, the patient should be sitting

with his or her head and arms resting on a supporting bedside table in to order facilitate a posterior approach (Figure 13–8). The entry site is determined by measuring the fluid level within the lungs using percussion. The needle should be passed through one interspace lower than this level (but no lower than the eighth intercostal space to avoid puncture of the liver or spleen) superior to the margin of the rib in order to avoid the intercostal bundle. The needle should infiltrate just through the pleura (a slight "give" will be felt after it has been penetrated).

Infiltrate the local anesthetic, then aspirate in order to confirm the presence of fluid or air. Use the clamp to mark the needle at the level of dermal entry. The needle should then be withdrawn with the clamp in place. The thoracentesis needle should be marked to the same depth with a clamp. This precaution helps to prevent laceration of the lung with the needle. Interpose a three-way stop-

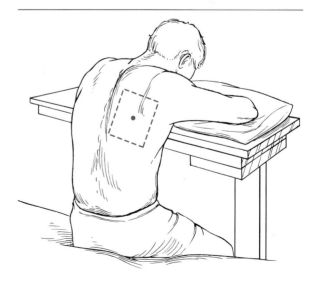

Figure 13–8. Positioning for a thoracentesis using the posterior approach.

cock between the needle (15-gauge for liquid or 18-gauge for air) and the 50-mL Luer-Lok syringe. Take care not to open the needle to atmosphere through the stopcock. Aspirate the specimen through the three-way stopcock, and send it to the laboratory for the appropriate laboratory studies. Remove the needle and apply a sterile dressing. Obtain an upright portable chest radiograph in order to assess the amount of fluid removed and to check for any signs of a pneumothorax.

It is generally acknowledged that thoracentesis should be used only to evaluate the initial pleural effusion and to relieve acute onset of respiratory problems. Repeated procedures may lead to hypoproteinemia and a decrease in osmotic pressure, which may lead to a rapid recurrence of pleural fluid collection.

Complications from this procedure include laceration of an intercostal vessel, pneumothorax (either from lung laceration or opening of the three-way stopcock, which leaves the lung cavity open to the atmosphere), and hepatic or splenic puncture.

LUMBAR PUNCTURE

Indications for this procedure include examination or therapeutic removal of cerebrospinal fluid (CSF) and administration of diagnostic or therapeutic agents. The equipment for this procedure is available in most hospitals as a pre-packaged, disposable, sterile kit that includes a three-way stopcock, manometer, collection tubes, 22-gauge (1.5-inch) and 25-gauge (5/8-inch) needles (for anesthetic), 18-gauge (3-inch) and 20-gauge (3-inch) spinal needles (with stilette), local anesthetic (10 mL of 1% lidocaine), towels, sponges, Betadine, and a sterile dressing.

Procedure

The correct position for this procedure is the lateral decubitus with the patient's back at the very edge of the bed and the knees, arms, and neck pulled toward the body (Figure 13–9). It may be helpful to instruct the patient, "Push your back towards me," in order to get maximum exposure. The puncture site is located between the L4 and L5 or L5 and S1 vertebrae.

Aseptic technique in this procedure is of the utmost importance to avoid contamination of the CSF. Any type of infection near the puncture site is a contraindication to this procedure. To avoid infection, the puncture site should be prepped thoroughly and draped in a sterile fashion.

A wheal of local anesthetic is infiltrated into the site between the chosen vertebrae. The spinal needle should then be introduced between the same vertebrae, but not at the same location where the skin was perforated by the infiltrating needle. This is a precaution to prevent red cells from being picked up from the earlier puncture site. The spinal needle should be advanced slowly with a 30-degree cephalad inclination. If bone is encountered at a shallow depth, the needle should be redirected in a more cephalad fashion. When bone is encountered at a deeper level, the needle should be redirected in a more caudal direction. Advance the needle until the "give" of the ligamentum flavum is felt. At this point, ask the patient to carefully stretch out the neck and legs and begin carefully removing the stilette at 2-mm intervals to check for flow of CSF. If intracranial pressure is suspected, the stilette should be removed with excessive caution to avoid a sudden gush of CSF. However, in most cases, increased intracranial pressure is a contraindication to this procedure.

Once the flow of CSF begins, check the opening pressure with the manometer. The normal range is 70–180 mm CSF. The CSF should then be collected into the sterile containers. Before dressing the wound, measure the closing pressure. Instruct the patient to remain lying down for the next 12–24 hours in order to avoid what is commonly referred to as a "spinal headache."

There are a number of complications associated with this procedure, including meningitis, subdural hematoma, spinal epidural hematoma, dry tap, and spinal headache (usually transient).

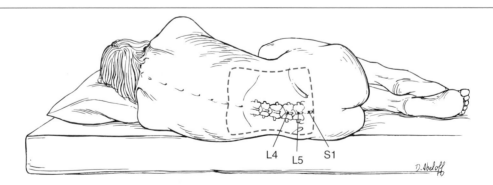

Figure 13–9. Lateral decubitus position for lumbar puncture.

NASOGASTRIC INTUBATION

Indications for nasogastric intubation include gastric decompression, sampling of gastric contents for analysis, placement of a feeding tube, or lavage of gastric contents. The equipment for this procedure includes a tube (16 French for adults and 12 French for children), bulb syringe, stethoscope, suction or feeding device (if necessary), water-soluble lubricant, anesthesia spray or gel, cup with water and straw, and tape.

Procedure

For this procedure, the patient who is awake should be in a sitting or semi-sitting position with the head slightly back and supported. Cooperation is very important to the success of the procedure, therefore, you should approach the patient with confidence and reassurance.

Nasogastric intubation is best performed with an assistant who will hold the water and the patient, if necessary. For a more comfortable passage, apply an anesthetic spray or gel to the posterior pharynx and nasal passage. While the anesthetic is taking effect, lubricate the tip of the tube to make passage through the nose easier.

Ask the assistant or the patient to place the straw between the patient's lips. Instruct the patient to drink when asked and keep drinking as quickly as possible. This is a very effective way to prevent coughing and gagging, as it actually lubricates the tube as it passes through the hypopharynx. Keep in mind that if gagging occurs it is usually transitory, and once the tube enters the esophagus it will stop.

While holding the tube, inspect the nares for any obstructions or deviations. The tube should be passed gently along the floor of the nasal passageway. This is almost directly posterior (Figure 13–10). A common error is to direct the tube posteriorly and superiorly. The tube may then be lost in the turbinates, causing pain or bleeding. Occasionally, an unforeseen obstruction may necessitate switching to the opposite side.

The patient should be told to drink, and keep drinking, when the tube begins to curve downward toward the pharynx. The average distance to the esophagogastric junction in the adult should be marked on the tube (~ 50 cm in adults). In most instances, it is best to advance beyond this point, then withdraw the tube slowly with aspiration until the ideal position is located. The other option is to insufflate the stomach with 50–100 mL of air while listening with a stethoscope for the sound of bubbling gastric contents.

When the tube is appropriately positioned, secure it with tape in such a manner that it does not rest against the nares, as pressure necrosis can occur. The tube should then be attached to the proper suction or feeding device.

Possible complications of this procedure include gagging and vomiting, airway occlusion, epistaxis, and injury to the mucosa of the posterior pharynx or esophageal perforation (virtually eliminated by softer tubes). Complications such as laryngeal edema, sinusitis, and pharyngeal or

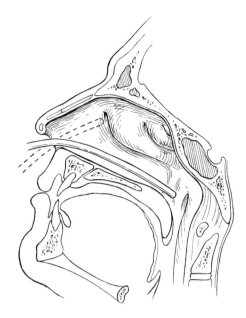

Figure 13–10. Proper course for a nasogastric tube is shown with a solid line. The tube passes almost directly backward along the floor of the nasal passage. A common mistake of angling the tube superiorly is indicated by the dotted lines.

esophageal erosion occur with greater frequency in the pediatric population. These patients should be monitored carefully.

URETHRAL CATHETERIZATION

Indications for urethral catheterizations include relief of urethral obstruction or postoperative retention, continuous monitoring of urinary output, decompression of the bladder (including preoperative decompression to ensure that the bladder will not be incised when opening the wound), and collection of an uncontaminated specimen for analysis or culture. Although catheters are often suspected of being the cause of serious urinary tract infections, allowing the bladder to become overly distended may cause prolonged dysfunction and infection. The equipment for this procedure is available in most hospitals as a pre-packaged, disposable, sterile kit, which includes a 16 French Foley catheter attached to tubing and specimen bag, syringe with 10-mL sterile saline, water-soluble lubricant, Betadine, towels, sponges, tongs, and adhesive tape.

Procedure

For this procedure the patient should be in the supine position. Females should be in a "frog-leg" position. Take time to explain the procedure to the patient and give the patient the maximum degree of privacy. The patient should be prepped and draped in a sterile manner. Exposure in females may require an assistant to spread the labia or hold the thighs apart.

In males, if a foreskin is present, pull it back carefully with the left (or non-dominant) hand while holding the shaft of the penis firmly. In females, pull back the labia to expose the meatus. Cleanse the area with sponges moistened in prep solution held in the right (or dominant) hand with sterile tongs or a clamp to prevent contamination. If the dominant hand remains sterile, the catheter may be advanced with the fingers. In males, the penis is held in an upright position to straighten the prostatic urethra (Figure 13–11). Lubricate the distal two thirds of the catheter, then pass it following the anterior wall of the urethra. Advance the catheter until urine is returned, then continue to proceed for about 2–3 cm to ensure that the balloon will not be inflated in the urethra. Gently inflate the catheter balloon with sterile water. If any resistance is encountered, stop immediately. This may mean the balloon is still within the urethra. Advance the catheter further and proceed with inflation. Slowly withdraw the catheter until the balloon rests against the bladder neck. The tubing, not the catheter, should be taped to the patient's leg in such a way as to prevent tension on the bladder neck. In uncircumcised males, reposition the foreskin over the glans to prevent paraphimosis.

Complications from this procedure include creation of a false passage, sepsis, urethral disruption or tear, and hematuria. In elderly males, rapid decompression of a distended bladder following catheter placement has been reported as a cause of shock. In cases of severe distension, it is best to drain off urine in smaller increments until the bladder is emptied.

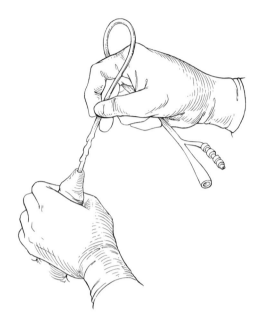

Figure 13–11. The left hand immobilizes the penile shaft for male urethral catheterization. The right hand (or dominant hand) should touch nothing but the catheter in order to ensure a sterile field.

SUGGESTED READING

Calman KC, Hanning CD: *Basic Skills in Clinical Medicine: A Guide to Ward Procedure for Students and House Officers.* Churchill Livingstone, 1984.

Vander-Salm TJ, Cutler BS, Wheeler HB: *Atlas of Bedside Procedures*, 2nd ed. Little, Brown, 1988.

Zimmerman CE: *Techniques of Patient Care.* Little, Brown, 1970.

Critical Care & Burn Management

14

Basic Considerations in Critical Care

Adam Seiver, MD

▶ Key Facts

- ▶ Two types of surgical patients are admitted to the Intensive Care Unit (ICU): (1) those who have undergone major operations without complications but require close monitoring, and (2) surgical patients who require organ support through a period of multiple organ dysfunction.

- ▶ The basic physiologic needs of the critical care patient are oxygen transport, maintenance of milieu intérieur, nutrition, host defense, and cellular regulation.

- ▶ Optimal care in the ICU requires excellent teamwork, which results from physicians, nurses, and other clinicians working together in a collegial fashion with the good of the patient as the foremost concern.

- ▶ A "command and control" management style between the physician and nurse in a critical care setting is out-of-date and ineffective. A better role for the critical care physician to assume is that of "coach."

- ▶ Because the critically ill patient will frequently be unable to communicate with the care team, it is important to initiate a conversation with the patient's family to gain insight into patient preferences for clinical decision making.

- ▶ To formulate an assessment and plan, a thorough evaluation of body systems, phase of care, and interventional requirements (ie, surgical, radiologic, medical, and nutritional) is required.

Skill in caring for the critically ill patient, like all surgical skills, requires immersive experience. There is no substitute for time at the patient's bedside, gaining direct exposure to the applied physiology encountered with the use of ventilators, inotropes, fluids and electrolytes, total parenteral nutrition, and the various monitoring technologies. One's first exposure to critical care, however, may seem like trying to drink from a fire hydrant. The goal of this section is to provide a framework that gives educational structure to the experience of caring for critically ill surgical patients.

PATIENT TYPES

Surgical patients admitted to critical care units start with a wide variety of diagnoses and follow unique clinical paths. Within this apparent inhomogeneity, however, we may distinguish recurrent patterns. Indeed, the clinical courses tend to follow two distinct trajectories.

HISTORICAL FACTS

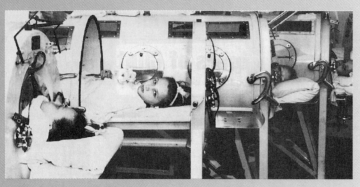

Children in iron lungs in 1950.

Today's critical care has been woven together from several different lines of development. As early as 1923 at Johns Hopkins, a special postoperative room was instituted. In 1942, a special ward was set up at the Massachusetts General Hospital to care for the victims of a fire at the Coconut Grove nightclub. The development of respirators in the 1950s led to a centralization of patients, staff, and equipment in specialized respiratory care units. This trend was accentuated by the polio epidemic of the early 1950s in Los Angeles and in Scandinavia.

In 1958, Peter Safar, one of the leaders in the development of cardiopulmonary resuscitation, organized a special care unit at the Baltimore City Hospital and introduced the term "intensive care unit." The heading "intensive care" first appeared in the Index Medicus in the 1955–9 edition.

The 1960s and 1970s saw the rapid development of monitoring technologies. Telemetry developed in the space program was applied to civilian electrocardiographic monitoring with the development of coronary care units in the 1960s. Cardiac catheterization was pioneered by Werner Forsman, a young German surgeon who catheterized himself in 1929. This work was rediscovered by André Counand and Dickinson Richards, who used cardiac catheterization to study traumatic shock in 1940. In the 1970s, balloon technology developed for the embolectomy catheter by a vascular surgeon, Thomas Fogarty, was combined with cardiac catheterization techniques to produce the flotation pulmonary artery catheter introduced by Swann and Ganz.

In the 1980s, critical care units proliferated with the development of subspecialty areas for cardiac surgery, neonatology, neurosurgery, and shock/trauma. There are now over 7,400 units in the United States, which consume approximately 1% of the gross national product in annual resources.

OBSERVATION & MONITORING

The first trajectory is typically traced by patients who have undergone major operations and who have not experienced complications, but who are admitted to the ICU to facilitate close observation and timely management of any complications that might develop. For these patients, the ICU functions as an extended recovery area postoperatively. Complications for which these patients are monitored include airway problems, respiratory failure, fluid and electrolyte abnormalities, oliguria, postoperative bleeding, and arrhythmias.

Until recently, the monitoring equipment that helped the clinical team provide close observation—including ECG monitors, pulse oximeters, and blood pressure transducers—was expensive and bulky. Patients requiring this equipment were managed in centralized ICU areas. This equipment is now much cheaper and portable. This makes it possible for any bed in the hospital (or even perhaps in outpatient areas) to serve as a monitored bed.

It is likely that changes in practice triggered by pressure to reduce costs will continue to reduce the number of intensive care bed days used for simply monitoring postoperative patients. Over the next 5–10 years, selected patients may be managed completely outside of the traditional ICU setting.

MULTIPLE ORGAN DYSFUNCTION

The second group of patients are surgical patients managed in the ICU to allow the provision of organ support through a period of multiple organ dysfunction. The common feature of these patients is that they suffer from an insult that provokes generalized inflammation. The most common stimuli are shock and infection, but tissue injury—operative, traumatic, or thermal—or processes such as pancreatitis can trigger the response as well. The clinical signs and symptoms of generalized inflammation are recognized as the Systemic Inflammatory Response Syndrome. Patients with this syndrome experience generalized cellular dysregulation, immune-mediated endothelial injury, and ultimately organ dysfunction, including immune system compromise.

It is possible for the significant organ dysfunction of this syndrome to be reversed and the patient saved. Typically, however, this requires a stay of several weeks in the ICU. Furthermore, with current approaches, in about half of such patients, the organ failure becomes progressive and the patient dies.

Unlike the patients admitted solely for monitoring, patients with multi-organ failure are not likely to be displaced from the ICU by cost-driven practice pattern changes. Indeed, extrapolation of current trends suggests that as more and more conditions are managed on an ambulatory basis, inpatient hospitals will evolve into large intensive care units and that multi-organ failure patients will dominate the census in these future units.

GOALS OF MANAGEMENT IN THE ICU

Critical care results when a physician assumes responsibility for ensuring that a patient's basic cellular needs are met. These needs can be organized into the following categories: oxygen transport, maintenance of the milieu intérieur, nutrition, host defense, and cellular regulation.

OXYGEN TRANSPORT

A cell requires energy to maintain its integrity by offsetting the flux of solutes and metabolites across its permeable membrane. This energy is derived from the metabolism of glucose and fat and stored with the creation of high-energy phosphate bonds in adenosine triphosphate (ATP). Because aerobic metabolism produces far greater energy than anerobic metabolism, a ready supply of oxygen is essential for the survival of cells. Nerve cells are particularly dependent upon oxygen and become irreversibly injured if oxygen is not available for more than 10 minutes.

Ensuring adequate availability of oxygen to cells is, therefore, the most critical obligation of the critical care physician. Oxygen transport is a complex process and involves multiple organ systems, with the pulmonary, cardiovascular, and blood systems each contributing essential components. The pathophysiology, identification, and treatment of inadequate oxygen delivery is presented in Chapter 15.

MAINTENANCE OF THE MILIEU INTÉRIEUR

The physiologist Claude Bernard used the term "milieu intérieur" to describe the fluid bathing the cells of an organism. He recognized that many physiologic mechanisms were aimed at maintaining this internal environment. In critical illness these homeostatic mechanisms are lost, and maintenance of the milieu intérieur becomes, in part, the responsibility of the physician. As in oxygen transport, a number of organ systems are normally involved, with primary roles played by the pulmonary, renal, and gastrointestinal systems. The pathophysiology, identification, and treatment of disturbances in the milieu intérieur are presented in Chapter 19, which includes acid-base disturbances.

NUTRITION

Cells not only require a finely tuned internal environment, but they also need to consume substrates drawn from that environment, including glucose, protein, fats, vitamins, and trace elements. In critical illness, the physician has an essential responsibility to ensure that adequate nutrition is provided. Critically ill surgical patients are usually physiologically stressed by wounds or infection, or both, and nutritional requirements are frequently altered and increased. Additionally, the gastrointestinal system may be unable to serve adequately in its usual primary role. The provision of nutrition, including both parenteral (intravenous) nutrition and enteral (gut) nutrition, is presented in Chapter 20.

HOST DEFENSE

In health, the human body maintains a vigilant defense against invasive organisms, including viruses, bacteria, fungi, and parasites. The defense mechanisms include physical barriers as well as the many cellular and humoral components of the immune system. In fact, these "good fences" make "good neighbors" of many microorganisms. In the gastrointestinal tract, for example, the body maintains a symbiotic relationship with a wide variety of bacterial species. In the critically ill patient, the defense mechanisms are altered and the body becomes vulnerable to infection, even from organisms that are ordinarily non-threatening.

Infection is often the initiating factor for critical illness. For example, abdominal infection with peritonitis often results from delayed surgical management of the acute abdomen (as with appendicitis, cholecystitis, or diverticulitis) or from surgical complications, such as an anastomotic breakdown; this typically leads to hospitalization in an intensive care unit, particularly in the elderly.

Additionally, infection frequently complicates intensive care management of other conditions, such as shock. The usual physical barriers that defend the blood, lungs, kidneys, and soft tissue from infection are often breached by surgical wounds and by standard management procedures in the critically ill, including intravascular monitoring lines (particularly those in the central veins), endotracheal tubes, and bladder catheters. Altered patterns of perfusion may weaken mucosal barriers, such as tissue lining the gut, and make the patient susceptible to direct invasion by normally symbiotic organisms in a process called **translocation**.

The critical care physician, thus, needs to assume responsibility for the patient's defense against microorganisms. The management of surgical infections and the appropriate use of antibiotics is presented in Chapter 16.

CELLULAR REGULATION

In health there is exquisite coordination of cellular function at many levels—between components within cells, between cells in organs, between organs in organ systems, and between organ systems in the human as a whole. A complex neurohumoral network supports intricate information flow to accomplish this coordination. It now appears that much of critical illness may be viewed as an inability to maintain homeostasis because of loss of coordination mechanisms. The result is altered cellular regulation—or cellular dysregulation—that leads to gene expression within cells of products that do not meet the basic physiologic needs for oxygen transport, for maintenance of the milieu intérieur, for nutrition, or for host defense. Even worse, this deleterious gene expression may communicate signals that lead to further dysregulation of other cells, organs, and organ systems. This self-perpetuating dysfunctional network is frequently triggered by shock or infection. It underlies the systemic inflammatory response syndrome and its dreaded complication, the multi-organ dysfunction syndrome. These are discussed in Chapter 17.

WORKING IN THE ICU: TEAM MANAGEMENT OF PATIENTS

Critical care is delivered round-the-clock, 365 days per year. Additionally, the complexity of critically ill patients requires a wide range of skills, experience, and knowledge that is frequently beyond the scope of a single clinician. Therefore, critical care is provided by a health care team.

Achieving effective teamwork in the ICU is challenging. Continuity of care is easily disrupted by handoffs occurring during transitions in staff coverage, such as change of nursing shift or physician on-call. Conflicting viewpoints about the patient's condition or about management strategy are inevitable, particularly given the narrow disciplinary perspective that is an unfortunate consequence of the fragmentation of medical care into subspecialties and micro-professional domains. Some tension between viewpoints is desirable because it leads to open discussion and prevents important patient care issues from being overlooked. In the extreme, however, it can lead to dysfunctional practices that are deleterious to patient care.

Excellent teamwork is encouraged when physicians, nurses, and other clinicians work together in a collegial fashion with the good of the patient as the foremost concern. Good working relationships require a substantial investment in communication. Listening is as important as speaking. Detailed orders that have a consistent format are extremely important. Examples of orders for each phase of care are illustrated in Figure 14–1.

A mistake that inexperienced physicians frequently make is to use the written physician orders as the primary means for communicating patient care plans. This casts the relationship between physician and nurse as one of "order-giver" and "order-taker." Such an approach evokes a "command-and-control" management style that is out-of-date and ineffective. A better approach is for the critical care physician to assume the role of "coach."

The emphasis should be on identifying and communicating the big picture, focusing attention on the key management issues, providing continuing education appropriate to the patient's evolving problems, and coordinating the activities of the many bedside team members. Clear and succinct orders are, of course, necessary, but they are but one element of an open, extended conversation among team members that leads to high-quality patient care.

The patient and the patient's family need to be part of this conversation. Family members are highly appreciative of efforts to keep them appraised of the patient's progress. Any constraints of confidentiality imposed by the patient must, of course, be respected. The critically ill patient will frequently be unable to communicate with the care team. This may create issues of guardianship when important decisions are encountered, such as whether to continue to provide intensive care in the face of a poor prognosis. In these situations, the family may provide important insight into the patient's preferences so that these can be incorporated into the decision.

Resuscitation Phase

Admit ICU

Diagnosis:
High risk for MODS because of Shock and/or Infection and/or Tissue Injury and/or Inflammation

Activity:
Bedrest

Diet:
NPO

Monitoring:
CVP, Pulmonary Art Cath—CCO/SvO$_2$ Art Line

IV:
Macrodrip NS TKO (blood line)

Meds:
Sedation/Analgesia/Muscle relaxation
Versed _____ bolus IV then _____ mg/h IV drip
Fentanyl _____ bolus IV then _____ mg/h IV drip
Vecuronium _____ bolus IV then _____ mg/h IV drip titrate to 1–2 twitches

Inotropes
Use after wedge 12 to 15 or _____ to _____
Goals: SvO$_2$ > 75 or _____ ; CI > 4.5 l/m^2 _____ ; MAP 75–85 or _____

Dopamine 3 mcg/kg/min or _____ to _____ mcg/kg/min
Epinephrine _____ to _____ ng/kg/min
Dobutamine _____ to _____ mcg/kg/min

Vasopressors
Norepinephrine titrate to keep MAP _____ to _____

Vasodilators
Nitroprusside titrate to keep MAP _____ to _____
Nitroglycerin 0.5 or _____ mcg/kg/min

Antibiotics

Other Meds:

Nutrition:
See TPN orders/Enteral feeding protocol

Vent Orders:
SIMV: Rate _____ ; TV _____ ; PEEP _____ ; FiO$_2$ _____ ; Pressure Support 10 or _____
Pressure Control: Rate _____ ; Pressure above PEEP _____ ; PEEP _____ ; FiO$_2$ _____

Special Care:
Bed: EfficaCC, Flexicare, Other _____
Splint extremities prn

Labs:
CBC, PT, PTT, Plts, CSP, q am
Lactate q 12 h until normal, then q 24 h
CXR q am
ABG q am and 20 min p vent change

Call HO T > 40°C. No cooling blanket or Tylenol unless specifically ordered.

A

Figure 14–1. Examples of detailed physician's orders for each phase of management of the critically ill patient. **A:** Resuscitation phase. **B:** Hypermetabolism phase. **C:** Weaning. **D:** Rehabilitation.

Hypermetabolism Phase

Diagnosis:
  High risk for MODS or
  Early MODS with ARDS and/or Brain and/or Hepatic and/or Renal Dysfunction
  Adequately resuscitated—lactate, SVO$_2$, CI ok and drips with infrequent adjustments

Monitoring:
  CVP, Pulmonary Art Cath—CCO/SvO$_2$, Art Line

IV:
  Macrodrip NS TKO (blood line)

Meds:
  Sedation/Analgesia
  Use transition protocol to switch to maintenance with methadone/Valium.

  Inotropes
    Dopamine   3 mcg/kg/min or _____ to _____ mcg/kg/min
    Epinephrine   _____ to _____ ng/kg/min
    Dobutamine   _____ to _____ mcg/kg/min

  Vasopressors
    Norepinephrine   titrate to keep MAP _____ to _____

  Vasodilators
    Nitroprusside   titrate to keep MAP _____ to _____
    Nitroglycerin   0.5 or _____ mcg/kg/min

  Antibiotics

Other Meds:
  Lasix _____ mg IV qd

Nutrition:
  See TPN orders/Enteral feeding protocol

Vent Orders:
  SIMV: Rate _____ ; TV _____ ; PEEP _____ ; FiO$_2$ _____ ; Pressure Support 10 or _____
  Pressure Control: Rate _____ ; Pressure above PEEP _____ ; PEEP _____ ; FiO$_2$ _____

Special Care:
  Bed: EfficaCC, Flexicare, Other _____
  PT/OT for ROM prn
  Splint extremities prn

Labs:
  Hct, CSP, lactate q am
  CXR q am
  ABG q am

Call HO T > 40°C. No cooling blanket or Tylenol unless specifically ordered.

B

Figure 14–1. Continued

Weaning

Diagnosis:
MODS improving with resolution of _____
ARDS, hepatic dysfunction, and renal dysfunction

Meds:
Sedation/Analgesia
Use protocol to wean off methadone/Valium
Propofol _____ to _____ mcg/kg/min for nighttime sedation 10 pm to 7 am

Inotropes
Dopamine   3 mcg/kg/min or _____ to _____ mcg/kg/min
Epinephrine   _____ to _____ ng/kg/min
Dobutamine   _____ to _____ mcg/kg/min

Vasopressors
Norepinephrine titrate to keep MAP _____ to _____

Vasodilators
Nitroprusside   titrate to keep MAP _____ to _____
Nitroglycerin   0.5 or _____ mcg/kg/min

Antibiotics

Other Meds:
Lasix _____ mg IV qd

Nutrition:
See TPN orders/Enteral feeding protocol

Vent Orders:
Use pressure support weaning protocol

Special Care:
Bed: EfficaCC, Flexicare, Other _____
PT/OT for ROM prn
Splint extremities prn

Labs:
Hct, CSP, lactate q am
CXR q am
ABG q am

Call HO T > 40°C. No cooling blanket or Tylenol unless specifically ordered.

C

Rehabilitation

Diagnosis:
MODS resolved and patient extubated or on trach collar

VS q 2 hr

Activity:
OOB at least tid

Diet:
Swallowing evaluation
If swallowing evaluation ok, then advance from soft to regular diet.

Special Care:
Regular bed
PT/OT consult

Meds:

Labs:

D

Figure 14–1. Continued

Table 14–1. Elements of typical case presentation.

Patient ID	
Hospital day, postoperative day, age, sex	Key elements of ICU course
Presenting problems and diagnoses, operative procedure	Significant events of last 24 hours

System-By-System Status	
Neurologic	
Glasgow Coma Scale—eye opening, verbal, and motor responses	Analgesics and sedative medications—drips, epidural, other
Respiratory	
Respiratory rate, spontaneous and total minute volume	Nasal canula, face mask
Maximal inspired force, vital capacity	Ventilator: mode, rate, tidal volume, PEEP, pressure support,
Arterial blood gas results, SaO_2	FiO_2
Cardiac	
Heart rate and rhythm	Cardiac output
CVP, PA pressures, wedge pressure, systemic arterial	Lactate measurement
pressure	Inotropes, vasopressors, balloon pump
Gastrointestinal	
Abdominal physical exam	Liver function tests, including bilirubin
Status of enteral feedings—diarrhea, residuals	Serum albumin
Renal	
Intakes and outputs—intravenous, enteral, urine, tubes, drains	Electrolytes, creatinine, BUN
Nutritional support—protein, calories, fats	
Hematologic	
CBC, coagulation tests	
Immunologic	
Culture results	Antibiotic therapy

Assessment and Plans	
Organ dysfunction status and trajectory	Resuscitation
Underlying surgical problem	Nutrition

BUN = blood urea nitrogen; CBC = complete blood count; CVP = central venous pressure; PA = pulmonary artery; PEEP = positive end-expiratory pressure.

CASE PRESENTATION

When making a case presentation, either orally or in the form of a written progress note, it is useful to use a consistent framework (Table 14–1). Remember that the depth of presentation is dependent on the context. The presentation on formal rounds will be much more detailed than the "bullet" presentation expected on work rounds.

The presentation should begin with an identification of the patient that briefly summarizes the key aspects of the patient's present illness and ICU course. Next, each of the major organ systems is reviewed. It is helpful for the subjective and objective findings to be presented together with the current therapy relevant to each organ system.

The neurologic status of the patient can be quickly summarized using the distinctions from the Glasgow Coma Scale. There are three dimensions: eye opening response, best verbal response, and best motor response. Eye opening is judged to be either *spontaneous, to voice, to pain, or none*. Best verbal response is graded as either *oriented, confused, inappropriate words, incomprehensible sounds, or none*. Best motor response ranges from *obeys command, localizes pain, withdraws to pain, flexion to pain, extension to pain, or none*. In the presentation, it is essential to mention any analgesic or sedative therapy to put the neurologic assessment in perspective.

Similarly, evaluation of respiratory measurements, such as blood gases, requires knowledge of concurrent therapy for evaluation. A PaO_2 of 80 mm Hg, for example, would suggest good gas exchange if the patient is breathing room air. If the patient is receiving an FiO_2 of 80%, however, the gas exchange would be quite poor.

When formulating the assessment and plan it is useful to make sure that the following questions are answered, since they address recurrent issues relevant to the critically ill surgical patient:

- Is the patient at risk for multiple organ dysfunction? If so, what is the status and trajectory of this dysfunction?
- Is the patient in the initial resuscitation phase, the period of stable hypermetabolism, the recovery phase, or the phase of rehabilitation?
- Have the patient's underlying surgical problems been addressed? Does the patient need imaging studies or operative intervention?
- Is resuscitation optimal? If not, what cardiorespiratory interventions are necessary to eliminate the shock?
- Is nutrition optimal? Is the patient receiving appropriate calories, protein, fats, vitamins, and trace elements? Can the patient be fed into the gut (enterally), or is intravenous (parenteral) nutrition necessary?

SUGGESTED READING

Covey SR: *Principle-Centered Leadership.* Summit Books, 1991.

Covey SR: *The Seven Habits of Highly Effective People: Restoring the Character Ethic.* Simon & Schuster, 1989.

Hammer M: *Engineering the Corporation: A Manifesto for Business Revolution.* Harper Business, 1993.

Seiver A: *Decision Analysis: A Framework for Critical Care Decision-Making.* Doctoral Dissertation, Dept. of Engineering-Economic Systems, Stanford University, 1992.

Sivak ED, Higgins TL, Seiver A: *The High Risk Patient: Management of the Critically Ill.* Williams & Wilkins, 1995.

Wilmore DW et al: *Care of the Surgical Patient: A Publication of the Committee on Pre and Postoperative Care.* Scientific American, 1988–1993.

15

Shock & Resuscitation

Adam Seiver, MD

▶ Key Facts

- ▶ A primary responsibility of the critical care physician is ensuring oxygen transport, which is essential for maintaining adequate cellular energetics.

- ▶ Shock may be defined as the pathological condition that develops when the cellular requirement for oxygen is not satisfied.

- ▶ Oxygen deficit is defined as the sum over time of the difference between oxygen demand and oxygen consumption.

- ▶ Oxygen demand is the total amount of oxygen per unit time that the body's cells require to maintain optimal metabolic activity.

- ▶ Surgical patients are likely to have a substantially increased demand for oxygen, as injury (operative or traumatic, especially burns) increases the metabolic rate.

- ▶ Oxygen consumption should be differentiated from oxygen demand in that it is defined as the amount of oxygen per unit time the patient actually consumes.

- ▶ Cardiac output is a product of heart rate and stroke volume. Decreased cardiac output is often a key component of shock syndromes.

- ▶ Four important shock syndromes are hypovolemic, cardiogenic, septic, and obstructive shock.

- ▶ The management of shock involves addressing the following seven control points in a systematic fashion: partial pressure of oxygen in the alveoli (PAO_2), ventilation–perfusion ratio ($\dot{V}/\dot{Q}$ relationship), hemoglobin, left ventricular filling pressure, left ventricular compliance, contractility, and afterload.

- ▶ Resuscitation proceeds in three phases: (1) primary resuscitation: airway, ventilation, oxygen; (2) secondary resuscitation: optimization of oxygen transport; and (3) monitor and titrate resuscitation.

A primary responsibility of the critical care physician is ensuring oxygen transport. Oxygen transport is essential for maintaining adequate cellular energetics. Without a constant supply of energy, cells are unable to maintain intracellular processes necessary for life. For example, loss of active ionic transport across membranes leads to cellu-

lar swelling and cell death. Cells can maintain some energy production in the absence of oxygen using anaerobic glycolysis. Anaerobic glycolysis, however, produces only 2 moles of adenosine triphosphate (ATP) per mole of glucose consumed, while aerobic glycolysis combined with oxidative phosphorylation through the Krebs cycle produces 38 moles of ATP. Oxygen is, thus, necessary to provide enough energy to ensure the survival of cells and ultimately the health of the entire body.

Shock may be defined as the pathological condition that develops when the cellular requirement for oxygen is not satisfied. Therefore, it is important to examine the pathophysiology of oxygen transport.

PATHOPHYSIOLOGY

A simple, aggregated, and holistic view of oxygen transport is presented in Figure 15–1. It shows oxygen transport to be the consequence of the interaction of three key components that can be somewhat arbitrarily labeled tissue, pulmonary, and cardiac. Let us consider each of these components and their subsidiary physiologic elements.

TISSUE

OXYGEN DEBT

As shown in Figure 15–1, **oxygen deficit** depends upon both oxygen demand and oxygen consumption. More specifically, it is defined as the sum over time of the difference between oxygen demand and oxygen consumption.

It is well accepted that large oxygen deficits that develop over minutes—such as in massive hemorrhage—lead to anoxic injury in vital organs, such as the brain and the heart, and result in death. While further investigation is required, current evidence strongly suggests that less clinically obvious oxygen deficits, including ones that develop over a longer period of hours to days, can play an important role in the development of organ failure. Organ failure, in turn, accounts for much of the surgical morbidity and mortality that occurs in the period of days to weeks following major injury or operation (see Chapter 17).

OXYGEN DEMAND

Oxygen demand is the total amount of oxygen per unit time that the body's cells require to maintain optimal metabolic activity. Oxygen demand tracks the patient's need for energy, which depends upon several factors. A heavier, taller, and younger patient will require more energy than a lighter, shorter, and older one. These factors are reflected in the Harris-Benedict equations for resting energy expenditure.

Temperature affects oxygen demand. For each degree Celsius increase (or decrease) in patient temperature, the patient's energy and oxygen requirements increase (or decrease) approximately 10%. Another key factor is the amount of work that a patient is doing—whether it involves large muscle groups, such as in a patient who is combative, or the diaphragm, such as in a patient with stiff lungs who works harder at breathing. This work directly translates into energy requirements and, thus, into oxygen demand. Sedation, analgesia, muscle relaxation, and mechanical ventilation can markedly reduce energy requirements and oxygen demand in such patients.

Injury, whether operative or traumatic, and especially thermal (burns), increases the metabolic rate. Surgical patients, thus, are likely to have a substantially increased demand for oxygen when compared to nonsurgical patients.

OXYGEN CONSUMPTION

Oxygen consumption is the amount of oxygen per unit time that the patient actually consumes. The concept of oxygen consumption must be clearly differentiated from the concept of oxygen demand. Except for brief periods, such as when oxygen deficits are being repaid, oxygen consumption is less than or equal to the oxygen demand. Because oxygen demand places an upper limit on oxygen consumption, Figure 15–1 indicates that oxygen demand is one determinant of oxygen consumption.

The other major determinants of oxygen consumption are oxygen delivery and maximal extraction. Figure 15–1 illustrates graphically the complex relationship between consumption and delivery, demand, and maximal extraction.

As oxygen delivery is increased, oxygen consumption typically will increase up to a point, known as the **critical delivery**, at which oxygen consumption will plateau. The slope with which consumption increases with delivery initially is equal to the maximal extraction. The value at which the consumption plateaus is equal to the oxygen demand.

At points below the critical delivery, oxygen consumption will be less than oxygen demand and the patient will be generating increases in the oxygen deficit. In other words, at deliveries below the critical delivery the patient is in shock.

MAXIMAL EXTRACTION

Normally, the patient is at a point on the curve well past the critical delivery. Note that **extraction** is simply the ratio of oxygen consumption to oxygen delivery. On the graph, it is the slope of a line drawn from a point on the curve back to the origin. If delivery should diminish, the patient compensates by increasing extraction to maintain the same consumption. In graphical terms, the

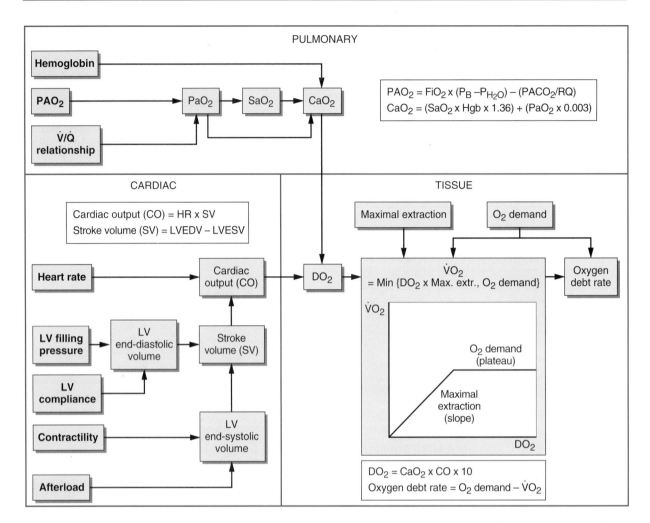

Figure 15–1. Diagram of oxygen transport. CaO_2 = arterial oxygen concentration; DO_2 = oxygen delivery; FiO_2 = fractional inspired oxygen; Hgb = hemoglobin; LV = left ventricular; PaO_2 = partial pressure of arterial oxygen; PAO_2 = partial pressure of oxygen in alveoli; P_B = barometric pressure; PH_2O = partial pressure of water vapor; SaO_2 = oxygen saturation of arterial blood; VO_2 = volume of oxygen consumption per unit of time; $\dot{V}/\dot{Q}$ = ventilation–perfusion ratio.

slope of the line back to the origin increases as the delivery decreases, keeping consumption equal to demand.

As delivery falls still further, the patient eventually reaches a point where the extraction cannot be increased further. This is where the slope equals the maximal extraction: it is at a delivery equal to the critical delivery. At this point, the patient can no longer increase extraction to compensate for decreased delivery. The drop in delivery is now associated with a drop in consumption below the oxygen demand, and the patient develops an oxygen deficit and shock.

In a critically ill surgical patient, the relationship between oxygen consumption and delivery may be altered in two important ways. First, the oxygen demand may be markedly increased because of injury, fever, and other metabolic stimuli that increase energy requirements and, thus, the need for oxygen. This is reflected by an oxygen consumption curve that plateaus at a higher value for oxygen consumption.

Second, maximal oxygen extraction may be reduced. This is reflected by an oxygen consumption curve that rises much more slowly as oxygen delivery increases. The initial slope to the curve is reduced.

There are multiple reasons for there to be a reduced ability of the tissues to extract oxygen. Most important is probably the loss of vasoregulation—particularly in cases of systemic inflammation or systemic infection.

Ordinarily, the body precisely matches blood flow and, thus, oxygen supply, to match the oxygen demand of individual tissue beds. This is accomplished by an intricate regulatory system that includes both local neuronal and local humoral components. Endothelium-derived relaxing factor, now known to be nitric oxide, probably is the key humoral factor involved in both normal vasoregulation as well as the abnormal vasoregulation of systemic inflammation and infection.

When oxygen delivery and oxygen need are not matched, then the ability of the tissues to unload oxygen becomes impaired. This is conceptually similar to the impairment of gas exchange that occurs in the lungs with mismatching of ventilation and perfusion. The inability of the lungs to exchange gas in the face of poor matching of ventilation to perfusion is analogous to the inability of the tissues to extract oxygen in the face of poor matching of perfusion to local tissue metabolic requirements.

Peripheral edema can reduce tissue extraction by increasing the diffusing distance from capillary to cells. A shift of the oxygen dissociation curve to the left can decrease extraction by increasing the hemoglobin affinity for oxygen at tissue partial pressures more than it increases the hemoglobin affinity for oxygen at alveolar partial pressures. A leftward shift can be produced by alkalemia, hypocapnia, decreased 2,3-diphosphoglycerate (2,3-DPG), decreased temperature, and carbon monoxide.

Critically ill surgical patients frequently will have both increased oxygen demand as well as decreased maximal extraction. In other words, the patient's tissues require more oxygen at the same time that their ability to utilize delivered oxygen efficiently is impaired, through limitations on extraction. The body could compensate by increasing delivery, but frequently surgical patients have cardiopulmonary dysfunction that prevents delivery from exceeding the critical threshold. The result is an accumulating oxygen deficit—shock.

HISTORICAL FACTS

The concept of oxygen deficit dates back at least to the work of Hill in the 1920s. He noted that study subjects undergoing intensive exercise would accumulate large amounts of lactic acid, which allowed the accumulation of an "oxygen debt." This was later "paid off" with an elevated oxygen consumption that continued after exercise was stopped. This oxygen consumption was associated with metabolism of the lactic acid to carbon dioxide.

The work of Guyton and his associates in the 1960s extended the concept of oxygen deficit. They noted that dogs subjected to hemorrhage experienced a marked decrease in oxygen consumption from baseline measurements. The baseline value was assumed to be the oxygen demand, and the amount of decrease was assumed to represent the rate at which an oxygen deficit was accumulating. After re-infusion of blood the oxygen consumption was increased over baseline, representing some diminution of the accumulated oxygen deficit. Some residual deficit, however, persisted. This deficit was found to be a good predictor of the dogs' survival from the hemorrhage. All dogs that developed less than 140 cc/kg of oxygen deficit survived while all dogs that developed greater than 160 cc/kg of deficit died.

Shoemaker, in the 1980s, related oxygen deficit to the development of complications in surgical patients. In a series of high-risk surgical patients for whom oxygen transport measurements were made in the perioperative period, calculated oxygen deficit was lowest for survivors without organ failure, greater for survivors with organ failure, and greatest for patients who died.

PULMONARY

OXYGEN DELIVERY

Oxygen delivery is defined to be the product of arterial oxygen content and cardiac output. Oxygen delivery represents the consequence of the combined performance of the pulmonary and the cardiac systems.

OXYGEN CONTENT

Arterial oxygen content is the concentration of oxygen in arterial blood. There are two components of the arterial content—oxygen that is dissolved and oxygen that is bound to hemoglobin. The amount of oxygen that is dissolved is directly proportional to the partial pressure of oxygen in arterial blood. The amount of oxygen that is bound to hemoglobin depends upon the affinity of hemoglobin for oxygen, described by the P_{50}, the concentration of hemoglobin, and the arterial saturation of oxygen. Factors that increase the binding of oxygen (decrease the P_{50} or shift the curve to the left) were listed above with the discussion of maximal extraction. Note that the increase in arterial content that might by accomplished by a leftward shift may increase delivery, but this is more than offset by the simultaneous decrease in extraction that a leftward shift entails.

PARTIAL PRESSURE OF ARTERIAL OXYGEN

The arterial partial pressure of oxygen represents a gradient in partial pressure below the alveolar partial pressure of oxygen. The size of the gradient depends upon a complex set of factors, principally the extent of the ventilation-perfusion abnormality, of which shunt may be viewed as an extreme case, and the partial pressure of oxygen in the venous blood that is returned to the lungs.

Ventilation-perfusion abnormality is closely related to the **functional residual capacity (FRC)** of the lungs. The FRC is the volume of the lungs at the end of a normal expiration. As this volume diminishes a point is reached where alveoli will collapse at the end of expiration. These alveoli will be perfused but not ventilated, contributing to ventilation perfusion abnormality. As FRC increases, alveoli become over-distended, leading to alveoli that are ventilated but not perfused. Thus, there is an optimal intermediate volume where alveoli are both perfused and ventilated.

In critically ill patients, the lung endothelium frequently becomes damaged, leading to a capillary leak of fluids into the pulmonary interstitium and eventually the alveoli. This increased intravascular volume leads to a decreased lung compliance. This decreased compliance can lead to a decreased FRC and the associated mismatching of ventilation and perfusion, impaired gas exchange, and decreased partial pressure of arterial oxygen.

PARTIAL PRESSURE OF ALVEOLAR OXYGEN

The partial pressure of alveolar oxygen is determined by the inspired oxygen fraction, the barometric pressure, and the partial pressure of carbon dioxide competing for "space" in the alveolus, as described by the alveolar gas equation. Thus, hypoventilation, by allowing accumulation of carbon dioxide in the alveolus, can lead to a lowered partial pressure of alveolar oxygen and, ultimately, to a decreased partial pressure of arterial oxygen.

CARDIAC

CARDIAC OUTPUT

Cardiac output is the blood flow generated by the heart. It is the product of heart rate and stroke volume. The stroke volume, in turn, may be thought of as the difference between the left ventricular end-diastolic volume and the left ventricular end-systolic volume.

LEFT VENTRICULAR END-DIASTOLIC VOLUME

The left ventricular end-diastolic volume is determined by two key factors: the left-ventricular filling pressure and the left ventricular compliance at diastole. The filling pressure is the consequence of the dynamic interplay of a large number of circulatory factors. The key determinants are the intravascular volume and the state of the venous capacitance vessels.

Hemorrhage clearly decreases intravascular volume. Fluid losses from the intravascular compartment—such as seen with sepsis, pancreatitis, and operative and nonoperative trauma—can also produce decreased intravascular volume, decreased left-ventricular end-diastolic volume, and ultimately low-cardiac output. The common factor in these processes is a systemic inflammatory response that leads to endothelial injury and capillary leak with expansion of the extracellular space, but contraction of the intravascular component of the extracellular space.

Loss of venous tone will increase the size of the venous capacitance vessels and reduce the peripheral, and thus central, venous pressures. This reduces venous return, reduces right-sided cardiac output, and ultimately leads to lower left-ventricular filling pressures. Spinal cord injury leads to loss of sympathetic tone and can produce decreased cardiac output by this mechanism. Nitroglycerin, and other nitrates, operate through a nitric oxide mechanism to produce decreased venous tone with the potential to decrease cardiac output by increasing venous capacitance and decreasing filling pressures.

LEFT VENTRICULAR END-SYSTOLIC VOLUME

The left ventricular end-systolic volume is also determined by two key factors: left ventricular contractility and left ventricular afterload. The former largely depends upon the inotropic state of the myocardium and the latter upon the compliance of the arterial vessels.

Pre-existing cardiac disease, such as ischemic, alchoholic, or idiopathic cardiomyopathy, are associated with a reduced inotropic state of the heart. More acutely, myocardial infarction, cardiopulmonary bypass, or negative inotropic drugs, such as most antiarrhythmics, can depress cardiac contractility. One of the most important negative inotropes is the so-called "myocardial depressant factor." This circulating humoral factor—still not fully characterized biochemically—appears to be responsible for the significant myocardial depression seen in systemic inflammatory processes, particularly sepsis.

Patients with hypertension or peripheral vascular disease may have alterations in arterial vessel compliance that increase the impedance to left-ventricular emptying. This abnormality in afterload may lead to an increased left ventricular end-systolic volume, a decreased stroke volume, and a decreased cardiac output. A transient cause of increased afterload is the aortic cross-clamping that is performed intraoperatively, for example, during abdominal aortic resection and grafting.

SHOCK SYNDROMES

Defects in one or more of the components of the oxygen transport model can lead to shock. Some of these defects or combinations of defects are relatively common and are specifically identified as shock syndromes. Four important shock syndromes are: hypovolemic, cardiogenic, septic, and obstructive shock.

HYPOVOLEMIC SHOCK

Hemorrhagic hypovolemic shock begins with bleeding and a decrease in intravascular volume. This leads to decreased left-ventricular end-diastolic volume, decreased stroke volume. Initially the heart rate may increase to compensate for the decreased stroke volume with maintenance of cardiac output. With severe volume loss, however, limits of compensation are exceeded, and cardiac output drops. This produces a decrease in delivery.

Compensation for decreased delivery may be achieved by an increase in extraction. When the maximal extraction is attained, however, any further decrease in delivery is accompanied by a decrease in consumption. This leads to the development of oxygen debt.

Bleeding, however, represents not just loss of volume but also loss of red cell mass. Initially, there will be no change in the hemoglobin concentration even though the hemoglobin amount will be decreased. The decreased oxygen-carrying capacity becomes apparent when intravascular volume is restored by the administration of asanguineous fluids, such as crystalloid. This hemodilution, however, may take hours to become fully manifest, so it is important not to be misled by early hematocrits or hemoglobins taken before equilibration has occurred. Red cell transfusion can simultaneously correct both oxygen transport defects caused by hemorrhagic shock—decreased intravascular volume and decreased hemoglobin concentration.

Hypovolemic shock can occur from losses of fluid from the vascular compartment that do not involve bleeding—for example, from dehydration resulting from gastrointestinal losses, or from capillary leaks, such as that associated with pancreatitis. In these cases, the loss of intravascular volume produces the same alterations in stroke volume, cardiac output, delivery, and extraction as seen in hemorrhagic shock. Unlike hemorrhagic shock, red cell mass is not lost is these cases and there may actually be hemoconcentration—an increase in hemoglobin concentration. The increase in arterial oxygen content, however, is never sufficient to compensate for the decrease in cardiac output. The resulting hypovolemic shock can be corrected with the infusion of asanguineous fluids—usually, crystalloid.

CARDIOGENIC SHOCK

In cardiogenic shock, cardiac contractility is depressed, leading to increased end-systolic volume. This leads to decreased stroke volume and decreased cardiac output. This further leads to decreased delivery and compensatory increased extraction. When the limit to increasing extraction is encountered, further decreases in delivery are associated with consumption that falls below demands and the development of oxygen debt.

Myocardial infarction with loss of functioning muscle mass or myocardial dysfunction secondary to ischemia in the still viable myocytes are typical settings for cardiogenic shock.

SEPTIC SHOCK

In septic shock, defects affect multiple components of oxygen transport in a characteristic dynamic progression. The initiating factor may be a bacteremia, a fungemia, or even an endotoxemia with translocation of endotoxin from the gut. This triggers a network of humoral cascades that produces altered vasoregulation. Abnormal vasodilatation, apparently mediated by nitric oxide, leads to mismatching of perfusion and metabolic need at the tissue level. This lowers the maximal extraction and leads to a less favorable relationship between consumption and delivery. The altered vascular tone, however, leads to decreased afterload so that, initially, cardiac output and, thus, delivery, may even be increased. On exam the patient may be warm, with prominent distal pulses.

Later, however, other defects become more prominent. Venous dilatation may lead to decreased filling pressures and decreased cardiac output. Myocardial depressant factors may further depress cardiac output. Capillary leak in the lung may lead to increases in extravascular lung water and ventilation perfusion mismatching and to decreases in arterial oxygen content. Delivery falls. The decreased capacity for extraction provides less capacity for compensation. Additionally, the inflammatory response to infection or endotoxemia is associated with increased energy demands. Thus, there is an increase in oxygen demand at the same time that oxygen delivery and maximal extraction are reduced. The combination of these three factors leads to the oxygen deficit of septic shock. Ultimately, the cardiogenic component of the septic shock syndrome will dominate, and the patient may present cold with decreased pulses.

OBSTRUCTIVE SHOCK

In obstructive shock, which includes tamponade, tension pneumothorax, and pulmonary embolism, the pathophysiology is primarily inadequate left-ventricular end-diastolic volume. This is similar to hypovolemic shock, but, unlike hypovolemic shock, right-sided filling pressures typically are high, not low. The defect involves a pressure gradient or obstruction that prevents venous return from making its way to the left heart.

In tamponade, fluid fills the pericardial sac and lowers the transmural gradient that distends the ventricles in diastole. Even though filling pressures may appear high, the transmural filling pressures are low, and thus end-diastolic volumes are reduced. This leads to decreased stroke volume and cardiac output.

In tension pneumothorax, pleural air under high pressure leads to high intrathoracic pressures, pulmonary collapse, and mediastinal shift. This reduces the pressure gradient that promotes venous return from the periphery. Additionally, torque of mediastinal structures may present further obstruction to flow. Again, the transmural filling pressures are low and end-diastolic volume, stroke volume, and cardiac output are reduced.

In pulmonary embolism, the clot in the pulmonary artery produces increased afterload on the right ventricle, which fails, and is unable to convey venous return to the left heart. Although right-sided pressures are high, left-sided pressures are typically low. Left-ventricular end-diastolic volume and, thus, cardiac output, are reduced.

APPROACH TO THE PATIENT WITH SHOCK

The oxygen transport diagram provides a conceptual framework, not only for understanding but also for managing shock (Figure 15–2). Typically, clinical shock consists of one or more defects in the oxygen transport mechanism. Resuscitation from shock involves correcting or compensating for these defects. The key points for clinical intervention on the oxygen transport mechanism are indicated by the ovals in the diagram highlighted in blue. The management of shock involves addressing these control points in a systematic fashion, with a sequence that respects temporal priorities. Figure 15–2 shows a step-by-step approach to the management of shock. In this figure the arrows connect the interventions with the affected elements of oxygen transport.

ASSESSMENT OF SHOCK

First, the clinician must assess shock. Clues to shock are generated by the abnormalities of blood flow and vascular tone, by the body's compensatory adrenergic responses, and by the fundamental inadequacy of tissue oxygenation. The following signs should serve to alert the physician to the possible presence of shock: cool and clammy skin, tachycardia, decreased peripheral pulses and hypotension, mental status changes, and oliguria.

In the young patient, pronounced compensatory vasoconstriction may delay the appearance of hypotension and tachycardia until the point of cardiac arrest. In young patients, therefore, particular attention must be paid to skin evidence of vasoconstriction, to confusion, to lethargy, to combativeness, to the loss of distal pulses, and to oliguria, even if the blood pressure and heart rate are normal. In shock from sepsis or from spinal cord injury, or in shock where the patient is intoxicated with alcohol, the vasoconstriction may be absent. In these cases, however, hypotension is typically present.

PHASES OF RESUSCITATION

Once shock is recognized, resuscitation proceeds in three phases. The first phase—primary resuscitation—addresses the pulmonary component of oxygen transport as

Assess for Shock
- Vasoconstriction
- Decreased peripheral pulses
- Hypotension
- Oliguria

Primary Resuscitation
- Airway, oxygen, ventilation
- Correct dysrhythmias
- Neck veins flat:
  - 30 cc/kg IV bolus crystalloid
  - Stop bleeding
- Neck veins distended:
  - Correct pneumothorax or tamponade
  - For pulmonary edema, give furosemide

Secondary Resuscitation
- Insert pulmonary catheter
- Optimize preload
  - Crystalloid
  - Packed cells
  - Diuretics or vasodilators
- Optimize contractility with inotropes
- Optimize afterload with vasodilators

Monitor and Titrate Resuscitation
- Monitor filling pressures, cardiac output, mixed venous saturation
- Assess $\dot{V}O_2$ to DO_2 relationship
- Obtain serial lactate levels
- Monitor organ dysfunction

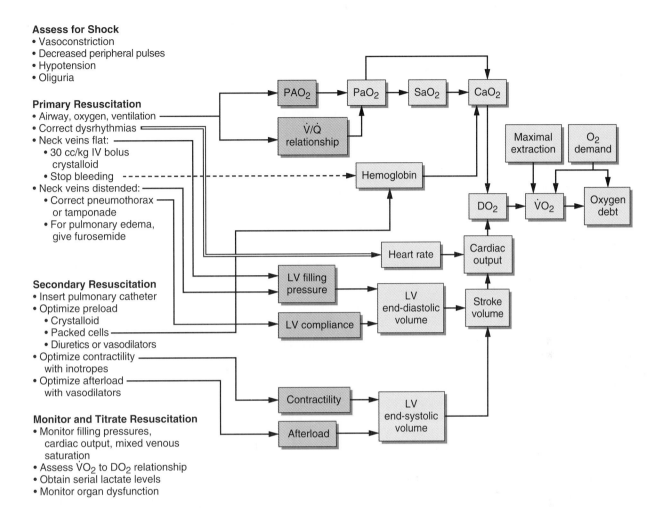

Figure 15–2. Algorithm of shock management. CaO_2 = arterial oxygen concentration; DO_2 = oxygen delivery; PaO_2 = partial pressure of arterial oxygen; PAO_2 = partial pressure of oxygen in alveoli; SaO_2 = oxygen saturation; $\dot{V}/\dot{Q}$ = ventilation–perfusion ratio.

well as the immediately life-threatening and immediately reversible defects that can reduce cardiac output. The second phase—secondary resuscitation—is entered if shock does not resolve with the interventions of primary resuscitation. In this phase, a pulmonary artery catheter is used to direct the correction of more complex defects affecting cardiac output. In the third phase, the patient's response to resuscitation is monitored and therapy is continually titrated to balance the potentially detrimental and potentially advantageous effects of the shock therapies.

PRIMARY RESUSCITATION: AIRWAY, VENTILATION, OXYGEN

The first step is to ensure adequacy of airway and ventilation. Airway and ventilation are initially managed by use of the head-tilt or jaw-thrust maneuvers, by the use of oral or nasal airways, and by bag-mask–assisted breathing, as needed (if a neck injury is possible, such as in the trauma patient, the neck must be left in a protected, neutral position). Supplemental oxygen is provided to raise the alveolar partial pressure, improving arterial oxygen content.

If the patient will need assisted ventilation for more than a short period, endotracheal intubation and mechanical ventilation is preferred. This allows for the maintenance of higher inspired oxygen fractions. Additionally, a patient on a ventilator can receive positive end-expiratory pressure (PEEP), which can help improve ventilation perfusion relationships—again, improving arterial oxygen content.

Dysrhythmias

Simultaneously, with the management of airway and ventilation, the clinician addresses rapidly reversible defects in cardiac output. Physical exam and electrocardiographic monitoring will identify the most common dysrhythmias. The Advanced Cardiac Life Support (ACLS) guidelines of the American Heart Association provide a guide to the management of common dysrhythmias associated with shock.

Other than arrhythmias, the rapidly reversible defects in cardiac output typically involve inadequate preload, that is, inadequate left-ventricular end-diastolic volume. Evaluation of the neck veins guides the restoration of preload in this part of primary resuscitation.

Neck Veins Not Distended

If the neck veins are not distended, then a decreased intravascular volume leading to decreased filling pressure is at least partly responsible for the shock. This is by far the most common situation on a surgical service. Large-bore intravenous access is obtained and a 30-cc/kg fluid bolus of crystalloid is administered. Our preference is to place a 7- to 8-French sheath into the femoral vein using a percutaneous puncture and guide-wire technique. This enables a flow rate of several hundred cc's per minute, which greatly facilitates timely fluid resuscitation.

For general surgical and trauma patients, expansion of intravascular volume requires not only intravenous fluid, but also control of the factors leading to vascular compartment fluid loss. Frequently, this means control of bleeding in the operating room. Controlling the bleeding further contributes to oxygen transport by maintaining red cell mass and ultimately maintaining hemoglobin concentration and, thus, arterial oxygen content.

An important point is that the hemoglobin concentration drops, not with the initial bleeding, but only after the reduced residual red cell mass is diluted by asanguineous fluid. This fluid may come from intravenous replacement during resuscitation or fluid shifts from the intracellular, or from both. The time course of hemodilution varies from patient to patient but generally takes hours to days for full equilibration. Consequently, hemoglobin concentrations are not a reliable guide to the extent of red cell mass loss in acute bleeding.

Neck Veins Distended

If the neck veins are distended—either initially, or following volume resuscitation—then two classes of rapidly reversible defects in cardiac output should be considered. The first includes mechanical problems such as tension pneumothorax or pericardial tamponade. These reduce preload even though central venous pressures are elevated by reducing the transmural filling pressure or by effectively altering ventricular compliance, or both. Treatment of these conditions involves drainage of the pleural or pericardial spaces. Fluid administration that generates very high central venous pressures can be a temporizing measure to compensate for the obstruction while the mechanical problem is corrected.

Congestive Heart Failure

Patients with primary cardiac disease may present with shock and distended neck veins, indicating congestive heart failure. In this case, preload is reduced by administration of diuretics (usually furosemide) or by using vasodilators, such as nitroglycerin or nitroprusside. By lowering pulmonary pressures, the frequently associated pulmonary edema is also corrected.

SECONDARY RESUSCITATION: OPTIMIZATION OF OXYGEN TRANSPORT

Frequently, the presenting signs of inadequate oxygen transport will improve promptly with primary resuscitation. For example, oliguria in a postoperative patient will usually resolve with an intravenous fluid bolus. In many cases, however, the interventions of primary resuscitation to do not produce unambiguous evidence of adequate oxygen transport. This is particularly the case where multiple defects may be present. In these cases our approach has been to use place a pulmonary artery catheter to provide further information to guide resuscitation.

Pulmonary Artery Catheter

The pulmonary catheter is a multilumen tube that is placed in the superior vena cava through a sheath inserted with percutaneous guide-wire venipuncture of the internal jugular or subclavian veins. A balloon at the tip of the catheter is inflated, allowing the catheter to be advanced with flotation into the pulmonary artery.

Pulmonary Artery Occlusion Pressure. One of the catheter lumens, with an opening that is positioned in the right atrium is filled with saline and connected to a manometer that measures central venous pressure. A lumen at the tip of the catheter distal to the balloon measures pulmonary artery pressures. When the balloon is inflated, the catheter floats out into a progressively smaller pulmonary artery branch. Ultimately, the balloon becomes wedged against the pulmonary artery wall and blocks forward blood flow. The pulmonary circulation distal to the balloon, including the pulmonary capillary and the pulmonary veins, thus become an extension of the lumen at the catheter tip, allowing manometry to measure the left-ventricular filling pressures. Because there is no flow through these branches of the circuit there is no pressure gradient between the distal catheter tip and the left atrium. In many cases this allows the pulmonary artery occlusion pressure—the PAOP, or "wedge" pressure, to be a useful approximation to the left-ventricular end-diastolic pressures.

This approximation will be good only if it is correct to assume that there is equilibration of pressure between the catheter tip and the left ventricle. One circumstance that voids this assumption is a break in the continuity of the fluid column that projects the manometery from the distal catheter tip into the left atrium. If the catheter is positioned in a portion of the lung in which pulmonary pressures exceed pulmonary vascular pressures, collapse of the pulmonary vessels may interrupt this necessary continuity. This argues for positioning the tip in a vessel that is in a dependent portion of the lung, where hydrostatic forces added to hemodynamic pressures maintain the vessel pressures greater than the pulmonary pressures throughout the cardiac cycle.

Cardiac Output Monitoring. One of the lumens of the pulmonary artery catheter contains a wire that runs to a thermistor placed in the tip of the catheter. If cold saline is injected into another lumen that empties into the right atrium, the saline will mix with blood in the right atrium, producing a temperature deflection in the pulmonary artery. This deflection is measured by the thermistor to be of a magnitude that is inversely proportional to blood flow. In practice, this approach—the thermodilution technique—is implemented using a bedside microprocessor that records the time course of temperature deflection and derives the cardiac output.

The thermodilution method has limitations in that it is somewhat operator-dependent, requiring a consistent injection technique to produce reproducible results. Furthermore, because the measurements require an operator intervention, it is very labor-intensive to obtain measurements more frequently than every 2–4 hours.

A new approach that allows cardiac output measurements to be made more frequently and without operator intervention has recently become commercially available. This technique for continuous (actually continual) cardiac output is a modification of the standard thermodilution approach. A heating coil is wrapped around a segment of the pulmonary artery catheter that is positioned in the right atrium. Under microprocessor control, a patterned sequence of heating pulses is applied to the blood. These pulses are too small to injure the blood, but register temperature deflections that are sensed by a thermistor at the catheter tip. Unlike the traditional thermodilution technique, where the deflections may register on the order of a degree Celsius, the continuous technique produces deflections on the order of a hundredth of a degree. Sophisticated digital signal processing is used to recover the induced temperature variation from the surrounding noise of spontaneous temperature variation in the pulmonary artery produced by ordinary activities, such as breathing. A microprocessor then converts the temperature signal to an estimate of cardiac output. Because the output measurement is updated approximately every 3 minutes, this technique provides timely feedback that is very useful for titrating shock therapies.

Mixed-Venous Monitoring. Still another lumen of the pulmonary artery catheter can be used for a fiberoptic bundle that allows a multi-wavelength light beam to be directed at the mixed-venous blood flowing through the pulmonary artery. The relative absorption of each of the wavelengths is proportional to oxygen saturation. By measuring these absorptions, a microprocessor-based device can provide continuous measurement of the oxygen saturation of mixed-venous blood—the SvO_2.

Optimizing Preload

If the pulmonary artery occlusion pressure is low, further crystalloid is administered. If the red cell mass is decreased, red cell infusions are used to both increase the filling pressures and increase the arterial oxygen content.

If the pulmonary artery occlusion pressure is high, further diuretics or vasodilators may be used.

Optimizing Contractility

If the patient remains in shock after optimization of preload, therapeutic agents are usually added to augment contractility. In our practice, dopamine is usually added initially at doses up to 10 µg/kg/min. If further inotropy is required, we then add epinephrine. In septic shock, epinephrine is frequently required. Starting doses may be as low as 25 ng/kg/min, but doses as high as 500 ng/kg/min may be needed to support patients through severe systemic inflammatory states in general and bacteremias in particular. If the patient requires additional inotropic support, then trials of dobutamine (if the patient is not hypotensive) or norepinephrine (if the patient is hypotensive) are instituted.

Optimizing Afterload

If the patient remains in shock after optimization of both preload and contractility, sometimes decreasing afterload will produce increases in cardiac output. This is a situation that is much more likely in patients with primary myocardial problems than in patients with multiorgan systemic disease, such as occurs with sepsis. In the former case, the patient may be hypertensive, while the septic patient in shock is likely to be too hypotensive to tolerate afterload reduction. Agents such as nitroprusside have been used for afterload reduction. In extreme cases, an intra-aortic balloon pump may be used.

MONITORING & TITRATION OF RESUSCITATION

Once the patient has been resuscitated, therapy is continually adjusted to maintain the patient in the resuscitated state. The challenge in this phase is the same one faced when optimizing preload, contractility, and afterload in the phase of secondary resuscitation—using information from the physical examination, monitoring, and laboratory to ensure that the best balance of risks and benefits is maintained in the use of powerful shock therapies. How is this balance ascertained?

Some clinicians advocate the use of specific measurement end points and the adjustment of therapies to meet these specific goals. For example, many clinicians will optimize preload by seeking to keep the pulmonary artery occlusion pressure between 12 and 18 mm Hg. Below 12 mm Hg, there is simply inadequate left-ventricular end-diastolic volume; above 18 mm Hg, hydrostatic pulmonary edema is likely. Pulmonary edema, however, is also a consequence of capillary leak, a common circumstance in patients in shock. Thus, the increased preload and cardiac output from any elevation in pulmonary artery occlusion pressure must be balanced against decreased gas exchange that may result from increased capillary leak in the lungs.

Similarly, some clinicians will aim for specific values for cardiac output, delivery, and consumption that have been reported to be associated with improved survival. Specifically, the goals of resuscitation for these clinicians are: a cardiac index of 4.5 L/min/m^2, an oxygen delivery of 600 cc/min/m^2, and an oxygen consumption of 167 cc/min/m^2. These goals may be adjusted to take into account the presence of sepsis (cardiac index goal is increased to 5.0) or myocardial ischemia (cardiac index goal is decreased to 2.5).

Our approach is to continually test and re-test each patient's individual and evolving dose-response to the various shock therapies. We attempt to identify how each therapy affects the oxygen transport system and reduces tissue oxygen debt, to ascertain any undesirable side effects that may be generated by the therapies, and to balance the benefit and harm. As shock is treated, peripheral vasoconstriction should diminish, with the return of warm, dry extremities, normal capillary filling, and normal peripheral pulses. Blood pressure should rise, and tachycardia, tachypnea, and confusion should abate. Urine output should increase to at least 0.5 cc/kg/h.

Because lactate is the end product of anaerobic metabolism, lactate levels in the blood are sometimes used to supplement vital signs in assessing the adequacy of resuscitation. The concentration of lactate, however, is a function not only of the rate at which it is created, but also the rate at which it is taken up by the liver and kidneys. Furthermore, an elevation of lactate may simply reflect what has been termed **aerobic glycolysis**. This occurs when there is down-regulation of pyruvate dehydrogenase by reduced nicotinamide adenine dinucleotide phosphate (NADH). Pyruvate, thus, is unable to enter the Krebs cycle and is converted to lactate, despite adequate tissue oxygenation. Under these circumstances, both lactate and pyruvate levels will be elevated; the lactate to pyruvate ratio will be normal. Pyruvate levels, however, are not routinely available.

SUGGESTED READING

Boyd O, Grounds RM, Bennett ED: A randomized clinical trial of the effect of deliberate perioperative increase of oxygen delivery on mortality in high-risk surgical patients. JAMA 1993;270:2699.

Committee on Trauma: Advanced Life Support Course for Physicians. American College of Surgeons, 1989.

Hayes MA et al: Elevation of systemic oxygen delivery in the treatment of critically ill patients. N Engl J Med 1994;330: 1717.

Lugo G et al: Relationship between oxygen consumption and oxygen delivery during anesthesia in high-risk surgical patients. Crit Care Med 1993;21:64.

Shoemaker WC, Appel PL, Kram HB: Role of oxygen debt in the development of organ failure sepsis and death in high-risk surgical patients. Chest 1992;102:208.

16

Surgical Infections & Antibiotics

Jeffrey P. Salomone, MD, & Ronald Lee Nichols, MD, MS, FACS

► Key Facts

- ► Surgical infections differ from other infectious processes in that a procedure is required in order to effect a cure.

- ► When postoperative patients manifest symptoms of infection, the first focus should be on the operative site prior to invoking other explanations for the origin of sepsis.

- ► Host defenses against infection include physical and chemical barriers as well as the immune system, with its humoral and cellular components.

- ► The factor that differentiates surgical infection of the soft tissues from more easily treated cellulitis is the presence of purulent exudate and often necrotic tissue as well.

- ► Approximately 70% of all nosocomial infections occur in patients who have undergone surgical intervention; these include urinary tract infection, surgical site infection, bacteremia, and pneumonia.

- ► Prophylactic antibiotics are indicated for many clean and all clean-contaminated operations.

- ► Current research suggests that a single preoperative dose of antibiotics yields protection from surgical site infections similar to the standard multiple perioperative doses for operations lasting less than 2–3 hours.

- ► Present data indicate that health care workers are far more likely to contract blood-borne infections from their patients than are the patients from their health care professionals.

- ► Epidemiologists estimate that during a surgeon's career, the risk of infection with hepatitis approaches 50% while the risk of contracting HIV in an area of high prevalence of AIDS ranges from 0.01–0.11%.

- ► In recent years, research has focused on the observation that certain nutrients, when supplied in quantities greater than nutritional requirements, seem to have pharmacologic activities and may well improve immune system functioning.

Throughout the ages, infectious diseases have challenged clinicians. Along with the successful development of anesthesia, the introduction of antiseptic principles into surgical practice were the two accomplishments of the late 19th century that led to dramatic advances in surgical practice. Louis Pasteur, after realizing that microorganisms were responsible for fermentation, studied bacteria as a cause of disease in man and identified the first pathogenic anaerobe, *Clostridium septicum*. Prior to Joseph Lister's conceiving the initial principles of surgical antisepsis in 1865 (see Chapter 2), surgeons performed few intracranial, intrathoracic, or intra-abdominal operations because of the significant mortality, primarily due to infectious complications. While surgeons quite rapidly accepted anesthesia techniques, more than 2 decades passed before most surgeons embraced listerism.

The decrease in infection resulting from adherence to antiseptic practices set the stage for the development of the "radical" operations introduced in the 1880s: appendectomy, mastectomy, herniorrhaphy, and gastric resection. While the identification of penicillin and the scores of other antibiotics in the 20th century have contributed to the decreased rates of infection seen in surgical patients, infection remains a challenging problem for the surgeon.

Surgical infections differ from other infectious processes in that a *procedure* is required in order to effect a cure. With many problems, such as a cutaneous abscess, an incision alone may suffice, and *antibiotics may not be necessary to adequately treat the condition*. In more complex cases, an operation may be required to remove a foreign body, evacuate pus, debride necrotic tissue, or repair or remove a damaged organ. Surgeons or interventional radiologists may employ percutaneous techniques to drain purulent material, namely, tube thoracostomies or image-guided drainage catheterization. Surgeons most frequently administer parenteral antibiotics to supplement the management of these conditions.

When postoperative patients manifest a deterioration in their condition, surgeons first focus on the operative site prior to invoking other explanations for the origin of the sepsis. Frequently, they will identify the need for further surgery in the form of additional debridement, drainage of a wound infection, or repair of an anastomotic leak. The best antibiotics cannot compensate for inadequate surgical intervention.

HOST DEFENSE MECHANISMS

Numerous bacteria, namely aerobic gram-positive cocci, colonize our skin, and remarkably high concentrations of aerobic and anaerobic gram-negative and gram-positive bacteria live in symbiosis in the human gastrointestinal (GI) tract. The fact that humans do not suffer from more infections speaks to the wonderful defense mechanisms found in the body. Only the most basic concepts will be reviewed in this section; students should refer to immunology and infectious disease texts for a thorough discussion of the complex host defenses.

These defenses include physical and chemical barriers and the immune system, with its humoral and cellular components. The mucous membrane linings of the aerodigestive tracts and the epithelial surface of the skin resist bacterial invasion. Mucus, secreted by specialized cells, contributes to the physical and chemical barriers, and cilia

aid in the removal of invading microbes. The sebaceous glands secrete substances that maintain bacteria levels in check by lowering skin pH.

Humoral immunity includes the various proteins of the classic and alternate complement pathways, as well as the antibodies found in the serum. Complement fixation on bacterial cell walls renders them more susceptible to phagocytosis. Immunoglobulins are produced by plasmacytes, B-lymphocytes that have been activated by T-lymphocytes. Neutrophils (the primary circulating phagocytic cells), macrophages, and killer T-lymphocytes comprise the significant components of cellular immunity. Macrophages can either present antigens to helper T-lymphocytes or phagocytic cells in tissues. Many of these immune cells produce cytokines, which activate other cells in the system. In recent years, medical researchers have realized that these substances are responsible for the manifestations of infections. Excessive activation of this system results in many of the detrimental aspects of sepsis, including third-space fluid loss and hypermetabolism.

Lastly, the aerobic and anaerobic bacteria of the GI tract live in symbiosis with their human hosts and contribute to host defense by challenging the developing immune system and limiting proliferation of invading organisms.

SURGICAL SOFT TISSUE INFECTIONS & TETANUS

SOFT TISSUE INFECTIONS

The factor that differentiates surgical infections of the soft tissues from the more easily treated cellulitis is the presence of purulent exudate and, often, necrotic tissue as well. Such soft tissue infections range from simple cutaneous abscesses, which may spontaneously rupture and heal, to the life-threatening problems of necrotizing fasciitis and clostridial myonecrosis.

Cutaneous Abscesses

Cutaneous abscesses are skin structure infections that contain a purulent, necrotic center. A physical examination reveals the classic signs of inflammation, including warmth (calor), edema (tumor), tenderness (dolor), and erythema (rubor). In the larger and more superficial abscesses, one may palpate fluctuation, however, this finding may be masked by a deep location. Aspiration of suspicious lesions will frequently yield pus. Examples include furuncles (boils), carbuncles (larger, multiloculated subcutaneous lesions), breast abscesses, and perianal or perirectal abscesses.

The gram-positive cocci species of *Staphylococcus* and *Streptococcus* predominate in abscesses of the head, neck, and trunk, while a polymicrobial aerobic and anaerobic flora are more commonly isolated from the axilla and groin. Incision and drainage frequently cures these lesions, and antibiotics are unnecessary unless the abscess is surrounded by a significant amount of cellulitis or if the infection has extended to the fascia.

Necrotizing Fasciitis

While necrotizing cellulitis implies a severe soft tissue infection with loss of skin and subcutaneous tissues, **necrotizing fasciitis** consists of a more severe infection that involves loss of muscle fascia and spreads along fascial planes. The infection is frequently seen in diabetic patients with preexisting local infections. Blisters, drainage, a woody consistency, and patches of necrotic skin in a region of cellulitis should compel the surgeon to thoroughly explore the wound, looking for evidence of a deep-seated infection, which commonly lacks a clear border. While streptococci and staphylococci have historically been the classic causative organisms, today this infection frequently harbors a flora of gram-negative aerobes or anaerobes, or a mixture of both. This process may extend from what is initially an innocent-appearing wound or a perirectal abscess.

Fournier's gangrene applies to a polymicrobial variant of necrotizing fasciitis of the perineum that is most frequently cryptogenic (ie, without predisposing infection). It may follow uncomplicated urologic or anal operations or, rarely, may extend from a perirectal abscess. The first manifestation is frequently the development of a black eschar on the scrotum. Advanced infections may require complete excision of the external genitalia.

In all of these cases of necrotizing fasciitis, the subcutaneous tissue and fascia appear gray-to-black at exploration and fail to bleed when cut. The deeper muscle usually remains unaffected. Wide debridement to viable tissue comprises the mainstay of treatment. Return visits to the operating room, daily for at least 3–5 days, permit careful inspection and further debridement. Antibiotics should be chosen that cover both aerobic and anaerobic flora, and adjustments to empiric therapy are made based upon the results of cultures and susceptibility testing of drainage or infected tissue (Table 16–1). Necrotizing fasciitis carries a 50% mortality rate in high-risk patients.

Clostridial Myonecrosis

Clostridial myonecrosis, or "gas gangrene," is a rapidly progressive soft tissue infection that results in necrosis of muscle tissue and that carries a 40–80% mortality rate. The overlying skin is edematous and firm, has a characteristic purplish hue, and may contain hemorrhagic bullae. Drainage from the involved tissue emits a foul-sweet odor. In advanced cases, radiographs of the affected area commonly demonstrate gas in the soft tissues, however, one should not forget that this finding is not specific for clostridial infection. Numerous other enteric aerobic and anaerobic organisms, including strains of *Escherichia coli* and *Klebsiella,* may also form gas. *Clostridium perfringens* accounts for more than 80% of myonecrosis, with other *Clostridia* species causing the remainder. These or-

Table 16–1. Recommended intravenous antibiotics for polymicrobial infections.

Combination Therapy
  Aerobic Coverage—to be combined with a drug having anaerobic activity
      Cephalosporins: cefotaxime, ceftriaxone
      Monobactams: aztreonam
      Quinolones: ciprofloxacin
      Aminoglycosides: amikacin, gentamicin, tobramycin
  Anaerobic Coverage—to be combined with a drug having aerobic activity
      Extended-spectrum penicillins: carbenicillin, mezlocillin, ticarcillin
      Others: chloramphenicol, clindamycin, metronidazole

Single-Drug Therapy
  Aerobic AND Anaerobic Coverage—single agents
      Beta-lactamase inhibitors: ampicillin/sulbactam; piperacillin/tazobactam; ticarcillin/clavulanate
      Cephalosporins: cefotetan, cefoxitin, ceftizoxime
      Carbapenems: imipenem/cilastatin

---

ganisms produce alpha toxin, which splits lecithin and spreads rapidly in tissues with compromised blood supplies, such as those in shock states or arterial insufficiency. More than two thirds of the cases involve extremities, while the other third involve the abdominal wall, chest wall, or pelvis.

Following inoculation, incubation occurs rapidly in only 8–48 hours. Radical debridement, including amputation if indicated, may be life-saving. Penicillin G, dosed at 3–4 million units intravenously every 4 hours, is the antibiotic regimen of choice. Frequent clinical assessment of the wound is mandatory, and any evidence of progressive infection requires a return to the operating room for additional debridement. If available, hyperbaric oxygen therapy may facilitate recovery.

While one most often associates gas gangrene with major traumatic tissue injury, this surgical emergency may even follow elective surgery. If faced with a patient in whom a high fever develops within 48 hours of an operation, the prudent surgeon will remove the dressing and examine the wound for evidence of crepitance or the skins changes as noted above. Delay in diagnosis or intervention may well contribute to the patient's death.

TETANUS

Clostridium tetani is a gram-positive, spore-forming, anaerobic bacillus that is found throughout our environment. Following an incubation of a few days to several weeks, the spores germinate and begin to liberate a toxin that causes the clinical syndrome in unprotected individuals. While several different manifestations of the disease are recognized, more than 80% of cases present with generalized tetanus. Patients have trismus (hence the nickname "lockjaw"), neck stiffness, abdominal rigidity, and spasms of the extremity musculature.

Like many anaerobes, *C. tetani* may be difficult to grow in bacterial culture. No satisfactory diagnostic tests exist, therefore, clinicians must make the diagnosis clinically.

Along with supportive care, the treatment of tetanus involves debridement of necrotic tissue, and the administration of tetanus immune globulin to bind circulating toxin and parenteral penicillin G (3 million units intravenously every 6 hours) or metronidazole (500 mg intravenously every 6 hours). Muscular spasms are controlled with benzodiazepines.

Antibiotic therapy and surgical debridement do not adequately protect patients from tetanus. The physician should establish the immunization status of every patient presenting for treatment of a wound and administer proper immunization, as needed (Table 16–2). Tetanus-prone wounds include those: greater than 6 hours old; with stellate shape or tissue avulsion; deeper than 1 cm; associated with established infection or devitalized tissue; contaminated with soil or feces; and due to missiles, crush injury, thermal burn, or frostbite.

Patients with both a tetanus-prone wound and a history of three or fewer tetanus immunizations should receive both tetanus immune globulin and a tetanus/diphtheria toxoid injection. In patients who have had more than three immunizations, an injection within the previous 5 years is considered adequate protection for tetanus-prone wounds, while immunization within the previous 10 years should protect one with a non–tetanus-prone injury. The tragedy of this disease lies in the fact that virtually all cases are preventable with proper immunizations.

NOSOCOMIAL INFECTIONS

While some hospital-acquired (nosocomial) infections fail to satisfy our definition of surgical infection, namely, that a procedure is usually required in addition to or in place of antibiotic therapy, many clearly do. Urinary tract infections and intravascular catheter sepsis require removal of fomites, and wound infections and intra-abdominal abscesses need adequate drainage. While pneumonia, candidiasis, and pseudomembranous colitis do not commonly require such interventions, they deserve attention because of their impact on surgical patients.

About 70% of all nosocomial infections develop in patients who have undergone surgical intervention. Across the board, nosocomial infections occur in about 33.5 patients per 1000 hospital discharges, but when broken down by specialty, surgical services predominate, with an incidence of 46.7 per 1000 discharges. These infections account for a significant portion of health care costs and represent about 8 million extra hospital days and over 1 billion dollars of hospital charges annually. A listing of the incidences of various nosocomial infections on surgical services is offered (Table 16–3).

While fever accompanies virtually all nosocomial infections, it can also develop in the absence of active infection. One should resist the temptation to immediately begin empiric antibiotics in the febrile postoperative patient lacking a diagnosis, unless severe sepsis is encountered. Atelectasis is the most common cause of immediate postoperative fever; aggressive pulmonary toilet and early mobilization, not anti-infective agents, should be initiated. Reflex actions, such as "pan-culturing," that is, obtaining blood, urine, sputum, and wound cultures on febrile postoperative patients, often fail to yield significant results and is clearly not cost-effective. Instead, a thorough history and physical examination is more useful, with specific cultures being ordered for problems suggested by the subjective and objective findings.

URINARY TRACT INFECTIONS

Urinary tract infections (UTIs) represent the most common nosocomial infection on surgical services. Urethral catheterization predisposes patients to this problem, and the rate of infection begins to increase following 5 days of indwelling catheterization. While this problem can develop at any time during hospitalization, it classically presents between the third and fifth postoperative day.

Table 16–2. Guidelines for active and passive immunization against tetanus.

Wound Status	History of Tetanus Toxoid Injections	
	Unknown or < 3 Injections	> 3 Injections
Tetanus-prone wound[1]	Td plus TIG	Td, if > 5 years since last dose
Non–tetanus–prone wound	Td only	Td, if > 10 years since last dose

[1]Tetanus-prone wounds include those: > 6 hours old; with stellate shape or avulsions; > 1 cm in depth; with established infection; with devitalized tissue; contaminated with soil or feces; due to missiles, crush injury, thermal burn, or frostbite.
Td = Tetanus and diphtheria toxoids, 0.5 ml injected intramuscularly; TIG = tetanus immune globulin, 250 units injected intramuscularly.
Adapted and reproduced, with permission, from: Committee on Trauma, American College of Surgeons: Advanced Trauma Life Support Manual. American College of Surgeons, 1993.

Table 16–3. Nosocomial infections on surgical services.

Infection	Incidence (per 1000 discharges)
Bacteremia	1.3 – 4.2
Cutaneous infections	1.4 – 3.3
Other	2.0 – 6.1
Pneumonia	5.4 – 11.2
Surgical site infection	8.5 – 15.0
Urinary tract infection	12.1 – 19.5
All	30.8 – 59.3

Adapted and reproduced, with permission, from: Horan TC et al: Nosocomial infection surveillance, 1984. CDC surveillance summaries. MMWR 1986;35:17SS.

Patients may initially complain of urgency and frequency of urination or dysuria. Fever greater than 38 degrees C and a cloudy appearance to the urine are common. A urine culture is considered positive if more than 10^5 colonies/mL (100,000) of no more than two organisms grow from a clean catch, catheterized, or aspirated specimen. Fewer than 10^5 colonies/mL may be significant in a patient with a urinary tract obstruction or foreign body (ie, stent), or if certain virulent pathogens such as *Pseudomonas* species are cultured. A positive culture of less than 10^5 colonies/mL may indicate colonization rather than infection, especially in a patient who has an indwelling urinary catheter. Pyuria, more than three leukocytes/high-power field of unspun urine, supports the diagnosis of infection.

Most nosocomial UTIs are caused by coliforms, namely, *Escherichia coli*, and *Klebsiella, Enterobacter, Proteus*, or *Pseudomonas* species. Rarely, cystitis can ascend to the renal pelvis, leading to pyelonephritis or perinephric abscess.

Treatment includes antibiotics and the removal of the catheter, if possible. While community-acquired UTIs frequently respond to many drugs, including ampicillin or trimethoprim/sulfamethoxazole, empiric agents for serious nosocomial UTIs in critically ill patients include extended-spectrum penicillins, aztreonam, third-generation cephalosporins, and aminoglycosides.

SURGICAL SITE (WOUND) INFECTIONS

Surgical site infections (SSIs) generally present between the fourth and eight postoperative day and are the second most common nosocomial infection found in surgical patients. As noted previously, high fever within the first 48 hours following operation should prompt the surgeon to assess the wound for evidence of a quickly advancing beta-hemolytic streptococcal infection or clostridial gangrenous infection. In general, an inoculation of more than 10^5 microorganisms is required for the usual SSIs to develop, however, in tissues with compromised blood supply (eg, shock), foreign bodies, necrotic tissue, or hematoma, far fewer organisms can induce infection.

Many other factors have been implicated as predisposing to SSI. Proven factors include: more than 1 week of hospitalization prior to surgery (colonization by antibiotic-resistant nosocomial organisms), shaving the operative site the day before surgery (skin trauma), remote active infection (eg, upper respiratory tract, urinary, or skin infection), the routine use of prophylactic drains (especially latex Penrose drains), and operations lasting longer than 2 hours. Far less convincing evidence for the predisposition to SSI exists for different types of preoperative scrub techniques, operating room laminar-flow air systems, or surgical glove-changing protocols.

Classically, surgical procedures have been classified into four categories, each with an increasing incidence of wound infection:

- **Class I—Clean:** Elective operation wherein the GI or respiratory tracts are not opened. Examples include craniotomies, herniorrhaphy, mastectomy, and orthopedic operations. Causative organisms are frequently the patient's own skin flora (*Staphylococcus*) or exogenous contamination. Historical SSI rate: 2–3%.
- **Class II—Clean-contaminated:** Elective operations involving the GI and respiratory tracts. Examples include: pulmonary, esophageal, and intestinal resection. Infections are from exogenous sources or the patient's endogenous bacteria. Historical SSI rate: 5–15%.
- **Class III—Contaminated:** Elective operations of the respiratory or GI tract with gross contamination of the wound, or resection of acutely inflamed organs. Examples include: colon resection with gastrointestinal content spillage (Table 16–4) and appendectomy for perforated appendicitis. Historical SSI rate: 15–30%
- **Class IV—Dirty:** These cases involve gross pus, feces, and necrotic tissues. Examples include: perforated appendicitis with peritonitis or intra-abdominal abscess and gunshot wounds to the colon. Historical SSI rate: over 30%.

In 1985, workers from the Centers for Disease Control and Prevention (CDC) published their review of nearly 60,000 nosocomial SSIs. They identified four primary risk factors for the development of SSI: abdominal operation; operation lasting more than 2 hours; contaminated or dirty case as defined above; and patients with three or more diagnoses. Using this data, they identified low-, medium-, and high-risk groups for clean and clean-contaminated cases and medium- and high-risk groups for contaminated and dirty cases. Interestingly, the infection rates were not statistically different between those cases classified as clean and clean-contaminated (low risk, about 1%; medium risk, about 3–4%; and high risk, about 15%) and those classified as contaminated or dirty (medium risk, 5–6%; and high risk, 24–27%).

In 1991, CDC researchers, assessing the data from the Study on the Efficacy of Nosocomial Infection Control (SENIC) project, created a risk index score (0 to 3) based upon three components: American Society of Anesthesiologists (ASA) preoperative score of 3, 4, or 5; operation classified as contaminated or dirty; and operation lasting longer than "T" hours. The ASA score separates patients by underlying medical problems: ASA 1, a normal healthy patient; ASA 2, mild systemic disease (eg, hypertension); ASA 3, severe systemic disease that is not incapacitating; ASA 4, life-threatening systemic disease; and ASA 5, a moribund patient not expected to survive more than 24 hours. The T time is based upon the 75% percentile duration of each surgical procedure; patients whose operations exceed this time are at risk for developing postoperative infections (Table 16–5).

This risk index score is attractive, as it both considers the patient-related factors (underlying health problems) and the specific surgery being performed. Using this score, the overall SSI rates were: no risk factors—1.5%;

Table 16–4. Gastrointestinal microorganisms.

Location	Concentration (per g of stool or mL of aspirate)		Predominant Microorganisms	
	Aerobes	Anaerobes	Aerobes	Anaerobes
Oropharynx	10^4–10^5	10^5–10^7	Streptococcus Haemophilus Neisseria Diphtheroids	Peptostreptococcus Fusobacterium Bacteroides melaninogenicus
Proximal small intestine	10^2	10^1–10^2	Streptococcus Escherichia coli Klebsiella Enterobacter	Peptostreptococcus Bacteroides oralis
Distal ileum	10^4–10^6	10^5–10^7	Escherichia coli Klebsiella Enterobacter	Bacteroides fragilis Peptostreptococcus Clostridium
Colon	10^6–10^8	10^9–10^{11}	Escherichia coli Klebsiella Enterobacter	Bacteroides fragilis Peptostreptococcus Clostridium

one risk factor—2.9%; two risk factors—6.8%; and three risk factors—13.0%. Not suprisingly, a patient's risk of developing nosocomial infections other than SSI also directly increased in proportion to the number of risk factors present.

The treatment of surgical site infections is generally straightforward. Wounds with suspected or established in-

Table 16–5. Duration of surgery cut point times for selected operations.

	T (h)
Cardiothoracic/vascular procedures	
Vascular surgery	3
Thoracic surgery	3
Cardiac surgery/aorto-coronary bypass	5
General surgery procedures	
Appendectomy	1
Cholecystectomy, splenectomy	2
Herniorrhaphy, mastectomy	2
Gastric, small bowel, or colon surgery	3
Biliary, hepatic, or pancreatic surgery	4
Gynecologic/obstetrical procedures	
Cesarean section	1
Hysterectomy (vaginal or abdominal)	2
Neurosurgical procedure	
Craniotomy	4
Orthopedic procedures	
Open reduction/fixation	2
Joint prosthesis	3
Otolaryngologic procedures	
Head and neck surgery	4
Urologic procedures	
Nephrectomy	3
Prostatectomy	4
Transplantation	
Organ transplantation	7

Adapted and reproduced, with permission, from: Culver DH et al: Surgical wound infection rates by wound class, operative procedure, and patient risk index. Am J Med 1991;91:3B-152S–157S.

fection should be opened and pus evacuated. Necrotic tissue should be debrided. Once opened, most SSIs will readily heal with good local wound care, however, topical agents, such as Betadine, contribute minimally and may be harmful to granulation tissue. Systemic antibiotics are unnecessary unless one observes significant local spread or systemic signs of infection. If antibiotics are indicated and the case was classified as clean, a first-generation cephalosporin or nafcillin will suffice; otherwise, a broad-spectrum antibiotic, such as a second- or third-generation cephalosporin, a beta-lactamase inhibitor, or combination therapy, should be utilized (Table 16–1). Adjustments in therapy are then based upon clinical response and culture and susceptibility reports.

PERITONITIS/INTRA-ABDOMINAL SEPSIS

Intra-abdominal infections may be classified as either primary, secondary, or tertiary peritonitis. While the first two of these are often community-acquired, tertiary peritonitis is a serious nosocomial infection. Because the diagnostic and therapeutic principles for these problems are similar, they will be considered together in this section. Primary peritonitis, results from hematogenous bacterial contamination of ascites. While gram-positive diplococci predominate in children with nephrotic syndrome, facultative gram-negative rods are the common species isolated from adults with cirrhosis, and anaerobes are quite unusual. Management consists of supportive care and antibiotics that cover the suspected microorganism. Surgical intervention is rarely required.

Secondary peritonitis, contamination of the abdominal cavity from a diseased or injured portion of the GI tract or anastomotic leakage, represents a true surgical emergency. Presenting symptoms and signs include abdominal pain and tenderness, fever greater than 38 degrees C, and diminished or absent bowel sounds. Evidence of peritoneal irritation, such as pain on cough, tenderness to percussion, and involuntary guarding ("board-like" abdomen) are found. The patient often assumes a fetal position to decrease the stretch on his abdominal wall and lessen the discomfort.

Laboratory findings include a moderate-to-marked leukocytosis (white blood cell count [WBC] > 15,000 cells/mm^3). Plain abdominal radiographs may demonstrate free intraperitoneal air. In cases where no clear cut indication for surgery exists and the diagnosis is difficult, a diagnostic peritoneal lavage may be performed. One liter of crystalloid solution (eg, normal saline) is infused through a catheter placed either percutaneously or by cutdown into the peritoneum. After draining the fluid, a WBC count exceeding 500 cells/mm^3 suggests peritonitis. Most often, the causative organisms are those bacteria found in the particular part of the GI tract that is leaking. The more common endogenous bacteria and their concentrations from various locations in the digestive system are listed in Table 16–4. Intraperitoneal collections of adjuvants, such as blood, ascites, bile, and barium, dramatically diminish the number of organisms required to initiate infection.

Management includes fluid resuscitation, parenteral antibiotics, and timely operative intervention. Some authors have compared generalized peritonitis to a 50% body surface area burn, stressing the dramatic fluid requirements necessary to compensate for third-space losses. Therefore, the treatment of shock and optimization of oxygen delivery to the tissues assumes a primary role in the treatment of peritonitis.

Appropriate doses of antibiotics directed at gastrointestinal flora should be administered, keeping in mind that both aerobic and anaerobic organisms must be covered. This can be achieved using two agents, one with activity primarily against aerobes and a second with activity against anaerobes. Some antimicrobials inherently provide sufficient coverage of both aerobic and anaerobic enteric pathogens, and these may be selected for single-drug therapy (Table 16–1). Surgical intervention involves the repair or resection of the diseased or injured organ combined with saline irrigation to remove all collections of purulent or particulate material.

Tertiary peritonitis, comprising persistent or suprainfection of the original intra-abdominal infection or abscesses, may complicate any abdominal surgery. Such problems usually present after the fifth to seventh postoperative day, unless the abscess formation is in the subphrenic or subhepatic spaces, which may delay the presentation until the seventh through tenth days. Worsening abdominal pain and tenderness, elevated temperature, and other local and systemic signs should lead the surgeon to consider anastomotic leak or intra-abdominal abscess. An intra-abdominal source should likewise be considered if a patient who has undergone abdominal surgery develops postoperative respiratory failure (ie, acute respiratory distress syndrome [ARDS]). Ultrasonography and computed tomography (CT) can identify more than 50% of abscesses, but prompt reexploration should ensue for postoperative patients with frank peritonitis.

Tertiary peritonitis will rarely resolve with efficacious parenterally administered antibiotics alone, and further surgical intervention is often necessary. In recent years, image-guided percutaneous drainage of an intra-abdominal abscess have saved many patients the discomfort of an additional operation. This technique, while tremendously useful, should not be utilized when two or more abscess collections exist; when the abscess is in close approximation with the pancreas; when septations are present; or when percutaneous drainage would involve traversing bowel or an uninfected body cavity. Severe intra-abdominal infections often require repeated reexplorations to ensure that the infection is under control. Some surgeons insert a piece of mesh containing a zipper or similar device to facilitate reexploration, while others opt to simply pack the abdomen open and manage the peritoneum as one large abscess cavity. Secondary closure of both the fascia and skin are accomplished when the intraperitoneal purulence has resolved.

POSTOPERATIVE PNEUMONIA

Nosocomial pneumonia represents a significant problem for surgical patients. The incidence in hospitalized patients is 0.5–5%, however, as many as 20% of patients admitted to a surgical intensive care unit (SICU) will develop a pneumonia. Many of these infections result from resistant gram-negative bacilli and the mortality rate approaches 50%.

Factors predisposing to pneumonia include thoracic and upper abdominal incisions, prolonged preoperative hospitalization, mechanical ventilation longer than 48 hours, and underlying lung injury (ARDS or pulmonary contusion). Pain commonly seen in the early postoperative course further compromises the patient's ability to cough and take deep breaths.

In many hospitalized patients, the diagnosis of nosocomial pneumonia is relatively simple to make. Findings of fever greater than 38°C, productive cough, pleuritic chest pain, leukocytosis, and new or increasing infiltrates on radiograph confirm the diagnosis. Gram's stain of the sputum should show numerous leukocytes with few epithelial cells while cultures grow a predominant pathogenic organism.

Diagnosis in critically ill patients in the SICU is more challenging. Chest radiographs frequently have preexisting abnormalities (atelectasis, ARDS, etc,) and cultures obtained by suctioning through an endotracheal tube or tracheostomy may well represent colonization rather than infection. In these circumstances, the intensivist must fall back on sputum WBCs, sputum production, leukocytosis, and fever to identify pneumonia. Bronchoscopy using a protected specimen brush (extended in bronchus after passage though the endotracheal tube) increases diagnostic yield and minimizes misinformation from contamination. In unusual circumstances, transtracheal aspiration, or even open lung biopsy, may be performed.

Gram-negative bacilli are the causative agent in more than three-quarters of nosocomial pneumonia, while *Staphylococcus* accounts for 15–20%. *Klebsiella* produces significant inflammation and blood-tinged sputum, while *Pseudomonas* results in greenish sputum. *Staphylococcus aureus* often manifests itself with a patchy appearance on the chest radiograph while others tend to produce lobar infiltrates. All three of these organisms may lead to lung necrosis and abscess formation.

Treatment of nosocomial pneumonia involves aggressive pulmonary toiletry and parenteral antibiotics. Bronchodilators are most useful in patients with reactive airway disease. Most experts treat severe *Pseudomonas* or *Enterobacter* pneumonia with two antibiotic agents to which they are sensitive, while single agents (imi-penem/cilastatin, aztreonam, ciprofloxacin, or a third-generation cephalosporin) may be used for less virulent microbes. Resistant forms of *Staphylococcus aureus* are treated with either oxacillin or vancomycin. As many as 75% of ICU patients develop colonization of their upper airways with gram-negative bacilli. Attempts at selective gut decontamination, where antibiotics are administered locally in the oropharynx and stomach to control colonization, have not significantly altered the mortality.

EMPYEMA

Strictly speaking, **empyema** represents a collection of pus in any body cavity. In modern usage, this term refers to an infection of the pleural space. When one considers all cases of empyema, about half of these result from direct seeding of a parapneumonic pleural effusion and about one third follow thoracic surgery. Transdiaphragmatic extension of intra-abdominal infection and chest trauma account for probably less than one fifth of cases. While many are not hospital-acquired, most cases encountered on surgical services follow thoracotomy for lung or esophageal resection, or placement of chest tubes for hemothorax. A smaller percentage result from nosocomial pneumonia.

While chest x-ray may reveal a pleural effusion, the return of foul-smelling purulent material upon thoracentesis or tube thoracostomy confirms the diagnosis. In situations where only cloudy fluid is obtained, laboratory analysis is indicated. Pleural fluid from empyema generally possess the following characteristics: WBC greater than 25,000 cell/mL, with a predominance of neutrophils; pH below 7.3 and often below 7.0; and glucose less than 40 mg/dL. As the pleural space is usually sterile, the presence of bacteria on Gram's stain or culture assure the diagnosis. *Streptococcus*, *Staphylococcus*, anaerobes, and gram-negative bacilli are among the predominant microorganisms.

Surgical drainage of the pleural space utilizing a large-bore tube thoracostomy is the first step in the management. Appropriate intravenous antibiotics are administered, with agents selected initially based upon the Gram's stain and altered, if necessary, after culture and suscepti-

bility reports are available. CT of the chest may reveal loculations. Failure to adequately achieve satisfactory re-expansion of the affected lung or residual loculation not drained by chest tubes requires more aggressive surgical intervention. Choices of procedures include open drainage of the pleural space, with resection of a rib to ensure continued drainage, and formal decortication, wherein the fibrotic peel that has entrapped the lung is removed. In most series, mortality rates range from 10–20%. When empyema follows thoracic surgery, one should be suspicious of a leaking esophageal anastomosis or bronchial stump, if they were part of the original procedure.

INTRAVASCULAR CATHETER SEPSIS

Approximately 5–10% of all vascular catheters become infected. More significant systemic manifestations are usually associated with central venous or pulmonary artery catheters, however, infection of venous and arterial catheters or needles, in any location, can cause generalized sepsis. *Staphylococcus aureus* and *S. epidermidis* are more frequently cultured, however, gram-negative rods and *Candida* also contribute.

Indwelling catheters may become infected via three routes. The most common involves skin flora tracking along the catheter from the puncture site. Hematogenous seeding of the device from a remote site and, most rarely, from the infusion of contaminated fluids also contribute. Surgeons should entertain this diagnosis in all patients with intravascular catheters who manifest fever over 38°C) and leukocytosis.

Of interest is that multilumen catheters have a higher incidence of infection than single-lumen ones. Central lines placed in the femoral vein are at highest risk for line sepsis, followed by internal jugular and subclavian sites, respectively. Strict aseptic technique as well as masks, hair covers, and sterile gowns and gloves should be utilized when placing central lines, especially in the intensive care setting.

Treatment involves removing the infected catheter. If skin puncture site demonstrates erythema or purulent discharge, the infected line should be removed and reinserted at a different site if continued vascular access is needed. In a febrile patient in whom catheter sepsis may be the source, a central venous catheter can be exchanged over a guide-wire and the tip of the old catheter cultured. A semiquantitative ("Maki") technique is utilized and the tip of the catheter is rolled on a culture plate. Fifteen or more colonies is considered positive, and the catheter should be moved to a new site. Rare complications of central vascular lines include septic thrombophlebitis requiring surgical excision of the involved vein.

In general, fever and leukocytosis should resolve within 24 hours following removal of the catheter. Continued signs of sepsis should encourage one to seek other possible etiologies or, if the catheter tip culture was positive, administer appropriate antibiotics. A culture positive for

S. aureus, associated with signs of systemic infection, should prompt one to consider both consultation with an infectious disease specialist and 10–14 days of parenteral antibiotic therapy. This has been shown to reduce the incidence of late metastatic infections, such as osteomyelitis or endocarditis. Penicillin-allergic patients and those with methicillin-resistant *S. aureus* should receive parenteral vancomycin.

PSEUDOMEMBRANOUS COLITIS

Virtually all cases of pseudomembranous colitis result from an overgrowth of *Clostridium difficile*. The use of almost all antibiotics predisposes patients to this problem. *Clostridium difficile* are normally found in 3–10% of the adult population and 30–40% of neonates. When they overgrow, they can produce symptoms ranging from mild diarrhea to frank toxic colitis. As most cases involve the left and sigmoid portions of the colon, flexible sigmoidoscopy may demonstrate pseudomembranes consisting of mucosal cells and fibrin. While *C. difficile* may be cultured, most clinicians depend on a stool assay for the toxin it produces. The toxin is found in the stool of about 90% of infected persons. Several case reports have documented isolated distal ileal involvement. Today, most patients are treated with ampicillin, cephalosporins, or clindamycin. This trend will no doubt change as antibiotic prescription practices are altered.

Treatment includes discontinuing the offending antibiotic and resisting the temptation to administer narcotic antidiarrheal agents. Previously, oral vancomycin was used because it is slowly absorbed. While doses as high as 500 mg enterally, four times daily for 7 days, have been recommended, the trend in the last decade has been toward lower doses, and many now use 125 mg enterally four times daily for 7 days. Out of concern for selecting out vancomycin-resistant strains, most experts currently recommend metronidazole, 500 mg every 8 hours for 7 days, as the initial drug of choice. While relapses of infection may be slightly higher with metronidazole, its advantages include the option of parenteral or enteral dosage and significantly lower cost.

CANDIDIASIS

Disseminated *Candida* infections pose significant risk to critically ill surgical patients, with mortality rates ranging from 33–75%. Severe candidal infections develop in catastrophically ill postoperative patients, most of whom have been in the ICU for 2–3 weeks before candidemia is first noted. Microabscesses with *Candida* lead to organ dysfunction, including cardiac dysrhythmias, decreased glomerular filtration, and visual disturbances from chorioretinitis. The fungus is believed to gain access to the body from the GI tract, where it is part of the normal flora, or via an intravascular catheter. Broad-spectrum antibiotics predispose to colonization of the oropharynx, respiratory tract, bladder, and surgical sites (eg, peritoneal cavity). The risk for candidemia and, therefore, disseminated candidiasis is directly related to the number of colonized sites.

Though the role for prophylactic agents remains unsettled, many experts recommend prophylactic fluconazole in patients in whom *Candida* colonization has been identified in two locations. Amphotericin B, in doses of at least 0.5 mg/kg/d, is recommended for patients with candidemia, or those with either persistently positive urine cultures or disseminated candidiasis.

ANTIBIOTIC PROPHYLAXIS

Surgeons have achieved great advances in lowering wound infection rates in elective surgical procedures. Altering those practices that put patients at risk for surgical site infections, such as treating remote infections prior to surgery, minimizing preoperative hospitalization, and abandoning the use of prophylactic drains, has contributed to the decrease in infections, but the appropriate use of prophylactic antibiotics has had the greatest effect. Authoritative committees have standardized issues of timing and route of administration as well as choice of antibiotic.

Prophylactic antibiotics are indicated for many clean procedures and all clean-contaminated operations. To ensure adequate tissue levels, these medications should be administered intravenously in the operating room just prior to incision. While experts have discouraged the use of prophylactic anti-infective agents for longer than 24 hours postoperatively, most current research suggests that a single preoperative dose yields protection from SSI similar to the standard multiple perioperative doses. Should the operation last more than 2 or 3 hours, an additional dose of antibiotic should be administered. The use of preoperative antibiotics in contaminated and dirty cases is, by definition, therapeutic and not prophylactic.

CLEAN OPERATIONS

Prophylactic antibiotics are not generally recommended unless the operation involves implanting foreign material, such as vascular grafts, artificial valves, orthopedic prostheses, or mesh. In these cases, a preoperative dose of a first-generation cephalosporin is administered, unless the hospital has a high rate of methicillin-resistant *Staphylococcus*, in which case vancomycin may be given. Some recent data supports the use of a single preoperative dose of cephalosporin for breast and hernia surgery (clean procedures without prostheses), especially in high-risk patients.

CLEAN-CONTAMINATED OPERATIONS

Gastric Surgery

Patients undergoing gastric surgery can be divided into two risk groups based upon their preoperative acid level and indication for surgery. Low-risk patients, such as those undergoing surgery for chronic nonobstructing duodenal ulcer, have normal preoperative gastric acid levels and have less than a 5% risk for SSI. No prophylactic antibiotics are indicated in these patients.

Those in the high-risk group have impairment of normal gastric acid secretion and gastric motility and, as a result, tend to have increased concentrations of gastric organisms. Patients in this category include those receiving surgery for chronic obstructive gastric and duodenal ulcers, malignancy, and hemorrhage, as well as those who were taking H_2 antagonists or proton pump inhibitors prior to operation. A first- or second-generation cephalosporin should be used preoperatively for patients in this group.

Cholecystectomy

Between 15% and 30% of patients with chronic calculous cholecystitis have colonization of their biliary tree with enteric pathogens. Risk factors for such colonization include age greater than 70 years, diabetes mellitus, and prior biliary tract surgery. Some believe that patients having one or more of these risk factors should receive a single prophylactic dose of a first- or second-generation cephalosporin prior to incision, while most others feel that every patient undergoing cholecystectomy should receive a single dose of antibiotic, regardless of the absence of risk factors. Patients with acute cholangitis or acute cholecystitis should receive therapeutic, not prophylactic, antibiotics.

Colon Surgery

The colon houses tremendously high concentrations of bacteria. Combinations of mechanical and antibiotic bowel preparation have enabled surgeons to perform colonic surgery safely and with a small risk of SSI (Figure 16–1). Two days prior to surgery, the patient limits his oral intake to a liquid or low-residue diet and may use an oral dose of magnesium citrate (or magnesium sulfate) cathartic or Fleet Phospho-Soda. The day before surgery, the patient cleanses the colon using oral polyethylene glycol/electrolyte solution, or additional doses of magnesium citrate (or sulfate) or Fleet Phospho-Soda.

While mechanical preparation reduces the total fecal mass, it fails to significantly reduce the number of organisms in the residual stool. To this end, an oral antibiotic preparation, involving doses of agents active against aerobes and anaerobes, is given at 1:00 PM, 2:00 PM, and 11:00 PM, when surgery is scheduled at 8:00 AM the following day. The most popular combination during the last 20 years has been neomycin (antiaerobe) and erythromycin base (antianaerobe). If the colon resection is scheduled for later in the day, the antibiotic schedule

should be readjusted to maintain the 19-hour interval before operation. An optional dose of second- or third-generation cephalosporin is most often given just before incision and repeated during the operation if the procedure lasts longer than 2 or 3 hours.

Appendectomy

In cases of suspected acute appendicitis, a single dose of a second- or third-generation cephalosporin should be given preoperatively. If the appendix is normal or simply inflamed, additional postoperative doses are unnecessary. Additional postoperative doses administered for perforated or gangrenous appendicitis are therapeutic and not prophylactic.

Small Bowel Resection

Little data exist to evaluate the risk of SSI following small bowel resection. In cases where the terminal ileum may be opened, one might consider using preoperative oral neomycin and erythromycin base, however, no mechanical preparation seems necessary. A parenteral second- or third-generation cephalosporin should be used just prior to incision in suspected small bowel obstruction.

Obstetrics/Gynecologic Surgery

A single dose of first-generation cephalosporin should be given following clamping of the umbilical cord in emergency Cesarean sections and preoperatively for abdominal or vaginal hysterectomy.

Urologic Surgery

Prophylactic antibiotics are generally not indicated for those undergoing transurethral prostatectomy unless a preoperative urine culture is positive. An agent effective against the organism isolated should be chosen. Most often, a first-generation cephalosporin will accomplish these ends.

TRAUMA SURGERY

Thoracic Trauma

Data suggest that, in patients undergoing placement of tube thoracostomies for traumatic hemopneumothorax, a first- or second-generation cephalosporin (eg, cefazolin or cefonicid) does decrease the incidence of subsequent empyema and pneumonia. Unlike older studies wherein a great number of doses were administered, current studies limit the total usage to around five doses.

Abdominal Trauma

Risk of SSI in victims of penetrating abdominal trauma has been shown to correlate with increasing age, injury to the left colon necessitating colostomy, transfusion of multiple units of blood products, and the number of organs injured. However, as one might predict, the risk factor that correlates best with the development of SSI following abdominal trauma is the presence of an enterotomy with

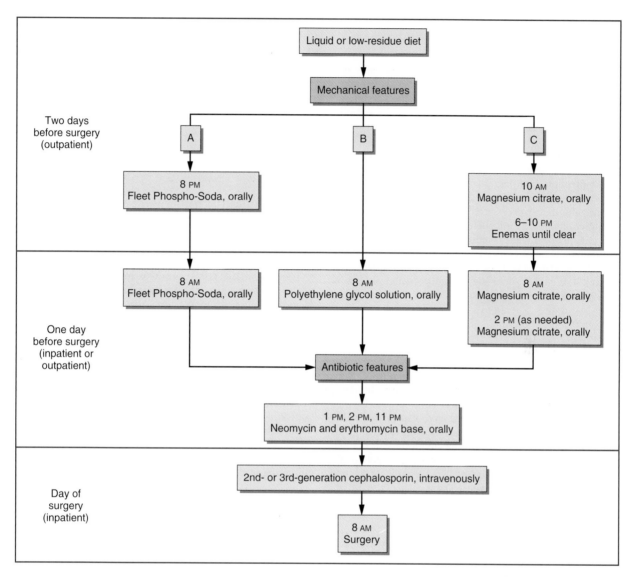

Figure 16–1. Alternative methods of bowel preparation for elective colon resection. Mechanical and antibiotic bowel preparation can be performed on an outpatient basis, however, high-risk elderly patients may require inpatient observation and intravenous therapy to prevent dehydration. ***A:*** Two doses of Fleet Phospho-Soda, each of 45 mL in 4 oz of water, are given 12 hours apart. Because of electrolyte abnormalities, Phospho-Soda should not be used in patients with congenital megacolon, congestive heart failure, or renal insufficiency. ***B:*** Polyethylene glycol solution is consumed at a rate of 1 L/hr for 2–4 hours, until the fecal effluent is clear. ***C:*** If magnesium citrate is selected, at least two doses of 10 oz each should be taken. The third dose is unnecessary if the fecal effluent is clear. Once mechanical preparation is completed, all patients should receive antibiotic preparation. Neomycin and erythromycin base, 1 g each, are given at 1:00 PM, 2:00 PM, and 11:00 PM the day prior to an 8:00 AM operation. If surgery is earlier or later, the dosages of the oral antibiotics must be adjusted to maintain the 19-hour schedule prior to surgery. A 1-g dose of parenteral cephalosporin is optional. If given, the agent should possess activity against aerobes and anaerobes (see Table 16–1) and be administered in the operating room just prior to skin incision.

contamination of the peritoneal cavity by gastrointestinal contents. Several agents, including cefoxitin, ceftizoxime, and ampicillin/sulbactam have all been shown to significantly decrease postoperative SSI in this clinical setting. A single preoperative dose of antibiotic is adequate when no GI perforation is identified at surgery, while 1–2 days of prophylaxis are usually employed when perforation is found. In the high-risk patients, the operative incision should be initially packed open and later closed secondarily.

BLOODBORNE ILLNESS

The recogniton of the acquired immune deficiency syndrome (AIDS) in the early 1980s focused new attention on the patient as a vector of bloodborne disease. Though initially conceived to protect the patient from the surgeon, operating room attire found a new purpose—to also protect the surgeon from the patient. Attempts have been made by both surgeons and patient's rights organizations to have the other group undergo mandatory testing for viral infection, but these attempts have not succeeded on either front. Of significance is that present data indicate that health care workers (HCWs) are far more likely to contract bloodborne infection from their patients than are the patients from their health professionals. While human immunodeficiency virus (HIV) disease has been the center of concern because of its universally fatal outcome, hepatitis B and C pose significantly greater threats to HCWs and deserve appropriate attention.

VIRAL HEPATITIS

Both hepatitis B virus (HBV) and hepatitis C virus (HCV) can be transmitted via human blood and, therefore, can potentially infect surgeons and other HCWs. Prior to the mandatory offering of preventative vaccination, HBV infected about 12,000 HCWs yearly. Up to 300 HCWs die annually from either fulminant hepatic failure or complications of chronic HBV infection. More than half of infected persons are asymptomatic and a significant fraction will develop a carrier state. Those patients who are seronegative for hepatitis B early antigen (HB_eAg) are less likely to transmit HBV to HCWs than those who are Hb_eAg-positive.

Hepatitis B immune globulin (HBIG) can provide passive protection from a low-volume inoculation, such as a percutaneous injury or mucous membrane exposure, but cannot provide adequate protection from the volume of virus transmitted by contaminated blood. A recombinant vaccine, derived from the hepatitis B surface antigen (HB_sAg), is available for hepatitis B, and all HCWs who have patient contact should be vaccinated. Surprisingly, studies have documented that up to 26% of surgeons have not received immunization. The Occupational Safety and Health Administration (OSHA) now requires employers to offer vaccination for employees in high-risk environments. Serologic testing should confirm antibody response following immunization.

Once identified, hepatitis C virus (HCV) accounted for about 85–90% of non-A, non-B hepatitis. Like HBV, HCV infection can range from an asymptomatic course to fulminant hepatic failure. More worrisome is that about two thirds of patients develop persistent elevations of liver enzymes, and in many the chronic active hepatitis progresses to cirrhosis and predisposes them to hepatocellular carcinoma. New developments in the HCV screen have improved the safety of blood supplies; current tests possess a specificity of over 99% and a sensitivity of 60–73%. No vaccine is yet available, and the efficacy of HBIG remains unproven for HCV inoculation. Most recent estimates place the risk of contracting hepatitis C from a unit of blood as about one in 10,000, still more frequent than the reported risk of one in 150,000 for a hemolytic transfusion reaction. Epidemiologists estimate that during a surgeon's career the risk of infection with hepatitis approaches 50%.

HUMAN IMMUNODEFICIENCY VIRUS

Though the risk of contracting hepatitis is much greater, more HCWs worry about HIV infection because of its uniformly fatal prognosis. Two serotypes of HIV have been identified: HIV-1 accounts for virtually all AIDS in the US and equatorial Africa, while HIV-2 is found almost exclusively in Western Africa. While early victims were male homosexuals, intravenous drug users, or hemophiliacs, HIV disease has now found its way into teenage and adult heterosexual populations, with concentrations in many minority communities.

The ELISA screening test has a low rate of false positives; all positive tests should be confirmed with the more sensitive Western Blot electrophoresis technique. The risk of contracting HIV from a unit of blood that passes all screening tests is currently estimated to be about one in 500,000, but this may vary according to the local prevalence. Prevalence rates of HIV infections in patients presenting to emergency departments vary with the community (eg, 4.3% in Chicago and 6% in Baltimore).

While most HCWs recognize that blood and semen of HIV-positive individuals can transmit the disease, vaginal secretions and pericardial, peritoneal, pleural, amniotic, and cerebrospinal fluids are all considered potentially infected. Tears, urine, sweat, feces, and saliva are generally not considered infectious unless they are grossly bloody. The highest risks of exposure to HIV occur in emergency Cesarean sections and cardiac, trauma, and emergency surgery.

To date, fewer than 50 HCWs have confirmed occupational infection with HIV, and most of these followed percutaneous injury by a hollow needle or other sharp; only a handful are felt to have occured from mucocutaneous contact. Of note, no seroconversions have been documented following puncture by a contaminated solid (suture) needle. Only 0.3–0.5% (about one in 250) of needlestick exposures to HIV-positive blood lead to infection, a figure much lower than infection from an HBV-infected needle (6–30%). Seroconversion following a needlestick contaminated with HCV falls somewhere in between. One explanation for this is the relative concentration of virus particles in the infected blood: HBV-positive blood contains 10^{8-109} virus particles/mL; HCV-positive blood, 106 particles/mL; and HIV-positive blood, 102–104 particles/mL.

These data may also explain why seroconversion has been documented from percutaneous inoculation by solid suture needles with both HBV and HCV, but not HIV. Thus, when seroconversion rates and prevalence of disease are considered, a susceptible surgeon exposed to HBV has a greater risk of dying than a surgeon exposed to HIV. Epidemiologists have estimated that the lifetime risk of contracting HIV to a surgeon practicing in an area with a high incidence of AIDS is in the range of 0.01–0.11%.

Following accidental exposure to potentially contaminated blood, an injury should be washed with a germicidal soap, and adequate tetanus coverage should be ensured. The event should be thoroughly documented, including the type of injury and an estimation of the volume of inoculate. OSHA requires each institution to have an individualized control plan for such exposures, however, one appropriate protocol includes the following steps. A baseline HIV screen is performed on both the involved patient and HCW. If the patient is seronegative for HIV and has no evidence of HIV disease, no further workup is indicated. If the patient is seropositive for HIV or refuses testing, the HCW should be retested at 6 weeks and 3, 6, and 12 months following exposure. Most seroconversions occur 6 to 12 weeks after exposure. Experts now recommend the prophylactic use of zidovudine (AZT), lamivudine (3TC), and indinavir for HCWs who suffer a high-risk exposure (deep inoculation of blood with a high titer of HIV). HCWs who suffer a low-risk exposure should be offered both AZT and 3TC, however, the protective effect of these agents in this setting is less substantiated. The long-term toxicity of these agents remains unknown.

The role of HCWs infected with HIV remains controversial. Although no documented case of HIV infection from an infected surgeon to a patient exists, six patients apparently contracted HIV disease from their infected dentist. But this transmission, if it, in fact, occurred, is the only example of HCW-to-patient transmission in over 10 years. HBV and HCV infection has been documented to occur from HCW to patient. The CDC recommends that HIV-positive physicians not perform exposure-prone, invasive procedures, but the President's Commission on AIDS concluded that HIV-infected HCWs need not curtail their practices nor inform their patients.

UNIVERSAL PRECAUTIONS

Since the identification of HIV disease, much emphasis has been placed upon practicing universal precautions– treating all patients as if they are potentially infected with bloodborne illness. Such precautions have been adopted because clinical examination cannot reliably identify all patients who pose a threat to HCWs. These guidelines, when followed, dramatically minimize a HCW's exposure to blood and body fluids of potentially infected patients. Despite the obvious benefit and federal regulations mandating such safe practices in the health care workplace,

studies have often documented poor compliance with universal precautions. Universal precautions include:

- **Needles and other sharps:** Because more than 80% of occupational HIV infection in HCWs occurs from needlesticks and injury from sharp instruments, extraordinary care must be taken when handling these items. Needle should never be reused or recapped. Following use, they should be immediately placed in protective containers. Scalpels should not be handed back and forth, but rather passed in a metal container. Surgeons should learn to operate with a minimal touch technique, holding the suture needle in one hand and and an instrument in the other hand to handle tissues, resisting temptation to use the fingers of the nondominant hand. Care should also be exercised when manipulating wires and bone fragments.
- **Gloves:** Gloves should be worn when touching nonintact skin, mucous membranes, or contaminated body fluids. Because perforations have been documented in more than 33% of surgeon's gloves during operative procedures, many opt for routine double-gloving. Gloves should be changed immediately after a glove is noted to be defective.
- **Masks:** Masks serve to protect the HCW's oral mucous membranes from exposure. They should be changed immediately if they become wet or soiled. Aerosolized transmission of HIV particles created by surgical power tools has not been documented.
- **Gowns:** Disposable gowns with impervious plastic liners offer the best protection, however they can be extremely uncomfortable to wear. Disposable gowns should provide proven protection and should be changed immediately if they become significantly soiled.
- **Eyewear:** Eye protection must be worn in circumstances where droplets of infected fluid may be splattered. Standard eyeglasses are not considered adequate, as they lack sideshields.
- **Handwashing:** Handwashing is a fundamental principle of infection control. Hands should be washed immediately if contaminated with blood or body fluids or as soon as gloves are removed following completion of an examination or procedure.
- **Resuscitation equipment:** Areas in which resuscitation might be predicted to occur should have resuscitation bags or mouthpieces for the protection of rescuers.

IMMUNONUTRITION

For more than 50 years, surgeons have recognized the relationship between malnutrition and perioperative infections and death. In 1936, Studley found a strong association between preoperative weight loss and increased mortality following gastric resection for chronic peptic ulcer.

Surgeons, therefore, have played significant roles in developing nutritional support for patients unable to eat. In recent years, research has focused on the observation that certain nutrients, when supplied in quantities greater than nutritional requirements, seem to have pharmacologic activities and may well improve immune system functioning.

The amino acids glutamine and arginine, omega-3 fatty acids, nucleic acids, and vitamins A, D, and E fall into this category. Glutamine, an essential amino acid in times of stress, serves as an important substrate for enterocytes and lymphocytes and improves neutrophil killing. Arginine, another conditionally essential amino acid, reduces protein catabolism during stress, stimulates T-lymphocyte proliferation, and improves macrophage functioning. It also stimulates the secretion of many hormones, including pituitary growth hormone and insulin-like growth hormone, and may improve wound healing. The omega-3 polyunsaturated fatty acids (PUFAs) are precursors for many eicosanoids, and their administration is believed to enhance cell-mediated immune response. The omega-6 PUFAs appear to have immunosuppressive effects, namely, through the production of PGE_2. Because a diet free of nucleic acids results in suppression of cellular immunity, some authorities believe that nucleotide supplementation could improve natural killer cell activity. The fat-soluble vitamins A, D, and E possess important antioxidant properties and thereby counteract oxygen-derived free radicals and peroxide.

Mounting evidence seems to support that seriously ill, hypermetabolic patients suffering from trauma, immunosuppression, or preexisting malnutrition from malignancy may well benefit from specialized nutrition. A recent multicenter, prospective, randomized clinical trial compared an enteral formula supplemented with arginine, glutamine, omega-3 PUFAs, and ribonucleic acids (Impact) to another commonly use enteral product. This study documented a statistically significant reduction in both hospital stay and frequency of acquired infections in the patients who received the specialized formula. The role of immunonutrition in surgical infections is yet to be fully defined.

SUGGESTED READING

Abramowicz M (editor): Antimicrobial prophylaxis in surgery. Med Lett Drugs Ther 1995;37:79.

Bohnen JM et al: Guidelines for clinical care: Anti-infective agents for intra-abdominal infection; A Surgical Infection Society Policy Statement. Arch Surg 1993;127:83.

Committee on Trauma, American College of Surgeons: Tetanus immunization. In: *Advanced Trauma Life Support Manual.* American College of Surgeons, 1993.

Culver DH et al: Surgical wound infection rates by wound class, operative procedure, and patient risk index. Am J Med 1991;91:3B–152S.

Gardner JS et al: CDC definitions for nosocomial infections, 1988. Am J Infect Contr 1988;16:128.

Grant JP: Nutritional support in critically ill patients. Ann Surg 1994:220;610.

Haley RW et al: Identifying patients at high risk of surgical wound infection. A simple multivariate index of patient susceptibility and wound contamination. Am J Epidemiol 1985; 121:206.

Horan TC et al: CDC definitions of nosocomial surgical site infection, 1992: A modification of CDC definitions of surgical wound infections. Infect Control Hosp Epidemiol 1992;13: 606.

Kelly CP, Pothoulakis C, LaMont JT: *Clostridium difficile* colitis. N Engl J Med 1994;330:257.

Nichols RL: Surgical wound infection. Am J Med 1991;91: 3B–54S.

Nichols RL: Bowel preparations. In: Wilmore DW et al (editors): *Scientific American Surgery.* Scientific American, 1995.

Nichols RL: Surgical antibiotic prophylaxis. Surg Clin North Am 1995;79:509.

Nichols RL et al: Prospective alterations in therapy for penetrating abdominal trauma. Arch Surg 1993;128:55.

17

Multiple Organ Dysfunction Syndrome

Adam Seiver, MD

▶ Key Facts

▶ The multiple organ dysfunction syndrome (MODS) is a temporal sequence of symptoms and signs associated with abnormal function in two or more organ systems.

▶ Patients in whom MODS develops have a high probability of dying (> 50%).

▶ It is now believed that MODS is a consequence of generalized inflammation.

▶ The patient in whom MODS develops has almost always experienced a major insult (shock, infection, tissue injury, or a combination of these), after which major organ systems (central nervous, pulmonary, cardiac, hepatic, gastrointestinal, immune, renal) begin to fail.

▶ If the patient recovers from critical illness, comprehensive rehabilitation is often required to return him or her to a baseline level of function.

▶ Nutrition is an essential part of the supportive care of MODS. It now appears that enteral nutrition is superior to parenteral nutrition.

▶ Future therapies for MODS may address the pathophysiology at a fundamental level, perhaps at the level of cellular and humoral mediators.

The **multiple organ dysfunction syndrome (MODS)** is a temporal sequence of symptoms and signs associated with abnormal function in two or more organ systems. Usually, MODS is triggered by a major insult—shock, infection, or tissue injury occurring singly or in combination. At an interval after the insult that varies from hours to days, respiratory, neurologic, hepatic, cardiac, gastrointestinal, and renal functional abnormalities become evident.

Frequently, these abnormalities become severe enough to require significant life-support, which may include mechanical ventilation, inotropes, parenteral nutrition, transfusion, and even dialysis. In some cases the organ dysfunction reaches a peak, regresses, and the patient survives. In other cases, however, the patient's organ dysfunction progresses. The patient ultimately dies of cardiopulmonary collapse—often, as life-support is withdrawn because of the grim prognosis.

Patients who develop MODS have a high probability of dying—typically, greater than 50%. Additionally, a large fraction of the patients on a surgical service that die following operation or trauma die with MODS. The daily cost (not charge) for managing an MODS patient requiring multi-organ life-support averages approximately $4000 per day. Because the syndrome may require 3 weeks of critical care and several more weeks of inpatient rehabilitation, the average cost for managing a surviving patient will frequently total more than $200,000. MODS is, thus, highly lethal and expensive, making its prevention and management an important challenge for the general surgeon.

PATHOPHYSIOLOGY

The pathophysiology of MODS is not completely understood, but is beginning to be elucidated with techniques from molecular biology. It appears that MODS is the consequence of generalized inflammation. The precipitating event—whether it is shock, infection, tissue injury, or pancreatitis—produces a local inflammatory response. Ordinarily, this is a welcomed occurrence, since the local inflammation is part of the healing response. In MODS, however, this local inflammation becomes generalized and is associated with injury and abnormality remote from the original site.

What causes the local inflammation to progress to persistent, generalized inflammation? One theory proposes that "two hits" are actually required. The precipitating event primes the immune system. Then a second event, which may be a much smaller insult than the first, triggers this primed immune system to produce widespread injury. Other theories stress the importance of ischemia and reperfusion or the translocation of microbes or endotoxin from the gut in causing persistence of inflammation. Still other theories focus not on abnormality in the inflammatory onset, but on a failure of inflammation to turn off. It is likely that multiple factors play a role in producing the damaging immunological response.

Much of the study of MODS recently has focused on the cellular and humoral mediators of the inflammation. These include macrophages, polymorphonuclear leuko-

HISTORICAL FACTS

MODS was first recognized in the 1970s with the description of "sequential systems failure" by Tilney and the report of "multiple, progressive, or sequential systems failure" by Baue. A key observation was that a severe physiologic insult—such as shock from a ruptured abdominal aortic aneurysm— could lead to failure of organ systems that were remote from the original insult and initially uninvolved. In the 1980s, the role of uncontrolled infection was highlighted by Eiseman, Polk, and Fry.

In the context of multiple organ failure following abdominal surgery, this often led to exploratory laparotomy to look for an intra-abdominal abscess in need of surgical drainage. The broad availability of computed tomography (CT) body scanning by the late 1980s shifted practice somewhat, with imaging and percutaneous abscess drainage substituting, in many cases, for laparotomy.

By the 1990s, the role of infection underwent reevaluation. While uncontrolled infection clearly produced organ failure, it appeared to be an incomplete explanation. There were many cases of multiple organ failure in which infection could not be identified. The focus, thus, has shifted to generalized inflammation, which might be triggered by infection, but which might also be initiated by tissue injury, by local inflammation such as pancreatitis, or by shock. Molecular biological tools have helped to characterize this inflammatory response in terms of humoral and cellular mediators.

The challenge for the next decade is to sort out the apparently extraordinarily complex network of interacting inflammatory pathways and gain insight into the key underlying processes. This insight may lead to recognition of practical intervention points. Perhaps these will enable definitive control of the inflammatory response and allow us to either prevent MODS, or to at least reduce its morbidity, mortality, and cost.

cytes, cytokines, such as tumor necrosis factor (TNF), interleukins (IL-1, IL-6, and IL-8); platelet activating factor; leukotrienes; bradykinin; and histamine. The mechanisms are complex, with intricate interactions and feedback.

Ultimately the immune activation leads to activated polymorphonuclear leukocytes, which cause endothelial injury. For example, this is the mechanism for acute respiratory distress syndrome (ARDS). Injured pulmonary capillary endothelium leads to leak of fluid into the interstitium in excess of what can be returned to the circulation by Starling forces or by lymphatics. This produces reduced compliance and impaired gas exchange. Ultimately, the fluid escapes from the interstitium into the alveoli, producing the characteristic diffuse infiltrates seen on chest roentgenograms.

The endothelial injury and "capillary leak" can be quite generalized and lead to extreme loss of intravascular volume. The MODS patient may require large amounts of intravenous fluids to maintain preload. Much of the fluid accumulates in the subcutaneous tissues, producing the characteristic edema of MODS, which may be massive.

There is an element of organ dysfunction, however, that may not be simply the result of injury to component cells, such as to the endothelium. The cells may, in fact, be uninjured, but may be expressing genes for enzymes or cellular products that do not serve to maintain general body homeostasis. This dysregulation is thought to result from neurohumoral messages linked to the generalized inflammatory response.

MODS FOLLOWING TRAUMA, SHOCK, & TISSUE INJURY

CASE DESCRIPTION

The following case description illustrates a clinical course typical for a patient with MODS.

Mechanism

A 28-year-old man was the unrestrained driver in a semi-truck accident at 4:30 AM. He was found off-road down a 5-foot embankment. The truck cabin was heavily damaged, with 2 feet of intrusion into the passenger space. The patient was airlifted to the trauma center, arriving 90 minutes after the accident.

Initial Evaluation

In the emergency department, the patient was awake and responded appropriately to commands. He was in obvious pain from his legs. There were bilateral lower leg deformities. Vital signs revealed a heart rate of 105 beats/minute, blood pressure of 140/80 mm Hg, and respiratory rate of 36 breaths/minute. Initial laboratory findings were: hematocrit, 27.3%; urinalysis, 3+ blood.

Initial Management

Initial management in the emergency department included the following radiographic studies: plain films of the cervical spine, chest, pelvis, and legs; CT of the cervical spine and abdomen/pelvis. Injuries identified included intra-abdominal hemorrhage, bilateral femur fractures, and an open left tibia-fibula fracture. The patient was treated with an infusion of 3.5 liters of crystalloid and 2 units of packed red blood cells. A catheter was placed to drain the bladder.

Operative Management of Abdominal Injuries

The patient was taken to the operating room. Abdominal exploration revealed a jejunal transection just distal to the ligament of Treitz with a tear to the base of the mesentery and a retroperitoneal hematoma. Additionally, there was a mid-jejunal avulsion and perforation. The devascularized bowel was resected and two anastomoses were created.

Operative Management of Orthopedic Injuries

Orthopedic repairs started immediately following the abdominal operation. Intramedullary nailing was performed for both femurs. Additionally, the orthopedic surgeons debrided and irrigated the left tibia-fibula fracture and performed intramedullary nailing of the left tibia.

Intraoperative Course

The patient's intraoperative course is illustrated in Table 17–1. The patient's abdominal procedures were started at 9:00 AM, at which time his blood gases showed a significant metabolic acidosis. PaO_2 was satisfactory, however, as were the vital signs of heart rate, mean arterial blood pressure, and temperature.

The abdominal repairs were concluded at noon and the orthopedic procedures were then started. By 4:00 PM the patient's arterial oxygenation was beginning to deteriorate, with drops in arterial saturation to 94%. The patient had persistent metabolic acidosis, and mean arterial pressure dropped slightly to 80 mm Hg. The patient's hypoxemia was managed by increasing the FIO_2 to 100%.

Over the next 90 minutes the patient's respiratory status markedly worsened. Despite being on 100% oxygen, the patient's SaO_2 dropped to values between 60 and 80%. This was confirmed by a blood gas measurement showing PaO_2 down to 49 mm Hg. The acidosis, both metabolic and respiratory, also progressed. The pH dropped to 7.08. The heart rate increased to 130 beats/minute and mean arterial pressure dropped to 70 mm Hg.

By 8:25 PM, after the orthopedics procedure ended, the patient had developed extreme pulmonary and hemodynamic derangements. Despite administration of sodium bicarbonate, the patient had a persistent acidosis with a still worsening respiratory component. $PaCO_2$ was up to 64 mm Hg.

PaO_2 was down to 42 mm Hg. Heart rate increased to 165. Mean arterial pressure was down to 60 mm Hg.

Operative blood losses were estimated to be 2.5 liters.

Table 17–1. Intraoperative course of MODS in a sample patient.

	Abdominal Procedures Started	Ortho Procedures Started				Ortho Procedures Completed
	9:00 AM	12:00 PM	4:00 PM	5:30 PM	7:00 PM	8:25 PM
PaO$_2$ (mm Hg)	502		97	237	49	42
pH	7.29		7.27	7.24	7.08	7.15
PCO$_2$ (mm Hg)	41		42	46	58	64
Base excess	–5.5		–6.1	–6		
FiO$_2$ (%)	100		48	100	100	100
SaO$_2$ (%)	100		94		60–80	
HR (bpm)	100		100	110	130	165
Mean arterial pressure (mm Hg)	90		80	90	70	60
Temperature (°C)	36.7		36.9	38.2		

MODS = multiple organ dysfunction syndrome.

The patient received the following fluids: crystalloid 10 L, bicarbonate 7 A, hetastarch 1 L, albumin 1 L, packed cells 5 U, blood from the cell saver 500 mL, fresh frozen plasma 2 U, platelets 6 U.

Initial Intensive Care Unit Course

The patient was transferred from the operating room to the intensive care unit (ICU). Arterial oxygen saturation (SaO$_2$) was 73% on an FiO$_2$ of 100%. Heart rate was 152, mean arterial pressure was 69 mm Hg. Bilateral chest tubes were placed to ensure drainage of any pneumothoraces. Blood gases, however, did not improve following tube placement. PaO$_2$ was 35 mm Hg. A mixed-venous pulmonary artery catheter was placed. Pulmonary artery occlusion pressure (wedge) was 15. Cardiac output was 5.0 L/minute. SvO$_2$ was 35%. Hematocrit was 26%.

The patient was placed on increased positive end-expiratory pressure (PEEP). At a PEEP of 28 cm, H$_2$O PaO$_2$ increased to 71 mm Hg and SvO$_2$ reached 60%. The patient was given 2 units of packed cells and was managed with sedation and pharmacologic paralysis. Inotropic support was provided with dobutamine and epinephrine.

Over the next 24 hours the PaO$_2$ increased to 226 mm Hg, and the PEEP was decreased to 18. FiO$_2$ was reduced to 70%. The epinephrine was discontinued and the dobutamine was continued at 13 μg/kg/min.

Subsequent Hospital Course

Week 1. Over the first week in the ICU the patient's respiratory status markedly improved. Figure 17–1 shows the rapid improvement over the first week in gas exchange as measured by the PaO$_2$/FiO$_2$ ratio. PEEP was weaned to 10 mm Hg. The patient, however, had spiking fevers to 39°C and was started on broad-spectrum antibiotics empirically. Tube feedings were begun.

Week 2. By the second week, the patient began to open his eyes to verbal stimuli. He continued to spike fevers to 39°C. During this time, the patient developed a leukocytosis above 20,000 cells/mm^3. Figure 17–2 shows the course of the leukocytosis. During the second week, he also devel-

oped significant hepatic dysfunction, as marked by clinical jaundice as well as an elevation of the serum bilirubin. The course of this hyperbilirubinemia is shown in Figure 17–3. *Pseudomonas* was cultured from the sputum.

Antibiotic coverage was adjusted accordingly.

Week 3. During the third week the patient became more alert. He continued to spike fevers, and the leukocytosis persisted (Figure 17–2), but the hepatic dysfunction began to resolve (Figure 17–3). He was weaned from the ventilator and extubated. Chest tubes were removed.

Week 4. The patient was transferred to the ward. His fever abated and he became oriented to name and place. He was advanced to a regular diet. On hospital day 33 he was discharged to a comprehensive rehabilitation facility, where he has made substantial recovery.

CLINICAL PRESENTATION OF MODS

The clinical presentation of MODS is variable, but certain patterns predominate. The typical clinical patterns have been clarified with the definition of commonly used

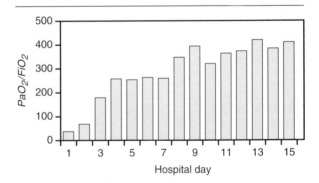

Figure 17–1. Improvement in gas exchange. PaO$_2$ = partial pressure of arterial oxygen; FiO$_2$ = fractional inspiratory oxygen.

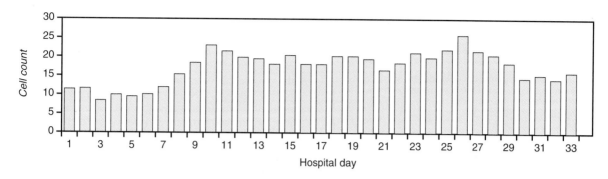

Figure 17–2. White blood cell (WBC) count shows persistence of inflammation.

clinical descriptors, such as infection, the systemic inflammatory response syndrome (SIRS), and the adult respiratory distress syndrome (ARDS). These definitions are given in Table 17–2.

Almost always, the patient who develops MODS experiences a major insult, which may involve shock, infection, tissue injury, or some combination of the three. On a surgical service, shock might occur from trauma or from hemorrhage during a surgical procedure. Infections that lead to MODS are often severe abdominal infections. These may result from delayed management of surgical abdominal conditions, such as appendicitis, peptic ulcer, diverticulitis, or mesenteric ischemia—particularly if there is bowel rupture and peritonitis. The infection may also be a complication of an abdominal procedure, such as failure to heal a bowel anastamosis, with resulting peritoneal contamination. Major burns and multiple fractures can produce enough tissue injury to lead to MODS, as can the tissue inflammation associated with pancreatitis.

Following the insult, major organ systems—central nervous, pulmonary, cardiac, hepatic, gastrointestinal, immune, and renal—begin to fail. The failure may appear right away, but frequently it is delayed and the patient may appear to be doing well. Usually, by 7 days after the insult, however, the MODS patient will develop brain dysfunction, manifested by confusion, and respiratory dysfunction, manifested by ARDS.

The patient's blood gases deteriorate, chest radiography shows bilateral infiltrates, and the patient frequently requires the initiation of mechanical ventilation. The patient's respiratory status may stabilize with the provision of mechanical ventilatory support, but hemodynamic instability will frequently then appear. The patient may require significant fluid volume to maintain blood pressure and cardiac output. Inotropic support is often required at this stage as well.

Over the first week to 10 days the patient develops jaundice, which can be documented by a rising serum bilirubin. The patient becomes significantly hypermetabolic, with oxygen consumption increased over normal by 30%, and occasionally as much as 100%. The patient may develop an ileus or gastrointestinal bleeding, although these appear to be less common if good perfusion is maintained.

The patient will spike fevers and demonstrate a persistent leukocytosis. If the initiating factor was infection, then a persistent infection may be identified and a specific organism cultured. If the initiating factor was shock or tissue injury, blood cultures may be negative despite the

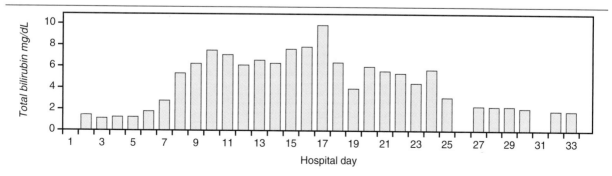

Figure 17–3. Bilirubin measurements monitor hepatic dysfunction.

Table 17–2. Definitions relevant to MODS.

Infection

Infection is the presence of microbes in a normally sterile tissue bed.

Systemic Inflammatory Response Syndrome (SIRS)

SIRS is a set of signs or symptoms meeting two or more of the following conditions:
- Temperature > 38°C or < 36°C
- Heart rate > 90 beats/min
- Respiratory rate > 20 breaths/min or $PaCO_2$ < 32 torr
- WBC > 12,000 cells/mm^3, < 4000 cells/mm^3, or > 10% immature forms

Sepsis

The generalized inflammatory response of SIRS may be triggered by a number of insults, including infection, necrotic tissue, uncontrolled local infection (such as pancreatitis), or shock. When infection leads to SIRS, the situation is termed sepsis.

Adult Respiratory Distress Syndrome (ARDS)

Patients with ARDS suffer from a severe defect in arterial oxygenation resulting from pulmonary edema. This pulmonary edema does not stem from elevated hydrostatic pressure, as in congestive heart failure, but rather from pulmonary capillary endothelial injury that increases permeability. The diagnostic criteria, therefore, for ARDS are:
- PaO_2/FiO_2 < 200
- Bilateral infiltrates on chest radiography
- Absence of left atrial hypertension

FiO_2 = fractional inspiratory oxygen; $PaCO_2$ = partial pressure of carbon dioxide in arterial gas; PaO_2 = partial pressure of arterial oxygen.

fever and leukocytosis. Sputum cultures, however, are very frequently positive for nosocomial organisms, such as *Pseudomonas, Serratia*, or *Enterobacter*. Distinguishing infection from inflammation and colonization when these organisms are cultured is extremely difficult.

Over the next 3 weeks the patient's ARDS usually improves. If the jaundice peaks and improves, then the patient may survive. If the jaundice progresses without plateau, however, the prognosis is extremely poor. Typically, the patient's renal function will then deteriorate, as manifested by an increase in blood urea nitrogen (BUN) and, ultimately, creatinine. Initially, the patient may have normal urine flows, or even be polyuric. Later, the urine flow rather abruptly decreases and the patient becomes rapidly oliguric and then anuric.

At this point, the prognosis is so poor that life-support is frequently withdrawn. In some patients—a young trauma victim, for example—it may be appropriate to offer continued life-support therapy. Renal replacement therapy is started, usually in the form of continuous veno-venous hemofiltration. Occasionally, patients can be salvaged from renal failure with recovery of kidney function, or survive to make the transition to chronic dialysis.

If the patient survives the period of recovery from critical illness (which may take weeks or months), comprehensive rehabilitation is required. Patients can frequently be returned to a baseline level of function.

MANAGEMENT

Clearly, it is best to prevent MODS by avoiding the precipitating events. This implies timely management of the surgical abdomen, prompt resuscitation of the injured patient, and excellent surgical technique. When prevention fails, management then focuses upon minimizing further inflammatory stimuli and ensuring good nutrition.

The inflammatory stimuli include injured tissue and infection. It is essential to drain abscesses, debride necrotic tissue, and immobilize long-bone fracures. Imaging studies, such as ultrasonography and CT are often utilized to ensure that no undrained infection is present.

Although there is generalized inflammation, the patient with MODS may be viewed as immunocompromised. Sputum cultures will frequently be positive for nosocomial organisms, such as *Pseudomonas, Enterobacter*, or *Enterococcus*. Because the patients will frequently have ARDS, chest radiography may not be useful in the evaluation for pneumonia. Distinguishing between pulmonary infection and colonization in MODS patients can, thus, be very difficult. Decisions about antibiotic use must balance the risks of leaving a pulmonary infection untreated against the possibility for selection of more virulent, resistant organisms. Shock is another potential stimulus for persistent inflammation. In MODS, systemic inflammation tends to be associated with loss of vasoregulation and inefficient utilization of oxygen delivery. Additionally, hypermetabolism leads to increased oxygen demands. The inadequate oxygen delivery may become self-perpetuating as respiratory and cardiac dysfunction leads to decreased oxygen delivery, which leads to shock, which leads again to further respiratory and cardiac dysfunction. Chapter 15 outlines a general approach to supportive oxygen delivery that can minimize the tissue hypoxia, despite these factors.

Nutrition is an essential part of the supportive care in MODS. Outcomes analyses suggest that enteral nutrition is superior to parenteral nutrition. Enteral nutrition in the mechanically ventilated patient is typically provided through a feeding tube. If there is a gastric ileus, the feeding tube needs to be placed distal to the pylorus, which can be accomplished fluoroscopically. The patient's hypermetabolism needs to be recognized in the prescription of caloric intake. Metabolic monitors built into the ventilator can now aid the assessment of caloric requirements.

Future therapies for MODS may address the pathophysiology at a fundamental level, perhaps at the level of cellular and humoral mediators. Unfortunately, clinical trials of agents designed to modulate the inflammatory response have been unsuccessful so far. It may be necessary to combine several agents to address the pathophysiology, which appears to be more a network than a cascade. Alternatively, hemofiltration techniques are now being proposed to remove undesirable cytokines by binding them to or excreting them through the filter.

SUGGESTED READING

Beal AL, Cerra FB: Multiple organ failure syndrome in the 1990's. Systemic inflammatory response and organ dysfunction. JAMA 1994;271:226.

Bone RC et al: Definitions for sepsis and organ failure and guidelines for the use of innovative therapies in sepsis. Chest 1992;101:1644.

Cerra FB: Nutrient modulation of inflammatory and immune function. Am J Surg 1991;161:230.

Marshall JC, Christou NV, Meakins JL: The gastrointestinal tract. The "undrained abscess" of multiple organ failure. Ann Surg 1993;218:111.

Moore FA, Moore EE: Evolving concepts in the pathogenesis of postinjury multiple organ failure. Surg Clin N Am 1995; 75:257.

18

Burn Trauma & Surgery

David W. Mozingo, MD, & Basil A. Pruitt, Jr, MD

▶ Key Facts

- ▶ There are approximately 5450 burn-related deaths in the United States each year, and 70% of them occur in house fires. Flame burns are the most common thermal injuries in adults, and scald burns predominate in children.

- ▶ The depth of a burn is determined by the extent of dermal destruction caused by heat-induced coagulation necrosis. Burns are commonly classified as partial-thickness burns (first- and second-degree burns) if some of the skin appendages (hair follicles, sweat glands, and sebaceous glands) in the dermis survive. If protected from infection, those structures provide a source of epithelial cells that will proliferate and resurface the burn. A full-thickness burn (third-degree burn) has no surviving skin appendages and skin grafting is required for closure.

- ▶ Loss of intravascular volume due to burn edema results in hypovolemic shock. Therefore, when airway patency and ventilation are assured, fluid resuscitation is an immediate priority.

- ▶ The most readily available clinical guide to the adequacy of fluid resuscitation is the hourly urinary output.

- ▶ Smoke inhalation injury is frequently observed in patients with thermal injury and is present in one third of the patients admitted to burn centers. Fiberoptic bronchoscopic examination of the upper airway and tracheobronchial tree is the most commonly used and most accurate method of diagnosing inhalation injury.

- ▶ Circulation may be impaired by circumferential full-thickness burns; to prevent secondary ischemic necrosis of distal and underlying tissues an escharotomy may be required to relieve the constriction caused by edema beneath the eschar.

- ▶ The delivery of nutritional support to the burn patient is best accomplished using the enteral route. Most patients tolerate this as soon as the early postburn ileus relents and gastrointestinal motility is reestablished.

- ▶ Effective topical antimicrobial chemotherapy with prompt burn wound excision and split thickness skin grafting reduces the risk of invasive burn wound infection and its attendant mortality, decreases the duration of hospital stay, and accelerates rehabilitation.

Thermal injury is estimated to affect more than 1.4 million individuals in the United States annually; however, the precise incidence of this injury is unknown. The majority of burn patients have minor burns and can be adequately cared for as outpatients. Approximately 54,000 burn patients require hospitalization, with about 16,000 of those patients having injuries of such significance that care is best undertaken in a burn center. The American Burn Association has developed guidelines by which those patients requiring treatment in a burn center can be identified. These criteria utilize the extent, depth, and location of the burn; the cause of injury; the presence of pre-existing co-morbid factors and associated injuries to guide in referral of those patients requiring multispecialty medical care; burn-specific intensive care units and specialized laboratory support unique to burn centers (Table 18–1).

Deaths from burn injury occur in approximately 5450 persons per year. House fires are responsible for more than 70% of all deaths; one fourth of these are due to burns and three fourths result from smoke inhalation or asphyxiation. House and structure fires are responsible for only 4% of burn admissions. Flame burns and ignition of clothing are the most common causes of injury in adults, whereas scald burns predominate in children.

PATHOPHYSIOLOGY OF BURN INJURY

Cutaneous burns cause direct cellular damage manifested by coagulation necrosis; the magnitude of tissue destruction is determined by the duration of contact and by the temperature to which the tissue is exposed. The histopathologic changes resulting from burn injury may be depicted as three concentric tissue zones radiating from

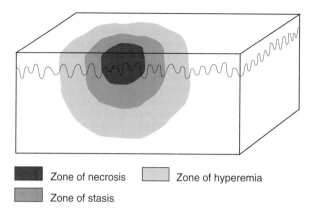

■ Zone of necrosis ☐ Zone of hyperemia
■ Zone of stasis

Figure 18–1. Early histopathologic changes may be depicted as concentric tissue zones about the point of thermal contact. The zone of stasis may be converted to necrosis by prolonged inadequate perfusion, infection, or dessication.

the point of thermal contact (Figure 18–1). The region in which immediate protein coagulation and cell death has occurred is referred to as the **zone of necrosis**. If the necrosis destroys all dermal elements, a full-thickness injury or third-degree burn is produced. Extending radially from the zone of necrosis, the zone of stasis is next encountered. This zone is characterized by decreased microvascular blood flow which, with successful resuscitation, may be restored to normal or converted to necrosis following inadequate perfusion, infection, or desiccation. The periphery of the wound, the **zone of hyperemia**, is caused by minimal thermal injury and characterized by an immediate inflammatory response and an increase in microvascular blood flow.

In clinical practice, the depth of burn is classified with respect to the extent of dermal destruction by coagulation necrosis and is defined as a **partial-thickness** or **full-thickness** burn injury (Figure 18–2). First- and second-degree burns are considered partial-thickness injuries and third-degree burns full-thickness injuries. Partial-thickness burns heal spontaneously by epithelial migration from preserved hair follicles, sweat glands, and sebaceous glands within the uninjured dermis. The rate at which partial-thickness wounds heal is governed by the depth of dermal destruction. More superficial wounds heal rapidly, since viable skin appendages are abundant. Deeper partial-thickness wounds may require many weeks to heal since only few viable dermal appendages remain; these wounds are typically treated by skin grafting to reduce the time required for closure and improve functional outcome. Full-thickness burns contain no viable dermal elements and require cutaneous autografting for wound closure.

The clinical criteria in Table 18–2 permit differentiation between the different depths of burn injury. First-degree burns only involve the epidermal layer and do not result in injury to dermal structures. As a consequence,

Table 18–1. American Burn Association burn center referral criteria.

- Second- and third-degree burns of more than 10% of the total body surface area in patients younger than 10 or older than 50 years of age
- Second- and third-degree burns of more than 20% of the total body surface area in other age groups
- Significant burns of face, hands, feet, genitalia, or perineum and those that involve skin overlying major joints
- Third-degree burns of more than 5% of the total body surface area in any age group
- Smoke inhalation injury
- Significant electric injury, including lightning injury
- Significant chemical injury
- Burns with significant preexisting medical disorders that could complicate management, prolong recovery, or affect mortality (eg, diabetes mellitus or cardiopulmonary disease)
- Burns with significant concomitant mechanical trauma (may require initial treatment in a trauma center)
- Burn injury in patients who will require special social and emotional or long-term rehabilitative support, including cases of suspected child abuse and neglect

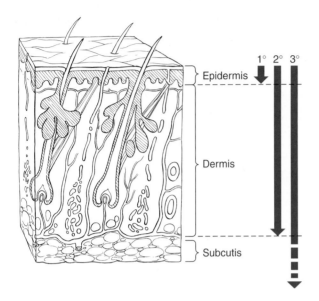

Figure 18–2. Diagram of the skin and subcutaneous tissues demonstrating the depth of burn and relationship to the location of the cutaneous adnexa. First- and second-degree burns are considered partial thickness. Spontaneous healing by epithelial cell migration requires preservation of the hair follicles and sweat glands. Full-thickness or third-degree burns will not re-epithelialize and require skin grafting for closure.

these burns are not associated with significant metabolic alteration or edema foundation. Full-thickness burns, in addition to destroying the dermal appendages, also coagulate peripheral cutaneous sensory nerve endings. As a result, full-thickness burns are typically insensate and not painful when compared to partial-thickness wounds, a particularly useful finding on physical examination.

Structural changes in burned tissues and the liberation of inflammatory mediators result in a loss of integrity of the vascular endothelium, leading to increased capillary permeability and edema formation. The edema, which may be massive, forms most rapidly in the first 6 hours following injury and continues to a lesser extent for the first 24 hours postburn. Postcapillary venular constriction, which causes a marked increase in capillary hydrostatic pressure, has been shown to occur with a maximal effect in the first 30 minutes following injury. An increase in the interstitial fluid colloid osmotic pressure with subsequent reversal of the transcapillary osmotic pressure gradient also contributes to early edema formation. Following these initial changes in the physical characteristics of burned tissue, the ongoing changes in microvascular permeability have been attributed to the effects of humoral factors liberated from burned tissue and cytokines produced by activated leukocytes. Many inflammatory mediators, including histamine, activated proteases, prostaglandins, leukotrienes, fibrin degradation products, and substance P, are liberated following burn injury and

Table 18–2. Clinical characteristics of burn wounds.

| First-Degree Burns | Partial-Thickness Burns | | Full-Thickness or Third-Degree Burns |
| | Second-Degree Burns | | |
	Superficial	Deep Dermal	
Cause			
Sun	Hot liquids	Hot liquids	Flame
Minor flash	Flashes of flame	Flashes of flame	High-voltage electricity
	Brief exposure to dilute chemicals	Longer exposure to dilute chemicals	Exposure to concentrated chemicals
			Contact with hot metal
Color			
Pink or light red	Pink to bright red	Dark red or yellow-white	Pearly white or charred
			Translucent and parchmentlike
Surface			
Dry or small blisters	Blisters and bullae	Large bullae often ruptured	Dry with shreds of nonviable epidermis
		Slightly moist	
Texture			
Soft with minimal edema and later superficial exfoliation	Thickened by edema but pliable	Moderate edema with decreased pliability	Inelastic and leathery
Sensation			
Hypersensitive	Hypersensitive	Decreased pinprick sensation	Insensate
		Intact deep-pressure sensation	
Healing			
3–6 days	10–21 days	> 21 days	Skin grafting required

increase microvascular permeability. Products of activated leukocytes, including lysosomal enzymes, increased xanthine oxidase activity, oxygen radicals, products of complement activation, and cytokines, may also perpetuate edema formation in burned tissue. Edema also forms in unburned tissues following a major burn. Although the exact mechanism by which this occurs is controversial, it is at least in part due to a decrease in plasma oncotic pressure resulting from the infusion of large volumes of crystalloid fluid required for burn resuscitation and the loss of circulating oncotically active proteins, namely albumin, into burned tissues.

This loss of intravascular fluid into the interstitial space results in a significant decrease in blood volume and an increase in blood viscosity. Cardiac output falls and systemic vascular resistance is increased. When uncorrected, this loss of intravascular volume due to burn edema results in hypovolemic shock. Therefore, fluid resuscitation is initiated in the immediate postburn period to maintain the circulating blood volume at a level that will ensure adequate organ perfusion.

Burn injury alters the function of all organ systems, and the extent and duration of dysfunction are proportional to the extent of burn. In patients with burns of more than 25% of the body surface area, this is clinically manifested by early depression, and later hyperfunction, of organ systems (Table 18–3). Patients with burns of less than 25% of the total body surface usually do not manifest clinically significant changes in organ function or metabolic rate.

CARDIOVASCULAR SYSTEM

The initial cardiovascular response to burns is manifested by a decrease in cardiac output and an increase in peripheral vascular resistance. The decrease in cardiac output is proportionate to the extent of burn and is caused by loss of fluid and protein from the intravascular into the extravascular compartment. Peripheral vascular resistance increases reflexively in response to this hypovolemia and to an increase in systemic catecholamine release. A circulating myocardial depressant factor has been implicated as a contributing factor in the initial impairment of myocardial performance; however, identification of this factor has not been made with certainty. Clinical studies have indicated that the initial depression of cardiac output could

be explained by hypovolemia as measured by a decreased left ventricular end-diastolic volume.

As the plasma volume deficit is replenished in the second 24 hours postburn, the cardiac output increases to supranormal levels. Peripheral vascular resistance decreases below normal, and the postburn hypermetabolic state, which typically peaks in the second postburn week and slowly diminishes thereafter, is established. The postresuscitation increase in cardiac output is primarily directed toward the burn wound and is increased in proportion to the extent of injury.

RENAL SYSTEM

The renal response following burns parallels that of the cardiovascular response. Renal blood flow and the glomerular filtration rate are initially reduced in proportion to the size of the burn and the extent of the intravascular volume deficit. Following a successful resuscitation phase, renal blood flow is increased as edema fluid is resorbed. Despite the markedly increased cardiac output and renal blood flow seen in the flow phase of burn injury, the total blood volume remains at only 80% of the predicted value. Plasma renin activity and antidiuretic hormone levels remain elevated and may, in part, explain the propensity for sodium retention during the course of treatment for thermal injury. The increase in renal blood flow and glomerular filtration rate cause drugs excreted by the kidneys to have markedly shortened half-lives and necessitate appropriate dosing adjustments. As in other organ systems, the duration of change in renal physiology is related to the timing of burn wound closure.

PULMONARY SYSTEM

Following burn injury, minute ventilation may be unchanged or slightly increased as a result of pain and anxiety-induced hyperventilation. During fluid resuscitation, respiratory rate and tidal volume progressively increase and minute ventilation increases proportionate to the extent of burn, reaching two to two-and-one-half times normal with severe injury.

Pulmonary vascular resistance increases immediately following thermal injury. The release of vasoactive amines and other mediators may be responsible for this pulmonary vasoconstriction, a process that may exert a protective effect during fluid resuscitation by decreasing pulmonary capillary hydrostatic pressure and preventing pulmonary edema. Neutrophil activation and release of oxygen free radical species, release of platelet-derived factors, and activation of the complement cascade have all been implicated in the pathogenesis of pulmonary dysfunction following burns.

Table 18–3. Organ system response to burn injury.

Organ System	Early Change	Later Response
Cardiovascular	Hypovolemia	Hyperdynamic state
Pulmonary	Hypoventilation	Hyperventilation
Endocrine	Catabolic effects	Anabolic effects
Gastrointestinal	Ileus	Hypermotility
Renal	Oliguria	Diuresis
Integument	Hypoperfusion	Hyperemia

IMMUNOLOGIC SYSTEM

Infection remains the major cause of death among burn patients. Almost every aspect of immunoregulation is affected following injury, with the dysfunction of the cellular and humoral immune response occurring proportionate to the extent of burn. For the first week following injury, the total white blood cell count is elevated, although peripheral blood lymphocyte counts are decreased. Alterations in lymphocyte subpopulations, including reversal of the normal ratio of T helper cells to T suppressor cells, have been described, which normalize during the second postburn week. Delayed hypersensitivity reactions may be attenuated or even absent in patients with extensive burns (those involving over 30% of the total body surface area).

Serum immunoglobulin levels decrease following burn injury, but gradually return to normal over 2–4 weeks coincident with patient recovery. Pharmacologic restoration of IgG levels to normal by exogenous administration has been found to exert no effect on subsequent morbidity or mortality. Circulating immunosuppressive factors in the serum of burn patients as well as immunosuppressive agents recovered from burn blister fluid have been identified and include immunosuppressive polypeptides, complement degradation products, prostaglandins, and immunoglobulin fragments.

Burn injury induces alterations in granulocyte function, including chemotaxis, adherence, degranulation, oxygen radical production, and complement receptor expression. Granulocytes from burned patients exhibit increased cytosolic oxidase activity and greater than normal oxidase activity following in vitro stimulation, suggesting that neutrophils from burned patients have an increased oxidative burst potential capable of producing increased tissue and organ injury.

ENDOCRINE SYSTEM

The metabolic response to burn injury also reflects the extent of burn and follows the typical biphasic response documented in other organ systems. Immediately following burn injury, the metabolic rate decreases in response to hypovolemia and diminished tissue perfusion; however, as resuscitation progresses, a catabolic or hypermetabolic hormonal pattern is observed. Serum levels of catecholamines, cortisol, and glucagon increase, whereas insulin and triiodothyronine levels are decreased. Activation of the hypothalamic pituitary axis results in increased release of antidiuretic hormone, adrenocorticotropic hormone (ACTH), and beta endorphins.

Glucose metabolism is also altered following thermal injury. There is an increase in net glucose flow, with relative peripheral insulin resistance. Hepatic gluconeogenesis also increases; however, glucose uptake by insulin-dependent tissues is decreased due to the relative insulin insensitivity. An exaggerated fraction of nutrient flow is directed to the burn wound. Large quantities of glucose are required to support the immune cell functions of microbial containment and necrotic tissue removal through anaerobic, insulin-independent metabolism. The predominance of anaerobic metabolism in the burn wound results in increased lactate production, with subsequent hepatic conversion of lactate to glucose via the Cori cycle.

Marked catabolism resulting in muscle protein breakdown and loss of lean body mass is observed following burns. Significant nitrogen loss occurs, with a markedly negative nitrogen balance.

OTHER SYSTEMS

Nonspecific neurologic changes, such as increased anxiety and disorientation, are observed in patients with extensive burns. These changes are most likely due to the neurohumoral stress response and may be exacerbated by isolation in the intensive care unit. Infection and sepsis as well as electrolyte and fluid disturbances may further alter central nervous system function.

Gastrointestinal dysfunction also is related to the magnitude of thermal injury. In patients with burns exceeding 25% of the total body surface area (TBSA), gastroparesis is often observed in the early postburn period. Gastric motility usually returns by the third to fifth postburn day, at which time nasogastric drainage can be discontinued and enteral feeding initiated. Later in the postburn course, gastrointestinal hyperactivity and diarrhea may occur due to the combined effect of increased gastrointestinal blood flow and excessive nutrient administration.

The hematopoietic system is also affected in direct proportion to the extent of burn injury. Destruction of red blood cells following burn injury occurs in proportion to the size and depth of burn. Immediate red blood cell destruction occurs by coagulation within the microvasculature in areas of full-thickness burn. During the first week postburn, a continuing loss of red blood cells occurs, presumably from reticuloendothelial clearance of damaged cells and repeated blood sampling. Platelets and serum levels of fibrinogen and factors V and VIII rapidly increase following resuscitation. Erythropoietin levels are also increased coincident with the anemia that develops following burn injury.

CARE OF THE BURN PATIENT

PREHOSPITAL MANAGEMENT

At the accident scene, the primary concern is to stop the burning process. Burning and smoldering clothing should be extinguished and patients with electrical injury should be separated from points of electrical contact. If the burn was caused by contact with a chemical agent, all contaminated clothing (even underclothes) should be removed and copious water lavage initiated. In all cases, extreme care should be taken to avoid injury to medical personnel.

The primary concern, as with all trauma patients, is maintenance of cardiopulmonary function. Airway patency and adequacy of ventilation must be maintained and supplemental oxygen administered as necessary. Placement of an intravenous cannula is not necessary if transport to a treatment facility can be accomplished within 45 minutes, unless associated mechanical trauma or need for cardiopulmonary resuscitation exists. With the exception of chemical burns, for which prompt water irrigation to remove the offending agent is required, no specific treatment of the burn wound is needed in the prehospital setting. The patient should be covered with a clean sheet and blanket to conserve body heat and minimize burn wound contamination during transport to the hospital. The application of ice or cold water soaks, when initiated within 10 minutes after burning, may reduce tissue heat content and lessen the depth of thermal injury. If cold therapy is used, care must be taken to avoid causing hypothermia; this is accomplished by limiting this form of therapy to 10% or less of the body surface and only for the time required to produce analgesia.

EMERGENCY DEPARTMENT CARE

Upon arrival, the patency of the airway and the adequacy of breathing should be reassessed and endotracheal intubation performed if necessary. Indications for endotracheal intubation include severe smoke inhalation with respiratory insufficiency and the presence of upper airway edema. Upper airway edema is usually not present immediately following burn injury, but develops as fluid resuscitation progresses. A history should be obtained, with special attention paid to the mechanism of injury, presence of preexisting disease, allergies, medications, and the use of alcohol or illicit drugs prior to injury. The primary survey of thermally injured patients proceeds in the same orderly manner advocated for other trauma patients, with particular attention given to the occurrence of associated mechanical injuries. Baseline laboratory data should include an arterial blood gas, pH analysis, serum glucose, electrolytes, blood urea nitrogen, and creatinine. A complete blood count and urinalysis should also be performed.

When airway patency and ventilation are assured, fluid resuscitation takes priority. For burns greater than 20% of the body surface area, two large-bore intravenous cannulae should be inserted. In addition, a urethral catheter should be inserted and the urine volume measured and recorded hourly. Since ileus is common in burn patients with greater than 20% TBSA burn, a nasogastric tube should be inserted to minimize gastric distention, emesis, and risk of aspiration. Also, the ambient temperature of the room should be increased and the patient covered with blankets to prevent hypothermia.

The administration of intravenous fluid for resuscitation is initiated by infusing a physiologic salt-containing solution (usually lactated Ringer's), with the initial rate estimated on the basis of extent of injury and patient weight (see Fluid Resuscitation). The extent of burn, expressed as the percent of the TBSA involved with second- and third-degree burns, can be quickly estimated using the "rule of nines" (Figure 18–3). This method assigns 9% or 18% of the TBSA to specific anatomic regions. The surface area of small or irregularly shaped burns may be estimated by considering the size of the patient's hand to represent 1% of his or her body surface area and then estimating how many "hands" would cover the burn wounds. Infants and children have a significantly different body surface area distribution, resulting from their relatively larger head and smaller legs compared to adults. More detailed burn diagrams, such as the Lund and Browder burn diagram, which more precisely define the surface area contribution of specific anatomic regions, have been developed to determine more accurately the TBSA burned in patients of different ages (Figure 18–4). Following initial stabilization, any gross contamination of the burn wound should be removed and the wound covered with a clean dry sheet and blanket to await inspection by a surgeon trained in the

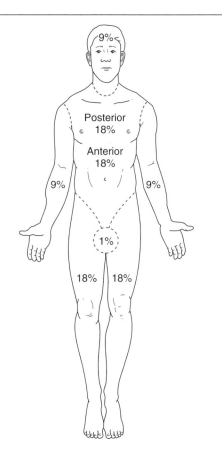

Figure 18–3. The "rule of nines" recognizes that specific anatomic regions represent 9% or 18% of the total body area.

UNIVERSITY OF FLORIDA BURN CENTER **Burn Evaluation Form**

ADMITTED

Date: _____ Hour: _____

Age: _____ Sex: _____ Race: _____

Date & Time Burned: _____

Secondary Diagnosis: _____

_____

ETIOLOGY OF BURN (Circle)

Flame	Indoors-Outdoors Flash
Hot Liquid	Immersion - Splash
Contact	Chemical - Electrical

CONDITION: Good Fair Poor

Weight (KG): _____ % Burn: _____

Burn Fluid Budget: _____

Colloid: _____

Electrolyte: _____

Insensible Loss: _____

TREATMENT PRIOR TO ARRIVAL

Date: _____ Time: _____

Nature of Rx: _____

_____

_____

_____

CALCULATION OF % OF BURN

AREA	AGE 0–1	1–4	5–9	10–15	Adult	% 2°	3°	% Total
Head	19	17	13	10	7			
Neck	2	2	2	2	2			
Ant. Trunk	13	13	13	13	13			
Post. Trunk	13	13	13	13	13			
R. Buttock	2.5	2.5	2.5	2.5	2.5			
L. Buttock	2.5	2.5	2.5	2.5	2.5			
Genitalia	1	1	1	1	1			
R. U. Arm	4	4	4	4	4			
L. U. Arm	4	4	4	4	4			
R. L. Arm	3	3	3	3	3			
L. L. Arm	3	3	3	3	3			
R. Hand	2.5	2.5	2.5	2.5	2.5			
L. Hand	2.5	2.5	2.5	2.5	2.5			
R. Thigh	5.5	6.5	8	8.5	9.5			
L. Thigh	5.5	6.5	8	8.5	9.5			
R. Leg	5	5	5.5	6	7			
L. Leg	5	5	5.5	6	7			
R. Foot	3.5	3.5	3.5	3.5	3.5			
L. Foot	3.5	3.5	3.5	3.5	3.5			
					Total			

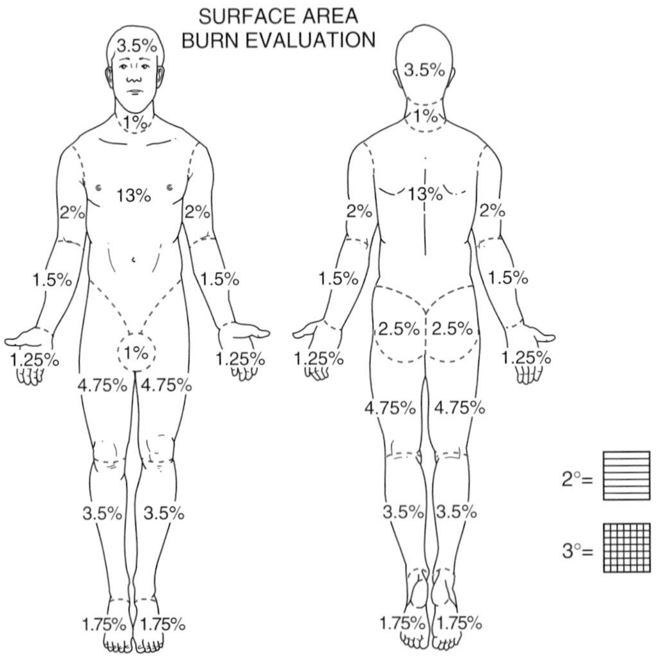

NOTES

SURFACE AREA BURN EVALUATION

Figure 18–4. A more exact estimation of the extent of burn is possible by using a burn diagram. The body area distribution changes with age, particularly the head and lower extremities.

HISTORICAL FACTS

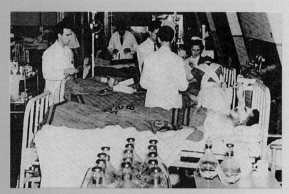

The burn ward at Massachusetts General Hospital. The victims of the Coconut Grove fire were housed here and cared for by staff organized into teams for dressing changes, fluid therapy, pain medicine, and other care. In the foreground are bottles of plasma awaiting infusion. (AP/Wide Photos)

In November of 1942, one of the worst civilian disasters in American history occurred in a popular Boston nightclub known as the Coconut Grove. It took only a few minutes before a devastating fire consumed the entire building, killing 491 persons and sending hundreds more to local hospitals. This incident stunned the entire nation, which was still adjusting to the shocks and losses of World War II. It also served to mobilize and modernize the medical community, which was already beginning to focus on the care of burn injuries as a result of the war. There is no doubt that this was a pivotal event in the treatment of burns in the United States.

The majority of the victims were sent to two local hospitals, Boston City Hospital (BCH) and Massachusetts General Hospital (MGH). The fire began at 10:15 PM, and by 10:30 PM the first casualties began to arrive at both facilities. BCH received more than 300 victims and MGH approximately 114. It was calculated later that in the first few hours a new victim arrived at BCH every 11 seconds. By the next morning only 171 of the 414 patients admitted to both hospitals remained alive, and three of those died shortly thereafter, leaving 129 to be cared for at BCH and 39 at MGH.

Although many of the victims were severely burned, a far more startling number died as a result of inhalation injury. The respiratory complications were so severe that authorities believed an unknown toxic gas must have been present in the building. It was later discovered that prolonged exposure to smoke often causes upper airway edema and inflammation, necrotizing tracheobronchitis, and obliterative bronchitis, which lead to the secondary changes of atelectasis and pneumonia. Those treating the victims noted the apparent ineffectiveness of bronchodilators and expectorants and emphasized the importance of humidification of the inspired air or oxygen and the use of suctioning or other measures, such as laryngoscopy and tracheostomy, to relieve the obstruction caused by bronchial casts. Inhalation still remains a powerful co-morbid factor in burn patients. It is widely acknowledged that the modern understanding of inhalation injury began with this disaster.

The standard treatment of burn injuries in 1942 consisted of coverage with tannic acid (a "tanning" technique) or antibiotic dyes (the "triple-dye" technique) to "neutralize toxins" produced by the burn, prevent infection, and arrest fluid loss. These techniques, which also required an initial wound cleansing and debridement (not burn wound excision as practiced today), usually under anesthesia, were considered by many to be ineffective in controlling burn wound infection and impractical in combat situations. Accordingly, new techniques of burn wound care were evaluated at both MGH and BCH.

The burn team at MGH, which included the young Francis D. Moore and Champ Lyons, was headed by Oliver Cope, then 40, who was well known for his studies of the metabolic response to injury and burn treatment. Cope had made a number of observations concerning the treatment of burns before the Coconut Grove tragedy. He noted that burn wounds healed much faster with less inflammation when treated with sterile boric acid ointment strips and bulky gauze wraps as pressure dressings than when treated with tannic acid or triple dye. This new protocol, which included the intravenous administration of sulfadiazine to offset infection, met with great success at both hospitals and thereafter was widely used in both military and civilian burn treatment. The MGH team also studied the hemodynamic and fluid compartment response to burn injury and used their findings to develop the "Burn Budget" formula used to estimate fluid resuscitation needs during the first 48 hours following injury on the basis of body weight and the extent of burn.

The incredible advances and observations made in treating the victims of the Coconut Grove fire influenced wound care, antibiotic usage, metabolic response to injury, the organization of burn units within hospitals, and almost every other aspect of the care of burn patients. In addition to promoting such important medical developments, this terrible tragedy must also be recognized for mobilizing the public to make advances in disaster planning, fire safety regulations, and public safety administration, which have been invaluable in the effort to prevent burn injuries.

treatment of such injuries. Debridement and the initiation of topical antimicrobial therapy can safely wait until referral to the definitive treatment facility.

The burn patient who has been immunized against tetanus should be given a booster dose of tetanus toxoid if the last dose was administered more than 5 years previously. Patients without prior active immunization should receive hyperimmune human antitetanus serum in addition to the initial dose of tetanus toxoid. Active immunization is subsequently completed according to the routine dosage schedule.

Pain control during the early care of the thermally injured patient may be achieved by administration of appropriate (usually 3–5 mg) intravenous doses of morphine on a frequent basis. Subcutaneous and intramuscular injections must be avoided due to decreased absorption during wound edema formation and the potential for subsequent mobilization during the period of edema resorption, which may produce respiratory depression. Extensive full-thickness burns are usually not painful due to the destruction of cutaneous nerves; patients with such injuries usually require little pain medication.

Burn patient transfers from a referring hospital to a specialized care facility require early physician-to-physician contact, appropriate patient stabilization with frequent reassessment of the patient's condition, and careful documentation of the care provided at the referring facility. At present, 135 specialty centers in the United States have self-designated expertise in burn care. All efforts should be directed at stabilization and prompt transfer of patients meeting the burn center referral criteria (Table 18–1) to one of those centers.

SMOKE INHALATION INJURY

Smoke inhalation injury is frequently observed in patients with thermal injury and is present in one third of the patients admitted to burn centers. The inhalation of smoke or toxic gases may induce chemical damage to the respiratory epithelium. Though uncommon, direct thermal injury to the tracheobronchial tree, usually associated with the inhalation of steam, may occur. Additionally, inhalation of cytotoxic gases, such as carbon monoxide and cyanide, may produce systemic sequelae rather than local injury.

Smoke consists of small aerosolized particles, usually with various cytotoxic chemicals or irritants adherent to their surface. The anatomic location of lung injury is dependent on the size of the inhaled particle; particles < 0.05 μm typically injure the bronchiolar airways or cause severe alveolar damage whereas particles of greater size deposit in the larger airways causing inflammation, mucosal ulceration, or necrosis of respiratory epithelium.

The diagnosis of smoke inhalation should be considered in patients who have been burned in a closed space, or who demonstrate facial burns, singed facial hair and nasal vibrissae, carbonaceous deposits in the oropharynx, or intraoral burns, along with altered mental status and signs of respiratory distress. The classic signs and symptoms of inhalation injury, however, have a poor predictive value in either excluding or assuring the diagnosis. Fiberoptic bronchoscopic examination of the upper airway and tracheobronchial tree is the most commonly utilized and most accurate method of diagnosing inhalation injury. The presence of carbonaceous material, erythema, edema, or mucosal ulcerations below the level of the true vocal cords confirms the presence of smoke inhalation injury. False-negative bronchoscopic examinations rarely occur and are due to the inability to detect inflammation or edema in the hypovolemic patient with impaired perfusion of the tracheal mucosa. When the clinical suspicion of inhalation is high but the bronchoscopic examination of the tracheobronchial tree is normal, [133]xenon ventilation lung scans may be performed. Following intravenous injection of 10 μCi of [133]xenon, retention of the gas in the lungs for over 90 seconds on serial chest scintigraphs is considered diagnostic of inhalation injury. False-negative studies may result from marked hyperventilation. Preexisting obstructive pulmonary disease, atelectasis, or bronchitis may cause false-positive examination results.

Patients with mild smoke inhalation injury require only administration of humidified oxygen-enriched air and noninvasive pulmonary physiotherapy. Those with copious secretions, severe smoke inhalation, or sloughing of the tracheobronchial mucosa may require endotracheal intubation for adequate pulmonary toilet. Mucolytic agents or bronchodilators may be useful to clear secretions and relieve bronchospasm. Frequent flexible fiberoptic or rigid bronchoscopy to clear the airways of sloughed mucosal debris or inspissated secretions may be required in severe cases. The use of steroids in patients with inhalation injury should be avoided; this treatment is appropriate only in patients with unrelenting bronchospasm.

A recent advance in the management of patients with inhalation injury has been realized through the use of high-frequency percussive mechanical ventilation. This mode of ventilation delivers a sub-dead space volume of inspired gas into the airway at a rate of about 600 breaths per minute, during which inhalation is active and exhalation is passive. In order to minimize gas trapping, the cycling mechanism is interrupted and airway pressure is returned to baseline positive end-expiratory pressure at regular intervals (usually every 4 seconds). Alveolar ventilation is controlled by adjusting peak inspiratory pressure and the rate at which the airway pressure is allowed to return to baseline. Though the exact mechanism by which high-frequency percussive ventilation exerts its beneficial effect is not known, the ability to maintain oxygenation and ventilation at lower peak airway pressures and inspired oxygen concentrations may reduce the iatrogenic injury associated with the use of volume-controlled ventilators. The high-frequency percussive breaths also improve clearance of secretions and mucosal debris. With this form of ventilation, the occurrence of pneumonia and mortality associated with inhalation injury has decreased by approximately one half that predicted on the basis of historical experience.

Bronchopneumonia remains the most common cause of morbidity in patients with inhalation injury. The daily chest roentgenograph should be carefully examined. Appropriate antimicrobial therapy, based on the presence of sputum leukocytosis, the detection of microorganisms on Gram's stain, and the evolution of pulmonary infiltrates, should be initiated. Pneumonia occurring after inhalation injury is usually caused by gram-positive organisms; gram-negative pneumonia, which occurs infrequently, usually develops later in the hospital course.

In the absence of cutaneous burn, smoke inhalation injury is almost always successfully treated by supportive measures. The tracheobronchial mucosa usually heals completely in 2–3 weeks. When smoke inhalation occurs in the presence of moderate to severe burn injury it exerts a comorbid effect. Mortality rates in patients with the combined injuries are increased by as much as 20% over that predicted on the basis of extent of burn injury and age of the patient. When complicated by pneumonia, the mortality rate rises even higher.

Smoke inhalation may also be associated with carbon monoxide poisoning, which impairs tissue oxygenation. Mild carbon monoxide poisoning may be manifested by headache whereas moderate exposure may cause restlessness and confusion. More severe exposure will produce obtundation and coma. Carbon monoxide displaces oxygen from oxyhemoglobin, producing carboxyhemoglobin. In addition, carbon monoxide produces chemical alterations of the cytochrome oxidase system, further impairing tissue oxygenation. The amount of dissolved oxygen in the blood is not affected, thus, the PaO_2 will remain normal. However, saturation of hemoglobin by oxygen will be markedly reduced. Carbon monoxide poisoning is treated by the administration of 100% oxygen by non-rebreathing mask or endotracheal tube to accelerate the dissociation of carboxyhemoglobin. Patients with altered mental status or those who are comatose should be presumed to have carbon monoxide poisoning and receive treatment with 100% oxygen. One hundred percent oxygen should be administered until the measured level of circulating carboxyhemoglobin is less than 7%.

Cyanide may also be produced by the combustion of common materials such as nylon, polyurethane, wool, and silk; trace levels of cyanide have been detected in smoke from house fires and in the blood of patients with smoke inhalation injury. Prompt detoxification of cyanide occurs with adequate hepatic circulation and function, thus, the trace levels in the patient's blood are of little consequence. Rarely, a persistent metabolic acidosis that is unresponsive to fluid or oxygen administration may suggest the diagnosis of cyanide poisoning. Elevated levels of cyanide in the absence of significant carbon monoxide poisoning are extremely uncommon and should prompt a reassessment of the patient for other causes of acidosis. Administration of cyanide antidotes such as sodium thiosulfate, which promotes the conversion of cyanide to thiocyanate, or hydroxocobalamin, a chelating agent, should be considered when a severe metabolic acidosis is present and other causative factors have been discounted.

FLUID RESUSCITATION

The goal of burn resuscitation is the maintenance of vital organ function by the administration of fluid in such a volume to minimize the occurrence of immediate or delayed physiologic complications. By knowing the extent of burn, the patient's weight, and the time elapsed since injury, one can calculate the volume of resuscitation fluid required to initiate resuscitation in these patients. Several clinically successful formulae exist for estimating the

fluid requirement and are displayed in Table 18–4. The various burn formulae differ considerably with respect to the volume and composition of the resuscitation fluid; however, each formula has been found to be clinically effective. A central theme is that the volume of fluid required is dependent on the patient's weight and the extent of burn and that, most often, it is recommended that half of the calculated requirement be infused over the first 8 hours following injury, the time of maximal vascular permeability, and the remainder of the first 24-hour resuscitation volume delivered over the ensuing 16 hours.

The **Modified Brooke Formula**, which is recommended by the authors, employs a physiologic salt solution in the form of lactated Ringer's during the first 24 hours without the addition of colloid or electrolyte-free crystalloid solutions until the second 24 hours. Lactated Ringer's is the preferred solution because the concentration of chloride ion is more physiologic compared to that of normal saline. Fluid needs in adults are estimated as 2 mL of lactated Ringer's solution per kilogram body weight per percent TBSA burn. One half of the calculated estimate is administered in the first 8 hours and the second half over the subsequent 16 hours postburn. When the initiation of fluid resuscitation is delayed, that amount of fluid calculated to be administered in the first 8 hours should be infused at a rate such that half of the estimated 24-hour fluid requirement will be infused by 8 hours postburn. However, any resuscitation formula serves only to guide the initiation of fluid therapy, and the actual amount of resuscitation fluid delivered is guided by each patient's physiologic response. Frequent reassessment, on at least an hourly basis, and adjustment of the fluid infusion rate,

Table 18–4. Formulas used to estimate resuscitation fluid requirements for burn patients.

Formula	Electrolyte-Containing Solution	Colloid-Containing Fluid Equivalent to Plasma (ie, 5% Albumin in Normal Saline)	5% Dextrose in Water
First 24 hours postburn			
Evans	Normal saline—1 mL/kg/% burn	1 mL/kg/% burn	2000 mL
Brooke	Lactated Ringer's—1.5 mL/kg/% burn	0.5% mg/kg/% burn	2000 mL
Parkland	Lactated Ringer's—4mL/kg/% burn	—	—
Modified Brooke	Lactated Ringer's—2 mL/kg/% burn	—	—
Consensus formula	Lactated Ringer's—2–4 mL/kg/% burn	—	—
Second 24 hours postburn			
Evans	50% of first 24 h requirement	50% of first 24 h requirement	2000 mL
Brooke	50–75% of first 24 h requirement	50–75% of first 24 h requirement	2000 mL
Parkland	—	20–60% of calculated plasma volume	As necessary to maintain urinary output
Modified Brooke	—	0.3–0.5 mL/kg/% burn	As necessary to maintain urinary output
Consensus formula[1]		0.3–0.5 mL/kg/% burn	As necessary to maintain urinary output

[1]American Burn Association: Advanced Burn Life Support Course.

is essential to ensure adequate tissue perfusion. Failure to reevaluate the patient's response to resuscitation on a scheduled basis may lead to either over- or under-resuscitation. Inadequate fluid administration results in organ dysfunction or failure while excessive administration of resuscitation fluids may cause pulmonary, cerebral, or excessive burn wound edema.

In the second 24 hours following injury, a solution of 5% albumin in physiologic saline is administered in an amount proportionate to pre-burn body weight and the extent of burn to aid in correction of the plasma volume deficit. In burns involving less than 30% of the body surface, the plasma volume deficit is not profound and routine colloid replacement is unnecessary. The following formulae are used to estimate colloid replacement based on the extent of burn injury: 30–50% burn, 0.3 mL per kilogram body weight per percent burn; 50–70% burn, 0.4 mL per kilogram body weight per percent burn; greater than 70% burn, 0.5 mL per kilogram body weight per percent burn. These formulae calculate the total volume of 5% albumin solution to be infused at a constant rate over the second 24 hours following injury. Additionally, the lactated Ringer's infusion is discontinued and 5% dextrose in water (D5W) is delivered to maintain urine output between 30 and 50 mL per hour during the second 24 hours.

FLUID RESUSCITATION IN CHILDREN

Several important differences must be considered in the fluid resuscitation of the burned child. Children have a greater body surface area per unit of body mass and, thus, require more resuscitation fluid relative to adults. Fluid needs in children weighing less than 30 kg are estimated as 3 mL of lactated Ringer's solution per kilogram body weight per percent TBSA burn. The addition of supplemental intravenous fluid to account for metabolic water requirements in the form of 5% dextrose in 0.45% saline is also necessary. This is essential because, in patients with small to moderate burns, the volume of fluid calculated on the basis of the extent of burn may not meet maintenance fluid requirements. As burn size increases, the contribution of the additional maintenance fluid to the overall resuscitation fluid volume becomes less significant. Also, the addition of dextrose in this maintenance fluid ensures that infants, who have limited hepatic glycogen reserves, do not become symptomatically hypoglycemic during the initial phase of resuscitation.

During the second 24 hours following injury, the plasma volume deficit is replaced using the same calculations as for adult patients. However, D5½ normal saline is used instead of D5W and titrated to maintain adequate urine output. The use of D5W in burn children should be avoided to prevent the occurrence of symptomatic hyponatremia, which may be accompanied by the rapid development of cerebral edema and profound neurologic sequelae, including brain death.

MONITORING RESUSCITATION

The most readily available clinical guide to the adequacy of resuscitation is the hourly urinary output, which should be maintained between 30 and 50 mL per hour in patients weighing more than 30 kg and 1 mL per kilogram per hour in patients weighing less than 30 kg. Oliguria in the first 48 hours postburn is rarely caused by acute renal or cardiac failure; it is initially treated by increasing fluid administration and not by pharmacologically inducing a diuresis. Assessment of the hemodynamic response and the status of mental function indicating the adequacy of cerebral perfusion is also helpful in monitoring fluid resuscitation therapy. Patient anxiety, restlessness, and disorientation may be early signs of hypovolemia or hypoxemia that require immediate assessment and correction. A resting tachycardia between 100 and 120 beats per minute is common following burn injury; heart rates above this level may reflect inadequate fluid resuscitation or inadequate pain control. Blood pressure measurements, even when obtained by an indwelling peripheral arterial cannula, may not be indicative of the true hydration status. The presence of circumferential burns on the extremities may impair arterial perfusion, resulting in blood pressure measurements not reflecting the true central arterial pressure. Additionally, markedly elevated circulating levels of catecholamines and other vasoactive materials may cause vasospasm and compromise the utility of blood pressure monitoring to guide the adequacy of resuscitation. Invasive hemodynamic monitoring with a pulmonary artery catheter is reserved for those patients who do not respond to fluid resuscitation as expected or whose fluid administration in the first 6 hours exceeds three times the volume predicted by the modified Brooke formula.

Pulmonary function must be continually reassessed throughout the resuscitative phase. Tachypnea may indicate the presence of acidemia from under resuscitation, hypoxemia, or restriction of chest wall motion due to circumferential burns or massive edema. Serial evaluation of chest roentgenograms and arterial blood gases are useful in patients with significant burn injury. Serum chemistry profiles, complete blood count, and other baseline blood studies are obtained upon admission, with further tests ordered depending upon the clinical situation. The patient's weight should be measured upon admission and followed daily as an indicator of fluid balance.

As blood flow to the burn wound increases following the resuscitative phase, the evaporative water loss from the wound increases and persists until the burn wound is healed or grafted. The insensible water losses, which include the evaporative wound losses, may be estimated according to the following formula:

insensible water loss in millimeters per hour =
(25 + % body surface area burn) × TBSA in m².

This formula provides a useful estimation of the insensible loss, however, replacement of fluid losses in the postresuscitation phase should be guided by monitoring the patient's weight, serum osmolality, and serum sodium concentrations.

ESCHAROTOMY/FASCIOTOMY

Circumferential full-thickness burns of the limbs may impair the circulation to the distal and underlying tissues. To prevent secondary ischemic necrosis of these tissues, an escharotomy may be required to relieve the constriction caused by edema beneath the eschar. To identify the need for escharotomy, the adequacy of circulation must be assessed at no less than hourly intervals. The detection of pulsatile arterial flow in the palmer arch and digital vessels in the upper extremities, and in the pedal vessels in the lower extremities, is made with a Doppler flow meter. Progressive decrease or absence of pulsatile flow is an indication for escharotomy. The development of cyanosis, impaired capillary refilling, progressive paresthesias, or deep tissue pain are extremely difficult to assess in an extensively burned extremity but may also indicate the need for escharotomy.

The escharotomy procedure is performed at the patient's bedside without the need for anesthesia, since only insensate full-thickness burn is incised. The first escharotomy incision is placed in the midlateral line of the involved extremity (Figure 18–5). If vigorous, pulsatile flow is not detected within 5–10 minutes following the initial incision, a second escharotomy is made in the midmedial line of that limb. The escharotomy incision must be performed along the entire length of the full-thickness burn to provide adequate release of vascular and neural compression. The incision must be carried across the involved joints where there is a relative lack of subcutaneous tissue, permitting ready compression of nerves and vessels. The escharotomy incises just the eschar and immediate subjacent thin connective tissue to permit expansion of the edematous subcutis. Blood loss from the escharotomy incision is minimal and readily controlled by application of pressure or electrocoagulation when performed at this level. When deeper incisions are made, excessive bleeding often ensues.

Patients with circumferential truncal burns may also require escharotomy incisions along the anterior axillary lines to relieve restriction of chest wall movement and ensure effective ventilation. An incision along the costal margin may be required in patients with full-thickness burns extending onto the upper abdominal wall. In mechanically ventilated patients, a progressive rise in peak inspiratory pressure or increase in arterial carbon dioxide tension may indicate the need for chest escharotomy. In spontaneously breathing patients, the development of restlessness, agitation, or tachypnea may signal the need for chest escharotomy.

Fasciotomy is rarely necessary to restore circulation in a limb with typical thermal injury. However, in patients

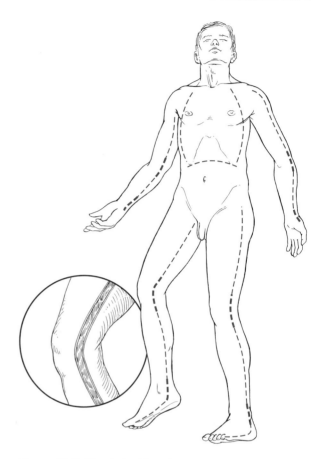

Figure 18–5. The dashed lines demonstrate the preferred sites for escharotomy incisions. The bold segments of the lines and the exploded view of the knee emphasize the importance of extending the incisions across joints with full-thickness burns.

with extensive deep burns involving fascia and muscle, or in patients with associated traumatic injuries, fasciotomies may be required to ensure adequate tissue perfusion. Additionally, in patients with high-voltage electric injury, fasciotomy is often required. The need for fasciotomy is evident when escharotomy fails to restore pulsatile arterial flow to an extremity in an otherwise successfully resuscitated patient.

ELECTRIC INJURY

Tissue damage from electric injury results from the heat generated by the passage of electric current through the body and direct thermal injury caused by flash burns or the ignition of clothing. **High-voltage** and **low-voltage injuries** are arbitrarily defined as those above or below 1000 V, respectively. The severity of injury is influenced by the voltage, the type of current, the duration of contact, and the path of current through the body.

The estimation of resuscitation fluid requirements in patients sustaining electric injury is difficult because of extensive subcutaneous or deep tissue involvement accompanied by limited areas of cutaneous injury. This "iceberg" effect often necessitates the performance of a fasciotomy rather than escharotomy to ensure viability of the distal, uninjured extremity and to evaluate the viability of underlying subcutaneous tissue and muscle. With extensive muscle necrosis, hemochromogens may be liberated, resulting in the production of a pigmented urine. In this case, intravenous fluids are administered in the volume required to produce a urine output of 100 mL/h. If the urinary pigments do not clear with this rate of urine output, additional treatments are directed towards the prevention of acute tubular necrosis resulting from circulating hemochromogens. Sodium bicarbonate (50 meq) should be added to each liter of intravenous fluid to promote alkalinization of the urine and decrease tubular pigment accumulation. An osmotic diuretic, such as mannitol, may be administered to force an increase in urine output if alkalinization of the urine does not result in pigment clearing.

Patients with electric injury are more likely to have associated injuries due to falls or tetanic skeletal muscle contractions induced by the electric current. The patient's spine should be immobilized until cervical, thoracic, and lumbar radiographs and physical examination exclude spinal fractures. Cardiac dysrhythmias occur in a small percentage of patients with electric injury. Thus, these patients should have continuous electrocardiographic monitoring for at least 24 hours and dysrhythmias treated promptly, if they occur. Neurologic changes are common in patients with electric injury. A thorough neurologic examination must be performed on admission and at scheduled intervals in these patients. Neurologic changes may be early or late in onset. Early peripheral deficits due to the damaging effects of electric current may be irreversible; however, early deficits in a distribution where there is no clear tissue damage often resolve (sensory nerves more often recover than do motor nerves). Symptoms of delayed onset, often resembling upper motor neuron disease, tend to be progressive and permanent and may be related to progressive thrombosis of nutrient vessels of the spinal cord or nerve trunks.

About one third of patients with significant electric injury of the extremities will require amputation. Conservative operations are performed according to the principles of limb salvage and only obviously necrotic tissue is debrided. It is often difficult to distinguish nonviable from viable tissue with certainty during the initial debridement, and patients with these injuries are frequently returned to the operating room at 24–48 hour intervals to reevaluate the extent of injury. Occasionally, unrelenting hyperkalemia, acidosis, or hemochromogenuria force early amputation to prevent systemic organ failure.

CHEMICAL BURNS

The depth and severity of chemical burns are related to the concentration of the chemical agent and the duration of contact with the tissues. These burns, dissimilar to other thermal injuries, require immediate care of the burn wound. The caustic agent must be thoroughly washed from the surface of the skin as soon as possible. All clothing, including shoes, must be removed and the wounds copiously irrigated with water. When the chemical agent is present in the form of a dry powder, this should be brushed from the skin prior to dilution with water. If ocular injury is suspected, prompt and prolonged irrigation with saline or water should begin, with care taken not to contaminate an unaffected eye by careful positioning of the patient's head.

The amount of tissue damage incurred is dependent on the nature of the specific agent. Strong alkalis react with tissues to produce saponification and liquefaction necrosis, whereas acids are water-soluble and penetrate easily into subcutaneous tissues, causing coagulation necrosis soon after contact. Cutaneous absorption of certain chemical agents may cause systemic toxicity, which may complicate subsequent therapy; therefore, identification of the causative agent is required. Initial wound management is not dependent on the nature of the specific agent, and prompt and thorough water lavage is employed for all chemical exposures. Time spent searching for specific antidotes is unnecessary and may delay the initiation of adequate water lavage.

Assessing the depth of injury in chemical burns is often difficult, since many agents produce a tanned or bronzed appearance of the skin. The skin may remain pliable to the touch but may represent extensive full-thickness tissue necrosis. With the exception of the initial attention given to the burn wound and possible systemic toxicity due to absorption of the causative agent, fluid resuscitation and later treatment of chemical injury follow that of thermal burns.

NUTRITIONAL SUPPORT

Extensive thermal injury can raise the resting metabolic rate to one-and-a-half to two times normal levels. The hypermetabolic response is related to the extent of burn, with the actual physiologic response influenced by environmental temperature, physical activity, pain and anxiety, the presence of infection, and the patient's age. Much like the hypermetabolic response common to other forms of trauma and critical illness, postburn hypermetabolism is driven by the neurohumoral milieu produced by the autonomic nervous system and hypothalamic–pituitary responses. Increased circulating levels of catecholamines, glucagon, and cortisol are the primary neurohumoral mediators of hypermetabolism, which result in increased oxygen consumption, a hyperdynamic circulation, wasting of lean body mass, increased core temperature, and increased urinary nitrogen excretion. The persistence of the hypermetabolic response in the flow phase of thermal injury may be caused, in part, by the presence of proinflammatory cytokines and other inflammatory mediators.

Blood flow to the burn wound is markedly increased when compared with the blood flow to other tissues. Through anaerobic, insulin-independent means, large amounts of glucose are required to support the immune cell functions of microbial containment and destruction and removal of necrotic tissue at the burn wound-viable tissue interface. Cellular proliferation and wound healing are also glucose-dependent functions.

Marked catabolism resulting in muscle protein breakdown and loss of lean body mass is also observed following burns. Breakdown of muscle protein provides amino acids for gluconeogenesis and for the synthesis of acute phase proteins. Consequently, the provision of nutritional support to thermal injured patients is an integral part of burn center care.

The delivery of nutritional support is best accomplished using the enteral route. Most patients tolerate enteral feeding beginning in the first postburn week, and their metabolic demands can be successfully met with nutritional supplementation provided through a nasoduodenal tube. When the gastrointestinal tract cannot be utilized effectively, the parenteral route may be used as well. The metabolic requirements of burn patients may be minimized through effective pain control with parenteral dosing of narcotics, nursing in a warm environment to prevent excessive thermogenesis, and timely treatment of infection. Many formulas exist for the estimation of caloric needs following burn injury. The more common ones are based on body size, age, sex, and extent of cutaneous burn. One such formula developed at the U.S. Army Institute of Surgical Research predicts resting energy expenditure (REE) as follows:

$$\text{REE (in kcal/m}^2\text{/h)} = \text{BMR} (0.8914 + 0.01355 \times \% \text{ burn}),$$

where BMR is the expected normal basal metabolic rate based on age, sex, and body surface area in noninjured humans.

The resting energy expenditure can also be measured at the bedside by indirect calorimetry.

Careful monitoring of nutritional therapy is necessary if the high metabolic demand is to be met and adequate nutrition maintained throughout the hospital course. Serial body weight, calorie counts, nitrogen balance studies, and indirect calorimetry studies are used to evaluate the adequacy of nutritional support following burn.

MANAGEMENT OF THE BURN WOUND

Following the initial wound assessment and thorough cleansing and debridement, the burn wound should be treated with topical antimicrobial agents to limit bacterial

proliferation on the wound and to prevent bacterial wound invasion. Three commonly employed topical agents, mafenide acetate cream, silver sulfadiazine cream, and 0.5% silver nitrate soaks, have been used extensively in burn patients and are effective in controlling bacterial proliferation. The development and clinical use of the effective topical antimicrobial agents has significantly decreased the incidence of invasive burn wound infection and subsequent sepsis. Each agent has specific advantages and limitations with which the physician must be familiar to ensure optimal benefit and patient safety (Table 18–5). All three agents are effective in the prevention of invasive burn wound infection; however, because of their lack of eschar penetration, silver sulfadiazine burn cream and silver nitrate soaks are most effective when applied within 48 hours of injury. After this time the proliferating bacteria on the wound begin to invade the eschar and become inaccessible to these poorly penetrating agents. On the other hand, mafenide acetate readily penetrates the burn eschar, thus exerting its antimicrobial action at the wound, within the eschar, and at the viable-nonviable tissue interface. Silver nitrate solution is delivered in multilayered occlusive gauze dressings that are changed twice daily and moistened every 2 hours to limit evaporation, which may increase the silver nitrate concentration to cytotoxic levels within the dressings.

Patients with greater than 30% TBSA burns should receive twice-daily applications of topical therapy, preferably mafenide acetate cream in the morning, and silver sulfadiazine cream in the evening. Due to the high osmolality of mafenide acetate cream, its application causes pain in the areas of partial-thickness burn, which persists for approximately 20 minutes. Therefore, daytime application is advised to limit patient discomfort prior to bedtime. Either cream is applied as a ⅛-inch-thick layer to the entire burn wound in an aseptic manner following initial debridement and reapplied at 12-hour intervals to ensure continuous topical chemotherapy. Once each day, all of the topical agent should be cleansed from the wounds using a surgical detergent disinfectant solution.

The presence of the avascular, nonviable eschar provides an excellent culture medium for microbial proliferation. When confined to the nonviable eschar, the bacteria merely colonize the burn wound, whereas invasion beneath the eschar into viable tissue constitutes bacterial burn wound infection. The early colonizing organisms are indigenous bacteria, usually gram-positive organisms. Gram-negative bacteria and fungi appear in the wound later in the postburn course.

The clinical signs of invasive burn wound infection are often indistinguishable from those observed in uninfected hypermetabolic burn patients or burn patients with other sources of infection. These signs include hyperthermia or hypothermia, tachycardia, tachypnea, glucose intolerance, ileus, and disorientation. The tinctorial and physical changes in the burn wound are more reliable signs of inva-

Table 18–5. Topical antimicrobial agents for burn wound care.

	Mafenide Acetate	Silver Sulfadiazine	Silver Nitrate
Active component concentration	11.1% in water-miscible base	1.0% in water-miscible base	0.5% in aqueous solution
Spectrum of antibacterial activity	Gram-negative—good Gram-positive—good Yeasts—minimal	Gram-negative—selectively good Yeasts—good	Gram-negative—good Gram-negative—good Gram-positive—good Yeasts—good
Method of wound care	Exposure	Exposure or single-layer dressings	Occlusive dressing
Advantages	Penetrates eschar No gram-negative resistance	Painless Greater effectiveness against yeasts	Painless
Disadvantages	Painful on partial-thickness burns Acidosis as a result of inhibition of carbonic anhydrase Hypersensitivity reactions in 7% of patients	Neutropenia Hypersensitivity—infrequent Limited eschar penetration Resistance of certain gram-negative bacteria, clostridia	Deficits of sodium, potassium, calcium, and chloride No eschar penetration Staining of environment and equipment

sive infection and include focal dark brown or black discoloration of the wound, unexpectedly rapid eschar separation, hemorrhagic discoloration of subcutaneous fat, erythema and edema of the wound margin, and the appearance of metastatic septic lesions in unburned tissue. The development of clinical signs and symptoms of sepsis in the thermally injured patients should prompt a thorough examination of the burn wound to identify areas of invasive infection.

Cultures of the burn wound do not differentiate colonization from invasive infection, and quantitative bacteriologic cultures of burn tissue correlate poorly with the presence of invasive burn wound infection. The most reliable means of diagnosing burn wound infection involves histologic examination of a biopsy of the burn wound and underlying viable tissue. When bacteria are present in the subjacent viable tissue, the diagnosis of burn wound infection can be made with certainty. If only colonization (the presence of bacteria in nonviable tissue) is present, no specific change in therapy is warranted.

When the diagnosis of invasive burn wound infection is made, changes in local wound treatment and the initiation of systemic antibiotic therapy is indicated. Twice-daily applications of mafenide acetate cream to the affected wounds is recommended because of the superior eschar penetrating ability of this agent. Systemic antibiotic therapy based on prior cultures or burn center organism prevalence is initiated, with further refinements in therapy based on biopsy, culture, and sensitivity results. Subeschar antibiotic clysis of the infected area with a broad-spectrum penicillin is performed at 12-hour intervals and immediately prior to operation to minimize the risk of precipitating florid septic shock at the time of eschar exci-

sion. Half of the daily dose of a broad-spectrum penicillin delivered in 1 liter of normal saline is injected into the subeschar tissues with a No. 20 spinal needle. The burn wound is thereafter excised to the level of the investing fascia to ensure removal of all nonviable tissue. The wound is usually treated with moist dressings and the patient returned to the operating room in 24–48 hours for wound inspection, redebridement if necessary, or split-thickness skin grafting.

CARE OF PARTIAL-THICKNESS BURNS

Partial-thickness burns re-epithelialize from uninjured epidermal elements in hair follicles, sweat glands, and sebaceous glands residing within the dermis. The healing of partial-thickness burns generally requires 2–3 weeks; however, deep partial-thickness injuries may require up to 6 weeks before epithelial coverage is complete. These deeper wounds are best managed by burn wound excision and split-thickness skin grafting, which hastens wound closure and decreases hospital stay. The rapidity with which partial-thickness burns heal is dependent not only on the depth of injury but the area involved, the general condition of the patient, and the density of the microbial flora. Daily wound cleansing and debridement of partial-thickness burns should be employed to remove the fibrinous coagulum that accumulates on the surface of these wounds. When the wound is free of exudate, a petrolatum-impregnated gauze may be applied to the wound and left in place until spontaneous healing is complete. At this point, the gauze may be sequentially trimmed as it separates from the healed wound. Alternatively, clean wounds may be covered in biologic dressings (to be discussed) which markedly decrease pain and promote re-epithelialization.

SURGICAL MANAGEMENT OF BURNS

Excision of burn tissues by several techniques is frequently employed as a means of effecting early closure of the burn wound. Prompt burn wound excision and split-thickness skin grafting decreases the duration of hospital stay and accelerates rehabilitation. Current operative management utilizes tangential excision, which entails sequential excision of thin layers of eschar until viable dermis is exposed, multiple applications of tangential excision technique to reach deeper viable tissue, or scalpel excision to the level of the investing muscle fascia for burn wound removal (Figure 18–6). These surgical procedures may be performed early in the postburn course, once the patient is hemodynamically stable and resuscitation is complete. The depth of excision in tangential, and sequential burn wound removal is governed by the appearance of healthy tissue and punctate bleeding from dermal or subcutaneous beds. Scalpel excision of burns involves removal of the wound and underlying subcutaneous tissue to the level of the investing muscle fascia.

This is accomplished more rapidly and with significantly less blood loss than the tangential or sequential wound excisions. In general, the operative procedure is limited to excision of 20% of the body area, which generally corresponds to an area of excision producing a blood loss equal to the patient's blood volume, or 2 hours of operating time. Careful anesthetic management is necessary to avoid hypotension and hypothermia. When a viable wound is obtained and hemostasis assured, wound coverage is accomplished with split-thickness cutaneous autograft or biologic dressings.

Cutaneous autografts, 0.008–0.012 inches thick, are usually obtained using an electric or compressed nitrogen-powered dermatome. As a general rule, the thinner the autograft the more certain the take, and the thicker the graft the better the cosmetic result. Thicker autografts result in slower donor site healing and a poorer cosmetic result at the donor site. Skin grafts may be applied as sheet grafts or meshed to provide expansion ratios ranging from 1.5:1 to 9:1. Expansion ratios of 4:1 or greater require prolonged time for interstitial closure and have a greater propensity for scar formation. Therefore, large expansion ratios are only utilized in patients with massive burns and limited donor sites. Following autografting, occlusive dressings moistened with topical antibacterial agents are usually applied. The wounds are kept moist to prevent

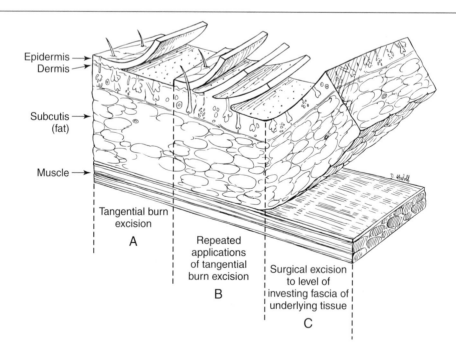

Figure 18–6. Diagram of the skin and subcutaneous tissues demonstrating the techniques of burn wound excision. **A:** Tangential burn wound excision exposing a viable dermal bed with punctate capillary bleeding in a medium-depth partial-thickness burn wound. **B:** Repeated applications of the tangential excision technique required for areas of deeper burns. **C:** Burn excision to the level of the investing muscle fascia, a technique useful to limit blood loss and expeditiously remove the burn wound.

desiccation until the interstices of the graph have epithelialized.

SKIN SUBSTITUTES
& BIOLOGICAL DRESSINGS

In the massively burned patient, the disparity between donor site availability and burn wound area requires the use of temporary skin substitutes or biological dressings to accomplish temporary wound closure while awaiting donor site healing and subsequent donor site reharvesting. The application of biological dressings to an excised wound bed prevents wound dessication, reduces wound pain, facilitates patient movement, limits bacterial growth, functions as a barrier against bacterial contamination, and reduces evaporative water and heat losses from the wound. Additionally, application of these dressings to partial-thickness burns improves subsequent healing quality, reduces wound edema, and permits prompt and orderly regeneration of the wound. Currently, the gold standard of biological dressings is viable human cutaneous allograft, which derives a temporary blood supply through direct vessel-to-vessel connection from the underlying wound bed. Successful engraftment produces a temporarily healed burn wound until the allograft is lost to rejection, usually occurring in 2–3 weeks. At this point, the allograft may be replaced with autograft, if available, or new allograft reapplied. Other less effective but commonly available biological dressings include porcine xenograft, which is available as a fresh, frozen, or lyophilized preparation. Advantages include an abundant supply and lower cost. This biological dressing does not become vascularized and adheres to the wound bed by fibrin bonding and partial penetration of the xenograft dermis by the fibrovascular tissue of the host. The underside of the graft is nourished by the plasmatic circulation, and desiccation and necrosis of the outer surface usually occurs within 1 week.

Several synthetic skin substitutes have been developed in an attempt to avoid the problems of disease transmission and storage requirements common to biologic dressings. Bilayer membranes composed of a dermal and an epidermal analogue have been developed. The outer layer mimics the epidermis, allowing water vapor transmission and preventing bacterial contamination, whereas the inner dermal layer is designed to promote adherence and fibrovascular ingrowth from the wound bed. Biobrane, a commonly used synthetic skin substitute, is composed of an epidermal layer of pliable silastic and a dermal component derived from porcine collagen. This product is removed in its entirety prior to subsequent cutaneous autografting. Integra is a synthetic dermal substitute that is unique in that a neodermis is formed by fibrovascular ingrowth into a glycosaminoglycan-enriched collagen fibril dermal analogue. The epidermal component is also made of silastic and is removed once the dermal analogue is vascularized, allowing definitive closure of the wound with ultrathin split-thickness skin grafts. Common problems encountered with all biologic dressings in general, and synthetic skin substitutes in particular, include incomplete adherence, submembrane suppuration, and technical problems with premature separation due to shearing or submembrane fluid collections.

Successful in vitro cultivation of human keratinocytes has led to recent evaluation of cultured autologous keratinocytes for coverage of wounds in massively burned patients. Current culture techniques require 3 or more weeks of preparation for a product 6–8 epidermal cell layers in thickness. These grafts are quite fragile and susceptible to bacterial colonization of the recipient wound bed. Additionally, minimal shear forces may dislodge these cells from the wound. Application of cultured autologous keratinocytes has resulted in a disappointingly small average extent of body area closed in the larger reported series. The percent take is inversely proportional to the extent of burn: an unfortunate relationship. The lack of a transplantable dermis, the 3- to 4-week delay from skin biopsy to the availability of cultured skin, and the lack of long-term durability of skin that does engraft are also limiting features. This technology has the potential for providing timely coverage of large areas, and active research to improve engraftment is ongoing.

THE MULTIDISCIPLINARY TEAM
APPROACH TO BURN CARE

The complexity of care required to manage patients with extensive thermal injury successfully requires the coordinated effort of a team of dedicated specialists spanning diverse disciplines. The concept of a multidisciplinary team was paramount in the development of a hierarchical regionalized system of burn centers throughout North America. The relatively prolonged acute hospitalization, when compared to other forms of injury or illness, necessitates the input of specialists in nutrition, physical and occupational rehabilitation, respiratory therapy, clinical psychology and psychiatry, social work, anesthesiology, medical laboratory sciences, nursing, critical care, and surgery. Assessment and treatment by all team members begins on admission and continues throughout the acute hospitalization in preparation for the transition to the rehabilitative phase of burn care. This team approach to patient care and to the timely solution of clinical problems through effective clinical and basic science research has been responsible for the advancements in the care of thermally injured patients that have been realized over the past 40 years.

SUGGESTED READING

Advances in Understanding Trauma and Burn Injury: June 21–23, 1990, Washington, DC. J Trauma 1990;30(Suppl 12): S1–211.

Cioffi WG et al: Prophylactic use of high-frequency percussive ventilation in patients with inhalation injury. Ann Surg 1991;213:575.

Demling RH: Burns. In: Wilmore DW et al (editors): *Care of the Surgical Patient*. Scientific American, 1991.

Graves TA et al: Fluid resuscitation of infants and children with thermal injury. J Trauma 1988;28:1656.

Hansbrough JF: Current status of skin replacements for coverage of extensive burn wounds. J Trauma 1990;30(Suppl 12):S155.

Mozingo DW, Barillo DJ, Pruitt BA: Acute resuscitation and transfer management of burned and electrically injured patients. Trauma Q 1994;2:94.

Mozingo DW, Pruitt BA Jr: Infectious complications after burn injury. Curr Opin Surg Inf 1994;2:69.

Pruitt BA Jr, Mason AD: Lightning and electric shock. In: Weatherall DJ, Ledinghan JGG, Warrell DA (editors): *Oxford Textbook of Medicine*, 2nd ed. Oxford University Press, 1987.

Pruitt BA Jr et al: Evaluation and management of patients with inhalation injury. J Trauma 1990;30(Suppl 12):S63.

Pruitt BA Jr, McManus WF, McDougal WS: Surgical management of burns. In: Nora FP (editor): *Operative Surgery: Principles and Techniques*. Saunders, 1990.

Shirani KZ et al: Undate on current therapeutic approaches in burns. Shock 1996;5:4.

19

Fluids, Electrolytes, & Acid-Base Balance

Lori J. Morgan, MD, & John E. Niederhuber, MD

▶ Key Facts

- ▶ In healthy individuals, water comprises 50–70% of total body weight.

- ▶ Total body water is comprised of 60% intracellular fluid and 40% extracellular fluid. Extracellular fluid is further divided into intravascular fluid (plasma) and extravascular fluid (interstitium).

- ▶ Control of osmolality is primarily dependent upon water intake and excretion, with the kidney acting as the chief regulator of this system affecting fluid shifts to keep osmolality balanced.

- ▶ The most common cause of water excess in the surgical patient is iatrogenic, caused by an excess of water in intravenous solutions. It is best treated by withholding water.

- ▶ Saline depletion is the most common abnormality in surgical patients and can be caused by diarrhea, nasogastric suction, vomiting, enteric fistulae, intraluminal sequestration, and other abnormalities. Treatment should be rapid resuscitation with an isotonic fluid (usually saline).

- ▶ Edema develops with saline excess, usually caused by overzealous maintenance or replacement therapy. Diuretics are the primary form of treatment.

- ▶ Electrolyte abnormalities include hypernatremia, hyponatremia, hyperkalemia, hypokalemia, hypercalcemia, and hypocalcemia.

- ▶ Acid-base balance is an extremely important factor in homeostasis. The physiologic pH of extracellular fluid is tightly maintained between 7.35 and 7.45. Extremes in pH (6.9–7.9) are poorly tolerated.

- ▶ Acid-base disorders are usually diagnosed by obtaining an arterial blood gas analysis and include metabolic acidosis, metabolic alkalosis, respiratory acidosis, respiratory alkalosis, and mixed acid-base disorders.

Water and electrolyte balance abnormalities commonly occur with many surgical diseases and as a result of surgical intervention and the process of recovery. In surgery, these disorders may produce life-threatening derangements of cardiovascular, pulmonary, and neurologic function. The homeostatic mechanisms in the body that maintain the correct quantity distribution and composition of total body water are complex and involve several organ systems and hormones. It is a process that must function despite diseases or tissue injuries that have the potential for rapid and large changes in solutes and water within the body.

The first task in evaluating the patient is to determine whether the current condition is the result of water and electrolyte losses or gains. Usually, it will be some of both. That is, there will be specific losses and some effort at replacement. The examining physician must determine the quantity of losses as well as the composition of the losses; the physician will then analyze the replacement water and electrolytes administered to determine further replacement and maintenance requirements.

The second task in surgery is almost always the assessment of the nature of the injury process to determine how it may be affecting the mechanisms that maintain water and electrolyte homeostasis. Finally, on occasion, the surgeon is faced with patients who also have underlying disorders of water and electrolyte homeostasis, such as inappropriate antidiuretic hormone production, hyperaldosteronism, diabetes, or impaired renal function.

The majority of every day surgical problems, fortunately, will be quite simple. They will generally be straightforward issues regarding the extracellular fluid compartment, abnormalities of volume osmolarity, and sodium and potassium concentration. Evaluation of patients begins with a clinical history (how did the patient get to this point in time?) and also includes an assessment of the patient's symptoms and physical findings. The latter includes body weight, blood pressure, pulse, and, often, central venous pressure. These carefully noted observations are integrated with a laboratory assessment of serum electrolytes, blood glucose, urea nitrogen, and creatinine. In addition, determinations of serum hematocrit, arterial blood pH, PCO_2, HCO_3^-, and so forth are indicated in more complex illnesses.

BODY WATER DISTRIBUTION & COMPOSITION

In healthy individuals, water composes 50–70% of total body weight. This percentage varies with age, sex, and adiposity. Overall, total body water (TBW) decreases with age. Infants are composed of approximately 80% water, with this percentage decreasing to adult levels by the age of 10. Men generally have more lean muscle mass than women, resulting in a higher percentage of total body water. Obese individuals have a lower percentage of body water by weight, as adipose tissue contains virtually no water.

Total body water is composed of 60% intracellular fluid (ICF) and 40% extracellular fluid (ECF). In an average 70-kg man, TBW equals 42 L, with 28 L of ICF and 14 L of ECF (Figure 19–1). Extracellular fluid is further divided into intravascular fluid (plasma) and extravascular fluid (interstitium). The interstitial fluid also includes transcellular fluid, which is comprised of the fluid from

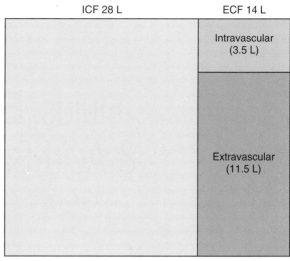

Figure 19–1. Total body water (42 L) divided into its components. ICF = intracellular fluid; ECF = extracellular fluid; TBW = total body water.

specialized tissue compartments, such as synovium, joint fluid, and cerebral spinal fluid. Extravascular fluid is approximately 11 L and intravascular fluid 3.5 L in the average person; thus, the ratio of intravascular to extravascular fluid is 1:3.

The various fluid compartments have different electrolyte and protein compositions. Electrical neutrality within compartments is maintained by balancing anions and cations. Extracellular fluid solutes are primarily sodium, chloride, and bicarbonate (Figure 19–2). This is true for both plasma and interstitium. Plasma, however, has a higher concentration of proteins because uninjured capillary membranes are generally impermeable to these

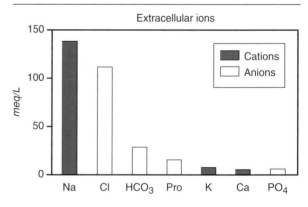

Figure 19–2. Extracellular ion distribution. PO_4 includes other organic anions.

moieties. The proteins have a net negative charge, which requires an increase in plasma cations in order to maintain electrical neutrality. The negatively charged plasma proteins also repel other anions from the intravascular space. The balance of anions are, therefore, found in greater abundance in the interstitium. This balance is referred to as the **Gibbs-Donnan equilibrium**.

The primary intracellular solutes are potassium, phosphates, sulfates, magnesium, and proteins (Figure 19–3). The protein content of the intracellular compartment is four times that of plasma. Again, a higher protein content requires an increase in cations to balance the net negative charge. There is an overall higher concentration of ions (not solutes) in the intracellular compartment. This difference creates the electrical potential seen across cell membranes and is maintained by active cell membrane transport systems. Ion concentrations are defined as milliequivalents (electric charge), which reflect electrical, not osmotic, activity.

OSMOLALITY & WATER SHIFTS

Osmotic activity is dependent upon the concentration of solutes (not their electrical combining capacity) in each fluid compartment. Cell and capillary membranes pass solutes selectively, but water is freely permeable throughout the compartments described above. This keeps the osmolality the same in both the ECF and ICF. For example, 1 millimole of glucose (a non-ionizable substance) equals 1 millimole of solute; 1 millimole of sodium chloride in solution creates 2 milliosmoles of solute. Control of osmolality is primarily dependent upon water intake and excretion. The kidney acts as the chief regulator of this system (see Chapter 44), effecting fluid shifts to keep osmolality balanced at approximately 290 milliosmoles in each compartment.

A non-ionic fluid shift in either the ECF or ICF will move water from the hypotonic to the hypertonic compartment in order to regain osmolal balance. For example, a patient given a solution of 5% dextrose in water (D5W) intravenously will quickly metabolize the glucose, and the intravascular compartment will be hypo-osmolar (increased water content) compared to the interstitium and the intracellular compartment. Water will diffuse across both cell and capillary membranes until the osmolarity in all compartments is again equal. Water is distributed across compartments according to the relative size of the compartment; for example, two thirds becomes intracellular and one third extracellular. The extracellular water is further divided with three fourths moving into the interstitium and one fourth remaining in the plasma. The rapid redistribution of D5W makes this solution a poor fluid for intravascular resuscitation.

Clinical Scenario: A hypotensive patient is given 1 liter of D5W as part of his volume resuscitation. This is delivered intravascularly by venous infusion. Promptly, approximately 666 mL diffuses intracellularly and 333 mL remains extracellular. This is distributed across the extracellular fluid compartment, with 250 mL diffusing into the interstitium and 83 mL remaining intravascular. Thus, less than 10% of the original volume remains intravascular for cardiovascular support.

An isotonic fluid (normal saline) has the same osmolality as the intracellular, plasma, and interstitial fluids. A transfusion of isotonic fluid does not change cell volume and will not shift water intracellularly. Normal saline given intravenously, however, is distributed throughout the extracellular compartment (ie, both plasma and interstitium) as sodium and chloride freely diffuse across capillary membranes and water "follows" these osmoles in order to balance the solute content. Thus, a transfusion of normal saline is distributed with one fourth in plasma and three fourths in the interstitium.

Clinical Scenario: A hypotensive patient is given 1 liter of normal saline as part of his volume resuscitation. This is delivered intravenously, where 250 mL of saline remains and 750 mL diffuses into the interstitium. When compared to D5W, more than three times the volume of saline remains intravascular, making it a much more appropriate solution for resuscitation.

A hypertonic change in the extracellular fluid (loss of water or increase in solutes) will correspond to a shift of water from the intracellular to the extracellular compartment (unless the solute itself is diffusible across cell membranes, such as ethanol). Non-diffusible solutes across the cell membrane, such as mannitol, glucose, or sodium, that

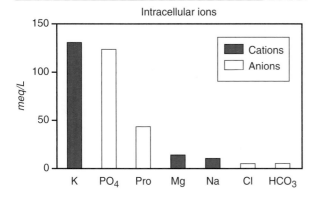

Figure 19–3. Intracellular ion distribution. PO_4 includes other organic anions.

cause this extracellular shift of water are referred to as **effective osmols**, as they determine the intracellular volume. Clinically, this is seen when the serum glucose (Glu_s) is elevated and water is shifted into the ECF, resulting in the dilution of other solutes, such as sodium. For each 100 mg/dL of increase in serum glucose above normal, there is an effective reduction in measured serum sodium (Na_s) of 1.6 meq/L. The true serum sodium content can be calculated as:

$$\frac{[Glu_s - 100 \text{ mg/dL}]}{100 \text{ mg/dL}} (1.6 \text{ meq/L}) + (Na_s) = \text{corrected } (Na_s)$$

Clinical Scenario: A patient with diabetic ketoacidosis presents with a measured serum glucose of 414 mg/dL and a measured serum sodium of 130 meq/L. The serum sodium is calculated first by subtracting a normal glucose (100 mg/dL) from 414 mg/dL, which equals 314 meq/dL. The serum sodium is adjusted for every 100 mg/dL increase in glucose above normal. In this case, that figure is 3. The serum sodium is then calculated as: 3.1 (1.6 meq/L) + 130 meq/L = 136 meq/L.

Sodium is the primary osmotic agent in plasma along with glucose, urea and other plasma salts. The sum total of all osmotic agents is approximately two times the sodium concentration. Plasma osmolality can be measured with an osmometer, but it is well estimated using the following formula:

$$P_{osm} \approx 2[Na_s] + Glu_s/18 + BUN_s/2.8$$

If the measured plasma osmolality is different from the calculated, another effective osmol, such as mannitol or ethanol, must be present in the plasma.

Clinical Scenario: A patient with a severe closed head injury is admitted to the intensive care unit. She is initially treated in the emergency room with intubation, mild hyperventilation, and mannitol, among other therapies. On arriving in the intensive care unit, her plasma osmolality is calculated from her serum electrolytes (Na 142, glucose 157, BUN 9) as: 2(142) + 157/18 + 9/2.8 = 296 mOsm/L. Her measured serum osmolality is 329 mOsm/L, indicating the presence of an unmeasured osmol, such as the mannitol that she was given.

Osmolality, as discussed above, is maintained by water movement between the fluid compartments. Water movement is governed by colloid osmotic pressure (oncotic pressure) and hydrostatic pressure. The net balance of the plasma and interstitial oncotic pressures and the permeability and area of the capillary membrane determines the direction of water flux (**Starling hypothesis**). Overall, the net flux is into the interstitium, which is balanced by lymphatic drainage. Lymphatic drainage prevents the accumulation of excess fluid in the interstitial space (edema) unless the balance is upset by a change in oncotic pressure or capillary permeability.

NORMAL FLUIDS & ELECTROLYTES

A healthy individual's fluid and electrolyte balance is maintained by renal and neuroendocrine control. In general, intake is equal to output in the steady state. The average water intake per day is 2–3 L, with approximately 1.5 L ingested as liquid and 0.5 L ingested as solids. An additional 150–400 mL of water is gained by oxidative metabolism. Sodium intake is approximately 100 meq/d and potassium intake averages 60 meq/d. Output varies with intake with the kidney, conserving sodium and water as necessary.

Water loss through urine is in the range of 1.5 L/d. Approximately 250 mL/d is lost in stool, with insensible losses (via skin and lungs) of 600–900 mL/d. An additional 100 mL of water is lost per day in sweat, but this is highly variable depending upon the environment and the acclimatization of the individual. Daily sodium losses are 50–150 meq/d, with 50–90 meq lost in urine, 10–60 meq lost in sweat, and 0–20 meq lost in stool. Sodium excretion is tightly regulated by the kidney; however, sodium conservation occurs at the expense of potassium wasting. Daily potassium losses are 50–100 meq in urine and 0–10 meq in sweat. Virtually no potassium is lost in stool.

Normal water, sodium, and potassium balance must be maintained. Excretion is usually balanced by oral intake. If patients are unable to tolerate oral intake, intravenous therapy must be provided to preserve fluid and electrolyte balance. Intravenous (IV) therapy must provide daily basal requirements, correct volume deficits or excesses, and replace ongoing losses. Basal water requirements are calculated as 25–35 mL/kg/d. Obligatory sodium losses are usually replaced by 1–2 meq/kg/d, and potassium is replaced as 0.5–1.0 meq/kg/d.

Clinical Scenario: Maintenance fluid for the 70-kg person who has no oral intake and no ongoing losses or deficits other than normal metabolism can be calculated for intravenous infusion. Water is replaced as: 35 mL/kg (70 kg) = 2450 mL/d. Sodium is 2 meq/kg (70 kg) = 140 meq/d. Potassium is 0.5 meq/kg (70 kg) = 35 meq/d. If a maintenance solution of 0.5 normal saline with 30 meq/L of potassium is given at 100 mL/h, over 24 hours the patient will receive 2400 mL of water, 178 meq of sodium, and 48 meq of potassium. This closely approximates basal requirements.

Deficit replacement depends upon the nature of the fluid lost. The first step in IV replacement therapy is to decide if there is a volume abnormality that needs to be corrected. Volume abnormalities can be seen as either saline or water excess or depletion. Water excess or deficiency is calculated as:

$$\Delta \text{ in water} = [(\text{measured Na}_s/\text{normal Na}_s) (0.6 \times \text{weight [kg]})] - (0.6 \times \text{wt [kg]}).$$

> **Clinical Scenario:** An elderly, 70-kg patient is brought to the emergency room slightly confused and weak. A serum sodium is measured at 125 meq/L. Her water excess is calculated as: Δ in water = (140/125) (0.6)(70) − (0.6)(70) = 5 L.

FLUID ABNORMALITIES

Water excess causes hyponatremia due to an increase in total body water. The most common cause is iatrogenic due to an excess of water in IV solutions. When water excess is calculated, the serum sodium must be corrected for abnormal glucose concentration. **Water excess** is an excess in total body water that is distributed across the ECF and ICF. Hypo-osmolality of the intracellular compartment results in muscle cramps, weakness, fatigue, confusion, disorientation, convulsions, and coma. The central nervous system (CNS) symptoms are a result of cerebral edema. Water excess is most effectively treated by withholding water. Water excess can be associated with saline excess as well as saline deficiency. Changes in a patient's weight can indicate associated volume problems, that is, if the patient with an excess of water of 4.5 L has an associated weight gain of 6 kg, there is an excess of 1.5 L of saline.

Water deficit is also associated with CNS dysfunction due to cell shrinkage. It is usually caused by an inability to obtain water. These patients become confused, combative, and eventually comatose. Symptoms of intravascular depletion are not seen because two thirds of the water loss is from the intracellular compartment. Treatment is slow replacement in order to avoid rapid changes in cell volume. The length of time that the deficit has been present dictates the speed of correction. If a deficit has occurred over a short period of time, it can be corrected fairly rapidly. Long-standing deficits need to be corrected slowly. Total deficit should be calculated and replaced over 24–48 hours. If there is an associated saline depletion, that should be corrected first, following with water replacement.

Saline depletion is synonymous with volume depletion. It is the most common abnormality in surgical patients and can be caused by a multitude of abnormalities. These include gastrointestinal (GI) losses secondary to diarrhea,

> **Clinical Scenario:** A patient normally weighing 70 kg is brought to the hospital after being stranded in the desert for 2 days. The patient's serum sodium is measured as 170 meq/L and his weight is noted to be 60 kg. His body water change is calculated as: 170/140 (0.6)(70) − (0.6)(70) = 9 L. He has lost 10 kg, therefore, he has additional saline depletion of 1 liter. The patient's hypovolemia and saline deficit is corrected by first using normal saline. Then, the serum sodium is remeasured and water deficit is recalculated. A deficit of 9 L replaced over 24 hours is 375 mL/h. This does not include maintenance fluid, which will need to be included in the total IV rate. After saline repletion is accomplished, any one of several hypotonic fluids can be used for replacement; however, the key to this therapy is frequent monitoring of serum sodium, with replacement adjusted according to the rate of change of serum sodium. In general, the serum sodium should not decrease more than 1–3 meq/h.

nasogastric suction, vomiting, enteric fistulae, and intraluminal sequestration. Urine losses occur due to excessive use of diuretics, osmotic diuresis, adrenal insufficiency, or postobstructive uropathy. Saline is also lost with sweat, burns, and third-space losses due to trauma (operative and mechanical), hemorrhage, and loss of ascites. Saline depletion is identified by weight loss and intravascular symptoms of hypotension, low central venous pressure (CVP) pulmonary capillary wedge pressure (PCWP), and urine output. Laboratory studies may indicate a contracted blood volume (high hematocrit), an elevated blood urea nitrogen (BUN)-to-creatinine ratio, or a low urine sodium. Saline is lost exclusively from the ECF. Treatment of saline depletion should be rapid resuscitation with an isotonic fluid—usually saline—with the goal of stabilizing the blood pressure and improving urine output. Hypotonic solutions should not be used because two thirds of the fluid will flux intracellularly and only one third will be available to the entire extracellular space (interstitium and plasma).

Saline excess is also a frequent abnormality seen in surgical patients. It is often associated with patients that have other comorbid disease processes, such as congestive heart failure or renal failure. Frequently, the excess is iatrogenic caused by overzealous maintenance or replacement therapy. Edema develops with saline excess as the excess is distributed only in the extracellular compartment. Other symptoms may include an elevated CVP or PCWP, distended jugular veins, a cardiac gallop, and pulmonary edema. The plasma and interstitium may both have excess volume or the patient may have a low oncotic pressure, resulting in intravascular depletion. This is seen in patients with liver disease (cirrhosis), renal disease (nephrotic syndrome), and hypoalbuminemia. Septic patients with abnormal capillary membrane permeability (allows protein to cross the capillary membrane) often have

HISTORICAL FACTS

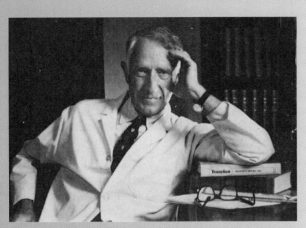

Francis D. Moore, MD (Reprinted, with permission, from Weiss AB: Conversations in Medicine: Francis Daniels Moore, MD. Hosp Pract 1988;189.)

The outstanding number of academic and clinical contributions bestowed upon the field of surgery by Francis D. Moore has led to his being called the "thinking man's surgeon." Moore completed his undergraduate and medical school training at Harvard. After a period of concentrated laboratory investigations as a National Council Research Fellow in 1942, he went on to complete his surgical residency training. By the age of 35, he was made surgeon-in-chief at Peter Bent Brigham Hospital and the Moseley Professor of Surgery at Harvard Medical School.

Early in his career, Moore became interested in the metabolic responses seen in surgical patients, and he incorporated a new area of study that used radioactive isotopes to determine fluid constituents within the body. In 1948, he published a landmark article in *Science* on the determination of total body water and solids by isotope dilution.

Moore is also well known for his contributions in the field of burn trauma and fluid resuscitation. In 1941, he was working with Oliver Cope at Massachusetts General Hospital when the Coconut Grove fire broke out (see Chapter 18). The two were able to use research they had begun almost 18 months earlier on extracellular fluid, based on the isotope dilutions, to save hundreds of lives. In 1952, he published his exceptional book, *Metabolic Response to Surgery*. In 1959, he extended his initial concepts in *Metabolic Care of the Surgical Patient*, which has been a standard work since it was originally published. In short, Moore has made remarkable contributions to the knowledge and treatment of metabolic derangements in patients undergoing elective surgery, as well as in those who have suffered traumatic injuries, such as burns.

saline excess (after resuscitation) associated with intravascular depletion.

Diuretics are the primary treatment for saline excess across the entire extracellular space (plasma and interstitium). The use of diuretics requires good renal function, and in patients with renal failure dialysis will be required. Saline infusions are restricted, and occasionally ionotropic agents are required to improve cardiac output and renal blood flow. Where saline excess is present but the intravascular compartment is depleted (indicated by edema and increased weight with hypotension and low central

pressure), the most effective therapy is to eliminate the underlying cause. Saline is used for resuscitation but it is rapidly distributed across the entire ECF. Diuretics make the hypotension worse, as they deplete the intravascular compartment quickly with a slower equilibration from the interstitium. Products with hyperoncotic pressure (albumin, hetastarch) transiently improve the intravascular oncotic pressure, but with leaky membranes these proteins can traverse the capillaries and actually increase the interstitial oncotic pressure. Blood may be useful to increase intravascular volume, oncotic pressure, and oxygen-carrying capacity; however, the transfusion of blood products has risks that must be evaluated carefully (see Chapter 6).

ELECTROLYTE ABNORMALITIES

HYPERNATREMIA

Hypernatremia is defined as a serum sodium greater than 145 meq/L. Patients with hypernatremia are always hyperosmolar. As discussed above, it may occur associated with volume depletion, volume excess, or euvolemia. It is caused by excessive salt intake, reduced water intake, or excessive water output. Excessive salt ingestion can usually be diagnosed by history. Decreased water intake usually is seen in patients who are unable to ingest water, as a result of either a comatose state or gastrointestinal (GI) intolerance without appropriate replacement. Excessive water output can be due to fever, skin losses (excessive sweating, burns, rashes), GI losses (diarrhea, nasogastric suction), lung losses (tachypnea, ventilation without humidification), or urinary losses (diuresis secondary to osmotic agents, diabetes insipidus). The diagnosis is made by taking a thorough history, conducting a physical examination, and evaluating the serum electrolytes, BUN, creatinine, urine sodium, and osmolality.

Symptoms of this disorder are primarily neurologic, with agitation, lethargy, and confusion the most common. In severe states there may be ataxia, seizures, stroke, and death. It is important to evaluate the overall volume status to see if there is also saline depletion. Treatment is dependent upon the volume status. If the hypernatremia is associated with saline depletion, then saline should be replaced first. Saline repletion can be done rapidly, then the water repletion should be done more slowly, correcting the serum sodium over 24–48 hours to decrease the serum sodium no more than 2 meq/h. This is particularly important for severe chronic deficits, which are at risk for cerebral edema with rapid water repletion. (A more conservative correction of 0.5 meq/h may be indicated for chronic deficits.) Acute deficits can be replaced quickly. Hypernatremia associated with volume expansion can be treated primarily with loop diuretics unless the patient has renal failure, which would necessitate dialysis. Patients that are euvolemic can usually be treated with slow replacement via hypotonic solutions (D5W, 0.2 normal saline [NS]). All replacement plans must include replacement of ongoing losses as well as deficits.

Patients with diabetes insipidus (DI) need to be considered separately. DI can be either neurogenic (trauma, surgery, CNS pathology, idiopathic) or nephrogenic (drugs, nephritis, pyelonephritis, obstructive uropathy, multiple myeloma, hypercalcemia, sickle cell disease). DI is diagnosed by hypernatremia with a low urine osmolality. Neurogenic DI is treated with fluid replacement and desmopressin or chlorpheniramine. Nephrogenic DI is treated by replacing urinary losses, giving thiazide diuretics (increases water resorption but will cause mild saline depletion), and treating the underlying cause.

HYPONATREMIA

Hyponatremia is defined as a serum sodium of less than 135 meq/L. It is indicative of excess water relative to sodium. As with hypernatremia, it can be associated with hypovolemia, hypervolemia, or euvolemia. It is generally caused by excessive water intake (psychogenic or inappropriate transfusion of hypotonic solutions), impaired renal excretion of water with normal secretion of antidiuretic hormone (ADH), renal failure, impaired renal dilution of urine secondary to inappropriate ADH secretion (both appropriate and inappropriate have multiple causes), and abnormal urine concentrating ability secondary to low blood flow to the kidney. Pseudohyponatremia may be seen with elevated serum proteins or lipids.

The diagnosis is made with a thorough history and physical, measurement of serum electrolytes, BUN, creatinine, osmolarity, and urine osmolarity. Symptoms include anorexia, lethargy, nausea, vomiting, coma, and seizures, but they do not generally appear unless the hyponatremia is very severe (Na_s < 120 meq/L) or has been very rapid. Treatment depends upon the cause and associated serum osmolality and volume status. As with hypernatremia, the serum sodium needs to be corrected slowly. Rapidly correcting hyponatremia can lead to central pontine myelinolysis, which is a dangerous complication of therapy. Hypertonic hyponatremia is present when there are other active osmoles in serum (glucose, mannitol). Therapy should be aimed at correcting the underlying cause, and the true serum sodium should be calculated, correcting for the additional solutes. Isotonic hyponatremia is seen with elevated serum proteins, lipids, and isotonic glucose or mannitol solutions; again, the primary treatment is correcting the underlying cause.

Treatment of hypotonic hyponatremia depends upon the patient's associated volume status. If hypovolemic, saline resuscitation is undertaken first. Further correction can usually be obtained with water restriction and, if necessary, the use of a loop diuretic. Patients that are hypervolemic often need therapy tailored to their comorbid conditions. Patients with renal failure may need dialysis; those with congestive heart failure will require water restriction, loop diuretics, and possibly ionotropes to improve glomerular filtration rate. Hyponatremia associated with hyperthyroidism is treated primarily with thyroid replacement therapy and fluid restriction.

Patients with impaired urine dilution secondary to increased ADH are also treated according to the underlying cause. ADH is released in response to low arterial volume (sensed by baroreceptors and the kidney) and increased serum osmolality (sensed in the neurohypophysis). ADH stimulates the resorption of solute-free water in the distal tubules of the kidney. ADH-induced hyponatremia is evidenced by a low serum sodium and osmolality with a high urine osmolality. If a patient has a normal or high volume status with a low serum sodium and a urine osmolality higher than serum osmolality, inappropriate ADH secretion, SIADH, is present (syndrome of inappropriate secretion of antidiuretic hormone). SIADH is caused by CNS trauma or tumors, surgery, pulmonary dysfunction, prostaglandin inhibitors, many medications, and several types of malignant tumors. Again, therapy is aimed at the underlying cause and fluid restriction.

Fluid restriction is effective for almost all causes of hyponatremia because of the obligate losses of water in normal body metabolism. With this therapy, the sodium is usually increased approximately 3 meq/d. If patients are symptomatic, more rapid correction may be required. Aggressive therapy is indicated for patients with CNS disturbances and also for those with a serum sodium less than 120 meq/L. The sodium deficit is calculated as:

$$\text{Desired serum sodium} - \text{measured serum sodium} \\ \times \text{weight} \times 0.6$$

Sodium levels should not be changed more than 2 meq/h or 20 meq/d. Three percent sodium and furosemide are used for rapid serum sodium correction. The diuretic is given, then the urine sodium and output are measured. Based on the urine output, the amount of sodium excreted is calculated (urine sodium meq/L × urine output mL/h) per hour, and this is replaced with 3% NS (0.45 meq/mL). The serum sodium is followed closely and adjustments are made according to the speed of the changes. Serum potassium is also followed and replaced, or serious hypokalemia can occur. When a serum sodium of greater than 125 meq/L is reached, the remainder of the replacement is done with isotonic saline, diuretics, and fluid restriction.

Clinical Scenario. A 70-kg patient presents comatose to the emergency room. On evaluation, her serum sodium is measured at 112 meq/L. Her total Na deficit is calculated as $(140 - 112)(6)(70) = 1176$ meq. Complete replacement over 24 hours would change her serum sodium far too rapidly, therefore, it needs to be done incrementally. To increase the sodium from 112 to 120 will require $(120 - 112)(0.6)(70) = 336$ meq of sodium over 24 hours. If 3% sodium is used (513 meq/L, only indicated for very low sodiums), then 336 meq/513 meq/L is 650 mL over 24 hours. Thus, initial replacement is with 3% saline at 27 mL/h. The serum sodium is rechecked every 4–6 hours, and adjustments are made according to the rate that the serum sodium is changing. The urinary sodium can be measured to help in guiding replacement therapy. This is useful when a combination of diuretics and hypertonic fluids are used for correction.

HYPERKALEMIA

Hyperkalemia is defined as a serum potassium (K) of greater than 5.0 meq/L. It occurs when there is increased K intake, decreased excretion, or redistribution from the intracellular compartment. Increased K intake is commonly iatrogenic via parenteral solutions, antibiotics, or blood transfusions. Oral intake of excessive fruit, vitamins, or salt substitutes can elevate serum K. Renal dysfunction is the most frequent cause of decreased K excretion. However, decreased excretion can be caused by hyperaldosteronism and many different pharmacologic agents. Redistribution of potassium from the intracellular compartment is seen with acidosis, where each 0.1 decrease in pH increases the serum K by 0.6 meq/L. Redistribution is also seen in insulin deficiency, rhabdomyolysis, and as a side effect of several drugs (digoxin, succinylcholine). Pseudohyperkalemia can occur secondary to a hemolyzed blood sample, thrombocytosis, or leukocytosis, and these must be considered before embarking on therapy.

Hyperkalemia is diagnosed by an elevated serum potassium and an ECG that shows peaked T waves. Cardiac dysrhythmias are the major complication and can lead to cardiac arrest. Neuromuscular symptoms of tingling, lethargy, paresthesias, or paralysis may occur but are rare. If measured, insulin and aldosterone levels will be elevated. Treatment depends on the level of potassium, the chronicity of the elevation (patients with renal failure tolerate much higher K than normal subjects), and any associated ECG changes. A mild elevation without ECG changes can be treated with potassium restriction and restriction of any drugs that can precipitate hyperkalemia. An elevated K with peaked T waves is treated with K restriction, restriction of drugs, furosemide, or potassium binders (sodium polystyrene sulfonate), insulin with glucose, sodium bicarbonate, and a repeat serum K and ECG after therapy is given.

An elevated K with an ECG showing a prolonged PR interval, peaked T waves, and U waves is a precursor to severe cardiac dysrhythmias and needs aggressive correction. Calcium is given rapidly as a cell membrane stabilizer (preventing abnormal depolarization of cell membranes), and sodium is given to increase conduction velocity in conducting cells. Bicarbonate is given to increase pH and shift K intracellularly. Insulin and glucose will also cause an intracellular shift of K. Insulin must be given, however, as glucose alone will shift K extracellularly and increase serum K. In critical situations, hemodialysis can be performed and will remove approximately 40 meq/h of potassium.

HYPOKALEMIA

Hypokalemia is defined as a serum K less than 3.5 meq/L. Hypokalemia occurs secondary to inadequate intake, intracellular redistribution, and excess excretion.

There are daily obligate potassium losses though the kidney, skin, and GI tract. Conservation mechanisms for K are not like those for sodium, and obligate losses are 15–35 meq/d. If there is no intake of potassium, either orally or parenterally, hypokalemia will occur. Intracellular redistribution of potassium occurs with the administration of bicarbonate, insulin, and glucose, and with alkalosis. Several drugs can also cause the intracellular redistribution of K (folate, barium poisoning), as can thyrotoxicosis. Renal potassium excretion is stimulated by increased volume and sodium in the distal tubules, diuretics, hyperaldosteronism, mineralocorticoid excess, drug effects (lithium toxicity, poorly resorbable anions like penicillin and carbenicillin), magnesium deficiency, or hypercalcemia. Excess excretion is also seen with GI losses (diarrhea, vomiting, nasogastric suctioning), burns, and excessive sweating.

Laboratory studies needed for evaluation are serum levels of potassium, magnesium, calcium, pH level, an ECG, and a 24-hour urine potassium level. Patients may have symptoms of muscle cramping, weakness, and paralysis. GI symptoms include ileus and constipation. At very low K levels (< 2 meq/L), respiratory arrest can occur. Cardiac dysrhythmias are also seen and can progress to refractory ventricular tachycardia or fibrillation. Hypokalemic patients are predisposed to digoxin toxicity. The ECG may show ST segment or T wave depressions. U waves may also be seen.

Treatment is directed at the cause. Hypomagnesemia is treated with magnesium, then potassium. Drugs that cause hypokalemia are withheld. K can be replaced either orally or parenterally. The maximum 1-hour replacement is 40 meq. Because the majority of K is intracellular, the serum K is a poor measure of total body K, and much more K may be required for replacement than is anticipated. For this reason, serum K levels should be checked frequently during replacement therapy. Ongoing losses must also be replaced.

HYPERCALCEMIA

Hypercalcemia is defined as a serum calcium of greater than 10.5 mg/dL or an ionized serum calcium of greater that 1.23 mmol/L. Serum calcium reflects approximately 1% of total body calcium. The remainder is stored in bones and teeth. Calcium is filtered by the kidney each day, and the majority is reabsorbed. Dietary calcium is absorbed in the intestine, and bone calcium resorption provides an additional source of calcium. Calcium levels are tightly controlled by parathyroid hormone, calcitonin, and vitamin D levels. Elevated albumin or serum proteins (multiple myeloma) can elevate serum calcium levels 0.8 mg/dL for each additional gram increase in protein above normal.

Hypercalcemia results from excess intake, decreased excretion, increased bone resorption, or decreased bone formation. Excess intake of calcium is usually excreted easily by the kidney, but renal dysfunction, which can be caused by hypercalciuria, can contribute to hypercalcemia. Vitamin D toxicity causes enhanced intestinal uptake of calcium as well as increased bone resorption, leading to hypercalcemia and hypercalciuria as well as hyperphosphatemia. Sarcoidosis and other granulomatous cells (and lymphoma) can activate vitamin D extrarenally and lead to hypercalcemia.

Increased bone resorption is the most common cause of hypercalcemia. Patients with primary hyperparathyroidism have elevated levels of parathyroid hormone (PTH), stimulating increased resorption. Malignancies stimulate resorption by local action of metastases, production of osteoclast activating factors, and secretion of ectopic hormones. Prolonged bedrest may stimulate increased resorption, as can thyrotoxicosis and vitamin A toxicity.

Decreased renal excretion of calcium contributes to hypercalcemia. The most common cause is decreased effective volume seen by the kidney. Volume depletion causes increased renal sodium resorption and calcium, as an additional cation, is also reabsorbed. Thiazide diuretics act directly on the tubule and stimulate renal calcium reabsorption. Calcium metabolism in the renal failure patient is beyond the scope of this discussion but can be difficult to manage in this population.

Symptoms of hypercalcemia are varied but may include lethargy, weakness, confusion, headache, anorexia, nausea, vomiting, constipation, nephrocalcinosis, nephrolithiasis, renal dysfunction, bradycardia, and heart block. Serum levels of calcium, phosphate, PTH, albumin, and protein are helpful in the differential diagnosis. Bone scans and x-rays can help diagnose malignancies. Treatment is usually supportive until the underlying cause is treated. Primary hyperparathyroidism is best treated by parathyroidectomy. Normal saline will decrease serum calcium by increasing the effective volume seen by the kidney. Furosemide is added to increase renal excretion of calcium. Potassium and magnesium levels are followed closely with this therapy. Bone metabolism is inhibited by etidronate disodium, calcitonin, and mithramycin. All of these substances are useful for hypercalcemia, particularly when it is caused by increased bone resorption. Phosphate induces the deposition of calcium in the extravascular tissues and can be effective in reducing serum calcium if the serum phosphate is low. Steroids decrease intestinal absorption of calcium and may decrease bony reabsorption stimulated by malignancies. Dialysis is necessary for hypercalcemia associated with severe renal dysfunction.

HYPOCALCEMIA

Hypocalcemia is defined as a serum calcium below 8.5 mg/dL or an ionized calcium below 1.12 mmol/L. Less than 50% of the calcium in serum is free or ionized. The remainder is bound to plasma proteins and cations. Hypocalcemia must be diagnosed by ionized calcium or by correcting for any protein deficiencies that would give a falsely reduced calcium (calcium falls 0.8 mg/dL for each 1 g/dL decrease in serum albumin). True hypocalcemia is caused by decreased calcium intake, increased calcium binding, decreased bone resorption, or increased bone formation. Decreased intake is seen in patients with poor nutrition and vitamin D deficiency. Pancreatitis is associated with increased calcium binding. Citrate in dialysate and blood transfusions can also bind calcium.

Hypoparathyroidism causes hypocalcemia by decreasing bone resorption. This is usually seen as a complication of parathyroid surgery but can also be caused by hypomagnesemia (low magnesium inhibits parathyroid hormone secretion). An increase in bone formation after subtotal parathyroidectomy for hyperplasia results in hypocalcemia. Many medications can also cause hypocalcemia (fluoride, calcitonin, phosphates).

Symptoms are primarily musculoskeletal with circumoral and acral paresthesias, hyperreflexia, tetany, and myopathy. Confusion, seizures, and cardiac dysrhythmias may also be seen. The diagnosis is made by a decreased serum calcium. Measuring serum phosphate, magnesium, amylase, and PTH can help differentiate the cause. Patients with neuromuscular symptoms are treated with IV calcium acutely, and oral calcium chronically. Other electrolyte deficiencies are replaced as needed and all drugs that can contribute to the hypocalcemia are withheld.

ACID-BASE BALANCE

Acid-base balance is an extremely important factor in homeostasis. The physiologic pH of extracellular fluid is tightly maintained between 7.35 and 7.45. This control maintains the optimal pH for the function of numerous enzymes, clotting factors, and proteins. A pH between 7.35 and 7.45 represents a hydrogen ion concentration $[H^+]$ of 35–45 nmol/L. pH is calculated as: $pH = 1/\log[H^+]$. The relationship of pH to $[H^+]$ is logarithmic, thus, small changes in pH represent rather large changes in $[H^+]$. Extremes in pH (6.9–7.9) are survivable for short periods of time but they are poorly tolerated. Derangements in pH are ameliorated by intrinsic buffering systems as well as by pulmonary and renal mechanisms.

Cell metabolism generates a continuous production of acids that are buffered (Figure 19–4) immediately to prevent the accumulation of free hydrogen ions. **Nonvolatile acids** are produced by the incomplete metabolism of proteins, carbohydrates and fats, organic phosphorus compounds, and nucleoproteins, which produce sulfuric acid, organic acids, inorganic phosphates, and uric acid, respectively. Systemically produced nonvolatile acids are buffered by the $NaHCO_3{:}H_2CO_3$ buffer system. The salt of the nonvolatile acid is then excreted by the kidney.

Volatile acids are those created by oxidative metabolism producing CO_2. The CO_2 is in equilibrium with its hydrated form, H_2CO_3. The balance is:

$$CO_2 + H_2O = H_2CO_3 = H^+ + HCO_3^-$$

The CO_2 in this equilibrium is continually removed during ventilation, thus the term "volatile" acid. Volatile acids are also buffered by sodium bicarbonate ($NaHCO_3$) and carbonic acid (H_2CO_3). The ratio of this buffer pair is maintained at 20:1. This is important for maintaining normal pH (7.40) as:

$$pH = pK + \log (NaHCO_3/H_2CO_3)$$

The pK (pH at which the buffer pair works most effectively) is 6.1. The calculation of pH at a 20:1 ratio is:

$$pH = 6.1 + \log (20/1) = 6.1 + 1.3 = 7.4$$

H_2CO_3 is also in equilibrium with CO_2 and H_2O. At equilibrium, the CO_2 concentration in the ECF (measured as its partial pressure of CO_2 in arterial blood [$PaCO_2$]) is a close approximation of H_2CO_3. This is formulated as:

$$pH = pK + \log ([HCO_3^-]/[0.03] PaCO_2)$$

The variables in the above equation are all easily measured with arterial blood gas analysis. The pulmonary and extracellular buffering systems are coordinated to maintain pH. As can be seen by examining the buffer pair of $NaHCO_3$ and H_2CO_3, bicarbonate (HCO_3^-) is continually used up by this system. Regeneration of HCO_3^- is a critical component of pH balance.

Renal mechanisms are used to regenerate bicarbonate and to excrete the salts of the nonvolatile acids. The kidney replaces systemic bicarbonate via several mechanisms. The first is by resorption of bicarbonate into the proximal tubule. This process is active as long as plasma bicarbonate is less than 26 meq/L. At plasma levels greater than this, bicarbonate is excreted into the lumen of the tubule. The H^+ binds with the acid salt. The sodium produced then moves into the cell to form $NaHCO_3$, regenerating that originally used for buffering. The nonvolatile acid is then excreted in the urine. The free hydrogen ion secreted into the tubular lumen also reacts with Cl^-, creating HCl, a strong acid. This is buffered by NH_3^+ secretion (generated by the metabolism of glutamine), which forms an ammonium compound and is excreted into the urine. Adjustments in glutamine metabolism and NH_3^+ production are one way that the kidney can compensate for derangements in pH; however, this process takes several days to be fully effective and it is not able to affect pH immediately.

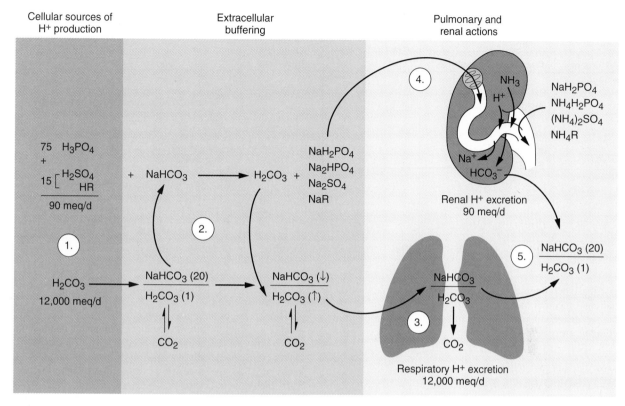

Figure 19–4. Normal buffering and excretion of acid by the lungs and kidneys. *1:* Cell metabolism produces acid, almost all as carbonic acid (H_2CO_3). H_2CO_3 is quickly removed by the lungs as CO_2. Only about 90 meq of all the acid generated per day is in the form of strong, nonvolatile acids. These strong acids cannot exist at physiologic pH; hence, they require immediate buffering. R = the anion of any nonvolatile acid besides H_3PO_4 and H_2SO_4 (eg, citrate). *2:* When strong acids enter the extracellular fluid, they immediately lower the bicarbonate (HCO_3^-) concentration by producing H_2CO_3 and sodium salts of the acids. *3:* The H_2CO_3 is excreted by the lungs as CO_2, thus lowering the H_2CO_3 concentration. *4:* The nonvolatile anion portion of the sodium salts can be excreted by the kidney along with hydrogen ion (H^+) or with ammonium ion. (NH_4^+). Secretion of H^+ or NH_4^+ leads to reabsorption of an equimolar quantity of sodium bicarbonate ($NaHCO_3$). *5:* This $NaHCO_3$ is returned to the blood and restores the $NaHCO_3$:H_2CO_3 ratio to the normal 20:1, thereby restoring the buffering capacity of body fluids. (Reprinted, with permission, from Stobo JC et al: *The Principles and Practice of Medicine,* 23rd ed. Appleton & Lange, 1996, p. 374.)

ACID-BASE DISORDERS

Acid-base disorders are usually diagnosed by obtaining an arterial blood gas (ABG) analysis. Measurements of pH, PaO_2 (partial pressure of oxygen in arterial blood), and $PaCO_2$ (partial pressure of carbon dioxide in arterial blood) are obtained from an ABG. Using the Henderson-Hasselbalch equation, HCO_3^- is calculated from the pH and $PaCO_2$. A true serum bicarbonate is measured as part of the electrolyte analysis from a venous sample. The partial pressures of gases measured in ABGs are affected by the presence of air bubbles in the specimen, temperature, delay in measurement, and the presence of heparin. All of the above can induce inaccurate results. Specimens for ABG analysis should be drawn from an artery after all heparin is cleared from the line. Air in the sample syringe should be removed immediately and the specimen placed on ice and measured as quickly as possible (less than 1 hour).

As noted previously, the normal range of pH is 7.35–7.45. The normal $PaCO_2$ in arterial blood ranges from 36–44 mm Hg. The bicarbonate is usually calculated as 24–26 meq/L. Once the ABG analysis has been performed, the results are evaluated. First, the pH is determined. Is the patient acidemic (pH < 7.35) or alkalemic (pH > 7.45)? Next, it is determined whether the derangement is respiratory or metabolic. This is most simply done by checking the $PaCO_2$. If the patient is acidemic and the $PaCO_2$ is greater than 40 mm Hg, there is respiratory acidosis. A $PaCO_2$ less than 40 mm Hg indicates that the acidemia is due to metabolic causes and the measured decrease in $PaCO_2$ is due to respiratory compensation. If the patient is alkalemic with a decreased $PaCO_2$, this suggests a respiratory alkalosis. Primary acid-base derangements are quite characteristic (Table 19–1); however, mixed

Table 19–1. Primary or single disturbances of acid-base balance: Clinical and laboratory characteristics.

Primary Disturbance	Acute Primary Change	Partial Compensatory Response	Arterial pH	Serum K+	Unmeasured Anions (Anion Gap)	Clinical Features
Respiratory Acidosis	CO_2 retention	↑ HCO_3^-	↓	↑	Normal	Dyspnea, respiratory outflow obstruction, ↑ anteroposterior diameter of chest, rales, wheezes; in severe cases, disorientation, stupor, coma
Alkalosis	CO_2 depletion	↓ HCO_3^-	↑	↓	Normal	Anxiety, occasional complaint of breathlessness, frequent sighing, lungs usually clear to exam, positive Chvostek's and Trousseau's signs
Metabolic Acidosis	HCO_3^- depletion	↓ PCO_2	↓	↑ or ↓	Normal or ↑	Weakness, air hunger, Kussmaul respiration, dry skin and mucous membranes, poor skin turgor; in severe cases, coma, hypotension, death
Alkalosis	HCO_3^- retention	↑ PCO_2	↑	↓	Normal	Weakness, positive Chvostek's and Trousseau's signs, hyporeflexia

Reprinted, with permission, from Stobo JC et al: *The Principles and Practice of Medicine,* 23rd ed. Appleton & Lange, 1996, p. 376.

acid-base derangements are evaluated in the context of the patient's medical history and current condition and recognizing discrepancies between anticipated and measured compensatory responses.

METABOLIC ACIDOSIS

A metabolic acidosis is an arterial pH less than 7.35 due to a reduction in the plasma bicarbonate (HCO_3^-) to less than 22 meq/L. The reduction can be the result of a loss of HCO_3^- or the addition of excess nonvolatile acids (due to increased production or decreased renal excretion). The result of either of these is an increase in the plasma concentration of free hydrogen ion and a decrease in plasma pH. A decrease in pH will stimulate an attempt at respiratory compensation. For each decrease of 1 meq/L of HCO_3^- the $PaCO_2$ should fall by 1.3 mm Hg. If the $PaCO_2$ is higher than anticipated, a concomitant respiratory acidosis exists. If the $PaCO_2$ is lower than expected, the patient also has a respiratory alkalosis.

A metabolic acidosis is usually categorized as a **gap** or **non-gap acidosis**. This refers to the anion gap calculated by the measurement of serum electrolytes. The **anion gap** is defined as:

$$\text{anion gap} = Na^+ - (Cl^- + HCO_3^-)$$

A normal anion gap is 8–16 meq/L. If the anion gap is greater than 18, there are unmeasured ions in the serum causing the acidosis. The common causes of gap and non-gap acidosis are listed in Table 19–2. The most common cause of perioperative metabolic acidosis is a lactic acidosis usually secondary to impaired tissue perfusion. Therapy is directed at correcting the underlying problem. Metabolic acidosis can also be caused by renal failure, renal tubular acidosis, GI loss of bicarbonate, and poison-

ing, among other things. All need to be treated in a problem-specific fashion.

Though the treatment is problem-specific, clinical findings of patients with a metabolic acidosis vary more with the severity of the acidosis rather than with the cause. A mild acidosis generally results only in a modest amount of tachypnea. As the severity of the acidosis increases, severe tachypnea, confusion, lethargy, stupor, and coma ensue. Patients may also develop decreased myocardial function, arrhythmia, and hyperkalemia. Therapy with $NaHCO_3$ may be indicated in a more severe acidosis. In general, it should only be given for a pH less than 7.2 with

Table 19–2. Causes of metabolic acidosis.

Anion Gap	Non-Anion Gap
Ketoacidosis Starvation Diabetes Alcoholic	**Renal tubular dysfunction** Renal tubular acidosis Hyperaldosteronism Potassium-sparing diuretics Addison's disease
Renal failure	
Lactic acidosis Shock Circulatory failure Hepatic failure Respiratory failure Neoplastic tissue Vigorous exercise	**Gastrointestinal losses** Pancreatic/biliary fistulae Diarrhea Ureterosigmoidostomy **Massive blood transfusion (citrate)**
Drugs or toxins Pressors Fructose Sodium nitroprusside	**Ammonium chloride** **Hyperalimentation**
Enzyme defects	**Carbonic anhydrase inhibitors**
Poisoning Ethylene glycol Methanol Salicylates	

a low HCO_3^- (< 16 meq/L). There are many undesirable side effects of bicarbonate administration, including ECF volume overload, hypernatremia, congestive heart failure, pulmonary edema, hypokalemia, metabolic alkalosis, and hyperosmolarity. The $NaHCO_3$ given must eventually be converted to CO_2 for excretion, and if there is inadequate ventilation a paradoxical worsening of the acidosis will ensue. If bicarbonate is given, it should be based on a calculation of the base deficit.

$$\text{Base deficit} = (\text{weight})\,(0.4) \times \text{desired } HCO_3^- - \text{actual } HCO_3$$

(where 0.4 is two times the ECF, and the desired bicarbonate should not be a normal bicarbonate but in the range of 15–16 meq/L).

Clinical Scenario. A 60-year-old, 70-kg man develops renal failure after a colectomy and colostomy for a perforated diverticular abscess. He is fully ventilated in the intensive care unit. The nurse calls to report recent laboratory values and notifies the physician of nonsustained ventricular arrhythmias. An arterial blood glass reveals a pH of 7.15, a $PaCO_2$ of 40 mm Hg, and a calculated HCO_3^- of 11 meq/L. Serum electrolyte analysis reveals a Na^+ of 137, a Cl^- of 104, and an HCO_3^- of 12. Analysis of his arterial blood gas indicates that he is acidemic (pH 7.15) with a normal $PaCO_2$ (there is no respiratory compensation from his current ventilator settings). The bicarbonate is less than 22 meq/L, indicating a metabolic acidosis. His anion gap is: $137-(104 + 12) = 21$ meq/L, indicating a gap metabolic acidosis. His acidosis is likely multifactorial, but a major cause is his renal failure. Other possibilities include a lactic acidosis, inadequate nutrition, or poorly controlled diabetes. His systemic bicarbonate can be replaced by giving enteral sodium citrate-citric acid; however, his cardiac instability indicates the need for more aggressive intervention. Intravenous $NaHCO_3$ can be used to improve his acidosis. His base deficit is calculated as $(70)(0.4) \times (15 - 12) = 84$ meq/L. A standard ampule of sodium bicarbonate contains 44 meq/L, therefore, two ampules of bicarbonate should be given. Further therapy will be dictated by noted clinical and serologic changes

---

METABOLIC ALKALOSIS

A metabolic alkalosis is a pH greater than 7.45 with an elevated HCO_3^- (> 26 meq/L). The elevation in pH causes a compensatory hypoventilation and secondary hypercarbia resulting in an improved pH. The $PaCO_2$ should increase 5–7 mm Hg for each 10 meq/L increase in HCO_3^-. Greater increases in $PaCO_2$ indicate a respiratory acidosis, and $PaCO_2$ levels below that expected indicate a respiratory alkalosis. At HCO_3^- levels greater than 26 meq/L, the kidney does not resorb bicarbonate unless stimulated to do

so by another abnormality, such as hypochloremia, hypokalemia, or mineralocorticoid excess.

The causes of metabolic alkalosis are categorized into those that are chloride-responsive and those that are chloride-unresponsive (Table 19–3). Those that are chloride-responsive can be resuscitated and corrected with normal saline. The determination of the type of alkalosis is made by history, physical examination, serum electrolytes, and urinary Cl^-. Chloride-responsive patients have a urinary Cl^- of less than 10 meq/L and have signs of volume depletion. Chloride-unresponsive patients have a urinary Cl^- greater than 10 meq/L and are either euvolemic or have volume excess. Chloride-responsive patients may have symptoms associated with hypovolemia. Other symptoms are usually attributable to the associated electrolyte abnormalities, such as hypophosphatemia, hypokalemia, or hypocalcemia.

Therapy is dependent upon the type of alkalosis. Chloride-responsive patients are resuscitated with saline, and serum electrolyte abnormalities are corrected. These patients are often very hypokalemic and require aggressive replacement therapy. Chloride-unresponsive patients need to have the source of excess mineralocorticoid removed. If that is not possible, then the action should be blocked with amiloride or spironolactone. Electrolyte abnormalities are aggressively corrected. In severe alkalosis, acetazolamide 250–500 mg IV is given per day. This drug causes renal bicarbonate wasting. It should be given only for a limited number of doses, as it can result in acidosis if used too vigorously. Life-threatening metabolic alkalosis (pH > 7.6 with an HCO_3^- of > 40) can be treated with 0.1N HCl intravenously. It is given based on the chloride deficit. The chloride deficit is calculated as:

$$0.2\ \text{L/kg} \times \text{weight} \times 103\ \text{meq/L (normal } Cl^-) - \text{measured } Cl^-$$

Replacement is begun at approximately 2 meq/kg/h. Serum electrolytes and ABGs are checked frequently, and further therapy is predicated on the correction that occurs.

Table 19–3. Causes of metabolic alkalosis.

Saline-Responsive	Saline-Unresponsive
Gastric drainage	Bartter's syndrome
Diuretics	Magnesium deficit
Post-hypercapnea	Potassium deficit (severe)
Bicarbonate therapy	
	Excess mineralocorticoid
Organic salt metabolites	Cushing's syndrome
Lactate	Hyperaldosteronism
Citrate (blood)	ACTH-secreting tumors
Acetate	Licorice
	Renal artery stenosis
Milk-alkali syndrome	Steroids (exogenous)
Congenital chloridorrhea	
Vomiting	

ACTH = adrenocorticotropic hormone.

> **Clinical Scenario.** A patient has been vomiting for 3 days prior to coming to the emergency room. He has been unable to keep down any food or liquids. He now complains of nausea, dizziness, dry mouth, and weakness. When asked, he says he last urinated a small amount 12 hours ago. An arterial blood gas reveals a pH of 7.50 with a PCO_2 of 48 mm Hg and a bicarbonate of 36 meq/L. The urinary chloride is 5 meq/L. The patient is alkalemic, and the elevated HCO_3 indicates a metabolic alkalosis. The $PaCO_2$ is elevated because of a compensatory response, and the compensation is as expected (40 + 7 = 47). The low urinary chloride indicates that this is a saline-response alkalosis that is compatible with the patient's history and presentation. The examination is consistent with volume depletion. The treatment is saline resuscitation, antiemetics, and electrolyte replacement.

RESPIRATORY ACIDOSIS

A respiratory acidosis is defined as a low pH combined with an elevated $PaCO_2$. It is caused by decreased alveolar ventilation due to either pulmonary or central nervous system disease (Table 19–4). Respiratory acidosis can be acute or chronic, as determined by the amount of renal compensation that has occurred (increased HCO_3^- retention).

Table 19–4. Causes of respiratory acidosis.

Acute	Chronic
Capillary gas exchange defect	**Capillary gas exchange defect**
Acute respiratory distress syndrome	Chronic obstructive pulmonary disease
Cardiogenic pulmonary edema	Cystic fibrosis
Asthma	
Pneumonia	**Respiratory muscle dysfunction**
Pneumothorax	Polio
Hemothorax	Multiple sclerosis
	Hypothyroid myxedema
Respiratory muscle dysfunction	Acute myelogenous leukemia
Myasthenia gravis	Obesity (severe)
Quadriplegia	Scoliosis
Hypokalemia	
Hypophosphatemia	**Medullary inhibition**
Antibiotics	Obesity (severe)
Prolonged chemical paralysis	Central nervous system tumor
Medullary inhibition	
Sleep apnea	
Cardiac arrest	
Drugs (alcohol, narcotics, sedatives)	
Upper airway obstruction	
Foreign body	
Laryngospasm	
Trauma	
Edema	
Obstructive sleep apnea	

Acute compensation is by buffering with HCO_3^-. For each 10 mm Hg rise in $PaCO_2$, the HCO_3^- will increase by 1 meq/L (the HCO_3^- will rarely increase above 30 meq/L as a compensatory response). As the kidney adapts, the serum HCO_3^- can increase 3–4 meq/L for each 10-mm rise in $PaCO_2$. The compensation never returns the pH to normal or overcorrects. If this occurs, a mixed disorder is present.

The pulmonary causes of decreased alveolar ventilation are usually due to airway obstruction, gas exchange abnormalities across the capillary membrane, or respiratory muscle dysfunction. Neurologic dysfunction is at the level of the medulla. The respiratory center is inhibited by many drugs, cardiac arrest, sleep apnea, obesity, and CNS tumors. In acute respiratory acidosis, patients usually appear uncomfortable with marked respiratory effort. As the $PaCO_2$ rises they become confused, disoriented, and then comatose. Chronic respiratory acidosis is often surprisingly well tolerated.

Treatment for both types of respiratory acidosis is the same—improved alveolar ventilation. However, in acute respiratory acidosis the goal is to return the $PaCO_2$ to normal. Chronic respiratory acidosis is often due to structural abnormalities that are not correctable, thus, the goal should be to achieve a steady state of compensated respiratory acidosis. Ventilation is improved with a variety of mechanisms, including improved pulmonary toilet, noninvasive ventilation, or endotracheal intubation. Bicarbonate therapy is contraindicated in patients with a respiratory acidosis, as it increases the CO_2 load that must be excreted by an already overtaxed ventilatory system.

> **Clinical Scenario.** A 28-year-old surgery resident is eating with colleagues in the cafeteria when he laughs suddenly and aspirates a piece of steak, causing an upper airway obstruction. He struggles to breathe and eventually loses consciousness. Heimlich maneuvers are unsuccessful in ejecting the foreign body. An emergency code is called. When the code cart arrives, the foreign body is located and removed under direct vision, and the resident is intubated. An arterial blood gas drawn at the time of intubation reveals a pH of 7.10, a $PaCO_2$ of 80 mm Hg, and a calculated HCO_3^- of 24 meq/L. His pH indicates that he is acidemic with an elevated $PaCO_2$ and a normal HCO_3^-; therefore, he has a pure respiratory acidosis. He is mechanically ventilated until his pH is normal and he is awake and responsive. He is then extubated without further sequelae.

Clinical Scenario. An elderly gentleman with a long history of chronic obstructive pulmonary disease presents to the surgery clinic for repair of a hernia. As part of his perioperative workup he has an arterial blood gas drawn. His pH is 7.32 with a $PaCO_2$ of 65 mm Hg and a calculated bicarbonate of 33 meq/L. Should you cancel his case and treat his acidosis? By analysis he is acidemic and his $PaCO_2$ is also elevated, suggesting a respiratory acidosis. He has documented pulmonary disease, which can affect his ventilatory capability. His calculated bicarbonate is 33 meq/L, suggesting a metabolic compensation. The expected compensation is 3 meq/L for every 10 mm Hg increase in the $PaCO_2$ above 40 mm Hg. The expected compensation is $2.5 \times 3.0 = 7.5$ meq/L; $7.5 + 26$ meq/L (normal $HCO_3^- = 33.5$ meq/L. He has a well-compensated chronic respiratory acidosis, and his surgery should proceed.

Table 19–5. Causes of respiratory alkalosis.

Acute	Chronic
Acute hypoxemia	Sepsis
Pneumonia	Cirrhosis
Atelectasis	Prolonged mechanical hyper-
Pulmonary embolism	ventilation
Pneumothorax	
	Prolonged hypoxemia
Drugs	Altitude
Salicylates	Congenital heart disease
Catecholamines	Anemia
Theophylline	
Progesterones	**Central Nervous System**
	Tumor
Central nervous system	Abscess
Tumor	Cerebrovascular accident
Abscess	Trauma
Cerebrovascular accident	
Trauma	
Pregnancy	
Hepatic encephalopathy	
Sepsis	
Hyperventilation syndrome	
Overzealous mechanical ventilation	

RESPIRATORY ALKALOSIS

Respiratory alkalosis is caused by alveolar hyperventilation resulting in a primary decrease in $PaCO_2$ below normal values. This can be caused by one of several processes, such as increased hyperventilation secondary to hypoxemia, a decreased cerebrospinal fluid pH stimulating the receptors in the medulla, and other stimuli, like pulmonary disease (Table 19–5). Respiratory alkalosis can also be acute or chronic, and the magnitude of compensation depends upon the chronicity of the derangement.

Acutely, the HCO_3^- will fall 1–2 meq/L for every 10 mm Hg decrease in $PaCO_2$. The bicarbonate will rarely fall below 18 meq/L when it is dropping as a compensatory response. If HCO_3^- is lower than this in the face of a respiratory alkalosis, there is a concomitant metabolic acidosis. Chronic renal compensation decreases the excre-

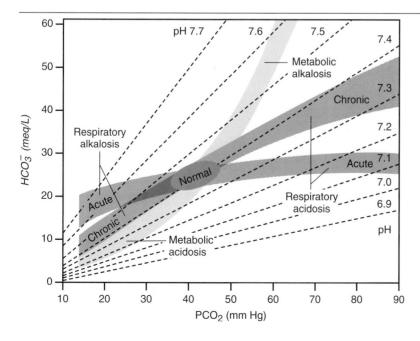

Figure 19–5. Nomogram for mixed acid-base disorders. (Reprinted and modified, with permission, from Graber M: Kidney Kard. Division of Nephrology, SUNY at Stony Brook, and the VA Medical Center, Northport, NY, 1990.)

tion of free hydrogen ion. Serum HCO_3^- can then decrease 4–5 meq/L for every 10 mm Hg drop in $PaCO_2$. If the HCO_3^- is greater than expected (ie, less compensated), then a metabolic alkalosis must also be present. If the HCO_3^- is lower than anticipated, a metabolic acidosis is present.

Alkalosis is relatively asymptomatic. However, in severe cases confusion, agitation, dizziness, cramps, circumoral numbness, and acral paresthesias may be noted. Treatment is aimed at the underlying cause rather than the alkalosis. The most common cause of perioperative respiratory alkalosis is inappropriate ventilator settings. These need to be corrected immediately by adjusting the ventilator (usually a decrease in the minute ventilation is all that is required).

Patients with hyperventilation syndrome due to anxiety also need treatment. The simplest therapeutic maneuver is to have the anxious person breathe into a paper bag. The inhalation of the previously excreted CO_2 is usually enough to raise the $PaCO_2$ and normalize the pH. For severe anxiety, anxiolytics may be needed for sustained control.

Clinical Scenario. A third-year medical student is starting her first surgical clinical rotation. She is to present a complex patient to the chairwoman of the department during rounds. Ten minutes before rounds begin, the student starts to hyperventilate and complain of shortness of breath, numb lips, and dizziness. The team obtains an arterial blood gas, which reveals a pH of 7.50, a $PaCO_2$ of 25 mm Hg, and a calculated HCO_3^- of 24 meq/L. The pH indicates that she is alkalemic and the low $PaCO_2$ indicates a respiratory cause. The bicarbonate is normal (uncompensated), therefore, this is identified as an acute process. The student sits down and breathes into paper bag for 5 minutes until she relaxes and her breathing slows. When rounds begin, the case presentation goes well.

MIXED ACID-BASE DISORDERS

Many patients have mixed acid-base disorders. These patients are identified when the expected compensatory mechanisms to normalize pH are not seen with a primary disorder. This is depicted graphically in Figure 19–5, where the arterial pH, $PaCO_2$, and HCO_3^- intersect outside of the 95% confidence limits of the primary acid-base disorder. The best way to analyze the information available is to look at the pH to decide if the patient is alkalemic or acidemic. The $PaCO_2$ is then inspected and an anion gap calculated. It is important to know the expected amount of compensation for a given primary abnormality. If the compensation deviates from expected, then a second abnormality is identified.

Clinical Scenario. A 68-year-old woman with severe chronic obstructive pulmonary disease (COPD) is in a motor vehicle accident and sustains multiple injuries, including a scalp laceration, a closed head injury, and a femur fracture. Her blood pressure, due to blood loss (scalp and femur laceration), is 75/50. On examination, she is cool and clammy with shallow respirations. An arterial blood gas reveals a pH of 7.10, a $PaCO_2$ of 70, and a HCO_3^- of 21 meq/L. Examination of the pH reveals that she is acidemic. The elevated $PaCO_2$ could be normal if she has compensated respiratory acidosis due to her COPD; however, this is not consistent with her clinical status and HCO_3^-. The expected HCO_3^- for a compensated patient (4 meq/L for each 10 mm Hg > 40), would be $26 + (3 \times 4) = 38$ meq/L. The actual HCO_3^- us 21 meq/L, leaving a deficit of 17 meq/L between expected and calculated HCO_3^-. Thus, she has a mixed acute metabolic acidosis with a chronic respiratory acidosis. Therapy is directed towards correcting the metabolic acidosis (volume resuscitation, warming, possible mechanical ventilation, possible transfusion) without overcorrecting her chronic respiratory acidosis.

SUGGESTED READING

Civetta J et al: *Critical Care*. Lippincott, 1988.

Guyton A, Hall J: *Guyton's Textbook of Medical Physiology*, 9th ed. Saunders, 1994.

Haber R: A practical approach to acid-base disorders. West J Med 1991:155;146.

Lyerly HK, Gaynor JW: *The Handbook of Surgical Intensive Care*. Mosby-Year Book, 1992.

Sivak E et al: *The High Risk Patient: Management of the Critically Ill*. Williams & Wilkins, 1995.

Nutritional Support

Michael D. Lieberman, MD, & John M. Daly, MD, FACS

▶ Key Facts

- ▶ A comprehensive nutritional assessment is the first step in effective nutritional support.

- ▶ The history, physical examination, and clinical evaluation should be used to identify high-risk patients who require a more detailed nutritional assessment.

- ▶ Current body weight < 90% of "usual" body weight is a marker of significant nutritional depletion. However, the absence of weight loss does not rule out the need for clinically relevant nutrition.

- ▶ Body weight changes must be evaluated in the context of alterations in body composition (ie, serial monthly measurements of skinfold thickness

and circulating protein stores to determine body fat and lean body mass).

- ▶ The final step in nutritional assessment is the evaluation of the demands on the patient: the rate of overall metabolism or energy expenditure and caloric balance, and the rate of protein catabolism and protein balance.

- ▶ Nutrient needs in the critically ill patient are defined by indirect calorimetry and nitrogen balance studies.

- ▶ In nutritionally depleted patients, daily weights, weekly determination of nitrogen balance and serum visceral proteins, and monthly measurements of anthropometrics are recommended.

Nutritional assessment is the comprehensive objective evaluation of nutritional status. The clinical need for nutritional assessment with subsequent appropriate nutritional intervention is justified by the high prevalence of nutritional deficits in hospitalized patients. "Malnutrition" has been identified in 15–50% of hospitalized patients, depending upon the patient's disease and the hospital population. More importantly, substantial nutritional depletion has an adverse affect on morbidity and mortality. For example, severely malnourished cancer patients undergoing surgery have a higher incidence of complications and mortality than well-nourished patients with the same disease and therapy. Recognition of the importance

of nutritional status has defined the need for objective, reliable, clinically relevant methods of nutritional assessment.

Nutritional assessment is the first step in effective nutritional support, which should not be undertaken without this proper diagnostic effort. Nutritional assessment quantitates clinically relevant malnutrition and is necessary to decide whether to initiate nutritional intervention. This chapter will review the nutritional parameters often used in assessment and define which are clinically relevant.

The ability to recognize and quantify clinically relevant malnutrition requires the rational collation of a variety of objective nutritional measures in an individual patient.

High-risk patients can be recognized by screening factors in the history and physical examination and by clinical circumstances.

SCREENING FACTORS

PATIENT HISTORY

The patient history (Table 20–1) should survey the following areas:

1. Past nutrient intake
2. Weight loss: etiology and rate
3. Gastrointestinal disorders, such as chronic diarrhea, gastrointestinal fistula, inflammatory bowel disease, pancreatitis, peptic ulcer disease, short gut syndrome, nausea and vomiting
4. Critical organ failure (pulmonary, cardiac, hepatic, renal)
5. Malignancy
6. Alcoholism, diabetes mellitus, and neurologic and psychological disorders
7. Treatment plans, including chemotherapy, immunotherapy, radiotherapy, and surgery

PHYSICAL EXAMINATION

The physical examination must be complete in order to uncover the signs of micronutrient (vitamins and trace elements) and macronutrient (calories and protein) deficiencies (Table 20–2). In general, micronutrient and macronutrient deficiencies coexist in malnutrition. Furthermore, a deficiency in one nutrient typically affects multiple organ systems phenotypically. For example, a patient with a thiamine deficiency (beriberi) will present with physical signs of encephalopathy, peripheral neuropathy, muscle atrophy, and congestive heart failure. A patient with severe protein-calorie nutritional depletion will present with signs of fat loss, muscle wasting and weakness, edema, glossitis, neuropathy, and skin rashes. Physical signs are usually not pathognomonic, but common to multiple nutrient deficiencies and non-nutrient etiologies. For instance, peripheral neuropathy is a common physical finding with niacin, thiamine, vitamin B_6, and vitamin B_{12} deficiencies.

FUTURE CLINICAL COURSE

A knowledge of the natural history of the patient's primary disease is indispensable in predicting its catabolic effects. For instance, patients with major trauma, burns,

Table 20–1. Disease states and historical features associated with micronutrient deficiencies.

Disease State/Historical Features	Associated Nutrient Deficiency
Gastrointestinal disorders	
Pancreatic insufficiency	Vitamins A, D, E, K
Gastrectomy	Vitamins A, D, E, B_{12}, folic acid, iron, calcium
Liver disease, alcoholism	Vitamins A, D, C, riboflavin, niacin, thiamine, folic acid, magnesium, zinc
Short bowel syndrome, ileal resection	Vitamin B_{12}, folic acid, calcium, magnesium
Blind loop syndrome	Vitamin B_{12}
Sprue, gluten enteropathy	Vitamin A, folic acid
Bile salt depletion, cholestyramine ingestion	Vitamins, A, K
Obstructive jaundice	Vitamins A, K
Prolonged antacid therapy, peptic ulcer disease	Vitamin C, thiamine
Endocrine disorders	
Thyrotoxicosis	Vitamins A, B_6, B_{12}, C, thiamine, folic acid
Diabetes mellitus	Magnesium, chromium
Cardiorespiratory disorders	
Chronic obstructive pulmonary disease	Vitamin A
Congestive heart failure	Vitamins A, C, thiamine
Cystic fibrosis	Vitamin A
Hematopoietic disorders	
Sickle cell anemia	Folic acid
Leukemia	Folic acid
Renal disorders	
Chronic renal failure	Magnesium, calcium, vitamin D[1]
Miscellaneous disorders	
Prolonged antibiotic therapy	Vitamin K
Fever	Vitamins A, C, thiamine, riboflavin, folic acid

[1]Inability of renal tissue to synthesize the metabolically active form of vitamin D.

Table 20–2. Physical and laboratory findings associated with micronutrient deficiencies.

Abnormal Physical or Laboratory Finding	Associated Nutrient Deficiency
Mucocutaneous/hair	
Angular stomatitis; cheilosis; magenta tongue	Riboflavin
Glossitis; pellagrous dermatitis; atrophic papillae	Niacin
Xerosis; follicular hyperkeratosis	Linoleic acid
Acneiform forehead rash; nasolabial seborrhea; stomatitis	Vitamin B_6
Conjunctival & corneal xerosis; follicular hyperkeratosis; Bitot's spots; kerotomalacia	Vitamin A
Petechiae; ecchymoses; swollen, hemorrhagic gums; prominent hair follicles; corkscrew hair	Vitamin C
Petechiae; ecchymoses	Vitamin K
Parakeratosis; alopecia	Zinc
Dystrophic nails (koilonychia); pale conjunctiva	Iron
Neurologic	
Peripheral neuropathy; Wernicke's encephalopathy	Thiamin
Peripheral neuropathy; convulsive seizures; depression	Vitamin B_6
"Burning feet" syndrome	Pantothenic acid
Peripheral paresthesias; spinal cord symptoms	Vitamin B_{12}
Peripheral neuropathy; myelopathy; encephalopathy (pellegra)	Niacin
"Night blindness"	Vitamin A
Hematologic	
Hemolytic anemia	Vitamin E
Macrocytic anemia	Vitamin B_{12}, folic acid
Microcytic; hypochromic anemia	Iron, copper
Microcytic anemia	Vitamin B_6
Coagulopathy	Vitamin K
Sideroblastic anemia; neutropenia (infants)	Copper
Thrombocytopenia	Linoleic acid
Musculoskeletal	
Osteomalacia; tetany; rickets	Vitamin D
Tender, atrophic muscles	Thiamin
Joint pain; muscle weakness	Vitamin C
Osteopenia (infants)	Copper
Visceral disorders	
Cardiac: congestive heart failure	Thiamin
Gastrointestinal: diarrhea	Folic acid, zinc, niacin
Goiter	Iodine
Hypogonadism; hepatosplenomegaly	Zinc
Other	
Anorexia; hypogeusia	Zinc

and septicemia have dramatically increased nutrient demands. Patients with malignancy frequently have altered nutrient requirements on the basis of unique changes in host intermediary metabolism. A thorough understanding of the primary disease process enables the physician to prognosticate and to determine if nutritional intervention will currently or ultimately benefit the patient. Nutritional care must be an adjunct to and supportive of the primary treatment plan.

DETAILED NUTRITIONAL ASSESSMENT

The history and physical examination of the patient combined with the physician's clinical judgement should serve as a screening mechanism to identify high-risk patients who require more detailed assessment.

ANTHROPOMETRIC MEASURES & BODY COMPOSITION

Current body weight is compared to ideal body weight and to usual body weight. Ideal body weight has been determined by population studies that control for height and gender and are based on the weight range with the lowest mortality, the ultimate outcome criteria (Table 20–3). **"Usual" body weight** is the patient's pre-morbid body weight. The patient's estimate of "usual" body weight is generally reliable and may be confirmed by medical records. Current body weight less than 90% of "usual"

Table 20–3. Ideal weight for height.

Males						Females					
Height (cm)	Weight (kg)	Height (cm)	Weight (kg)	Height (cm)	Weight (kg)	Height (cm)	Weight (kg)	Height (cm)	Weight (kg)	Height (cm)	Weight (kg)
145	51.9	159	59.9	173	69.7	140	44.9	150	50.4	160	56.2
146	52.4	160	60.5	174	69.4	141	45.4	151	51.0	161	56.9
147	52.9	161	61.1	175	70.1	142	45.9	152	51.5	162	57.6
148	53.5	162	61.7	176	70.8	143	46.4	153	52.0	163	58.3
149	54.0	163	62.3	177	71.6	144	47.0	154	52.5	164	58.9
150	54.5	164	62.9	178	72.4	145	47.5	155	53.1	165	59.5
151	55.0	165	63.5	179	73.3	146	48.0	156	53.7	166	60.1
152	55.6	166	64.0	180	74.2	147	48.6	157	54.3	167	60.7
153	56.1	167	64.6	181	75.0	148	49.2	158	54.9	168	61.4
154	56.6	168	65.2	182	75.8	149	49.8	159	55.5	169	62.1
155	57.2	169	65.9	183	76.5						
156	57.9	170	66.6	184	77.3						
157	58.6	171	67.3	185	78.1						
158	59.3	172	68.0	186	78.9						

body weight or ideal body weight is a marker of significant nutritional depletion.

Body weight changes must be evaluated in the context of alterations in body composition. Body composition is broadly divided into two compartments, fat mass and lean body mass. Fat mass normally represents approximately 25–35% of total body weight and serves as the primary energy source during prolonged, adapted starvation. It rarely is dangerously depleted and is less important than lean body mass. Normal-weight individuals carry a 60-day supply; obese patients carry even more. Determination of the magnitude of fat stores may permit one to estimate the duration and severity of caloric intake deficits and provides a measure of a patient's current caloric reserve. Lean body mass represents the critical cellular mass necessary for cellular structure as well as function. Lean body mass is subdivided into the extracellular mass and a cellular component, the body cell mass. The lean body cell mass comprises 40% of the body weight of a normal adult and is composed of skeletal muscle (60%), red blood cells and connective tissue (20%), and visceral cell mass (20%). Depletion of lean body cell mass as opposed to fat mass is a much more severe insult defining patient morbidity and mortality.

Anthropometric measurements are utilized for clinical determination of total body fat and skeletal muscle store. This simple, inexpensive, noninvasive technique utilizes calipers to measure skinfold thickness over one or more anatomic sites (triceps, biceps, subscapular, abdominal, suprailiac, medial calf, and anterior thigh). Triceps skinfold thickness should be measured and compared to percentile standards (Table 20–4). Measurements below the 35th to 40th percentile imply mild depletion, those below the 25th to 35th percentile indicate moderate depletion, and measurements below the 25th percentile denote severe depletion.

This method represents a reasonable estimate of adipose caloric reserves, since 50% of total body fat is located subcutaneously and adipose tissue losses from subcutaneous and central depots during caloric deprivation occur proportionally, as determined by the research techniques of isotope dilution and inert gas uptake. Estimation of total body fat stores from such skinfold measurements is subject to inaccuracies due to age, race, gender, and habitus-specific variability in topographic distribution and interobservor errors. Only serial monthly measurement of skinfold thickness is useful for determining semi-quantitative changes in adipose stores.

Lean body mass is assessed clinically by determining skeletal muscle stores and circulating protein stores. Sixty percent of total body protein is contained in skeletal muscle; this is the major site of protein catabolism during illness and/or starvation. Measurement of skeletal muscle mass provides an approximation of the major protein reserve. The most widely used anthropometric measures of skeletal muscle protein are the midarm muscle circumference (MAMC) and the midarm muscle area (MAMA). Both measures are derived from mid-upper arm circumference (MAC) and triceps skinfold (TSF):

$$\text{MAMC (cm)} = \text{MAC (cm)} - \text{TSF (mm)} \frac{\pi}{10}$$

$$\text{MAMA (cm}^2) = (\text{MAMC})^2 / 4\pi$$

These measurements are compared to reference standards (Table 20–5) with the same qualitative percentile guidelines for determination of severity of depletion as previously described for adipose reserves. This technique gives only a crude estimate of skeletal muscle protein, since several inaccurate anatomic assumptions are made in these equations.

The excretion of creatinine and 3-methyl histidine estimates the size of the skeletal muscle mass, assuming a steady state without imbalance between synthesis and catabolism. The most widely used biochemical marker of muscle mass is the 24-hour urinary creatinine excretion. Creatinine is a degradation product of creatine, an energy storage compound located in skeletal muscle. Creatinine

Table 20–4. Reference standards for sum of triceps and subscapular skinfolds.[1,2]

Age Group (Yrs)	Percentile						
	5	10	25	50	75	90	95
American Men							
18–74	11.5	13.5	19.0	26.0	34.5	44.0	51.0
18–24	10.0	12.0	15.0	21.0	30.0	41.0	51.0
25–34	11.5	13.5	19.0	26.0	35.5	45.0	54.0
35–44	12.0	15.0	21.0	28.0	36.0	44.0	48.5
45–54	13.0	15.0	21.0	28.0	37.0	46.0	53.0
55–64	12.0	14.0	20.0	26.0	34.0	44.0	48.0
65–74	11.5	14.0	19.5	26.0	34.0	42.5	49.0
American Women							
18–74	18.5	22.0	28.5	39.0	53.0	65.0	73.0
18–24	17.0	19.0	24.0	31.0	41.5	54.5	64.0
25–34	18.5	20.5	26.5	35.0	48.0	64.0	73.0
35–44	20.0	23.0	30.0	40.5	55.0	68.0	75.0
45–54	22.0	25.0	33.5	45.0	58.0	69.5	78.5
55–64	19.0	25.0	33.0	46.0	58.0	68.0	73.0
65–74	20.0	25.0	32.0	41.0	52.2	63.0	70.0

[1]Developed from data collected during the Health and Nutrition Examination Survey of 1971–1974.
[2]Values are in millimeters.

cannot be reutilized, and its excretion in urine is proportional to muscle creatine content if renal function is stable. The measured 24-hour urinary creatinine excretion is compared to expected creatinine excretion controlled for age, gender, and height to obtain the creatinine-height index (CHI), with 100% being normal. A CHI less than 80% of predicted defines skeletal muscle depletion. This technique requires normal renal function and patient abstinence from meat-containing diets during the test period. Similar to creatinine, 3-methyl histidine (3-MH) is found predominately in skeletal muscle. 3-MH is released with muscle degradation, is metabolically inert, and is excreted in the urine. The rate of 3-MH excretion is more a measure of skeletal muscle breakdown rate rather than the size of the skeletal muscle mass.

Visceral protein mass is estimated by determination of serum proteins synthesized by the liver. Serum levels are dependent upon the availability of adequate nutrient precursors, synthetic rates, catabolic rates, and distribution forces. A decline in precursor intake will rapidly decrease hepatic synthetic rates of the serum protein, and the rate of normal catabolism varies with the specific protein. Various diseases affect both synthetic and catabolic rates. It is currently recommended to measure serum albumin, transferrin, and prealbumin weekly (Table 20–6).

Albumin is a 65-kilodalton (kd) protein produced by the liver and has a serum half-life of 18–20 days. Albumin maintains plasma oncotic pressure and is a carrier protein for enzymes, drugs, hormones, and trace elements. Chronic protein intake insufficiency (kwash-

Table 20–5. Reference standards for midarm muscle circumference.[1,2]

Age Group (Yrs)	Percentile						
	5	10	25	50	75	90	95
American Men							
18–74	26.4	27.6	29.6	31.7	33.9	36.0	37.3
18–24	25.7	27.1	28.7	30.7	32.9	35.5	37.4
25–34	27.0	28.2	30.0	32.0	34.4	36.5	37.6
35–44	27.8	28.7	30.7	32.7	34.8	36.3	37.1
45–54	26.7	27.8	30.0	32.0	34.2	36.2	37.6
55–64	25.6	27.3	29.6	31.7	33.4	35.2	36.6
65–74	25.3	26.5	28.5	30.7	32.4	34.4	35.5
American Women							
18–74	23.2	24.3	26.2	28.7	31.9	35.2	37.8
18–24	22.1	23.0	24.5	26.4	28.8	31.7	34.4
25–34	23.3	24.2	25.7	27.8	30.4	34.1	37.2
35–44	24.1	25.2	26.8	29.2	32.2	36.2	38.5
45–54	24.3	25.7	27.5	30.3	32.9	36.8	39.3
55–64	23.9	25.1	27.7	30.2	33.3	36.3	38.2
65–74	23.8	25.2	27.4	29.9	32.5	35.3	37.2

[1]Developed from data collected during the Health and Nutrition Examination Survey of 1971–1974.
[2]Values are in centimeters.

Table **20–6.** Serum proteins.

Protein	Function	Serum Half-Life (Days)	Normal Range	Limitations
Albumin	Carrier protein for hormones, drugs, and enzymes. Plasma oncotic pressure	18–20	> 3.5 g/dL	Long half-life
Transferrin	Iron carrier protein	8–9	200–260 mg/dL	Fluctuates with Fe stores
Prealbumin	Thyroxine carrier protein	2–3	15–25 mg/dL	Sensitive to acute changes in nutrient intake

iorkor), in contrast to chronic caloric intake insufficiency (marasmus), is characterized by hypoalbuminemia. Serum albumin concentrations greater than 3.5 g/dL are normal, levels of 3.0–3.5 g/dL indicate mild depletion, concentrations of 2.5–2.9 g/dL point to moderate depletion, and levels of less than 2.5 g/dL indicate severe depletion.

Transferrin is a 76-kd glycoprotein synthesized by the liver and has a serum half-life of 8 days. Transferrin serves as a carrier protein for iron. The normal transferrin level is greater than 22 mg/dL, and a concentration less than 180 mg/dL is considered metabolically significant. Prealbumin, a serum protein with a half-life of 2–3 days, is also produced by the liver and functions as a transport protein for thyroxine and retinol-binding protein. The normal range for prealbumin level is 15–25 mg/dL; a concentration less than 12 mg/dL indicates clinically significant nutritional depletion. The sensitivity of prealbumin to acute changes in nutrient intake requires the simultaneous measurement of serum proteins with longer half-lives for a more balanced assessment.

Some clinical nutritionists utilize immune response as a gross functional marker of nutritional status. Many studies have associated malnutrition with host predisposition to infection and sepsis. Defects in cellular, humoral, and nonspecific immunity have been identified in patients with protein-calorie malnutrition as well as in patients with certain micronutrient deficiencies, such as deficiencies in zinc, iron, copper and selenium.

Generally, cell-mediated immunity is affected earlier and to a greater extent than the other components of the immune system. Some clinicians measure total lymphocyte count and delayed hypersensitivity (DH) as initial assays of lymphocyte function. Lymphopenia, when not attributable to confounding etiologies, suggests clinically relevant malnutrition. The DH assay measures the patient's ability to respond to an intradermal challenge with one or more antigens to which the host has been previously sensitized (eg, tuberculin, trichophytid, mumps, and streptodornase). Anergy (absence of skin reactivity) suggests clinically significant malnutrition if other factors are not contributors to anergy, including immunosuppressive drugs, age, and concurrent diseases, such as infection, renal or hepatic failure, and cancer. Such widespread and diverse confounding factors have pushed

immunologic evaluation out of routine nutritional assessment.

METABOLISM & CATABOLISM

The final step in nutritional assessment is the evaluation of the demands on the patient: the rate of overall metabolism or energy expenditure and caloric balance, and the rate of protein catabolism and protein balance.

CALORIC BALANCE

Resting energy expenditure (REE) may be estimated with questionable validity from a patient's height, weight, age, and gender, utilizing the Harris-Benedict equation:

Male: REE (kcal) = 66 + 13.7 × weight (kg) + 5 × height (cm) − 6.8 × age (y)

Female: REE (kcal) = 655 + 9.6 × weight (kg) + 1.7 × height (cm) − 4.7 × age (y)

The Harris-Benedict predictions of REE are accurate for healthy individuals, as they assume a normal body composition. However, the Harris-Benedict prediction will not adequately reflect actual REE for many patients, such as those with burns, endocrine disorders, fever, neoplasia, sepsis, and trauma who do not have normal body composition or metabolism. In these patients, a more accurate assessment of metabolic rate is required and provided by bedside indirect calorimetry. A widely available portable indirect calorimeter is used to measure oxygen consumption ($\dot{V}O_2$) and carbon dioxide production ($\dot{V}CO_2$) in liters per minute. The modified Weir formula is used to calculate REE:

REE (kcal/day) = 1440 (3.9 × $\dot{V}CO_2$) + 1.1 × $\dot{V}CO_2$)

The measured REE can be normalized as a percent of predicted based on the Harris-Benedict equation. A measured REE between 90 and 110% of predicted is normometabolic, less than 90% hypometabolic, and greater than 110% hypermetabolic.

The patient's caloric requirement is dependent upon energy expenditure and the size of fat stores. When caloric intake is less than total energy expenditure, a loss of total body fat occurs. Conversely, when caloric intake is greater than total energy expenditure, accumulation of total body fat results. The typical hospitalized patient requiring nutritional intervention has a total daily energy expenditure (TEE) that is 130% of the measured REE. The clinician, by measuring caloric fat stores, determines whether the patient requires caloric fat store repletion, depletion, or maintenance. As a general guideline, patients requiring caloric fat store repletion receive calories greater than TEE; for caloric fat store maintenance, calories are equal to TEE; and for caloric fat store depletion, calories are less than TEE.

PROTEIN BALANCE

In addition to static measurements of skeletal and visceral protein, determination of protein turnover and catabolism is critical. The most commonly employed measure of protein turnover is nitrogen balance. Nitrogen balance equals nitrogen intake minus nitrogen losses. A positive value indicates that the patient is in a net state of anabolism (anabolism greater than catabolism), and a negative value indicates that the patient is in a net state of catabolism (catabolism less than anabolism).

Whole body nitrogen balance is the sum of compartmental nitrogen balances, which may individually demonstrate disparate results when compared to overall nitrogen balance. For instance, net positive visceral protein nitrogen balance may occur at the same time net negative skeletal muscle nitrogen balance is occurring. The whole body nitrogen balance may be either positive or negative.

Measurement of nitrogen balance is relatively simple when medical records and laboratory specimens receive proper attention. Nitrogen intake is easily measured and includes both enteral and parenteral nutrients. Calculation of nitrogen output requires determination of nitrogen losses from the urine, gastrointestinal tract, and skin. Renal excretion of nitrogen is measured from 24-hour urine urea measurements, and extrarenal losses of nitrogen are estimated at 2–4 g/d.

Utilization of this correction factor for extrarenal nitrogen non-measured losses may result in erroneously low levels in patients with malabsorption, large draining wounds, and gastrointestinal fistulas. Furthermore, patients with progressive renal insufficiency may retain urea, and this amount must be considered as output. An equation is used to make corrections for such incomplete urinary excretion of nitrogen:

$$\text{Adjusted nitrogen (N) balance} = \text{N intake} - \text{urinary N} - \text{change in body urea N}$$

Nitrogen excretion varies from a normal level of 5–8 g/day to low levels of 2–4 g/day after several days of unstressed starvation, to as high as 30–50 g/day in sepsis and trauma. One gram of urinary nitrogen excretion represents a loss of 30 g of lean tissue mass. In stressed patients with urinary N losses of 33 g, 1 kg of lean tissue is being lost daily.

Net protein utilization, the amount of dietary nitrogen retained by the body, is determined by illness severity, level of energy intake, and degree of recent nutritional depletion. Malnutrition, high energy intake, and low stress increase the efficiency of dietary protein retention. Conversely, "normal" nutritional status, low energy intake, and high stress decrease the efficiency of dietary protein retention.

The severity of lean body mass catabolism can be estimated by the measurement of 24-hour urinary urea excretion and calculation of the catabolic index. Total urinary urea excretion equals dietary protein intake not retained as well as endogenous protein catabolism. The catabolic index balances these sources of urinary urea to quantify severity of metabolic stress. The catabolic index equals 24-hour urine urea nitrogen excretion minus (0.5 dietary nitrogen intake + 3 g) where an index of less than zero represents no significant stress; an index of 0–5, moderate stress; and an index greater than 5, severe stress.

SUMMARY

The ability to recognize clinically relevant malnutrition is sometimes easy but often difficult. No single test will define clinically relevant malnutrition that predicts nutritionally based clinical outcomes. It is important to clinically evaluate the patient with respect to the natural history of the disease process, physical examination, and treatment plan to not only assess present nutritional status, but to predict future course of nutritional status. The body weight and composition data are then used to better define current deficits in fat mass and lean body mass as suggested by the clinical examination. Finally, nutrient needs are then defined by indirect calorimetry and nitrogen balance studies.

Serial assessment of nutritional status is critical in evaluating both short-term and long-term nutritional goal achievement. Most parameters do not show consistent change with nutritional intervention of less that 2–3 weeks duration. However, nitrogen balance may be improved after 3 days, and increases in prealbumin may be detected after 4–7 days. Changes in anthropometric measurements or serum albumin levels may not be detected until several weeks after the patient receives adequate nitrogen and caloric intake. Thus, nutritionally depleted patients should receive daily weight measurements, weekly determination of nitrogen balance and serum visceral proteins, and monthly anthropometric measurements.

SUGGESTED READING

Grimble G, Silk D: *Artificial Nutritional Support in Clinical Practice.* Edward Arnold, 1995.

Rombeau L, Rhoads JE: *Atlas of Nutritional Support Techniques.* Little, Brown, 1989.

Roubenoff R, Roubenoff RA: Nutritional issues in acute illness. In Stobo JD et al (editors): *The Principles and Practice of Medicine,* 23rd ed. Appleton & Lange, 1996.

Principles of Surgical Oncology

21

Cancer Biology

Ronald J. Weigel, MD, PhD

▶ Key Facts

▶ At the most fundamental level, neoplasia results from abnormal regulation of the cell cycle.

▶ The normal cell cycle is divided into five phases: G0 (growth arrested), G1 (first growth phase), S (DNA-synthesis), G2 (second growth phase), and M (mitosis).

▶ After mitosis, the daughter cells will normally enter a prolonged G1 or G0 phase. However, in cancer the daughter cells proceed with another cycle of replication.

▶ The process of "programmed cell death" is called apoptosis and involves characteristic cellular changes that result in the physiologic demise of the cell.

▶ Mutations that activate proteins involved in cell growth represent a gain of function and are classified as oncogenes.

▶ Mutations that disrupt proteins that normally suppress growth represent a loss of function and are classified as tumor suppressor genes.

▶ In familial cancers, genetic mutations are inherited which predispose an individual to cancer development.

▶ The identification of inherited cancer genes has relied upon modern techniques of molecular biology called "positional cloning." In positional cloning, the cancer gene is located by a laborious technique of searching through large regions of a chromosome identified through linkage analysis.

▶ Oncogenesis involves the abnormal regulation of the cell cycle, which results in derangements of mechanisms established for quiescence or apoptosis.

The last several decades have witnessed an unprecedented expansion of our understanding of cancer biology. The study of cancer oncogenesis and metastasis is now being addressed at the molecular level with the hope that a better understanding of the molecular details of these cellular events will lead to more effective treatments. This chapter is intended to provide a brief overview of our current understanding of cancer biology.

CELL CYCLE

At the most fundamental level, neoplasia results from abnormal regulation of the cell cycle. In normal cells, mitosis is tightly regulated and most cells have a limited capacity to replicate. All cancer cells have the ability to divide continuously and are not responsive to signals that are designed to induce **quiescence** (growth arrest) or **apoptosis** (programmed cell death).

The normal cell cycle is divided into phases, as shown in Figure 21–1. Terminally differentiated cells normally exist in the G0 (growth arrested) phase of the cell cycle. Certain signals can cause the cell to enter a growth phase (G1), during which the cell synthesizes proteins needed for DNA synthesis. After reaching a critical point, the cells enter S-phase characterized by DNA synthesis. At the completion of S-phase the cell enters a second growth phase (G2) prior to cell mitosis (M). The two resulting daughter cells will normally enter a prolonged G1 phase or G0. However, in cancer the daughter cells proceed with another cycle of replication. The progression of a cell through the cell cycle is regulated by two closely related families of proteins—the cyclins and the cyclin-dependent kinases (CDKs). There are two main points at which the cell cycle is regulated. One is at mid to late G1 and the second during G2.

G1 BOUNDARY

There is a point during G1, called the **restriction point** (R), at which a cell becomes committed to cell division or quiescence. Control at R is regulated primarily by the action of cyclin D1 and related D-type cyclins. Cyclin D binds to a number of CDKs, including CDK2, CDK4, CDK5, and CDK6. The cyclin D-CDK4 complex has been shown to modulate the activity of a number of regu-

latory proteins involved in transcriptional control, including E2F and Rb. Rb is underphosphorylated in early G1 and sequesters several proteins, including E2F. At R, Rb is phosphorylated, releasing E2F, which then is free to activate transcription of a number of proteins required for S-phase, including DNA polymerase, thymidine kinase, dihydrofolate reductase, myc, and cdc2.

The p53 protein also plays a critical role in regulating the cell cycle at the G1 boundary. One function of p53 is to arrest the cell cycle prior to S-phase in response to DNA damage caused by radiation. This gives the cell time to restore the DNA prior to replication. If the damage cannot be repaired, p53 induces apoptosis. Many cancer cells have lost wild-type p53 and do not arrest in G1 in response to irradiation. Under these conditions, DNA replication occurs with a high rate of mutation.

Late in G1 there is an increase in cyclin E, which forms an active complex with CDK2. This complex is essential for cells to enter S phase. Once the cell enters S phase the predominant cyclin is cyclin A, which remains active through G2. It is likely that cyclin A is involved in regulating DNA synthesis.

G2 BOUNDARY

The mitotic cyclins are involved in regulating the transition of cells from G2-phase into M-phase. Cyclin B complexed with cdc2 plays a dominant role in regulating mitosis. The activity of cyclin B-cdc2 is closely regulated through phosphorylation by wee1/mik1 and the cdc25c phosphatase. Cyclin B-cdc2 targets many proteins necessary for mitosis, including microtubule-associated proteins, nuclear lamins, and actin-binding proteins. Cyclin B is destroyed by proteolysis induced by ubiquitination. Cyclin B is rapidly destroyed when cells reach anaphase. The rapid activation and destruction of cyclin is critical to normal progression through the cell cycle.

APOPTOSIS

Normal processes of differentiation and growth involve the orderly destruction of cells. Cells can also be killed by T cells in response to viral infection or rejection. The process of "programmed cell death" is called **apoptosis** and involves characteristic cellular changes that result in physiologic demise of the cell. The process of apoptosis can be divided into four phases. The first phase involves the stimulus, which induces cell death. The stimulus then results in a signal that is transmitted to the apoptosis machinery. In the third phase, proteases and protease regulators are activated. In the final phase, chromatin becomes condensed and DNA is degraded.

The process of apoptosis involves activation of the ICE-related protease family. These proteins are synthe-

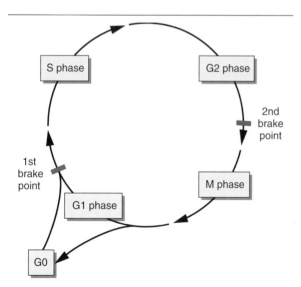

Figure 21–1. Diagram of a typical cell showing mitosis (M), the possibility to enter a resting phase (G0), the first growth phase (G1), the period of DNA synthesis (S), and the second period of growth in preparation for cell division (G2). Note the positions of the two brake points, which must be overcome for cell division to be achieved. (Reprinted, with permission, from Leake R: The cell cycle and regulation of cancer cell growth. Ann N Y Acad Med 1996;784:252.)

sized as pro-enzymes and are activated within a network of autoproteolysis and transproteolysis. The ICE proteases normally cleave substrates after an aspartate residue. ICE-protease targets include the nuclear enzymes poly(ADP-ribose)polymerase, DNA-dependent protein kinase, U1 ribonucleoprotein, and nuclear lamins.

TNF receptor 1 (TNFR1) can trigger apoptosis following binding to the ligand, tumor necrosis factor (TNF). TNFR1 contains a conserved intracellular domain known as the "death domain" (DD). TNFR1 activation results in the recruitment of other DD-containing proteins with eponymic names such as MORT1, RIP, and reaper. It has recently been determined that cell surface activation of TNFR1 is linked to activators of the ICE-proteases through activation of another ICE-related protein called FLICE. As more is learned about the molecular details of apoptosis, we have also gained a greater appreciation of the role apoptosis plays in cancer biology.

ONCOGENES & TUMOR SUPPRESSOR GENES

Mutations involved in oncogenesis can generally be characterized as one of two types. Mutations that activate proteins involved in cell growth represent a gain of function and are classified as **oncogenes**. Mutations that disrupt proteins that normally suppress growth represent a loss of function and are classified as **tumor suppressor genes**. Since there are two alleles of every gene, oncogenesis occurring from mutation of a tumor suppressor gene requires disruption of both copies of the gene.

The oncogenes were originally identified as cellular homologs of transforming genes found in retroviruses. Oncogenes have also been identified by transfecting DNA from cancer cells into certain types of tissue culture cells. The oncogene, ras, was identified in such an assay. A plethora of oncogenes have now been identified and each appears to be associated with specific types of cancer.

The identification of tumor suppressor genes has been more difficult. Transfection assays cannot be used since introducing a tumor suppressor gene would make the cell stop growing. However, many of these genes have been found by studying chromosomes from tumors. If a cancer is caused by mutation of a tumor suppressor gene, then both copies of that gene must be lost. As it turns out, deleting the second copy of a gene is most likely to result from a large chromosomal deletion or a duplication of that area of the chromosome. For this reason, there is commonly a loss of heterozygosity (LOH) at that locus. Identifying consistent LOH at a locus in a specific type of cancer can locate a tumor suppressor gene involved in oncogenesis of that type of cancer. Many tumor suppressor genes have been identified by studying LOH in primary cancer.

INHERITED CANCER

A great deal has been learned about the molecular biology of cancer from a study of familial cancer syndromes. In familial cancers, genetic mutations are inherited that predispose an individual to cancer development. With genetic techniques, the genes involved in hereditary cancers have been identified and, in many instances, these genes have been found to be involved in oncogenesis of the sporadic cancer counterpart. Table 21–1 shows a summary of the common inherited cancer syndromes. Many of the genes mutated in hereditary cancer syndromes are tumor suppressor genes. The first genetic cancer for which the molecular mechanism was identified was retinoblastoma. Retinoblastoma serves as a useful paradigm for a study of inherited cancers.

Retinoblastoma is a malignant eye tumor, and approximately 40% of cases are hereditary. Retinoblastoma results from deletion or mutation of both copies of the retinoblastoma susceptibility gene, Rb. In this regard, Rb is a tumor suppressor gene and oncogenesis requires that both Rb alleles be deleted in the developing retinoblasts. Sporadic retinoblastoma requires a somatic mutation of the Rb gene, which is a rare event. In hereditary retinoblastoma there is a germline mutation of one copy of Rb (Figure 21–2). The second copy is lost by deletion or recombination, which can occur with a much higher frequency than local mutation. Because of this, Rb mutations transmitted through the germline result in a higher frequency of cancer risk in offspring.

The identification of inherited cancer genes has relied upon modern techniques of molecular biology called **positional cloning**. In positional cloning, the cancer gene is located by a laborious technique of searching through large regions of a chromosome identified through linkage analysis. Recent insight into mechanisms of cancer development resulted in the identification of the gene responsible for hereditary non-polyposis colon cancer (HNPCC) by a direct approach.

It had been determined that tumors of patients with HNPCC demonstrated instability of repetitive DNA known as microsatellite DNA. The microsatellite DNA from the tumors was found to lose or gain numbers of repetitive elements. Normally, the cell replicates the number of repetitive elements precisely and, hence, the cancer cell demonstrated a loss of this replication fidelity. Researchers working on yeast genetics identified mutants that demonstrated the same microsatellite instability. The genes involved in the yeast defect were one of a number of DNA repair genes related to the mutHLS DNA repair pathway. They reasoned that HNPCC resulted from a mutation of the human homolog of this yeast repair gene. Based upon conserved domains of the mutS gene with the yeast MSH2 gene, these researchers cloned the human homolog, hMSH2. This gene was confirmed by linkage analysis to be the gene responsible for one form of HNPCC. An additional gene, hMLH1, was also found using an identical approach.

Table 21–1. Summary of familial cancer syndromes.

Syndrome	Tumor	Associated Traits/Cancer	Chromosome Location	Cloned Gene	Proposed Mechanism of Action
Familial retinoblastoma	Retinoblastoma	Developmental retardation Osteosarcoma	13q14	*Rb*	Cell cycle regulation Binds viral oncogenes Transcriptional regulation Modulates E2F

Familial Wilms	Wilms' tumor	WAGR
		  Wilms' tumor
		  Aniridia
		  Go abnormalities
		  Mental retardation
		Denys-Drash
		Beckwith-Wiedemann
		  Organomegaly
		  Adrenocortical
		    carcinoma
		  Hepatoblastoma
			11p13
			
			11p15
				WT1	Zinc finger transcription
					  factor
					Cell cycle regulation

Multiple endocrine neoplasia type 1 (Werner syndrome)	Pancreatic islet cell	Parathyroid hyperplasia Pituitary adenonas	11q13	*MEN 1*	

Multiple endocrine neoplasia type 2 (Sipple's syndrome)	Medullary thyroid carcinoma	Type 2A
		  Pheochromocytoma
		  Parathyroid
		    hyperplasia
		Type 2B
		  Pheochromocytoma
		  Mucosal neuromas
		  Martanoid habitus
		Familial medullary thyroid
		  carcinoma
			10 cen–10q11.2	*Ret*	Receptor tyrosine kinase

Xeroderma pigmentosum	Skin cancer	Pigmentation abnormalities Hypogonadism CNS defects	Eight complementa-tion groups	*ERCC*	Helicases Nucleotide excision repair
Fanconi's anemia	AML	Pancytopenia Skeletal abnormalities	Four complementa-tion groups	*FACC*	DNA repair
46BR	Lymphoreticular	Sun sensitivity Immunodeficiency Growth retardation		*DNA ligase I*	DNA ligation
Bloom's syndrome	Solid tumors	Telangiectasias Impaired immunity			
Ataxia telangiectasia	Lymphoma	Cerebellar ataxia Telangiectasias Immunodeficiency	Five complementa-tion groups 11q22–q23	*ATM*	PI-3 kinase

Familial adenomatous polyposis	Colon cancer	Colonic polyposis
		Congenital hypertrophy of
		  retinal pigment
		  epithelium
		Gardner's syndrome
			5q21	*APC*	Binds catenins

Hereditary non-polyposis colon cancer (Lynch syndrome)	Colon cancer
	Colon cancer
		HNPCC type I
		HNPCC type II-
		  endometrial CA
		  (others)
			3p21
			2p16
				hMLH1
				hMSH2
					DNA mismatch repair
					DNA mismatch repair

Li-Fraumeni syndrome	Sarcomas	Breast cancer
		Adrenocortical
		  carcinomas
		Brain tumors
			13q	p53
				Probably
				  others
					Cell cycle regulation
					Transcription factor
					Ultraviolet arrest

Neurofibromatosis type 1 NF1 (von Recklinghausen's disease)	Neurofibromas, neurofibrosarcoma	Café-au-lait spots Lisch nodules Optic gliomas	17q11.2	*NF1*	GAP related control of p21-ras Microtubule association
Neurofibromatosis type 2 NF2	Acoustic neuromas	Meningioma Glioma Schwannoma	22q12	Meriin	Linds cell membrane to cytoskeleton
Familial breast cancer	Breast carcinonoma Breast carcinoma	Ovarian carcinoma	17q21.1 13q12–13	BRCA1 BRCA2	Transcription factor

Reprinted and modified, with permission, from Abeloff MD et al: *Clinical Oncology*. Churchill Livingstone, 1995, p. 171.

Presumably, mutations of DNA repair genes result in mutations of other genes involved in colon carcinoma oncogenesis. There are also a set of recessive inherited cancer syndromes that result from mutations of genes involved in DNA repair. These syndromes include xeroderma pigmentosum, Fanconi's anemia, Bloom's syndrome, and ataxia telangiectasia. Each of these cancer syndromes is caused by mutations that result in hypersensitivity to DNA damage caused by radiation or chemical mutagens.

Multiple endocrine neoplasia 2A and 2B are examples of inherited cancer caused by activation of a proto-oncogene. In MEN2A and 2B, the ret proto-oncogene, which is a tyrosine kinase receptor, becomes activated. In MEN2A and familial MTC, one of a number of cysteine residues is targeted. It has also been shown that specific mutations are more likely to result in hyperparathyroidism. In MEN2B, the catalytic core of ret is targeted. This same mutation has also been shown to result in Hirschsprung's disease. These molecular findings now allow identification of affected family members at birth and also offer the possibility of greater insight into the oncogenesis of medullary thyroid carcinoma.

Genes involved in familial breast cancer have also been identified. Mutations of the *BRCA1* or *BRCA2* genes result in a greater predisposition to developing breast cancer. Unfortunately, these genes do not seem to be directly involved in the oncogenesis of sporadic breast cancer. However, it is likely that common sporadic mutations in breast cancer target the same metabolic or differentiation pathway involved with the *BRCA* genes.

SUMMARY

Studies of the molecular biology of cancer have revealed the intricacies of the regulation of cell growth and differentiation. The cell cycle is controlled by a complex network of proteins, many of which are regulated by phosphorylation. Oncogenesis involves the abnormal regulation of the cell cycle, which results in derangements of mechanisms established for quiescence or apoptosis. The molecular targets of these mutations involve either the activation of oncogenes or the deletion of tumor suppressor genes. In some instances these mutations can be inherited as a germline mutation, resulting in a familial cancer syndrome.

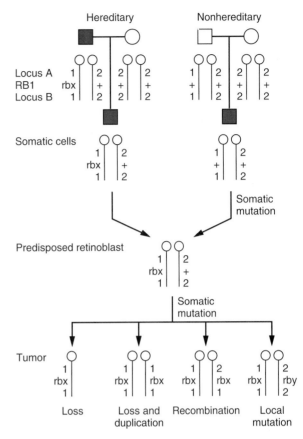

Figure 21–2. Schematic representation of retinoblastoma inheritance. In hereditary retinoblastoma, an affected parent transmits retinoblastoma susceptibility to his son through inheritance of allele rbx. Within the predisposed retinoblast, inactivation of wild-type retinoblastoma allele (rb) is accomplished by the loss of the allele with the wild-type copy of rb, loss with duplication of disease allele, mitotic recombination between disease allele and homologous chromosome, or local mutation (rby) of the wild-type allele. Each of these steps occurs at the somatic level within the predisposed retinoblast. In nonhereditary retinoblastoma, the first step involves a somatic mutation of one retinoblastoma locus in the predisposed retinoblast. The second mutation occurs in a fashion identical to hereditary retinoblastoma. (Reprinted and modified, with permission, from Horsthemke B: Genetics and cytogenetics of retinoblastoma. Cancer Genet Cytogenet 1992;63:1.)

SUGGESTED READING

Fearon ER: Oncogenes and tumor suppressor genes. In: Abeloff MD et al (editors): *Clinical Oncology.* Churchill Livingstone, 1995.

Leake R: The cell cycle and regulation of cancer cell growth. Ann NY Acad Sci 1996;784:252.

Weigel R: Inherited cancer. In: Abeloff MD et al (editors): *Clinical Oncology.* Churchill Livingstone, 1995.

Principles of Radiotherapy

Joseph C. Poen, MD

▶ Key Facts

- ▶ Radiation therapy is an integral component of treatment for 60% of all cancer patients.

- ▶ Curative radiotherapy is usually administered in daily increments over the course of 4–7 weeks.

- ▶ External beam radiotherapy is the administration of a measured dose of high-energy photons or electrons directed to a target volume within the patient, typically from a distance of 1 meter.

- ▶ Brachytherapy is the treatment of lesions using radioactive materials at short distances, often within the tumor itself, or within the affected or adjacent body cavity.

- ▶ The accepted units of radiation dosage are the Gray (1 joule of energy per kilogram of tissue) and the rad (0.01 Gray or 1 centigray [cGy]).

- ▶ For most carcinomas, a total dose of 4500–5000 cGy for microscopic disease and 6000–7000 cGy for clinically apparent disease is administered.

- ▶ Preoperative radiotherapy may enhance the surgeon's ability to completely resect locally advanced malignancies, while postoperative radiotherapy will often improve local disease control and overall outcome in a number of tumor sites.

- ▶ Intraoperative radiotherapy is a technique that allows for the delivery of tumoricidal radiation doses during a surgical procedure in order to avoid irradiation of critical normal tissues.

- ▶ Radiosurgery is a high-dose, single-fraction, stereotactically directed radiotherapy.

Soon after the discovery of x-rays and radioactivity in 1895–1896, physicians observed the beneficial effects of exposing otherwise untreatable tumors to the energy of the x-ray beam and the radioisotope. Early treatment techniques were crude and radiobiologic principles poorly understood; however, the responses and complete clinical remissions following these exposures were unmistakable.

In the century that has passed since these seminal events, the science of radiation oncology has evolved dramatically. With a better understanding of the biologic effects of ionizing radiation and the technical advances of the 20th century, modern radiotherapy has become a well controlled and easily quantified treatment modality that is now an integral component of treatment for 60% of all cancer patients. For some patients, radiation therapy is the single best treatment for achieving relief from pain and suffering. For many others, radiotherapy offers an opportunity for complete eradication and cure of their disease.

BIOLOGIC EFFECTS OF IONIZING RADIATION

Benign and malignant tumors share the property of having lost the capacity for normal growth regulation. Replication of neoplastic cells leads to tumor expansion and, in the case of malignancy, eventual tumor cell dissemination. The process of tumor expansion and dissemination accounts for the morbidity and mortality associated with disease progression. Cancer therapies are aimed at either removing the abnormal cells (**surgical therapy**) or rendering them incapable of further reproduction by chemical disruption (**chemotherapy**) or physical disruption (**radiotherapy**).

MECHANISM OF PHYSICAL DISRUPTION

When ionizing radiation interacts with tissues, the predominant result is the intracellular production of hydroxyl free radicals. If this interaction occurs within the nucleus, the hydroxyl radical may in turn interact with an adjacent DNA molecule, resulting in a single-strand or double-strand break. DNA disruptions occurring within a redundant or nonfunctioning portion of the chromosome produces little or no functional detriment to the cell. Conversely, a double-strand break within a critical gene region may alter life-sustaining intracellular biochemical processes, resulting in programmed cell death (**apoptosis**). Alternatively, the injury may become apparent only after an attempt to replicate the genetic material (**mitotic cell death**), rendering the cell incapable of further proliferation.

RADIOSENSITIVITY & RADIATION RESPONSE

The ability of a given radiotherapy dose to irreversibly injure a critical organ or permanently eradicate a specific tumor is determined by the inherent radiosensitivity of the tissue or tumor in question and may be affected by a number of factors, such as tissue vascularity or tumor oxygenation. This inherent "radiosensitivity" is well known for most normal and neoplastic tissues so that tables of normal tissue tolerances and tumoricidal doses can be constructed (Table 22–1). When conditions permit the administration of a tumoricidal dose without exceeding the tolerance of the surrounding normal tissues, a favorable clinical outcome may be expected.

The radiosensitivity or radioresistance of a specific tissue or tumor should not be inferred from the rapidity of the clinical response to ionizing radiation. The time course of the clinical response in any tissue, normal or malignant, is determined by the rate of tissue turnover. Rapidly proliferating normal tissues (eg, bone marrow and gastrointestinal mucosa) and neoplasms (eg, small cell lung cancer and lymphoma) manifest cell loss and injury within days of the first dose of radiation. However, normal tissues (eg, hepatocytes and nerves) and tumors with slow turnover rates (eg, sarcomas and prostate cancer) may not exhibit the effects of cell loss for months or years after a course of radiotherapy. The rate of response is a function of the cellular kinetics rather than the radiosensitivity and may not reflect the eventual outcome. For example, the highly sensitive pulmonary parenchymal cell will show little or no functional abnormality several weeks after a potentially lethal whole lung dose of 2500 cGy, whereas the more resistant dermis (tolerance > 7000 cGy) will express reversible injury in the form of erythema and desquamation within days to weeks of a tolerable radiation dose.

IMPROVED THERAPEUTIC INDEX WITH FRACTIONATION

Delivery of a tumoricidal dose of radiation in a single treatment session would, in most cases, cause unacceptable normal tissue injury. Consequently, potentially curative radiotherapy is administered in daily increments over the course of 4–7 weeks. Throughout a typical course of fractionated radiotherapy, several important biologic events help to preserve the integrity of normal structures and enhance the probability of malignant tumor control. Repair of sublethal single-strand radiation damage in noncycling normal cells helps to maintain the viability and preserve function of normal tissues. In general, malignant tumors have less capacity for repair than do normal tissues. In addition, as the tumor responds to treatment and the tumor volume is reduced, the relatively hypoxic core of the tumor mass is exposed to increasing blood flow and

Table 22–1. Inherent radiosensitivity of normal tissues and malignant tumors.

	Dose (cGy)	Normal Tissue Tolerance	Tumoricidal Dose
Radiosensitive	1000	Bone marrow	Leukemia
	2000	Lung, kidney	Seminoma
	3000	Liver	Hodgkin's lymphoma
	4000	Heart	Non-Hodgkin's lymphoma
	5000	Gastrointestinal organs	Carcinoma (subclinical)
	6000	Central nervous system	Carcinoma (< 1 cm^3)
	7000	Skin	Carcinoma (> 1 cm^3)
Radioresistant	8000	Connective tissues	Sarcoma

reoxygenation, thereby enhancing its radiosensitivity. Furthermore, because malignant cells are moving through the cell cycle more rapidly than normal cells, the opportunity exists for each malignant cell to be exposed to ionization during the particularly vulnerable G2-phase and M-phase of the cell cycle. The more quiescent normal cell population is generally not affected by this redistribution into radiosensitive phases of the cell cycle.

RADIATION TECHNIQUES

A variety of techniques have been developed to optimize the delivery of potentially tumoricidal radiation doses while maintaining the integrity of the surrounding normal tissues.

TELETHERAPY (EXTERNAL BEAM RADIOTHERAPY)

External beam radiotherapy involves the administration of a measured dose of high-energy photons or electrons directed to a target volume within the patient, typically from a distance of 1 m (source to target distance). The radiation beam is shaped to conform to the relevant tumor and normal tissue anatomy and is precisely targeted with the assistance of external laser light sources. The most widely used radiation source is the medical linear accelerator, which can produce high-energy x-rays or electrons for radiotherapy. X-ray energies in the range of 4–25 million volts (MV) are generally employed, with the higher energy beams reserved for treating tumors located deep within the body (eg, pancreas and prostate). Lower energy x-ray beams are appropriate for treating more superficial structures, such as the larynx and breast.

Electron beams are less penetrating than x-rays and are useful in treating tumors within the first few centimeters of the skin surface. Their dose deposition characteristics are particularly advantageous for eradicating skin lesions (eg, mycosis fungoides or basal cell carcinoma) and treating the superficial lymphatics of the posterior neck while avoiding the underlying cervical spinal cord. Less commonly, teletherapy is delivered from a high-activity external radioisotope, such as [60]cobalt, or from a low-energy x-ray orthovoltage unit. These predecessors of the modern linear accelerator remain useful in certain clinical situations.

A few specialized centers in the United States utilize dedicated cyclotrons for the production of high-energy neutrons, protons, and other charged particles for radiation therapy. By virtue of their mass, neutrons are a densely ionizing radiation with an enhanced radiobiologic effect. Because of their positive charge, protons exhibit superior physical dose deposition characteristics. The complexity and cost of maintaining these particle accelerators prohibit their widespread use.

BRACHYTHERAPY

Brachytherapy is the treatment of lesions using radioactive materials at short distances, often within the tumor itself (**interstitial**) or within the affected or adjacent body cavity (**intracavitary**). Solid radioisotopes ([137]cesium, [192]iridium, [125]iodine) with moderate photon energies can be inserted directly into a lesion with the guidance of specially designed interstitial needles or intracavitary applicators that ensure a uniform dose distribution throughout the target tissue (Figure 22–1). Interstitial or intracavitary brachytherapy is typically used in conjunction with external beam therapy to deliver an additional "boost" dose of radiation within a high-risk tumor volume. Doses of several thousand centigray (cGy) may be administered within the high-dose treatment area in a matter of hours. Since the radiation exposure to surrounding tissues is proportional to $1/distance^2$, normal structures at a greater distance from the implanted tissue are relatively spared.

The **activity** of a radioisotope is a measure of the magnitude of its rate of decay. The basic unit of activity, the **curie** (Ci), is defined as 3.7×10^{10} disintegrations per second. Historically, brachytherapists utilized low-activity sources to deliver doses at a rate of 30–80 cGy/h. A standard 3000-cGy implant would often require a 2- to 3-day hospital admission. Newer high-activity sources are becoming increasingly available for high dose rate (HDR) brachytherapy. Comparable doses can now be administered in a matter of minutes to hours in an outpatient setting.

RADIATION DOSES, SCHEDULES, & TREATMENT VOLUMES

The most widely accepted unit of absorbed radiation dose is the **Gray**, which is defined as the absorption of one joule of energy per kilogram of tissue. An older unit of radiation dose, the **rad**, is equal to 0.01 Gray or 1.0 cGy. Daily radiation doses of 180–200 cGy are standard. For purposes of palliation in the setting of advanced

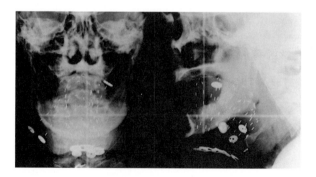

Figure 22–1. Anterior and lateral radiographs demonstrating a [192]iridium interstitial implantation of a bulky squamous cell carcinoma of the tongue.

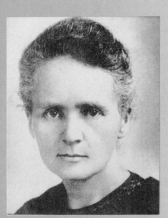

Marie Curie (1867–1934) shared the 1903 Nobel Prize for physics for the discovery of radioactivity with her husband, Pierre Curie, and won the 1911 Nobel Prize for chemistry for the isolation of pure radium metal.

Marie Curie (1867–1934) is not only one of the most famous women in physics, she is one of the single greatest contributors to radiation therapy. She shared the 1903 Nobel Prize in physics for the discovery of radioactivity with her husband, Pierre Curie (1859–1906). Unfortunately, Pierre Curie died soon after, when he was struck by a truck on a Paris street.

After Pierre's death, Marie threw herself into her work and was offered his position as a lecturer and head of the laboratory at the Sorbonne. In 1908, she was appointed as a full professor. While examining pitchblende, a uranium ore, she discovered radium and polonium. In 1911, she won the Nobel Prize for chemistry for the isolation of pure radium metal. The rest of her life was dedicated to research concerning the chemistry of radioactive materials and their medical applications. In 1934, Marie Curie died of leukemia, thought to have been brought on by her extensive exposure to high levels of radiation. In her honor, the basic unit of radioactivity, the curie (Ci), bears her name.

metastatic disease, the daily dose may be increased to 300–400 cGy so that the overall treatment time can be reduced to 1–2 weeks.

Alternatively, the radiation oncologist may choose to increase the number of treatment fractions to achieve a higher total dose and improve the probability of local tumor control. In one example, smaller fractions are given twice daily (eg, 120 cGy twice a day) over several weeks. This technique, called **hyperfractionation**, has been shown to permit higher total doses, producing higher rates of tumor control with comparable long-term side effects. For rapidly proliferating malignancies, tumor cell repopulation during a prolonged course of radiotherapy can be avoided by accelerating the course of treatment. In this example, a slightly reduced fraction is administered twice daily (eg, 160 cGy twice a day) to achieve the standard total tumor dose in a reduced overall treatment time. This treatment scheme has been appropriately termed **accelerated fractionation**.

The total dose for a course of radiation therapy is a function of the clinical setting, tumor histology, and amount of disease to be controlled. For most palliative therapy, the goal of treatment is to achieve a relatively durable tumor response rather than permanent eradication of the focus of disease. Lower total doses and shorter overall treatment schedules are employed. For most curative therapy, the total dose is a function of the tumor type and its inherent radiosensitivity, as well as the amount of residual disease or number of malignant clones to be sterilized.

For most carcinomas, a total dose of 4500–5000 cGy is administered to control microscopic disease and 6000–7000 cGy to eradicate clinically apparent disease. Lower doses may be appropriate for unusually radiosensitive cancers, such as lymphoma, leukemia, and seminoma; considerably higher doses may be required for more resistant tumors, such as soft tissue sarcomas.

Radiation doses are applied to a target volume or treatment volume. The total radiation dose must not exceed the tolerance of any of the critical normal structures within that volume. Radiotherapy fields are two-dimensional representations of treatment volumes. Multiple fields are treated daily (eg, anterior, posterior, lateral, and oblique) to ensure the homogeneity of dose deposition throughout a given volume. Examples of standard radiation therapy fields for the treatment of rectal cancer are shown in Figure 22–2.

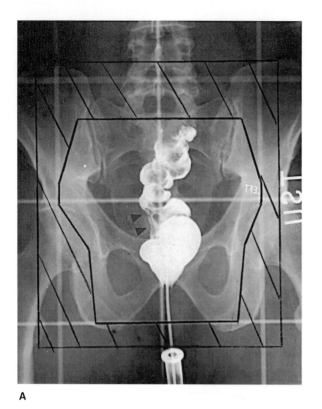

A

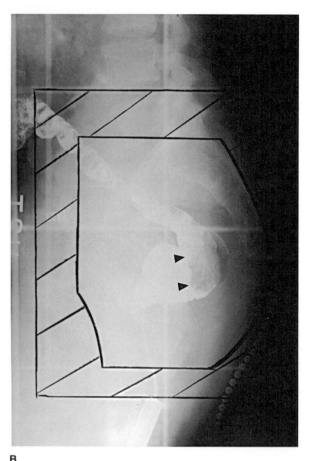

B

Figure 22–2. Posterior *(A)* and lateral *(B)* radiotherapy fields for preoperative treatment of rectal carcinoma and the regional pelvic lymphatics. The barium filling defect *(arrows)* reveals the location of this cancer.

SURGERY & RADIOTHERAPY

Radiotherapy, like surgery, is a local and regional treatment modality. In many instances, a single treatment modality will achieve local tumor control, and the choice of surgery or radiation therapy is based upon the results of either approach. For other cancers, both local modalities must be employed to ensure adequate tumor eradication. Still other clinical scenarios call for all three oncologic modalities (surgery, radiation therapy, and chemotherapy) in order to obtain the optimal local results.

Concurrent chemotherapy for radiosensitization is commonly recommended in the treatment of malignancies of the gastrointestinal tract. The mechanism of action, biologic effects, and clinical results of concurrent chemotherapy and radiotherapy are beyond the scope of this text. For further information, the reader is referred to the general oncology text.

SINGLE-MODALITY THERAPY

Single-modality therapy is appropriate when one treatment modality alone provides a high probability of local tumor control with an acceptable functional and/or cosmetic outcome. For many cancer patients the selection of the most appropriate local treatment modality is clear. One form of treatment may offer clearly superior local tumor control (eg, surgical resection for lung adenocarcinoma; radiotherapy for Hodgkin's disease) or may yield a better functional result (eg, surgery for a pituitary microadenoma; radiotherapy for a T_1 laryngeal cancer). In other clinical settings, the effectiveness of the two local treatment options may be equivalent, and the decision to proceed with one modality or the other may be determined by convenience or patient biases (eg, as in prostate cancer). Several examples of appropriate treatment options are shown in Table 22–2.

Table 22–2. Examples of tumors for which a single local treatment modality therapy is appropriate.

Surgery Alone	Radiotherapy Alone	Either Modality Alone
Pituitary adenoma	T1 glottic carcinoma	Ocular melanoma
Pilocystic astrocytoma	Hodgkin's lymphoma	Oral mucosa carcinoma
Cutaneous melanoma	Non-Hodgkin's lymphoma	Cutaneous squamous carcinoma
Colon carcinoma	Small cell lung cancer	Prostate carcinoma
Bladder carcinoma	Anal carcinoma	Uterine cervix carcinoma

COMBINED-MODALITY THERAPY

Combinations of surgery and radiation therapy are appropriate when either modality alone fails to meet the criteria for single-modality therapy. The indications for combined surgical resection and radiotherapy are: (1) either modality alone results in unacceptably high rates of local or regional recurrence (eg, advanced head and neck cancers, pancreatic cancer); (2) the addition of radiotherapy allows for a more limited surgical resection, thereby preserving organ function or cosmesis (eg, breast cancer, extremity soft tissue sarcomas); or (3) the tumor has advanced to a stage where surgical resection alone is not technically feasible (eg, locally advanced rectal cancer).

In the combined-modality setting, the goal of surgery is to remove the bulk of the tumor and to achieve clear surgical margins. Radiation therapy is then administered to eradicate microscopic extensions of the disease in the surrounding tissues or draining lymphatics.

Combined-modality therapy has impacted dramatically on the quality of cancer survival. The evolution of local therapy for breast cancer and extremity sarcomas illustrates this point. As recently as the 1960s, medical dogma established radical mastectomy including resection of the pectoralis major and extremity amputation as the standard surgical treatments for breast cancer and extremity sarcomas, respectively. Prospective randomized trials in the 1970s and 1980s eventually proved that equivalent or improved results could be obtained with simple local excisions and postoperative radiation therapy. The impact of organ and limb preservation on quality of life for many of these cancer patients was profound. By offering improved quality of survival without compromising the probability of cure, breast conservation for breast cancer and limb salvage therapy for extremity sarcomas have since become the standard of care in most university medical centers.

PREOPERATIVE RADIOTHERAPY

Preoperative radiotherapy may enhance the surgeon's ability to completely resect locally advanced malignancies. This effect has been well documented in carcinoma of the rectum, where preoperative treatment has permitted subsequent curative resections in patients with otherwise inoperable tumors. In cases of marginal resectability, preoperative radiotherapy has been shown to increase the probability of complete resection and local disease control. Furthermore, by permitting a narrower margin of resection, preoperative treatment may improve the likelihood of a function-preserving surgical resection. Other potential advantages of preoperative irradiation include sterilization of cancerous cells prior to surgical manipulation, thereby avoiding possible wound contamination and treatment of tumors under maximally oxygenated conditions when cells are most radiosensitive. Patients with cancers of the bladder, head and neck, esophagus, pancreas, and endometrium may also benefit from preoperative radiotherapy.

Doses in the range of 4500–5000 cGy are generally targeted to the primary site, surrounding tissues, and draining lymphatics. In designing treatment fields, the radiation tolerance of normal structures must be respected. After a 3- to 5-week delay, surgical resection is undertaken. All tissues known to be involved with measurable disease should be completely resected, since 5000 cGy will completely eradicate only microscopic extensions of the disease. With the addition of concurrent chemotherapy, complete pathologic responses may be seen in cases of measurable or bulky disease.

Operating in the radiation therapy field will not pose a significant challenge to the experienced surgical oncologist. Operative complications are uncommon following doses of 4500–5000 cGy, provided adequate time has been allowed for recovery from radiotherapy. Tensile strength of the unirradiated wound increases rapidly from 4–10 days following incision and reaches near maximum tensile strength by day 15. Preoperative irradiation in moderate doses delays this process by approximately 5 days. Since radiation-induced tissue fibrosis typically becomes apparent 6–8 weeks after preoperative treatment, unnecessary surgical delays are not advised. The optimum surgical window appears to be 3–6 weeks following the completion of radiotherapy with 4500–5000 cGy.

POSTOPERATIVE RADIOTHERAPY

Postoperative radiotherapy will improve local disease control and overall outcome in a number of tumor sites. Indications for postoperative radiotherapy include: (1) treatment of tumors with a high risk for local recurrence following surgery alone; (2) eradication of disease in regional lymphatics; (3) use of a limited surgical resection for functional organ preservation; (4) use of a limited surgical resection for cosmetic purposes; and (5) tumor transection/positive surgical margins. Since nearly all malignant tumors have the capacity to invade adjacent critical structures and create a narrow margin of resection, postoperative radiation therapy is potentially applicable to all malignant neoplasms.

The postoperative radiotherapy dose is dependent upon the histology of the neoplasm, its inherent radiosensitivity, and the extent of residual disease following surgery. For example, 5000 cGy will eradicate residual subclinical microscopic disease for the vast majority of squamous cell carcinomas and most adenocarcinomas. Doses approaching 6000 cGy must be administered when carcinomas are transected surgically, and 7000–7500 cGy are appropriate following incomplete resections of soft tissue sarcomas.

The time interval between surgery and postoperative therapy is also important. In the absence of surgical complications and for patients in good general health, wound healing is complete by postoperative day 21. Since regrowth of residual cancer cells will begin within hours of surgery, radiation therapy should commence as soon as the healing process has been completed. Inordinate delays have been associated with increased rates of local tumor recurrence.

INNOVATIVE RADIOTHERAPY TECHNIQUES

In the laboratory, all tumors are radiocurable, given sufficient radiation doses. In clinical practice, normal tissue tolerance often limits the dose that may be safely administered. If the radiation dose required for tumor eradication exceeds the dose that produces normal tissue complications, conventional radiotherapy cure cannot be accomplished without unacceptable morbidity. Innovative techniques have been developed in an effort to permit higher radiotherapy doses and to circumvent the major obstacles of normal tissue injury and treatment-related complications.

INTRAOPERATIVE RADIOTHERAPY

For many gastrointestinal and pelvic malignancies, radiotherapy doses are limited by the tolerances of the kidneys (2000 cGy), liver (3000 cGy), and small intestine (4500 cGy). A technique that allows for the delivery of tumoricidal radiation doses while avoiding irradiation of these critical normal tissues is **intraoperative radiotherapy** (IORT). Several comprehensive oncology treatment

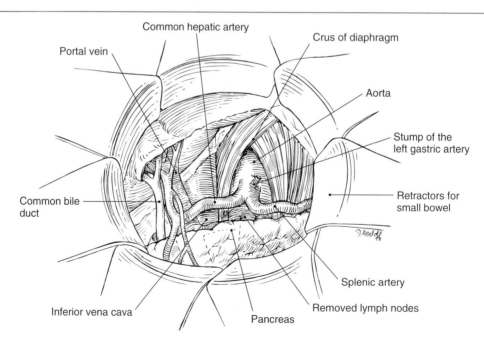

Figure 22–3. Intraoperative radiation field following gastrectomy for adenocarcinoma of the stomach. Two-millimeter lead plates are used to retract the liver, gall bladder, duodenum, colon, and small intestine. The common sites of recurrence around the celiac and portal vessels are treated with little exposure to the adjacent critical structures. (Reprinted and modified, with permission, from Ogata et al: A 10-year experience of intraoperative radiotherapy for gastric carcinoma and a new surgical method of creating a wider irradiation field for cases of total gastrectomy patients. Int J Radiat Oncol Biol Phys 1995;32:342.)

centers have equipped operating suites with radiation therapy units where a single large dose of radiotherapy can be administered during an operation. Following wide exposure of the operative field, critical normal structures are physically displaced, and the radiation beam is directed onto either the surgically exposed unresectable tumor or the area of resection where recurrence is most likely to occur (Figure 22–3). Intraoperative single-fraction doses of 1500–3000 cGy may be safely administered. When used in conjunction with conventional fractionated external beam radiotherapy, total doses in the range of 6000–7500 cGy may be achieved.

The greatest clinical experience to date with IORT has been in the treatment of carcinoma of the pancreas. By virtue of its propensity to encase the celiac, mesenteric, and portal blood vessels and to access the extensive regional lymphatic network, carcinoma of the pancreas has proven to be one of the most difficult malignancies to eradicate. The majority of patients have locally unresectable tumors at the time of diagnosis. For patients with tumors amenable to potentially curative resection, local tumor bed recurrence and regional nodal relapse remain a significant problem. Ultimately, only 20% of patients with the most favorable pancreatic cancers have been cured of their disease.

In an effort to improve the outlook for these patients, several investigators have employed IORT in combination with conventional fractionated radiotherapy and chemotherapy with encouraging local and regional control results. More aggressive treatment strategies incorporating chemotherapy, IORT, and whole liver irradiation are under investigation.

Other locally advanced or recurrent abdominal and pelvic cancers are potentially amenable to high-dose IORT. Several investigators have reported improved survival rates with surgery and IORT for locally advanced gastric cancer. For patients with surgically incurable rectal, gynecologic, and genitourinary malignancies, aggressive combination regimens of neoadjuvant chemoradiotherapy followed by surgery and IORT have yielded long-term salvage rates of approximately 30%.

HIGH-DOSE STEREOTACTIC RADIOTHERAPY (RADIOSURGERY)

High-dose single-fraction stereotactically directed radiotherapy has been called "radiosurgery." Radiosurgery was first described by the Swedish neurosurgeon Lars Leksell in 1951. Using a conventional low-energy x-ray beam and stereotactic guidance, Dr. Leksell was able to deliver a highly focused dose of ionizing radiation to destroy specific intracranial targets that were otherwise inaccessible by conventional techniques. In 1968, the prototype Gamma Knife employing 179 stereotactically focused [60]cobalt sources was used for functional neurosurgery (thalamotomies for intractable pain syndromes) at the Karolinska Institute in Stockholm. By the mid-1980s,

linear-accelerator–based radiosurgery was available in North America, and in 1993 nearly 200 radiosurgery facilities were in operation throughout the United States.

Although radiosurgery was originally developed for benign intracranial lesions (arteriovenous malformations, meningiomas, pituitary adenomas, and acoustic neuromas) and functional neurosurgery (pain center ablation), recent advances in high-resolution imaging have permit-

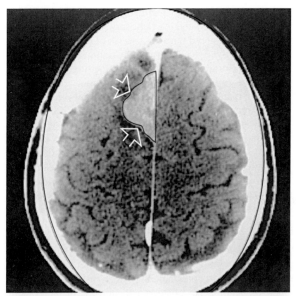

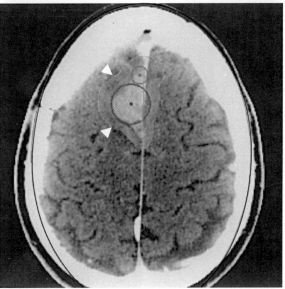

Figure 22–4. Radiosurgery treatment plan for recurrent parafalcine meningioma. The tumor *(top, large arrows)* receives a minimum dose of 2000 cGy while the surrounding normal brain *(bottom, small arrows)* is exposed to less than 600 cGy.

ted an expansion of the treatment indications to include primary malignancies of the central nervous system (eg, glioblastomas) and brain metastases. Under local anesthesia, a stereotactic localizing frame is fixed in four locations to the external skull. With the frame and attached fiducial reference system in place, angiography, computed tomography scanning, or magnetic resonance imaging is performed, and the intracranial target lesion is identified.

The fiducial reference allows for precise localization of the target isocenter within a three-dimensional coordinate system. Target coordinates are determined and a dose/volume treatment plan is formulated. The stereotactic frame is fixed into position on the treatment table, appropriate target coordinates are set, and the radiosurgery dose (1800–3000 cGy) is administered through a series of dynamic arc rotations. The entire procedure typically requires 4–5 hours and may be performed in the outpatient setting. A recurrent parafalcine meningioma and multicenter radiosurgery treatment plan (2000 cGy) are shown in Figure 22–4.

Until recently, stereotactic radiotherapy has been limited to the brain, base of skull, and upper head and neck, where rigid frame fixation is possible. Newer frameless radiosurgical systems are under development at Stanford University. The Neurotron 1000 (Figure 22–5) was designed to deliver precision stereotactic radiosurgery or to allow for fractionated stereotactic radiotherapy without the relative inconvenience of the current frame-based technology. It consists of a compact linear accelerator mounted on a computer-controlled robotic arm that permits a much wider range of beam orientations than exists with conventional radiosurgery systems. Continuous computer analysis of real-time fluoroscopic imaging permits instantaneous feedback of beam-target position and allows for stereotactic millimeter precision without rigid target fixation. Such a system will eventually permit stereotactic radiosurgical ablation of tumors located throughout the body.

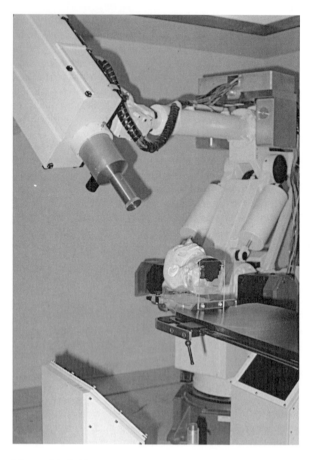

Figure 22–5. The Neurotron 1000, a 6MV linear accelerator mounted on a computer-controlled robotic arm, permits precision radiosurgery without rigid frame immobilization.

SUGGESTED READING

Bagne FR, Dobelbower RR, Milligan AJ: Radiation therapy in cancer management: History and basic principles. In: Moossa AR, Schimpff SC, Robson MC (editors). *Comprehensive Textbook of Oncology*, 2nd ed. Williams & Wilkins, 1991.

Devita VT Jr, Hellman S, Rosenberg SA: *Cancer: Principles and Practice of Oncology*. 4th ed. Lippincott, 1993.

Dobelbower RR et al: Radiation therapy in cancer management: new frontiers. In: Moossa AR, Schimpff SC, Robson MC (editors). *Comprehensive Textbook of Oncology*, 2nd ed. Williams & Wilkins, 1991.

Fisher B et al: Five-year results of a randomized clinical trial comparing total mastectomy and segmental mastectomy with or without radiation in the treatment of breast cancer. N Engl J Med 1985;312:665.

Forastiere AA et al: Preoperative chemoradiation followed by transhiatal esophagectomy for carcinoma of the esophagus: final report. J Clin Oncol 1993;11:1118.

Gunderson LL: Rationale for and results of intraoperative radiation therapy. Cancer 1994;74:537.

Loeffler JS et al: The role of stereotactic radiosurgery in the management of intracranial tumors. Oncology 1990;4:21.

Perez CA, Bredy LW: *Principles and Practices of Radiation Oncology*, 2nd ed. Lippincott, 1992.

Rich TA et al: Preoperative infusional chemoradiation therapy for stage T3 rectal cancer. Int J Radiation Oncology Biol Phys 1995;32:1025.

23

Principles of Chemotherapy

Helen Collins, MD

► Key Facts

► The guiding principle behind the development and use of chemotherapeutic agents is that the drug must be both cytotoxic and deliverable to the tumor cell.

► The most important factor in determining whether to recommend chemotherapy to a particular patient is the responsiveness of the histological cell type to chemotherapy.

► Four terms define the different goals and timing of chemotherapy: (1) primary chemotherapy (primary use); (2) adjuvant chemotherapy (use after surgery); (3) induction or neoadjuvant chemotherapy (use before surgery); (4) palliative chemotherapy (relief of symptoms).

► Resistance of tumor cells to chemotherapy, caused either by a lack of exposure to adequate concentrations of effective drugs or by resistance to the drug itself, is one of the primary reasons chemotherapy fails.

► Dose intensity is the amount of chemotherapeutic drug given over a specific time, or in pharmacological terms, the area under the curve.

► Immunotherapy is an attempt to stimulate the immune response against tumor cells. Active immunization is the process of injecting an antigen to stimulate an immune response. Passive or adoptive immunotherapy is the process of injecting patients with the actual immune effector cells.

► Gene therapy is the technique of introducing a specific gene into a target cell to produce an antineoplastic response.

► The most common toxicities to chemotherapeutic drugs include hematologic and gastrointestinal side effects.

The majority of solid tumors are not curable with surgery alone. Frequently, the surgeon is the first physician to inform a patient that he or she will require further treatment, and it is the surgeon who refers the patient to a medical oncologist for chemotherapy. The indications for chemotherapy, the timing of chemotherapy in relation to surgery, its potential side effects, and the methods of chemotherapy delivery are essential knowledge if the maximum benefit for the patient is to be achieved.

The guiding principle behind the development and use of chemotherapeutic agents is that the drug must be both cytotoxic to the tumor cell and deliverable to that tumor cell. Historically, drugs have been developed that take advantage of a narrow therapeutic range between effectiveness against tumor cells and toxicity to normal cells, and these drugs have been the cornerstone of treatment. Recently, increased effort has been aimed at developing biological and gene therapies, finding mechanisms to reverse chemotherapy resistance, and predicting which patients will respond to specific treatment modalities.

INDICATIONS FOR CHEMOTHERAPY

The decision to treat or not treat an individual patient with chemotherapy is dependent on several factors, including: the histological type of tumor, the patient's individual characteristics, and the goals of treatment (Table 23–1). The most important factor in determining whether to recommend chemotherapy to a particular patient is the responsiveness of the histological cell type to chemotherapy. Histological type and grade are the most important predictors of response. Certain malignant cell types, such as leukemias, lymphomas, and germ cell tumors, tend to be very sensitive and potentially curable with chemotherapy alone. Some malignancies, such as ovarian, breast, and prostate cancer, have moderate chemotherapy responsiveness, and other malignant tumors, such as renal cell cancer and melanomas, are extremely resistant to all types of chemotherapy (Table 23–2).

Characteristics of the individual patient that affect the decision to give chemotherapy and determine the choice of drugs include the patient's medical history, performance status, and age. A history of a comorbid medical condition, such as cardiac, hepatic, renal, or pulmonary dysfunction, may preclude the use of certain drugs or predict for a life expectancy shorter than the life expectancy if the malignancy was left untreated.

It is important to note, however, that simply the presence of comorbidity does not necessarily infer a worse prognosis. For example, in colorectal cancers a history of hypertension, diabetes, or chronic obstructive pulmonary disease may increase the surgical complication rate but not influence overall survival. Before the decision is made

Table 23–2. Tumor responsiveness to chemotherapy.

Sensitive to chemotherapy (chemotherapy alone can potentially cure)

Germ cell tumors
Lymphoma
Leukemia
Wilms' tumor
Embryonal rhabdosarcoma

Some chemotherapy responsiveness (response rate > 50%, no cures with chemotherapy alone)

Ovarian
Breast
Small cell lung cancer
Prostate
Bladder
Thymoma

Resistant to chemotherapy (response rate < 50%, rare complete responses and no cures)

Non-small cell lung cancer
Melanoma
Hepatocellular carcinoma
Central nervous system
Renal cell
Pancreatic
Gastric
Sarcoma
Endometrial
Carcinoid
Biliary
Adrenal
Esophageal
Thyroid
Head and neck
Neuroblastoma

to withhold chemotherapy, a distinction must be made between medical conditions that predict for a shorter life expectancy versus conditions that just increase the complication rate of chemotherapy. A patient should never be denied treatment purely because of the presence of a co-morbid medical condition.

The patient's ability to perform the usual activities of daily living is another factor that correlates with tolerance and response to chemotherapy. Because of its prognostic importance, functional status, or "performance status," has been translated into standardized scales. The two most commonly cited performance status scales are the Eastern Cooperative Oncology Group (ECOG) and Karnofsky (KPS) scales, which stratify a patient's functional status from fully functional to bedridden (ECOG scale, 0–4), or no symptoms of disease to death (KPS scale, 100%–0%) (Table 23–3).

The importance of age as a separate predictor of chemotherapy tolerance is unclear. Being older than age 70 years is a poor prognostic indicator in some cancers, such as intermediate-grade lymphomas, but has no influence on survival in other cancers, such as small cell lung cancer. In other tumors, such as breast and prostate cancers, younger

Table 23–1. Decision to administer chemotherapy to an individual patient.

Patient characteristics	Performance status and age
	Comorbid medical conditions: cardiac, renal, hepatic, hematologic, pulmonary
	Social factors
Tumor characteristics	Histology
	Grade
	Stage
	Bulk of disease
	Site of disease
Goal of chemotherapy	Cure
	Palliation
Toxicity of chemotherapy	Acute
	Long-term

Table 23–3. Performance status scales.

ECOG (0–4)
0 = Asymptomatic
1 = Normal activity with some symptoms
2 = Symptoms, in bed < 50% of day
3 = Symptoms, in bed > 50% of day
4 = Bedridden

Karnofsky (0–100%)
100% = Normal, no evidence of disease
 90% = Able to carry on normal activity, minor symptoms of disease
 80% = Normal activity with effort, some symptoms or signs of disease
 70% = Cares for self, unable to carry on normal activity or do active work
 60% = Requires occasional assistance but is able to care for most of needs
 50% = Requires considerable assistance and frequent medical care
 40% = Disabled; requires special medical care and assistance
 30% = Severely disabled; hospitalization is indicated, although death not imminent
 20% = Very sick; hospitalization necessary, active supportive Rx needed
 10% = Moribund, fatal
  0% = Dead

ECOG = Eastern Cooperative Oncology Group.

patients tend to present with higher-grade, more advanced tumors, but, stage-for-stage, patients have the same prognosis, and age is not an independent risk factor.

The difficulty evaluating published data concerning chemotherapy in the elderly population is that prospective studies have tended to exclude elderly patients, and retrospective chart reviews find chemotherapy doses in older patients are often decreased because of, and in anticipation of, increased toxicity. Elderly patients do have more adverse side effects from chemotherapy, but until more studies are completed, treatment in elderly patients needs to be individualized, and performance status is the better predictor of chemotherapy tolerance.

The final factor in deciding whether chemotherapy is indicated for a specific patient is determining if the goal of chemotherapy is curative or palliative. The following terms—induction, adjuvant, neoadjuvant, and palliative chemotherapy—have been developed to reflect the different goals and timing of chemotherapy.

Primary chemotherapy is the use of chemotherapy to treat a tumor that is responsive to chemotherapy, such as lymphoma. Chemotherapy is frequently the only treatment used for these malignancies, and the objective in this setting is usually curative. Although important, the role of surgery is often only to obtain tissue for diagnosis.

Adjuvant chemotherapy is the use of chemotherapy after surgery has removed all macroscopic disease. In some types of malignancies, surgery alone will cure some patients; another group of patients will relapse, even with the addition of adjuvant chemotherapy; and a third group of patients will have a survival benefit from treatment with

chemotherapy. Since, at present, there is no way to predict which group a particular patient will fall into, all patients are recommended for adjuvant chemotherapy; it is inherent, therefore, in the principle of adjuvant chemotherapy that some patients receive chemotherapy unnecessarily.

Again, to decide whether to recommend chemotherapy to a specific patient, it is necessary to know the disease-free and overall survival rates with surgery alone and the improvement of these rates with chemotherapy. It is also important to determine the patient's life expectancy with regard to other comorbid diseases and the toxicities and adverse effects on quality of life that chemotherapy will bestow. For example, an 88-year-old man with stage III adenocarcinoma of the colon and congestive heart failure has an expected 5-year disease-free survival from his colon cancer of approximately 40% with surgery alone. His disease-free survival would increase to approximately 60% with a year of adjuvant chemotherapy with fluorouracil (5-FU). However, his life expectancy from his cardiac disease is less than 5 years, and the potential toxicities of 5-FU include neutropenia, diarrhea, and mucositis. Therefore, adjuvant therapy would not be indicated for this patient. On the other hand, a 35-year-old woman with the same presentation of a stage III adenocarcinoma of the colon and no other medical conditions would certainly be recommended for adjuvant treatment.

Induction or **neoadjuvant chemotherapy** is the use of chemotherapy, radiation therapy, or a combination of the two as the initial treatment prior to surgery. The theoretical advantage of induction treatment is to "downstage" the tumor: either make an unresectable tumor resectable, or decrease the extent of the surgery.

For example, induction chemotherapy and radiation is successful in advanced laryngeal squamous cell cancers where the larynx can be preserved without changing the survival rate. A second potential benefit of induction treatment is to determine whether a particular chemotherapy regimen is effective while there is still measurable disease and to use these findings to guide postsurgical chemotherapy. For example, in osteogenic sarcomas, neoadjuvant methotrexate is followed by tumor resection, the specimen is evaluated microscopically for response to the methotrexate, and the decision to undergo further chemotherapy is guided by the histopathologic findings.

The criticism against using chemotherapy or radiation therapy before surgery is that nonsurgical staging is less accurate, and postoperative recovery may be slower or more difficult. Another criticism is that if a tumor is not responsive to induction treatment, and actually grows throughout the treatment, the surgery may have to be more extensive, or will no longer be possible to perform.

Induction chemoradiotherapy has become the standard of care in some cancers, such as certain stages of laryngeal carcinoma, anal cancer, bladder cancer, locally advanced breast cancer, and osteogenic sarcomas. Further trials are underway in several neoplasms, including rectal, nasopharyngeal, esophageal, and non-small cell lung cancers, to determine if there is benefit to this approach.

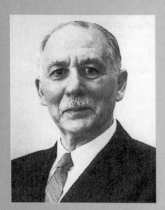

Sidney Farber (1903–1973).

Sidney Farber (1903–1973) is considered one of the founding fathers of modern chemotherapy. He had a special interest in cancer in children and was committed to efforts to combat it. Immediately after World War I, he devoted himself to a study of the stimulating effects of folic acid on bone marrow.

In 1948, he reported the first induction of a complete hematological remission in children with acute leukemia following treatment with a chemical agent (an antimetabolite of folic acid and aminopterin synthesized with Dr Y Subba Row of Lederle Laboratories). Around the same time (1947/1948) he also founded the Children's Cancer Research Foundation in Boston, which became the first institution in the world devoted solely to the study, treatment, and care of children with cancer, especially those with acute leukemia. By 1952, Dr Farber was able to describe a complete, persistent 5-year remission in a group of 50 children with leukemia. He believed strongly that "total care," including physiologic and psychologic care of the patient, was an important component in the success of any regimen.

Sydney Farber was the first chairman of the Cancer Chemotherapy National Committee and also served as president of the American Cancer Society. He was frequently called in as a consultant to Congress on cancer and served as an expert in cancer in the World Health Organization and the US National Program for the Conquest of Cancer. He was awarded three honorary doctor of medicine degrees, four doctor of science degrees, and one doctorate in humane letters, and received more than 20 scientific awards. While at work in his office, he died on March 20, 1973.

Palliation alone may also be a goal of chemotherapy treatment. Palliative chemotherapy implies that reduction of tumor volume and relief of symptoms are the only goals of treatment. Since cure is not a possibility in this setting, the risks and side effects of chemotherapy and the effect on overall quality of life are relatively more important.

PRINCIPLES OF CHEMOTHERAPY

No malignant tumors are curable with a single dose of a single chemotherapy drug. Although certain tumors that are extremely sensitive to chemotherapy (such as leukemia) may have an initial dramatic response to single-drug treatment, the patient will inevitably relapse. Through in

vitro and in vivo observations, theories have been developed to explain the presence of resistance to chemotherapy, tumor growth kinetics, and chemotherapy-induced cell death kinetics. These theories are the basis upon which chemotherapy scheduling, dosing, and administration have been developed (Table 23–4).

Table 23–4. Principles of chemotherapy.

Goldie-Coldman hypothesis	The probability of a tumor having a resistant cell is proportional to the mutation rate and the total number of cells.
Gompertzian kinetics	The growth rate of a tumor decreases exponentially with time.
Log-kill kinetics	A drug kills a constant proportion, not an absolute number, of remaining tumor cells.

Resistance of tumor cells to chemotherapy is one of the primary reasons chemotherapy fails. Resistance is either present before treatment (**intrinsic resistance**) or develops in response to treatment (**acquired resistance**). The **Goldie-Coldman hypothesis** proposes that clinically observed resistance occurs because of "intrinsic resistance." A chemotherapy drug kills all sensitive cells and leaves remaining tumor cells that are resistant to that drug, and these cells have become resistant because of the inherent genetic instability of tumor cells.

The Goldie-Coldman hypothesis is actually a mathematical model predicting the probability of a resistant cell being present as proportional to the total number of tumor cells and the tumor's spontaneous mutation rate. For example, if a 0.5-cm ovarian tumor (approximately the limits of detection) is composed of approximately 10^9 cells and the mutation rate is one in 10^5, then there will be 10^4 resistant cells in this tumor. The patient with this tumor will clinically appear to be in remission after all the sensitive tumor cells are killed, however, 10^4 resistant cells (below the level of clinical detection) remain, and as these cells divide, the tumor will clinically recur and now be resistant to the drug to which it was sensitive before.

The Goldie-Coldman hypothesis also explains why "adjuvant" treatment, which treats patients at a time when there are a minimal number of tumor cells and less chance of a resistant clone, will cure some patients. The same patients would not be curable with chemotherapy if they had lesions of clinically detectable size because the probability of a resistant clone would be essentially 100%. A third, practical implication of the Goldie-Coldman hypothesis is that a combination of drugs with different mechanisms of action (and hence different mechanisms of resistance) will be more effective than single-drug treatment.

A second important concept in understanding why chemotherapy is more effective at a lower tumor burden is the tumor's growth kinetics. The growth rate of a tumor varies depending upon its size, and over time the growth rate decreases. The reasons for this decrease in tumor growth rate are several. First, when a tumor is small, a higher percentage of cells are in an actively dividing phase, or "S phase." As the tumor grows, limits to the growth rate develop, such as a need for its own blood supply to provide nutrients and oxygen. Without the necessary nutrients for growth, more tumor cells die, and a greater proportion of tumor cells enter into a nondividing phase, or "resting phase" (G0) of the cell cycle.

Gompertzian kinetics is a mathematical description of this change in growth rate over time. The Gompertzian curve is S-shaped, with an initial slow rate of growth, then a linear fast rate of growth, and finally a plateau where the growth rate slows down again. Since most chemotherapy drugs are cell-cycle–specific, preferentially working in S phase, chemotherapy will be relatively more effective on tumors that are in the fast growth phase. Like the Goldie-Coldman hypothesis, this principle implies that chemotherapy given in the adjuvant setting, at a time of low

tumor volume, can be curative, but the same chemotherapy regimen given in the setting of gross measurable disease will not be curative.

Another implication of an exponentially decreasing tumor growth rate is that a clinically large difference in tumor volume between patients treated with a particular chemotherapy drug can give similar survival times. For example, suppose two patients with tumors 3.0 cm in diameter are treated with the same chemotherapy drug, and one patient has a partial response (greater than 50% reduction in tumor volume) and the other patient has no response to this drug. After chemotherapy is discontinued, the tumor that has responded to the chemotherapy has a smaller volume, but it is now on a steeper part of the growth curve. Because it is on a steeper part of the growth curve, the tumor now grows more quickly than the tumor in the second patient (that did not respond to the chemotherapy). Therefore, both patients end up with nearly equal survival times.

The initial studies evaluating tumor growth kinetics were performed in murine leukemia models, and recent data from solid tumors suggest that growth rate is more irregular, with periods of tumor growth alternating with periods of dormancy. The smooth Gompertzian growth curve probably does not reflect solid tumor growth rate.

The concept that chemotherapy drugs exhibit a constant log-kill kinetics explains the necessity of administering chemotherapy in repeated "cycles." Skipper published several studies in the 1960s using murine leukemia models to evaluate the rate at which chemotherapy drugs killed tumor cells. He showed that a given chemotherapy drug exhibits specific, constant log-kill kinetics. For example, if a tumor has 10^{11} cells, and the chemotherapy drug has a log-kill rate of 3, after one cycle of chemotherapy there will be 10^8 cells remaining (Figure 23–1). If there is one log growth of the tumor before the next cycle of chemotherapy, there will be 10^9 cells. After a second cycle of drugs with the same log-kill rate of 3, there will be 10^6 cells, and so forth. After two cycles of chemotherapy, disease is no longer detectable, but if treatment was stopped at this time the patient would relapse.

This theory presumes a linear growth rate and the presence of no resistant cells. Even with these limitations, the clinical implication of this model is that multiple courses of therapy will be needed to eradicate a tumor, since each time the same *proportion* of cells, not the same *number* of cells, is killed. Patients must continue treatment, even when there is no clinically detectable disease. Delays in dosing allow the tumor to grow between cycles.

Unfortunately, in real life, tumors do not grow at a constant rate, and tumor cells exhibit intrinsic resistance to, and acquire resistance to, chemotherapy drugs. Therefore, an initial response to chemotherapy is often followed by a relapse, even if there are no unnecessary delays or dose reductions of chemotherapy drugs. Nonetheless, the Goldie-Coldman hypothesis, the Gompertzian growth model, and the concept of a constant log-kill explain the development of the classic method of administering

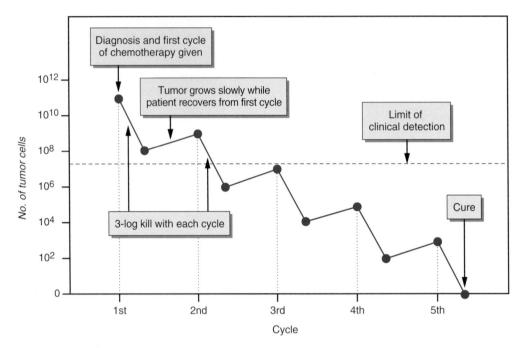

Figure 23–1. Graph showing the concept of constant log-kill kinetics. In this hypothetical patient, the tumor is diagnosed when there are 10^{11} tumor cells. The drug being used to treat the patient has a 3 log-kill rate, so that after one cycle there are 10^8 cells. As the patient recovers from the first cycle of chemotherapy, 1 log cell growth occurs, such that the tumor is composed of 10^9 cells at the time of the second cycle of chemotherapy. After the second cycle, the tumor size is reduced to 10^6 cells, and the disease is no longer clinically detectable. However, if treatment is stopped at this time, the patient will relapse **(dotted line)**. Only if treatment is continued beyond the point of clinically detectable limits is there a potential for cure.

chemotherapy: combining drugs with different mechanisms of action, different mechanisms of resistance, and non-overlapping toxicities, given over repeated cycles.

CHEMOTHERAPY RESISTANCE

Drug resistance is responsible for most chemotherapy treatment failures, and the mechanisms of resistance are multiple. Tumors can be resistant, either by lack of exposure to adequate concentrations of effective drugs or through resistance to the drug itself. With acute leukemias, high-grade lymphomas, and germ cell tumors, patients can relapse because tumor cells are protected from the effects of chemotherapy in sanctuary sites, such as the central nervous system and testes. This pattern of reoccurrence can be avoided if treatment is directed to these anatomically protected sites.

Whereas resistance to chemotherapy drugs because of anatomic location can be observed in vivo, other mechanisms of chemotherapy resistance are much more difficult to evaluate and prove their relative importance in vivo. Therefore, most of our knowledge about cellular mechanisms of drug resistance comes from in vitro and animal models. Through in vitro models, multiple cellular mecha-

nisms of drug resistance are observed, such as decreased uptake of the drug, increased efflux of the drug, decreased activation of the drug, altered target enzymes, cellular repair of drug-induced damage, or inactivation of the drug (Table 23–5).

As discussed earlier, Goldie and Coldman showed that the probability of preexisting, or intrinsic, chemotherapy resistance exponentially increases with tumor size. Unfortunately, in addition to intrinsic resistance, tumor cells can also acquire resistance, as shown through DNA transfer studies where drug-resistant cells confer resistance to previously drug-sensitive cells.

Gene amplification is also an "induced" type of chemotherapy resistance. For example, cells grown in gradually increasing concentrations of methotrexate gradually amplify the gene that produces dihydrofolate reduc-

Table 23–5. Mechanisms of drug resistance.

1. Decreased uptake
2. Increased efflux
3. Decreased activation
4. Altered target enzyme
5. Inactivation of drug
6. Gene amplification
7. Increased repair of drug-induced damage

tase. The alteration of target proteins is another form of "induced" resistance. Cells grown in increasing concentrations of vincristine alter their tubulin structure.

Development of resistance to one chemotherapy drug can lead to cross-resistance to structurally unrelated drugs. One of the most widely studied types of cross-resistance is the multidrug resistance (MDR) phenotype. MDR clinically presents as cross-resistance to anthracyclines, taxanes, epipodophyllotoxins, and vinca alkaloids: all "natural product" chemotherapy agents. One cause of MDR are *mdr 1* genes that encode for P-glycoprotein, which functions as an efflux pump that actively transports the antineoplastic drugs out of the cells. Interestingly, normal cells of the biliary tract and renal tubules express high levels of P-glycoprotein, suggesting that P-glycoprotein's normal function is to excrete environmental toxins from the body. Attempts at blocking these efflux pumps have been successful in vitro with verapamil, quinidine, cyclosporine, and newer cyclosporine analogues, and in hematologic malignancies early clinical studies are encouraging. Other mechanisms of multidrug resistance have been described: alterations in topoisomerase II activity (that infer cross-resistance to anthracyclines, etoposide, and mitoxantrone), alterations of drug-conjugating enzymes, such as glutathione S-transferase (an enzyme used to detoxify hydrogen peroxide), alterations in components of the cytochrome P-450 enzyme, and alterations in drug transport enzymes, like glucuronyl transferase. Mutation in the tumor suppressor gene p53 inactivates the gene and decreases chemotherapy-induced apoptosis.

There are certainly many more mechanisms of resistance that have not yet been elucidated; again, the relative importance of many of these mechanisms in vivo is still unknown. However, continued improvement in our understanding of the mechanisms of chemotherapy resistance will lead to more rational drug combinations and the development of methods to counteract resistance.

DOSE INTENSITY

Dose intensity is the amount of chemotherapy drug given over a specific time, or, in pharmacological terms, the area under the curve. The importance of avoiding unnecessary delays and unnecessary dose reductions is shown in the concept of log-kill kinetics: between consecutive cycles of chemotherapy the tumor grows, therefore, the time between cycles should be as short as possible. In vitro studies of murine leukemia cells support the importance of dose intensity by showing that a 20% decrease in dose leads to a 50% decrease in cure. As discussed earlier, there are also in vitro data showing that sublethal chemotherapy doses induce drug resistance.

Retrospective reviews of chemotherapy dosing in lymphomas and in ovarian, colon, and breast cancer have shown lower complete response rates and cure rates in patients who receive reduced doses. Since lower doses of chemotherapy are not as effective as standard doses, these

findings have raised the question of whether a higher-than-standard dose of chemotherapy may be even more effective. With the utilization of growth factors and bone marrow and stem cell support, very high doses of chemotherapy have become feasible. In acute leukemias, Hodgkin's disease, and certain non-Hodgkin's lymphomas, high doses of chemotherapy with bone marrow support definitely cure some patients who are not cured with standard chemotherapy doses. Several early trials suggest there may be benefit to high-dose chemotherapy and stem cell support in solid tumors such as breast, testicular, and ovarian cancer, and further trials are underway.

CHEMOTHERAPY TRIALS

Bringing a promising new drug from the laboratory into a patient is accomplished through a specific order of trials designed to evaluate toxicity, optimum dosing, and efficacy (Table 23–6). First, a drug that is suspected in vitro to have activity against tumor cells is screened against several human tumor cell lines. If the drug has antitumor activity, then toxicology testing in mice is performed to determine the dose that is lethal to 10% of mice (LD10). Confirmatory toxicology studies are usually performed on larger animals, and the drug is cleared for human use.

Chemotherapy trials are divided into phases as a new drug is brought from animal testing into human trials and eventually compared to the standard treatment. Phase I trials are dose-finding toxicity trials. Only patients for whom there is no standard approved treatment may be enrolled in Phase I trials. Because they are dose-finding studies, the patients usually must have essentially normal renal and hepatic function and a several-months life expectancy, as side effects need to be referable to the drug being tested and not to the underlying disease. In Phase I trials, the dose of the experimental drug is usually started as low as 1/10th of the mouse LD10 and gradually increased, either with each cycle or with each cohort of patients, until a dose-limiting toxicity determines the maximum tolerated dose.

If the drug shows any suggestion of response in a Phase I study and is well tolerated, a Phase II trial will treat a

Table 23–6. Chemotherapy trials.

Preclinical trials
1. Screen or develop a new drug
2. In vitro trials on tumor cell lines
3. Determine the LD10[1] in mouse toxicology studies
4. Confirmatory large animal toxicology studies

Clinical trials
1. Phase I—dose-finding
2. Phase II—determine response rate
3. Phase III—randomized trial to compare new drug to standard treatment

[1]LD10 is the dose that is lethal in 10% of mice.

group of patients (anywhere from 14–90) with the maximum tolerated dose to determine a response rate. (If there are no responses in the first 14 patients, the drug statistically has less than the 20% response rate necessary to be a potentially beneficial drug, and usually the trial is discontinued). If the response rate with the new drug appears to be better than standard treatments with similar or less toxicity, a prospective, randomized, Phase III trial can be done to directly compare the new regimen to the standard "best available" treatments.

Several problems are inherent in testing new drugs with this method. A frequently observed phenomenon is that results in Phase II trials are better than what is eventually observed in the final Phase III trial. This finding has been attributed to Phase II patients tending to be younger, healthier, and more compliant. Also, Phase II trials are usually done at one institution, and adherence to dosing and scheduling criteria may be better. It can be tempting to treat patients with a new, unproven regimen that has good preliminary Phase II results and not enroll the patients in the subsequent and necessary Phase III trials. Unfortunately, the medical literature is filled with promising Phase II drugs that turned out to be no better, or even worse, than standard treatments once the direct randomized comparison was done.

Another psychological obstacle in randomized trials is encountered when the experimental treatment appears so much more effective than the standard treatment that patients resist enrollment (such as in the present trial evaluating adjuvant treatment for gastric cancer that randomizes patients to no treatment versus treatment with radiation and chemotherapy). Although such obstacles exist, it is imperative that physicians continue to encourage patients to enroll in appropriate clinical trials whenever possible.

ANTINEOPLASTIC DRUGS

ALKYLATING AGENTS

Alkylating agents were among the first nonhormonal drugs found to be cytotoxic when, in World War II, nitrogen mustard was found to cause myelosuppression. The alkylating agents exert their effect by producing a positively charged alkyl group capable of attacking a negatively charged nucleophilic site. These negatively charged nucleophilic groups can be the nitrogen, oxygen, or phosphorous groups found in DNA, as well as proteins and RNA. DNA alkylation produces a variety of defects, such as double- and single-stranded breaks and interstrand crosslinks, which all disrupt DNA replication and transcription. If the cell cannot efficiently repair these defects, cell death or mutation occurs.

Alkylating agents are most effective in rapidly dividing cells. However, since they react with preformed nucleic acids, they are active throughout all phases of the cell cycle and are, therefore, effective in slowly dividing tumors as well, such as multiple myeloma. Because of their cell cycle nonspecificity, increasing the dose increases cellular damage; for this reason, high-dose alkylators are an integral part of the preparative regimens for bone marrow transplantation. Many of the drugs in this category can be given orally as well as intravenously, although gastrointestinal absorption is not always reliable.

The nitrogen mustards include mechlorethamine, melphalan, chlorambucil, cyclophosphamide, ifosfamide, and the nitrosoureas. Mechlorethamine is the parent compound, used in the "MOPP" (mechlorethamine, vincristine, prednisone, procarbazine) regimen against Hodgkin's disease. Other drugs in this category are all derivatives of mechlorethamine. The dose-limiting toxicity of most of the alkylating agents is generally bone marrow toxicity; taken over prolonged periods of time or at high doses, alkylating agents cause prolonged or permanent marrow failure. The alkylators are also leukemogenic, with mechlorethamine (the worst offender) causing a nearly 100-fold increase in leukemia. Other long-term side effects include permanent sterility, with amenorrhea in women and oligospermia in men. Most of the metabolites of alkylating agents are excreted by the kidney, and doses need to be adjusted for renal insufficiency.

Melphalan is used to treat multiple myeloma, acute myelogenous leukemia, breast cancer, Ewing's sarcoma, melanoma, neuroblastoma, and ovarian cancers. Chlorambucil is effective in chronic lymphocytic leukemia and some non-Hodgkin's lymphomas. Busulfan is an oral agent used in chronic myelogenous leukemia and bone marrow transplant regimens.

Cyclophosphamide and ifosfamide are unique in requiring liver metabolization through the microsomal P-450 system to change to their active forms. Cyclophosphamide is widely used in lymphomas and breast and ovarian cancer regimens. Ifosfamide is used in regimens for testicular cancer, sarcomas, and lung cancer. Cyclophosphamide and its analogue ifosfamide cause sterile hemorrhagic cystitis, which can occur at any dose level but is generally dose-related. Very high doses of cyclophosphamide (> 1.5 g/m^2) cause cardiac necrosis. High-dose ifosfamide causes a reversible change in mental status in approximately 30% of patients.

Because of their lipid solubility, the nitrosoureas (bischloroethyl-nitrosourea [BCNU, or carmustine], and chloroethylcyclohexylnitrosourea [CCNU, or lomustine]) have better central nervous system penetration and are used in the treatment of brain tumors, non-Hodgkin's and Hodgkin's lymphomas, melanoma, multiple myeloma, and gastrointestinal tumors. Thiotepa is a second-line drug for ovarian and breast cancers and is locally instilled for superficial bladder tumors.

Less commonly used alkylators include hexamethylmelamine, dacarbazine (dimethyl triazeno imidazole carboxamide, or DTIC), and procarbazine. Hexamethylmelamine also methylates DNA, although it is not completely cross-resistant with other alkylators. It can be taken orally, making it attractive as a second-line treatment primarily used in ovarian cancer, but nausea and vomiting is frequently the dose-limiting toxicity. Dacarbazine is used in Hodgkin's disease, melanoma, and sarcomas. Given intravenously, its most significant side effect is nausea and vomiting, but it can also cause a flulike syndrome, photosensitivity, and, according to several reports, fatal hepatic veno-oclusive disease. Procarbazine is an oral drug used in Hodgkin's disease and brain tumors that is related structurally to monoamine oxidase inhibitors, so foods containing tyramine (wine, bananas, yogurt, cheese) must be omitted from the diet to avoid a hypertensive crisis. Tricyclic antidepressants and sympathomimetic drugs should also not be combined with procarbazine. Procarbazine causes nausea and vomiting and can cause a hypersensitivity reaction manifested by dermatitis and pulmonary infiltrates.

ANTIFOLATES

In 1948, it was found that an analog of folic acid, aminopterin, induced short-term remissions in leukemia. The development of **methotrexate** (MTX), a 4-amino, 10-methyl analog of folic acid, followed. As purine and pyrimidine synthesis was better understood, other antimetabolites, such as fluoropyrimidines and nucleoside analogs, were developed.

Folate pools are stored intracellularly in a reduced tetrahydrofolate form and serve as carbon carriers, which are needed for the synthesis of pyrimidines and purines. These tetrahydrofolates are formed by the reduction of dihydrofolates by the catalyst dihydrofolate reductase (DHFR) (Figure 23–2). Along with helping in the synthesis of pyrimidines and purines, tetrahydrofolates also provide a methyl group so that deoxyuridylate (dUMP) can be converted to thymidylate (dTMP) using thymidylate synthase as the catalyst. When MTX is actively taken up by the cell, it binds to DHFR, and the intracellular concentration of tetrahydrofolates decreases, inhibiting the production of purine, pyrimidines, and dTMP. Methotrexate can bind to DHFR in its native state or after transforming to its polyglutamate form, which has a slower dissociation rate. The polyglutamate form of MTX also directly inhibits other enzymes, such as thymidylate synthase, glycineamide ribonucleotide transformylase (GAR), and aminoimidazole carboxamide ribonucleotide transformylase (AICAR), used in the production of purine synthesis. Reduced folates, such as 5-foryltetrahydrofolate (leucovorin), replete the tetrahydrofolates and also compete with methotrexate to override the inhibition of thymidylate synthase and AICAR, thereby "rescuing" the cell from the toxic effects of MTX.

MTX is used in the treatment of leukemia, breast cancer, head and neck cancers, lymphomas, osteogenic sarcoma, and choriocarcinomas, as well as non-neoplastic

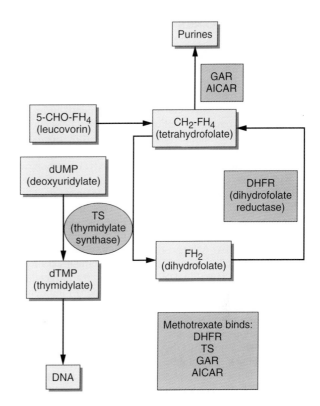

Figure 23–2. Diagram of the formation of tetrahydrofolates. AICAR = aminoimidazole carboxamide ribonucleotide transformylase; GAR = glycineamide ribonucleotide transformylase; TS = thymidylate synthase.

processes, such as rheumatoid arthritis and graft-versus-host disease.

MTX is distributed into third-space fluid collections, such as pleural fluid and ascites, and must be significantly dose-reduced, or the fluid removed before treatment. MTX elimination is through the kidneys, and if given in high doses, adequate hydration and urine alkylination is essential to avoid intratubular precipitation. Some lymphomas, osteogenic sarcoma, gastric cancer, and acute leukemia regimens use doses of MTX (500 mg/m^2) that would be lethal without leucovorin rescue. Leucovorin should be administered at the end of the MTX infusion and continued until the plasma concentration is less than 5×10^{-8}.

The primary toxicity of MTX is myelosuppression and gastrointestinal mucositis. It can cause hepatotoxicity, pneumonitis, and, when given intrathecally (for certain lymphomas and acute leukemias), an acute arachnoiditis. Months to years later, children can develop a demyelinating encephalopathy.

A new antifolate entering clinical trials is trimetrexate, a lipophilic antifolate that avoids MTX resistance caused by transport deficiencies. There are also new thymidylate synthase inhibitors and inhibitors of GAR in Phase I and II trials.

FLUOROPYRIMIDINES

The fluoropyrimidine **5-fluorouracil** (5-FU) was synthesized when it was noted that rat hepatoma cells used uracil more efficiently than normal rat intestinal mucosa. All the fluoropyrimidines require intracellular activation to be cytotoxic. 5-FU is converted to fluorodeoxyuridine (FUDR) by thymidine phosphorylase, then FUDR is phosphorylated by thymidine kinase to make fluorodeoxyuridylate (FdUMP) (Figure 23–3). In the presence of tetrahydrofolates, FdUMP inhibits thymidylate synthase activity, which depletes deoxythymidine triphosphate (dTTP), which in turn is a precursor for DNA synthesis. 5-FU has other mechanisms of action; it can be converted to fluorouridine (FUR) or fluorouridine monophosphate (FUMP), which is converted to a triphosphate and incorporated into DNA. As opposed to methotrexate, in which leucovorin "rescues" the cell, leucovorin augments the cytotoxicity of 5-FU and FUDR by increasing the intracellular pool of tetrahydrofolates, thereby increasing binding to thymidylate synthase.

Dipyridamole is a nucleoside transport inhibitor that inhibits the uptake of thymidine, so that dTTP pools are decreased (required for DNA synthesis), and it increases the intracellular formation of FdUMP. One randomized trial in colorectal cancer found that dipyridamole increased the serum concentration of 5-FU, but there was no correlating clinical benefit.

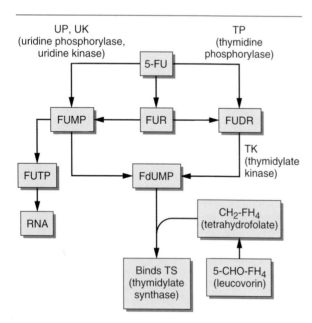

Figure 23–3. Metabolism of 5-fluorouracil (5-FU). 5-FU is converted to fluorodeoxyuridine (FUDR) by thymidine kinase to make fluorodeoxyuridylate (FdUMP). FUDP = fluorouridine diphosphate; FUMP = fluorouridine monophosphate; FUR = fluorouridine; FUTP = fluorouridine triphosphate.

FUDR is available as a separate drug, but it is rapidly degraded and, therefore, only used in hepatic artery infusions. 5-FU and its derivatives have activity in gastrointestinal cancers, head and neck cancers, and breast and ovarian cancers. It appears to be synergistic with irradiation and other drugs and, therefore, is frequently used in combined-modality regimens.

5-FU produces toxicity to the gastrointestinal tract and bone marrow, which varies by dosing, schedule, and route of administration, with bolus causing more myelosuppression and the continuous infusion more stomatitis and diarrhea. Stomatitis and diarrhea occur 8–12 days after treatment and can be life-threatening if the drug is not discontinued or support therapy is delayed. When given through the hepatic artery, continuous infusion 5-FU or FUDR causes biliary sclerosis. Reversible hand-foot syndrome, cerebellar ataxia, blepharitis, and conjunctivitis are other side effects of the fluoropyrimidines.

Ongoing studies are evaluating oral preparations of 5-FU and combining 5-FU with immune modulators, such as interferons and interleukin-2, and PALA (N-(phosphonacetyl)-L-aspartate), a drug that inhibits the enzyme aspartate transcarbamylase, which is needed in pyrimidine synthesis.

NUCLEOSIDE ANALOGS

Cytarabine is an arabinose nucleoside isolated from the sponge *Cryptothethya crypta*. As an analog of nucleoside 2π-deoxycytidine, an inhibitor of DNA polymerase-alpha, it inhibits DNA synthesis. It is also incorporated directly into DNA, inhibiting template function and causing ligation defects in newly synthesized DNA. Cytarabine is a standard drug in the treatment of acute myelogenous leukemia (AML), childhood acute lymphocytic leukemia (ALL), and some high-grade lymphomas. Its major toxicities are myelosuppression, nausea, vomiting, and diarrhea, reversible intrahepatic cholestases and reported cases of pancreatitis. With high-dose cytarabine, there can be cerebral dysfunction. Cytarabine can be given intrathecally where, rarely, it can cause fever, seizures, and a change in mental status.

PURINE ANALOGS

The **purine analogs** are a group of drugs that include 6-mercaptopurine (6-MP), 6-thioguanosine (6-TG), deoxycoformycin, fludarabine, and 2-chlorodeoxyadenosine (2-CdA). In the same class of drugs are the non-chemotherapy drugs: azathioprine, allopurinol, and acyclovir. The oldest drugs are 6-MP and 6-TG, which are inhibitors of guanine synthesis. These drugs exert their cytotoxicity in three ways: by inhibiting de novo purine synthesis, inhibiting purine interconversion reactions, and incorporating their nucleotide metabolites into nucleic acids. 6-MP is used in the maintenance therapy of ALL, and 6-TG is used in AML. The primary toxicities are myelosuppression and gastrointestinal side effects.

Fludarabine and 2-CdA are analogs of adenosine used in the treatment of low-grade lymphomas and chronic lymphocytic leukemia. Fludarabine undergoes phosphorylation into an active triphosphate form that inhibits DNA polymerase and ribonucleotide reductase and, therefore, DNA synthesis. 2-CdA is resistant to adenosine deaminase, so it accumulates in cells in its triphosphate form; feedback inhibition decreases the other deoxynucleotide precursors necessary for DNA synthesis. Both drugs are excreted by the kidney and are myelosuppressive. Fludarabine also causes a peripheral sensorimotor neuropathy. 2P-deoxycoformycin is an adenosine deaminase inhibitor that induces remissions in hairy cell leukemia and is also effective against T-cell ALL, T-cell CLL, and mycosis fungoides. Like 2-CdA, it also increases intracellular concentrations of deoxyadenosine triphosphates, leading to decreased levels of the deoxynucleotide precursors necessary for DNA synthesis. Toxicities include central nervous system dysfunction, elevated liver enzymes, decreased renal function, nausea, vomiting, conjunctivitis, and immunosuppression.

L-ASPARAGINASE

L-asparaginase is an enzyme isolated from *Escherichia coli* or *Erwinia carotovora* used in the treatment of childhood ALL. The enzyme lowers L-asparagine concentrations, which are needed for protein synthesis. Its primary toxicity is the development of hypersensitivity to the drug in approximately half of patients. The other adverse effects are related to the inhibition of normal protein synthesis, with the development of hypoalbuminemia, decreased anticoagulant and clotting factors (causing thrombosis of the major vessels 6–10 days after treatment), decreased serum insulin levels, and acute pancreatitis.

ANTINEOPLASTIC ANTIBIOTICS

This group of chemotherapy drugs, which includes bleomycin, the anthracyclines, mitoxantrone, mitomycin C, dactinomycin, and mithramycin, are structurally diverse but all isolated from the fungus *Streptomyces*.

The **anthracyclines**—doxorubicin, daunorubicin, epirubicin, and idarubicin—are characterized by an anthraquinone ring attached to an amino sugar. There are several ways anthracyclines exert their cytotoxicity: by inhibiting topoisomerase II, intercalating DNA, and creating free radicals. Topoisomerase II controls the degree of supercoiling of DNA by creating double-strand breaks so that one strand of DNA can pass through another strand. Anthracyclines allow topoisomerase II to bind to the DNA and cause the intended double-strand breaks, but inhibit the topoisomerase II from ligating the broken strands back together. Anthracyclines also intercalate between base

pairs of DNA to produce single- and double-stranded DNA cuts that impair DNA repair. Finally, the third mechanism of action is for the anthracycline to reduce ferric iron to ferrous iron, and in its oxidized form the anthracycline reacts with O_2 to make the free radical, superoxidase (O_2-). Superoxidase attacks DNA and disrupts cell membranes.

Anthracyclines are used against many tumor types. Doxorubicin is used in breast cancer, ovarian cancer, sarcomas, and lymphomas. Daunorubicin and idarubicin are doxorubicin analogs used in the treatment of AML.

Anthracyclines cause bone marrow suppression, alopecia, and nausea and are potent vesicants, but their major toxicity is the production of an irreversible cardiomyopathy. Free radicals are thought to be the cause of the cardiac damage, because heart tissue does not have the necessary catalase enzyme system to detoxify free radicals. The cardiac toxicity is cumulative, with a lifetime maximum dose of doxorubicin of 550 mg/m^2. In practice, doxorubicin is usually discontinued after 450 mg/m^2, or continued past this point only with close cardiac monitoring.

The gold standard to determine the extent of cardiac damage is an endocardial biopsy, but for obvious reasons it is impractical. Radionuclide cineangiography (MUGA scanning) is used, therefore, to follow cardiac function. Below 450 mg/m^2 the development of cardiomyopathy still sporadically occurs (1–2%). The cardiotoxic effects of the anthracycline are increased in the setting of long-standing hypertension or radiation to the heart, or with the co-administration of cyclophosphamide or mitomycin C. Prolonging the infusion of doxorubicin from its usual intravenous push to 72 hours decreases the cardiotoxic effects. The EDTA (ethylenediaminetetraacetic acid) analog, dexrazoxane, decreases cardiac toxicity by chelating iron but may also reduce its effectiveness.

Mitoxantrone is a synthetic drug based on the anthracycline structure with the same mechanism of action, except that the mitoxantrone semiquinone free radical is unreactive. Therefore, it still causes DNA cleavage through inhibition of topoisomerase II, but it does not produce the same extent of cardiac toxicity. It is used in lymphomas and breast cancer, usually as second-line treatment. Hematologic and cardiac toxicities as well as mucositis are dose-limiting.

Mitomycin C is the only chemotherapy agent that is more active in a hypoxic environment. It is used primarily in gastrointestinal tumors and in non-small cell lung cancer. Its hematologic effects are cumulative such that, usually, only 3–4 doses can be given before the dose must be reduced. A rare complication is the development of hemolytic uremic syndrome (renal failure, hemolytic anemia, thrombocytopenia, or mental status changes). Treatment is generally not effective, but plasmapheresis may help. Mitomycin C can also cause a dose-related pneumonitis and cardiomyopathy.

Bleomycin is used in the treatment of germ cell tumors and lymphomas. Unusual among chemotherapy drugs, it has essentially no gastrointestinal or bone marrow toxicity. Bleomycin forms a complex with iron and oxygen that binds to DNA, causing single- and double-stranded DNA breaks through oxygen-mediated free radical formation. It can be given by subcutaneous, intramuscular, intravenous, or intrapleural (sclerosis of malignant effusions) administration.

Its primary toxicity is a pneumonitis, thought to be caused by the stimulation of collagen synthesis, a direct effect on pulmonary arteriole and veins, and the release of nitric oxide. Toxicity is more frequent in older patients (over 70), in patients who have a history of underlying lung disease, and in patients who have a history of radiation therapy to the lungs. It is important to note that a history of bleomycin exposure predisposes patients to respiratory failure after high concentrations of inspired oxygen (such as during surgery to remove residual masses in nonseminomatous germ cell tumors). A non–life-threatening, but common, transient side effect is fever (sometimes greater than 40°C) and chills the first 24 hours after administration, which should be treated with prophylactic acetaminophen and diphenhydramine.

Less commonly used drugs derived from *Streptomyces* are dactinomycin and mithramycin. Dactinomycin is used in Wilms' tumors, Ewing's sarcomas, rhabdomyosarcomas, choriocarcinomas, testicular carcinomas, Kaposi's sarcomas, and lymphomas. Its side effects are nausea and vomiting, and it causes a "recall" effect if given after radiation therapy. Mithramycin works by inhibiting RNA synthesis and is used in testicular carcinoma and also to treat hypercalcemia caused by any malignancy.

Mithramycin causes renal and hepatic toxicity as well as nausea, vomiting, myelosuppression, and mucositis and can affect clotting enzymes and platelets, causing a bleeding diathesis.

TAXANES

Paclitaxel is extracted from the bark of the Pacific yew *Taxus brevifolia*. Paclitaxel and its analog, docetaxel, can now can be semisynthesized from needles of other yew species. Paclitaxel is first-line treatment for ovarian cancers, and both paclitaxel and docetaxel are used in breast cancer and non-small cell lung cancer.

The **taxanes** work by binding to microtubules and promoting and stabilizing microtubule assembly. Paclitaxel can be given over 1–24 hours, with the shorter period causing less myelosuppression. The taxanes are excreted through bile. The toxicities include neutropenia, alopecia, myalgias, and a hypersensitivity reaction. The hypersensitivity reaction, which is manifested by significant bronchospasm, urticaria, diaphoresis, and hypotension, occurs only 5–10% of the time if the patient is premedicated with steroids, diphenhydramine, and H_2 antagonists. Docetaxel has the added toxicity of fluid retention.

PLATINUM DRUGS

This group of drugs was discovered when it was found that platinum electrodes inhibited the growth of bacteria. Their cytotoxicity appears to be related to the platinum creating interstrand crosslinks to DNA. Cisplatin-based regimens can cure most nonseminomatous testicular cancers, are first-line treatment for ovarian cancers, and are used in head and neck, esophageal, gastric, non-small cell and small cell lung cancers.

Renal toxicity is dose-limiting for cisplatin given as a single dose, and ototoxicity is dose-limiting for cisplatin given as a continuous infusion over several days. A 24-hour creatinine clearance is obtained prior to dosing the drug, and close monitoring of patients is imperative to ensure adequate hydration and the avoidance of nephrotoxicity.

Cisplatin is also among the most emetic drugs used in oncology, causing both acute and delayed (up to 3–4 days later) nausea and vomiting. Cisplatin can be used intraperitoneally, because peak peritoneal concentrations are 21 times higher than peak plasma concentrations.

Carboplatin is a cisplatin analog that has less renal toxicity, but more myelotoxicity. Because there is less nausea and it does not require the high intravenous fluid rate that cisplatin does, carboplatin is better tolerated by patients, but in vitro data suggest that it may not be quite as effective as cisplatin. Results from clinical trials are conflicting about its comparative effectiveness. Because carboplatin is an easier drug for the patient to receive, if renal function precludes cisplatin use, or if palliation is the goal, carboplatin is sometimes substituted for cisplatin.

VINCA ALKALOIDS

The **vinca alkaloids** are extracts of the periwinkle plant, originally found to cause myelosuppression in rats, which led to the isolation of vincristine, vinblastine, vindesine, and vinorelbine. These drugs exert their cytotoxicity by binding to the protein tubulin. The normal function of tubulin is to polymerize and form the microtubular apparatus along which chromosomes migrate during mitosis. Tubulin also serves as a neurotransmitter transport along axons. Vinca alkaloids bind to tubulin and stop its polymerization. The cells are then arrested in metaphase and cell lysis follows.

Vincristine is used to treat ALL, Hodgkin's and non-Hodgkin's lymphomas, Wilms' tumor, Ewing's sarcoma, neuroblastoma, rhabdomyosarcoma, multiple myeloma, and breast and small cell lung cancer. Vinblastine is used in testicular cancer and Hodgkin's disease regimens. Vinorelbine is used in breast and lung cancer, and vindesine has similar activity to vincristine. The vinca alkaloids are eliminated primarily via the biliary tract. Their primary side effect is neurotoxicity, manifested by paresthesias in the fingers and toes, a loss of deep tendon reflexes, and constipation. With increasing cumulative dose, more severe neurotoxicity can occur, including motor neuron weakness and paralytic ileus. The drugs are all vesicants.

Etoposide is a semisynthetic derivative of the naturally occurring epipodophyllotoxin isolated from the root of the May apple plant. Epipodophyllotoxin is a multi-ring agent that causes DNA strand breaks by interfering with the reunion reaction of topoisomerase II. Although its gastrointestinal absorption is not completely reliable, it can be taken orally as well as intravenously. It is used in lymphomas, in small cell lung cancers, and germ cell tumors. Etoposide is myelosuppressive, and higher doses cause mucositis and hypotension.

RETINOIDS

Retinoids are analogs of vitamin A (retinol). Proteins that bind retinoids in the cytoplasm appear to play a role in the control of differentiation and proliferation. All-*trans*-retinoic acid induces complete remissions in acute promyelocytic leukemia, and cis-retinoic acid decreases the incidence of second malignancies in head and neck cancers. Cis-retinoic acid is presently undergoing trials in the treatment of squamous cell cancer of the skin and cervical cancer.

The toxicities of the retinoids are similar to those seen with hypervitaminosis A: nausea, vomiting, anorexia, headache, dizziness, fatigue, irritability, and hyperostosis. In patients with acute promyelocytic leukemia, it can cause an initial leukocytosis due to differentiation of the leukemic cells in the marrow. This leukocytosis can be accompanied by fever, pulmonary infiltrates, and pleural and pericardial effusions and usually responds to high-dose steroids.

CAMPTOTHECINS

Topoisomerase I causes a break in a single strand of DNA, binds to the nucleic acid of the broken strand, then allows passage of the unbroken strand through the break site and re-ligates the cleaved DNA. **Camptothecin** is a heterocyclic alkaloid isolated from the stem of *Camptotheca acuminata* that inhibits the re-ligation step of topoisomerase I, but is too toxic to use as a chemotherapy drug. The analog of camptothecin, CPT-11, has produced response rates in colorectal, lung, ovarian, and cervical cancer and in non-Hodgkin's lymphoma. Topotecan has produced early reports of responses in non-small cell lung cancer. The dose-limiting toxicity for both drugs is neutropenia and, with CPT-11, some gastrointestinal toxicity.

HORMONAL THERAPY

With the discovery of cortisone, hormones became the first drugs found to be useful in the treatment of malignant disease. The most clinically useful hormones have continued to be steroid hormones, which work by binding to intracellular receptors and stimulating or repressing specific mRNAs, thereby altering cell function and growth. Their specific mechanisms of action are not completely understood, but they are only effective in tumors that have retained part of the hormonal sensitivity of their tissue of origin, such as breast, prostate, endometrial, and ovarian cancers.

For example, blocking the androgen receptor produces a response in 80% of patients with metastatic prostate cancer. Flutamide blocks the androgen receptor from the androgens secreted by the adrenal gland, and luteinizing hormone-releasing hormone (LHRH) analogues (leuprolide, cetrorelix) suppress pituitary release of luteinizing hormone (decreasing androgen production). Unfortunately, except for tamoxifen in the adjuvant treatment of breast cancer, no hormonal therapy cures any malignant tumor. Furthermore, over time, tumors that are initially controlled with hormonal therapy gradually become more poorly differentiated, less dependent upon hormonal stimulation, and resistant to hormonal therapy.

BIOLOGICAL AGENTS

Immunotherapy was developed as an attempt to either increase the host immune response or make the tumor appear "more foreign." Simplified, B lymphocytes secrete antibodies in response to foreign antigens, and T lymphocytes secrete cytokines (interferons and interleukins) in response to the combination of a foreign antigen and the major histocompatibility antigens (MHC). There are multiple levels of interactions, with both negative and positive feedback loops between the cells of the immune system; there are also other cells (such as endothelial cells and monocytes) involved in cytokine production and modulation that are proving to be more intricate. Only the information necessary to understand present clinical trials is presented here. The interested reader is referred elsewhere for an extensive review.

To achieve antitumor effects, the immune system can be altered either actively or passively. **Active immunization** is the process of injecting an antigen to stimulate an immune response. **Passive**, or **adoptive, immunotherapy** is the process of injecting patients with the actual immune effector cells themselves.

The first attempts at immunization against tumors were through active, nonspecific immunization using antigens, such as the bacillus Calmette-Guérin (BCG), *Corynebac-*

terium, and levamisole. BCG is successful at decreasing the recurrence of superficial bladder cancers. Levamisole was originally developed as an antihelminthic drug that was found in vitro to improve the function of macrophages and T lymphocytes. It is still used in conjunction with 5-FU in the adjuvant treatment of colon cancer. Alone, levamisole as an anticancer drug is ineffective, and whether it actually contributes to the effects of 5-FU is controversial.

The **interferons** (IF) and **interleukins** (IL) are cytokines that have been used in an attempt to actively stimulate the immune system in a more specific fashion. The interferons (α, β, ω, γ, with IF-α further subtyped into 1, 2, etc) are a family of proteins that are produced in response to the presence of infections, double-stranded RNA, and antigens. The functions of interferons include immune modulation, inhibition of angiogenesis, reduction of cell proliferation, and enhancement of expression of certain cell surface antigens.

Interferon-α-2 is the clinically available drug. It produces response rates of nearly 90% in hairy cell leukemia and chronic myelogenous leukemia, and an equally high response rate in some local malignant processes, such as cervical intraepithelial neoplasia and epidermal basal cell and superficial bladder cancers.

The interleukins (1, 2, 3, etc) include IL-2 as the commercially available drug; 1, 4, 6, and 12 are in clinical trials. IL-2 appears to activate and cause proliferation of T lymphocytes and natural killer cells. In turn, these IL-2–activated cells secrete secondary cytokines, such as IL-1, tumor necrosis factor (TNF), and IF-γ. Used alone, IL-2 produces a response rate of 10–15% in melanoma and renal cell cancers. Its toxicity comes from increased vascular permeability with decreased systemic vascular resistance, pulmonary edema, nausea and vomiting, diarrhea, azotemia, and hyperbilirubinemia.

Unfortunately, active immunization has not been very successful in disseminated solid tumors, presumably because of our limited understanding of the interactions within the immune system as well as impairments in immune responsiveness in oncology patients. Malignant tumors secrete suppressive factors, tumor antigens are heterogeneous, and even the MHC antigens on tumor cells are altered, impairing recognition by the immune system.

Passive immunotherapy is the process of injecting patients with stimulated immune cells. Lymphocytes stimulated in vitro with IL-2 are transformed into lymphocyte-activated killer cells (LAK cells) that are non-MHC–restricted killer cells. Response rates of 20% have been seen in renal cell cancer and melanomas with this therapy. T cells can also be extracted from the host's tumor (tumor infiltrating lymphocytes, or TILs) and then stimulated in vitro with IL-2 and injected back into the patient. In vitro studies suggest that these IL-2–stimulated TIL cells are 50 times more tumor-specific than LAK cells, but the early clinical studies have not shown any improvement over IL-2 alone in renal cell carcinoma or melanoma.

Another method of passive immunotherapy under investigation is the use of monoclonal antibodies (usually mouse antibodies against human tumor antigens such as carcinoembryonic antigen [CEA] or beta human chorionic gonadotropin [βHCG]) that can be given alone or conjugated with toxins or radioactive compounds. The development of human anti-mouse antibodies (HAMA) frequently limits the number of doses a patient can tolerate. Passive immunotherapy with anti-idiotype monoclonal antibodies and radiolabeled monoclonal antibodies have been tried in low-grade lymphomas with some anecdotal success. A specific anti-idiotype antibody must be created for each individual (Table 23–7).

Although all of these immunotherapy methods sound promising, and measurable response rates have been observed, no overall change in survival with immunotherapy alone has been demonstrated in any solid tumors, except in the case of BCG in superficial bladder cancers. However, most of these early trials have been small studies, frequently performed on patients with large tumor bulk. Trials are underway using these biological modifiers in an adjuvant setting, where they may prove to be more effective.

GENE THERAPY

Gene therapy is the idea of introducing a specific gene into a target cell. As an antineoplastic technique, there are several ideas under investigation including: (1) inserting a gene that makes cytokines (eg, IL-2) into a tumor cell or into a normal immune cell; (2) inserting genes (such as *mdr 1*, encoding for multidrug resistance) into normal blood stem cells to protect against cytotoxic therapy; (3) providing genes that give only tumor cells the ability to activate a nontoxic prodrug into a cytotoxic drug; (4) "vaccinating" patients with plasmids that produce tumor antigens; (5) correcting the genetic defects that cause the cancer, such as inserting a tumor suppressor gene or inserting an antisense sequence against the oncogenic mutation.

There are multiple barriers to overcome before gene therapy can be successful. Success requires both knowledge of the defect in question and the ability to clone the normal functioning gene, but the biggest obstacle has been the ability to place the gene in the desired target tissue.

Table 23–7. Immune therapies.

Active immunotherapy	Nonspecific: Bacillus Calmette-Guérin (BCG), levamisole Specific: Interleukins and interferons
Passive immunotherapy	Monoconal antibodies Activated tumor infiltrating lymphocytes (TILs) Lymphocyte activated killer (LAK) cells

Retrovirus, adenovirus, and herpes virus vectors and direct injection with plasmids have all been attempted. Finally, presuming insertion of the genetic sequence into the proper target cells, the target cell must still be able to promote, transcribe, and process the gene product correctly.

COMMON TOXICITIES

Most chemotherapy drugs have a very narrow therapeutic range between their effectiveness against tumor cells and their toxicity to normal cells. In general, the degree of toxicity is dependent upon the peak concentration of drug, the concentration of the drug over the time of exposure, and the host response. Chemotherapy drugs, especially those that are cell-cycle–specific, tend to cause damage to those normal cells with the highest proliferation rates: hair follicles, cells lining the gastrointestinal track, and bone marrow stem cells.

HEMATOLOGIC TOXICITY

In the surgical patient who is receiving chemotherapy, knowledge of the expected degree, onset, and length of marrow toxicity for different drugs is important to the timing of a surgical procedure. For most drugs, the usual white blood cell count nadir occurs 7–14 days after the chemotherapy drug is given, but several drugs, such as mitomycin C and the nitrosoureas, have delayed nadirs (occurring 3–4 weeks later). Some drugs, such as bleomycin and vincristine, have essentially no myelotoxicity. Concomitant irradiation or a history of past irradiation (especially to the marrow-containing spine and pelvis) will often synergistically affect the decrease of white cell count as well as delay recovery.

The **myeloid growth factors**—filgrastim (granulocyte colony-stimulating factor, or G-CSF) and lenograstim (granulocyte-macrophage colony-stimulating factor, or GM-CSF) decrease the duration and the degree of the nadir. The drawback to the routine use of growth factors are cost, inconvenience to the patient, and transient bone pain. There are theoretical, but unproven, concerns about repeated cycles of marrow stimulation followed by more chemotherapy, since the chemotherapy preferentially kills dividing cells.

A fever occurring in any patient on chemotherapy, even if the patient feels entirely well and the physical examination is entirely normal, should be considered a medical emergency until it is proven that the absolute neutrophil count is greater than $1000/mm^3$. If the patient is neutropenic, the immediate institution of intravenous antibiotics with adequate antipseudomonal coverage is required. Gram-positive bacterial coverage, particularly for *Staphylococcal aureus*, must be added if the patient has an indwelling catheter, develops mucositis, or the fever does not resolve within 2–3 days. Febrile and neutropenic patients who have failed to respond within 4–7 days of broad-spectrum antibiotics should be considered for antifungal coverage. Frequently, in neutropenic patients, a specific etiology for the fever is never found.

The granulocyte growth factors (G-CSF, GM-CSF) do not improve the platelet count. Thrombocytopenia of less than $5000/mm^3$ or clinical evidence of bleeding requires platelet transfusions until the marrow recovers from the chemotherapy insult. In certain settings, erythropoietin can be used for chemotherapy-induced anemia. It is successful in approximately 50% of patients but takes several weeks to show effects. Iron supplementation does not usually help chemotherapy-induced anemia unless the patient has a reason to be iron-deficient, such as a history of recent surgery.

GASTROINTESTINAL TOXICITIES

The vinca alkaloids can cause a paralytic ileus, which can be exacerbated by the frequent use of narcotics in oncology patients. If a patient is neutropenic as well, then attempting to treat the obstipation with oral laxatives is preferable to giving enemas or suppositories. Obviously, recurrent or progressive malignancy can cause a similar clinical picture due to a mechanical bowel obstruction. Usually, the two can be differentiated by history, physical examination, and a flat abdominal radiograph.

Mucositis and diarrhea are other frequent side effects of chemotherapy drugs that usually occur between the first and second weeks after chemotherapy. This condition may require the discontinuation of chemotherapy and prompt treatment with antidiarrheal medication (loperamide, diphenoxylate, or octreotide) and intravenous fluids. Again, if the patient develops diarrhea at a time not coinciding with the chemotherapy, other causes of diarrhea need to be investigated, such as infections or a partial bowel obstruction.

A number of drugs have been tried for mucositis. Filgrastim and lenograstim lessen the duration of mucositis; topical mixtures of sucralfate, viscous lidocaine, diphenhydramine, and vitamin E have all been reported to help.

Nausea and vomiting have become much less of a problem in recent years since the development of the 5-HT3 inhibitors: granisetron and ondansetron. Glucocorticoids increase the antiemetic effect of these drugs. The exact mechanism of nausea and vomiting is still not known. Other effective drugs, including the phenothiazines, butyrophenones, metoclopramide, benzodiazepines, and cannabinoids, can be used. The primary side effect of these drugs (except the 5-HT3 inhibitors) is sedation.

Nausea associated with chemotherapy should not last longer than 3–4 days; any nausea or vomiting that persists beyond that should be evaluated to rule out other causes, such as a bowel obstruction, metabolic disturbance, infection, or brain metastases.

VESICANTS

Anthracyclines, mitomycin C, vinca alkaloids, and the nitrogen mustard drugs are the major **vesicants**. Vesicants cause a severe, progressive ulceration if there is any subcutaneous leakage into the skin at the intravenous site. In a few patients, continued ulceration to the underlying bone has been reported. If extravasation is suspected, there should be an immediate attempt to aspirate as much drug as possible and elevate the arm. There is anecdotal evidence that antidotes may be useful, including dimethylsulfoxide (DMSO) applied topically to an anthracycline extravasation, topical hyaluronidase to a vinca alkaloid extravasation, or sodium thiosulfate to mechlorethamine extravasation. A plastic surgeon should be consulted, especially if blistering or ulceration is noted.

SUGGESTED READING

Curt GA, Clendeninn NJ, Chabner BA: Drug resistance in cancer. Cancer Treat Rep 1984;68:87.

DeVita Jr V, Hellman S, Rosenberg SA (editors): *Cancer, Principles and Practice of Oncology*, 4th ed. Lippincott, 1993.

Hentges D (editor): *Microbiology and Immunology*, 2nd ed. Little, Brown, 1995.

Hortobagyi GN: Multidisciplinary management of advanced primary and metastatic breast cancer. Cancer 1994;74(1 Suppl): 416.

Levine RJ: Ethics of clinical trials. Do they help the patient? Cancer 1993;72(9 Suppl):2805.

Skipper HE: Dose intensity versus total dose of chemotherapy: an experimental basis. Important Adv Oncol 1990;43.

Traynor A. Recent advances in hormonal therapy for cancer. Curr Opin Oncol 1995;7:572.

Trimble EL et al: Neoadjuvant therapy in cancer treatment. Cancer 1993;72(11 Suppl):351.

24

Chronic Vascular Access

John E. Niederhuber, MD

▶ Key Facts

▶ The most common indications for central venous catheterization in the oncologic setting include the need to administer chemotherapeutic agents, provide nutritional support, and obtain multiple blood tests to monitor a patient's condition.

▶ Vascular access devices are placed in the largest veins in the body, where there is a greater flow of blood; this results in an increased rate of intravascular dilution.

▶ Several types of vascular access devices are available, including standard central venous, PICC, Hohn, and tunneled (Hickman, Broviac) catheters, as well as implantable ports.

▶ A detailed history and physical examination will greatly reduce the risk of placement and post-placement complications but may not be possible in an emergent situation.

▶ The most common method of central venous catheter placement is the Seldinger technique, which involves introducing a catheter using a narrow needle to enter the vein, passing a guide-wire through the needle, and then passing the catheter over the guide-wire into the vein.

▶ Catheter removal should be carefully explained to the patient to reduce anxiety. If any resistance is encountered, excessive force should not be applied, as this could cause the catheter to break.

▶ Regimens designed to maintain catheter patency for extended periods of time without thrombosis include low-dose Coumadin and high-dose heparin flushes.

▶ Complications of catheter placement with a closed technique include pneumothorax, arterial perforation, venous laceration, hemothorax, and pericardial tamponade. In an open procedure, the main concern is an air embolus entering the vein during catheter insertion.

▶ Long-term complications of catheter placement include infection, thrombosis, device damage and fracture, and dislodgement.

Chronic vascular access is an important, and sometimes essential, component of modern patient care. Several remarkable advances are responsible for the increased number of vascular access devices placed during the last 2 decades, including the advent of a soft, cuffed, silicone elastomer catheter first used to deliver total parenteral nu-trition to children in the early 1970s. Since that time, larger-bore, higher-volume devices and totally implantable infusion ports have been developed. In the past, these devices were often placed in the operating room with direct exposure of the vein. Cost containment issues have moved many of these procedures out of the operating room setting into the ambulatory clinics and minor surgery suites, almost always utilizing a percutaneous technique (Seldinger technique) for placement. New vascular access devices and improvements to existing catheter systems continue to be developed. Such medical devices are subject to pressures of manufacturers desiring to sell their products, and physicians must look carefully for the best device by weighing patient safety, ease of use, and product reliability.

INDICATIONS FOR CHRONIC VASCULAR ACCESS

Modern-day management of the cancer patient most often involves effective administration of chemotherapeutic agents, nutritional support, and the ability to obtain multiple blood tests for monitoring the patient's condition. Other indications for central venous catheterization include the continuous infusion of antibiotics, blood products, or other medications, as well as hemodynamic pressure monitoring and vascular access for hemodialysis or apheresis.

By far, the most common use of vascular access devices in the oncologic setting is intravenous drug delivery and total parenteral nutrition (TPN). With these devices, cytotoxic drugs and highly concentrated glucose solutions can be infused continuously (rather than intermittently through a peripheral venous cannula). Such drugs and solutions would quickly sclerose smaller peripheral veins, rendering routine venipuncture access impossible and causing significant patient discomfort. Vascular access devices are placed in central locations in the largest veins in the body where there is a greater flow of blood, resulting in an increased rate of intravascular dilution. Unfortunately, this does not always prevent vessel wall inflammation and irritation, localized thrombosis, or even vessel occlusion.

VASCULAR ACCESS DEVICES

Chronic vascular access via an external arteriovenous shunt was first developed for patients undergoing renal dialysis in the early 1960s. Although this concept was rapidly assimilated into practice, it was ultimately limited by high infection and thrombosis rates as well as nursing care issues. The first widely used central venous catheters were employed in the critical care setting for central venous and arterial pressure monitoring as well as the rapid infusion of fluids into trauma and burn victims. These catheters were initially made of firm biomaterials (eg, polyurethane) and were ultimately injurious to venous endothelium when used for long-term access.

Central venous access lines have evolved to include a more pliable version known as "transition" or "long-line"

central access devices. These catheters are similar to the acute care central venous catheters but consist of a silastic material, which makes them acceptable for a number of short-term to intermediate-duration indications. These devices include the peripherally inserted central catheter (PICC) and the Hohn catheter (Bard Access Systems, Salt Lake City, Utah) (Table 24–1). They are often referred to as transition devices because they facilitate the transition of patient care from the inpatient setting to the home care setting, which significantly reduces the cost of treatment. These "long" central lines are placed percutaneously via the antecubital, brachial, or cephalic veins into a central venous position. Although these devices are not considered suitable for long-term use, they have the positive characteristic of being relatively easy to insert in an outpatient setting, which only adds to their cost-effectiveness.

It was the advent of TPN that led to the development of a pliable catheter (Silastic; Dow Corning Corporation, Midland, Michigan) suitable for long-term TPN treatment in children (Broviac, 1973). A key feature of this device, known as the Broviac catheter (Bard Access Systems, Salt Lake City, Utah), was a cuff of material that anchored it to the soft tissues. The cuff is placed inside of a subcutaneous tunnel formed to separate the venous insertion site from the catheter skin exit site. Theoretically, this subcutaneous tunnel decreases the risk of externally derived infection. For this reason the Broviac and Hickman catheters (Hickman, 1979) (both Bard Access Systems, Salt Lake City, Utah) are often referred to as "tunneled" catheters. The cuff develops a fibrous barrier, preventing bacteria from tracking back to the site of catheter entrance into the vein. Remember that the normal healing process of the body creates a smooth, glistening fibrous sheath around the catheter through which bacteria can course from the skin or port pocket to the wall of the vein.

The final type of device to be discussed in this chapter is the implanted port (Figure 24–1). The Infuse-A-Port (Infusaid Corporation, Sharon, Massachusetts) was first developed in the early 1980s (Niederhuber, 1982). Several types of implanted ports are now available. The most common design includes a plastic reservoir, a self-sealing access septum, and an attached venous catheter. The ports are implanted beneath the skin with no external catheter. A noncoring (Huber) needle is used to access the im-

Table 24–1. List of commonly used vascular access devices.

Device	Material Used	Potential Length of Use
Standard central	Polyurethane	< 2 weeks
PICC	Long-line silastic	< 3 months
Hohn	Silastic	< 3 months
Tunneled (Broviac, Hickman)	Silastic (implantable)	1–12 months
Ports	Silastic/ polyurethane	< 6 months

PICC = peripherally inserted central catheter.

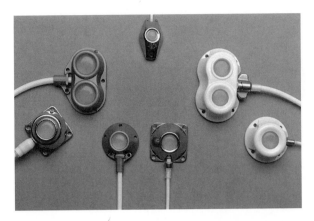

Figure 24–1. Examples of a number of different implantable infusion devices. **Top center:** Low-profile titanium ports. **Bottom center:** Peripheral access port used in the arm. **Left:** Single and dual polysulfone-titanium ports. **Right:** Single- and double-lumen standard profile ports. (Reprinted, with permission, from Abeloff MD et al: *Clinical Oncology.* Churchill Livingstone, 1995, p. 566.)

Table 24–2. Preoperative evaluation for placement of venous access devices.

Vascular access history
  Side(s) used and pneumothorax history
  Previous deep venous thrombosis
  Previous line infection
Anatomic pitfalls
  Clavicle fracture
  Cervical or mediastinal adenopathy
  Chest wall tumors
  Previous chest or breast surgery
  Known venous anomalies
  Rotation flaps as part of head and neck reconstructive surgery
Unilateral lung cancer or pneumonia
Complete blood count
Coagulation studies (only in patients receiving anticoagulant medicines)
Body habitus

Reproduced, with permission, from Whitman ED: Complications associated with the use of central venous access devices. Curr Probl Surg 1996;33:323.

planted port for the administration of drugs and blood products, or for blood sampling. The Huber needle is normally no more than 22 gauge, as repeated use of a larger needle could lead to permanent damage and leakage from the self-sealing silicone rubber port septum. Unfortunately, the small-gauge needle limits both the rate of infusion and aspiration that can be obtained from the implanted port, so there is often limited advantage of the port compared to a larger-bore catheter. The advantages are that the system is totally implanted and the smaller-bore catheters often have fewer complications. The decision of using a port versus a larger-bore tunneled catheter is, thus, based on the device characteristics needed to perform the planned therapy. An important consideration regarding implanted ports is the increased risk of infection created by the closer proximity of the needle hole in the skin and the entrance of the device catheter in the central vein. Bacteria from the skin can be introduced along the needle tract unless there is optimum skin care at the insertion point and strict sterile technique. The port also has no external drainage point, in contrast to the tunneled catheter, and the presence of a foreign body in a pocket of fibrous tissue makes an infection difficult to resolve without removal of the port.

TECHNICAL ASPECTS OF DEVICE PLACEMENT

A careful history and physical examination focuses on the details outlined in Table 24–2 and should be undertaken before any venous access device is placed. Of course, in some cases, venous access is required emergently and the need to proceed with catheter placement may limit the extent of preoperative evaluation. However, if possible, keep in mind that appropriate questioning will greatly reduce the risk of both placement and postplacement complications.

A complete blood count, prothrombin time, and platelet count should be obtained for elective placement. A chest radiograph is helpful to identify any lesions or anatomic abnormalities. If there is a question of venous patency, the patient should be evaluated using venous duplex ultrasonography.

Catheter insertion can take place at the bedside, in an ambulatory surgical setting, or in the operating room. As mentioned previously, transition catheters are usually placed at the bedside or in the clinic because they are relatively simple to insert. Unfortunately, significant patient discomfort has been associated with the placement of these devices through the antecubital veins. Concerns regarding cost issues have led to a trend of placing tunneled catheters and ports in minor procedure or ambulatory surgical rooms with local anesthesia, rather than formal operating rooms under general anesthesia, as was the case in the past.

The most commonly used method for the placement of traditional central lines, PICCs, tunneled catheters, and ports is the percutaneous or Seldinger technique. This method involves introducing the catheter using a narrow needle to enter the vein, passing a guide-wire through the needle, then passing the catheter over the guide-wire into the vein. A second method for larger catheters requires a dilator and a tear-away sheath (Figure 24–2). The patient should be placed in the Trendelenburg position with the head tilted down 20–30 degrees to allow the neck veins to distend and to minimize the risk of air embolism. The skin of the neck and upper anterior thorax is prepped and draped in a sterile fashion for either internal jugular or subclavian vein access.

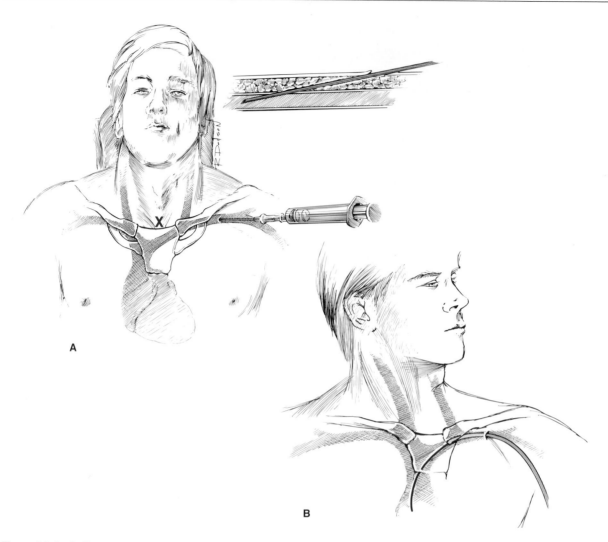

Figure 24–2. **A:** Placement of catheter using Seldinger technique. Long insertion needle shown entering the subclavian vein through skin and subcutaneous tissues. **B:** Demonstration of catheter passing over guide-wire. (Reprinted and modified, with permission, from Abeloff MD et al: *Clinical Oncology.* Churchill Livingstone, 1995, p. 573.)

When the subclavian vein is used, the skin should be punctured approximately 1 cm below the lateral one third of the clavicle. The long insertion needle is aimed at a point approximately one finger-breadth above the sternal notch. When the veins in the neck are used, the right internal jugular vein provides more direct access to the superior vena cava and right atrium. The insertion site is just lateral to the carotid and approximately two finger-breadths above the head of the clavicle.

One develops a "feel" for the needle puncture of the vein, and the syringe begins to immediately fill with venous blood. This should not be done applying vigorous and constant negative pressure. The syringe should be carefully removed (a thumb over the hub of the needle while one

reaches for the guide-wire will prevent any transient blood loss). The guide-wire is immediately fed through the hub of the needle. Correct positioning will be checked by fluoroscopy. The correct intravascular length can be estimated using the necessary chest wall landmarks that place the catheter along its imagined path to a point four finger-breadths below the sternal notch. Using fluoroscopy, with the patient now prone, position the tip approximately 1 cm below the caval-atrial junction. When the patient is upright, the catheter will rise to a point just at the caval-atrial junction. The catheter is fed over the guide-wire, which is then promptly removed. A chest radiograph should be obtained to ensure proper catheter placement and the absence of unsuspected pneumothorax or hemothorax.

For tunneled silastic catheters, the patient should be given an intravenous antibiotic before the procedure begins. A guide-wire is placed in the appropriate vein by the technique discussed above. An incision is then made for the exit site approximately 3–10 cm distant from the venous insertion site, usually at the level of the fourth or fifth interspace, approximately 3–4 cm lateral to the nipple-areola complex (Figure 24–3). The course of the planned "tunnel" is injected with 1% lidocaine. A tunneler device is passed from the lower incision to the upper incision where the guide-wire exits. A large suture is pulled through the tract as the tunneler is withdrawn and tied securely around the end of the catheter. The catheter is then brought through the subcutaneous tunnel in a caudad to cephalad fashion until the cuff rests 4–5 cm above the skin exit site within the subcutaneous tract.

The intended internal end of the catheter should be trimmed and cut straight across at an appropriate length. A tear-away sheath with an introducer obturator is placed into the subclavian vein over the previously inserted guide-wire. The guide-wire and obturator are removed, and the catheter is carefully threaded into the subclavian vein through the tear-away sheath. The sheath is removed by the assistant as the catheter is held firmly in position. The catheter should be secured with a 3-0 nylon suture at the exit site. The suture should secure the catheter without occluding the lumen. The suture can be removed 2–3 weeks after placement, once healing has secured the cuff to surrounding tissue within the tract. A chest radiograph should be obtained to confirm proper catheter placement.

Ports are placed in a similar fashion as the tunneled catheters, but a subcutaneous pocket is created surgically for the port chamber to rest under the skin and on the upper chest wall (Figure 24–4). The port is then anchored to the subcutaneous fascia to prevent dislodgement or twisting. The pocket is closed using skin or subcuticular sutures. A postoperative radiograph should be used to confirm catheter position and absence of complications resulting from placement.

CATHETER REMOVAL

Begin by carefully explaining the catheter removal procedure to the patient, to reduce anxiety. The dressing should be removed carefully. Scissors should never be used, as the catheter could be cut accidentally. Central venous catheters should be withdrawn in short segments without any pressure on the insertion site until it is completely withdrawn from the vein. If any resistance is encountered, excessive force should not be applied, as this could cause the catheter to break. Possible reasons for resistance include venospasm or constriction, inflammation, thrombophlebitis, fibrin sheath, and venous thrombosis.

Recent studies suggest that tunneled catheters should be removed via a surgical cutdown around the cuff to completely excise that structure and any tissue ingrowth surrounding it. Port removal also requires a minor surgical procedure, which can be accomplished in an outpatient setting. Port removal should include the reservoir, catheter, and all suture material in order to avoid leaving behind any foreign bodies that might become sites of chronic infection or irritation. The pocket containing the port is incised and the port removed, slowly withdrawing the catheter from the vein. It is a good idea to close the fibrous catheter track opening in the pocket with a figure-of-eight or purse string suture of 3-0 Dexon.

Incidents of difficulty removing PICCs have been reported. It has been suggested that this may be related to the smaller size of the arm veins in which the PICC becomes lodged. As the phenomenon of a "stuck PICC" is usually caused by a venous spasm, a warm compress to the arm is the first line of treatment. If the PICC does not loosen, a venous cutdown should be performed on the insertion site to remove it.

POSTPLACEMENT MANAGEMENT

Several regimens are designed to maintain catheter patency for extended periods of time without thrombosis. These regimens include both low-dose Coumadin and high-dose heparin flushes. Another recent study suggests low-dose warfarin administration (1 mg administered orally each day) to prevent thrombosis. Unfortunately, at least 20% of catheters still eventually present with this complication. One of the most troublesome outcomes of this particular complication is that the site is then eliminated for future catheter placements. The major threat of catheter-associated venous thrombosis is, of course, pulmonary embolism.

When malfunction of a catheter is suspected, a venogram should be performed to confirm that the catheter is still intravascular. If a fibrin sheath is found to surround the catheter tip, or if a clot is discovered in the venous lumen or catheter lumen, thrombolytic therapy through the catheter with agents such as streptokinase, urokinase, or tissue plasminogen activator may be used. The dosage of these agents should be small enough to only occupy the catheter itself, as larger systemic doses are not necessary.

In most cases, the initial wound dressing will be sterile gauze maintained for the first 7–10 days. This dressing should be changed every day and used with an antibacterial ointment such as Betadine, Tribiotic, or Silvadene. The skin should be prepped and allowed to dry for each dressing change. After the initial period, a transparent permeable or semipermeable membrane dressing such as Tegaderm, Opsite 3000, Vigilon, or Tegasorb may be used. These dressings should be changed according to manufacturers' directions.

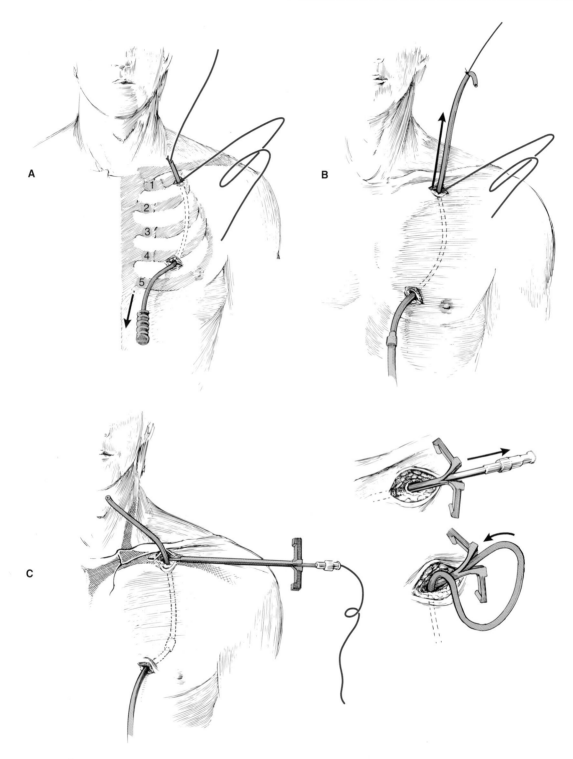

Figure 24–3. Placement of a permanent silastic catheter (such as a Hickman). ***A:*** The first and second incision sites are shown, as well as the path of the tunneler. ***B:*** The catheter is pulled through the tract using a heavy suture. The catheter cuff is secured 3–4 cm from the skin exit site. ***C:*** The catheter is trimmed and positioned 1 cm below the superior vena caval-right atrial (SVC-RA) junction. Introducer and tear-away sheath are shown passing over the guide-wire. The catheter is inserted into the sheath, and the sheath and introducer are removed. (Reprinted and modified, with permission, from Abeloff MD et al: *Clinical Oncology.* Churchill Livingstone, 1995, pp. 574-575.)

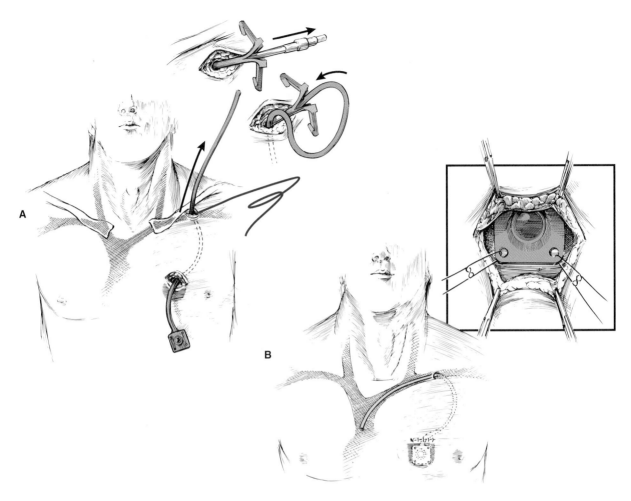

Figure 24–4. **A:** Placement of an implanted injection port. First and second incision sites are shown, as well as dissected pocket to accommodate port. **B:** Demonstration of placement of port into subcutaneous pocket. (Reprinted and modified, with permission, from Abeloff MD et al: *Clinical Oncology.* Churchill Livingstone, 1995, pp. 576–577.)

COMPLICATIONS

COMPLICATIONS OF DEVICE PLACEMENT

Catheter insertion is accomplished by either a closed (Seldinger) or open (cutdown) technique. The **closed technique** has specific hazards associated with a blind venipuncture, including pneumothorax, arterial perforation, venous laceration, hemothorax, and pericardial tamponade. The incidence of pneumothorax is approximately 1–4%. Fortunately, most pneumothoraxes from catheter insertion are small and do not represent a significant threat to the patient. A small (< 30%) pneumothorax can generally be treated by observation without a tube thoracostomy, if it is not enlarging on subsequent chest radiographs over a 24-hour period.

The most likely culprits of venous laceration by a closed technique are the guide-wire or the introducer, which is made of a fairly inflexible material and may fail to correspond to the shape of the venous structure. The catheters have become far more flexible and do not present a significant risk for this complication. Intrathoracic venous perforation can be manifested as either a hemothorax or pericardial tamponade. A hemothorax may necessitate a tube thoracostomy and requires immediate consultation by an experienced thoracic surgeon.

Although rare, pericardial tamponade has the highest mortality rate (65–90%) of any complication associated with catheter insertion. The symptoms of this complication include hypotension, muffled heart sounds, distended neck veins, and cardiorespiratory arrest. Once again, this situation calls for immediate consultation by an experienced cardiothoracic surgeon, however, urgent surgical intervention is often required and may involve emergent pericardiocentesis, creation of a pericardial window, or a median sternotomy.

In the **open technique**, the main concern is that an air embolus will enter the vein during catheter insertion. The internal jugular vein is the most common site of this complication, and only those skilled in open techniques should attempt surgical placement of a catheter in this vein. While an open procedure is a safer technique, it requires more training, experienced operative personnel, and a larger incision.

LONG-TERM COMPLICATIONS

Long-term complications associated with venous access devices include infection, thrombosis, device damage and fracture, and dislodgement. Catheter-related infections can progress rapidly from a local problem to a systemic life-threatening situation. Infections localized at the exit site or within the subcutaneous tunnel of the catheter are best treated with oral antibiotics. A systemic line sepsis confirmed with qualitative blood cultures must be treated with broad-spectrum intravenous antibiotics, which can initially be given through the device itself. If the patient continues to have symptoms of sepsis after 48 hours, the device should be removed. After removal, the venous access device should be sent to the laboratory for culture.

As mentioned earlier, thrombosis is the most common long-term complication associated with venous access devices. Fortunately, in the majority of cases this is a preventable occurrence with appropriate catheter maintenance. The venous access device itself may become damaged, either internally or externally. An internal catheter fracture can be caused by neighboring bony structures, such as the clavicle or ribs, while external damage may include a hole or tear. If the catheter has a pinched appearance on radiography (known as the "pinch off" sign) the catheter is at risk for compression and should be removed as soon as possible. External damage can often be repaired using commercially available repair kits, which contain replacement tubing, connectors, and silicone cement for holes. Dislodgement most often occurs in pediatric patients. If dislodgement is suspected, a chest radiograph is necessary to check the exact placement. Dislodgement is usually the result of excessive force applied to the external portion of the catheter and may require complete removal of the device.

SUGGESTED READING

Broviac JW, Cole JJ, Schribner BH: A silicone rubber atrial catheter for prolonged parenteral alimentation. Surg Gynecol Obstet 1973;136:602.

Dooley WC et al: Establishing and maintaining vascular access. In: Abeloff MD et al (editors): *Clinical Oncology.* Churchill Livingstone, 1995.

Hickman RO et al: A modified right atrial catheter for access to the venous system in marrow transplant recipients. Surg Gynecol Obstet 1979;92:706.

Niederhuber JE et al: Totally implanted venous and arterial access system to replace external catheters in cancer treatment. Surgery 1982;92:706.

Whitman ED: Complications associated with the use of central venous access devices. Curr Probl Surg 1996;33:313.

Section 5

Surgical Presentations

25

The Esophagus

Danny O. Jacobs, MD

▶ Key Facts

- ▶ The esophagus is a stratified, squamous, epithelial-lined, muscular tube that extends from the lower end of the pharynx to the upper end of the stomach.

- ▶ Patients with upper esophageal sphincter dysfunction are generally elderly and complain of dysphagia. Treatment includes myotomy of the cricopharyngeus muscle in the posterior midline.

- ▶ Miscellaneous diseases of the esophagus include diffuse esophageal spasm, congenital abnormalities, upper esophageal webs, midesophageal webs, and lower esophageal webs. Treatment ranges from antacids, antireflux procedures, repeated dilatation of strictures, or Roux-en-Y gastrojejunostomy for patients with delayed gastric emptying.

- ▶ Pharyngoesophageal pulsion (Zenker's) diverticula are the most common of all diverticula and are more likely to require surgical intervention.

- ▶ Esophageal tears and perforations classically occur after heavy eating, drinking, and alcohol consumption.

- ▶ Patients who are thought to have ingested a caustic substance should be immediately evaluated, as they are at risk for airway obstruction secondary to pharyngeal edema.

- ▶ There are two types of hiatal hernia. Type I is considered a normal finding in most individuals, but type II is much more likely to strangulate and infarct.

- ▶ Left untreated, patients with severe esophagitis may progress to fibrosis, scarring, and stricture formation and may develop iron deficiency anemia secondary to chronic blood loss.

- ▶ The most common type of benign tumor of the esophagus is a leiomyoma.

- ▶ Esophageal cancer in the United States occurs three times more frequently in men than in women and three times as frequently in African-Americans than in Caucasians.

- ▶ Standard surgical approaches to esophageal carcinoma include the left thoracoabdominal incision, a laparotomy and right thoracotomy, and the transhiatal esophagectomy.

ANATOMY & PHYSIOLOGY

The esophagus is a stratified, squamous, epithelial-lined, muscular tube. Secretions from submucosal glands help lubricate the lumen and protect it from irritants. The esophagus extends from the lower end of the pharynx near the sixth cervical cartilage to the upper end of the stomach within the peritoneal cavity (Figure 25–1). In the process, it passes through the thorax in the mediastinum behind the aortic arch and the left main stem bronchus. It enters the abdomen through the esophageal hiatus. Normally, about 2–4 cm of the esophagus lie within the peritoneal cavity.

A unique feature of the anatomy of this organ is that it traverses three major areas of the body—the neck, thorax, and abdomen. It is intimately related to a number of other organs, including the tracheobronchial tree and lungs, the heart and great vessels, the phrenic and vagus nerves, and the thyroid gland and associated structures.

The esophagus has a thick muscular coat that consists of an outer longitudinal and an inner circular layer. It does not have a serosal covering layer like the stomach and other gastrointestinal organs. The muscular layers are striated in the upper third but undergo transition to become exclusively composed of smooth muscle in the lower half of the esophagus. This allows voluntary control of the inlet to the esophagus, while control of the outlet is involuntary.

A strong circular band of striated muscle called the **cricopharyngeus** creates a high-pressure zone in the upper esophagus. The activities of this muscle are normally carefully orchestrated with the larynx to avoid aspiration. The lower end of the esophagus does not have a true sphincter but does have a high-pressure zone that can be detected manometrically. The high-pressure zone is known as the **lower esophageal sphincter**. Resting pressures in this region normally exceed the pressure within the stomach by 15–25 cm of water (Table 25–1). Sphincter competence is enhanced by the presence of the distal portion of the esophagus within the peritoneal cavity. The lower esophageal sphincter prevents the reflux of gastric contents into the esophagus but also must relax to allow food to pass. The gastroesophageal sphincter also is normally incompetent during vomiting. During this process, the gastroesophageal junction rises above the level of the diaphragmatic hiatus. Gastric contents are then expelled by sharp contractions of the gastric antrum and the abdominal wall.

Liquids and solids normally pass very quickly from the mouth to the stomach. The activities of the upper and lower esophageal sphincters are coordinated such that they relax and contract appropriately. A peristaltic wave is not required for passage of substances through the body of the esophagus unless they are very large pieces of food.

Three different **wave forms** can be identified, however. Primary waves occur after swallowing and represent sequential contractions of the circular muscle. Secondary waves occur after the food bolus has passed into the stomach and are believed to strip the esophagus of any debris remaining after the primary wave. Tertiary contractions

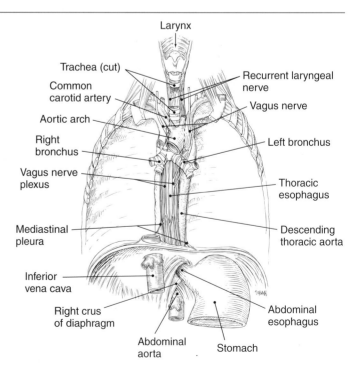

Figure 25–1. Anatomy of the esophagus.

Table 25–1. Normal manometric pressures in the esophagus.

Region	Pressure (cm of water)
Esophageal body	−5 to −10
Lower esophageal sphincter	+15 to +25
Stomach	+5 to +10

have no known function but are frequently detected in elderly asymptomatic patients.

Blood supply to the upper esophagus is derived from thyroid vessels, while arterial supply in the thorax is derived from both the aorta and from bronchial arteries. The arterial supply to the distal esophagus is primarily derived from the left gastric artery. Venous drainage is highly variable but ultimately is collected into the azygos system. Lymphatic drainage occurs along the left gastric artery to the celiac axis, as well as to various periesophageal nodes and then to the thoracic duct that lies between the esophagus and the thoracic vertebral column.

The esophagus is also subject to neurohormonal control. Autonomic innervation is provided via the vagus and thoracic sympathetic nerves. A vagal nerve plexus is closely intertwined about the upper esophagus and coalesces to form the anterior and posterior vagal nerves distally. The vagus nerves only appear to supplement native esophageal function, since central vagal denervation does not normally result in measurable abnormalities in lower esophageal function or motility. The motor for progression of muscular contractions lies within the body of the esophagus and most likely involves the myenteric plexus. Peristaltic contractions are mediated cholinergically. Inhibitory nerves also play a major role in esophageal motility, because a period of relaxation is required before each normal contraction, and spontaneous contractions do not occur in normal esophageal smooth muscle. The lower esophageal sphincter is responsive to parasympathetic stimulation, since its pressure will increase after the administration of acetylcholine or its esters.

The **esophageal hiatus** is normally encompassed by fibers of the right crus of the diaphragm. Another important structure in this region is the **phrenoesophageal ligament**. It is formed by the fusion of the mediastinal and diaphragmatic pleura with the peritoneum and transversalis fascia in the region of the gastroesophageal junction. The ligament is very well developed posteriorly and normally tethers the distal esophagus to the base of the right crus in the region of the first lumbar vertebrae.

UPPER ESOPHAGEAL SPHINCTER DYSFUNCTION (CRICOPHARYNGEAL ACHALASIA)

Some patients will present with dysfunction of the upper esophageal sphincter of uncertain etiology. These patients are generally elderly and complain of dysphagia. Abnormalities of the cricopharyngeus muscle may not be specifically identified. Upper esophageal sphincter dysfunction may also occur in association with a Zenker's diverticulum (see below). **Oculopharyngeal muscular dystrophy** is a hereditary syndrome described in patients of French-Canadian ancestry. The syndrome consists of ptosis, dysphagia, and cricopharyngeal dysfunction.

The cervical dysphagia that patients with cricopharyngeal achalasia experience is typically more pronounced for solids than for liquids. The sphincter dysfunction and secondary minor aspiration of saliva and ingested foods may lead to a chronic cough and, occasionally, episodes of aspiration pneumonia.

Diagnosis

A barium swallow characteristically demonstrates a prominent ridge running across the pharynx—the so-called **cricopharyngeal bar**. It may be so prominent as to suggest the presence of luminal obstruction. The endoscopic findings may be subtle as no mucosal abnormalities should be observed, however, endoscopy is important to rule out esophageal malignancies or other co-morbid conditions. There may be a suggestion of extrinsic compression of the upper pharynx that relaxes as the endoscope is passed. Esophageal manometry will detect incomplete relaxation of the upper esophageal sphincter during swallowing or impaired coordination and relaxation of the proximal esophagus after swallowing. Some patients have both abnormalities.

Management

Once the diagnosis is established, patients with upper esophageal sphincter dysfunction are treated by performing a myotomy of the cricopharyngeus muscle in the posterior midline that includes 3–4 cm of the proximal esophagus. The operation is usually performed by exposing the esophagus via a left-sided cervical incision that parallels the anterior border of the sternocleidomastoid muscle.

LOWER ESOPHAGEAL DYSFUNCTION (ACHALASIA)

Dysfunction of the lower esophageal sphincter occurs uncommonly, with an incidence of less than one case per 100,000 patients per year in western industrialized countries. The disease occurs approximately equally in men and women and is most often diagnosed between the third and sixth decades of life. Esophageal carcinoma in association with achalasia is rare but appears to occur more frequently in patients with lower esophageal dysfunction, as compared to the general population.

The etiology of achalasia is unknown, however its pathophysiologic features are well described. Achalasia is a neuromuscular disorder characterized by a failure of propagation of peristalsis through the esophagus and an inability of the lower esophageal sphincter to relax in response to swallowing. The disease is typically progressive. Thus, over time the esophagus dilates and the outer circular muscle layer hypertrophies, whereas the inner longitudinal coat does not. Early findings in the esophagus of patients with achalasia include abnormalities of parasympathetic ganglia in Auerbach's plexuses and a decrease in the number of these cells in the esophageal body and in the region of the lower esophageal sphincter. Recent experiments have shown that postganglionic inhibitory neurons in the circular layer of the lower esophageal sphincter are selectively impaired. Some investigators have detected changes similar to Wallerian degeneration in fibers of the vagus nerve in association with a decreased number of nerve cells in the dorsal motor nucleus of the vagus nerve in the brainstem. This and other experimental and clinical observations suggest that the autonomic nervous system is the primary target of the disease.

The greater the duration of symptoms, the more pronounced are the histologic findings. Late in the course of disease the wall of the esophagus may be thickened and its lumen enlarged and tortuous. Narrowing in the region of the lower esophageal sphincter may be observed over a distance of several centimeters. Diverticula may also develop, as well as mucosal ulcerations or inflammation secondary to chronic stasis.

Dysphagia is the most prominent symptom of patients with achalasia but is usually a late finding. Patients may initially sense a sticking sensation after the ingestion of solids or liquids. Cold fluids may be especially problematic. These symptoms may be tolerated for years, and patients do not typically seek medical attention until dysphagia interferes with their eating patterns or lifestyles. Despite the presence of functional obstruction, significant weight loss is usually not a prominent feature of achalasia, although 60% of patients will lose some weight. Patients may regurgitate retained esophageal contents, especially at night if they are sleeping in a recumbent position. These aspiration events may cause recurrent pneumonia, tracheobronchitis, or even asphyxiation. Although shallow ulcerations may be seen in some patients late in the course of disease, pain is rare. Only approximately one third of patients will complain of substernal or epigastric pain.

Occasionally, a few patients will complain of severe pain, and this is a different variant of the disease known as **vigorous achalasia**. Their discomfort is usually severe, localized to the substernal area, and may last for several minutes. These individuals have severe chest pain secondary to esophageal spasms that generate nonpropulsive high-pressure waves in the body of the esophagus. In this variant, lower esophageal sphincter dysfunction is still present. These patients are more likely to seek medical assistance early in the course of their disease.

Patients with scleroderma and those with benign or malignant strictures near the gastroesophageal junction may have symptoms that closely mimic achalasia. Further-

more, patients with infiltrating intramucosal cancers near the cardia may have all of the cardinal features of achalasia if the malignancy interferes with neural control of esophageal motility.

Diagnosis

In all instances fluoroscopy, manometry, and upper endoscopy should be performed to confirm the diagnosis of achalasia and to determine if other diseases are present that mimic its effects (Table 25–2). Esophageal cytological examinations or biopsies should also be performed to diagnose cancer.

On upper endoscopy, small ulcerations may be seen in the esophagus that are caused by irritation from retained food and secretions. However, true peptic ulceration or hemorrhage is very rare in achalasia. One should be able to pass the scope into the stomach beyond the high-pressure lower esophageal sphincter. Once in the stomach, the scope should be retroflexed to ensure that a tumor is not present high in the cardia.

Radiologic findings may be characteristic, even in the early stages of achalasia. Classically, the esophagus is linearly narrowed over a distance of 3–6 cm in the region of the cardia, like a bird's beak (Figure 25–2). The body of the esophagus is dilated, blending into the narrowed region. Fluoroscopy may reveal weak, irregular, or uncoordinated contractions. The diameter of the esophageal body mirrors the severity of the disease. A diameter of less than 4 cm is considered mild, 4–6 cm is intermediate, and greater than 6 cm is considered severe. Late in the course of disease, the esophagus may be so dilated as to be tortuous or even sigmoid in shape.

Manometric studies may be used to confirm the diagnosis of achalasia. A hallmark of these studies is increased pressure measured at the gastroesophageal sphincter and incomplete relaxation during swallowing. The upper esophageal sphincter functions normally. No primary peristaltic waves are present in the body of the esophagus, and occasionally peristalsis is completely absent (Table 25–3). When bethanechol is administered subcutaneously, patients with achalasia, and some with diffuse esophageal spasm (see below), experience a forceful sustained contraction of the lower two thirds of the esophagus that may be momentarily painful. It is believed to occur because of autonomic denervation. The response is not observed in normal subjects.

Table 25–2. Diagnosis of achalasia.

Etiology	Abnormalities of myenteric ganglia
	Failure of lower esophageal sphincter to relax on swallowing
Diagnosis	Dysphagia
	Dilatation of the esophagus above the lower esophageal sphincter
Treatment	Balloon dilatation or myotomy of the lower esophageal sphincter

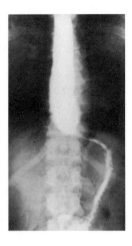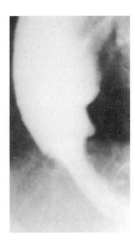

Figure 25–2. Barium study of the esophagus in a patient with achalasia. The film on the left demonstrates a dilated body of the esophagus and a smooth, tapering "bird's beak" of the lower portion. The film on the right shows expansion of the lower esophageal sphincter region after esophageal myotomy. (Reprinted, with permission, from Way LW: *Current Surgical Diagnosis & Treatment,* 9th ed. Appleton & Lange, 1991, p. 405.)

Management

The purpose of therapy is to relieve the functional obstruction at the gastroesophageal sphincter. Some patients obtain relief with the use of calcium channel blockers that decrease pressure in the sphincter and improve swallowing. Most patients are treated with either forceful balloon dilatation or direct surgical division of the muscle fibers of the lower esophageal sphincter (**myotomy**).

Balloon dilatation, or **bougienage**, is accomplished by forcibly expanding a balloon with air or water after it is placed across the gastroesophageal junction. The balloon may be passed over a thread, olive-tipped bougie, or under radiographic control. The balloon is inflated to a pressure of 300 torr for 15 seconds. This is painful, but disrupts the circular layer of smooth muscle within the lower esophageal sphincter. Patients are premedicated with an analgesic and tranquilizer. Usually 3 or 4 dilatations are made with balloons that inflate to 3–4 cm in diameter. Forceful dilatation of the lower esophageal sphincter is successful in approximately 75% of patients but has a 5% risk of perforation. Additional dilatations are needed in about 15% of patients. If esophageal manometry is re-

Table 25–3. Manometric diagnostic criteria for achalasia.

Elevated lower esophageal sphincter pressure
Incomplete or absent relaxation of the lower esophageal sphincter with swallowing
Absence of peristalsis in the body of the esophagus
Elevated intraesophageal pressure

peated in patients who are treated successfully, lower esophageal pressure falls significantly. Approximately 20% of patients will develop significant gastroesophageal reflux after treatment.

Patients with advanced achalasia, where the esophagus has become very dilated and tortuous, may be best treated surgically. About 15–20% of patients will eventually come to surgical operation and should receive a Heller myotomy. This longitudinal myotomy extends from the level of the inferior pulmonary vein down and across the gastroesophageal sphincter to a distance of no greater than 1 cm on the stomach. Thus, the length of the incision is normally 10–12 cm. If it extends too far onto the stomach (> 1 cm), patients may develop significant esophageal reflux after operation. Furthermore, when the myotomy is performed through the abdomen, the phrenoesophageal ligament must be divided. The resultant weakening of the lower esophageal sphincter and dissection of the esophageal hiatus may be followed by a high incidence of reflux. For this reason, some surgeons perform an antireflux procedure after the myotomy is completed. The vagus nerves should, of course, be preserved, and gastric drainage procedures, therefore, should not be needed.

The majority of patients (75–85%) report good to excellent results after operation. Those who still have difficulty may have had an incomplete myotomy or had extensive preexisting esophageal paralysis. All of the circular smooth muscle fibers must be divided if the myotomy is to be successful. Patients who are perforated during forceful dilatation are best treated by immediate operation, with closure of the perforation and a myotomy on the opposite side of the esophagus.

The results of operation can be assessed using radioisotopically labeled meals, if needed, to follow transit through the esophagus and stomach. Esophagoscopy should be performed periodically to monitor for the development of esophageal cancer. Laparoscopic and thorascopic approaches to the procedure are being studied. These approaches are less painful and may shorten recovery times.

MISCELLANEOUS DISEASES OF THE ESOPHAGUS

A variety of systemic diseases may affect esophageal motility, including diabetes and various collagen vascular diseases, such as scleroderma and progressive systemic sclerosis. The diagnosis of these conditions may be difficult if esophageal symptoms are predominant.

Most patients with scleroderma will manifest esophageal dysfunction at some point in their illness. These individuals may complain of esophageal reflux with regurgitation, heartburn, and, occasionally, bleeding. Dysphagia is not usually a common symptom unless stricturing occurs. Symptoms typically are noted once patients develop skin changes and Raynaud's syndrome, but changes in esophageal motility may antedate other findings. Atrophy and fibrosis of the smooth muscle layer progressively weakens contractility, especially in the region of the lower esophageal sphincter. Esophageal manometry reveals weak primary peristaltic waves that attenuate as they approach this area.

The natural history of the disease is that peristalsis becomes weaker and weaker as the disease progresses. Eventually, shortening of the esophagus may displace the gastroesophageal sphincter above the diaphragmatic hiatus, producing a hiatal hernia. At this time, radioisotopic emptying studies will document delayed gastric emptying of solids. However, these changes as well as abnormalities seen on fluoroscopy are not specific and may be observed in patients with rheumatoid arthritis, systemic lupus erythematosus, or the diseases alluded to previously.

Treatment options are limited in patients with nonspecific motility disorders. Control of the underlying disease process may be of some benefit, especially if treatment is begun early in the course of disease, except for patients with scleroderma, for whom there is no known therapy to prevent or delay the deterioration of their esophageal function. Esophageal reflux may be controlled using antacids and elevation of the head of the bed during sleeping. Occasionally, patients may benefit from antireflux procedures if their native esophageal function is sufficiently preserved. Strictures can often be repeatedly dilated. Patients with delayed gastric emptying may benefit from Roux-en-Y gastrojejunostomy.

CONGENITAL ABNORMALITIES

A number of congenital anomalies affect the esophagus, including vascular rings and various webs, cysts, and duplications. **Vascular rings** usually cause symptoms in young adulthood. Patients typically present in their late teens with symptoms of dysphagia. Barium studies will show constriction of the esophagus at the level of the obstruction. Angiography or other vascular imaging studies will demonstrate which, if any, arterial vessels are involved. If the symptoms are persistent or progressive, patients are treated by dividing the vascular ring.

Thin, membranous areas of narrowing within the lumen of the esophagus are called **webs**. These are atrophic mucosal folds that may extend partially or completely into the lumen of the esophagus. Most are acquired and cause symptoms in adulthood. However, congenital webs may cause symptoms shortly after birth and should be suspected when newborns fail to nurse properly or regurgitate frequently.

UPPER ESOPHAGEAL WEBS (PLUMMER-VINSON SYNDROME)

Plummer-Vinson syndrome is a disease that tends to affect middle-aged or older women of Anglo-Saxon descent. It is a cluster of signs and symptoms, including the presence of webs in the upper or cervical esophagus, fissured lips, dry skin, a smooth tongue, flat brittle nails, weight loss, dysphagia, and iron deficiency anemia. The iron deficiency anemia is somehow responsible for the development of the esophageal webs, though the mechanism by which this occurs is unknown. However, the webs will typically disappear once the iron deficiency anemia is corrected. Furthermore, the risk of developing cervical esophageal carcinoma decreases when the iron deficiency anemia is diagnosed and treated early.

The diagnosis should be considered when the constellation of signs and symptoms occur in an anemic woman with dysphagia. A thick barium swallow will demonstrate the presence of one or more webs within the esophagus that never extend below the level of the aortic arch. Upper endoscopy will identify the thin flimsy webs that are easily ruptured by the passage of the scope.

MID-ESOPHAGEAL WEBS

Midesophageal webs may occur congenitally or secondary to esophagitis and the development of Barrett's epithelium. The two can usually be distinguished by the presence of chronic reflux symptoms in the latter. Barium studies may reveal a short stricture in the mid-esophagus and an associated hiatal hernia. If the abnormality is secondary to gastroesophageal reflux, changes associated with esophagitis rather than a true membranous web are identified on upper endoscopy.

LOWER ESOPHAGEAL WEBS (SCHATZKI'S RING)

Rings involving the lower esophagus may be commonly detected radiographically and are different from congenital webs that may also involve the lower end of the esophagus. The exact etiology of Schatzki's rings is unknown but they may occur secondary to reflux esophagitis, as a normal variant of the gastroesophageal junction, as radiographic evidence of a hiatal hernia that is only occasionally seen, or as a result of these three factors combined. The ring itself identifies the boundary between the epithelial lining of the esophagus and the stomach.

Lower esophageal webs become clinically significant if the lumen of the esophagus is reduced to less than 10–20 mm. Patients with significant narrowing may complain of dysphagia, especially to solids. True webs rings may be identified endoscopically as a white membrane narrowing the lumen of the esophagus. As mentioned previously, they are often seen on barium swallow. Webs are easily treated. They may be serially dilated using mercury-weighted bougies, incised using electrocautery, or ruptured by balloon tamponade. Surgical correction via an open approach is rarely needed.

DIVERTICULA

Esophageal diverticula are acquired lesions of two types. Pulsion type diverticula result from the protrusion of mucosa and submucosa through a defect in the esophageal musculature. Pulsion type diverticula result from increased intraluminal pressure and are more likely to cause symptoms because they typically interfere with esophageal function. Traction type diverticula are full-thickness herniations that occur secondary to inflammation and scarring, typically from a peribronchial mediastinal lymph node, which pulls outward on the esophageal wall. Diverticula may occur anywhere in the esophagus between the pharyngoesophageal junction and the lower esophageal sphincter but are most commonly identified at the cricopharyngeal sphincter, in the mid-esophagus, and in the lower esophagus just above the diaphragm. Adults are most commonly affected, and the incidence increases with age.

PHARYNGOESOPHAGEAL (ZENKER'S) DIVERTICULUM

Pharyngoesophageal pulsion diverticula are the most common of all diverticula and also are more likely to require surgical intervention. High pressures generated during swallowing are observed in all patients in the upper cricopharyngeal sphincter that fails to relax. Coordination of swallowing is poor, and many patients have abnormal esophageal motility patterns and hiatal hernias. The excessive pressures generated force the mucosa and submucosa through an area between the inferior pharyngeal constrictor muscle. This region of the esophagus has no muscle covering posteriorly. About a third of patients will have an associated functional disorder of the esophagus, including other diverticula, achalasia, or diffuse esophageal spasm.

When small, these lesions are usually asymptomatic. However, they can be expected to gradually increase in size with time. Zenker's diverticula are rarely seen in individuals under the age of 30 years. Most patients are over the age of 60 when they present. As the sac enlarges, it usually projects laterally into the left paravertebral region.

Patients will report dysphagia and gurgling noises during swallowing. Retained food in the pouch may be regurgitated into the mouth, especially when the patient is recumbent, and cause halitosis. Some patients will massage their necks after eating in an effort to empty the pouch manually. They may also report repeated episodes of aspiration that sometimes cause pneumonia and pulmonary abscess formation. Other patients may complain of asthma or hoarseness if the enlarged sac compresses the recurrent laryngeal nerve.

Spontaneous perforation of a Zenker's diverticulum is rare, however, perforation can easily be induced iatrogeni-

cally. When perforation does occur it may cause mediastinitis, a paraesophageal abscess, or generate fistulas between the trachea and the pouch.

Diagnosis

A barium swallow will reveal a rounded balloon-like sac extending from the esophagus in the posterior midline (Figure 25–3). These radiographic studies are usually sufficient to examine the rest of the esophagus. Upper endoscopy can be hazardous and lead to perforation of the diverticulum. However, endoscopy is indicated when there is complete esophageal obstruction of if a malignancy is suspected. Manometry is performed if symptoms suggest the presence of motility disorders that require investigation.

Management

Even patients with small diverticula should be offered operative correction. No other therapies are successful and, if left alone, the sacs will increase in size and place the patient at risk for significant respiratory complications. There are two surgical treatment options available, depending on the size of the sac. If the sac is less than 2 cm in diameter, cricopharyngeal myotomy alone is sufficient to relieve symptoms and prevent further enlargement. Larger diverticula are best treated by cricopharyngeal myotomy and excision. If excision alone is done for larger diverticula, the patients may complain of persistent dysphagia.

The operation is usually performed through an incision that parallels the anterior border of the left sternocleidomastoid muscle. The left lobe of the thyroid gland is carefully mobilized and the recurrent laryngeal nerve is dissected free and avoided. The diverticulum is dissected free from the surrounding structures and divided at least 2 cm from its origin to avoid constricting the esophagus. A two-layered closure of the resulting defect is typically performed. If the diverticulum is not dissected, it can be pexed superiorly to the inferior sphincter. Patients with gastroesophageal reflux should also have antireflux operations performed to reduce the risk of aspiration and other complications.

EPIPHRENIC DIVERTICULA

These pulsion diverticula can occur at any point but are usually found below the mid-esophagus. Epiphrenic diverticula on the whole are relatively rare. They represent only about 10–20% of all esophageal diverticula and are more common in males. Usually, only those that occur just above the diaphragm are symptomatic and only about half of all epiphrenic diverticula have associated symptoms. Common complaints include dysphagia, regurgitation, epigastric or chest pain, choking, or coughing. When these symptoms are present, patients should be evaluated for associated esophageal motility disorders.

Epiphrenic diverticula grow larger than other esoph-

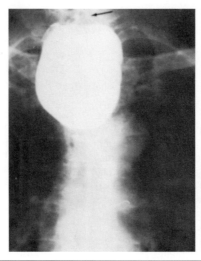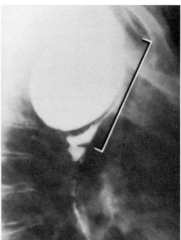

Figure 25–3. A large pharyngoesophageal (Zenker's) diverticulum is demonstrated. The arrow in the left panel indicates the place of origin in the midline. The bracket in the panel on the right indicates compression of the esophagus by the diverticulum. (Reprinted, with permission, from Way LW: *Current Surgical Diagnosis & Treatment,* 9th ed. Appleton & Lange, 1991, p. 408.)

ageal diverticula and can measure as much as 10 cm in diameter. The neck of these diverticula is often very narrow. If there is associated reflux, esophagitis may develop at the opening of the sac. Mediastinitis may also be observed secondary to inflammation.

Diagnosis

These diverticula are readily detected by barium studies of the esophagus. Manometry is also important to identify commonly associated esophageal motility disorders. Endoscopy should be performed with care to avoid entering and rupturing the diverticular sac.

Management

Appropriate treatment follows principles similar to those outlined for cricopharyngeal diverticula. Thus, a myotomy and excision of the diverticulum are performed when this can be accomplished. The myotomy performed varies according to whether other disease processes or motility disorders are present. The esophagus is usually approached through a left posterolateral thoracotomy. Typically, myotomy extending from the diverticulum to the lower esophageal sphincter is indicated. If diffuse spasm is present, a long myotomy extending from the lower esophageal sphincter to the aortic arch is indicated. Similarly, a short myotomy extending distally from the diverticulum works well when there is associated achalasia. If an associated hiatal hernia is present, it should be repaired cautiously, else the patient may have obstructive symptoms postoperatively. Often, therapy must be individualized to meet a particular patient's clinical circumstances. Surgical treatment works wells in most cases, with an 80–90% response rate.

TRACTION DIVERTICULA

Traction diverticula are most often seen in the midthoracic esophagus. They are thought to arise from the effects of inflamed lymph nodes on the esophageal wall. Inflamed nodes near the bifurcation of the trachea adhere to the esophagus. As contraction and fibrosis occur during healing, the esophageal wall is distorted. This forms a sac that is initially cone-shaped with its apex attached to the lymph node. Ultimately, the sac may become more rounded due to the pulsion effects of intraluminal pressure.

Most often, these diverticula occur because of granulomatous necrosis of tracheobronchial lymph nodes, such as is seen with tuberculosis or histoplasmosis. The sacs formed are true diverticula (all layers of the esophagus are involved), have broad necks, are typically located on the left side of the thorax, and point upward. For these reasons, they are rarely symptomatic. They may occasionally bleed and rarely fistulize. They are usually found in patients over the age of 40 and occur with equal frequency in both sexes. Often, they are found incidentally during routine x-ray examinations.

Diagnosis

As with the other diverticula, traction diverticula are readily detected and diagnosed using barium studies of the esophagus. If there is evidence of narrowing of the esophageal lumen in the vicinity of the diverticulum, endoscopy is needed to rule out the presence of a carcinoma.

Management

Surgical therapy is rarely indicated. If a patient does develop clear-cut symptoms, then excision is warranted, although the risk of leakage may be high because of peridiverticular scarring and inflammation.

ESOPHAGEAL TEARS & PERFORATIONS

MALLORY-WEISS SYNDROME

Diagnosis

Patients who develop upper gastrointestinal bleeding after vomiting and who are found to have stomach or esophageal lacerations on endoscopy have the Mallory-Weiss syndrome. Classically, these episodes occur after heavy eating, drinking, and alcohol consumption. Emergency endoscopy will demonstrate the location of the bleeding and rule out other causes of hemorrhage.

Management

Most patients can be controlled using conservative measures. Ice water (36°F) lavage though a large-bore nasogastric tube will often control the bleeding. Balloon tamponade is contraindicated. Patients without coronary artery disease can be treated with vasopressin infusion at 0.3–0.4 units per hour. When patients do not stop spontaneously or respond to conservative measures, surgical treatment is necessary. The site is best approached through a high gastrostomy. The bleeding vessels can usually be seen and oversewn using this approach. Occasionally, a left thoracotomy will be needed for access.

BOERHAAVE'S SYNDROME

Spontaneous perforation of the esophagus is known as Boerhaave's syndrome. There may be underlying disease of the organ that predisposes the patient to the disease. It is five times more common in males than females. Often times, as is the case for patients with esophageal tears, there is a history of excessive alcohol and food intake. The syndrome can also occur after coughing, heavy lifting, defecation, forceful swallowing, childbirth, or other events that rapidly increase intraesophageal pressure when gastric contents reflux into the esophagus while the upper esophageal sphincter is closed.

All layers of the esophagus are involved in the rupture. Patients experience violent vomiting and then develop severe pain in the epigastrium and lower anterior thorax. They may also complain of pain in the left shoulder secondary to diaphragmatic irritation. The tears are most often found in the left posterior aspect of the esophageal wall, 3–5 cm above the gastroesophageal junction. The second most common site of perforation is in the midthoracic esophagus on the right side at the level of the azygos vein.

Diagnosis

Critically ill and septic patients who present with dyspnea and air in the mediastinum or left hydropneumothorax should be suspected of having complete rupture of the esophagus. Water soluble contrast studies of the esophagus will help to confirm the diagnosis.

Management

The principles of treatment include fluid resuscitation, broad-spectrum antibiotic coverage, drainage of the mediastinum and pleural cavity, and suture closure of the esophagus, if this is technically feasible. If the diagnosis has been delayed it may not be possible to close the tear because the esophageal wall becomes friable and inflamed. A portion of the stomach wall can be mobilized (Thal gastric patch) and used to buttress the repair if the surrounding tissues can be sutured. When the esophagus cannot be repaired, the best approach may be to close the esophageal lumen above and below the tear and divert the patient's secretions through a cervical esophagostomy. A gastrostomy tube should also be placed.

IATROGENIC PERFORATION

Iatrogenic perforation may occur after upper endoscopy, esophageal dilatation, or other therapeutic or diagnostic procedures involving the upper gastrointestinal tract. Most iatrogenic perforations occur after diagnostic esophagoscopy. During upper endoscopy, perforation is most likely to occur in the region of the cervical esophagus near the upper sphincter. This occurs because a fair amount of pressure may have to be exerted in order to force the endoscope past the high-pressure zone in this region. This pressure may give suddenly and lead to injury of the esophageal wall distally. For example, the esophagoscope may lacerate the esophagus against osteoarthritic vertebral spurs. Perforations occur about once every 1000 procedures and are most common in the region of the cricopharyngeus muscle. Injuries to the intrathoracic esophagus are most likely to occur at areas where the esophagus narrows anatomically, such as near the left mainstem bronchus or at the diaphragmatic hiatus.

The risk of perforation after pneumatic dilatation of the esophagus for achalasia is approximately 4%, whereas the risk of perforation is only approximately 1% after esophagomyotomy. Dilatation using semiflexible bougies with hollow centers that can be threaded onto an endoscopically placed guide wire or with mercury-filled bougies is much safer and carries a risk of perforation of only 0.5%.

Other procedures that may be associated with iatrogenic esophageal perforation include the placement of Celestin tubes for palliation of unresectable esophageal carcinomas, and the placement of Sengstaken-Blakemore tubes to control variceal bleeding when the latter are overinflated or left inflated for too long. Endotracheal intubation can lead to esophageal perforation if the tube is misplaced. Esophageal sclerotherapy and endoscopic laser treatments can also perforate the esophagus. Other rarer causes of perforation include the traumatic placement of esophageal stethoscopes, or obturator airways. Lastly, the esophagus can, of course, be injured during any mediastinal or intrathoracic surgical procedure.

PENETRATING ESOPHAGEAL INJURY

Penetrating injury to the esophagus is rare, largely because of the organ's central, protected location. Only 2–3% of penetrating chest wounds caused by stabbing or gun shots will perforate the esophagus. The mortality rate for penetrating wounds of the thoracic esophagus is much higher than that observed after cervical injury.

Most patients will complain of severe cervical or thoracic pain, depending on the location of the perforation. The severity of symptoms that the patient experiences depends on the site and size of the perforation and the inflammatory response that is generated. Pain is followed shortly thereafter by fever, dysphagia, mediastinal and cutaneous emphysema, and dyspnea. The presence of mediastinal air can often be heard as a "mediastinal crunch" as the heart beats against air-containing tissues. This is known as **Hamman's sign**. Hyperapnea is common, whereas true dyspnea usually indicates that the perforation has occurred in the thoracic esophagus and the pleura has been lacerated. This injury causes a pneumothorax and pleural effusion, usually in the left hemithorax.

Patients who are not treated rapidly experience systemic sepsis, shock, and death. Patients are much sicker after perforation of the intrathoracic esophagus, and shock develops more promptly because of the rapidity with which infections spread in the pleural cavity. Transudative and exudative fluids may accumulate in the chest at the rate of 1 liter per hour. The physician should maintain a high index of suspicion when patients develop any signs or symptoms after the esophagus has been instrumented.

Patients who have perforations of the cervical esophagus complain of neck pain and dysphagia shortly after the injury. Mediastinitis may occur from high cervical perforations because the prevertebral fascial space in the neck is contiguous with the mediastinum.

Diagnosis

A number of tests may be useful for diagnosing esophageal perforation. Plain films of the chest may show evidence of mediastinal or cutaneous emphysema, which should increase the index of suspicious. Plain films of the neck may demonstrate air in the prevertebral space that indicates a cervical site of perforation. Other findings of note that may be seen on cervical radiography include: the loss of normal spinal lordosis, anterior displacement of the esophagus or upper airway, and a widened retropharyngeal space seen on the lateral film. Contrast films obtained using the water-soluble contrast medium Gastrografin (meglumine diatrizoate) will confirm the presence of esophageal perforation (Figure 25–4). Occasionally, a barium study may be required if the Gastrografin study is negative because small tears may be missed unless barium is used. However, barium spillage into closed spaces may aggravate bacterial infection if it is not removed promptly. Computed tomography (CT) of the esophagus using contrast media may also detect and localize small esophageal leaks.

Chest films may reveal widening of the mediastinum, mediastinal emphysema, and a hydropneumothorax if the thoracic esophagus is perforated. Patients who are noted to have hematemesis or bloody nasogastric tube drainage after chest trauma should have Gastrografin swallows to rule out the presence of esophageal perforation.

When thoracentesis is performed, the fluid returned may be cloudy or grossly purulent, depending upon how much time has elapsed since the injury occurred. An elevated amylase level and low pH of the pleural fluid support the diagnosis of esophageal perforation.

Management

Surgical options vary according to the location, extent, and age of the lesion. There are five basic options for the treatment of esophageal perforations: nonoperative con-

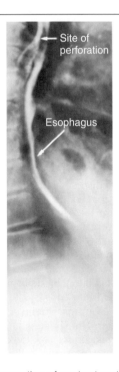

Figure 25–4. Extravasation of contrast material from the thoracic esophagus is noted after instrumental perforation. Air and fluid loculated anterior to the esophagus indicate that mediastinitis has already developed. (Reprinted, with permission, from Way LW: *Current Surgical Diagnosis & Treatment*, 9th ed. Appleton & Lange, 1991, p. 418.)

servative management, drainage alone, suture repair of the esophagus with or without local tissue flap coverage, esophagectomy, or esophageal exclusion (Table 25–4). The indications for conservative treatment are controversial. Nonoperative management can be attempted in selected hospitalized patients who are diagnosed immediately or, perhaps, more than 72 hours after instrument perforation. The ideal patients for this approach are those who were fasting, have minimal systemic symptoms, have no signs of sepsis, and have small perforations high in the cervical esophagus.

Treatment includes broad-spectrum antibiotic therapy and nasogastric (carefully placed) drainage. These patients are kept NPO and often require parenteral or tube feedings. Although conservative management can be successful, it is riskier than direct surgical repair and most likely should be reserved for patients who can not tolerate a general anesthetic. Patients who are managed conservatively should be monitored carefully to be certain that a tiny perforation does not contaminate the pleural space and lead to shock and adult respiratory distress syndrome (ARDS).

Absolute indications for operation include hydropneumothorax, pneumoperitoneum, empyema, systemic sepsis, shock, and ARDS. Traumatic cervical wounds that penetrate the platysma should be explored to rule out the presence of cervical injury. Thus, the overwhelming majority of patients who suffer esophageal perforation will require surgical operations.

Cervical perforations can often be handled by primary repair, with or without local muscle flap coverage, and drainage using closed suction. Abdominal perforations are treated by primary closure and drainage of the upper abdomen. Perforations of the intra-abdominal esophagus can easily be buttressed using the wall of the stomach.

Thoracic perforations have a high mortality and morbidity rate, regardless of the type of surgical repair that is performed. Nonoperative treatment of thoracic perforations is extremely hazardous. The mortality rate after simple chest tube drainage is 50%. Early thoracotomy and primary repair of the esophagus with drainage is the preferred method of treating thoracic esophageal perforations. The principal cause of postoperative morbidity and mortality is leakage at the site of closure. As mentioned previously, inflammatory changes around the perforation in the esophageal wall may prevent secure closure, especially if the diagnosis has been delayed. The suture line can be buttressed using local tissue flaps of pericardium,

diaphragm, intercostal muscles, the stomach wall, or a pedicled pleural flap. Decompression of the stomach with a gastrostomy tube may be indicated as well as the placement of a feeding jejunostomy tube. Patients with obstructing lesions of the thoracic esophagus who perforate should be treated definitively, if possible, by esophagectomy and reconstruction using the stomach or colon. Appropriate reconstructive procedures are chosen according to the level where the perforation occurred. Lower (distal one third) lesions of the esophagus can be approached through the right chest, whereas higher lesions are better exposed using a right thoracotomy. Obviously, it is preferable to perform this major operation within hours of the perforation, else the postoperative morbidity and mortality can be prohibitive. Patients who rupture at the point of preexisting stricture can be treated by opening the stricture to the point of the laceration and sewing the anterior wall of the stomach to the peripheral esophagus around the laceration. In all instances where a primary repair or reconstruction has been performed, the patient should not be fed until water-soluble contrast studies show that there is no leak. Similarly, chest tubes and other drains should not be removed until it is certain that the perforation is closed.

Exclusion and diversion procedures may be needed if the diagnosis is delayed or if other treatment options have failed. The esophageal perforation is sutured closed, and the esophagus is stapled or otherwise ligated above the repair. Oral secretions are diverted using a cervical esophagostomy. A gastrostomy is usually placed for feeding. Patients who are diagnosed early in the course of illness and have the appropriate surgical therapy can be expected to survive. The overall mortality rate is 50%. Only about a third of patients are diagnosed early.

FOREIGN BODY OBSTRUCTION

Coins and bones are the most commonly ingested foreign bodies that become lodged in the esophagus. However, chunks of meat may also become impacted, especially in edentulous patients, and swallowed dental prostheses may obstruct the esophageal lumen. Most foreign body obstruction occurs in children and in mentally disturbed patients. Ingested foreign bodies or other substances tend to lodge where the esophagus narrows anatomically, such as at the thoracic inlet, at the level of the aortic arch, at the left main stem bronchus, and just above the gastroesophageal junction.

The diagnosis usually can be made from the patient's history. Pain is a common complaint and may roughly indicate the level of obstruction. Some patients may also complain of dyspnea and dysphagia.

Diagnosis
Plain films and oral contrast studies may indicate the

Table 25–4. Treatment options for esophageal perforation.

Nonoperative, conservative management
Drainage
Suture repair of the esophagus with or without local tissue flap coverage
Esophagectomy
Esophageal exclusions

presence of a foreign body and rule out the presence of other coexisting abnormalities. Lateral films of the cervical esophagus are especially useful for detecting the presence of foreign bodies trapped in this region. These films are performed with the neck hyperextended so that the clavicle does not obstruct the view of the lower portion of the cervical esophagus. Radiolucent foreign bodies not seen on plain radiographs but trapped in the esophagus can sometimes be seen when the patient ingests a thin solution of barium. These studies may demonstrate perforation and will show if stricturing has occurred.

Management

Most foreign bodies, especially if they are round and smooth, will pass spontaneously. Some will have to be removed endoscopically. Endoscopic removal is normally performed under general anesthesia. Foreign bodies that are difficult to remove are often impacted in preexisting strictures.

CAUSTIC INJURY TO THE ESOPHAGUS

Diagnosis

Sodium hydroxide (lye) and hydrochloric acid, when swallowed, can severely injure the esophagus. Lye ingestion is more common. The extent and severity of injury depend on the concentration of toxin ingested and the length of time that the agent remains in contact with the mucosa. Acid ingestion typically induces the greatest injury to the stomach, whereas the esophagus remains intact over 80% of the time. Most adults will have evidence of extensive injury, as compared to children, because they typically will ingest a much larger amount—often as part of a suicide attempt. Usually, but not always, affected patients will show evidence of external injury around the mouth.

Management

Patients who are thought to have ingested a caustic substance should immediately be evaluated in an emergency room. All are at risk for airway obstruction secondary to pharyngeal edema. After a careful physical examination is performed, baseline plain films are obtained. Patients should not be induced to vomit, and gastric lavage is not indicated. Contrast studies are also not helpful initially and may be harmful. Flexible upper endoscopy should be performed as soon as it is safe, usually within the first 48 hours after injury. The scope need only be passed to the point where significant injury to the esophageal mucosa is observed. Complete esophageal obstruction secondary to edema, inflammation, and mucosal sloughing may develop within a few days.

Prolonged therapy is not usually necessary for patients with mild injuries. Patients with severe ulcerations and exudates will be prone to develop esophageal fibrosis and strictures. Patients with moderate to severe injuries will heal over a period of 4–6 weeks. There may be some substernal discomfort initially. Some patients with moderate injury are still able to take liquids and can maintain a normal nutritional status in this manner until healing has occurred. A small nasogastric tube can be carefully placed and used for enteral feeding in patients with severe injuries. Antibiotics should also be administered to these patients to decrease the risk of septic mediastinitis. The use of corticosteroids in an effort to reduce the risk of stricture formation is controversial.

Careful follow-up of patients with moderate and severe injury is needed to monitor for the development of stenosis and fibrosis. Early fibrosis can be treated by sequential bougienage. Barium contrast studies are obtained at 2-week intervals beginning after the initial injury over a period of 6 weeks, and then decreasing to every 3 months. If strictures are not detected early, then the best therapeutic approach is fiberoptic endoscopy with passage of filiform catheters and followers to gradually dilate the esophagus. Patients with extensive injuries should have large-bore nasogastric tubes left in place, as stenosis of the esophagus can be expected to occur early. Dilatation can begin early in the postinjury repair period. Some patients can be trained to swallow dilators so that therapy can continue at home. Esophageal resection with colonic or jejunal interposition will occasionally be indicated if conservative therapy fails. Even if bougienage therapy is successful, patients must be followed for life because of the risk of developing cancer in the healed esophagus.

TRACHEOESOPHAGEAL FISTULA

Diagnosis

Tracheoesophageal fistulas may occur secondary to cancer, infection, or trauma. In the past, many of these fistulas occurred secondary to tuberculosis or other granulomatous disease of the lung. Patients have symptoms that reflect the underlying disease process as well as the presence of the esophageal fistula. A characteristic symptom is coughing after the ingestion of food or liquids. Contrast studies are diagnostic if they demonstrate the tracheobronchial tree. Esophagoscopy will often not detect the presence of a small fistula but will detect esophageal cancer if this is the underlying etiology. Bronchoscopy should be performed in all patients to determine the extent of tracheal involvement or to diagnose primary pulmonary or bronchial disease.

Management

Treatment of tracheobronchial fistula may be difficult. Often only palliative measures can be instituted if the fistula occurs secondary to malignancy. Cervical esophagostomies may be helpful in severely symptomatic patients when all other measures fail. Celestin tubes or other stents can sometimes aggravate the problem by inducing pressure necrosis in the esophageal wall. Definitive surgical procedures are of limited success.

Greater success may be achieved with benign fistula. Patients with fistulas secondary to infection should be treated with antibiotics. Patients with fistulas secondary to endotracheal tube or cuff erosion or from blunt or penetrating injury can have these corrected surgically after nutritional rehabilitation. The trachea is dissected from the esophagus, and both openings are repaired. The sutures lines are then separated using a leaf of pleura. This operation has a 90% success rate for benign disease.

HIATAL HERNIAS & REFLUX ESOPHAGITIS

HIATAL HERNIAS

All or a portion of the stomach may extend into the mediastinum through the esophageal hiatus of the diaphragm. These are of two types (Figure 25–5). The passage of the cardia of the stomach together with the esophagogastric junction directly through the esophageal hiatus into the mediastinum is known as a **type I hiatal hernia**. It is not clear if a type I hernia is a true pathophysiologic condition. The gastroesophageal junction can be forced to pass

cephalad in most normal subjects during a Valsalva maneuver. This can be easily visualized on barium swallow. Therefore, it can be considered a normal finding in most individuals. Most patients with type I hiatal hernias have normal lower esophageal pressures and function, even when a large portion of the stomach herniates into the mediastinum.

In **type II hiatal hernias** the gastroesophageal junction remains within the abdominal cavity while a portion or all of the stomach protrudes into the mediastinum between the fibers of the right crus of the diaphragm.

However, type I hiatal hernias may be associated with reflux esophagitis. Most patients with significant esophageal reflux have a large hiatal hernia. The normal intra-abdominal location of the gastroesophageal junction is believed to facilitate the function of the lower esophageal sphincter. Increases in intragastric pressure, such as after eating, increase intra-abdominal pressure, which tends to prevent gastroesophageal reflux.

Type II hernias are rarely associated with gastroesophageal reflux and, in fact, may be entirely asymptomatic. However, they are much more likely to strangulate and infarct. These hernias are common in the elderly. Patients with type II hernias may also develop respiratory, gastrointestinal, and cardiac symptoms after meals when the dilated stomach compresses adjacent structures. Some patients complain of intermittent epigastric or chest pain after meals that is occasionally accompanied by shortness of breath. Acute gastric dilatation or volvulus may occur. Sudden severe epigastric and chest pain accompanied by cardiovascular instability should suggest the presence of gastric volvulus and impending infarction and perforation. Furthermore, ulceration of the displaced stomach is described. Gastric perforation into mediastinal structures, such as the aorta or pericardium, has dire consequences.

Diagnosis

Type II hernias are typically diagnosed when chest radiographs are obtained for other reasons. These films will show a gastric bubble and air fluid level in the retrocardiac space. Barium swallows or CT may confirm the diagnosis but are not necessary unless one is concerned about the presence of other abnormalities.

Management

The natural history of type II hiatal hernias is uncertain. Current dogma is that surgical correction is the only way to treat patients with type II hiatal hernias and should be performed electively in patients who have no contraindications to operation. Emergent repair is indicated for patients who have symptoms or who are acutely ill. Fluid replacement, nasogastric tube decompression, supplemental oxygen, and antibiotic therapy are all important aspects of the preoperative preparation. The elective operation is performed through an upper midline abdominal incision. The stomach is reduced, the hernia sac excised, and the crura of the diaphragm are reapproximated using nonabsorbable sutures. The stomach is fixed by suturing it to the

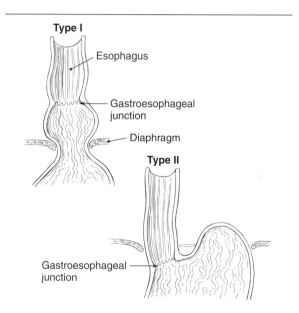

Figure 25–5. Types I and II hiatal hernias. The cardia of the stomach and the gastroesophageal junction pass directly through the esophageal hiatus into the mediastinum in type I hernia. In type II hernias, the gastroesophageal junction remains within the abdominal cavity.

anterior abdominal wall or by performing a gastroenterostomy.

Acutely ill patients, those who have the entire stomach herniated into the thoracic cavity or those with gastric ulcers, may be best served by a left thoracotomy through the seventh or eighth rib. Peptic ulcers may be removed using a wedge resection or partial gastrectomy. The intrathoracic approach is less well tolerated by frail elderly patients and has a higher complication rate.

Other hernias of the diaphragm can occur congenitally or secondary to blunt and penetrating trauma. Congenital hernias occur where the embryonic precursors of the diaphragm fail to fuse with each other or to the body side walls. Bochdalek hernias originate when the posterior pleuroperitoneal canal fails to obliterate. Anterior diaphragmatic hernias protrude through the foramen of Morgagni; they occur when the diaphragm fails to fuse with the sternal and costal margins.

REFLUX ESOPHAGITIS

Diagnosis

Esophagitis is a serious problem for patients who have gastroesophageal reflux, but not all patients have symptoms. Similarly, some patients with long-standing chronic symptoms may have only minimal evidence of esophagitis. Gastric and duodenal juices are more injurious together than either substance is alone, indicating that the damage caused by esophagitis is not solely pH-dependent. Changes observed during upper endoscopy may range from mild mucosal inflammation to friable hemorrhagic mucosa to deep ulceration and exudation. Patients with deep ulcerations usually have severe retrosternal pain that is aggravated by eating. Left untreated, patients with severe esophagitis will progress to fibrosis, scarring, and stricture formation. Some patients, especially the elderly, may present with strictures without ever having had other complaints. Patients with significant esophagitis may develop iron deficiency anemia because of chronic blood loss. However, bleeding is rarely massive unless there is coexistent variceal disease, for example, in patients with portal hypertension. Erosion into a submucosal vein may produce massive hematemesis.

The most common complaints are dyspepsia and pyrosis, or "heartburn." Nocturnal reflux may disturb sleep; patients may wake with regurgitated food or a foul taste in their mouths. Occasional subjects will complain of asthma. The etiology of this effect is unknown. Patients who complain of dysphagia and heartburn but who only have minimal or no evidence of esophagitis should have esophageal manometry to rule out the presence of a primary motility disorder. However, one should recall that patients with severe esophagitis may have altered secondary peristaltic waves.

The esophagus is normally lined by squamous epithelium. In some patients, the squamous epithelium may be replaced by columnar metaplastic cells. This is called **Barrett's change**. These metaplastic cells may have gastric or intestinal characteristics. It is not known why some patients develop strictures and others develop Barrett's esophagus. Barrett's changes are more likely to occur in younger patients who have severe daytime reflux, whereas strictures are more likely to occur in elderly patients who have nocturnal reflux and defective esophageal clearing mechanisms. Patients with Barrett's esophagitis are at risk for developing adenocarcinoma, especially if they have intestinal metaplasia. The risk is small but may merit repeated endoscopic surveillance.

Regurgitation of gastric contents, especially when the patient bends over or is supine, is clear-cut evidence of free esophageal reflux. Some individuals will have repeated episodes of aspiration pneumonitis. These episodes may be life-threatening in elderly subjects.

The history is extremely important. Endoscopy is important to document the presence of esophagitis or columnar transformation of the distal esophageal mucosa after barium contrast studies and fluoroscopy are obtained to rule out the presence of comorbid diseases. The severity of mucosal injury can best be determined endoscopically. Biopsy specimens demonstrating the presence of basal cell hyperplasia or an excessive number of neutrophils strongly suggest the presence of pathophysiologic reflux. A hiatal hernia may also be evident above the crura of the diaphragm.

A **provocative acid infusion test (Bernstein)** may be useful when symptoms are equivocal. The administration of 0.1 molar hydrochloric acid into the lumen of the esophagus may reproduce the patient's pain and give a clue as to its etiology. The symptoms should disappear when the infusion is changed to saline.

Reflux of gastric contents into the esophagus can be a normal physiological occurrence. **Pathological reflux** is that which is greater than the 95% confidence limit for the normal population and exists if the distal esophageal lumen has a pH below 4 for more than 4% of a day, or if there are more than 10 reflux episodes where the luminal pH falls below 4 in any 24-hour period. Alkaline reflux raises the luminal pH above 7.5. The normal esophagus rapidly clears alkaline or acid challenges until the pH is returned to normal (pH = 7).

Twenty-four-hour pH monitoring requires the insertion of a small probe through the nostril such that the tip of the instrument lies just above the lower esophageal sphincter. The probe records the number of episodes of esophageal reflux as well as the amount of time needed to clear the acid load. The patient keeps a diary that can be used to correlate symptoms and other activities with changes in esophageal pH. Esophagitis may result from frequent episodes of acid reflux, from less frequent episodes where large volumes enter the esophagus, when esophageal clearance mechanisms are inadequate, or from a combination of all three. Monitoring of pH is also useful because it may temporally correlate episodes of reflux with the patient's symptoms.

Esophageal manometry is performed to study esophageal motility and to measure pressure in the lower esophageal sphincter. Manometry is the most accurate method for determining the strength, timing, and coordination of esophageal peristalsis. Specific criteria exist to define the presence of significant abnormalities in esophageal function. Normal peristalsis must be present in the esophageal body if the patient is to benefit from antireflux procedures that obstruct the passage of materials through the gastroesophageal junction.

Management

The objectives of therapy are to reduce the incidence and severity of reflux. Treatment with antacid preparations may be sufficient for patients with mild esophagitis. Furthermore, H_2 antagonists or proton pump inhibitors play a primary role in reducing the severity of symptoms and decreasing mucosal inflammation. Seventy-five percent of patients can be expected to respond to a 6-week course of treatment with histamine receptor antagonists by healing of esophageal changes.

Lifestyle changes are helpful. Coffee and alcohol should be eliminated from the diet, and patients should not smoke because these factors decrease lower esophageal sphincter pressure. Anticholinergic medications should be discontinued. Patients should sleep with the head of the bed elevated at least 8 inches by placing the bed posts on blocks. They should also eat small meals and avoid eating dinner too close to bedtime. Obese patients should be encouraged to lose weight, which will decrease the incidence and severity of symptoms. Patients who continue to complain of reflux after adequate acid suppression is achieved may benefit from the use of prokinetic agents, such as metoclopramide or cisapride.

Most patients will respond to medical therapy. Surgical intervention is reserved for the patients who fail or who are unwilling to continue lifelong medical therapy. A number of antireflux procedures are used, including the **Nissen fundoplication**, the **Hill posterior gastropexy**, and the **Belsey Mark IV repair**. These different operations share some common features. All include wrapping a portion or all of the cardia of the stomach around the lower end of the esophagus, which is returned to and fixed in the abdominal cavity. The esophagus must be fully mobilized if the wraps are to be successful. The esophageal hiatus is narrowed by suturing the crura together.

The Nissen procedure can be performed through the abdomen or the chest. The greater curvature of the stomach is mobilized by taking down several short gastric vessels. The stomach is then sutured to itself around the lower esophagus, through which a large, at least 48F, bougie is passed. Thus, the standard Nissen fundoplication wraps the stomach 360 degrees around the esophagus. The Hill median arcuate ligament posterior gastropexy must be done via the abdomen, whereas the Belsey Mark IV procedure can only be performed through the chest. Hill's procedure fixes the gastroesophageal junction in the abdomen by suturing the phrenoesophageal fascia bundles to the dense arcuate ligament that lies anterior to the aorta. The crura of the diaphragm are approximated and the gas-

troesophageal junction is imbricated. The thoracic route is also preferable when a stricture is present because the entire esophagus can be mobilized. The Belsey procedure invaginates the esophagus into the fundus of the stomach and includes the diaphragm. This produces a 270-degree wrap of the stomach around the esophagus. Laparoscopic wraps and repairs are becoming popular. Short-term follow-up studies suggest that the laparoscopic procedures are as effective as the open approaches.

The success rates of the three operations are similar. The recurrence rates for each are about 10% over the first 5 years and 2% per year thereafter. The Nissen wrap may be slightly more successful in relieving heartburn, however, the wrap must be done loosely to avoid the "gas-bloat" syndrome. Patients with this syndrome cannot belch and have trouble vomiting. They may also develop aerophagia with gastric and intestinal distention. The best procedure is likely the one that will be best tolerated by the patient and with which the surgeon is most familiar.

STRICTURES

Diagnosis

Ninety percent of all benign strictures are caused by acid reflux from the stomach into the esophagus with chronic transmural esophagitis and fibrosis. Other causes include infection, trauma, and congenital malformations. A variety of systemic illnesses, such as Stevens-Johnson syndrome, Behçet's syndrome, and Crohn's disease, may also cause benign strictures. *Candida albicans* accounts for half of the cases of strictures caused by infection. Other pathogens or infections include the herpes simplex virus, cytomegalovirus, mucormycosis, histoplasmosis, and tuberculosis in immunocompromised patients or those infected with the acquired immunodeficiency syndrome (AIDS) virus (human immunodeficiency virus, HIV).

Treatment is directed at the organism responsible for the infection. Additional therapy, such as dilatation, may be needed once the infection is resolved. The risk of perforation may be higher in these patients, who do not typically develop thickening of the esophageal wall such as is found in patients with peptic strictures. Strictures caused by fungal infections may need to be resected.

Localized injury to the esophagus from acid or alkali ingestion as discussed previously, prolonged nasogastric intubation, and radiation therapy may cause transmural inflammation and stricture formation. Ingestion of potassium chloride or guanidine, aspirin, ascorbic acid, phenytoin, and tetracycline in pill form have also been reported to cause traumatic strictures. A variable number of patients will develop strictures after injection sclerotherapy for esophageal varices.

Painless dysphagia is the most common symptom. Reflux strictures typically occur just above the squamocolumnar junction. One third of patients with Barrett's

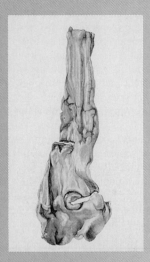

Figure that appeared in Barrett's 1950 report. It is a drawing made from an esophageal specimen "in which there is a chronic gastric ulcer situated in the lower part of the specimen ... found in the mediastinum above the level of the crura of the diaphragm." (Reprinted, with permission, from Barrett NR: Chronic peptic ulcer of the oesophagus and aesophagitis. Br J Surg 1957; 41:175–182.)

Norman Rupert Barrett (1903–1979), an influential British surgeon, published a report in 1950 (Barrett NR: Br J Surg 1950;38:175–182) that described a condition of the esophagus in which "a part of the stomach extends upwards into the mediastinum—or even to the neck—and that in this stomach a typical chronic gastric ulcer can form." The article was thoroughly investigated and researched by Barrett and his associates. Not only was the condition portrayed clinically, but the origins of his observations were carefully described. The original report included color representations of gross and endoscopic specimens, radiographs of strictures caused by "reflux esophagitis," and histologic slides to support Barrett's thesis, such as "gastric mucous membrane in the postcricoid region of the esophagus."

When Barrett's original paper was published, he believed this condition to be a congenital replacement of esophagus with stomach. However, he later became convinced that the columnar-lined organ was, in fact, esophagus and not stomach. Barrett called the condition "lower esophagus lined by columnar epithelium" (Barrett NR: Br J Surg 1957;41:881–894). He certainly recognized that hiatal hernia and severe reflux esophagitis were associated with the disorder, but he assumed that the columnar lining was congenital.

Although reports throughout the late 1950s and 1960s implied that the columnar lining might not be congenital in origin, by the 1970s there was little doubt of its association with gastroesophageal reflux disease and chronic injury to normal squamous epithelium. It is interesting to note Barrett's early recognition that patients with this disorder often do not experience symptoms: "On the contrary, the patients have come to the hospital because of emergencies such as massive bleeding, perforation, or carcinoma. They have died and typical gastric ulcers have been found." Thus, Barrett set the stage for what is recognized today as a chronic injury/repair process that can progress to atypical dysplasia and invasive cancer when left untreated.

changes will develop strictures. However, most patients with gastroesophageal reflux will not develop strictures. Patients who do will likely have had symptoms for many months or years. The spontaneous resolutions of symptoms of esophageal reflux may herald the development of a stricture. Fifty percent of patients will present with dysphagia and no prior history of reflux. Patients with scleroderma may be plagued by reflux strictures that are especially difficult to manage. These patients have abnormal motility and decreased esophageal clearance.

Management

Various tests may be performed to exclude malignancy, assess the severity of the stricture, and to search for other diseases. Barium contrast studies, endoscopy with biopsy and brushings, and esophageal manometry are all useful. Twenty-four–hour pH monitoring, as discussed earlier, is also important. Strictures longer than 20 mm, that are found in the upper or mid-esophageal region, or that are not associated with reflux, are suspicious for neoplasia. Esophageal manometry may be helpful in selecting patients for surgical correction and in determining which procedure should be performed. For example, patients with decreased lower esophageal sphincter pressures, a short intra-abdominal esophageal segment, and poor distal motility may be best served by a partial, Belsey Mark IV type, gastric fundoplication.

Very few patients with strictures can be successfully treated medically. Many patients with peptic esophageal strictures can be managed using endoscopic dilatation and long-term treatment with a proton pump inhibitor, like omeprazole. Such therapy appears to reduce the need for subsequent dilatations. However, about 50% of patients will need repeated dilatations, especially those who have transmural fibrosis. Female patients are more likely to respond than males. Most patients should be offered antireflux therapy to prevent relapse after successful dilatation if they are satisfactory candidates for operation. Patients with a shortened esophagus and esophageal stricture can be treated with gastroplasty to lengthen the esophagus. A fundoplication is then performed around the neoesophagus. Patients who have normal motility of the distal esophagus can be expected to do quite well with gastroplasty, with a long-term satisfaction rate of over 90%. Occasionally, resection of the strictured portion of the esophagus and intestinal interposition will be necessary. Antrectomy and Roux-en-Y diversion can also be considered for patients with intractable reflux whose strictures are resected. Esophageal resection includes a vagotomy by necessity, and a drainage procedure is needed to avoid gastric outlet obstruction. The duodenojejunal anastomosis must be constructed at least 45 cm distal to the gastrojejunostomy to avoid bile reflux gastritis and esophagitis.

BENIGN TUMORS

LEIOMYOMAS

The most common benign tumor of the esophagus is a leiomyoma. However, these benign tumors of the esophagus are actually rare, comprising only about 10% of all gastrointestinal leiomyomas. More than 90% of leiomyomas are found in the thoracic portion of the esophagus between the middle and third levels. They may also be found at multiple sites. Most measure 5–8 cm in diameter, are solitary, and are well encapsulated, although they can occasionally grow quite large. They likely originate from the muscular components of the esophageal wall, from the muscular component of blood vessels, or from embryonic cell rests.

Seventy percent of all leiomyomas of the esophagus occur in men between the ages of 20 and 50 years. Female patients tend to be older. A large number of esophageal leiomyomas are found incidentally. Half of the patients will have dysphagia or odynophagia as an initial symptom. Rarely, leiomyomas may cause weight loss, bleeding, or obstruction.

Diagnosis & Management

A barium swallow typically will detect a sharply defined, smooth-walled filling defect abutting on the lumen of the esophagus (Figure 25–6). Endoscopy will reveal the presence of a bulging, firm, mobile, intramural mass with a completely normal mucosal covering. These features are highly suggestive of the presence of a leiomyoma. Biopsy is contraindicated in this instance because this could prevent successful enucleation, should the patient come to operation.

Enucleation is the treatment of choice. Biopsies should be performed at the time of operation to rule out malignant degeneration. Esophagectomy is rarely needed.

POLYPS & OTHER BENIGN TUMORS

Diagnosis & Management

Polyps of the esophagus represent 20% of all benign tumors that affect this organ. Other rare benign tumors of

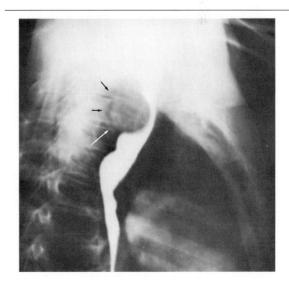

Figure 25–6. Leiomyoma of the esophagus. The film shows a smooth, rounded density compressing the esophageal lumen. (Reprinted, with permission, from Way LW: *Current Surgical Diagnosis & Treatment,* 9th ed. Appleton & Lange, 1991, p. 422.)

the esophagus include lipomas, fibromyomas, myxomas, various vascular growths, and neurofibromas.

Polyps are typically found in the cervical esophagus, and are usually long and cylindrical in shape. Older men are most often affected. Polyps may rarely regurgitate into the larynx and cause airway obstruction and asphyxia. They are composed of vascular fibroblastic tissue and, like leiomyoma, are covered by normal epithelium. They may also cause dysphagia.

Cysts and duplications receive their blood supply directly from the aorta and may rarely cause significant upper gastrointestinal bleeding. Pedunculated intraluminal lesions may cause pain, edema, infection, and bleeding if torsion occurs.

Barium contrast studies are typically diagnostic. Leiomyomas, cysts, and duplications have a distinct x-ray appearance that allows them to be distinguished from malignancies. Upper endoscopy and biopsies will confirm the diagnosis.

Small lesions can be removed endoscopically. Larger symptomatic polyps are removed through a esophagotomy opposite to the side of the lesion.

ESOPHAGEAL CANCER

Esophageal cancer in the United States occurs about three times as frequently in men as in women in persons 50–70 years of age. The median age of death is 66. It is three times more common in African-Americans than in Caucasians. Most malignancies are carcinomas. Tumors that arise proximal to the cardia are almost all squamous cell carcinomas. Those that occur in the distal esophagus near the gastroesophageal junction and cardia may be adenocarcinomas. Adenocarcinoma of the body of the esophagus occurs in only 3–10% of cases. The incidence of adenocarcinomas appears to be increasing. Esophageal cancers tend to be relatively evenly distributed along the length of the esophagus: 20% occurring in the upper third, 35% in the middle third, and 45% in the lower third. Squamous cell cancers occur slightly more often in the middle third of the esophagus.

Although the incidence of esophageal carcinoma is relatively small in the United States, it is much higher in other parts of the world. For example, in Northern China the risk of esophageal cancer may exceed 100 cases per 100,000 population. Heavy alcohol and tobacco use increase the risk of developing esophageal cancer.

The etiology of the esophageal carcinoma is unknown but is related to malnutrition itself and a number of dietary factors.

Nutrition-related risk factors include consumption of large amounts of hot tea, spices, and betel nuts, excess zinc intake, and various vitamin and trace element deficiencies (vitamins A and C, copper, manganese, magnesium). The presence of silica particles in bread that de-

posit in the wall of the esophagus, and nitrosamine contamination in the drinking water or fungal contamination of food, may also increase the risk of developing esophageal carcinoma. Plant foods contain elevated levels of nitrates and nitrites when there is a deficiency of molybdenum in the soil. Consumption of these foods then leads to elevated levels of nitrosamine.

Other risk factors for esophageal cancer include chronic iron deficiency, achalasia or other states that lead to esophageal stasis, Barrett's change, reflux esophagitis, and congential tylosis, which is a rare autosomal dominant disease of the esophagus. Patients with nontropical sprue also have an increased risk of developing esophageal cancer, for unknown reasons. Patients with severe dysplasia of the esophagus from any cause have a 15% chance of developing esophageal carcinoma.

Esophageal cancers typically present as fungating, ulcerated, intraluminal lesions. Most are at least 5 cm on presentation. They likely grow very slowly, taking years to progress from the in situ, asymptomatic stage to clinical presentation. However, survival without treatment is less than 9 months on average, once patients become symptomatic. The most common cause of death is bronchopneumonia. Cancers with annular growth patterns may obstruct the esophageal lumen earlier in the course of disease.

All esophageal tumors may directly invade surrounding mediastinal structures and metastasize through the blood or lymphatic system. Esophageal cancers also have a propensity to spread intramurally from the site of the primary lesion; this tends to occur proximally rather than distally. In over half the cases, intramural extension does not exceed 3 cm, however, 10% of the time tumor may be found 9 cm from the original tumor. Metastases to regional lymph nodes or to sites in the mediastinum, neck, or celiac region are found in 80% of patients with esophageal carcinoma at the time of diagnosis. The risk of lymph node metastasis correlates with the depth of tumor invasion. Only 14% of patients whose cancers are limited to the mucosa and submucosa (T1) have positive nodes. The incidence of nodal metastases is 30% when tumors are limited to the muscularis propria (T2), 50% for lesions that involve the adventitia (T3), and 75% when tumors invade periesophageal tissues (T4) (Table 25–5).

Many esophageal carcinomas involve other structures, such as the trachea, left main stem bronchus, or aorta at the time of presentation. Such transmural tumor penetration may be more rapid in cancers of the esophagus because the organ does not have a serosal layer. Distant sites of metastasis include the lung, liver, bones, kidneys, and brain. Thus, most patients are quite advanced when their disease is first diagnosed; almost no patients with Stage I disease are diagnosed in the United States. Most patients complain of dysphagia that may be severe. Initially, solid foods cause discomfort, but eventually even liquids may be difficult to swallow. Weight loss, weakness, and anemia are also common. Approximately 30% of patients will complain of persistent pain at presentation. Persistent pain implies that the tumor has extended beyond the

Table 25–5. TMN staging system for esophageal cancer.

T Primary Tumor
TX	Primary tumor cannot be assessed
T0	No tumor
Tis	Carcinoma in situ
T1	Tumor invades the lamina propria or submucosa
T2	Tumor invades the muscularis propria
T3	Tumor invades the periesophageal tissue
T4	Tumor invades adjacent structures

N Regional Lymph Nodes
NX	Regional nodes cannot be assessed
N0	No regional lymph node metastases
N1	Regional lymph node metastases

M Distant Metastases
MX	Distant metastases cannot be assessed
M0	No distant metastases
M1	Distant metastases

Staging Groups
Stage 0	Tis	N0	M0
Stage I	T1	N0	M0
Stage IIA	T2	N0	M0
	T3	N0	M0
Stage IIB	T1	N1	M0
	T2	N1	M0
Stage III	T3	N1	M0
	T4	Any N	M0
Stage IV	Any T	Any N	M1

esophageal wall. Hoarseness implies that the tumor has spread to involve the recurrent laryngeal nerve. Regurgitation and aspiration may occur when patients are supine.

Massive bleeding from esophageal cancers is rare but may occur if the tumor has invaded the superior vena cava or aorta. Other complications result from tumor invasion of other mediastinal structures, including the trachea or major bronchi or the pericardium. These include tracheal obstruction or fistula, pneumonitis bronchitis or lung abscess, and cardiac arrhythmias.

Diagnosis

The findings on chest radiographs are nonspecific. An air fluid level may be visible in the esophagus. Extensive disease may be associated with x-ray evidence of pneumonitis, abscess, or pleural effusion.

Barium contrast studies will show narrowing of the esophageal lumen in the region of the tumor. The esophagus may be dilated proximal to the lesion. The mass is visualized as an irregular shelf-like lesion or as a constriction involving the lumen (Figure 25–7). Mucosal irregularity is prominent in both instances. Angulation of the axis of the esophagus above and below the cancer suggests that the tumor has spread beyond the muscular wall.

Esophagoscopy and bronchoscopy are indispensable parts of the diagnostic evaluation. Esophagoscopy and biopsy will confirm the diagnosis of esophageal carci-

noma in over 95% of cases. If the tumor is not directly visible during endoscopy because the lumen of the esophagus is distorted, inflamed, or narrowed, brushings or washings should be obtained. Bronchoscopy is performed to determine if the cancer has invaded the tracheobronchial tree. Lesions of the upper and mid-esophagus are especially prone to invade and distort the bronchial lumen or carina. Occasionally, tumor may be visualized directly in the intrabronchial tree. CT, although very useful in assessing the esophageal wall and mediastinal wall as well as distant sites of metastasis, does not accurately predict invasion and, of course, does not provide tissue for pathological examination. For this reason, diagnostic laparoscopy and mediastinoscopy are also important components of the preoperative staging and evaluation of esophageal carcinoma. These tools, together with endoscopic ultrasound, may improve the preoperative assessment of patients with these malignancies.

Management

Esophageal carcinomas that involve the tracheobronchial tree or aorta, as noted by bronchoscopy or CT, are not resectable. Patients who have hoarseness associated with vocal cord paralysis or tracheobronchial fistulas are also not resectable. Even in the absence of specific evidence that suggests the esophageal cancer cannot be safely excised, only approximately 50–60% of tumors will actually be resected. Nevertheless, in the absence of distant metastases, most patients should be offered surgical resection if they are suitable operative candidates. Esophageal resection and reconstruction provides the best palliation for most patients. Radiotherapy or chemotherapy alone or in combination with operation also play important roles in the treatment of esophageal malignancies.

The average operative mortality is 13%. The survival rate is approximately 27% at 1 year, 12% at 2 years, and 10% at 5 years with standard therapy. Some centers report operative mortality rates under 5% and 5-year survival rates over 20% in patients with squamous cell carcinomas.

Preoperative radiation may improve the likelihood of successful resection, but has not yet been shown to significantly improve the overall cure rate. New regimens that use preoperative chemotherapy with radiation followed by operation are currently being evaluated. The initial results of these combined modality treatment programs are promising.

Patients who are operative candidates should stop smoking and undergo pulmonary function testing. Any reversible respiratory deficiencies should be addressed. Patients who have lost greater than 10–15% of their usual body weight are candidates for preoperative nutritional support, ideally via the enteral route. Gastrostomy or jejunostomy tubes can be inserted when diagnostic laparoscopy is performed for preoperative staging or as isolated procedures if the patient is significantly malnourished.

Many surgical techniques can be used to treat esophageal cancers. The techniques are usually selected

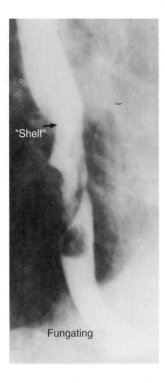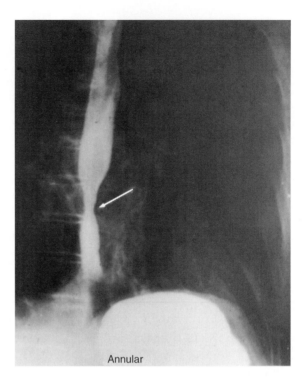

Figure 25–7. Two types of esophageal cancer. The film on the left shows an irregular mass with a "shelf-like" upper border and fungating distal components. The film on the right shows a constricting band about the esophagus, typical of annular carcinomas. (Reprinted, with permission, from Way LW: *Current Surgical Diagnosis & Treatment,* 9th ed. Appleton & Lange, 1991, p. 424.)

according to the level of the tumor and the surgeon's experience and preference. Standard approaches include the left thoracoabdominal incision (Sweet), a laparotomy and right thoracotomy (Ivor-Lewis), and the transhiatal esophagectomy (Grey Turner and Orringer).

The **Sweet left thoracoabdominal incision** was very popular in the past for carcinomas involving the lower esophagus or gastroesophageal junction. This approach offers the best exposure for abdominal lymphadenectomy. Its major disadvantage is that exposure is limited at the level of the heart and the aortic arch, which makes more proximal dissections and anastomoses very difficult. Thus, approaching esophageal lesions via a thoracoabdominal incision is more limiting. Less esophagus can be removed and the risk of local recurrence is probably higher.

At the present time, tumors involving the lower third of the esophagus or the gastroesophageal junction are usually resected using separate laparotomy and right thoracotomy incisions (**Ivor-Lewis**). Resection margins should include celiac lymph nodes and left gastric vessels and should also extend to the esophagus above the azygos vein. Classically, the spleen is preserved in patients with squamous carcinoma but is removed in patients who have adenocarcinoma. A pyloroplasty may be performed to avoid problems with gastric emptying postoperatively,

since the vagus nerves have been taken by necessity. The risk of dumping syndrome after pyloroplasty or pyloromyotomy is approximately 2%. Intestinal continuity is reestablished by pulling the stomach into the chest and anastomosing it to the residual esophagus. The Ivor-Lewis approach provides easy access to the thoracic esophagus. It is easier to obtain a wide margin on the tumor, and anastomoses can be performed with ease. However, exposure of the gastroesophageal junction and diaphragmatic hiatus can be very difficult, especially in obese patients.

Tumors of the middle and upper thirds of the esophagus require resection of the esophagus to the cervical region. However, most of the stomach can be preserved if it is present. Reanastomosis is performed to the stomach through a third incision made in the right or left neck. Ideally, 10 cm of esophagus is removed proximal to the esophageal cancer. Frozen sections of the resection margins obtained during surgery may be helpful in determining the limits of resection.

If the cancer does not involve the trachea, aorta, or bronchi, esophagectomy can sometimes be performed using just an abdominal and cervical incision (**Grey-Turner and Orringer**). The esophagus between the two incisions is removed bluntly. The stomach is passed through the posterior mediastinum and anastomosed to the cervical esophagus. Although this approach has been criticized, current survival rates are indistinguishable from those obtained using more aggressive operations. Furthermore, patients with chronic pulmonary disease may be more tolerant of blunt esophagectomy without thoracotomy. In general, it appears that postoperative mortality and morbidity may be decreased using blunt esophagectomy, except for the risk of cervical anastomotic leaks, but this has not been proved in prospective randomized trials. Other disadvantages of the Orringer esophagectomy include an increased risk of injury to nearby structures and, occasionally, troublesome bleeding.

If the stomach is not available or is otherwise unsuitable for reconstruction, then portions of the colon may be interposed between the cervical esophagus and the upper gastrointestinal tract. However, this operation is much more difficult and its morbidity and mortality rates are much higher.

Radiotherapy alone relieves dysphagia in only half of patients treated this way and the response is usually transient. Typical dosing regimens expose patients to 4500–6000 rads. Patients whose tumors involve the tracheobronchial tree should not be treated with preoperative radiation or chemotherapy becauses this significantly increases the risk of fistula formation. Patients with unresectable tumors are best treated by substernal gastric bypass and cervical esophagogastrostomy. The distal esophagus is drained using a Roux-en-Y esophagojejunostomy. Once the patients has recovered from this operation, the cancer may be treated with radiotherapy.

Palliative intubation of the tumor may be attempted in patients who cannot tolerate operative resection. Tubes can be inserted at laparotomy or endoscopically. The quality of life after tube placements is usually poor, so the procedure is best reserved for patients who have extensive disease and are not expected to survive more than a few months. Use of the YAG laser may be used in an effort to restore an adequate esophageal lumen. Several treatments may be necessary, but there is a low incidence of perforation and the ability to swallow usually returns promptly, if only transiently.

Patients with malignant tracheoesophageal fistulas may be treated using a substernal gastric bypass and cervical esophagogastrostomy. The ends of the thoracic esophagus are stapled to exclude them from the gastrointestinal tract. A tube is inserted into the thoracic esophagus to collect secretions.

Patients are monitored in an intensive care unit postoperatively until they are stable. In many instances, it is best to continue mechanical ventilation for the first 24 hours. Nasogastric suction is continued until bowel function returns and there is no evidence of an anastomotic leak. Chest physiotherapy is very important to decrease the risk of pneumonia. Jejunostomy tubes should be placed, especially in those patients who are nutritionally depleted.

Anastomotic leaks occur in 3–15% of cases. Cervical leaks present as fever and a swollen, painful neck incision. These are treated by opening the neck incision and establishing adequate drainage. These will normally heal as long as adequate nutrition support, drainage, and antibiotic coverage are provided. Strictures are treated with repeated dilatations. Intrathoracic leaks are far more serious, and mortality rates as high as 50% are reported after this dreaded complication. If the leak occurs within the first few days, then reoperation is mandatory to exclude gastric necrosis and to exclude the area and drain cervical secretions. Thus, infected or necrotic tissue is debrided, drainage of the mediastinum and pleural cavity is obtained, and a cervical esophagostomy is performed. The gastrointestinal tract is reconstructed at a later date. Leaks occurring later in the postoperative period also usually require reoperation to establish adequate drainage.

SUGGESTED READING

Moody FG, Devries WC: The esophagus and diaphragmatic hernia. In: Hardy JD (editor): *Hardy's Textbook of Surgery*. Lippincott, 1983.

Morris PJ, Malt RA: *Oxford Textbook of Surgery*. Oxford University Press, 1995.

Orringer MB et al: The esophagus. In: Sabiston DC (editor): *Textbook of Surgery*, 13th ed. Saunders, 1986.

Pellegrini CA, Way LW: Esophagus and diaphragm. In: Way LW: *Current Surgical Diagnosis & Treatment*, 10th ed. Appleton & Lange, 1994.

Willmore DW et al: *Scientific American Surgery*. Scientific American, 1996.

26

The Stomach, Small Intestine, & Appendix

J. Augusto Bastidas, MD, & Harry A. Oberhelman, Jr, MD

► Key Facts

- ► The stomach may be divided into four segments: the cardia, fundus, body, and antrum, while the small bowel is divided into three segments: the duodenum, jejunum, and ileum.

- ► The important peptides found in the stomach include gastrin, somatostatin, gastric-releasing peptides, vasoactive intestinal peptides, glucagon, and substance P.

- ► Gastric emptying of liquids is thought to be primarily controlled by the proximal stomach, whereas emptying of solids is controlled by the distal stomach.

- ► The duodenum functions to neutralize the acid content of particles delivered to it, achieve an isosmotic solution, and add the necessary components of bile and pancreatic juice.

- ► Intestinal contents are transported through the gut lumen in a complex process of peristalsis.

- ► An ulcer is the outcome of a disturbance of the balance between destructive factors—such as acid, pepsin, and infection—and the mechanisms protecting the gastric and duodenal mucosa, known as the mucosal barrier.

- ► Diagnosis of an ulcer may be confirmed by upper gastrointestinal endoscopy or by barium studies.

- ► Regional enteritis, or Crohn's disease, is the most common inflammatory disease of the small bowel that may require surgical intervention.

- ► Though the small bowel has a great capacity to adapt following massive bowel resection, one needs to remain aware that the jejunum and ileum do have specific functions that may be absent, depending on which segment of bowel has been eliminated and preserved.

- ► Small bowel obstruction is most frequently caused by adhesions and can often be managed without surgery.

- ► Appendicitis is the most common cause of the "acute abdomen." It occurs in approximately 6% of the United States population, primarily between the ages of 10 and 30.

- ► There are approximately 20,000 new cases of gastric cancer per year in the United States, and over 50% of these are amenable to tumor removal. Surgical resection is the only potentially curative treatment.

- ► Small bowel tumors are very rare.

ANATOMY & PHYSIOLOGY

ANATOMY

GROSS & MICROSCOPIC ANATOMY

The stomach lies between the gastroesophageal and pyloric sphincters and may be divided into the cardia, fundus, body, and antrum (Figure 26–1). The esophagogastric junction lies slightly below the diaphragmatic hiatus, which is at the level of the twelfth thoracic vertebra, while the pyloroduodenal junction is at the level of the first lumbar vertebra. The cardia extends several centimeters beyond the gastroesophageal junction and consists predominately of mucous-secreting simple columnar cells. The fundus and body (corpus) of the stomach are characterized by a relatively thin muscular wall, in contrast to the thick musculature of the antrum. The mucosa of the body contains the acid-secreting oxyntic or parietal cells and pepsin-secreting chief cells. The gastric pits themselves are lined with mucous cells that secrete a thick mucous gel over the surface of the mucosa (Figure 26–2). The acid-secreting cells contain large amounts of mitochondria in their cytoplasm, indicative of the high energy requirements of gastric acid secretion. They also produce intrinsic factor necessary for the absorption of vitamin B_{12}. The antrum of the stomach contains mainly mucous-secreting cells and the gastrin-secreting cells (G cells). In addition to the gastrin-secreting cells, the gastric mucosa is known to contain other cells, such as D cells that secrete somatostatin, EC cells that secrete serotonin, and other peptide-secreting cells.

The small bowel is divided into three segments: the duodenum, jejunum, and ileum. The **duodenum** begins at the pylorus and ends at the ligament of Treitz. This segment of bowel is located and fixed in the retroperitoneum. As the bowel passes behind the mesenteric vessels the jejunum emerges from the retroperitoneum at the ligament of Treitz. The jejuno-ileum ends at the ileocecal valve. The mesentery, through which course the mesenteric vessels, nerves, and lymphatics, runs from the ligament of Treitz toward the right lower quadrant (Figure 26–3).

Each of these segments of small bowel are histologically and physiologically distinct, though the overall microscopic anatomy is similar throughout the small intestine (Figure 26–4). The small intestine is covered by the **serosa**. This single layer of cells covers the muscular wall of the intestine, which consists of the outer longitudinal muscles and the inner circular layer of muscles. The myenteric plexus of nerves is located between the two muscular layers. A second neural plexus exists deep to the circular muscle layer.

The **submucosa** is the next layer of the gut. This layer is composed of a vast network of connective tissue, including vessels and nerves. Of note, this layer contributes significantly to the structural integrity of the wall of the small bowel and, hence, it is vital to include this layer in performing intestinal anastomoses. The submucosa is then separated from the true mucosal layer by the muscularis mucosa and the lamina propria.

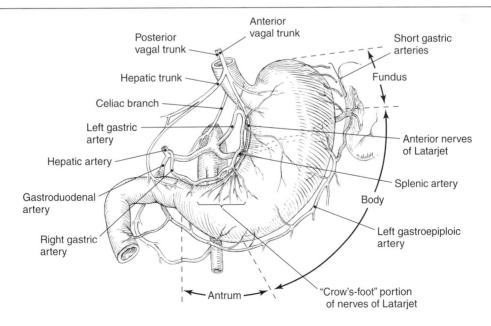

Figure 26–1. Anatomy of the stomach and duodenum.

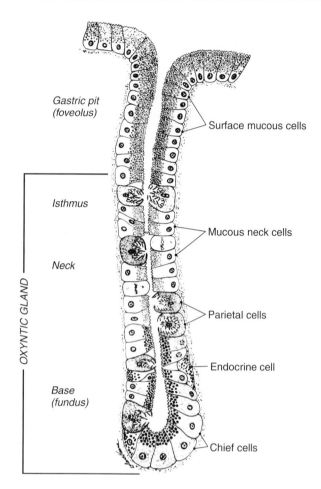

Gastric pit
(foveolus)

Surface mucous cells

Isthmus

Mucous neck cells

OXYNTIC GLAND

Neck

Parietal cells

Endocrine cell

Base
(fundus)

Chief cells

Figure 26–2. Oxyntic gastric gland. (From Ito S, Winchester RJ: The final structure of the gastric mucosa in the bat. Modified and reproduced from The Journal of Cell Biology, 1963;16:541, by copyright permission of The Rockefeller University Press.)

The intestinal mucosa protrudes into the gut lumen as **villi**. These villi significantly increase the available surface area of the small intestine. The mucosa has further folding that is seen grossly as the valvulae conniventes, which is a distinguishing feature of the small intestine. At the base of the villi there are crypts in the mucosa that penetrate the lamina propria. These crypts are composed of various cell types, including undifferentiated cells that are the precursor cells for the villus enterocytes. Other cell types that are found include enterochromaffin cells, goblet cells, and Paneth's cells. As cells mature and migrate from the crypt to the villus they differentiate from being secretory cells to the mature "absorptive" villus enterocytes.

EMBRYOLOGY

With the exception of parts of the mouth and anus, the entire alimentary tract is derived from cells of the endo-derm of the embryo. Early in development, the foregut and hindgut are enclosed within the embryo while the midgut remains in continuity with the yolk sac by way of the vitello-intestinal duct. The stomach develops as a dilation of the foregut tube, whereas the other foregut derivatives develop from diverticula of the foregut tube (liver and pancreas). All these structures remain "attached" to the posterior abdominal wall since their blood supply is derived from the foregut nutrient vessel, the celiac artery.

As the midgut develops and elongates, it separates from the posterior abdominal wall to which it remains attached by its dorsal mesentery. A long, looped tube is formed and actually passes out through the umbilical orifice to lie in the umbilical sac through week 6 of development.

The midgut continues to develop into the jejunum, ileum, appendix, and right colon. Following this process of rapid elongation, the vitello-intestinal duct disappears. The intestine is then returned to the abdominal cavity and during this process undergoes a counterclockwise rotation around the axis of the superior mesenteric artery (the artery of the midgut). With the exception of the most proximal segment of the intestine that develops into the horizontal part of the duodenum, the small bowel remains free in the peritoneal cavity, attached only by its dorsal mesentery. The appendix develops its own mesentery and usually remains free of the retroperitoneum, whereas the mesentery of the right colon fuses with the posterior abdominal wall and becomes retroperitoneal. Review of this embryology is essential to completely understand the congenital abnormalities seen in the neonate as well as other anatomic variants, such as Meckel's diverticulum and malrotation.

CIRCULATION

The stomach receives its blood supply from the right and left gastric arteries, the right and left gastric epiploic arteries, and the "short" gastric arteries (vasa brevia). These vessels penetrate the muscularis before ramifying extensively throughout the entire submucosa in a rich anastomotic plexus. The venous drainage parallels the arterial supply, draining directly into the portal vein or indirectly to the portal vein through the splenic or superior mesenteric veins. The lymphatic submucosal plexus is as extensive as the arterial and venous plexuses and transports lymph to the subserosal lymphatic plexus. Lymph drainage continues through extrinsic channels that follow the course of the arteries of the stomach, with the celiac nodes representing the primary collecting point. Accurate knowledge of the lymphatic supply is mandatory for gastric cancer surgery.

The duodenum receives an extensive blood supply from both the celiac and superior mesenteric (SMA) arteries. The **gastroduodenal artery** is a branch of the common hepatic artery that originates from the celiac axis. The gastroduodenal artery joins with branches of the inferior pancreaticoduodenal branch of the SMA through both an

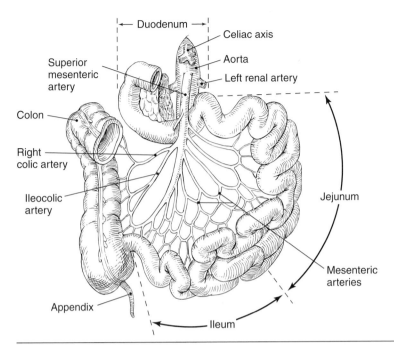

Figure 26–3. Anatomy of the small intestine and appendix.

anterior and posterior arcade supplying both the duodenum and the head of the pancreas. Venous drainage parallels the arterial supply, with branches draining into the superior mesenteric and portal veins, which then drain into the liver. The remainder of the small bowel receives its blood supply exclusively from branches of the SMA. The jejunoileal branches travel along the dorsal mesentery and are paralleled by their corresponding venous drainage and

lymphatics. The appendiceal artery is derived from the ileocolic artery, which is a branch of the SMA.

INNERVATION

The stomach receives its extrinsic innervation from the sympathetic nervous system via the greater splanchnic

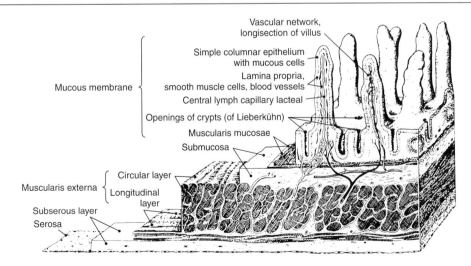

Figure 26–4. Layers of the small intestine: serosa, muscularis externa, submucosa, and mucous membrane. A large surface area is provided by the villi for the absorption of required nutriments. The stroma of the sectioned villi show the central lymph lacteal and the villous capillaries. (Reprinted, with permission, from Sobotta J, Figge FH: *Atlas of Human Anatomy.* Hafner Press, 1974, p. 103.)

nerves and celiac ganglia and from the parasympathetic nervous system via the terminal branches of the gastric vagi. Both components of the nervous system contain peptidergic and purinergic nerves. It should be noted that over 80% of the fibers in the vagi are afferent neurons carrying information to the brain. The left anterior and right posterior vagal nerve trunks descend along the esophagus to innervate the corresponding wall of the stomach, with the hepatic ramus from the left vagus and celiac ramus from the right posterior vagus. Both vagi give off their gastric branches to the proximal stomach and continue on to the antrum as the nerves of Latarjet (Figure 26–1).

The extrinsic innervation of the small bowel also includes sympathetic and parasympathetic fibers. The sympathetic input comes through postganglionic fibers from the celiac and superior mesenteric ganglia, whereas the parasympathetic inflow arises from preganglionic fibers from the vagus. These fibers travel along the vascular branches to eventually synapse with the enteric nervous system or other target cells.

The sympathetic preganglionic neurons from the fifth to twelfth thoracic segments reach the celiac and superior mesenteric plexuses through the greater splanchnic nerves. Their postganglionic fibers are distributed in the adventitia of the arterial supply to the stomach and small bowel. The gut contains two ganglionic plexuses. The myenteric (Auerbach's plexus) is between the circular and the longitudinal muscle layers, and the submucosal plexus (Meissner's plexus) is where the parasympathetic fibers synapse. This enteric nervous system contains cholinergic, serotoninergic, and peptidergic functions and is considered important in influencing gastric motility and gastrin release, and in modulating the control of the microcirculation. Additionally, afferent vagus fibers mediate various visceral reflexes while the afferent fibers that travel into the sympathetic system are responsible for the conduction of pain impulses.

PHYSIOLOGY

GASTRIC PHYSIOLOGY

Gastric Secretory Peptides

The important peptides found in the stomach include gastrin, somatostatin, gastric-releasing peptides, vasoactive intestinal peptides, glucagon, and substance P. **Gastrin** is the most important hormone in the control of gastric secretion. It is released from the gastric antrum by gastric distension, by the presence of luminal protein and amino acids, and by vagal stimulation. Its release is largely mediated by acetylcholine and blocked by atropine or when the pH of the antral lumen falls below 2.5. Gastrin stimulates the secretion of acid, increases lower esophageal sphincter pressure, and stimulates pepsinogen and intrinsic factor secretion. There is also a significant trophic effect on the parietal cell mucosa when gastrin levels are high.

Somatostatin is found both in the antrum and fundus of the stomach and is released by food, antral acidification, vagal stimulation, and the circulating gastrin. It is considered an important modulator of gastrin release as it exerts a paracrine inhibitory effect. Gastrin-releasing peptide is a potent releaser of gastrin and stimulant of acid secretion. Its main action is to act as a neurotransmitter by which vagal stimulation releases gastrin. Vasoactive intestinal polypeptide, substance P, and glucagon are also found in the stomach but their precise role in the physiology of gastric secretion is less well understood.

Exocrine Secretions

The secretion of hydrochloric acid by the parietal cell is in response to neurogenic or endocrine stimulation. The oxyntic or parietal cell has three distinct receptors for the stimulation of acid secretion, and these include acetylcholine, gastrin, and histamine (Figure 26–5). When these basolateral cell surface receptors are stimulated, H^+ K^+ ATPase (proton pump) is activated, resulting in the final step of hydrogen ion secretion.

Pepsin is secreted by the chief cells as pepsinogen, which is then converted to pepsin by acid. Intrinsic factor is secreted by the parietal cell and results in a mucoprotein that forms a complex with vitamin B_{12}, facilitating its absorption in the distal ileum. Two other exocrine secretory products of the stomach are mucus and bicarbonate, which both exert a protective effect on the gastric mucosa and maintain normal gastrointestinal flora.

Phases of Gastric Secretion

Gastric secretion may be divided into the interdigestive basal secretion and the digestive secretion that is produced in response to specific stimuli. Basal secretion of acid is usually intermittent and largely under the control of the vagus nerves. However, there appear to be other influences on basal secretion since the ablation of the vagi does not completely abolish it. These factors may include the presence of food in the intestinal tract, humoral substances, and extraneous stimuli. A normal subject secretes 1–3 meq of hydrochloric acid per hour under basal conditions. H_2 receptor antagonists have been found to reduce the basal acid secretion by up to 90%, thus demonstrating an important role for histamine.

The major digestive periods of gastric secretion include the cephalic or neural phase, the gastric or humoral phase, and the intestinal phase. The **cephalic phase** is stimulated by the thought, sight, smell, and taste of food, which stimulate several brain centers. The stimulus ultimately travels to the vagal dorsal nucleus where efferent stimulation of the parietal cells occurs via the vagus nerves. Vagal stimulation results in direct activation of the parietal cells by the release of acetylcholine. It is also known that vagal stimulation releases small amounts of gastrin from the antrum, which may potentiate the effects of acetylcholine.

The **gastric phase** of secretion is mediated by the hor-

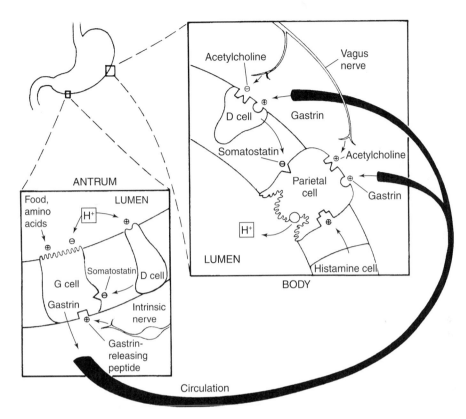

Figure 26–5. Regulation of gastric acid secretion. Major gastric mucosal ligand-receptor interactions regulate parietal cell HCl secretion. (D cell; somatostatin cell; G cell. Reprinted and modified, with permission, from Feldman M: Acid and gastrin secretion in duodenal ulcer disease. Regul Pept Lett 1989;1:1.)

mone gastrin produced by the mucosa of the gastric antrum when food enters the stomach. This stimulation of acid secretion is due both to distention of the gastric antrum as well to the chemical constituents of the food ingested. Protein digests and amino acids, but not carbohydrates or fats, stimulate the G cell to secrete gastrin. The inhibition of the gastric phase of secretion occurs when the intragastric pH reaches 2.5, inhibiting the release of gastrin by the gastric antrum. The mechanism by which luminal acids inhibit the release of gastrin probably involves somatostatin (Figure 26–5).

The **intestinal phase** of gastric secretion is thought to be caused by the release of entero-oxyntin, a stimulant originating from the intestine. This secretory response appears to be relatively unimportant in terms of the total acid production from the stomach.

Inhibition of Gastric Acid Secretion

A number of inhibitory mechanisms are activated when chyme enters the small intestine from the stomach. These include the presence of acid and hyperosmolar solutions as well as fat in the upper intestine, releasing enterogastrone. Other intestinal peptides would include secretin,

vasoactive intestinal peptide (VIP), glucagon, and cholecystokinin (CCK), all of which are capable of inhibiting acid secretion. It is not known what role these inhibitory peptides play in the normal physiologic regulation of gastric secretion.

Gastric Motility

The electrical phenomena of the stomach that control gastric motility are characterized by slow potential variations, basic electrical rhythm, and spike potentials occurring during depolarization in association with mechanical activity. The cyclic changes in potential occur at a frequency of three cycles per minute and are propagated distally from the pacemaker located high on the greater curvature to the stomach. This pacemaker controls the frequency, the direction of propagation, and the velocity of the contractions and is associated with mechanical contractions.

During fasting, interdigestive motor cycles occur every 1–2 hours and are characterized by three phases: (1) a quiescent period; (2) a period in which a regular contractile activity is seen, followed by (3) a sweeping burst of contractions that have the effect of clearing the stomach of its contents. During the ingestion of food there is a period of receptive relaxation of the muscle of the stomach. This is followed by regular peristaltic activity consisting of circumferential contractions of the muscle wall, propagated from the body to the antrum to the pylorus at a frequency of three per minute. The pressure in the antrum is 4–6 cm of water, whereas the pressure in the duodenum is 1–2 cm of water. Pressures of 15–30 cm of water are generated in the antrum by its contractions acting against the increased resistance of the duodenal bulb, providing a pressure gradient to move the food bolus through the partially contracted pyloric sphincter.

The control of gastric emptying is complex in that it is regulated by neural, humoral, and local factors. Gastric emptying of liquids is thought to be primarily controlled by the proximal stomach, whereas emptying of solids is under the control of the distal stomach and is associated with the strong antral and antral-pyloric contractions. It is of interest that only particles less that 1 mm in diameter are emptied into the duodenum. Other properties of gastric contents that influence emptying include the size of the particles, caloric density, acidity, and osmolarity. Peptides that affect gastric emptying include CCK, which has been shown to inhibit gastric emptying in physiologic doses. In the duodenum, pH and osmoreceptors are present, and activation of these receptors delay gastric emptying.

Following vagotomy there is a loss of receptive relaxation and accommodation of the proximal stomach and a loss of the relaxing effect of the pyloric sphincter. This results in an inhibition of emptying of both liquids and solids unless the pylorus is severed or bypassed, in which case gastric emptying of liquids is accelerated and relative normal emptying of solids occurs.

SMALL BOWEL PHYSIOLOGY

Gastric contents are delivered into the duodenum at a rate that is inversely related to caloric density. The duodenum functions to neutralize the acid content, achieve an isosmotic solution, and add the necessary components of bile and pancreatic juice. The duodenum also produces several important hormones, such as CCK, secretin, and motolin. These hormones have important gastrointestinal (GI) effects and, as in the case of CCK, may have regulatory effects on the central nervous system affecting appetite and satiety.

Appropriate mixing of the chyme with bile and pancreatic secretions allows the jejunoileus to proceed with efficient absorption of nutrients.

Nutrient Absorption

The jejunum and ileum are very efficient organs in that virtually all ingested nutrients are absorbed. Furthermore, there is massive absorption of water and electrolytes such that endogenous secretions (salivary, gastric, biliary, pancreatic, and intestinal) plus 1–2 L of exogenous fluid are absorbed. Though there is extensive overlap in the function of the jejunum and the ileum, there are some nutrients whose absorption is site-specific (Table 26–1).

Water & Electrolytes. Approximately 8–10 L of fluid is absorbed in the jejuno-ileum. Current understanding of this process centers on various mechanisms of electrolyte absorption with subsequent "passive" water transport. Sodium is the predominant ion, whose absorption is thought to drive water absorption. Sodium absorption is achieved either through electroneutral sodium absorption or electrogenic sodium absorption. Electroneutral absorption involves the coupling of sodium-hydrogen ion exchange in concert with sodium bicarbonate exchange. Electrogenic sodium absorption can be coupled with various co-transporter molecules, such as the sodium-glucose exchanger and the sodium amino acid exchanger. Energy-dependent absorptive mechanisms are driven by the sodium-potassium ATPase and the basal lateral membranes. This absorptive function of the small bowel occurs predominantly in the villus tips. In contrast, chloride secretion is predominant in the villus crypts. Following the transcellular absorption of sodium, water is thought to follow passively through paracellular pathways.

Carbohydrates. Carbohydrate is initially broken down by amylases from the salivary glands. This hydrolysis of starch is continued by amylases from pancreatic secretions to eventually create oligosaccharides. These oligosaccharides are then broken down into simple sugars by several brush border enzymes. The resulting glucose, galactose, and fructose are absorbed transcellularly by specific transport carrier proteins.

Fat. Fat is digested by pancreatic lipase, forming fatty acids, and two monoglycerides. These products are emul-

Table 26–1. Absorption in the small intestine.

	Duodenum	Jejunum	Ileum
Water	+	+++	++
Sodium	+	+++	++
Potassium	+	+++	+
Chloride	+	++	+++
Fats	++	+++	+
Proteins	++	+++	+
Carbohydrates	++	+++	+
Bile salts	0	0	+++
Fat-soluble vitamins[1]	+	+++	+
Water-soluble vitamins			
Vitamin B_{12}	0	0	+++
Folic acid	+	+++	++
Ascorbic acid	?	+	+++
Minerals			
Iron	+++	++	0
Calcium	++	+++	+
Magnesium	+	++	++
Zinc[2]	0	+	++

[1]Vitamin K (endogenously produced fraction) absorbed in colon.
[2]Based on animal studies.
Reprinted, with permission, from Wilson JAP, Owyang C: Physiology of digestion and absorption. In: Nelson RL, Nyhus LM (editors): *Surgery of the Small Intestine.* Appleton & Lange, 1987, p. 22.

sified by bile salts forming micelles. These micelles facilitate the diffusion of the monoglycerides and fatty acids through the brush border. Intracellularly, the triglycerides are reformed and then combined with cholesterol and phospholipids to form chylomicrons. These chylomicrons then pass through the basal lateral membrane into the lymphatic drainage system by way of the central lacteal in the villus. Fatty acids with chain links of less than ten may be absorbed directly into the portal circulation. The bile salts are maintained intraluminally; they are reabsorbed in the ileum and returned to the liver where they are re-excreted into the bile. Fat absorption occurs predominantly in the jejunum and is very efficient, such that less than 1–2% of ingested fat is passed into stool.

Protein. Pancreatic proteases are responsible for the majority of protein digestion. Protein hydrolysis is then completed by aminopeptidases and dipeptidases in the brush border. The resultant amino acids are then absorbed through specific transporters.

Vitamins & Minerals. Fat-soluble vitamins are absorbed by way of micelles. Water-soluble vitamins, on the other hand, generally have a specific carrier-mediated absorptive system and, therefore, tend to be more site-specific. For example, vitamin B_{12} requires binding with intrinsic factor. This complex binds to ileal receptors that exist only in the distal ileum. Vitamin C absorption is an energy-dependent, sodium-carrier–mediated process that exists predominantly in the ileum. In contrast, folate is predominantly absorbed in the jejunum.

Calcium is absorbed predominantly in the duodenum and jejunum through a process that is dependent on vitamin D. Iron is absorbed in the duodenum and jejunum. Transferrin is secreted into the gut lumen where it binds reduced iron. This complex is absorbed by endocytosis where the iron is then transported across the basal lateral membrane. Magnesium absorption appears to occur predominantly by passive diffusion. The remaining trace elements are absorbed either through passive diffusion or with specific transporter mechanisms.

Endocrine Function

Multiple **gut hormone peptides** are released in the small bowel and function as either hormones or paracrine agents. The most important of these include: motilin, a duodenal hormone that alters gastric and small bowel motility; secretin, which stimulates water and bicarbonate secretion from the pancreas; and CCK, which regulates biliary motility and may influence appetite.

Intestinal Motility

Intestinal contents are transported through the gut lumen through a complex process of **peristalsis**. The motility pattern of the small bowel changes in the fed and fasting states. During fasting, there is an intermittent migrating myoelectric complex (MMC). The frequency of the MMC seems to be influenced by levels of serum motilin, a hormone secreted by the duodenum. Luminal contents, extrinsic nerves, and local peptides alter the

MMC pattern after a meal. The fed pattern persists for 3–4 hours.

NON-NEOPLASTIC DISEASE

ULCER DISEASE

GENERAL CONCEPTS

An ulcer is the outcome of a disturbance of the balance between destructive factors, such as acid, pepsin, and infection, and the mechanisms protecting the gastric and duodenal mucosa known as the **mucosal barrier**. **Peptic ulcers** are usually associated with increased acid production. These ulcers are either duodenal ulcers or gastric ulcers (types II and III), which are usually prepyloric. Type I and IV gastric ulcers, on the other hand, are not usually associated with increased acid output, have several causes, and can occur throughout the stomach.

Patients may present with specific symptoms of epigastric pain relieved by food or antacids. Alternatively, the symptoms may be less specific and may be described as heartburn, gas, or indigestion. Patients can also present with acute or chronic blood loss. Diagnosis is confirmed by upper GI endoscopy or by barium studies.

PEPTIC ULCER

Diagnosis

The most common symptom for a peptic ulcer is abdominal pain in the midepigastric area. This pain can be mild to severe and can improve with eating, though occasionally eating exacerbates the pain. These patients are usually male and can have significant relief of symptoms with over-the-counter oral antacids, if taken frequently. Occasionally, patients may present with few pain symptoms but rather are found to have chronic GI bleeding or an acute GI bleed. Microcytic anemia or occult blood in the stool may be the first clue to the presence of a peptic ulcer. Alternatively, a duodenal ulcer can erode into a major artery, such as the gastroduodenal artery, and patients may present with hematemesis, melena, or shock. Occasionally, patients may present with an acute abdomen with pneumoperitoneum from a perforated anterior ulcer. Lastly, patients infrequently can present with gastric outlet obstruction from stricture formation.

Management

The medical treatment of peptic ulcers (duodenal and gastric ulcers, types II and III) has been primarily directed at controlling acid secretion. Widespread use of H_2 blockers, proton pump inhibitors, and surgical procedures are aimed at reducing the level of gastric acid secretion. Recently, the emphasis on *Helicobacter pylori* infestation of the stomach has required a reevaluation of therapeutic options in the management of peptic ulcer disease. It has been found in patients undergoing upper GI endoscopy that *H. pylori* is associated with duodenal ulcer disease in over 90% of patients. Eradication of this organism has become an important therapeutic goal in the management of peptic ulcer disease. Eradication of *H. pylori* prevents duodenal ulcer relapse in more than 90% of patients, with an extremely low rate of recurrence and reinfection. Commonly employed treatment regimens include "**triple therapy,**" a combination of bismuth subsalicylate, amoxicillin, and metronidazole or tetracycline in combination with the use of omeprazole, a proton pump inhibitor.

The surgical management of duodenal ulcer remains based on reducing acid secretion by severing the vagus nerves. Vagotomy may be performed in combination with a gastric drainage procedure (pyloroplasty or gastrojejunostomy) or with antrectomy, a procedure that is followed by a less than a 2% rate of recurrence. Highly selective, or parietal cell, vagotomy has become popular during the past decade; it denervates the acid-secreting portion of the stomach while preserving the vagal innervation to the gastric antrum, thus maintaining normal antral motility and avoiding the need for a drainage procedure. This procedure results in normal gastric emptying, although the rate of recurrence of ulcer is around 10%. The indications for surgery in patients with duodenal ulcer disease include intractability (failure of medical therapy), perforation, hemorrhage, and obstruction. In selected patients, surgical therapy may be limited to managing a complication, such as closing a perforation followed by medical management of the underlying disease (Table 26–2).

GASTRIC ULCER

Diagnosis

In contrast to patients with peptic ulcers, type I and type IV gastric ulcer patients tend to secrete normal or less-than-normal basal acid. It has been postulated that the antral or gastric phase of secretion is responsible for gastric ulceration, in contrast to the peptic ulcer patient in whom vagal hypersecretion is often demonstrated. Gastric ulcers are also seen in patients with hypochlorhydria and patients with altered mucosal protection and must be differentiated from gastric cancers (Table 26–3).

Table 26–3. Associated and predisposing factors for gastric ulcers (types I, IV).

Drugs
  Aspirin
  Nonsteroidal anti-inflammatory drugs (NSAIDS)
  Corticosteroids
Achlorhydria
Sepsis
Shock

As in peptic ulcers the symptoms of a gastric ulcer are often vague and nonspecific. These patients may present with epigastric symptoms that improve with eating, or with loss of appetite and weight loss. Again, a high index of suspicion is needed, and one can then investigate further with upper endoscopy or barium studies. Endoscopy has the advantage of more specificity in the diagnosis and allows one to biopsy the ulcers.

Management

Gastric ulcers are initially treated medically. If persistent, these ulcers are best treated by limited gastric resection that includes the ulcer, a procedure that results in a recurrence rate of less than 2% with a low morbidity. It is important to maintain a suspicion for occult carcinoma in an ulcer that has failed to heal after 6–8 weeks of medical therapy, even if biopsies were negative for carcinoma. When the ulcer is situated high on the lesser curvature, a limited gastric resection (antrectomy) will result in healing of the ulcer in over 95% of the patients. This approach, however, has the disadvantage of leaving the ulcer in-situ and potentially missing a malignancy.

ZOLLINGER-ELLISON SYNDROME

Diagnosis

The Zollinger-Ellison syndrome (ZES) is characterized by a hypersecretion of gastric acid secondary to an excess of circulating gastrin arising from a tumor, either in the pancreas or the duodenum. Though hypergastrinemia is essential to its diagnosis, ZES needs to be differentiated from other conditions causing hypergastrinemia (Table 26–4).

Patients with ZES usually present with intractable or complicated duodenal ulcer disease, esophagitis, or diarrhea. Gastrinomas tend to occur in an anatomic triangle

Table 26–2. Comparison of surgical procedures for the treatment of peptic ulcer disease.

	Mortality (%)	Morbidity	Recurrence (%)
Highly selective (parietal cell) vagotomy	< 1	low	10–20
Truncal vagotomy with drainage procedure	< 1	low	5
Truncal vagotomy with antrectomy	~ 1	low	< 2

Table 26–4. Causes of hypergastrinemia.

Precipitating Condition	Mechanism
Zollinger-Ellison syndrome	Gastrinoma
Antral hyperplasia	G cell hyperplasia
Vagotomy	Loss of vagal inhibition
Pernicious anemia	Loss of acid inhibition
Antral exclusion	Lack of acid inhibition
Chronic renal failure	Decreased catabolism
Pyloric obstruction	Chronic gastric distention
H_2 blockers	Loss of acid inhibition
Protein pump inhibitors	Loss of acid inhibition

Reprinted and modified, with permission, from Simmons RL, Steed DL: *Basic Science Review for Surgeons.* Saunders, 1992, p. 234.

location, bounded by the junction of the cystic and common ducts, the junction of the head and body of the pancreas, and the junction of the second and third portions of the duodenum. Recently it has been recognized that as many as 50% percent are malignant.

Management

Surgical management consists of local excision with removal of nodes for duodenal lesions to more radical resection, if necessary. Though gastrectomy was often necessary in the past to palliate patients with ZES, many patients are now controlled by proton pump blockers if the primary tumor or its metastases are not resectable.

ANTRAL HYPERPLASIA

Diagnosis & Management

Antral or G cell hyperplasia may result in hypergastrinemia associated with peptic ulceration. This condition is characterized by an increased number of gastrin-secreting cells in the antrum of the stomach and is thought to be inherited as autosomal-dominant disease. This condition may be distinguished from patients with ulcerogenic tumors (Zollinger-Ellison syndrome) by the intravenous injection of secretin. The latter results in a marked increase in the serum gastrin level, whereas, in those patients with G cell hyperplasia, there is no increase in the serum gastrin levels. However, those patients with G cell hyperplasia do show definitive increases in the serum gastrin level in response to the ingestion of a meal. This condition may be medically treated with omeprazole or surgically by antrectomy.

MOTILITY DISORDERS

Diagnosis

Chronic impairment of gastric emptying most often occurs in diabetes, particularly in individuals with insulin dependency or with elements of diabetic neuropathy. The symptoms of poor gastric emptying can be very vague and insidious. Eventually anorexia, nausea, vomiting, and upper abdominal pain can develop. Physical examination may reveal some epigastric or left upper quadrant fullness or a succussion splash. An upper GI series with barium can be useful to confirm delayed gastric emptying. However, sometimes it is necessary to use radionuclide scans to objectively quantify emptying of solids or liquids. Alternatively, a barium "motor meal" can be used for gross estimation of gastric emptying of solids.

Management

These patients often respond to metoclopramide or cisapride to improve gastric emptying. Delay in gastric emptying may be seen following truncal vagotomy. Although pyloroplasty overcomes this delay in emptying, it may be questioned whether the emptying of solids returns to normal, despite the fact that the emptying of liquids is accelerated. Other abnormalities in gastric emptying may occur following the Roux-en-Y gastrojejunostomy performed for bile gastritis. When this delay in emptying occurs, it may be treated with prokinetic agents; if surgery becomes necessary, further gastric resection may be required. Accelerated gastric emptying occurs following disruption of the pylorus or a resection of a portion of the stomach in which the dumping of gastric contents may occur, particularly those that are hyperosmolar. Such rapid gastric emptying may be managed by recommending solid foods without liquid at mealtime and a decrease in the consumption of carbohydrates.

SHORT BOWEL SYNDROME & MALABSORPTION

Diagnosis

Adequate absorption of nutrients is dependent on an adequate absorptive surface area, functional enterocytes, and adequate exocrine secretions from the foregut. Loss of adequate surface area is most often related to loss of bowel length. This state, known as **short bowel syndrome** (SBS), is most often due to surgical excision of diseased bowel. In adults, it is often due to multiple bowel resections in patients with inflammatory bowel disease or it occurs following vascular accidents. In children, intestinal atresias and surgical resection for various neonatal diseases may also result in SBS.

Fat malabsorption can be caused by pancreatic exocrine insufficiency from either pancreatitis or pancreatic resection. Untreated, this may result in significant diarrhea and weight loss. There are innumerable acquired and congenital disorders of nutrient transport. These are rarely seen in surgical patients. However, malabsorption due to bacterial overgrowth in the small bowel is an important consideration in patients with defunctionalized segments of small bowel (blind loop), small bowel diverticulosis, and dysmotility disorders. The altered flora in the small bowel contributes to consumption of nutrients as well as an to associated mucosal injury.

Management

The development of parenteral nutrition has allowed treatment of this disease and remains the cornerstone of therapy. Since the management of this syndrome is very difficult, special efforts should always be made to try to prevent inadequate bowel length. It is felt that as little as 40 cm of small bowel length associated with an intact ileocecal valve is the minimum length required to sustain enteral nutrition.

Though the small bowel has a great capacity to adapt following massive bowel resection, one needs to remain aware that the jejunum and ileum do have specific functions that may be absent, depending on which segment of bowel has been eliminated or preserved. New experimental therapies have included the increased use of glutamine and growth factors to try to increase total available surface area. Small bowel transplantation is now also being used clinically to remove the dependence on parenteral nutrition in these challenging patients.

The treatment of bacterial overgrowth consists of initial fluid and nutritional support, including replacement of vitamin deficiencies. The underlying cause is then identified, if possible. If the underlying lesion is not correctable, the primary treatment is antibiotics to suppress the bacterial overgrowth.

DIVERTICULA

Diagnosis

Diverticula of the stomach are uncommon and are usually of the pulsion variety located on the lesser curvature, near the esophagogastric junction. They are usually asymptomatic and are incidental findings on upper GI examination. On the other hand, diverticula of the duodenum are found in about 5–10% of patients undergoing upper GI radiographic examinations. They are usually asymptomatic but may result if situated near the ampulla of Vater in obstructive jaundice, pancreatitis, and inflammation. Enteroliths may form in the diverticula. Treatment for diverticula of the stomach is only required for complications of the disease. Care must be taken in excising duodenal diverticula, particularly those in close association with the ampulla of Vater.

Diverticula of the small bowel are uncommon. **Meckel's diverticulum** is the most common congenital diverticulum. It represents a remnant of the vitellin (omphalomesenteric) duct. These diverticula are true diverticula containing all layers of the bowel from serosa to mucosa. Acquired diverticula occur on the mesenteric margin of the bowel and are thought to be pulsion diverticula. These tend to be more common in the jejunum and are

most often multiple. These diverticula are similar to those seen in the colon in that they are hernias of the mucous membrane penetrating through the muscular wall at the point of entrance of the vessels.

Management

Diverticula of the stomach and small bowel are usually asymptomatic but can rarely present with serious complications, including acute inflammation, perforation, obstruction, and hemorrhage. These lesions can also have associated bacterial overgrowth requiring resection.

Meckel's diverticula may occur in 2% of the population, but is usually an incidental finding. These lesions may have associated ulceration, particularly when ectopic pancreatic or gastric tissue is present in the diverticulum. Resection is required only when there is clear evidence of inflammation from the diverticulum; prophylactic removal is not indicated.

INFLAMMATORY BOWEL DISEASE

Diagnosis

Regional enteritis, or **Crohn's disease**, is the most common inflammatory disease of the small bowel that may require surgical intervention. The etiology of Crohn's disease remains unknown. *Mycobacterium paratuberculosis* has been proposed as a possible infectious agent contributing to Crohn's disease. Possible immune mechanisms are receiving increased attention, since immunosuppressive agents have been found to be efficacious in the management of these patients. It is likely that several factors contribute to the development of Crohn's disease. Until these are more clearly delineated, the management of these patients will remain difficult.

Pathologically, Crohn's is characterized by transmural inflammation with eventual submucosal and subserosal fibrosis. Mucosal ulceration is found early. There is usually significant edema and a predominant lymphocytic infiltrate. Noncaseating granulomas are present in approximately half the patients. The gross appearance of the bowel is that of a thickened bowel wall and mesentery with extension of the mesenteric fat onto the bowel wall (fat creeping).

The clinical manifestations of Crohn's disease are not limited to the small bowel. Approximately one third of patients have Crohn's limited to the colon, one third have involvement of both the terminal ileum and colon, and one third have predominantly small bowel disease. In rare cases, patients will also demonstrate Crohn's disease in the stomach and duodenum. Approximately one third of patients will have involvement of the anal canal that presents with perianal abscesses and fistulas.

Patients often present with diarrhea and abdominal pain. They may often have signs and symptoms of partial bowel obstruction or an active inflammatory process.

Confirmation of the diagnosis is often made with a barium small bowel series. This study can demonstrate skip areas and strictures and is usually reliable in identifying the most common site of the disease in the terminal ileum. In addition to obstruction, patients may present with actual abscess formation and fistulas, since this disease is characterized by transmural inflammation and, hence, is associated with microperforation that is usually walled off by surrounding tissues. Because of chronic inflammation, patients can present with malnutrition and anemia. The anemia can be due to slow chronic blood loss or vitamin B_{12} deficiency. The peak age of onset of Crohn's is between 15 and 25 years of age. It can present during childhood and is often associated with growth retardation and delayed maturation.

Management

The initial management of Crohn's disease is medical, with an active program to manage the diarrhea, abdominal pain, and nutrition. Sulfasalazine, steroids, and immunosuppressive agents such as 6-mercaptopurine and azathioprine are often used in combination to control symptoms. Surgical intervention is indicated for complications of this disease, including obstruction, perforation, bleeding, abscess formation, refractoriness to medical management, and carcinoma. Exploration for obstruction usually occurs in the chronic setting. Occasionally, acute inflammation that is refractory to medical management will necessitate exploration.

Surgical resection is often indicated for grossly diseased segments. Free perforation is a rare event in Crohn's disease but requires urgent exploration. More often, fistulization to either other loops of bowel or viscera will require surgical resection if medical management is unsuccessful. Occasionally, exploration is necessary for adequate drainage of intra-abdominal abscesses. However, these often can be managed with antibiotics and percutaneous drainage. Chronic blood loss requiring a transfusion is an indication of failure of medical management. Major bleeding episodes are uncommon in Crohn's and rarely require surgical intervention. Most often, persistent active disease (in spite of medical management), failure to thrive, or an inability to work results in consideration of surgical resection of the diseased segments.

The danger in managing these patients surgically is the chronicity of this disease, with a high incidence of recurrence following surgical resection. This cycle can result in short bowel syndrome if too much bowel is sacrificed. Lastly, cancers can develop in areas of chronic Crohn's; though this is uncommon, it needs to be considered in patients with long-standing Crohn's disease with either chronic strictures or segments of surgically bypassed bowel.

As mentioned, excision of gross disease is the procedure of choice. Primary reanastomosis is usually achievable. Occasionally, bypass procedures are necessary when patients are severely compromised and resection of the acute inflammation is dangerous. For chronic strictures, the treatment options are resection or stricturoplasty, which is a technique that involves opening the bowel longitudinally and closing it transversely to eliminate the narrowed segment.

Enteritis has many causes, including several infectious processes that can mimic Crohn's. It is important to differentiate these diseases from Crohn's disease. *Tuberculous enteritis* is more common in the ileum and may require surgical resection as well as antituberculous drugs. Acute infections with agents such as *Yersinia bacterium* can also cause acute terminal ileitis. Other infections, such as typhoid enteritis, can require emergency surgery when their medical management is insufficient. Usually, this is either for free perforation or refractory hemorrhage.

FISTULAE

Diagnosis

Fistulae from the small bowel develop most often following surgical intervention. Initially, they may present in association with an abscess; hence, patients usually have fever and leukocytosis. These fistulae are usually enterocutaneous fistulas, though entero-enterofistulas and enterovesicular fistula can be seen in certain disease processes. The enterocutaneous fistulae have drainage of succus entericus (bowel contents) that may be low- or high-output. Internal fistulae may present with an inflammatory mass, they may be asymptomatic, or they can present with diarrhea, particularly if the fistula is between a segment of proximal bowel and a segment of distal bowel or colon. Enterovesicular fistulae present with pneumaturia and symptoms of urinary tract infection.

Management

The basic principles of the management of fistulae include control of sepsis and the assurance that any potential abscesses are completely drained. Once this is established, most fistulas will close spontaneously, provided the patient is maintained with good nutrition and there is no distal obstruction. Other factors that may deter fistula healing include persistent cancer, epithelialization of the tract, or high output. Only when conservative measures have failed should surgical resection be considered. Parenteral nutrition is an important adjunct in the management of these patients.

GASTRIC OUTLET OBSTRUCTION

Diagnosis

Peptic ulcer disease, either acutely with edema or chronically with stricture formation, is the most common cause of gastric outlet obstruction. Patients present with symptoms of poor gastric emptying, epigastric discomfort, nausea, and vomiting. An enlarged stomach can sometimes be elicited on examination by auscultating a succussion splash. Diagnosis can be confirmed by barium upper GI series. These patients can present with a hypochloremic metabolic alkalosis, severe hypovolemia, and possible malnutrition. Children with congenital hypertrophic pyloric stenosis often present with non-bilious vomiting.

Management

The management of these patients first centers on correction of the fluid and electrolyte abnormalities. Nasogastric decompression with a tube should be performed. Nutritional supplementation is also often necessary. If the outlet obstruction is due to edema of the pyloric channel in reaction to an active ulcer, this process may be resolved with medical management of the ulcer disease. On the other hand, in the more chronic setting a stricture may be present, in which case surgical intervention will be necessary. Treatment options include pyloroplasty, gastrojejunostomy, or partial gastric resection. These patients often benefit from the placement of feeding tubes, since gastric emptying of the chronically dilated stomach is impaired and recovers slowly. The treatment for children with congenital pyloric stenosis is a pyloromyotomy.

DUODENAL OBSTRUCTION

Diagnosis

Duodenal obstruction is uncommon in the adult. Patients may present with abdominal pain and non-bilious or bilious emesis. Postbulbar strictures from ulcer disease are possible. Strictures may also develop from Crohn's disease. Annular pancreas may present later in life, though it usually presents in the infant. Duodenal atresia also obviously presents in infancy. A rare disorder that is associated with significant weight loss, abdominal pain, nausea, and bilious vomiting is superior mesenteric artery (SMA) syndrome. In this disease, the third portion of the duodenum is narrowed between the SMA and the aorta. This entity is initially treated nonoperatively, but if nutritional supplementation fails, a duodenojejunostomy needs to be considered.

Management

The management of duodenal obstruction is not significantly different from that of gastric outlet obstruction. Correction of dehydration and electrolyte abnormalities is paramount. If the obstruction is distal to the papilla of Vater, bile is a component of the fluid loss. Stricturoplasty, duodenoduodenostomy, or duodenojejunostomy are the common procedures when surgical intervention is required.

SMALL BOWEL OBSTRUCTION

Diagnosis

Patients with small bowel obstruction present with colicky abdominal pain, abdominal distention, nausea, and vomiting. The most common cause of small bowel obstruction in the United States is intra-abdominal adhesions from previous surgery. In underdeveloped countries, hernias continue to be the predominant cause of bowel obstruction. Other potential causes for bowel obstruction are listed in Table 26–5. When patients present it is important to differentiate between a partial small bowel obstruction, complete bowel obstruction, and closed loop obstruction. This distinction is often made clinically in conjunction with plain films of the abdomen and sometimes with contrast studies.

Management

The initial management of small bowel obstruction consists of fluid resuscitation and nasogastric decompression with a nasogastric tube ("short tube"). Alternatively, a Cantor tube ("long tube") can be placed beyond the pylorus for direct decompression of the small bowel. There is no distinct advantage of one type of tube over the other, although the "short" tubes are usually easier to place and manage. Following the initial resuscitation and decompression, careful serial examinations need to be performed to assess improvement in the patient or to determine the need for surgical intervention. Since complete bowel obstructions and closed loop obstructions can be associated with strangulation and bowel ischemia, it is essential to be very attentive to these patients since they may require early exploration. Patients with incarcerated hernias and symptoms of bowel obstruction need to be explored urgently. Patients with malignancy tend to have more subacute presentations and can often be managed initially with rehydration and nasogastric decompression. Patients with partial or incomplete small bowel obstruction from adhesions can be managed nonoperatively and will often recover without surgery. In the absence of a previous history of intra-abdominal surgery, the presence of hernias, or known metastatic cancer, a patient with mechanical bowel obstruction will benefit from prompt laparotomy.

At surgery, incarcerated hernias can be reduced and bowel viability assessed. Patients with adhesive disease undergo lysis of adhesions or entero-enterostomy to bypass and decompress the obstructed segment. The urgency in exploring persons with bowel obstruction relates to the

Table 26–5. Common causes of bowel obstruction.

Cause	Percent
Adhesions from previous surgery	50–60
Hernias (internal or external)	20–25
Tumors (metastatic or primary)	10–15

possibility of bowel congestion and development of mesenteric ischemia. Following lysis of adhesions, any nonviable bowel is resected and primary reanastomosis is usually performed. The uncommon causes of small bowel obstruction listed in Table 26–6 are usually managed with small bowel resection or entero-enterostomy for proximal diversion if the obstruction is not resectable.

MESENTERIC ISCHEMIA

Diagnosis

Mesenteric ischemia can occur both acutely and chronically. Because of the extensive collaterals in the mesenteric circulation, chronic mesenteric ischemia is uncommon and requires severe atherosclerotic disease in multiple blood vessels. Isolated chronic SMA occlusion is often extremely well tolerated by patients because of the extensive collaterals with the celiac system and inferior mesenteric arterial system. The predominant collaterals are through the pancreaticoduodenal arcades and through the marginal artery in the colon. However, if two or three of the mesenteric vessels are diseased, symptoms of chronic ischemia may develop.

Patients with bowel ischemia often present with weight loss and postprandial abdominal pain (abdominal angina). Mesenteric angiography has been the standard diagnostic test. This diagnosis is now often confirmed with a high-resolution computed tomographic (CT) scan. More recently, MRI has been used to assess blood flow in the SMA and oxygen desaturization in the superior mesenteric vein in the chronic setting.

Acute mesenteric ischemia can be due to arterial thrombosis, arterial embolus, or venous thrombosis. Arterial thrombosis is usually seen in conjunction with underlying chronic arterial atherosclerosis. Often, the diagnosis of mesenteric ischemia is not made until patients are explored, because they present with severe pain suggesting an abdominal catastrophe. Furthermore, findings of abdominal pain, fever, leukocytosis, and acidosis are nonspecific and not sensitive. Patients with mesenteric emboli often have predisposing factors, such as chronic atrial fibrillation, and tend to present more acutely, since they have not developed increased collateral flow.

Management

Once the diagnosis of acute mesenteric ischemia is entertained, preoperative arteriography can be useful in making

Table 26–6. Uncommon causes of bowel obstruction.

Intussusception
Gallstone ileus
Crohn's disease
Meckel's diverticulum
Food debris (bezoar)
Volvulus

the diagnosis and potentially allowing one to initiate thrombolytic therapy. Arteriography is essential for the planning of arterial reconstruction for patients with bowel ischemia. Surgical treatment involves reestablishment of blood flow if possible, assessment of bowel viability, and resection of nonviable bowel. Since there are no good chemical parameters to assess bowel viability, direct inspection and multiple operations are often necessary. Patients with chronic bowel ischemia usually have a poor prognosis because of their diffuse vascular disease, which affects their cerebrovascular and cardiovascular systems.

APPENDICITIS

Diagnosis

Acute appendicitis is a bacterial infection whose origin is probably related to appendiceal luminal obstruction. This entity is the most common cause of the "acute abdomen." Appendicitis occurs in 6% of the US population, predominantly in the age group 10–30 years. However, appendicitis can occur at all ages and is particularly difficult to diagnose in the very young and very old, since both of these groups tend to have atypical presentations.

The clinical manifestations of acute appendicitis relate to the pathophysiology, beginning with luminal obstruction and ending with perforation. Early in the disease process, patients have vague abdominal pain that is usually periumbilical with associated anorexia. As inflammation spreads to the serosal surface of the appendix and involves the parietal peritoneum, the pain becomes more localized and is associated with peritoneal irritation. The progression of vague abdominal pain, anorexia, and nausea to focal right lower quadrant pain and tenderness usually occurs over a period of less than 24 hours.

The diagnosis of appendicitis is made by a history and physical examination and is usually straightforward in males. However, in young women the diagnosis is more complicated because of potential adnexal pathology or pregnancy. A careful gynecologic history is vital to an accurate diagnosis. Infrequently, the diagnosis remains unclear and additional imaging can be considered with either ultrasonography or CT scans. Often, the most useful technique in identifying early acute appendicitis is serial examinations performed by the same physician. There are no specific laboratory findings to assist in the diagnosis of appendicitis. The white blood cell count is not specific or sensitive; nor is an elevated temperature. Since a delay in diagnosis and treatment may result in perforation and diffuse peritonitis, early open exploration or diagnostic laparoscopy is warranted.

Management

Once the diagnosis of acute appendicitis has been entertained, prompt surgical consultation is indicated. Sometimes, the history and examination are not entirely clear and the patient is stable; it is useful to observe the patient over a short period and conduct serial examinations. If, however, there are signs of focal or diffuse peritoneal irritation, one should proceed to the operating room.

In women it is often useful to begin with diagnostic laparoscopy, which allows complete evaluation of the pelvis and confirmation of the diagnosis of acute appendicitis. One can then make the traditional right lower quadrant incision at McBurney's point (one third of the distance between the anterior superior iliac spine and the umbilicus) or one can proceed with a laparoscopic appendectomy. In men, the diagnosis is usually more clear, and it is simplest to proceed with a traditional open appendectomy. In older patients, if the diagnosis is unclear it is sometimes useful to begin with a lower midline incision that will allow adequate exploration of the abdomen. Patients with early appendicitis usually have a very short recovery period and often leave within 24 hours after surgery. Patients with perforated appendicitis may require a longer period in the hospital, antibiotics, and closer follow-up. Wound infections are common in this latter group; therefore, some surgeons prefer to leave the skin incisions open.

BENIGN NEOPLASTIC DISEASE

LEIOMYOMA

Diagnosis & Management

Leiomyomas usually arise from the proximal stomach and often are characterized by a central ulceration caused by necrosis from overgrowth of their blood supply. Although they are usually asymptomatic, they may result in gastrointestinal bleeding; if diagnosed, they should be removed by enucleation or wedge resection.

POLYPS

Diagnosis

Gastric polyps may occur as single or multiple lesions and have been classified etiologically as hyperplastic, adenomatous, or inflammatory. **Hyperplastic polyps** are the most frequently seen lesions and consist merely of an overgrowth of normal epithelium. **Adenomatous polyps**, although less common, may be considered premalignant in that 20–30% of these polyps contain foci of carcinoma. These polyps are characteristic in patients with multiple polyposis of the colon, and these patients must be screened for gastric involvement over time.

Management

Gastric polyps are usually asymptomatic, although they

may result in chronic blood loss and usually can be removed endoscopically. If cancer is suspected or diagnosed, operative intervention is indicated.

MALIGNANT NEOPLASTIC DISEASE

GASTRIC ADENOCARCINOMA

Diagnosis

Although the incidence of gastric carcinoma has dropped significantly over what it was 30 years ago, there are still about 20,000 new cases of gastric cancer annually in the United States. However, during this same period there appears to be an increasing incidence of gastroesophageal cancer, particularly of the adenocarcinoma type. The role of *H. pylori* and the cause of gastric cancer remains unknown. It appears to be a causative agent of chronic atrophic gastritis, which has always been considered a precursor of gastric adenocarcinoma.

Five morphologic categories of cancer have been recognized: ulcerating carcinomas, polypoid carcinomas, superficial spreading carcinoma, linitis plastica, and advanced carcinoma. As a result of mass screening programs in Japan, **early gastric cancer** has been defined as a primary lesion confined to the mucosa and submucosa. This early stage results in an excellent 5-year survival prognosis. The more malignant type of gastric cancer is known as **linitis plastica**, in which all layers of the stomach are involved with diffuse spreading of the tumor. Survival at 5 years for this type of cancer is extremely low.

Symptoms of gastric cancer include postprandial abdominal discomfort, dyspepsia, anorexia, weight loss, and epigastric pain that often is relieved with H_2 blockers or antacids. Lesions near the esophagogastric junction usually result in some degree of dysphagia and weight loss. Anemia is present in many of the patients, and the carcinoembryonic antigen (CEA) is elevated in about 60–70% of patients. Diagnosis is usually made by an upper endoscopy with biopsy, although upper GI barium examinations frequently show changes in the gastric wall suggestive of tumor.

Management

Surgical resection is the only curative treatment for gastric cancer, and over 50% of these lesions are amenable to removal. Surgical resection should be accompanied by removal of regional lymph nodes and any contiguous organs that are involved by the cancer. Reconstruction is usually performed by either a Billroth I or II procedure, though the latter is preferable since recurrence of the tumor may result in outlet obstruction following a gastroduodenal anastomosis.

Cancers of the esophagogastric junction are usually re-

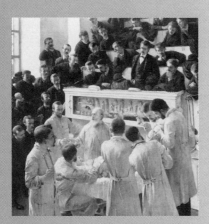

Theodor Billroth operating in the Auditorium of the Allgemeine Krankenhaus, Vienna (1889). This painting by Anton F. Seligman depicts Theodor Billroth at approximately 60 years of age. (Courtesy of the Osterreichische Galerie, Vienna.)

Theodor Billroth (1829–1894) was one of the most influential and celebrated surgeons of the nineteenth century and is still considered the father of gastric surgery. After receiving his medical degree in 1852, he was made a privatdocent in 1856 and a professor of clinical surgery in Zurich in 1860. His crowning achievement was an appointment to the prestigious Chair of Surgery at the University of Vienna in 1867, which he occupied for the next 27 years.

Billroth possessed extraordinary technical expertise as well as experimental genius. He firmly believed in the importance of imagination and felt it was necessary for great achievement in both art and science. In addition to his talent as a surgeon, he was also a gifted musician and enjoyed a lifelong friendship with Brahms.

Billroth performed the first successful gastrectomy on January 29, 1881. The entire procedure took only an hour and a half. The research he and his assistants conducted before attempting the procedure was extensive. Over 900 autopsy records dating back to 1817 were examined. The technique itself was perfected on dogs and cadavers in the laboratory. When Therese Heller appeared at the Allgemeine Krankenhaus (or general hospital) with a palpable, movable gastric mass, Billroth and his team were ready. By 1888 he and his assistants had developed the Billroth I and Billroth II gastric resections, anterior and posterior gastroenterostomies, and pyloroplasty.

Although Billroth is best known for his contributions to gastric surgery, he also developed daring new procedures for carcinoma of the tongue, larynx, esophagus, prostate, breast, and bladder. In 1873, Billroth performed the first successful laryngectomy and also fitted the patient with a prosthesis of his own design. It had a metal tongue analogous to that of an organ and sounded much like a modern artificial larynx. In addition to surgical therapy, Billroth also experimented with early chemotherapy in the form of arsenicals, copper, antimony, and manganese.

Billroth himself believed his greatest achievement was the establishment of his world-renowned surgical school and the publication of his surgical textbook, *Surgical Pathology and Therapy*. As a professor, he was justifiably proud of his outstanding students and insisted they publish their own experiments and be the main authors on reports from his clinic. One of Billroth's most quoted sayings is, "He who helps others contributes to his own happiness." Over a century after his death, his surgical contributions are still in use today and his inspiring spirit endures in his books, lessons, and wise advice.

moved via a left thoracolaparotomy or by an Ivor-Lewis technique, which is conducted through the abdomen and right chest. More recently, the transhiatal route has been used, particularly following neoadjuvant chemo-radiation. The overall 5-year survival rate in this country is around 10–12%, with a 90% percent cure rate for early gastric cancer as opposed to a 0% survival for stage IV lesions.

GASTRIC LYMPHOMA

Diagnosis & Management

Lymphomas of the stomach are the second most common primary cancer seen by these authors. They are generally classified as B cell lesions. Their symptoms are similar to those patients with carcinoma, and diagnosis may be made by gastroscopy, with biopsy or cytology preoperatively. Therapy consists of chemotherapy, radiotherapy, or both, or, in selected patients, subtotal gastrectomy. Disease-free survival at 5 years for these patients is around 50%, with most recurrences within 2–3 years.

GASTRIC LEIOMYOSARCOMA (SPINDLE CELL TUMORS)

Diagnosis & Management

Leiomyosarcomas, or gastric spindle cell tumors, frequently grow to a large size and are often associated with gastric bleeding. Spread is by direct invasion or bloodborne metastases, and the diagnosis is usually made by endoscopy, CT scan, or barium studies. Treatment consists of radical resection for these tumors, whose degree of malignancy is determined by the DNA ploidy pattern and number of mitotic figures.

DUODENAL CANCER

Diagnosis & Management

Tumors of the duodenum include adenocarcinoma, lymphomas, leiomyosarcomas, and gastrinomas. The lat-

ter results in gastric hypersecretion with intractable peptic ulceration or diarrhea, whereas the former lesions frequently produce pain, obstruction, bleeding, and obstructive jaundice. They may be diagnosed on barium x-ray studies, endoscopy, or CT scan. The surgical treatment usually consist of pancreaticoduodenectomy for curative resections. The 5-year survival rate is 30–40%.

SMALL BOWEL CARCINOMA

Diagnosis

Cancers of the small bowel are very rare, especially considering the overall length of the small intestine. Fewer than 3000 cases occur annually in the United States. Most of these cancers are duodenal and jejunal adenocarcinoma; less commonly, one can find carcinoid and lymphoma in the ileum or sarcoma throughout the small bowel. The clinical presentation is usually nonspecific and includes vague pain, change in bowel habit, nausea, anorexia, and occult fecal blood. Since these symptoms are very nonspecific, it is difficult to detect these tumors while they are small. Nevertheless, with a high index of suspicion, one can identify these tumors with a dedicated barium small bowel series (enteroclysis) or, occasionally, with a high-quality CT scan. In spite of the available imaging, many of these tumors are actually found at laparotomy.

Management

When tumors of the small bowel are identified, excision is usually indicated. Benign tumors such as leiomyomas, adenomas, and lipomas can cause symptoms and may not be differentiated from malignant tumors without excision. Since malignant tumors can remain fairly silent, symptoms may not develop until the tumors are very advanced and unresectable. In this setting, entero-enterostomy is sometimes required to palliate obstructive symptoms. The 5-year survival with small bowel carcinoma is 20% for adenocarcinoma, 50–80% for carcinoid, and 40–50% for lymphoma.

SUGGESTED READING

Cameron JL: *Current Surgical Therapy*. Mosby, 1995.
Jordan PH: Stomach and duodenum. In: Hardy JD (editor): *Hardy's Textbook of Surgery*, 2nd ed. Lippincott, 1988.
Moody FG et al: Stomach. In: Schwartz SI (editor): *Principles of Surgery*, 5th ed. McGraw-Hill, 1989.

Pass HI, Hardy JD: The appendix. In: Hardy JD (editor): *Hardy's Textbook of Surgery*, 2nd ed. Lippincott, 1988.
Townsend CM, Thompson JC: Small intestine. In: Schwartz SI (editor): *Principles of Surgery*, 5th ed. McGraw-Hill, 1989.
Yamada T: *Textbook of Gastroenterology*. Lippincott, 1995.

27

The Colon, Rectum, & Anus

James M. Stone, MD

▶ Key Facts

▶ The colon, rectum, and anus serve to transport intestinal contents from the ileum to the rectum where fecal material is stored, to be evacuated completely at the appropriate time.

▶ The colon wall consists of mucosa, submucosa, muscularis propria, and serosa.

▶ Transport of material through the colon is dependent on colonic motility described with measurements of wall motion, intraluminal pressure, electrical events in the muscular colonic tube, and the rate of transit of material through the colon.

▶ The goal of bowel preparation for surgery is the reduction of colonic bacteria achieved by emptying the colon of solid and liquid feces and initiating appropriate prophylactic antibiotic regimens.

▶ More than 50% of Americans over 70 years of age have colonic diverticula; however, only 10–20% become symptomatic.

▶ Diverticulitis refers to inflammation of one or more diverticula and is thought to occur secondary to luminal obstruction of the diverticular neck.

▶ Severe hematochezia is most often caused by diverticular disease, but may also have several other causes. The first priority should be to find the bleeding site.

▶ Severe ulcerative colitis requires hospitalization with maximal medical therapy. Failure to improve after 1 week is an indication for a colectomy.

▶ Although Crohn's disease cannot be cured surgically, timely operative intervention may dramatically palliate symptoms and improve quality of life. In some situations, it may be life-saving.

▶ The most important clinical decision to be made in the case of hemorrhoids, which are not a pathologic entity, is to balance the morbidity of treatment against the severity of symptoms.

▶ Anal fissure is by far the most common finding in patients with anal pain.

▶ The most common cause of fecal incontinence is perineal injury during childbirth.

▶ Adenomatous polyps of the colon and rectum are a particular source of concern, as 10–30% are believed to progress to carcinoma.

▶ Cancer of the colon and rectum is the third most common cause of cancer deaths for men and women in the United States. Approximately 60,000 people die annually from this disease.

▶ Surgical resection remains the mainstay of therapy for primary colon and rectum cancers. The goal of surgical therapy is to remove the primary tumor along with the lymphatics draining the involved bowel.

ANATOMY

The colon, rectum, and anus serve to: (1) transport the intestinal content from the ileum to the rectum; (2) store fecal material; and (3) evacuate it completely at the appropriate time. The colon also functions to absorb water and electrolytes, normally reducing approximately 1 L of water introduced into the cecum to about 150 mL/d.

The human intestinal tract begins as a simple tube extending from the stomach to the cloaca. It elongates to a hairpin-shaped primary intestinal loop supported by a dorsal mesentery. The cephalic limb develops into the proximal gut while the caudal limb becomes the distal ileum, cecum, and ascending and transverse colon. At the junction of the cephalic and caudal limbs is the vitelline duct, which may persist as a Meckel's diverticulum. As the loop further elongates, it herniates through the umbilicus and undergoes clockwise rotation around the axis of the superior mesenteric artery. Incomplete rotation is occasionally seen in adults and may result in atypical locations of various parts of the colon.

The colon wall consists of mucosa, submucosa, muscularis propria, and serosa. The muscularis propria consists of a complete inner circular layer and an incomplete outer longitudinal muscle layer, which is gathered into three continuous bands known as **taeniae coli**. Muscular activ-

ity of the colon wall creates sacculations of the colon known as **haustra**.

The **ileocolic junction** is typically located in the right lower quadrant and is marked by an antimesenteric fat pad (Figure 27–1). This pad is the only antimesenteric fat on the normal small intestine. The appendix, which is located at the junction of the three taeniae coli, may occupy a variety of positions but most commonly resides beneath McBurney's point (two thirds of the distance of the line drawn from the umbilicus to the anterior superior iliac spine). The ileocecal valve is the narrowest part of the colon and may serve as a site of obturation obstruction, particularly with gallstone ileus. The cecum has the greatest diameter within the colon, and as such is the segment most prone to distention. The ascending colon is fixed to the retroperitoneum while the transverse colon is freely mobile on an intraperitoneal mesentery. The splenic flexure is fixed in the left upper quadrant as is the descending colon. The lateral retroperitoneal attachments of the right and left colon are referred to as the **white line of Toldt**. The sigmoid colon is also freely mobile on an intraperitoneal mesentery. The discontinuous bands of longitudinal muscle (taeniae) coalesce into a continuous coat of longitudinal muscle at the rectosigmoid junction. The upper rectum is intraperitoneal, while the lower two thirds of the rectum is extraperitoneal.

The rectum begins at the level of the puborectalis mus-

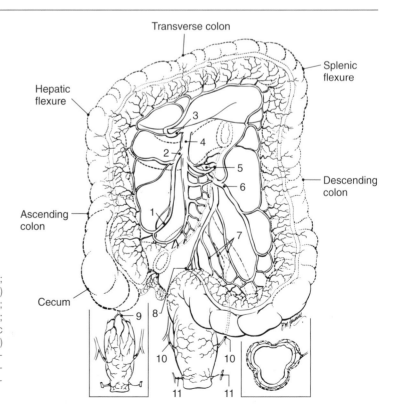

Figure 27–1. Anatomy of the colon: (1) ileocolic; (2) ileocolic artery giving off the right colic artery; (3) middle colic artery; (4) superior mesenteric artery; (5) inferior mesenteric artery; (6) left colonic artery; (7) sigmoidal branches of the inferior mesenteric artery; (8 and 9) superior hemorrhoidal artery; (10) middle hemorrhoidal artery; (11) inferior hemorrhoidal artery. (Modified and reprinted, with permission, from Schwartz SI, Ellis H: *Maingot's Abdominal Operations.* Appleton & Lange, 1989, p. 1050.)

cle and extends approximately to the level of the sacral promontory. It varies from 12 to 15 cm in length in the average adult. There are three submucosal folds, which create lateral curves known as the **valves of Houston**. The second valve is a useful indicator of the level of peritoneal reflection. Valves of Houston can only be seen endoscopically.

The dense presacral fascia of Waldeyer reflects back onto the posterior rectum and envelops the mesorectum as the fascia propria of the rectum. An areolar avascular plane exists between the fascia propria of the rectum and the presacral fascia. The reflection of this fascia at the rectosacral junction may be quite dense and must be sharply incised to expose the pelvic floor.

The anterior rectal wall is intraperitoneal except in its distal third, where it is covered by a condensation of endopelvic fascia known as **Denonvilliers' fascia**. The continuation of the endopelvic fascia laterally forms the lateral rectal stalks that contain the middle rectal artery.

The right and transverse colon arise off of the embryonic midgut and receive their blood supply from the superior mesenteric artery. The extrinsic parasympathetic nerve supply to the midgut comes from the vagus nerve, and the sympathetic supply comes through the superior mesenteric ganglion. The function of sympathetic nerves is generally to cause inhibition of motor and secretory activity and contraction of the gastrointestinal sphincters. The function of the parasympathetic nerves is complex, however, with regard to the colon the primary parasympathetic function is to increase motility.

The splenic flexure, descending colon, sigmoid colon, rectum, and anus are derived from the embryonic hindgut and receive their blood supply from the inferior mesenteric artery. In the lower third of the rectum and anus, the blood supply is received from the hypogastric arteries. The parasympathetic nerve supply to the rectum and anus arises off of the sacral plexus and is known as the **nervi erigentes**. The sympathetic supply comes from the paired presacral sympathetic nerves.

The sphincter mechanism consists of the tonically contracted, smooth muscle, internal sphincter as well as the striated external sphincter. The external sphincter is a unique striated muscle in that it demonstrates continuous tone even during sleep. The anal canal is lined with columnar epithelium in its proximal portion and squamous epithelium distally. The squamocolumnar junction is referred to as the **dentate line** (because, to someone, the corrugated folds resembled teeth).

There is a 1- to 2-cm zone of transitional mucosa located immediately above the dentate line. This zone is very rich in sensory receptors and plays an important role in the continence mechanism. At the dentate line, longitudinal folds known as the **columns of Morgagni** are visible. The bases of the columns of Morgagni are known as **anal crypts**. Each crypt may contain the duct of an anal gland. Anal glands reside in the intersphincteric space and their ducts traverse the internal anal sphincter muscle to

empty at the crypts. Obstruction of these ducts is felt to be the primary mechanism for perianal abscesses. Cancers that arise in the transition zone are referred to as **cloacogenic cancers**.

The lymphatic drainage of the colon and rectum parallels the segmental blood supply. The right and transverse colon drain toward the origin of the superior mesenteric artery. The left colon and upper rectum drain to the inferior mesenteric artery. The rectum and anal canal have a dual blood supply and lymphatic drainage. Lymph from the upper and middle rectum ascends along the superior rectal artery to the inferior mesenteric lymph nodes. The lower third of the rectum drains via the superior rectal lymphatics as well as laterally via the middle rectal lymphatics to the hypogastric nodes. Lymphatics from the anal canal proximal to the dentate line also drain via the superior rectal lymphatics and hypogastric lymphatics. Lymph from the anal canal below the dentate line drains to the inguinal lymph nodes. The lymphatic drainage of the lower rectum appears to be more diffuse than other portions of the gut. Dye injection studies in women demonstrate lymphatic flow from the rectum to the posterior vaginal wall, broad ligaments, and cul de sac.

The pelvic floor muscles consist of the iliococcygeus, pubococcygeus, and puborectalis muscles. The most important of these muscles, the puborectalis, arises off of the pubic bone anteriorly and encircles the anorectal junction posteriorly. In its normal, tonically contracted state, the puborectalis muscle creates a posterior angulation to the anorectal junction. Relaxation of the puborectalis muscle is necessary to effect bowel evacuation. Fecal incontinence is frequently associated with the loss of normal puborectalis function and the loss of the posterior anorectal angle. The anal canal high-pressure zone measure approximately 4 cm in length. The high-pressure zone is longer in men than in women.

Several potential spaces around the distal rectum and anus are filled with loose areolar tissue or fat (Figure 27–2). These spaces typically define the spread of perianal infections. The supralevator or pelvirectal space is located on each side of the rectum above the levator ani muscle. Both lateral supralevator spaces communicate posteriorly. The ischiorectal space is a triangular space below the levator ani muscle. Its medial boundary is the external sphincter, the lateral boundary is the ischium, and the inferior boundary is the perianal skin. The inferior rectal vessels traverse this space. The ischiorectal space communicates in the posterior midline with the deep postanal space, which lies between the levator ani muscle and the superficial external sphincter muscle. The perianal space is limited above by the subcutaneous external sphincter and below by the perianal skin and medially by the anal verge. The intersphincteric space lies between the internal and external sphincter. This space surrounds the anal canal. The submucosal space lies between the internal sphincter and the mucosa.

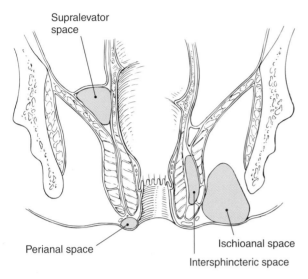

Figure 27–2. Perianal spaces.

PHYSIOLOGY

The colon functions as both a transport and storage organ as well as the site to absorb water and electrolytes. The transport of material through the colon is dependent on colonic motility. Motility may be described with measurements of wall motion, intraluminal pressure, electrical events in the muscular colonic tube, and the rate of transit of material through the colon. The most clinically useful index of motility is **colonic transit time**, the amount of time required for radio-opaque markers to pass from the cecum to the outside of the body.

The physiologic processes of continence and bowel evacuation depend on the relationship between the rectum and the anal sphincter mechanism. Those forces which tend to favor bowel evacuation are rectal contraction, increased intra-abdominal pressure, and straightening of the anorectal angle by relaxation of the puborectalis muscle. Those mechanisms that tend to promote continence are tone within the anal canal high-pressure zone (sphincter), maintenance of an acute anorectal angle, and rectal wall accommodation of stool volume. The majority of normal anal canal resting tone is provided by the internal anal sphincter, which is a specialized continuation of the circular smooth muscle of the rectum. Normal anal canal resting pressure ranges from 50 to 100 cm of water. The internal sphincter normally remains within a state of maximal contraction.

The nerve supply to the internal sphincter arises from the presacral sympathetic nerves and sacral parasympathetic plexus. The primary neurotransmitter within the internal sphincter is nitrous oxide. This neurotransmitter may be blocked and the internal sphincter muscle relaxed with topical nitroglycerin.

The external anal sphincter is comprised of three, ill-defined muscular segments (subcutaneous, superficial, and deep) that fuse with the puborectalis muscle of the pelvic floor. The external anal sphincter functions primarily to prevent incontinence during periods of transiently increased evacuation pressure, such as with rectal contraction or increased intra-abdominal pressure. Maximal contraction of the external sphincter approximately doubles the pressure within the anal canal, but can only be maintained for 1–2 minutes.

The area of specialized mucosa just proximal to the dentate line is known as the **transition zone**. This area is rich in sensory receptors and plays an important role in the continence mechanism. The rectal-anal inhibitory or sampling reflex occurs continuously at an unconscious level throughout the day and during sleep. The reflex is initiated by an acute stretch of the rectal wall from an incoming bolus. The internal sphincter relaxes by reflex action and the external sphincter contracts (holding reflex). A sample of the rectal content is allowed to come in contact with the transition zone in the proximal anal canal. The unique sensory receptors of this zone are capable of detecting minute differences in specific heat of the rectal bolus, thus determining whether the content is solid, liquid, or gaseous.

The external sphincter muscle is innervated via the pudendal nerve. This nerve frequently sustains traction injury during vaginal delivery and is an important cause of fecal incontinence in women. Pudendal nerve traction injury may also occur with rectal prolapse or as a result of pelvic floor descent from long-term constipation and straining during defecation.

BOWEL PREPARATION

Emptying the colon of solid and liquid feces is the most important step in reducing the risk of infectious complications after elective colon surgery. The combination of mechanical removal of stool and antibiotic suppression of the intrinsic colonic bacterial flora has made a substantial impact in this regard. Luminal antibiotics will not be efficacious in the presence of large amounts of stool. And an empty colon is less likely to spill contents on surrounding structures when it is opened.

Modern mechanical cleansing agents include nonabsorbed colon lavage solutions or cathartic/enema preps. The lavage type prep is preferred in patients to whom dehydration might be hazardous and in patients with partial bowel obstructions. The disadvantage of the lavage type agents is the need to ingest 4 L of liquid over a relatively short period of time. Cathartic type preps may be given in conjunction with enemas and a clear liquid diet over 1–2 days. Although the amount of material ingested is less, the resulting increased motility, dehydration, and hypo-kalemia may be hazardous to some patients.

The great majority of the dry weight of stool is made up by colon bacteria. Most of the fecal flora is anaerobic and *Bacteroides fragilis* is the most common bacterium. Other anaerobes, such as lactobacillus, clostridia, and pepto-streptococci, are common.

The goal of preoperative bowel preparation is reduction in the number of colonic bacteria. The most common aerobic organism cultured from infections arising from the colon is *Escherichia coli*. Other important aerobic coliforms include *Klebsiella*, *Proteus*, and *Pseudomonas*. The wide range of bacteria that normally reside within the colon is the basis for the broad-spectrum oral antibiotic prophylaxis typically used in colon surgery. A variety of regimens exist. The most common regimen uses neomycin and erythromycin in a dose of 1 g each given three times on the evening before surgery. Erythromycin is frequently associated with gastrointestinal upset and vomiting, therefore, some clinicians substitute metronidazole for erythromycin. Additional intravenous antibiotics (typically a second-generation cephalosporin) are often given at the time of surgery. These prophylactic parenteral antibiotics should not be continued for longer than 24 hours.

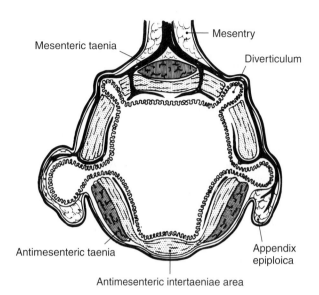

Figure 27–3. Diagrammatic representation of the relationship of diverticula and blood vessels of the taeniae coli. (Reprinted, with permission, from Schwartz SI, Ellis H: *Maingot's Abdominal Operations.* Appleton & Lange, 1989, p. 1008.)

NON-NEOPLASTIC DISEASE

DIVERTICULAR DISEASE

The basic abnormality in diverticular disease of the colon is herniation of the mucosa and submucosa through the muscular coat of the colon to form small outpouchings. Since all layers of the colon are not represented in the diverticula, they are referred to as **pseudodiverticula**. Diverticular disease of the colon is common in industrialized societies today but was rare before improved grain milling techniques caused a decrease in dietary fiber intake in the latter nineteenth century. More than 50% of Americans over 70 years of age have colonic diverticula.

Diverticula are thought to herniate through clefts between bundles of circular muscle fibers where nutrient arteries penetrate the colon wall (Figure 27–3). The close relationship between diverticula and the intramural arteries of the colon is an important factor in the pathogenesis of diverticular hemorrhage. Diverticula may form because of weakness in the bowel wall or because of an increased transmural pressure gradient between the colonic lumen and the abdominal cavity. Although diverticular disease is very common, only 10–20% of patients with diverticula become symptomatic.

Diverticula are classified as spastic, simple massed, right-sided, solitary, and giant. The most common type of diverticular disease in the United States is **spastic diverticulosis**. It occurs primarily within the sigmoid colon and

is associated with a thickened colon muscle wall with prominent haustration. The diverticula are thought to be formed by a process known as **myochosis**. With myochosis, the colon is divided into discontinuous chambers by muscular activity, and very high intraluminal pressures are generated in the small, closed chambers. The next most common type of diverticular disease is referred to as **simple massed diverticulosis**. It accounts for approximately 30% of diverticular disease in the United States. In this condition, there is little or no thickening of the circular muscle layer of the colon. The diverticula involve the more proximal colon as well as the sigmoid colon.

Diverticula confined to the right side of the colon, known as **right-sided diverticulosis**, is uncommon in Western countries but is the most common form of diverticular disease in Asia. Patients with right-sided diverticular disease tend to be younger than those with other types. Differentiating the condition from acute appendicitis may be difficult. **Solitary diverticula** typically form on the right side of the colon and are most commonly true diverticula. All walls of the colon are represented within the diverticula. On occasion, a solitary diverticula of the sigmoid colon will be greater than 10 cm in diameter and will be referred to as a **giant sigmoid diverticulum**.

1. DIVERTICULITIS

Diagnosis

Diverticulitis refers to inflammation of one or more diverticula and is thought to occur secondary to luminal obstruction of the diverticular neck. Some patients with diverticulitis-like symptoms probably have ischemic pain from persistent sigmoid muscle spasm. Diverticulitis may progress to microperforation, with local cellulitis and an inflammatory phlegmon, macroperforation with abscess formation, or free peritonitis. Surgical treatment and prognosis are determined by the type of perforation.

The most common symptom of diverticulitis is left lower quadrant pain. This is usually associated with low-grade fever, left lower quadrant tenderness, and, on occasion, a palpable, tubular mass. Mild diverticulitis is said to occur when there is no systemic toxicity or peritoneal signs and patients are able to take liquids by mouth.

Most diverticulitis occurs within the sigmoid colon, therefore, most localized symptoms occur in the left lower quadrant. On occasion, the pain and tenderness may be elsewhere because a very mobile sigmoid colon may be located outside of the left lower quadrant. With gross perforation and formation of a pelvic abscess, there are usually systemic symptoms, such as fever, tachycardia, and a decrease in urine output along with a tender mass. Sometimes the mass is best felt on rectal or vaginal examination.

Rupture of a pericolic or pelvic abscess results in diffuse peritonitis associated with profound systemic toxicity. On occasion, free intraperitoneal air is seen with perforated diverticulitis, although the amount of air is typically less than that seen with a perforated duodenal ulcer. A history of diverticulitis symptoms preceding the perforation by several days is typically elicited. Fecal peritonitis occurs when diverticular perforation is not walled off by the normal intraperitoneal defense mechanisms. This may occur because the diverticular perforation evolved too rapidly or host defense mechanisms are somehow impaired. Fecal peritonitis or a ruptured diverticular abscess are surgical emergencies (Table 27–1).

Management

Most episodes of mild diverticulitis are treated outside of the hospital with a clear liquid diet and broad-spectrum oral antibiotics. If patients are unable to eat or have complicating associated diseases, they are hospitalized for intravenous hydration, gut rest, and broad-spectrum intravenous antibiotics. The antibiotic should be directed at both gram-negative enteric organisms and anaerobes. Approximately 85% of episodes of diverticulitis will resolve

Table 27–1. Diverticulitis: clinical manifestations.

Fever
Change in bowel habit
Left lower quadrant pain or tenderness
Left lower quadrant mass
Left lower quadrant peritonitis (abscess)
Diffuse peritonitis (ruptured abscess or free perforation)
Leukocytosis
Decreased urine output

Table 27–2. Diverticular disease: indications for surgery.

Recurrent episodes of diverticulitis
Perforation
    Abscess
    Peritonitis
    Fistula
Bleeding
Stricture
Inability to differentiate from cancer

with nonoperative therapy. Approximately 20% of patients with resolved diverticulitis will go on to develop further episodes of acute diverticulitis, often requiring hospitalization. Those patients who develop recurrent episodes should undergo elective resection of the involved colon (Table 27–2).

Small (< 2.5 cm) pericolic or pelvic abscesses will generally resolve with antibiotic therapy. Larger abscesses may be drained percutaneously under computed tomographic (CT) or ultrasonographic guidance, followed by elective single-stage resection. With purulent or fecal peritonitis secondary to perforation, an urgent laparotomy with abdominal lavage, resection of the involved colon if at all possible, and diverting colostomy should be performed. Resection for sigmoid diverticular disease should be extended to the proximal rectum distally and to an area of proximal colon wall that appears and feels normal.

If local conditions in the abdomen are poorly suited to resection, or if the patient is very ill, a diverting colostomy may be the best choice. In some instances, the distal rectal segment may be oversewn and left in the pelvis (Hartmann's procedure) and the proximal colon brought out on a temporary colostomy (Figure 27–4) (Table 27–3).

The threshold for surgery is generally lower in younger patients (< 45 years) because recurrent episodes are more likely. The threshold should also be low in immunosuppressed patients in whom the consequences of diverticulitis are likely to be more severe.

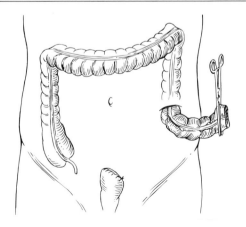

Figure 27–4. Hartmann's procedure.

Table 27–3. Surgical therapy of diverticulitis.

Situation	Procedure	Comment
Elective resection	Resection and primary anastomosis	Percutaneous drainage of pericolic abscess converts to elective resection
a) Diffuse peritonitis b) Anastomosis lies within abscess bed	a) Resection with Hartmann's procedure and colostomy or b) Resection with anastomosis and protecting loop colostomy or ileostomy	a) Closure of Hartmann's requires entering peritoneal cavity b) Simple to close, takes longer to perform, may leave column of stool above tenuous anastomosis
c) Patient in extremis	c) Proximal colostomy with drainage	c) Poor option; should rarely, if ever, be used

Repeated episodes of diverticulitis may result in fibrosis in and around the involved colon wall, eventually causing a stricture. Diverticular strictures occur exclusively within the sigmoid colon and almost never result in complete colonic obstruction. Diverticular strictures that are identified as incidental findings generally do not require resection if a careful history does not reveal convincing symptoms of partial colonic obstruction and if a high-quality colonoscopic examination carried above the area of stricture confidently excludes the possibility of cancer. Symptoms suggestive of partial colonic obstruction are a change in bowel habit, postprandial abdominal bloating and distention, and, perhaps, audible borborygmi. A plain abdominal radiograph that demonstrates colonic distention proximal to the sigmoid colon is strong supporting evidence of a functionally significant obstruction. When partial colonic obstruction occurs at the time of an acute episode of diverticulitis, edema may significantly contribute to the obstructive process. In this setting, a course of antibiotics and reevaluation in approximately 6 weeks is recommended, provided the patient does not have ongoing obstructive symptoms. If surgery is necessary, a gentle bowel prep can generally be tolerated, and a single-stage sigmoid resection and anastomosis is usually possible.

2. COLOVESICAL FISTULA

Diagnosis

Localized sigmoid perforations that resolve by perforation into an adjacent organ or through the abdominal wall result in internal or external colonic fistulas. The most common type of diverticular fistula is between the colon and urinary bladder (colovesical fistula). Colovaginal, coloenteric, and colocutaneous fistulas may also occur. Colovesical fistulas are more common in men than women because the uterus normally separates the sigmoid colon from the urinary bladder. Colovesical fistulas typically present with symptoms of cystitis, such as dysuria and urgency. The complaint of pneumaturia (air within the urine) is nearly pathognomonic of a colovesical fistula. Examination of the urine will often reveal pyuria, vegetable material, and polymicrobial infection. The evalua-tion should include cystoscopy and either colonoscopy or a double-contrast barium enema. It is unusual to demonstrate the fistula with these tests; their chief value is in ruling out bladder or colon neoplasms as causes for the fistula. A positive Bourne test, which consists of taking a voided urine sample after a barium enema (the urine is centrifuged and the sediment is radiographed for barium), may be reassuring in cases where the symptoms and findings are equivocal.

Management

The initial treatment consists of administering broad-spectrum antibiotics, draining the bladder with a catheter, and confirming that there is no residual abdominal or pelvic abscess with a CT scan. A one-stage sigmoid colon resection and anastomosis can usually be performed. The bladder side of the fistula will generally close spontaneously after the involved colon is separated. A Foley catheter is left in the bladder for approximately 1 week. Some patients with established colovesical fistulas and severe concurrent medical disease may be managed with intermittent bladder drainage and antibiotics alone.

3. LOWER GASTROINTESTINAL HEMORRHAGE

Diagnosis

Diverticulosis is the most common cause of massive (> 4 units of blood transfused) lower gastrointestinal hemorrhage. Angiodysplasia of the colon is perhaps a more common cause of chronic colonic blood loss, but is a less common cause of massive bleeding. Bleeding from diverticular disease is typically bright red and is usually painless. The best predictor of recurrent bleeding is the amount of blood shed during the initial episode. Patients who require more than 4 units of packed red cells for resuscitation very commonly have continued bleeding and need further transfusions. Patients who require 2 or fewer units of packed red blood cells have a less than 10% chance of further bleeding. In addition to diverticulosis, there are several other sources of severe hematochezia, several of which are outlined in Table 27–4.

Table 27–4. Source of severe hematochezia.[1]

Source	Percent
Diverticula	30
Angiodysplasia	15
Postoperative/postpolypectomy	12
Polyp or cancer	10
Colitis	10
Proximal to ligament of Treitz	10
Small bowel	8
No site found	5

[1] ≥ 4 units of blood loss.

Management

Patients with severe hematochezia should be admitted to an intensive care unit. The first priority is resuscitation and optimization of coagulation followed by a timely search for the bleeding site. It is far more important to know the source rather than the specific cause of the bleeding. Patients with hematochezia should have a nasogastric tube inserted because approximately 15% of patients with hematochezia have an upper gastrointestinal source. An anoscopy should be performed because hemorrhoid bleeding is occasionally massive and is usually not identified by other diagnostic tests done for lower gastrointestinal bleeding. The remainder of the workup depends primarily on the amount of ongoing bleeding. If bleeding stops or is minimal, a lavage type bowel prep is used to clear the colon, and colonoscopy is performed at the bedside or in the endoscopy unit. Recent studies suggest that colonoscopy is the most sensitive diagnostic test when used in this manner. If colonoscopy fails to reveal a source or there is continued ongoing bleeding, a dynamic CT or technetium 99-labeled red blood cell scan should be performed to localize the source.

Approximately two thirds of diverticular bleeding comes from right-sided colonic diverticula, and approximately 20% of patients with hematochezia have a bleeding source proximal to the ileocecal valve. Many patients with diverticular disease will be bleeding from a non-diverticular source (Table 27–4). Therefore, segmental colon resection without preoperative identification of the bleeding site is a poor strategy. In very unusual cases when bleeding is massive, the workup for hematochezia is unrevealing, upper endoscopy is unrevealing, and exploration in the operating room shows no discreet lesion, subtotal colectomy may be performed.

Most episodes of hematochezia are self-limited. Resection for bleeding diverticular disease is actually quite uncommon because bleeding is the presenting symptom in only 10–20% of patients with diverticular disease. Of those who bleed, only 5–10% go on to require surgery.

ULCERATIVE COLITIS

Diagnosis

Ulcerative colitis and ulcerative proctitis are descriptive terms indicating inflammation confined to the mucosal layer of the rectum that may extend contiguously through some or all of the colon. Some patients manifest symptoms outside of the intestinal tract, such as ankylosing spondylitis, migrating polyarthralgias, uveitis, sclerosing cholangitis, pericholangitis, and erythema nodosum.

The cause of ulcerative colitis remains unknown, although distinctive serum antineutrophilic cytoplasmic antibodies, an abnormal colonic mucosal glycoprotein, as well as certain genetic predispositions, seem to provide clues. Once the condition has been initiated, activation of many facets of immune response may be identified.

Ulcerative colitis always begins in the distal rectum. When the inflammatory process is limited to the rectum, it is referred to as **ulcerative proctitis**. Inflammation that stops at or before the splenic flexure is referred to as **left-sided ulcerative colitis**. Inflammation extending to the cecum is referred to as **ulcerative pancolitis**.

The diagnosis of ulcerative colitis generally requires colonoscopy with biopsy. The most striking histologic features of ulcerative colitis are abscesses in the colonic crypts of Lieberkühn (crypt abscesses). Other typical features are an inflammatory cell infiltrate with basally located lymphoid aggregates and distorted crypt architecture. The inflammatory infiltrate does not extend into the muscle layers of the colon.

Negative stool cultures and the appropriate clinical setting are required for initial diagnosis. Most patients with ulcerative colitis are treated successfully with medical therapy. The mainstays of treatment are anti-inflammatory agents, such as Azulfadine and 5-acetylsalicylic acid compounds as well as corticosteroids, and, less commonly, other immunosuppressive agents.

There is an increased risk of colorectal cancer in patients with long-standing ulcerative colitis. The risk is believed to be greatest in patients with pancolitis, intermediate in patients with left-sided ulcerative colitis, and indistinguishable from the general population in patients with ulcerative proctitis. The risk of cancer in patients with pancolitis is generally calculated at 0.5–1% per year starting 10 years after the onset of disease. A patient with a 20-year history of ulcerative colitis would, therefore, have a 5–10% risk of harboring a colorectal cancer. The activity of the colitis does not appear to correlate with the risk of cancer. It has been demonstrated that the great majority of patients with ulcerative colitis and colon cancer will have premalignant (dysplastic) changes elsewhere in the colon. This has given rise to the practice of colonoscopic surveillance for colon cancer. Patients who have had ulcerative colitis for more than 10 years undergo complete colonoscopy at 1- to 2-year intervals, with multiple biopsies taken at 10-cm intervals. If evidence of dysplasia is identified, a colectomy is recommended.

The clinical course and ultimate prognosis in ulcerative colitis is highly variable from patient to patient. Ulcerative colitis tends to run an exacerbating and remitting course. The initial presentation or subsequent exacerbations may be insidious or abrupt and severe. Typical symptoms include fecal urgency and frequent loose bowel movements that may contain increased mucous, pus, or blood. Crampy abdominal pain, dehydration, and weight loss may also occur.

Patients with more than seven bowel movements per 24 hours and associated systemic findings, such as tachycardia or fever, are said to have severe colitis. When severe colitis is accompanied by radiographic signs of colonic dilatation (transverse colon > 6.5 cm on a supine abdominal radiograph), the diagnosis of toxic megacolon is made. Severe colitis and toxic megacolon require hospitalization with maximal medical therapy and close surgical monitoring. Any deterioration under therapy or a failure to improve after 1 week of medical therapy is an indication for a colectomy.

Management

Surgical therapy is curative in ulcerative colitis, however, the price of a cure is a major surgical operation and the life-style changes that result from not having a colon. The indications for surgery in ulcerative colitis include inability to control symptoms with medical therapy, unacceptable side effects from needed medical therapy, growth failure in children, severe colitis or toxic megacolon unresponsive to therapy, colonic mucosal dysplasia, or colon cancer.

Four operations are currently performed for ulcerative colitis. Total proctocolectomy with a permanent end ileostomy (Brook ileostomy) is the oldest and simplest operation for ulcerative colitis. Total proctocolectomy with Brooke ileostomy has been performed for over 50 years and is known to be a durable operation. By removing all the colonic mucosa at risk, the operation cures ulcerative colitis and completely eliminates the risk of a subsequent colon cancer. Most younger patients, however, are unwilling to trade the requisite permanent ileostomy for a cure.

Total abdominal colectomy with anastomosis of the ileum to the remaining rectum was a popular operation 2–3 decades ago because it obviated the need for a permanent ileostomy. Patients who undergo this operation frequently have significant symptoms from their retained rectum and must continue to undergo endoscopic surveillance because the retained rectal mucosa remains at risk for cancer. More than half of the patients who have an abdominal colectomy and ileorectal anastomosis will go on to have their rectum removed at another operation because of continued symptoms or neoplastic changes. The indications for this operation currently are very limited but include special situations, such as patients with relative rectal sparing and sphincter function too poor for successful outcome with an ileoanal pull-through, or patients with relative rectal sparing in whom the diagnosis of Crohn's disease is as likely as the diagnosis of ulcerative colitis.

An early solution to the need for a permanent ileostomy was the creation of a continent ileostomy (Koch pouch). In this operation the colon, rectum, and anus are completely removed and a reservoir and artificial sphincter mechanism (nipple valve) are created out of the distal 50 cm of the terminal ileum. The opening to the pouch is placed inconspicuously low on the abdominal wall and is covered with a large adhesive bandage. The pouch is emptied four to five times per day by placing a catheter through the stoma into the pouch. In addition to the need to carry a non-disposable catheter to effect bowel evacuation, this operation has decreased in popularity because of a high need for re-operation. In particular, the nipple valve continence mechanism tends to leak with time.

In 1978, the technique of the colon pull-through operation as performed for Hirschsprung's disease, and pouch creation as developed for the Koch pouch, were used by Sir Allen Parks to create the ileoanal pull-through operation (Figure 27–5). In this operation, the entire abdominal colon and most of the rectum are excised through an abdominal incision. The mucosa in the most distal rectum is elevated with submucosal injections of saline and is stripped out of the rectum, leaving only a 2- to 3-cm segment of demucosalized or denuded rectal muscle tube attached to the anal sphincters. A reservoir created from the distal 30–50 cm of the terminal ileum is pulled through the rectal muscle tube and sewn to the sphincter mechanism in the region of the dentate line.

Many surgeons divert the fecal stream above the pouch with a temporary ileostomy, because the consequences of a leak from the pouch or the pouch-anal anastomosis can be devastating. In adequately nourished patients without technical problems, such as tension on the anastomosis, a temporary ileostomy is not routinely necessary. With the ileoanal pull-through operation, an average of six to seven

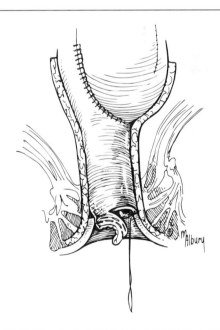

Figure 27–5. The stapled distal end of the ileum is excised to allow the anastomosis to be achieved. (Reprinted, with permission, from Schwartz SI, Ellis H: *Maingot's Abdominal Operations.* Appleton & Lange, 1989, p. 1085.)

bowel movements per 24 hours can be expected. Most men have perfect continence, although minor incontinence, particularly during sleep, occurs in approximately 20% of women. Most patients can defer bowel movements for over 1 hour.

Because this operation was first described in 1978, 10-year and 15-year follow-up studies are only now being published. The operation appears to be durable, and there is gradual improvement in pouch function over the first 18 months; the incidence of pouchitis (nonspecific inflammation of the neorectal reservoir), however, seems to increase with time. Follow-up studies show that more than 90% of patients who have this operation are able to return to their usual occupation or schooling, and that social, sexual, and recreational function is also excellent.

CROHN'S COLITIS

Diagnosis

Crohn's disease is a chronic inflammatory disorder of unknown etiology that affects the entire intestinal tract. In approximately one third of patients, Crohn's disease is limited to the small intestine. One half the patient popula-

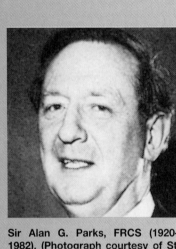

Sir Alan G. Parks, FRCS (1920–1982). (Photograph courtesy of St. Mark's Hospital, London, United Kingdom.)

Alan Guyatt Parks (1920–1982) received his BA degree from Oxford in 1943 and was awarded a Rockefeller Fellowship to Johns Hopkins University in that same year. He completed his medical training and internship at Johns Hopkins, returning to Guy's Hospital in London in 1949 after passing the FRCS examination. Early in his career, he dedicated himself to studies of the anatomy of the anal canal and to correlating his findings with improvements in surgery of the rectum, anus, and perineum. His extended list of publications is a lasting legacy to his amazing achievements and extraordinary creativity.

Parks obtained a Master of Surgery degree in 1954 for his work in specialized operations for the treatment of hemorrhoids. In 1959, he was appointed Consultant Surgeon to the staff at both St. Mark's Hospital and London Hospital. His name is closely associated with innovations in the area of colon and rectal surgery, which include the development of specialized surgical instruments, etiology and classification of fistula-in-ano, the treatment regimens for anal incontinence, as well as the application of ileal reservoir with ilioanal anastomosis for the surgical management of ulcerative colitis and familial polyposis. Parks was recognized with numerous honors, including Presidency of the Royal College of Surgeons, Presidency of the Section of Proctology of the Royal Society of Medicine, Fellowship in the Royal College of Physicians, and honorary fellowships from the American, Australian, Canadian, Edinburgh, and Glasgow Colleges of Surgeons. He was further recognized with a knighthood. He was regarded by all who knew him as an exceptionally gifted technical surgeon, a compassionate human being, and a superior academic researcher. Sir Alan Parks died after emergency cardiac surgery on November 3, 1982.

tion have both small and large intestinal disease while approximately one fifth have disease limited to the colon.

Crohn's colitis, in contradistinction to ulcerative colitis, is characterized by full-thickness inflammation of the colonic wall. In addition to the transmural inflammatory infiltrate, hyperplasia of the autonomic nerves, and characteristic discreet, noncaseating granulomas in the submucosa and lamina propria, may be found. The bowel wall itself is thickened and indurated. There is increased fat surrounding the serosal surface of the colon and thickening of the mesentery, with enlarged mesenteric lymph nodes. In advanced cases, the mucosal surface is cobblestoned because of a series of serpiginous, deep mucosal ulcerations.

In some patients, the transmural inflammation extends through the wall of an adjacent organ, creating an internal fistula. However, most patients with Crohn's disease and bowel perforation develop blind fistula tracts that end in intra-abdominal abscesses. Because bowel perforations with Crohn's disease tend to occur very slowly, it is uncommon for there to be free perforation and diffuse peritonitis with Crohn's disease. The risk of colon cancer in Crohn's colitis is felt to be about the same as in ulcerative colitis when the extent of colitis and the effect of early removal of the colon for symptoms are taken into account.

Management

Crohn's disease cannot be cured surgically, therefore, operative therapy is reserved for patients whose quality of life is significantly impaired despite appropriate medical treatment, or for those persons who have developed one or more disease complications. The indications for operative intervention in Crohn's disease include (1) failure of medical therapy to control symptoms; (2) unacceptable side effects from medication necessary to control symptoms; (3) small- or large-bowel obstruction; (4) symptomatic fistula; (5) intra-abdominal abscess; (6) growth retardation; (7) carcinoma; and (8) toxic megacolon.

Although Crohn's disease cannot be cured, timely surgical intervention will dramatically palliate symptoms and improve quality of life. In some situations, surgery may be life-saving. The theory that surgery should not be performed for Crohn's disease is emphatically incorrect.

Several empirically derived principles of Crohn's disease surgery should be followed. Surgical treatment for Crohn's disease should be directed only at symptomatic disease. Findings such as palpable, indurated bowel segments, radiographically impressive strictures, enteroenteral fistulas, or perianal ulceration should not be treated surgically unless they are causing troublesome symptoms. At the time of surgery, conservation of all possible macroscopically normal small intestine should be practiced. There is no need for frozen section confirmation of normal margins and no need to obtain wide, macroscopically normal margins as is done for cancer surgery. Such practice may contribute to short gut syndrome. It is also established that the removal of enlarged mesenteric lymph nodes does not improve outcome. Intra-abdominal ab-

scesses should be percutaneously drained prior to resection, unless it appears that the abscess can be completely resected along with the involved bowel.

When the colon is involved with Crohn's disease, total proctocolectomy with an end ileostomy gives the lowest recurrence rate (approximately 20%). If the Crohn's disease is limited to a specific segment of the colon, a segmental resection and anastomosis may be performed, although recurrence rates of 60–80% are common. Although the recurrence rate is much higher with segmental resection, most of these patients are spared from a permanent ileostomy for several years. Where there is colonic involvement and rectal sparing, an abdominal colectomy with ileorectal anastomosis may be performed.

ISCHEMIC COLITIS

Diagnosis

The most common setting for ischemic colitis is the early postoperative period after abdominal aortic surgery. When the portion of the abdominal aorta giving rise to the inferior mesenteric artery is separated from the circulation, the left colon is dependent on collateral flow. Unless adequate collateral flow is present, the distal end of the transected inferior mesenteric artery must be reimplanted into the aortic graft. Colon ischemia occurs in approximately 5% of patients after elective aortic surgery and 40–60% after surgery for ruptured aneurysm. Approximately 10% of operative deaths after abdominal aortic aneurysm surgery are from ischemic colitis.

Isolated right colon ischemia appears to be increasing in frequency and most commonly occurs in critically ill patients with sepsis or low flow states. Colonic distention with resulting increases in wall tension and decreases in lymphatic, venous, and, eventually, arterial flow, probably plays a significant role in right colon ischemia.

Symptoms vary with the degree of ischemia. Some episodes of left lower quadrant pain attributed to diverticular disease are more likely related to subclinical ischemia, perhaps brought on by sigmoid muscle spasm. More severe ischemia causes bloody diarrhea from sloughing of the ischemic mucosa. Ischemia involving the muscular layers of the bowel wall may heal with a dense, fibrotic stricture. Severe, full-thickness ischemia may result in frank necrosis of the colon with peritonitis and signs of sepsis.

Management

In the absence of symptoms of perforation or necrosis of the bowel wall, nonsurgical treatment is indicated. The primary goal of treatment is to increase oxygen delivery to the colon. This typically involves optimizing cardiac function, optimizing oxygen content, withdrawing medications that promote mesenteric vasoconstriction, such as digitalis or vasopressors, and decompressing distended colon. Gut rest, broad-spectrum antibiotics, and total parenteral nutrition may also be of value. Most patients improve significantly over 1–2 days on such a regimen. Surgery is indicated if there is deterioration during treatment, or if ischemic symptoms persist for more than 1 week. The extent of colonic ischemia may be difficult to judge at the time of surgery because the serosal surface can appear relatively normal, despite severe mucosal ischemia. The mucosal surface of the resection margins should be inspected, and the cut ends of the remaining bowel should bleed when they are cut. Anastomoses should rarely be performed when operating for acute colonic ischemia.

VOLVULUS OF THE COLON

Diagnosis

A volvulus is said to occur when a portion of the alimentary tract rotates about itself. The twisting movement kinks the gut, producing a closed loop mechanical obstruction and, occasionally, occluding the blood supply to the involved segment as it traverses the twisted mesentery. Sigmoid volvulus accounts for approximately two thirds of the cases and cecal volvulus accounts for approximately one third. A characteristic anatomic abnormality present in patients with sigmoid volvulus is a long, redundant sigmoid colon with a narrowly based mesenteric attachment to the retroperitoneum. Volvulus of the transverse colon is highly unusual.

Most patients who develop sigmoid volvulus are elderly or have been under long-term custodial care. Most patients have a history of chronic constipation. Cecal volvulus can only occur when the cecum and right colon are tethered by a mobile mesentery instead of resolving in the normal fixed retroperitoneal position. This may occur as the result of incomplete embryologic descent of the right colon into the right lower quadrant (malrotation). Upward displacement of the cecum with stretch of the cecal mesentery by a gravid uterus may also contribute to the problem. A condition known as **cecal bascule** occurs when the cecum folds anteriorly over the ascending colon. **Cecal volvulus** is said to occur when the cecum rotates medially and comes to lie within the left upper quadrant.

All types of colon volvulus present with signs and symptoms of colonic obstruction, such as distention, obstipation, crampy abdominal pain, and repeated emesis. The closed loop-type obstruction created by volvulus is especially prone to perforation, and in all cases the volvulus should be decompressed as soon as possible after diagnosis. When fever, localized abdominal tenderness, and elevated leukocyte count or metabolic acidosis are present, gangrenous bowel should be suspected. Immediate resuscitation along with broad-spectrum antibiotics should be undertaken, followed by an urgent laparotomy.

The characteristic radiographic finding in sigmoid volvulus is of a dramatically dilated loop of sigmoid colon that resembles a bent inner tube arising from the left lower quadrant. A cecal volvulus is suggested by a distended loop of colon arising from the right lower quadrant, which is said to resemble a coffee bean in appearance.

Management

In the absence of signs suggestive of colonic gangrene, patients with sigmoid volvulus should undergo preoperative decompression with either a 25-cm rigid proctoscope or a flexible sigmoidoscope. It is technically easier to traverse the area of twist with a flexible sigmoidoscope, however, the rigid proctoscope is preferred because it allows passage of a large-caliber decompression tube through its lumen up into the sigmoid colon. It is common for patients who undergo a simple detortion without internal stenting to re-establish their volvulus soon after decompression. With an internal stent in place, the patient may be given a bowel prep, and an elective, single-stage sigmoid resection and anastomosis may be performed.

Although colonoscopic decompression of cecal volvulus may be performed, it adds little besides risk to overall care. Patients with cecal volvulus should be taken to the operating room as soon as they have been physiologically stabilized because there is no need for bowel prep. In cecal volvulus the goal of surgery is to untwist, decompress, and fix the right colon in its normal right lower quadrant position. This may be accomplished by cecopexy, where the cecum is sewn to the parietal peritoneum in the right gutter with multiple, interrupted sutures. A cecostomy or appendicostomy, which consists of placing a tube through the abdominal wall and into the cecum or lumen of the appendix, may also be performed to ensure decompression. In cases where the viability of the cecum is unclear, a right hemicolectomy with anastomosis between the ileum and the transverse colon may be safely performed in unprepped bowel.

HEMORRHOIDS

Diagnosis

The hemorrhoidal cushions are normal vascular tissue that are present in the human fetus. There are three major vascular cushions located in the left lateral, right anterior, and right posterior positions of the anal canal. The presence of hemorrhoidal tissue, therefore, is not a pathologic entity. Age, gravity, shear forces, increased abdominal pressure, and other factors may cause degeneration of the connective tissue tethering the vascular cushions to the underlying sphincter mechanisms. Prolapse of the vascular tissue results in venous congestion dilation of precapillary sphincters, venous hypertension, and, ultimately, to development of high-pressure varicosities. Regardless of their size, the sole determinant of the clinical significance of hemorrhoidal tissues are the symptoms they cause. Hemorrhoids are classified as **internal** if the epithelial covering is columnar mucosa, **external** if the epithelial covering is squamous mucosa, or **mixed** if both types of epithelia are represented. Internal hemorrhoids are further classified by their degree of prolapse. The degree of prolapse is an important consideration because it determines the type of symptoms a hemorrhoidal cushion is capable of producing as well as the types of treatment that are available. A well-illuminated slotted anoscope is the best way to evaluate internal hemorrhoids. Little useful information can be gleaned from the use of forward-viewing colonoscopes or flexible sigmoidoscopies, even with retroflexed views of the anorectal junction.

Management

The clinical decision that must be made in each case involves balancing the morbidity of treatment against the severity of hemorrhoidal symptoms. Since most hemorrhoid symptoms are self-limited, reassurance, institution of a high-fiber, high-fluid diet, avoidance of straining, and, perhaps, sitz baths are usually sufficient treatment. Topical creams, ointments, and suppositories have little efficacy in treating true hemorrhoid symptoms, but they are relatively safe and inexpensive and may be of use in treating the patient who absolutely must have a prescription. When symptoms are persistent and troublesome to the patient, specific treatment is indicated. Small grade I and II internal hemorrhoids usually respond well to nonresectional treatments such as rubber-band ligation, infrared coagulation, or injection sclerotherapy. These treatments may only be applied to insensate tissue above the dentate line (Table 27–5).

ANAL FISSURE

Diagnosis

Anal fissure is by far the most common finding in patients with anal pain (Table 27–6). The diagnosis is strongly suggested by the typical history: pain brought on by defecation that lasts from minutes to hours and is associated with bright red blood on the toilet tissue. It is common to elicit a history of similar episodes of pain and bleeding in the past. Diagnosis is confirmed on physical examination by everting the skin of the anal verge in the posterior and anterior midlines. The great majority of fissures that occur in men are found in the posterior midline, whereas approximately 20% of fissures in women are found in the anterior midline. Fissures that occur off of the midline are suggestive of Crohn's disease, viral ulcers (herpes simplex virus, cytomegalovirus, human immunodeficiency virus), squamous cell cancer, tuberculosis, or syphilis.

Table 27–6. Causes of anal pain.[1]

Anal fissure
Thrombosed hemorrhoid
Abscess
Skin excoriation/pruritus ani
Levator spasm/proctalgia fugax
Viral dermatitis
Tumor

[1]In descending order of frequency.

Management

Most patients with fissure symptoms will improve with sitz baths and correction of constipation or diarrhea. Fiber supplements and fluid intake are titrated to produce one soft, bulky bowel movement per day. Recently, it has been discovered that topical nitroglycerin may relieve the pain of anal fissures and may even increase the healing rate.

If troublesome symptoms persist, a lateral internal sphincterotomy may be performed under local or regional anesthesia. In this procedure, the distal one half of the internal sphincter is sharply transected. Approximately 95% of patients who undergo lateral internal sphincterotomy will have their symptoms relieved. Minor incontinence may occur in up to 20% of patients who undergo lateral internal sphincterotomy. Forceful anal dilatation (Lord procedure) is an uncontrolled way of tearing the sphincter muscle to accomplish the same goal. Anal dilatation has a lower efficacy rate and a higher incidence of incontinence.

Anal fissure is commonly associated with anal stenosis. Recurrent cycles of fissuring, healing via scar contracture, and tearing of the scar with fissuring commonly result in anal stenosis. Lateral internal sphincterotomy may be sufficient treatment for anal stenosis. When the stenosis is significant, scar excision with advancement of anoderm into the anal canal to cover the defect may be necessary.

PERIANAL ABSCESS & FISTULA

Diagnosis

It is widely held that obstruction of the anal crypts results in bacterial overgrowth within the anal glands. An

Table 27–5. Grade description, symptoms, and treatments of hemorrhoids.

	Grade Description	Symptoms	Treatment
I	Protrudes into lumen, no prolapse	Bleeding	Nonresectional measures[1]
II	Prolapse with straining, spontaneous return	Bleeding, perception of prolapse	Nonresectional measures
III	Prolapse, requires manual reduction	Bleeding, prolapse, mucous soilage, pruritus	Consider trial of nonresectional measures; many require excision
IV	Prolapse cannot be reduced	Bleeding, prolapse, mucous soilage, pruritus[2]	Excision

[1]Nonresectional methods (rubber-band ligation, infrared coagulation, or injection sclerotherapy) can be used in insensate tissue only (above the dentate line).
[2]Pain if thrombosed or ischemic.

abscess is formed within the intersphincteric space. The pathway of spread of the cryptoglandular abscess determines the location of the abscess or fistula. In approximately one half of cases, the abscess dissects distally in the intersphincteric space and presents at the anal verge, forming a so-called perianal abscess. In approximately 20% of cases, the abscess remains in the intersphincteric space in the region of the dentate line. The **intersphincteric abscess** may be a difficult clinical problem because it presents no external findings. Intersphincteric abscesses should be suspected in cases of subacute anal pain when anal fissure, thrombosed hemorrhoid, or perianal abscess cannot be identified on physical examination. Many patients with intersphincteric abscess require examination under anesthesia to make the diagnosis.

Ischiorectal abscesses occur when the abscess penetrates through the external sphincter into the ischiorectal space. Abscesses that ascend within the intersphincteric space (supralevator abscesses) may be difficult to diagnose. They frequently are associated with pelvic pain and difficulty urinating. CT scan of the pelvis is performed to document the location and extent of abscess.

Management

Approximately 50% of the time when an abscess is either spontaneously or surgically drained, a perianal fistula is formed. The fistula arises at the original infected crypt and has its secondary opening at the site of abscess drainage. Fistulas are classified by their anatomic course (Table 27–7).

The treatment of anal fistula is surgical. The surgical principles include destroying the offending crypt and either widely opening or excising the entire tract. Unroofing of the tract (fistulotomy) is the simplest and most efficacious treatment, however, its use is limited when the fistula tract encompasses a substantial amount of internal and external sphincter. Where the amount of sphincter to be transected is likely to cause incontinence, several techniques have been devised. A **seton** is a suture, rubber band, or drain placed through the fistula tract. The seton is tied to itself and gradually tightened so it will cut through the tissue slowly enough that healing can occur on the backside of the seton. This frequently requires 6–12 weeks to occur.

Other techniques include complete excision of the fistula tract with surgical approximation of the cut edges of the muscle or the endoanal advancement procedure. In the endoanal advancement flap procedure, the internal fistula

opening is excised. The fistula tract is laid open from the external opening up to the area of the sphincter muscles, and the internal opening is covered by advancing the rectal wall over the internal opening.

Fistulas that arise in the posterior midline crypts have access to both ischiorectal spaces and may be known as **horseshoe fistulas**. Goodsall's rule states that fistulas with external openings anterior to the midcoronal plane have tracts that extend radially out from the anal canal, whereas external openings posterior to the coronal plane have their internal opening in the posterior midline. Goodsall's rule is accurate for fistulas located within 3 cm of the anal verge.

PILONIDAL SINUS

Diagnosis

Multiple causes for pilonidal disease have been advanced, ranging from congenital problems (midline fusion defect) to a completely acquired condition (jeep driver's disease). A popular theory today states that gravitational forces pulling between the sacrum and the gluteal cleft stretch the skin with its hair follicles. In some locations the hair follicle breaks, resulting in an abscess at the base of the follicle. Hair is thought to be a secondary invader.

Management

Regardless of the pathogenesis, the treatment involves excising or laying open the granulation tissue-lined tracts, removing all foreign material. Since wounds in the midline gluteal cleft tend to heal poorly, minimal skin excisions are used to core out the primary openings within the gluteal cleft and a larger, secondary incision is made lateral to the gluteal cleft for access to and drainage of the chronic abscess cavity or sinus tracts. This procedure can typically be done under a local anesthetic on an outpatient basis. Although healing of the open wound may take 4–6 weeks, most patients are able to return to work within 1–2 days after surgery.

FECAL INCONTINENCE

Diagnosis

Enteric continence is defined as the ability to defer defecation to a socially appropriate time. Multiple factors play a role in maintaining fecal continence, including the anal sphincter high-pressure zone, anorectal sensation, rectal distensibility, rectal tone, colon transit, and stool volume.

The prevalence of fecal incontinence in women over 65 years old is 7% for those living at home and 33% for those living in nursing homes. By far, the most common cause of fecal incontinence is perineal injury during childbirth. Recent prospective studies have demonstrated that 13% of primiparous women have clinical impairment of continence after a vaginal delivery, 30% have sonographic evi-

Table 27–7. Anal fistulas.

Type of Fistula	Frequency (%)
Intersphincteric	60
Transphincteric	30
Suprasphincteric	7
Extrasphincteric	3

dence of sphincter injury, and 16% have evidence of pudendal nerve injury (delayed nerve conduction velocity). Risk factors for obstetric injury include forceps delivery, prolonged second stage of labor, and high-birth-weight infants (Table 27–8).

Incontinence may be for flatus, liquid stool, or formed stool. It may occur on rare occasions or several times a day. A common complaint is of "diarrhea," which on closer questioning proves to be fecal urgency, the need to reach a bathroom rapidly to avoid an episode of incontinence.

Management

The treatment of fecal incontinence includes identifying any contributing factors, such as time of day, precipitating events, or foods. The addition of fiber without an increased water intake is of use in patients with chronic liquid bowel movements. Antimotility agents, such as loperamide, may also be of benefit. A standardized bowel program with, perhaps, a morning enema, may be useful. If there remains some residual voluntary motor function, patients often benefit from biofeedback with sphincter retraining. In patients with obvious anatomic defects, re-approximation of the sphincter muscle is generally helpful unless there is concomitant pudendal nerve damage.

BENIGN TUMORS

COLORECTAL POLYPS

Diagnosis

Polyp is a morphologic term used to describe any tissue protrusion above the normal, flat, colorectal mucosal surface. Polyps are typically classified as **sessile** (broad-based and flat) or **pedunculated** (rounded polyp adhered to the mucosa by an attachment or stalk thinner than the head of the polyp). Polyps may cause symptoms, such as bleeding, mucous discharge, or intussusception, but more commonly polyps are a source of concern for their potential for malignant transformation. On occasion, pedunculated polyps autoamputate with brisk bleeding from the polyp stalk. This is most common with juvenile polyps. Villous adenomas frequently secrete large amounts of mucus, which may be noted by patients as a change in their bowel habit. Large rectal villous adenomas occasion-

ally cause a syndrome of watery diarrhea, hyponatremia, and hypokalemia from this mucous discharge.

The long-held belief that most colon cancers begin as adenomatous polyps has recently been confirmed by molecular biology studies, which indicate that the genetic lesions in benign polyps are intermediate between normal mucosa and colon cancer, and by the empiric finding that colonoscopic removal of polyps reduces the incidence of colon cancer (Table 27–9).

Adenomatous polyps are believed to be the important premalignant lesion. Overall, 10–30% of adenomas are believed to progress to carcinoma. Malignant potential is highest in villous polyps, intermediate in tubulovillous polyps, and somewhat lower in tubular adenomas. In general, the larger the size of the adenoma the greater the risk of cancer. Polyps less than 1 cm in diameter have a less than 1% risk of harboring a carcinoma. Polyps greater than 2 cm in diameter have a greater than 33% risk of harboring a cancer.

Management

Polyps should be removed or destroyed when they are identified to diminish the risk of colon cancer. Whenever a colorectal adenomatous polyp is discovered, a complete colonoscopy is indicated because approximately 50% of patients will have a second, synchronous adenoma somewhere within the colon. The great majority of colorectal adenomas can be removed with a colonoscope. Large, sessile adenomas, particularly within the rectum or the cecum, occasionally require operative removal.

It is well known that malignant transformation may take place in only a small locus within a large adenomatous polyp. Endoscopic biopsies showing benign adenomatous tissue should not be interpreted as proof that malignant transformation has not already taken place. Since the presence or absence of malignant transformation and potential lymph node metastases are not known until the specimen is reviewed by a pathologist, some surgeons perform formal cancer operations (wide margins of normal colon and removal of mesenteric lymph nodes at risk) in case a malignant focus is present. Another optional pro-

Table 27–8. Classification of obstetric injury.

Sphincteric Class	Depth of Injury
I	Superficial to muscle
II	Intoperineal muscle but not sphincter
III	Sphincter muscles
IV	Injury into rectum

Table 27–9. Histologic classification of colorectal polyps.

Adenomatous polyps
   Tubular
   Tubulovillous
   Villous

Hyperplastic polyps

Hamartomatous polyps
   Juvenile polyps
   Peutz-Jeghers polyps

Inflammatory polyps

Submucosal polyps
   Lipoma
   Leiomyoma
   Carcinoid tumor

cedure that may be performed laparoscopically, or by a very small incision, is colotomy and polypectomy, including the entire polyp with its subjacent colonic wall. If an invasive cancer is identified in the specimen, a second, more inclusive, cancer operation is performed.

POLYPOSIS SYNDROMES

Diagnosis & Management

Familial adenomatous polyposis is an autosomal dominant syndrome. Patients develop innumerable adenomas diffusely throughout the colon and rectum. Polyps typically manifest themselves at some point between the second and fourth decades, and colon cancer is inevitable unless the entire colon is removed. Reconstruction with an ilioanal pull-through operation is commonly performed. An alternative solution is total abdominal colectomy with anastomosis of the ileum to the rectum. This is followed by lifelong surveillance of the retained rectum, with endoscopic removal or destruction of all identified polyps in the rectum. Awareness of the cancer risk in this population has greatly diminished the incidence of colorectal cancer, however, this does not cure the genetic lesion. Familial adenomatous polyposis patients frequently go on to die from adenocarcinoma of the duodenum or desmoid tumors. Genetic testing is now available for individuals in known kindreds.

The **hereditary nonpolyposis colon cancer syndrome** (HNPCC, or Lynch syndrome) is an autosomal dominant predisposition to colorectal cancer. Approximately 5% of all colon cancers are felt to be related to this syndrome. Two distinct presentations are recognized. Lynch syndrome I involves patients without multiple polyps who develop predominantly right-sided colon cancer in an autosomal dominant manner. Lynch syndrome II, sometimes known as "family cancer syndrome," involves the same risk of colon cancer, however, extracolonic adenocarcinomas, such as endometrial, ovarian, cervical, and breast cancers, also occur. Surveillance of all family members, beginning approximately 10 years from the age of the earliest diagnosed colon cancer in the family, should be performed. Since most colon cancers are right-sided, the operation of choice is total abdominal colectomy with an ileorectal anastomosis.

Patients with **Peutz-Jeghers** syndrome have multiple, predominantly small bowel hamartomatous polyps that may grow to a very large size. Bleeding may occur from these polyps, but, most commonly, the problem is of multiple small bowel obstructions from intussusception caused by the polyps acting as a lead point for the intussusception. Colonoscopic surveillance of Peutz-Jeghers patients is typically performed because there is an association of colon adenomas in this syndrome. Surgery is reserved for symptomatic polyps and very large small bowel polyps. A combined endoscopic and surgical procedure desiged to remove all identified small bowel polyps is generally attempted.

COLON & RECTAL CANCER

Cancer of the colon and rectum is the third most common cause of cancer death for both men and women in the United States. Approximately 60,000 people die annually from this disease. The incidence of colorectal cancer increases with age, however, 8% of colon cancers occur in patients before the age of 40. There is strong evidence that both environmental and genetic factors are important in the pathogenesis of cancer of the colon and rectum. The genetic predisposition to colorectal cancer is most clearly demonstrated in the familial adenomatous polyposis syndrome. Unless the colon and rectum are removed surgically, essentially 100% of people with this syndrome develop colon cancer. The genetic abnormality responsible for familial adenomatous polyposis has been mapped to a specific chromosome (5q). Recently, a sequence of genetic alteration (mutations and deletions) culminating in colorectal cancer has been outlined. The great majority of colorectal cancers are adenocarcinomas. Lymphoma, malignant carcinoid, melanoma, squamous cancer, or sarcoma on occasion, may also arise from the colon or rectum. There are multiple staging systems for colon cancer. The most widely used system was described by Cuthbert Dukes in 1932. In Dukes' system, tumors limited to the bowel wall were classfied as A, through the bowel wall as B, and tumors with regional lymph node metastases as C. The numerous modifications of Dukes' classification that are commonly used create a good deal of confusion. The **TNM classification** (tumor, nodes, metastasis) is a rational, universally applicable system for categorizing patients (Table 27–10).

Colorectal carcinoma may spread by direct extension, lymhatic metastases, hematogenous metastases, or transperitoneal seeding. The time course for transition from normal, flat mucosa to a neoplastic polyp is thought to be approximately 5 years. The time course from benign polyp to invasive carcinoma is approximately 5 more years. Lymphatic spread of colorectal cancers parallels that of the arterial blood supply. The most common location for hematogenous spread is via the portal circulation to the liver. Pulmonary metastases usually follow liver metastases. Bone metastases are generally an indication of end-stage, widespread disease. Cancers of the lower rectum have access to the systemic circulation via the presacral paravertebral plexus and the hypogastric veins. These tumors may, therefore, occasionally manifest early spread to the spine or lungs instead of the liver.

PREVENTION & SCREENING

The environmental factors believed to predispose an individual to the development of colon and rectum cancers include a diet low in fiber and high in fat, as well as a sedentary lifestyle. Several studies indicate that a diet that

Table 27–10. American Joint Committee on Cancer staging system for colorectal cancer.

Primary Tumor (T)

TX	Primary tumor cannot be assessed
T0	No evidence of primary tumor
Tis	Carcinoma in situ
T1	Tumor invades submucosa
T2	Tumor invades muscularis propria
T3	Tumor invades through the muscularis propria into the subserosa, or into nonperitonealized pericolic or perirectal tissues
T4	Tumor perforates the visceral peritoneum or directly invades other organs or structures

Regional lymph nodes (N)

NX	Regional lymph nodes cannot be assessed
N0	No regional lymph node metastasis
N1	Metastasis in 1 to 3 pericolic or perirectal lymph nodes
N2	Metastasis in 4 or more pericolic or perirectal lymph nodes
N3	Metastatis in any lymph node along the course of a named vascular trunk

Distant metastasis (M)

MX	Presence of distant metastasis cannot be assessed
M0	No distant metastasis
M1	Distant metastasis

Stage grouping

Stage				
Stage	0	Ms	N0	m0
Stage	I	T1	N0	m0 Dukes A
		T2	N0	m0
	II	T3	N0	m0 Dukes B
		T4	N0	m0
	III	Any T	N1	m0 Dukes C
		Any T	N2, N3	m0
	IV	Any T	Any N	mi

T = primary tumor; N = regional lymph nodes; M = distant metastasis.
Reprinted, with permission, from Beart RW: Colon and Rectum. In: Abeloff MD, et al: *Clinical Oncology.* Churchill Livingstone, 1995, p. 1274.

Table 27–11. Characteristics of persons at increased risk for colon cancer.

Personal history of colon or rectal cancer
Presence of adenoma
Ureterosigmoidostomy
Radiation therapy involving the colon
Ulcerative colitis > 10 years
Family history of two or more first-degree relatives with:
  Colorectal cancer
  Polyposis syndrome
  HNPCC[1]

[1]HNPCC = hereditary nonpolyposis colon cancer syndrome, also known as Lynch syndrome.

is high in fiber and low in fat leads to a decreased incidence of colon and rectum cancers. Current studies are focused on identifying the components of fiber that may be the chemopreventive agent, including calcium, ascorbic acid, vitamin E, and wheat bran.

While most colon and rectum cancers are sporadic, it is estimated that 5–10% of all colorectal malignancies are considered heritable. Patients with a family history of colon cancer or other factors that place them at increased risk should be tested regularly with colonoscopy (Table 27–11).

A controversy exists as to which method of screening is most appropriate for the general population. While it has been determined that colonoscopy is a far more sensitve test and includes the ability to obtain a biopsy if necessary, an air-contrast barium enema (in conjunction with sigmoidoscopy) is more cost-effective and may yield adequate results. Typical recommendations for screening of persons at normal risk include digital rectal examination at yearly intervals starting at 40 years of age, fecal occult blood testing at yearly intervals as part of the rectal exam, and flexible sigmoidoscopy at 3- to 5-year intervals beginning at 50 years of age. This is more cost-effective than

colonoscopy but is limited by a less than complete look at the colon. While this is currently considered adequate, the regular use of colonoscopy for screening is certainly the gold standard in prevention. If polyp(s) are identified and excised, the patient is brought back 1 year later for a repeat colonoscopy. If the colonoscopy is negative and no polyps are detected, the examination should be repeated at 3- to 5-year intervals.

Diagnosis

The probability of cure of a colorectal carcinoma is much less if the tumor is identified because of symptoms as compared to tumors that are identified by screening of asymptomatic individuals. Symptoms are determined by the location, size, and invasiveness of the primary lesion. Cancers of the right colon tend to be bulky, exophytic lesions. Occult blood loss and anemia are generally responsible for symptoms such as fatigue, light-headedness, dyspnea on exertion, atrial fibrillation, or congestive heart failure. Malignant obstruction of the cecum is uncommon unless the tumor is located at the ileocecal valve, in which case the patient presents with symptoms of a distal small bowel obstruction.

Tumors in the left colon tend to cause more obstructive symptoms because the lumen is narrower and the stool is more formed. Left colon tumors tend to cause subtle obstructive symptoms, such as postprandial bloating, abdominal cramps relieved by bowel movements, diarrhea, or constipation. These symptoms, generally referred to as "change in bowel habit," are a very important clue in the diagnosis of colorectal cancer in adults. Evaluation of the colon with either colonoscopy or barium enema should be performed whenever an adult has had a persistent change in the established bowel pattern.

Tumors of the rectum may cause bright red rectal bleeding or increased mucous in the stool. As the tumors grow, they may cause tenesmus, fecal urgency, or a sense of incomplete evacuation. Bright red blood per rectum should never be ascribed to hemorrhoids unless a minimal evaluation, consisting of a good-quality rigid or preferably flexible sigmoidoscopy, has been performed.

After the diagnosis of colon or rectum cancer is established, measurement of the hematocrit determines the

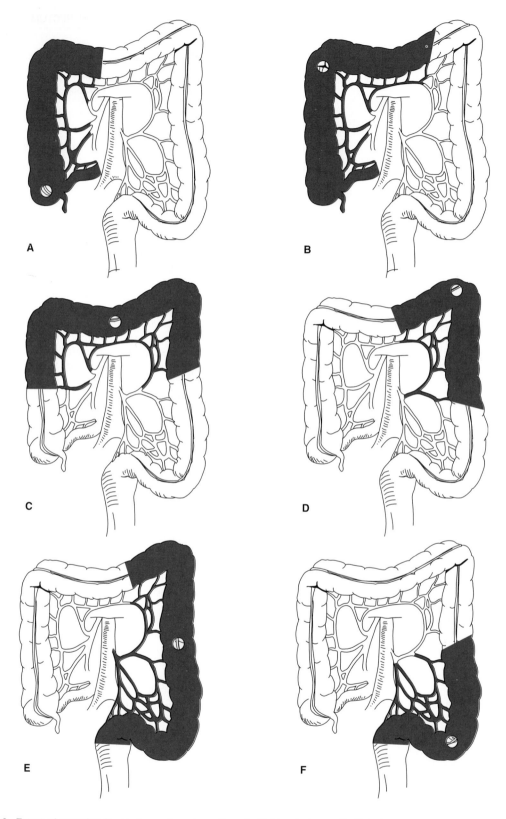

Figure 27–6. Extent of resection for carcinoma in various sites. **A:** Right colectomy. **B:** Right hemicolectomy with division of middle colic pedicle. **C:** Transverse colectomy. **D:** Resection of splenic flexure and ligation of left colic pedicle. **E:** Left hemicolectomy. **F:** Sigmoid colectomy sparing the left colic vessels. (Reprinted and modified, with permission, from Schwartz SI, Ellis H: *Maingot's Abdominal Operations.* Appleton & Lange, 1989, p. 1053.)

ability of the patient to donate autologous blood. Measurement of blood carcinoembryonic antigen (CEA) is important as a baseline and for ruling out the possibility of synchronous metastases, for early diagnosis of recurrent disease, or for following the effects of palliative chemotherapy. A chest radiograph is used to check for the presence of lung metastases. Abdominal and pelvic CT scanning provides information about invasion of the primary tumor into adjacent structures and the possible presence of liver metastases that can be removed at the time of resection of the primary tumor. A less expensive strategy, but one that is less sensitive, is preoperative ultrasonography of the liver instead of CT scan. The most sensitive test for identification of liver metastases is the combination of intraoperative ultrasonography with inspection and palpation of the liver.

Management

Surgical resection remains the mainstay of therapy for primary colon and rectum cancers. The goals of surgical therapy are removal of the primary tumor along with the lymphatics draining the involved bowel (Figure 27–6). An adequate margin of normal proximal and distal bowel naturally follows from the proximal vascular ligation involved in this technique. The adequacy of bowel margins is most at issue in low rectal cancers where preservation of the sphincter mechanism limits the distal resection margin. A 2-cm unstretched, distal margin is believed to be adequate. Radial margins of rectal cancers, which are often quite limited by the rigid, boney walls of the pelvis, are a better predictor of local recurrence than are distal margins.

The general trend with respect to cancers of the rectum is an attempt to match the aggressiveness of the therapy to the invasiveness of the primary tumor. Endorectal ultrasonography is the most sensitive test for determining depth of invasion of rectal cancers. Small (< 3–4 cm) tumors invading no deeper than the submucosal layer may be removed via a transanal excision. Tumors that invade the muscle coat are traditionally excised through a transabdominal approach, but transanal excision with postoperative adjuvant radiation and chemotherapy is gaining popularity. Tumors invading through the entire rectal wall should be excised through a radical, transabdominal approach. An adequate distal margin (2 cm) can be obtained in most patients without the need for excision of the sphincter muscles and creation of a permanent colostomy known as **abdominoperineal resection**. When an anastomosis is created below the peritoneal reflection, the procedure is termed a **low anterior resection**. Most low anterior resections are performed with a stapling device (Figure 27–7).

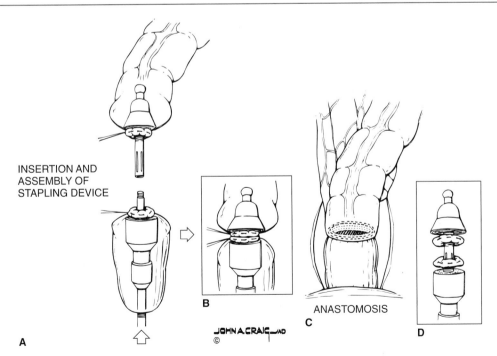

Figure 27–7. **A:** Purse string suture tied around anvil and proximal stapler shaft inserted via the anus. Instrument reconnected and re-approximated. **B:** Completed anastomosis. **C:** Donuts containing purse string sutures and resection margins. **D:** Completed low anterior resection. (Reprinted and modified, with permission, from Schwartz SI, Ellis H: *Maingot's Abdominal Operations.* Appleton & Lange, 1989, p. 1127.)

About 10–20% of colon and rectal cancers are associated with significant colonic obstruction. If the amount of intestinal distention does not preclude a standard resection and lymphadenectomy, resection with anastomosis and a proximal loop colostomy or ileostomy may be performed. The colostomy may be closed approximately 6 weeks later. If the ileocecal valve has protected the small intestine from the effects of distention, resection back to the terminal ileum with an ileosigmoid anastomosis may be performed. An anastomosis created with a massively dilated colon has a high likelihood of not healing and should be avoided.

Laparoscopic colectomy may be of benefit in some patients with benign colonic disease. The oncologic outcome after laparoscopic colectomy for colon cancer is unknown. Its effectiveness is currently being studied in a national trial. At this time, the use of laparoscopic resection for colon cancer should be limited to prospective trials.

An indication that microscopic metastases are frequently undetected is that 40–50% of patients with supposedly curative resections go on to die from colorectal cancer. The attempted elimination of these microscopic metastatic deposits via adjuvant therapy is useful in patients with colon cancer metastatic to lymph nodes or in rectal cancer with spread throughout the entire rectal wall. The standard adjuvant treatment of colon cancer consists of 5-fluorouracil (5-FU) and levamisol or 5FU and leucovorin. In rectal cancer, adjuvant pelvic radiation therapy, using 5-FU as a radiosensitizer, is used. The pelvic radiation is followed by 5-FU and leucovorin, usually for 6 months (six cycles). There is ongoing interest in developing adjuvant protocols that further improve the disease-free and overall survival of high-risk patients.

SUGGESTED READING

Beart RW: Colon and rectum. In: Abeloff MD et al (editors): *Clinical Oncology.* Churchill Livingstone, 1995.

Corman ML: *Colon and Rectal Surgery.* JB Lippincott, 1993.

Moody FG et al: *Surgical Treatment of Digestive Diseases.* Year Book Medical Publishers, 1990.

Schwartz SI, Ellis HE: *Maingot's Abdominal Operations.* Appleton & Lange, 1989.

28

The Liver

John E. Niederhuber, MD

▶ Key Facts

▶ Approximately 1500 mL of blood enters the liver each minute and 70–80% arrives via the portal vein.

▶ The liver has three major functions: (1) the filtering of incoming portal blood; (2) monitoring of hepatic arterial blood for proper plasma concentrations of glucose, lipids, and amino acids; and (3) synthesis of most of the plasma proteins, including albumin, carrier proteins, and clotting factors.

▶ Ultrasonography is the most common imaging procedure performed to evaluate the liver, but dual phase or dynamic CT is the ultimate imaging approach.

▶ The mortality of liver infections has declined in recent years and is most often cited at approximately 10%.

▶ Portal hypertension is defined as portal vein pressure that is elevated to 5 mm Hg or more above the patient's systemic venous pressure.

▶ Nonoperative methods for controlling bleeding secondary to portal hypertension are preferred, but when these fail it is imperative that a decision for operative intervention not be delayed.

▶ Improvements in the management of liver trauma have significantly reduced the mortality associated with these injuries to approximately 10%.

▶ Massive injuries to the liver, such as evulsive tears to the hepatic veins or vena cava, are hard to control and generally fatal. However, initial compression of the liver against the diaphragm, packing of bleeding liver surfaces, and the occlusion of arterial and portal inflow (Pringle maneuver) may provide the surgeon with an opportunity to deal with such injuries.

▶ In the United States, primary liver tumors are uncommon and occur at a rate of approximately 3 per 100,000 of the population. Cavernous hemangiomas are the most common benign hepatic tumor, with a quoted incidence of approximately 3–7%.

▶ Hepatocellular carcinoma is the most common primary malignant tumor. It tends to occur in the fifth and sixth decades of life and is associated with hepatitis B infection and cirrhosis.

▶ The most common mass lesion in the liver is a metastasis of tumor from another primary site in the body. Almost every solid tumor will, at some point in its course, involve the liver.

From the earliest time of written records, the liver has held a special place, along with the heart, as a vital organ of the body. It was mummified in Egyptian times and regarded by many early civilizations as the seat of life. It is the largest organ in the body, weighing 1200–1500 g, and has an especially complex anatomy and a somewhat overwhelming number of functions. It has only been in the past 15 years, and with the introduction of orthotopic liver transplantation, that significant advances have been made in the surgical management of diseases involving the liver. While still viewed as an organ to be respected, the morbidity and mortality associated with surgery of the liver has been dramatically reduced. This has extended the surgical options available and, as a result, liver surgery is becoming a distinct subspecialty of surgical practice.

SURGICAL ANATOMY

The liver is situated directly below the diaphragm and is entirely protected by the lower rib cage. On deep inspiration, the sharp edge of the normal liver can be palpated at the right costal margin. Upon entering the upper abdomen, the surgeon first encounters the round ligament of the liver at the inferior margin of the falciform ligament (Figure 28–1). The round ligament contains the vestige of the umbilical vein coursing to the left portal vein. Division of the round ligament early in exposure of the upper abdomen avoids tearing these structures within the liver fissure. Bleeding associated with such a tear can be difficult to control.

The visceral peritoneum adheres to the surface of the liver, forming a fibrous covering known as **Glisson's capsule**. This fibrous capsule reflects onto the diaphragm, forming the **coronary ligament**, sometimes referred to as the right and left triangular ligaments. Between the leaves of the coronary ligament is the so-called "bare area" of the liver surface, which is in direct contact with the diaphragm. The fibrous capsule also forms the falciform ligament, and within the liver hilum it is continuous with peritoneum, investing the hepatic arteries, common bile duct, cystic duct, and gallbladder.

The liver is distinguished for its dual blood supply consisting of the hepatic arterial circulation and the portal venous circulation. Approximately 1500 mL of blood enters the liver each minute, and 70–80% arrives via the portal vein. The portal vein is formed by the union of the superior mesenteric vein and the splenic vein. One fifth of the flow in the portal vein arises from the spleen.

The portal circulation has extrahepatic connections with the systemic circulation via the esophageal veins and the inferior rectal veins. These become important in disease states impairing portal venous flow within the liver and raising portal venous pressure. It should be remembered that the portal vein has no valves but does have a well-defined wall of unstriated muscle.

The hepatic artery supplies 20–30% of the blood entering the liver and provides oxygen to the hepatocytes. The portal and arterial blood mix within the hepatic sinusoids. The hepatic artery arises from the celiac axis and courses through the gastrohepatic ligament to the region of the gastric pylorus, where it gives off the gastroduodenal artery and a smallish right gastric branch (Figure 28–2). The proper hepatic artery turns in a superior direction toward the liver, coursing in the gastroduodenal ligament medial to the common bile duct and anterior to the portal vein. The proper hepatic artery divides into right and left hepatic arteries well below the hilum. The right hepatic artery courses behind the common bile duct and gives off the cystic artery to the gallbladder. A smaller middle hepatic branch is commonly identified. The surgeon must be aware of the frequent variations in the anatomy of the hepatic artery. For example, a hepatic artery replaced to the superior mesenteric artery is found as often as 16% of the time. The left hepatic artery may arise from the left gastric artery with a similar frequency. When a replaced right hepatic artery is present, it can be found coursing behind the pancreas as the first branch of the superior mesenteric artery in a groove to the right of the portal vein and posterior to the common bile duct as it proceeds toward the liver.

The venous drainage of the liver is via three major hepatic veins: the **right**, **middle**, and **left hepatic veins**. These are short and rather large and enter the inferior vena cava at the superior attachment of the liver just below the diaphragm. The middle and left hepatic veins usually join before entering the cava. In addition, there are a number of small veins from the liver that enter directly into the inferior vena cava throughout its course across the posterior liver.

SURGICAL LOBES & SEGMENTS

A clear understanding of the internal or surgical structure of the liver is critical to performing safe resections of

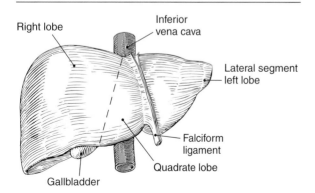

Figure 28–1. Anatomy of the liver.

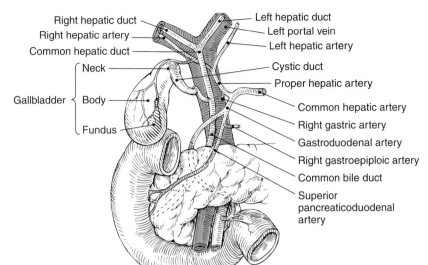

Figure 28–2. Relationship of the extra-hepatic biliary tree, portal vein, and arteries to the liver.

primary and secondary tumors. There are two descriptions in common use regarding the anatomic divisions of the liver, that of Couinaud (1957) and Goldsmith and Woodburne (1957). The nomenclature devised by Couinaud is more commonly used with the liver divided into eight segments—four in the right lobe and four in the left. The segments are numbered counterclockwise, starting with the caudate lobe. Each is supplied by a portal vein branch and has a segmental bile duct to drain the bile duct system (Figure 28–3A).

The right and left sides of the liver are divided along the course of the middle hepatic vein (Figure 28–3B). This plane of division is termed the main hepatic portal scissura and proceeds from the middle of the gallbladder bed anteriorly across the liver to the patient's left of the right hepatic vein and directly posterior to the left of the inferior vena cava. A right lobe portal scissura describes a plane that divides the right lobe into two sectors along the course of the right hepatic vein. Segments VI and VII are to the right and more posterior, while segments V and VIII are medial and more anterior.

The left portal scissura divides the left lobe into two sectors along the course of the left hepatic vein. The anterior medial sector is divided by the umbilical fissure into an anterior segment, segment IV, and an anterior lateral segment, segment III. The posterior sector of the left lobe is not divided into segments and is comprised of only one segment, segment II, which is the posterior aspect of the left lobe of the liver.

The caudate lobe, segment I, can be considered an autonomous segment of the liver receiving portal circulation and arterial blood supply from both the right and left main vascular arcades and draining its blood via independent veins directly into the cava.

Similar to the extrahepatic anatomy, the frequency of variations from normal by intrahepatic anatomy are at least 40%. It is for this reason that the surgeon must exercise caution and utilize available imaging technology in planning surgical resections. Intraoperative ultrasonography is an outstanding method of documenting the extent of tumor and the relationship of the plane of planned resection to major ducts and vascular structures. It should be utilized when performing major resections of the liver.

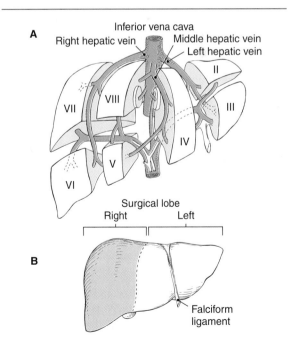

Figure 28–3. *A:* Segments of the liver. *B:* Surgical lobes of the liver.

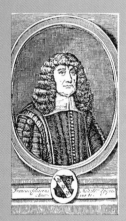

Francis Glisson (1598–1677).

Francis Glisson (1598–1677), in his classic text entitled *Anatomia Hepatis,* published in 1654, provided the first systematic description of the liver and biliary tract. This seminal treatise also included many original concepts regarding liver function. The first anatomic drawings of the distribution of veins and the bile ducts in the liver are contained in the pages of this remarkable text.

Glisson is believed to have been born in Bristol, England, although the records are somewhat unclear. He obtained a classical education in Greek before taking his medical degree in 1634 at Cambridge. Despite a late start, at age 36 he was elected a Regius Professor of Physic at Cambridge. Glisson held this professorship until his death in 1677 (longer than any Regius Professor before or since). He was one of the founding members of the Royal Society and was named President of the Royal College of Physicians in London, England, in 1667.

Glisson is eponymously remembered for his description of the thin connective tissue that encases the liver (Glisson's capsule). In *Anatomia Hepatis*, Glisson described this capsule as the "capsula communis." As defined in his text, it extended beyond the limits of the Glisson's capsule as it is defined today to include "the liver . . . enfolding the portal vein and bile ducts down to their last ramifications." The reason for this extension is clear; however, the connective tissue sheath surrounding the hepatoduodenal ligament does become more dense near the porta hepatis and may readily be considered the continuation of the capsule enclosing the liver.

SURGICAL PHYSIOLOGY

Blood flow through the liver is normally 40% of the cardiac output. During exercise this falls sharply to provide a greater flow to the brain, heart, and muscles. In the hepatic artery, pressures are 100–150 mm Hg; in the portal vein, from 8 to 12 mm Hg; and in the hepatic vein, 1–4 mm Hg.

Intrahepatic portal triads composed of branches of hepatic artery, portal vein, and biliary radicals are located at right angles to hepatic venous radicals (Figure 28–4). The hepatic sinusoids are lined by endothelium and Kupffer's cells and traverse a column of 12–20 hepatocytes. Therefore, blood does not come into direct contact with hepatocytes because of the endothelial layer and a porous basal lamina. The hepatocyte, instead, interfaces with a steady flow of plasma containing approximately 6 g protein/100 mL. The bile canaliculi lie along the outer side of the hepatocyte and collect the secretions that will become the bile. The hepatocytes divide frequently having a life span of some 300 days and, unlike other organs of the body, the liver can regenerate lost tissue rapidly by cellular hypertrophy and hyperplasia. The mechanisms that control this remarkable regenerative capacity are yet to be elucidated.

The liver has three major functions. It acts to filter incoming portal blood from the gastrointestinal tract, removing bacteria and processing substrates and vitamins. The reticuloendothelial system within the liver has a major role in removing and destroying bacteria. Vitamin B_{12}, vitamin A, iron, and copper are stored in the liver. Certain drugs and hormones are detoxified in the liver.

The liver also monitors hepatic arterial blood in order to maintain proper plasma concentrations of glucose, lipids, and amino acids. The hepatocytes have the capacity to capture specific substrates from the blood, leading to in-

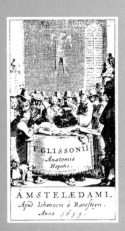

The title page of Glisson's *Anatomia Hepatis* **showing the anatomic theatre in London. (Reprinted from Glisson's** *Anatomia Hepatis* **1659 edition.)**

During his studies of hepatic vasculature, Glisson was able to demonstrate that an open communication existed between the portal venous system and the vena cava using a dye injection method. This same method was used to make the extraordinarily accurate figures contained in the text. He also described the flow of bile into the duodenum that was regulated by a "sphincter" similar to that of the rectum. This description long preceded that of Oddi.

Many of Glisson's observations sank into oblivion, only to be discovered later. He was one of the first to describe hemobilia. His discussion preceded any other by almost a hundred years:

> I believe that if the liver is injured by a contusion, it may lead to blood leaving the body by way of vomit or the stool for there is no doubt that the biliary tract takes unto itself (to the great good of the patient) some of the blood issuing into the liver and leads it down to the intestines. From there it is either impelled upwards through reverse peristalsis or downwards the normal way.
>
> ——from *Anatomia Hepatis*

Francis Glisson was one of the great intellects of the 17th century. It is somewhat unfortunate that this great anatomist, physiologist, physician, and philosopher has become associated with such a trivial anatomic structure, but it serves to keep his name present in the minds of all those who operate on the liver.

tracellular metabolism, storage, and eventual release as required. The most important of these tasks is the maintenance of glucose levels.

The liver is also involved in lipid metabolism and specific protein synthesis. In fact, the liver is responsible for the synthesis of most of the plasma proteins, including albumin, carrier proteins, and clotting factors. The production of albumin is important, as it is responsible for approximately one half of the colloidal osmotic pressure provided by the circulating plasma.

These processes within the hepatocyte require considerable energy derived from the conversion of adenosine triphosphate (ATP) to adenosine diphosphate (ADP) and aerobic oxygenation via the citric acid cycle. These metabolic mechanisms generate an excessive amount of heat, which the liver provides in the body.

MEASURES OF LIVER FUNCTION

The many and varied functions of the liver, as expected, require a battery of laboratory tests to investigate how well the hepatocellular tissue is working. It is important to remember that considerable liver damage can exist without altering specific individual tests, and patients with cirrhosis may have quite normal liver biochemistries. The standard screening panel is outlined in (Table 28–1).

In addition to the general tests for hepatocyte viability, synthesis, and excretion functions, there are a number of specific laboratory tests for different liver diseases. For example, alpha-fetoprotein is a protein marker of primary hepatocellular cancers and is essentially diagnostic of tumor when elevated. This marker can also be increased

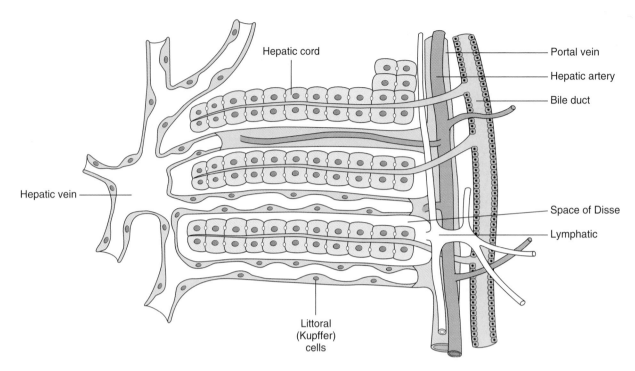

Figure 28–4. Portal triad structures are at a right angle to hepatic vein tributaries. Between portal elements and the central vein are the hepatic sinusoids, the units of hepatic function. (Modified and reprinted, with permission, from Merrell RC: Hepatic physiology. In: Miller TA (editor): *Physiologic Basis of Modern Surgical Care.* CV Mosby, 1988, p. 405.)

during significant liver regeneration following liver resection. Other specific tests are outlined in Table 28–2.

Specific immunologic tests are used to screen and diagnose active and chronic hepatitis. These tests, coupled with liver biopsy, provide considerable diagnostic information. Liver biopsy is only performed following laboratory assurance of normal or normalized coagulation capacity. Ascites and hydatid disease of the liver are contraindications to percutaneous biopsy. Ultrasonographic or computed tomographic (CT) guidance is used to direct the biopsy needle to specific suspicious masses within the liver; core samples are preferred to fine needle aspiration. Laparoscopy can also be used to provide direct visualization of the liver and to direct the biopsy. The latter involves anesthesia support and is more costly. Core biopsy is especially useful in determining the extent of liver diseases, such as cirrhosis and hepatitis. The major complications are intraperitoneal or subcapsular hemorrhage and bile leak with peritonitis.

IMAGING THE LIVER

Ultrasonography is the most common imaging procedure performed to evaluate the liver. It is safe, noninva-

sive, and easy to perform. Ultrasonography of the liver also provides useful information regarding the biliary tree—whether these ducts are of a normal size or dilated—and it may provide information regarding stone disease and tumors. One of the disadvantages of ultrasonography is the small field of view of a single image, which makes it difficult for consultants to review and interpret the results without the aid of real time display. The lack of bony structures on images also makes it difficult to compare to CT images. Finally, ultrasonography is highly dependent on the skill level of the radiologist performing the examination and interpreting the results.

Intraoperative ultrasonography is of specific value in determining the number and location of primary and secondary tumors. It is also very useful in assessing the relationship of the tumor(s) to important vascular structures, such as hepatic veins and portal veins, enabling the surgeon to determine the extent of resection and the margins that may be safely obtained. Intraoperative ultrasonography is currently the most sensitive imaging modality for detecting small tumors within the liver parenchyma.

CT has always been the mainstay of modern liver imaging. Today, the dual-phase or dynamic CT is the ultimate imaging approach. This provides for a 3-mm spacing of image slices, and, with the rapidity of scanning, allows imaging of both arterial and venous phases during dye in-

Table 28–1. Standard screening tests for liver function.

Test	Function/Event Measured
Serum bilirubin	Conjugation, excretion
Serum bile acids	Excretion, shunting
Alkaline phosphatase	Cholestasis
Gamma-glutamyl transpeptidase	Cholestasis, enzyme induction, alcohol abuse
5′-Nucleotidase	Cholestasis
Transaminases	Necrosis
Coagulation factors, prothrombin time	Synthesis
Albumin	Synthesis

Reprinted and modified, with permission, from Zimmerman H, Reichen J: Assessment of liver function in the surgical patient. In: Blumgart LH (editor): *Surgery of the Liver and Biliary Tract,* 2nd ed. Churchill Livingstone, 1994, p. 41.

jection. Computer-generated magnification views and 3-D reconstructions provide amazing detail.

Magnetic resonance imaging and positron emission tomography (PET) scanning are infrequently used because they have no real advantage over current CT technology. Similarly, radioactive scans using sulfur colloid are rarely used today.

Selective celiac and superior mesenteric artery retrograde angiography is occasionally useful in documenting the arterial blood supply to the liver, which can be quite variable. The venous phase of such studies provides accurate visualization of the portal system. The portal circulation can also be imaged directly using a variety of approaches, most commonly, transhepatic portography or transjugular portography. Angiography is used less frequently today because of the advances made in CT.

The biliary tract is imaged either by upper gastrointestinal endoscopy and cannulation of the duct via the ampulla of Vater or via the percutaneous transhepatic route. The former, known as **endoscopic retrograde cholangiopan-**

Table 28–2. Specific screening tests for liver disease.

Test	Disease/Condition Tested
Alpha-fetoprotein	Tumor marker
Hepatitis A IgM	Acute hepatitis A
HBs, anti-HBs, anti-HBc, etc	Hepatitis B
Anti-HCV	Hepatitis C
Antimitochondrial antibodies	Primary biliary cirrhosis
Antineutrophil antibodies	Primary sclerosing cholangitis
ANA, ASM, anti-LKM	Autoimmune hepatitis
Iron-binding capacity, ferritin	Hemochromatosis
Alpha-1-antitrypsin	Alpha-1-antitrypsin deficiency
Caeruloplasmin, urine copper	Wilson's disease

ANA = antinuclear antibodies; ASM = anti-smooth muscle; HBs = hepatitis B surface antigen; HBc = hepatitis B core antigen; LKM = liver-kidney microsome.
Reprinted and modified, with permission, from Zimmerman H, Reichen J: Assessment of liver function in the surgical patient. In Blumgart LH (editor): *Surgery of the Liver and Biliary Tract,* 2nd ed. Churchill Livingstone, 1994, p. 41.

creatography (ERCP), may provide adequate assessment of the intrahepatic biliary radicles but is most frequently used in assessing the extrahepatic biliary system (Figure 28–5). The transhepatic route is generally required when lesions are located at the bifurcation of the bile duct or higher within the liver.

Radiopharmaceutical agents, such as derivatives of iminodiacetic acid, termed HIDA, are occasionally used to determine bile excretion into the gallbladder and common bile duct. Ultrasonography and CT, however, have largely replaced such studies.

LIVER INFECTIONS

Surgery of the liver may involve the management of pyogenic and amoebic abscesses. In the United States pyogenic abscesses are relatively rare, having an incidence at autopsy of only 0.3–1.5%. Now that appendicitis management has improved to the point where perforation and pelvic abscesses are becoming rare events, this cause of liver abscess has been replaced by biliary tract disease as the underlying cause for most infections. As a result, liver abscesses have become a disease of the elderly instead of the young, with biliary calculi or malignancy as the primary etiology. The infections are either multiple, diffuse, and microscopic, or large single abscesses confined to one lobe. They are commonly categorized as to their cause.

The mortality of liver infections has declined in recent years and is most often cited at approximately 10%. Obviously, such estimates depend heavily upon the underlying disease that led to the development of microabscess(es) or macroabscess(es). Undoubtedly, a major factor in improved survival is the ability to accurately image the process for purposes of diagnosis, treatment, and ongoing follow-up of treatment results. Ultrasonographic and CT imaging have led to percutaneous catheter drainage of macroabscesses and, in some cases, has eliminated the need for operative intervention. The management of such patients requires considerable experience and relies heavily on good surgical judgement. Initial broad-spectrum antibiotic coverage is imperative until cultures direct more specific therapy. Intra-abdominal pathology must be corrected surgically.

PORTAL VEIN PYELOPHLEBITIS

Diagnosis & Management

As noted, in the past, a perforated appendix and or a pelvic abscess were the most common causes of liver abscess. Any intra-abdominal disease process with the potential for generating a major inflammatory response may lead to suppurative thrombophlebitis of veins feeding the portal circulation. Although bacteria frequently obtain ac-

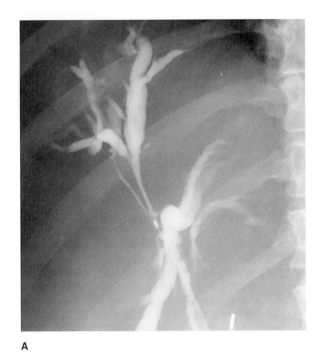

A

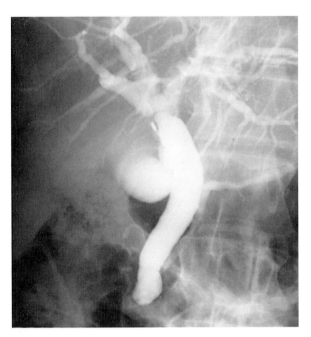

B

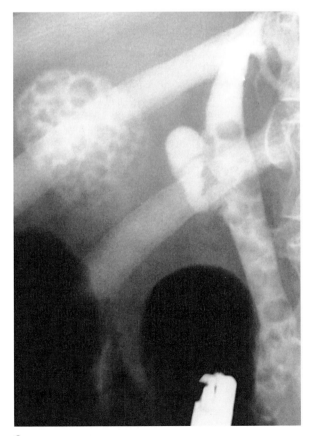

C

Figure 28–5. Endoscopic retrograde cholangiopancreatography demonstrating **(A)** cholangiocarcinoma; **(B)** ampullary stenosis; **(C)** common bile duct stones.

cess to the portal circulation, even in healthy individuals, the development of a hepatic abscess is virtually unheard of unless there exists a significant inflammatory process that causes thrombosis of veins and probably infected emboli to the liver. In severe cases, treatment consists of anticoagulation to decrease embolization, broad-spectrum antibiotics, and elimination of the intra-abdominal process.

INFECTIONS SECONDARY TO SYSTEMIC BACTEREMIA & HEPATIC ARTERIAL COMPROMISE

Diagnosis

The development of liver abscesses secondary to systemic bacteremia is generally seen in the setting of a compromised host. Patients that are immunocompromised because of an underlying disease or secondary to treatment of cancer are particularly at risk. Others with compromised granulocyte function are susceptible. Any condition that may result in hepatic artery thrombosis and areas of parenchymal infarct are at risk for secondary bacterial seeding and abscess formation. Patients with secondary malignant involvement of the liver may develop abscesses in areas of necrotic tumor. A history of recent liver trauma should also make one wary of the potential for liver abscesses in areas of necrotic or ischemic liver parenchyma. As might be expected, staphylococcus aureus and group A streptococci are cultured more often than are organisms common to the gastrointestinal tract.

Management

The management of these abscesses is similar to what has been described in previous sections and primarily centers on establishing adequate percutaneous drainage. Drainage can almost always be accomplished via an appropriate rigid percutaneous catheter placed by an interventional radiologist. Operative exploration and drainage are rarely required.

INFECTION BY DIRECT EXTENSION

Diagnosis & Management

Abscesses that develop in the subphrenic space and subhepatic spaces, including the gallbladder, may involve the liver parenchyma by direct extension. The resultant microabscesses are dealt with in conjunction with surgical management of the contiguous abscess. Occasionally, such processes may be the result of malignancy in the colon or stomach, resulting in malignant perforation. Such occurrences may require resecting liver parenchyma at the time the tumor is resected.

AMOEBIC LIVER ABSCESS

Diagnosis

While uncommon in the United States, where it is a disease of immigrants, travelers, and, occasionally, homosexuals, *Entamoeba histolytica* is estimated to infect 10% of the world's population. In Africa, India, Asia, and part of Central and South America an estimated 50% of the population is infected, with greater than 90% asymptomatic carriers. Only approximately 10% of infected individuals will develop liver abscess. The male-to-female ratio is often cited at 20:1. Immunocompromised individuals are more at risk, and often this is associated with malnutrition and other diseases.

Individuals become infected when ingesting cysts. In the small intestine, cysts release motile trophozoites that migrate to the colon. The cycle is perpetuated by the shedding of cysts in the stool. Amoebae in the colon may gain access to the veins through defects in the integrity of the colon. The amoebae pass via the inferior mesenteric vein to the portal venous circulation and the liver. The amoebae colonize in the liver, causing necrosis of surrounding hepatocytes. The abscess that forms is solitary in some 70%, and the indirect hemagglutination test is positive in 95%. Amoebic cysts may become secondarily infected with other bacteria.

Management

Initial treatment involves metronidazole 750 mg, three times per day for 10 days. Only a small percentage fail to respond, requiring therapy with emetine and chloroquine phosphate. The intestinal disease requires treatment with iodoquinol, diloxanide furoate, or paramomycin.

Drainage is reserved for very large abscesses with a risk of rupturing, those that involve other organs, and those that have failed to respond to metronidazole. The vast majority respond to medical therapy, and the risks of catheter drainage (secondary bacterial contamination) generally outweigh the potential benefits.

ECHINOCOCCUS GRANULOSUS & HYDATID CYSTS

Diagnosis

The *Echinococcus granulosus* and *Echinococcus multilocularis* tapeworms live in the intestine of carnivorous animals that serve as the definitive host. Humans are intermediate hosts, accidentally ingesting the excreted ova. The outer shell of the egg is digested in the duodenum and the embryo released; the embryo moves into the intestinal mucosa, enters small veins of the portal circulation, and is trapped in the liver. Embryos may also pass through the liver, reaching the lungs, spleen, and other organs. The embryos that survive in the liver develop over several days into the hydatid cysts.

The hydatid cyst has three layers: the germinal layer from which scolices (heads of parasites) develop, and two outer layers. Hydatid cysts tend to grow slowly at the rate of 1 cm per year, and cysts harbor thousands of scolices. The outer two layers of the cyst wall are absent in *E multilocularis*, allowing the scolices to develop in an uncontrolled manner, invading in a budding fashion into surrounding liver parenchyma, and forming a myriad of small cysts (Figure 28–6).

Hydatid cysts may cause biliary obstruction based on size and location. Cholangitis may be a secondary complication. Portal hypertension may develop if the disease is left untreated, and cysts may rupture. Free rupture into the peritoneal cavity can cause anaphylactic shock. Cysts are generally present for many years before causing symptoms or being diagnosed incidentally.

Management

Patients are treated with albendazole prior to intervention. This treatment is continued through surgery and for a period after surgery. When possible, if the cyst is not too large and is located appropriately, the involved liver is simply resected. When this is not possible, the cyst can be carefully enucleated. Every precaution is taken to avoid spilling any contents of the cyst.

OTHER HEPATIC INFECTIONS

There are a number of other causes of liver infection. In general, these organisms do not result in abscesses or other liver pathology requiring direct surgical intervention. Their importance to the surgeon comes from the common theme of such diseases, which is the secondary fibrosis and cirrhosis of the liver leading eventually to portal hypertension. Examples are hepatitis viruses, schistosomiasis, malaria, clonorchiasis and opisthorchiasis liver flukes, as well as other parasites.

PORTAL HYPERTENSION & CIRRHOSIS

Diagnosis

Portal hypertension occurs when there is obstruction to normal portal venous flow. The pressure in the portal vein is normally 5–10 mm Hg, slightly higher than systemic venous pressure. Portal hypertension is defined as a portal vein pressure that is elevated 5 mm Hg or more above the patient's systemic venous pressure. The oxygen content of the portal blood is also slightly higher when portal hypertension is present. The absence of valves in the portal vein means that portal vein pressure is more directly related to resistance of liver blood flow.

Eighty percent of all cases of portal hypertension are the result of intrahepatic obstruction to blood flow, and the cause is almost always cirrhosis. In this country, cirrhosis is most often secondary to viral hepatitis or alcohol abuse. However, worldwide, presinusoidal intrahepatic obstruction is the most common cause of cirrhosis and is the result of schistosomiasis infection.

The majority of other causes of portal hypertension (≈ 20%) are the result of prehepatic obstruction and presinusoidal obstruction. For example, portal vein thrombosis may be caused by malignancy, pancreatitis, and cirrhosis. Occasionally, thrombosis in the splenic vein may extend into the portal vein. In children, portal vein thrombosis may be the result of neonatal umbilical sepsis and umbilical vein catheterization. These children may present with cavernous transformation of the porta hepatis.

Posthepatic causes of portal hypertension are uncommon and are manifested by thrombosis of hepatic veins or the inferior vena cava (Budd-Chiari). Malignancy, myeloproliferative disease, constrictive pericarditis, and right heart failure have all been associated with posthepatic portal hypertension.

Obstruction to portal flow and the development of portal hypertension result in the opening of collateral communications between the portal and systemic venous circulations. The most common sites for the development of these engorged variceal communications are the plexus around the distal esophagus and upper stomach, and around the umbilicus (which may form what is known as a Caput Medusae on the anterior abdominal wall). Other sites include the plexuses around the distal rectum and anus, as well as communications from venous branches of the superior mesenteric vein and inferior mesenteric vein that communicate with veins of the systemic circulation around the surfaces of organs within the abdomen and retroperitoneum.

While bleeding of significance can occur from dilated veins around the anus, by far the only life-threatening hemorrhage occurs from erosion of esophageal varices, and

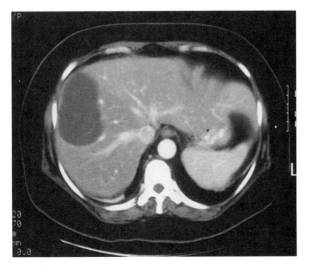

Figure 28–6. CT of *E multilocularis* cyst formation.

less commonly from associated gastric varices. These veins are exposed to the trauma of food passage and the erosive nature of acidic gastric secretions. It is estimated that only one third to one half of the patients who have portal hypertension and esophageal varices will bleed. The varices most likely to rupture are located at the esophagogastric junction and within a region extending an inch above and below. For significant bleeding, the portal circulation pressure must be increased by more than 12 mm Hg.

The diagnosis of bleeding esophageal varices is best made by upper endoscopy; 90% of bleeding is from the esophageal varices while 10% occurs on the stomach side of the esophagogastric junction. Even though the patient is known to have cirrhosis and portal hypertension, other causes of upper gastrointestinal bleeding can also be suspected in such patients. Approximately one third of the time, conditions such as peptic ulcers and portal hypertensive gastropathy are the cause. Obviously, the treatment of these would be different. Bleeding from esophageal varices is usually intermittent, and the diagnosis may be made on the basis of the bleeding history, the presence of varices, and the exclusion of other causes.

Management

It is important to have an understanding of the management of patients presenting with acute variceal hemorrhage. Of the patients who experience an acute bleed, it is estimated that about one third stop bleeding on their own prior to reaching the emergency department. Some arrive still bleeding, but slowly, and their condition is relatively easy to manage acutely. A significant number, however, arrive with a life-threatening massive hemorrhage.

For these patients, one must act quickly and effectively to initiate resuscitation. The first steps are control of the airway and rapid blood replacement. Airway management may require endotracheal intubation and appropriate sedation. Large-bore peripheral intravenous catheters are placed and usually a central venous line is helpful. For initial fluid resuscitation, normal saline solutions should be avoided in favor of Ringer's lactate. The goal is to eliminate sodium from the infusions as soon as the patient stabilizes.

Emergent laboratory studies are drawn at the time of line placement and include complete blood count (CBC), platelet count, prothrombin time (PT), partial thromboplastin time (PTT), electrolytes, blood urea nitrition (BUN), creatinine, and liver profile. A type and crossmatch for 6 units of packed cells should be requested, and the blood bank should have 6 units in reserve until the patient's condition is stabilized.

At this point, a decision on further management must be developed largely based on volume of ongoing blood loss and response to resuscitation. The decision is best made by physicians experienced in managing such patients. Ongoing massive blood loss and difficulty maintaining a hemodynamically stable patient requires the physician team to consider placement of a Sengstaken tube in an effort to tamponade the bleeding. In my experience, patients requiring this should be intubated to control their airway. Balloon tamponade is not required very often, but it may be lifesaving in an acute, uncontrolled hemorrhage from esophageal varices.

In patients responding to resuscitation and without evidence of ongoing massive bleeding, a nasogastric tube is placed and the stomach lavaged with saline. Packed red cells are administered when available and fresh frozen plasma as well as platelets are infused as indicated. Magnesium citrate, cathartics, and lactulose are given via the nasogastric tube in an effort to minimize the effect of blood in the gastrointestinal tract on liver function and the development of encephalopathy. Hypokalemic alkalosis must be treated expectantly with appropriate amounts of intravenous potassium chloride. Alkalosis will contribute to the development of encephalopathy and cause a shift in the oxyhemoglobin dissociation curve, impairing oxygen delivery to the critical organs of the body.

Vasopressin (20 U/200 mL) may be infused over 20 minutes, followed by a continuous infusion of 0.4 U/min to lower portal venous pressure. While vasopressin is estimated to stop bleeding in about half the patients, the patient must be monitored carefully and is usually given vasopressin in combination with nitroglycerin to avoid risks of coronary artery constriction.

Once the patient has been stabilized, the esophagus and stomach are evaluated endoscopically. In over 90% of patients, the bleeding can be quickly and safely controlled by sclerotherapy using sodium morrhuate and sodium tetradecyl sulfate. Generally, both intravariceal and paravariceal injections of the sclerosing agents are carried out, starting with the bleeding varix and including all varices from the esophageal gastric junction to approximately 5 cm proximal. Endoscopic ligation or banding of esophageal varices is another technique that has been effective.

In general, these direct approaches are only effective in the distal esophagus and are not helpful in treating bleeding from gastric varices and portal hypertensive gastropathy. Complications include re-bleeding, esophageal ulceration, perforation, stricture formation, and aspiration. Fifty percent of endoscopically treated patients experience significant re-bleeding.

In recent years, a new approach has been developed to non-operatively decompress the portal systemic varices termed percutaneous **transjugular intrahepatic portosystemic shunts (TIPS)**. This technique, developed by interventional radiologists, can be performed without anesthesia. Under fluoroscopy, the radiologist creates a tract, using a stiff guide-wire and catheter, between the right hepatic vein and right main portal vein within the liver parenchyma. A 10-mm expandable stent is fashioned to the appropriate length and passed through the tract. The stent is expanded and pressures measured to determine gradient and decompression (Figure 28–7). The procedure has a high rate of success in controlling bleeding. It is especially useful for patients with end-stage liver disease

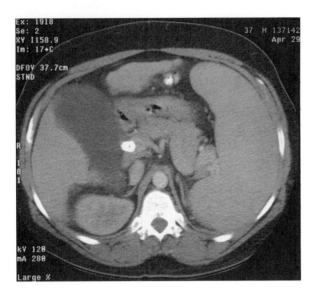

Figure 28–7. Transjugular intrahepatic portosystemic shunt (TIPS) stent in place.

who are candidates for liver transplantation and for high-risk Child-Pugh class C patients who would not be good operative risks (Table 28–3).

Nonoperative methods for controlling bleeding secondary to portal hypertension are preferred, but when these fail it is imperative that a decision for operative intervention not be delayed. While several emergency operations have been proposed, including those that involve devascularization of the esophagogastric junction (including transection and reconstruction with an end-to-end stapler), the preferred approach by experienced hepatic surgeons is the construction of a portasystemic shunt. In a truly emergent situation, an end-to-side or side-to-side portacaval shunt (or an interposition mesocaval shunt) can be rapidly established.

In elective situations, the most frequently used method

Table 28–3. Child-Pugh classification.

	No. of Points		
	1	2	3
Bilirubin (mg/dL)	< 2	2–3	> 3
Albumin (g/dL)	> 3.5	2.8–3.5	< 2.8
Protime (increased seconds)	1–3	4–6	> 6
Ascites	None	Slight	Moderate
Encephalopathy	None	1–2	3–4

Grade A	5–6	points
Grade B	7–9	points
Grade C	10–15	points

Reprinted, with permission, from Zimmerman H, Reichen J: Assessment of liver function in the surgical patient. In: Blumgart LH (editor): *Surgery of the Liver and Biliary Tract*, 2nd ed. Churchill Livingstone, 1994, p. 1718.

of decompressing the varices is the distal splenorenal shunt. The splenic vein is divided at the portal vein and anastomosed end-to-side to the left renal vein. An important feature of this operation is the direct interruption of all collateral veins that connect the superior mesenteric/portal circulation with gastrosplenic venous circulation. The distal splenorenal shunt gained popularity based on its lower risk (10–20%) of postshunt encephalopathy. A contraindication, however, is preexisting ascites, which is not managed well by the splenorenal shunt. Examples of various operative shunts are depicted in Figure 28–8.

The other complications of portal hypertension are the consequences of decreased blood flow to the liver, resulting in an impaired clearance of toxins, impaired liver synthetic functions (decreasing PT, PTT), splenic congestion with hypersplenism, and ascites. Hypersplenism causes thrombocytopenia, leukopenia, and anemia. This coupled with impaired synthetic functions may lead to severe coagulopathy.

Ascites can develop in patients with cirrhosis and elevated portal venous pressure. It results from a combination of factors that cause fluid to leak from the splanchnic bed, including a decrease in serum colloid osmotic pressure secondary to a drop in serum albumin, the retention of salt and, therefore, water by the kidneys, and obstruction of blood flow through the liver. Treatment involves countering the renal retention of sodium by restricting the intake of sodium and administration of diuretics. Diuresis of 0.5–1.5 lb/d (0.22–0.67 kg/d) is desired. Patients with normal renal function can be given aldactone (aldosterone antagonist), initially at 75–150 mg/d. It is usually necessary to add Lasix at 20–40 mg/d in order to decrease sodium reabsorption at the more proximal renal tubules. It may be necessary to also add hydrochlorothiazide at 25 mg/d.

Hepatic encephalopathy is another complication of cirrhosis and portal hypertension. While the exact cause of encephalopathy is unclear, the buildup of several substances in the circulation has been implicated, including ammonia, aminobutyric acid (GABA), and endogenous benzodiazepine receptor ligands. This complication, fortunately, remains subclinical in 50–80% of cirrhotics. Others have recurrent episodes of encephalopathy and a few develop chronic dysfunction. Treatment consists of dietary restrictions of protein to approximately 70 g/d and the oral use of lactulose (30–120 mL/d) to decrease ammoniagenesis by bacterial flora of the gastrointestinal tract. Occasionally, especially with acute hemorrhage, it may be helpful to administer neomycin (1–2 g) orally four times per day and metronidazole 250 mg orally three times per day to decrease bacterial flora in the gastrointestinal tract and, therefore, lower the bacterial breakdown of blood as it passes through. The drug flumazenil is a benzodiazepine receptor antagonist and is now being tested for its efficacy in treating hepatic encephalopathy.

Complications such as cirrhosis and portal hypertension remain extremely difficult to manage; a poor outcome is

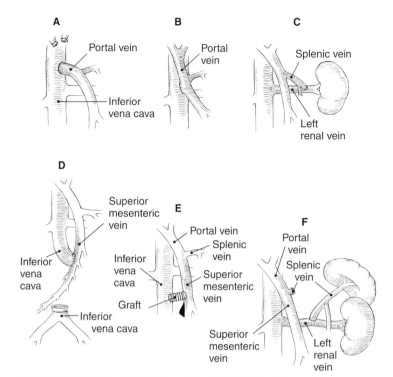

Figure 28–8. Examples of portosystemic shunts. **A:** Portacaval end-to-side; **B:** portacaval side-to-side; **C:** splenorenal; **D:** mesocaval; **E:** mesocaval h-graft; **F:** distal splenorenal.

usually predicted unless the liver can be replaced via orthotopic transplantation.

TRAUMA

The improvements in the resuscitation, and intraoperative and postoperative management, of patients admitted with liver trauma continues to reduce the mortality associated with these injuries. Today, it is anticipated that in-hospital mortality should be no more than 10%. Many factors have contributed to this improvement. Certainly, the experience gained in liver transplantation and in resectional therapy have been a significant factor. As a result of these surgeries, a new subspecialty of anesthesiologists has emerged with extensive expertise in managing the anhepatic patient.

Trauma to the liver comes in two forms: penetrating and blunt. A higher mortality rate is associated with blunt trauma ($\approx 25\%$), undoubtedly because there is a greater risk for potentially fatal injuries to associated organs, such as the brain, lungs, and skeleton (pelvis).

The rapid transfer from the field to a major trauma facility and the initiation of resuscitation while in the field is extremely important. The early use of blood transfusion in the unstable patient and the rapid transfer to the operating room for exploration have been responsible for saving many lives.

Diagnosis

CT imaging is reserved for selected patients who are suspected of having liver injury but are hemodynamically stable. Imaging enables the surgeon to select patients with relatively minor injuries (< 500 mL blood loss) for careful observation. The CT must confirm that no other injuries to the stomach, duodenum, pancreas, colon, kidney, and spleen exist and that no immediate surgical intervention is required. Interventional radiology has added immeasurably to the conservative management of liver trauma by coil embolization of bleeding arteries and the subsequent embolization of the vascular sequelae of trauma, such as intrahepatic aneurysms and arteriovenous fistula. It has also been effective in the percutaneous drainage of secondary abscesses and for control of bile leaks. There must always be a low threshold for moving quickly to the operating room if the patient's condition becomes unstable.

Management

For those patients who present with an unstable condition, rapid exploration is imperative. There is not time to obtain CT images. Bleeding can be massive in these cases and anesthesiologists familiar with both trauma and liver surgery, especially those experienced in liver transplantation, are a critical part of a team approach. Cell-savers and rapid infusers are essential equipment.

In the past few years there has been a renewed interest in packing for control of diffuse bleeding from liver parenchyma (assuming the absence of a major vascular injury). Debridement of devitalized tissue continues to be given a priority, but most trauma and liver surgeons have determined that anatomic resections neither improve survival nor decrease morbidity. Table 28–4 provides a useful liver injury scale.

Managing trauma to the liver can be one of the most challenging surgical exercises. A major premise of every operation is to proceed in a controlled manner with a carefully prepared plan. In the emergent setting of liver injury, this is generally not possible. A midline incision is helpful, as it can be extended to the chest. The patient should be placed in the Trendelenburg position to avoid an air embolism. As noted, operating on patients with major liver trauma, unfortunately, begins in a setting where the first challenge for the surgeon is to regain control and in so doing to assess the extent of injury in order to formulate a rational plan. It must be remembered that evulsive tears of the major hepatic veins and major tears of the intrahepatic vena cava are hard to control and generally fatal. Nevertheless, initial compression of the liver against the diaphragm, packing bleeding liver surfaces, and the occlusion of arterial and portal inflow (Pringle maneuver), may provide the surgeon with an opportunity to deal with such injuries.

Obtaining control of the caval above and below the liver requires time and dissection. Generally, total occlusion of the cava is not tolerated by the patient, since too much blood return to the heart is blocked in an already unstable patient. The exact length of time one can occlude the arterial and portal inflow is not known; clearly, it is not as long in the trauma setting as it is in controlled resections and transplantation, probably, about 20 minutes.

Table 28–4. Liver injury scale.

Grade		Injury Description
I.	Hematoma	Subcapsular, nonexpanding, < 10% surface area
	Laceration	Capsular tear, nonbleeding, < 1 cm parenchymal depth
II.	Hematoma	Subcapsular, nonexpanding, 10–50% surface area
	Laceration	Capsular tear, active bleeding; 1–3 cm parenchymal depth, < 10 cm in length
III.	Hematoma	Subcapsular, > 50% surface area or expanding; ruptured subcapsular hematoma with active bleeding; intraparenchymal hematoma > 2 cm or expanding
	Laceration	> 3 cm parenchymal depth
IV.	Hematoma	Ruptured intraparenchymal hematoma with active bleeding
	Laceration	Parenchymal disruption involving 25–50% of hepatic lobe
V.	Laceration	Parenchymal disruption involving > 50% of hepatic lobe
	Vascular	Juxtahepatic venous injuries; ie, retrohepatic vena cava/major hepatic veins
VI.	Vascular	Hepatic avulsion

Reprinted, with permission, from Moore EE et al: Organ injury scaling: Spleen, liver, and kidney. J Trauma 1989;29:1664.

Atriocaval shunts to assist in control of injuries involving the intrahepatic cava are frequently talked about and, as devised, would appear to be potentially a major help. However, in reality, atriocaval shunts are rarely used, even at major trauma hospitals. Veno-venobypass, which is used in liver transplantation, may prove lifesaving in major vessel injuries.

Once a degree of control has been obtained so that the parenchymal injuries can be viewed, resist the temptation to move or disrupt areas that seem relatively stable. Gently debride areas that have been clearly devitalized and do not attempt to re-approximate tears or crevices that have been generated by the trauma.

The argon beam electrocoagulator is useful in coagulating exposed parenchymal surfaces. Use of products that assist clotting are helpful, such as thrombin solution and Avitene. It is often helpful to compress areas of liver by placing Teflon felt strips 2.0 cm wide across the anterior and posterior surface of the liver. The felt strips are compressed together using mattress sutures of 0-chromic. This suture as well as other absorbable sutures come in a large, blunt-tipped liver needle. It is helpful to straighten the curved needle and to sew by hand. Hand-sewing gives one a better sense of direction and of structures within the parenchyma encountered as the needle is passed. The surgeon will avoid doing this too close to the portal triad for fear of compromising critical portal venous, arterial, or ductal structures. The Teflon strips help to distribute pressure and increase the amount of pressure that can be applied by the sutures without creating further tears in the liver. With any major liver injury, the surgeon must be aware of occult disruptions to the intrahepatic cava. This is especially true of penetrating injuries that appear to track in this direction. It may, therefore, prove necessary to completely mobilize the right lobe of the liver in order to completely assess the intrahepatic cava.

Finally, do not hesitate to firmly pack the liver and plan a return in 24–48 hours or a transfer of a stabilized patient to a major center. If packing is undertaken, the surgeon must be confident that in doing so the bleeding has been controlled. This approach often avoids the complications of hemodilution and hypothermia and provides an opportunity for continuing resuscitation and maintaining normal coagulation status. There is no substitute for experience and the judgement that accompanies it.

TUMORS OF THE LIVER

While primary liver tumors are relatively uncommon in the United States, on a worldwide basis they pose a serious health problem. For example, the incidence in areas such as Africa and Asia varies from 30 per 100,000 to more than 100 per 100,000 of the population. In the United States, primary liver tumors are estimated at a rate of 3 per 100,000 of the population. Tumors of the liver may be benign or malignant. Those that are malignant carry a grave prognosis. The most significant advances in the management of primary liver cancers relate to improvements in imaging technology that permit more accurate definition of the extent of tumor and the potential for resection. Advances in liver transplantation, anesthesia, and surgical critical care have lowered mortality rates for major hepatic resections. These advances have resulted in a more aggressive multidisciplinary approach to the management of these tumors.

BENIGN LIVER TUMORS

Diagnosis

Benign lesions of the liver are an important factor in the differential diagnosis of any mass lesion discovered while imaging the liver using ultrasonography or CT. Autopsy reports in this country indicate that 1–7% of adults have some type of benign liver tumor. **Hemangiomas** are the most common benign tumor and are classified as hemangioendotheliomas, capillary hemangiomas, and cavernous hemangiomas. Hemangioendotheliomas are almost always found in infants and young children. When these lesions are discovered within the first 6 months of life, they are associated in 50% of cases with a cutaneous vascular lesion. The presence of an infantile hepatic hemangioendothelioma should be looked for whenever there is a significant cutaneous hemangioma in a newborn. This is especially true if the cutaneous lesion rapidly increases in size or if there are signs of congestive heart failure, rapid heart rate, enlarged heart, systolic murmur, jaundice, or an enlarged liver. The presence of such lesions is confirmed by CT or magnetic resonance imaging (MRI) and, of course, these lesions should never be biopsied. The presence of high-output cardiac failure heralds a poor prognosis, and mortality rates as high as 70% have been reported in such infants. Thus, initial treatment is directed toward supporting cardiac function with digitalis and diuretics. The use of steroids (prednisolone 2–5 mg/kg/d) has been reported to reduce the size of cutaneous hemangiomas and to be helpful in treating hepatic lesions. Operative approaches to these lesions result in an unacceptably high mortality rate. In recent years, this has led to interventional radiologic approaches focused on embolization of selected feeding arteries. Hepatic transplantation may prove necessary and be the only hope for patient salvage. Histologically, these tumors must be differentiated from angiosarcomas and cholangiocarcinomas.

Capillary hemangiomas can be found in any age group and almost never are large enough to produce symptoms. A major difficulty is in differentiating such lesions when they are discovered by CT or MRI from primary or metastatic malignant lesions of the liver.

Cavernous hemangiomas are the most common benign hepatic tumor, with a quoted incidence of about 3–7%. These hemangiomas are primarily found in the adult population, with a mean age of 50 years. They are uncommonly symptomatic and infrequently multiple. The diagnosis of cavernous hemangiomas is usually made by contrast-enhanced dynamic CT or gadolinium-enhanced MRI. Since fewer than 15% of these tumors are large enough to produce symptoms, the treatment of choice is simply observation (usually by scanning at appropriate intervals). There is no tendency for adult cavernous hemangiomas to become malignant. Only approximately 1% of observed cavernous hemangiomas go on to become symptomatic.

Management

Resection is undertaken for the large, symptomatic lesions. Symptoms include pain, right upper quadrant fullness, jaundice, Kasabach-Merritt syndrome (hemangioma-thrombocytopenia syndrome), uncontrolled congestive heart failure, and, rarely, rupture with hemorrhage.

Embolization of feeding arteries may be helpful in situations of emergent hemorrhage, but it is otherwise not a useful therapy since there is rapid collateralization around occluded vessels. In recent years, a small number of patients have been treated, with excellent results by conformal radiation directed at the lesion.

In addition to hemangiomas, hepatic adenomas are a common benign tumor found in the liver. Their incidence is felt to be increased following the introduction of oral contraceptives. Hepatic adenomas are generally associated with patients who have a history of oral contraceptive use or chronic use of steroids. They are also associated with patients who have diabetes mellitus, glycogen storage disease, or other gastrointestinal adenomas. They are more commonly found in the right lobe of the liver and the average diameter is 8–10 cm at the time of diagnosis. Patients who harbor more than ten adenomas in their liver are diagnosed as having hepatic adenomatosis. The treatment for patients with solitary adenomas is liver resection. Surgery is recommended in order to eliminate the estimated 50% risk of rupture and hemorrhage.

In 1958, Edmondson described a rare benign liver lesion, which he termed "focal nodular hyperplasia." The lesions are composed of hepatocytes and Kupffer's cells. Such lesions more often occur at multiple sites within the liver and are often associated with hemangiomas. Focal nodular hyperplasia is most often diagnosed in women during their reproductive years. It is important to establish this diagnosis, especially to differentiate it from adenomas by biopsy. Whereas adenomas need to be resected because of the high risk of hemorrhage, there is no indication that focal nodular hyperplasia is associated with an increased risk of rupture and life-threatening hemorrhage. Thus, these lesions tend to be simply observed.

MALIGNANT LIVER TUMORS

Hepatocellular carcinoma is the most common primary malignant liver tumor. Hepatocellular cancer accounts for 75% of all primary malignant liver tumors. Tumors arising from the bile duct epithelium, cholangiocarcinomas, account for the remaining incidence of primary lesions. Of course, rare tumors, such as angiosarcoma and mixed cholangiohepatocellular tumors, are also seen.

1. HEPATOCELLULAR CANCER

Diagnosis

As noted previously, in some areas of the world hepatocellular tumors account for over half of the tumors seen in the population. There is a male predominance for hepatocellular cancer, with some areas of Asia reporting a ratio of four to seven males to every one female. In the United States, the ratio is 2:1, male to female. Hepatocellular cancers tend to occur in the fifth and sixth decades of life, and there is a common theme that associates the presence of cirrhosis with a high risk for development of hepatocellular cancers. The association between hepatitis B and the risk for developing hepatocellular cancer is especially strong. For patients who have cirrhosis secondary to hepatitis B infection, the risk of developing hepatocellular carcinoma is increased to greater than 20%. In areas of the world where hepatitis B is endemic, more than 70% of the patients developing hepatocellular cancer are found to be seropositive for hepatitis B.

Although, worldwide, hepatitis B has a stronger association with hepatocellular cancer, hepatitis C is also of major importance. This is particularly true in areas such as Japan, where the incidence of hepatocellular cancer is high, while rates of hepatitis B are only moderate. Hepatitis C is an RNA virus that is responsible for most cases of non-A and non-B hepatitis related to transfusion and other blood products. The development of symptoms and subsequent hepatocellular carcinoma is prolonged in patients with hepatitis C, usually taking approximately 30 years. The course of the disease usually runs as follows: (1) during the first 10 years, the patient develops chronic active hepatitis; (2) cirrhosis develops after 2 decades; and (3) the disease culminates in the development of hepatocellular carcinoma.

Alcohol-induced cirrhosis, aflatoxin-contaminated foods, and certain drugs, such as anabolic steroids, thorotrast, and immunosuppressive agents, are also known to cause cirrhosis. Certain chemicals, such as pesticides, chlorinated hydrocarbons, aromatic amines, and chorophinyls, can also induce liver injury and cirrhosis and, therefore, hepatocellular cancer. For example, the risk of developing hepatocellular cancer in the presence of hemochromatosis of the liver is approximately 13%. All of the cases are in cirrhotic livers. The risk is 40% in patients who have alpha-1 antitrypsin deficiency. The most significant risk, however, is the development of hepatitis B infection. In fact, prospective studies have shown a relative risk of 250:1 for development of hepatoma in patients that are asymptomatic hepatitis B antigen carriers, as compared to noninfected controls.

The most common presentation is one of vague abdominal discomfort or right upper quadrant pain. Patients also commonly complain of fatigue, general malaise, anorexia, and weight loss. Jaundice is occasionally a presenting symptom. Patients generally have had symptoms for several months prior to their presentation for evaluation.

The initial evaluation of these patients should include abdominal ultrasonography. This is relatively inexpensive, noninvasive, and highly accurate in screening the liver for hepatic masses. Alpha-fetoprotein is an excellent marker for the presence of hepatocellular cancer, being positive in more than 85% of patients with this tumor. False-positive alpha-fetoprotein results are rare but may be secondary to germ cell tumors or pregnancy. Patients with an elevated alpha-fetoprotein and a mass by ultrasonography can be considered as having hepatocellular cancer and do not require biopsy.

The initial evaluation should include a screen for the presence of hepatitis B and C and an evaluation of synthetic and excretory liver functions. A dynamic contrast CT provides valuable information regarding the presence or absence of metastatic tumor and the resectability of the tumor based on its relationship to the central hepatic veins and central portal circulation. Table 28–5 reviews the TNM staging of liver tumors. It should be noted that patients who are hepatitis B antigen positive, and, therefore, at high risk for developing cirrhosis and hepatocellular cancer, should be screened every 4 months with alpha-fetoprotein determinations and an ultrasonographic evaluation.

Hepatocellular cancer of the liver can present as a single mass or as diffuse, multiple, encapsulated tumors throughout the liver. The nodular presentation usually has multiple tumor lesions in both lobes of the liver. The majority of cases are of the diffuse or massive type and present as a single, large mass. Hepatocellular tumors and other malignant tumors of the liver are summarized in Table 28–6. Histologically, the tumor cells appear as normal liver cells except for the large, round, hyperchromatic nuclei and prominent nucleoli. The cytoplasm has abundant granular eosinophilic characteristics. Usually the cells are lined up as liver cords of two to eight cells surrounded by a basement membrane and endothelial cells. More poorly differentiated tumors tend to lose this organized pattern and show evidence of spindle cells and giant cells.

Management

Surgical Management. Resection of these tumors offers the only chance for cure. Unfortunately, these tumors tend to present when they are quite large and when it is difficult to obtain adequate surgical margins. They are also almost always associated with cirrhosis, and cirrhosis is most often the limiting factor regarding surgical resection. The cirrhotic liver has impaired function, does not tolerate the trauma of surgery or blood loss, and lacks the capacity to regenerate. A low white blood cell count and low platelet count may be early indications for the presence of cirrhosis and portal hypertension. In the presence of cirrhosis, operative mortality is still 3–15% and significant morbidity usually accompanies surgery on cirrhotic livers. Patient selection becomes extremely important in

Table 28–5. TNM staging.

Primary Tumor (T)

TX Primary tumor cannot be assessed
T0 No evidence of primary tumor
T1 Solitary tumor ≤ 2 cm in greatest dimension without vascular invasion
T2 Solitary tumor ≤ 2 cm in greatest dimension with vascular invasion; or multiple tumors limited to one lobe, none > 2 cm in greatest dimension without vascular invasion; or a solitary tumor > 2 cm in greatest dimension without vascular invasion
T3 Solitary tumor > 2 cm in greatest dimension with vascular invasion; or multiple tumors limited to one lobe, none > 2 cm in greatest dimension, with vascular invasion; or multiple tumors limited to one lobe, any > 2 cm in greatest dimension, with or without vascular invasion
T4 Multiple tumors in more than one lobe, or tumor(s) involving major branches of the portal or hepatic vein(s)

Regional Lymph Nodes (N)

NX Regional lymph nodes cannot be assessed
N0 No regional lymph node metastasis
N1 Regional lymph node metastasis

Distant Metastasis (M)

MX Presence of distant metastasis cannot be assessed
M0 No distant metastasis
M1 Distant metastasis

Stage Grouping

Stage I	T1	N0	M0
Stage II	T2	N0	M0
Stage III	T1	N1	M0
	T2	N1	M0
	T3	N0	M0
	T3	N1	M0
Stage IVA	T4	Any N	M0
Stage IVB	Any T	Any N	M1

Reprinted, with permission, from Beahrs OH et al: *Handbook for Staging of Cancer,* 4th ed. Lippincott, 1993, p. 108.

the management of hepatocellular tumors. The patients who are Child-Pugh class B or C are generally not candidates for major resection. In recent years, transplantation has become an option for patients with hepatocellular carcinoma. Survival is comparable to that of resection in good-risk patients. When patients have cirrhosis, transplantation has proved to be a safer option, especially for stage II and III tumors.

While surgery is the only treatment that offers the potential for cure, most series report that only 5–30% of incident cases are candidates for resection. Only stage I and II hepatocellular tumors (T1 or T2, N0) should be considered for surgery, and these patients must be carefully evaluated for hepatic reserve.

As mentioned above, cirrhosis is the major deterrent to surgical resection for stage I and stage II hepatocellular tumors. Thus, patients with cirrhosis and tumors less than 5 cm may be candidates for liver transplantation. Studies have reported a 5-year survival rate of 36% for patients treated with transplantation for their hepatocellular tumors. This figure is similar to the 33% 5-year survival rate reported for patients having curative resection. In addition, tumor recurrence is lower for stages II and III hepatocellular cancers after transplantation than after resection.

Radiation Therapy. The liver has a low threshold for external-beam radiation, tolerating only 2000–3000 cGy. With new technologies that permit direct targeting of the radiation to the mass, higher doses are possible, but it is not reasonable to expect to reach 4500–6000 cGy. As a result, radiation is generally used to palliate the pain of large masses and occasionally to treat diffuse liver involvement. Experimental protocols have tested external beam radiation combined with systemic chemotherapy and hepatic artery infusion therapy without benefit and with treatment toxicity that significantly limits the therapeutic efficacy.

Chemotherapy. The drugs most commonly used are 5-fluorouracil (5-FU), doxorubicin, and recombinant interferon-alfa. There are an extensive number of reports evaluating both single-agent and polychemotherapy. As expected, the number of patients studied in each report is usually small. Response rates rarely reach 20%, are of

Table 28–6. Malignant liver tumors.

Type	Affected Population	Distinguishing Characteristics	Therapeutic Options
Hepatocellular single mass, diffuse, multiple encapsulated	Adult	Most often associated with cirrhosis	Resection, transplantation, chemotherapy
Fibrolamellar histology		Not associated with cirrhosis	Transplantation
Cholangiocarcinoma	Adult	Frequently CEA-producing, indolent, and diffuse	Chemotherapy, ? transplantation
Cystadenoma	Rare in adults, more common in females	Nodular cyst wall	Resection
Epithelioid hemangioendothelioma	Adult	Multifocal in both lobes	Transplantation

Reprinted, with permission, from Niederhuber JE: Tumors of the liver. In: Murphy GP, Lawrence W, Lenhard RE (editors): *American Cancer Society Textbook of Clinical Oncology.* American Cancer Society, 1995, p. 274.

short duration, and do not significantly prolong survival. Cisplatin, etoposide, and mitoxantrone, as well as tamoxifen and megestrol acetate, are other agents that appear to have little benefit. Perhaps the most important fact to remember when considering multidrug chemotherapy is the observation that poor performance status has consistently proven to predict a lack of response to chemotherapy.

Percutaneous Intratumoral Ablation. Tumors less than approximately 5 cm that are not candidates for resection are more and more frequently being considered candidates for an attempt at ablation. The current methods include direct tumor injections of 95% ethanol using ultrasonographic or CT guidance and cryosurgery. The latter ablative method, at this writing, still requires open laparotomy to place the freezing probe within the tumor. Usually, three freeze-thaw cycles are used, monitoring the subzero zone of freezing by intraoperative ultrasonography. In one study, a 5-year survival rate of 37.5% for tumors 5 cm or less was reported.

Arterial Approaches. Hepatocellular tumors derive nearly their entire blood supply from the hepatic arterial circulation. This observation has fostered attempts at arterial embolization, especially for large bulky tumors, in an effort to palliate symptoms and to downstage the tumor. Two thirds of embolized tumors will demonstrate some degree of necrosis and shrinkage.

Chemoembolization involves embolizing the tumor's arterial blood supply with pellets of gelatinous sponge permeated with mitomycin C or doxorubicin. Survival rates of 44% at 1 year and 29% at 2 years have been reported. Fatty acid esters, such as Lipiodol and Ethiodol, have been shown to localize and be retained for 1–2 months in hepatocellular tumors. Studies have been developed to test the benefit of injecting doxorubicin-Lipiodol and I^{136} Lipiodol via the hepatic artery.

Hepatic Artery Chemotherapy. When hepatocellular cancer is unresectable but otherwise confined to the liver, hepatic arterial infusion (HAI) chemotherapy is an option. Response rates of 40% lasting a median 14.5 months have been reported with 5-fluorouracil deoxyribonucleoside (FUDR) and mitomycin C in combination. Patients with cirrhosis are more susceptible to drug-induced toxicity and must be monitored closely. In general, they do not respond as well and have shorter survival. Many clinical studies of HAI are done in combination with other therapies, such as embolization, making it difficult to accurately assess the contribution of HAI.

2. CHOLANGIOCARCINOMA

Diagnosis

The other major primary tumor of the liver is cholangiocarcinoma. These tumors arise from the lining cells of the bile ducts and ductules. They tend to be peripheral and multifocal or more central and solitary. The latter, often termed **Klatskin tumors**, are located at the bifurcation of the right and left bile ducts and usually present with jaundice. These are rare tumors, occurring with an incidence of 2.0–2.8 per 100,000 per United States population each year. The incidence is higher in Asia and in countries where biliary parasites are prevalent. There is a 3:1 male-to-female predominance, and most occur in the sixth and seventh decade.

A number of chronic diseases are associated with an increased risk of cholangiocarcinoma. These include: inflammatory bowel disease (even in the absence of sclerosing cholangitis); congenital biliary duct anomalies, including choledochal cysts, Caroli's disease, and polycystic liver disease; Oriental cholangiohepatitis (clonorchiasis sinensis); and chemical exposure, such as thorotrast, benzidine, 3,3 dichlorobenzidine, and m-tolunediamide. Primary sclerosing cholangitis has the strongest association.

Most of the tumors are adenocarcinoma and cause considerable fibrotic response. Anorexia, weight loss, epigastric distress, and diarrhea are common symptoms. Bacterial cholangitis as a presenting symptom is uncommon. Bilirubin may or may not be elevated, depending on tumor location and whether significant ductal obstruction is present. CA 19-9 and CEA are often elevated and serve as tumor markers. Dynamic contrast-enhanced CT will demonstrate dilated ducts, but it may not be helpful in demonstrating a specific mass unless the tumor is advanced. Since vascular invasion is a contraindication to resection of more central tumors, arterial and venous phases of the dynamic CT are meticulously studied, usually with magnification of critical areas. ERCP and percutaneous transhepatic cholangiography (PTC) are generally part of the evaluation in an attempt to demonstrate the site of the tumor. Brushings may provide cells for cytologic examination and will be positive in 60–70% of cases.

Management

Intrahepatic cholangiocarcinomas have a tendency to be slow growing and rarely present when resection is possible. In general, while aggressive resections are frequently attempted, cures and long-term benefit are uncommon. Similarly, transplantation has been disappointing, with 100% of patients developing recurrent disease after transplantation.

Systemic chemotherapy is uniformly ineffective, and the majority of effort is focused on palliation to maintain biliary enteric continuity or external drainage of bile to delay liver failure and septic complications. The 5-year survival rate is 4–10%.

METASTATIC LIVER TUMORS

The most common mass lesion in the liver is a metastasis of tumor from another primary site in the body. Almost every solid tumor will, at some time in its course, involve the liver. However, some tumors develop relatively isolated liver metastases as a first site of recurrent tumor, without evidence of dissemination to other sites in the body. The most common example of this is the spread of cancers from the colon and rectum. It is estimated that 80% of patients with metastases from colorectal cancer have only liver involvement at the time of initial recurrence. As a result, they form a special group.

Other tumors, such as ocular melanomas, have the liver as the sole site of initial failure. Neuroendocrine tumors of the gastrointestinal tract and pancreas are also known to involve the liver without evidence of other tumor spread and are usually slow growing. Metastases from other gastrointestinal tumors often appear first in the liver, perhaps because of the portal circulation, but have a more rapid progression than metastases from colorectal cancer. Other tumors, such as those originating in the breast or lung, may also appear first in the liver but are really indicators of more widespread disease.

Diagnosis

In most instances, the origin of metastatic liver lesions will be evident, but when this is not the case or a degree of uncertainty exists, the initial procedure is a CT-guided fine needle aspiration biopsy. Core needle biopsies are selectively employed when more tissue is required to make an accurate diagnosis, such as in cases when the primary tumor is unknown. CT imaging establishes the extent of disease and, when resection is indicated, is extremely important in planning the resection and determining the adequacy of planned margins. When the CT demonstrates 75% involvement of liver parenchyma, the mean survival is 3.4 months; when less than 25% involvement is present, the mean survival is 6.2 months. Liver function is assayed and tumor markers obtained. These are important in following therapy.

Management

Surgical Resection. Resection is reserved primarily for a special group of metastatic tumors, the major group being that of colorectal metastases. It has been estimated that only about 10% of patients with colorectal metastases to the liver are candidates for resection. The biology of colorectal cancer sets this tumor apart from others in that a great number of patients present with isolated recurrences that are amenable to resection. Their presence does not indicate an immediate threat of widespread tumor and, as a result, resection in many instances provides a significant prolongation of life.

The indications for liver resection have been well determined by many retrospective analyses and by a prospective evaluation by the Gastrointestinal Interinstitutional Tumor Study Group (GITSG). These indications are tumor resection margins no less than 1 cm and four or fewer lesions to be resected. Duke's B tumors appear to have a better prognosis than Duke's C. Tumors may be resected by a nonanatomic wedge approach or by a more formal lobectomy or segmental resection. Operative mortality of 1–2% has been reported in recent years, and 30–35% of patients can be expected to be alive at 5 years. This ability to provide long-term survival and even cure

despite metastasis to the liver clearly sets this type of tumor apart (Figure 28–9).

Other so-called special tumors where resection of liver metastases is indicated include ocular melanoma, Wilm's tumor in children, and metastases from carcinoid or neuroendocrine tumors of the gastrointestinal tract and pancreas. The latter group may have considerable morbidity from the secretion of biologically active peptides produced by the metastases and, therefore, benefit considerably from their removal. These tumors, similar to colorectal cancer, are often slowly progressive, are present as isolated recurrences, and, therefore, lend themselves to resection with a long-term benefit.

In general, resection of even isolated metastases from breast, lung, stomach, or pancreatic cancers has a poor prognosis and is, therefore, not justified. When such cases present themselves to the cancer surgeon, a very careful assessment of the indications and potential benefits must be undertaken.

Strategies for Unresectable Liver Metastases. In general, single-agent and polydrug chemotherapy of liver metastases have met with disappointing results. Since most liver metastases are gastrointestinal in origin, 5-FU is a mainstay of such therapies. Liver metastases from colorectal cancer that are unresected can be expected to have a 15–20% response rate to systemic 5-FU-based therapy. Recently, studies have indicated a greater benefit from giving the 5-FU as a continuous infusion.

Regional chemotherapy via hepatic artery infusion has proved efficacious in managing liver-only, unresectable colorectal metastases. HAI therapy has, however, not

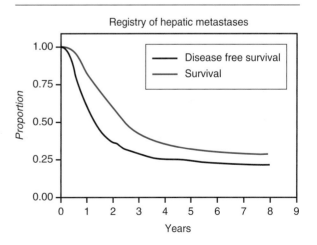

Figure 28–9. Survival and disease-free survival for patients who have undergone hepatic resection for colorectal carcinoma metastases to the liver. (Reprinted, with permission, from Registry of Hepatic Metastases: Resection of the liver for colorectal carcinoma metastases: A multi-institutional study of indications for resection. Surgery 1988;103:278–288, p. 281.)

proved to be beneficial in managing liver metastases from other sites.

Chemoembolization is also a useful approach for palliation. It has considerable associated toxicity primarily involving the liver, and 60% of treated patients experience some degree of transient liver failure. Nevertheless, this treatment can be performed safely in appropriately selected patients, with reports indicating significant palliative benefit.

Local ablative therapy, as with hepatocellular cancer, includes cryotherapy, injection of ethanol, hyperthermic necrosis, and, perhaps in the future, biologic therapies. Since most of these patients have their metastatic liver disease in an otherwise normal liver, there exists more opportunity for innovative and aggressive treatment. Unfortunately, for most tumors the liver metastases are part of a more disseminated spread of their cancer. It is, therefore, imperative that each case be considered carefully on its own merits with close scrutiny of the biology and growth characteristics of the patient's tumor.

SUGGESTED READING

Blumgart LH: *Surgery of the Liver and Biliary Tract*, 2nd ed. Churchill Livingstone, 1994.

Curley SA et al: Liver and bile ducts. In: Abeloff MD et al (editors): *Clinical Oncology*. Churchill Livingstone, 1995.

Johnson AG: The liver. In: Mann CV et al (editors): *Bailey and Love's Short Practice of Surgery*, 22nd ed. Chapman and Hall Medical, 1995.

Lebovic GS, Niederhuber JE: Colorectal cancer metastatic to the liver: Arterial infusion. In: Niederhuber JE (editor): *Current Therapy in Oncology*. Mosby-Year Book, 1993.

Niederhuber JE: Tumors of the liver. In: Murphy GP, Lawrence W, Lenhard RE (editors): *American Cancer Society Textbook of Clinincal Oncology*. American Cancer Society, 1995.

Warren KW et al: *Atlas of Surgery of the Liver, Pancreas and Biliary Tract*. Appleton & Lange, 1991.

Zinner MJ et al: *Maingot's Abdominal Operations*, 10th ed. Appleton & Lange, 1997.

29

The Biliary System

John E. Niederhuber, MD, & Mark Vierra, MD

▶ Key Facts

- ▶ Calculous disease of the gallbladder is the most common gastrointestinal disorder and one of the most prevalent problems for which the general surgeon is consulted.

- ▶ Several variations of anatomy in the extrahepatic biliary tree and adjacent hepatic arteries occur and must be clearly understood and appreciated before beginning any operation on the biliary tree.

- ▶ Vital factors believed to lead to actual stone formation are nucleation, poor gallbladder function, and the solubility of cholesterol in bile.

- ▶ The two types of gallstones are pigment, or "bilirubinate," and cholesterol, or "mixed."

- ▶ The most commonly used imaging study for evaluation of the biliary tract is transabdominal ultrasonography, although ERCP has become the dominant means of assessing the bile duct.

- ▶ Approximately 20 million Americans have gallstones, but only one in four will develop symptoms of biliary tract disease.

- ▶ Today, over 90% of cholecystectomies performed in the United States are done laparoscopically.

- ▶ Open cholecystectomy is now most often reserved for the most difficult cases, the sickest patients, and cases in which laparoscopic cholecystectomy is attempted but cannot be safely pursued.

- ▶ Pain associated with gallbladder disease is referred to as "biliary colic." It is often associated with nausea and vomiting and may present as a pressure sensation rather than pain.

- ▶ ERCP with sphincterotomy and stone extraction is performed for retained common bile duct stones, with a 90–95% success rate.

- ▶ Acute cholangitis is an infection of the bile ducts as a result of obstruction of the bile ducts. It should be treated with antibiotics and urgent drainage of the obstructed biliary tree.

- ▶ Benign biliary stricture is most often a result of iatrogenic injury sustained during cholecystectomy. Approximately 90% can be successfully repaired in the hands of an experienced surgeon.

- ▶ Sclerosing cholangitis is an inflammatory disease that causes chronic cholestasis, obliterative fibrosis, and multiple strictures of the bile ducts. Treatment is by Roux-en-Y hepaticojejunostomy or liver transplantation.

- ▶ Biliary tract carcinoma is relatively uncommon but, in general, these tumors are difficult to manage and have a high mortality-to-incidence ratio.

Calculous disease of the gallbladder is the most common gastrointestinal disorder and, therefore, is one of the most prevalent problems for which the general surgeon is consulted. While most patients are asymptomatic, cholelithiasis may result in acute and chronic inflammation of the gallbladder (**cholecystitis**), and, occasionally, stones may migrate to or form de novo in the common bile duct, causing more serious problems. The surgeon is also involved in managing other less common diseases of the biliary tract, including congenital defects, inflammatory diseases, infections, and malignant tumors. The management of biliary tract disease has been greatly impacted by recent technical advances, perhaps, more than any other disease process. The introduction of minimally invasive surgery (laparoscopic surgery) and fiberoptics, which led to the development of endoscopic retrograde cholangiopancreatography (ERCP), have dramatically changed surgical approaches to this disease. The latter has greatly reduced the need for surgical exploration of the common bile duct in patients with choledocholithiasis and has markedly enhanced the ability to accurately diagnose biliary and pancreatic disease processes.

BILIARY ANATOMY

The extrahepatic biliary tree is composed of the right and left hepatic ducts, which join to form the common hepatic duct (Figure 29–1). The gallbladder joins the common hepatic duct via the cystic duct, at which point the common hepatic duct becomes the **common bile duct**. The distal common bile duct descends behind the duodenum and traverses a portion of the pancreatic head before entering the second portion of the duodenum. It empties into the ampulla of Vater. The common duct is normally joined by the pancreatic duct before entering the duodenum. The entrance of the pancreatic duct to the duodenum can vary, however; it may enter the duodenum separately from the bile duct (Figure 29–2). It is thought that variations of this anatomy may be clinically relevant to the development of gallstone pancreatitis, which is more common in patients who have a common channel between the bile duct and pancreatic duct.

The **portal vein**, formed by the confluence of the splenic and superior mesenteric vein, lies just behind the common duct. It bifurcates to form the right and left portal veins as it enters the liver and is closely associated with the posterior wall of the left and right bile ducts.

The **common hepatic artery**, arising from the celiac trunk, gives rise to the right gastric and gastroduodenal arteries, continues as the proper hepatic artery, and bifurcates to form the right and left hepatic arteries. The right hepatic artery usually crosses behind the common or proper hepatic duct and gives off the cystic artery that supplies the gallbladder. There is no specific venous drainage of the gallbladder; most of the drainage is into the portal vein by unnamed small veins and veins that traverse the gallbladder bed and flow directly into intrahepatic veins. Lymphatic drainage is maintained via regional lymph nodes along the cystic duct and bile duct as well as

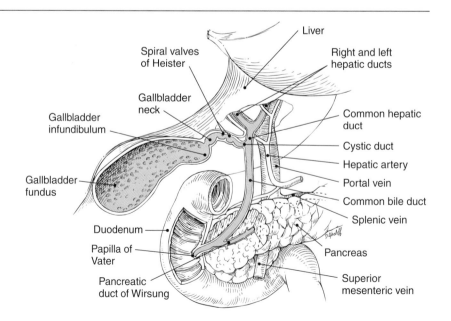

Figure 29–1. Anterior aspect of the biliary system.

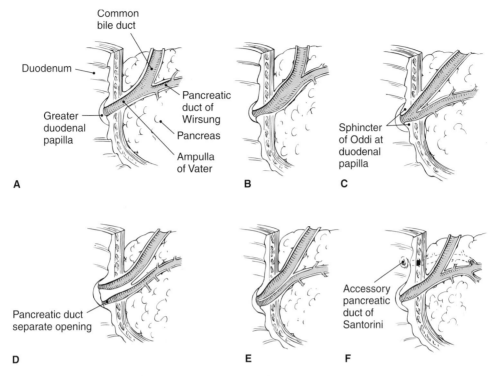

Figure 29–2. Variations in union of common bile duct and pancreatic duct. **A:** Pancreatic and common bile ducts join early, resulting in a long hepatopancreatic duct. **B:** A long hepatopancreatic duct is modified by an expanded ampulla. **C:** Pancreatic and common bile ducts join very close to the greater duodenal papilla, resulting in a short hepatopancreatic duct. **D:** Both pancreatic and common bile ducts open separately on a somewhat larger duodenal papilla. **E:** Pancreatic and common bile ducts drain through a single opening, but the ducts are separated by a septum. **F:** Long hepatopancreatic duct along with a well-developed accessory pancreatic duct, which opens through a lesser duodenal papilla. (Reprinted and modified, with permission, from Clemente CD: *Anatomy: A Regional Atlas of the Body.* Urban & Schwarzenberg, 1981, Fig. 249–254.)

through channels that flow directly into the liver. The **hepatoduodenal ligament** contains the portal vein, hepatic arteries, and common duct. Behind this structure is an opening termed the **foramen of Winslow**, which provides access to the "lesser sac."

The **hepatocystic triangle**, otherwise known as Calot's triangle, is defined today (though it was defined differently by Calot) as the triangle formed by the common hepatic bile duct, the cystic duct and gallbladder, and the liver. This area must be carefully dissected in order to perform a safe cholecystectomy. Failure to appreciate the anatomy and the frequency of anatomic variations in this region may lead to serious ductal or arterial injury. Important structures in this area include the common hepatic bile duct, right hepatic artery, cystic duct lymph node, cystic artery, aberrant right hepatic bile duct(s), and cystic duct.

The gallbladder holds only 30–60 mL of bile when fully distended. The normal gallbladder wall is approximately 2 mm thick and is composed of a mucosal layer, a thin layer with muscular fibers, and virtually no submucosa. One can speculate that the intimate proximity of the

mucosa to the muscular layers of the gallbladder, as well as the direct venous drainage of the gallbladder into the liver, may contribute to the poor prognosis of gallbladder cancer.

It is often stated that more variations in anatomy occur in the area of the porta hepatis than anywhere else in the body. Several of these variations are clinically important, especially those involving the extrahepatic biliary tree and the adjacent hepatic arteries. For example, the right hepatic bile duct or a segment of this may insert low on the hepatic duct or even onto the cystic duct, where it is at risk for injury during cholecystectomy. The same is true for the right hepatic artery. The right hepatic artery may arise from the superior mesenteric trunk (a replaced right hepatic artery) instead of the celiac axis/common hepatic artery. The replaced right hepatic artery occurs in approximately 16% of patients and can be found coursing behind the head of the pancreas, just lateral to the portal vein and posterior to the common bile duct. The right hepatic artery may also cross anterior to the common hepatic duct and course high through Calot's triangle, where it may be ligated by mistake during the performance of a cholecystec-

Table 29–1. Todani classification of choledochal cysts.

Type	Findings
I	Solitary fusiform extrahepatic cyst
II	Extrahepatic supraduodenal diverticulum
III	Intraduodenal diverticulum; choledochocele
IVA	Fusiform extrahepatic and intrahepatic cysts
IVB	Multiple extrahepatic cysts
V	Multiple intrahepatic cysts; Caroli's disease

Reprinted, with permission, from Todani T et al: Congenital bile duct cysts: classification, operative procedures, and review of thirty-seven cases including cancer arising from choledochal cyst. Am J Surg 1977;134:263–269.

tomy. In order to avoid serious consequences, all of these anomalies, and many more, must be clearly understood and appreciated before beginning any operation on the biliary tree.

In addition to the more common anatomic anomalies noted above, there are other congenital anomalies of the biliary system as well. Rarely, there may be a duplicated gallbladder or congenital absence of the gallbladder. **Choledochal cysts** represent a congenital dilatation of the extrahepatic or intrahepatic biliary tree. Table 29–1 describes the Todani classification of choledochal cysts, which has gained widespread acceptance. While choledochal cysts may be discovered at any age, typically they are diagnosed early in life. Two percent are discovered in infants, 60% present before age 10 years, and 75% present by age 20 years. Considerable debate exists regarding the cause of choledochal cysts. A longer than usual (≈ 2 cm) common channel between the bile duct and pancreatic duct has been observed in many patients. This has been postulated to permit the reflux of pancreatic secretions into the common bile duct, causing a weakening and dilatation of the duct wall. While this remains a well-known concept familiar to students of hepatobiliary diseases, it has not been proven.

Choledochal cysts are more common in Asians and are four times as likely to occur in females. Pain in the epigastrium (55%), jaundice (66%), and a palpable mass (60%) are the classic findings in at least one third of patients. These findings are similar to other causes of common bile duct obstruction that must be excluded. Such cysts may lead to stasis and stone formation, cholangitis, or pancreatitis. They also harbor a significant risk of future malignancy (≈ 15% of patients over age 20 years develop adenocarcinoma of the cyst wall) and may be associated with other anomalies, such as hypoplastic or polycystic kidneys and congenital hepatic fibrosis. Two percent of cases have an associated biliary atresia.

Treatment is by resection of the involved duct and Roux-en-Y hepaticojejunostomy, except for Type III (Table 29–1) choledochoceles, where the risks of subsequent carcinoma is low and where sphincterotomy will usually establish adequate drainage. Failure to resect all of the cyst or to exclude any remaining cyst from exposure to pancreatic secretions will increase a patient's risk for developing carcinoma in the residual duct.

BILIARY PHYSIOLOGY & GALLSTONE FORMATION

BILE COMPOSITION & SYNTHESIS

Bile is a mixture of the secretory product of hepatocytes and biliary duct epithelial cells. Approximately two thirds of the bile manufactured daily is formed directly in the hepatic canaliculus, which is then mixed with ductular bile (Figure 29–3). Bile is stored by the gallbladder and delivered at specific intervals into the duodenum to promote digestion, the absorption of fat and fat-soluble vitamins, the alkalinization of the duodenum, and the excretion of soluble bilirubin (bilirubin diglucuronide).

An average male (≈ 70 kg) produces 4 mg/kg body weight of bilirubin; 80–85% is derived from the breakdown of senescent red blood cells and catabolism of the hemoglobin heme group in the reticuloendothelial system. Bilirubin is a water-insoluble tetrapyrrole. The destruction of maturing erythroid cells in the marrow, termed **ineffective erythropoiesis**, contributes another 15–20% of the bilirubin pool. The remaining small contribution comes from hepatic hemoproteins, such as cytochrome P-450 and cytochrome c (Figure 29–4).

The rate-limiting step in bile production is the processing that occurs in the liver, where the bilirubin is made water-soluble by its conjugation with glucuronic acid. This occurs in the hepatocyte endoplasmic reticulum and is catalyzed by the enzyme uridine diphosphate-glucuronyl transferase. Only the conjugated bilirubin can be excreted in the urine. Thus, with sustained obstructive jaundice, conjugated bilirubin regurgitates back into the plasma where a proportion becomes covalently bound to albumin and cannot be excreted. In the intestine, a portion of the conjugated bilirubin is converted by bacteria into colorless urobilinogens (tetrapyrroles) and about 20% is reabsorbed. Diseases of the extrahepatic biliary tree, therefore, can be expected to present as conjugated hyperbilirubinemia but must be carefully evaluated to eliminate other causes of jaundice (Table 29–2). Complete obstruction of the ductal system can produce a conjugated hyperbilirubinemia that plateaus at 30–40 mg/dL.

Bile contains electrolytes in concentration that approximate those found in normal serum and in lactated Ringer's; lactated Ringer's is the solution of choice, therefore, to replace external biliary losses (Table 29–3). The average 70-kg man produces approximately 700–1000 mL of bile each day. The amount varies depending on the frequency of feeding and the presence or absence of ductal obstruction. Feeding causes the gallbladder to contract and empty its contents into the duodenum. This function is largely controlled by the action of the hormone **chole-**

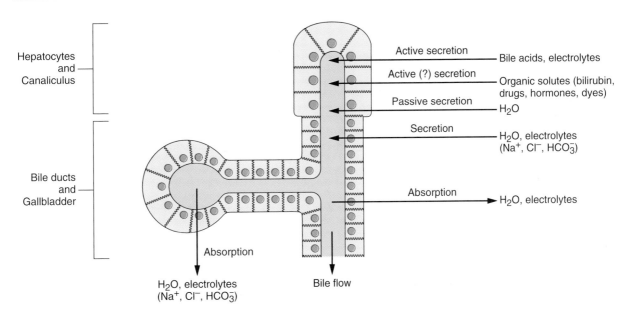

Figure 29–3. Schematic representation of the formation of bile. Bile secretion begins in the canaliculus with active transport of bile salts (acids), inorganic electrolytes, and possibly other organic solutes. Secretion of these substances is followed passively by water flow into the canaliculus. Bile is concentrated in the gallbladder by the isotonic absorption of water and electrolytes. (Reprinted, with permission, from Scharschmidt BF: Bile formation and cholestasis, metabolism and enterohepatic circulation of bile acids, and gallstone formation. In: Zakim D, Boyer TD (editors): *Hepatology.* WB Saunders, 1982, p. 307.)

cystokinin (CCK). CCK is released from the duodenal endocrine cells primarily by intraluminal fat and amino acids. In some individuals, in situations such as prolonged fasting or those who take certain drugs that inhibit gallbladder contractility (eg, somatostatin, octreotide), the formation of gallstones may be a result of the lack of CCK stimulation and subsequent gallbladder stasis. As mentioned earlier, the normal gallbladder holds only about 30–60 mL of bile and concentrates bile approximately fivefold under normal conditions. During fasting, however, bile may be concentrated 12- to 18-fold.

The total bile salt pool of the body is about 2–5 g. This pool circulates approximately six to eight times a day during fasting and even more frequently during feeding. The secreted bile salts are reabsorbed in the terminal ileum. Disease or resection of the terminal ileum will lead to a smaller bile salt pool as bile salts are not absorbed and are lost in the stool. This may account for the observation that loss of ileal function often leads to gallstone formation. In the presence of an external bile fistula (ie, a T-tube), the amount of bile declines as the bile salt pool is depleted and then increases as bile salt synthesis is induced.

FACTORS LEADING TO GALLSTONE FORMATION

The factors that cause gallstone formation are incompletely understood (Table 29–4). While gallstones are

commonly referred to as either cholesterol or pigment stones, they are rarely composed of only one component. Pigment stones, in fact, can be divided as black pigment stones and brown pigment stones. Black stones are composed of bilirubin polymers with a large component of mucin glycoproteins. Brown stones consist of calcium salts of unconjugated bilirubin termed calcium bilirubinate. In general, nucleation, gallbladder function, and the stability of solutes are all believed to be vital factors in actual stone formation. In any individual with gallstones, it may not be possible to describe the contribution of each of these factors, and a precise understanding of the mechanism of gallstone formation in the majority of patients is lacking.

1. NUCLEATION

Factors that promote the formation of a nucleus upon which stones may precipitate are now recognized as important. It is likely that certain types of gallbladder mucus may be more likely to act as a nidus for gallstone formation, and there is evidence in animal models that prostaglandin inhibitors, by altering the character of gallbladder mucus, may help to prevent gallstone formation. Bacteria may also act directly as a nidus, as bacteria have occasionally been demonstrated at the center of some gallstones. Biliary proteins, including mucous glycoproteins, play a role as promoters of nucleation of cho-

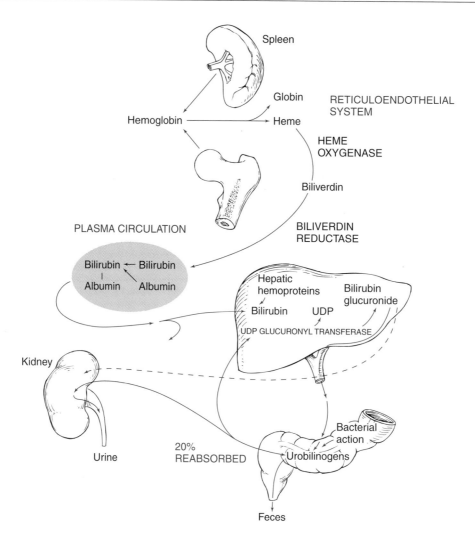

Figure 29–4. The metabolic pathway for bilirubin generation and excretion.

Table 29–2. Classification of jaundice.

Unconjugated ↑ Bilirubinemia	Conjugated ↑ Bilirubinemia
Overproduction	Impaired hepatic excretion (cholestatic jaundice)
Hemolysis	Drug (impaired canalicular transplant)
Impaired hepatic uptake	Cirrhosis (destruction of small bile ductules)
Drugs which compete	Sepsis (gram-negative)
Gilbert's syndrome	Postoperative
Impaired conjugation	15% heart surgery
Crigler-Najjar syndrome	1% elective abdominal surgery
Drugs (chloramphenicol)	Hepatitis
Neonatal jaundice	Extrahepatic biliary obstruction[1]
(Risk of kernicterus)	

[1]Diseases of the extrahepatic biliary system, therefore, can be expected to present as conjugated hyperbilirubinemia but must be carefully evaluated to eliminate other causes of jaundice. Complete obstruction of the ductal system can produce a conjugated hyperbilirubinemia that plateaus at 30–40 mg/dL.

Table 29–3. Composition of bile.

Component	Approximate Concentration
Bilirubin	1–2 mM
Bile acids	3–45 mM
Lecithin	150–800 mg/dL
Cholesterol	100–300 mg/dL
Sodium	145 mM
Potassium	4 mM
Chloride	90 mM
Bicarbonate	25 mM

Reprinted, with permission, from Mulvihill SJ: The biliary system. In: Sabiston DC, Lyerly HK (editors): *Essentials of Surgery,* 2nd ed. WB Saunders, 1994, p. 380.

lesterol crystals, and they may also impair gallbladder motility.

2. GALLBLADDER FUNCTION

Incomplete gallbladder emptying occurs in patients who are morbidly obese, patients who have undergone vagotomy, and women during pregnancy. All of these individuals are at increased risk for gallstone formation, and it is likely that poor gallbladder function is one factor that may lead to gallstone formation. There is some evidence that impaired gallbladder function may precede the development of gallstones, as in the case of impaired regulation of gallbladder function via inhibited CCK stimulation, rather than be a consequence of the gallstones themselves. Other gallbladder contributing factors include altered mucosal synthesis of prostaglandins.

3. STABILITY OF SOLUTES

The stability of solutes in solution has been an area of considerable interest regarding stone formation. In particular, the solubility of cholesterol by its metabolites, the bile salts, has been pursued as a possible explanation for the formation of cholesterol gallstones (Figure 29–5).

Table 29–4. Risk factors for the formation of gallstones.

Cholesterol Gallstones

Gender (higher ratio of women to men)
Pregnancy
Obesity
Rapid weight loss (especially with very low-calorie liquid diets)
Medications (clofibrate therapy, high-dose estrogens for men with prostate cancer)
Ileal resection or ileal disease
Vagotomy

Bilirubinate Gallstones

Hemolytic illness
Cirrhosis
Total parenteral nutrition
Infections (*Clonorchis sinensis,* etc)

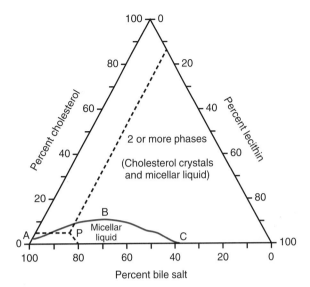

Figure 29–5. Solubility of biliary cholesterol. The components of bile are listed on separate axes. The area under the curved line ABC defines a solution in which cholesterol is soluble and stone formation will not occur. The area above line ABC represents a solution in which cholesterol may exist in several phases, including crystals. Point P contains 80 mol/dL of bile salts, 18 mol/dL of lecithin, and 5 mol/dL of cholesterol, and equilibrium that allows cholesterol solubility in a micellar phase. (Reprinted, with permission, from Small DM: Current concepts: Gallstones. N Engl J Med 1968;279:588.)

Normal bile has three main constituents: cholesterol, bile salts, and phospholipids (> 90% lecithin). Cholesterol is insoluble in aqueous solution and requires the formation of micelles containing cholesterol, bile acids, and lecithin to be soluble in bile. The majority of the cholesterol in bile is the result of hepatic synthesis and is not derived from dietary cholesterol. Chenodeoxycholic acid and cholic acid are conjugated in the hepatocytes with taurine and glycine before being secreted in the bile. These conjugated bile acids are reabsorbed in the terminal ileum (enterohepatic circulation). A small component of the bile acids are deconjugated by bacteria in the bowel and may be reabsorbed or excreted. If they are not resorbed they are usually dehydroxylated by colonic bacteria forming secondary bile acids–deoxycholic acid and lithocholic acid. It is important to remember that the quantity of bile acid actively circulating in the hepatoenteric pathway acts to regulate the level of hepatic bile acid synthesis.

Biliary sludge is comprised of very viscous mucoproteins containing cholesterol crystals. Sludge may be imaged by ultrasonography but may be a transient finding. When it is present at the time of other biliary-related diseases, especially pancreatitis, it must be taken seriously as a precursor lesion for stone formation.

GALLSTONE COMPOSITION

Approximately 80% of gallstones in the Western world are composed primarily of cholesterol, although most of these contain bile salts and other substances and are best termed "mixed stones." These stones are yellow, or yellow and greenish, and may be faceted, may be mulberry-shaped, or may appear as a single large stone. The remainder of stones contain primarily calcium bilirubinate and bilirubinate salts and are known as **bilirubinate stones** or **pigment stones**. These may be firm, smooth, and faceted; granular and black; or brown and earthy. Pigment stones are found in patients with hemolytic illnesses, with cirrhosis, and on long-standing total parenteral nutrition. Pigment stones are the predominant type in much of Asia. Their predominance in Asian countries is not well understood but appears to be environmental, as Asian immigrants to the West gradually acquire a pattern of stone disease more like that of the West. In Hong Kong, it has also been observed that the relative frequency of bilirubinate stones is declining. It is likely that infection plays a role, because certain types of bacteria contain beta-glucuronidases, which may deconjugate bilirubin glucuronide, allowing the bilirubin to precipitate as calcium bilirubinate. Excess secretion of unconjugated bilirubin is an important factor. Bacteria may also be important by acting as a nucleating agent, providing a nidus for stone formation. This is most clearly the case in the brown, earthy stones that are related to chronic infection of the biliary tree. Black pigment stones form in the gallbladder in patients with cirrhosis or chronic hemolytic anemia. In contrast, the brown pigment stones form either in the gallbladder or in the bile duct.

DIAGNOSTIC IMAGING & LABORATORY TESTS

By far the most commonly used radiographic study in the evaluation of biliary tract disease is transabdominal ultrasonography. Quick, safe, and relatively inexpensive, it supplies vital information regarding the bile duct system, gallbladder, and surrounding structures. It is approximately 95% reliable at demonstrating calculous disease of the gallbladder, although it may miss 50% or more of common duct stones. The characteristic ultrasonographic image of cholelithiasis is an echogenic focus that casts a shadow (Figure 29–6). In the proper clinical setting the demonstration of gallstones by ultrasonography is the only study beyond the history and physical examination necessary to establish the diagnosis of acute or chronic cholecystitis. Because of its sensitivity, transabdominal ultrasonography has essentially replaced oral cholecystography as a diagnostic test. Other signs of acute cholecysti-

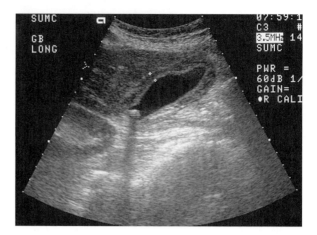

Figure 29–6. Ultrasonographic image of cholelithiasis.

tis, such as gallbladder wall thickening, pericholecystic fluid, discreet tenderness over the gallbladder during an ultrasonographic examination (a "sonographic Murphy's sign"), hyperemia of the gallbladder wall, or the presence of an impacted stone in the cystic duct provide additional evidence of acute inflammation.

The upper limit of normal for common duct diameter is approximately 8 mm. This can be reliably demonstrated by ultrasonography. Since choledocholithiasis (stones in the common duct) is only demonstrated about half the time, duct diameter serves as a better indicator for obstruction than the actual demonstration of stones. Even duct diameter, however, does not have a predictive value. In the acute setting, ductal dilatation may not yet have occurred or may not occur at all if the stone is not fixed at the ampulla, causing significant obstruction.

The **HIDA scan** (dimethylphenylcarbamylmethyl iminoacetic acid) is a more sophisticated study of gallbladder function and is occasionally helpful, especially when the clinical history is uncertain. In the HIDA scan, the radionucleotide is excreted by the liver into the biliary tree and backs up into the gallbladder within 30–45 minutes of injection. Failure to visualize the gallbladder, with tracer appearing in the intestine, suggests obstruction of the cystic duct. This does not necessarily imply acute cholecystitis, however, and the test must be interpreted within the clinical setting. Occasionally, morphine may be given to cause a spasm of the sphincter of Oddi and force the bile back up toward the gallbladder to exclude the possibility of a false positive study.

The computed tomography (CT) scan is seldom needed for benign biliary tract disease but is indispensable in the management of malignant disease. For example, cholesterol stones may be missed on a CT scan unless they contain some calcium. On the other hand, a CT scan may demonstrate inflammation of the gallbladder and is the procedure of choice for the staging and planning of treatment when biliary tract malignancy is present. CT is also a good choice in the critically ill or complicated patient in whom a number of diagnoses are being considered, as it surveys the entire abdomen.

Percutaneous transhepatic cholangiography is particularly useful in patients with proximal bile duct obstruction. In these patients, ERCP may be difficult and may not demonstrate the intrahepatic extent of the stricture or tumor adequately to assess resectability. The study is performed transhepatically as a diagnostic procedure and can be therapeutic for stone removal, balloon dilatation of strictures, or stenting of the ductal system to relieve obstruction.

ERCP has become the dominant means of assessing the common bile duct. Cholangiography may be performed to look for stones, stricture, or tumor. It may also be used to obtain biopsies of the biliary tree, the sphincter of Oddi may be incised (sphincterotomy) to allow improved bile duct drainage and the passage of small stones, and stents of various types may be placed endoscopically to achieve long-term relief of obstruction.

Oral cholecystography is seldom used anymore as a diagnostic test (at one time it was the most common study). It may, however, still be useful on those rare occasions when ultrasonography has been negative but the suspicion for gallbladder disease remains high. It is most commonly used in evaluating patients for nonsurgical treatment of cholelithiasis. It can provide information regarding gallbladder function, size, and number of stones and whether stones are calcified or float within the gallbladder.

Liver function tests are an important aspect of the evaluation of biliary tract diseases. Aspartate aminotransferase (AST) is the first enzyme to be elevated acutely in the presence of biliary tract obstruction, and the alanine aminotransferase (ALT) may also be elevated. While elevation of these enzymes is usually associated with hepatocellular injury, such as chemical or viral hepatitis, it is not uncommon for these enzymes to rise to levels above 1000 with acute, complete bile duct obstruction. The alkaline phosphatase, on the other hand, rises more slowly and usually represents long-standing obstruction of the biliary tree. Obstruction of a single biliary radicle, or sclerosing cholangitis without complete obstruction of any part of the functioning liver, may produce an elevation of the alkaline phosphatase. The bilirubin also rises more slowly, and even in the presence of complete obstruction usually does not rise more than 3 mg/dL per 24 hours.

CHOLECYSTECTOMY

INDICATIONS FOR SURGERY

Approximately 20 million Americans have gallstones, but only one in four will develop symptoms of biliary

tract disease. In general, it is felt that cholecystectomy is not indicated for incidentally discovered, asymptomatic stones. This recommendation is based on studies from the mid-1980s suggesting that about three out of four patients with asymptomatic stones are likely to remain asymptomatic indefinitely, and that the vast majority of patients who do develop symptoms will develop pain (biliary colic) before they develop complications of their stone disease, such as pancreatitis, cholangitis, or gallbladder cancer. In general, if patients are to become symptomatic they do so within the first 5 years following the development of their stones. Patients that do become symptomatic have a higher risk for future problems. For example, up to two thirds of patients who experience an attack of biliary pain will have recurrent episodes within 1 to 2 years. More importantly, at least 3% annually will develop significant biliary complications. Elective cholecystectomy in this group can be shown to result in a real increase in life expectancy of 3–4 months.

Recent reports suggest that cholecystectomy in some young patients who are asymptomatic may be indicated. As stones are probably most commonly discovered by "accident" in young women undergoing ultrasonography for pregnancy-related services, it would seem reasonable to offer prophylactic cholecystectomy to young women who plan to become pregnant. Biliary tract complications during pregnancy do not occur commonly, but if they occur may certainly be difficult to manage. Other groups of patients for whom cholecystectomy may be indicated in the absence of symptoms are children, transplant recipients, immunologically compromised patients, and, perhaps, patients with diabetes. Prophylactic cholecystectomy has also been commonly used in patients with sickle cell disease because of the high risk of pigment stones and the difficulties in distinguishing the pain of sickle cell crisis from that of acute cholecystitis.

Another reason for recommending therapy in otherwise asymptomatic patients with gallstones is the risk of gallbladder cancer. In general, for asymptomatic individuals, the risk of cancer is not considered great enough to justify gallbladder removal. The exceptions to this are those patients who develop a calcified gallbladder and Native Americans with gallstones. Both of these patient groups have a higher incidence of cancer of the gallbladder.

Since the introduction of laparoscopic cholecystectomy, the number of cholecystectomies has risen in this country by about 30%. This increase most likely represents the greater willingness of patients and referring physicians to consider an operation that is perceived as safer and less incapacitating than the traditional open cholecystectomy. There are, however, no large-scale studies to prove that the laparoscopic procedure is safer than an open cholecystectomy. Therefore, it is probably premature to broaden indications for cholecystectomy.

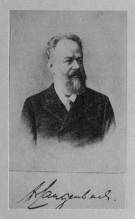

Carl Lagenbuch (1846–1901). (Reprinted, with permission, from Hardy KJ: Carl Langenbuch and the Lazarus hospital: Events and circumstances surrounding the first cholecystectomy. Aust NZ J Surg 1993;63:62.)

Although Carl Langenbuch (1846–1901) achieved much during his lifetime, he is best known for having performed the first cholecystectomy in July of 1882. He was born in Kiel, Germany, and orphaned at an early age. Having been trained as an organist, he supported himself with his music while he attended medical school. After fighting in the Franco-Prussian War, he moved to Berlin where he became an assistant to Professor Max Wilms at Bethany Hospital. Wilms arranged Langenbuch's appointment as Director of Surgery and Internal Medicine at Lazarus Hospital in 1873. Although he was only 27 years old, Langenbuch accepted the appointment, which presented a formidable challenge as the hospital served the poorest, sickest patients in the primarily industrial St. Elizabeth area of Berlin. At the time that Langenbuch was appointed, the hospital was not connected for local sanitation and had no electricity or operating rooms.

Langenbuch first became interested in gallstone disease in 1874 when an administrator at Lazarus Hospital died of chronic cholecystitis. As the head of both surgery and internal medicine at Lazarus, he was able to observe many patients with gallbladder disease. After several years of clinical study, cadaver studies, and experiments conducted in live animals, he concluded that a human could survive without a gallbladder, that the gallbladder could be safely removed, and that the only cure for cholecystitis was cholecystectomy.

In 1882, an opportunity to apply his investigations presented itself. A patient with chronic cholecystitis with a very poor prognosis due to weight loss, weakness, and morphine dependence for pain presented for evaluation. He was a 43-year-old male who had suffered from biliary colic for 16 years. The patient agreed to the operation despite the risks and on July 15th, 1882, the first cholecystectomy was performed using strict antiseptic techniques (introduced by Lister just 15 years earlier and not in widespread use). On the morning after the operation, Langenbuch found the patient smoking a large cigar and stating that his pain had gone.

HISTORICAL FACTS *continued*

Before Langenbuch, it was not believed that a patient could survive without a gallbladder and it was several years before cholecystectomy gained widespread popularity. By 1890, only 20 cholecystectomies had been performed worldwide. At a presentation in 1897, Langenbuch stated his disappointment that cholecystectomy had not become more popular. For years there were far more critics than proponents. The surgeon known for his expertise in cholecystostomy, Robert Larson Tait, said of cholecystectomy, "The proposal is intrinsically absurd, for there can be no reason for removing the gallbladder merely because it has some stones in it." Tait was also outspoken in his criticism of Listerian principles of antisepsis.

Langenbuch had a remarkably creative, inventive mind. His technical skill and thorough investigations allowed him to excel in the field of biliary and liver surgery. In addition to his renown for cholecystectomy, he is also known as one of the pioneers of hepatic resection. The first volume of his classic book entitled *The Surgery of the Liver and Gallbladder* was published in 1894 and the second volume in 1897. Ironically, as president of the Berlin Surgical Society, he addressed its members on how to properly manage peritonitis in 1901. He died later that year of peritonitis following acute appendicitis.

TECHNIQUE OF CHOLECYSTECTOMY

Today, over 90% of the cholecystectomies performed in the United States are done laparoscopically. This technique was first introduced in 1987. Generally, four trocars are used to perform the procedure, positioned through the umbilicus, the epigastrium, and two beneath the right costal margin (Figure 29–7). The camera is introduced through the umbilical port, and the gallbladder is grasped and elevated through the lateral-most port. The epigastric and second right upper quadrant port are used to perform the dissection. The cystic duct and arterial branches are skeletonized, serially clipped, and divided. Following division of the duct and vessels, the gallbladder is removed retrograde from the gallbladder bed and then extracted through the umbilical port.

Laparoscopic cholecystectomy is considered a safe procedure when performed by appropriately trained surgeons in properly selected patients. Major complications are said to occur in approximately 1–5% of cases. The incidence of biliary stricture is difficult to determine, however, reports suggest this may occur in up to 0.7% of patients. Strictures may present weeks or months after laparoscopic cholecystectomy and are thought to frequently be caused by diathermy and misplaced clips.

Intraoperative cystic duct cholangiography may be performed to look for stones or to assess biliary anatomy. Some surgeons suggest routine cholangiography in all cases. While cholangiography may document alterations in bile duct anatomy and common bile duct stones not otherwise recognized, some duct injuries may actually be incurred during the performance of the cholangiogram. In addition, the false positive identification of stones may exceed by a considerable margin real positives in patients who have no risk factors for the presence of choledocholithiasis.

The routine use of intraoperative cholangiography has been a debated issue among surgeons for nearly 60 years. Advocates of intraoperative cholangiography during laparoscopic cholecystectomy support their position by arguing that its routine use detects the presence of unsuspected common bile duct stones, delineates the anatomy of the bile ducts, helps to prevent injury to the biliary ductal system (especially injury to the common bile duct), and identifies other bile duct pathology. These supporters frequently site previous studies for open cholecystectomy that suggested routine intraoperative cholangiography de-

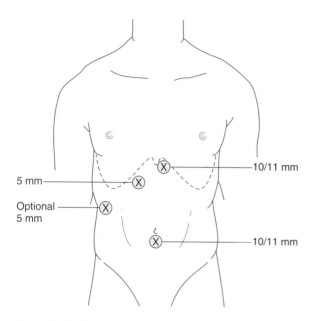

Figure 29–7. Diagram of port positions for laparoscopic chole-cystectomy. (Reprinted, with permission, from Rosin RD: Laparoscopic cholecystectomy. In: Zinner MJ et al (editors): *Maingot's Abdominal Operations,* 10th ed. Appleton & Lange, 1997, p. 1859.)

creased unnecessary common bile duct explorations from 66% to less than 5%. Clearly, however, their greatest concern is the avoidance of injuries to the common bile duct, as higher rates of common bile duct injury have been reported after laparoscopic cholecystectomy (0–1.8%) as compared to open cholecystectomy (0–0.5%).

Of importance to this debate is the ability today to successfully manage common bile duct stones endoscopically. The incidence of postcholecystectomy endoscopic procedures or sphincterotomy has been variously reported as 1.4% to as high as 3.5%. Very few (< 1%) would fail an endoscopic procedure and require a second operation. Thus, a selective approach to intraoperative cholangiography seems best. Commonly cited preoperative clinical data include elevated while blood cell count, elevated serum bilirubin, elevated alkaline phosphatase, a history of suspected gallstone pancreatitis, and, of course, demonstration of common bile duct calculi on preoperative imaging (usually ultrasonography). These preoperative indicators are combined with three intraoperative anatomic assessments: (1) a cystic duct less than 3 mm in diameter; (2) stones greater than 6 mm in diameter; and (3) a single stone. These intraoperative findings preclude a significant risk of choledocholithiasis.

Another important factor in this debate, as mentioned above, is the rate of false positive cholangiograms. Normal cholangiograms are essentially 100% accurate, but abnormal cholangiograms in a setting of routine cholangiography have been associated with false positive rates

as high as 16%. This high figure appears to be in marked contrast to studies using intraoperative cholangiography only on a selective basis. In these studies, the incidence of false positive radiographs was only 1–4%.

With routine, uncomplicated laparoscopic cholecystectomy, the majority of patients can be discharged on the first postoperative day following operation and many can be released the same day as surgery. Duration of disability varies considerably from country to country and is highly dependent on individual motivation to return to work, but most patients may return to unrestricted activity within a week. In the hands of a skilled surgeon, and with careful case selection, it can be expected that well under 5% of laparoscopic operations will need to be converted to an open procedure, but this figure for conversion rises to 25–35% in patients with acute cholecystitis.

Open cholecystectomy is most often reserved for the most difficult cases, the sickest patients, and cases in which laparoscopic cholecystectomy is attempted but cannot be safely pursued. It is also advocated for any patient in which gallbladder cancer is a consideration. In general, the abdomen is entered through a right subcostal incision (Kocher's incision) (Figure 29–8), although some prefer a right paramedian incision. The gallbladder is grasped with a clamp and elevated. The cystic duct and artery are looped. The cystic artery should be carefully dissected free as it passes from left to right within the triangle of Calot and ligated. Figure 29–8B demonstrates catheter placement in the cystic duct for an intraoperative cholangiogram. The cystic duct is ligated in close proximity to its junction with the common bile duct. The preference is to place a second suture ligature on the end of the cystic duct. The gallbladder is removed and the incision is closed. Drain placement is optional but generally not done.

The mortality rate for open cholecystectomy is approximately 0.17%. The morbidity rate of 14.7% is seemingly high, but this figure includes all reported complications, including minor problems such as electrolyte imbalances, atelectasis, urinary retention, and other minor difficulties. The risk of bile duct injury during open cholecystectomy is approximately 0.1%. The disadvantage, of course, is the increased period of patient recuperation and time in the hospital.

Following cholecystectomy, most patients notice no sustained change in dietary tolerance or bowel habits, and no medications or dietary restrictions are needed. Rarely, a patient may have persistent diarrhea that does not resolve. The mechanism for this is not well understood, but presumably relates to continuous flow of bile into the gastrointestinal tract. It is important to recall that repeated or sustained episodes of cholecystitis may also render the gallbladder nonfunctional, so that avoidance of cholecystectomy will not necessarily allow a symptomatic patient to avoid the loss of gallbladder function.

It is not at all clear that antibiotics are indicated for elective laparoscopic cholecystectomy in normal hosts. For normal hosts with early acute cholecystitis or who require prophylaxis for invasive procedures such as ERCP,

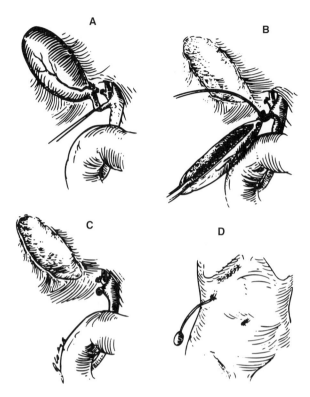

Figure 29–8. Technique of open cholecystectomy. **A:** Gallbladder in situ with the cystic duct isolated and the cystic artery ligated and divided. **B:** The gallbladder has been taken down from the liver bed and a catheter placed in the cystic duct for an intraoperative cholangiogram. **C:** Gallbladder completely removed with the cystic duct stump and proximal stump of the cystic artery remaining. **D:** The abdomen is closed with a closed-suction drain placed through a separate stab incision. (Reprinted, with permission, from Karam J, Roslyn JJ: Cholelithiasis and cholecystectomy. In: Schwartz SI, Ellis H (editors): *Maingot's Abdominal Operations,* 10th ed. Appleton & Lange, 1997, p. 1773.)

piperacillin or mezlocillin are the appropriate antibiotics. These provide good coverage of *Escherichia coli, Klebsiella,* and *Enterococcus* and achieve exceptionally high concentrations in the bile due to hepatic synthesis. In more complicated patients an aminoglycoside may be added, and in critically ill or complicated patients it may be appropriate to add metronidazole.

NONOPERATIVE MANAGEMENT OF GALLSTONE DISEASE

In the 1980s there was considerable interest in two nonoperative strategies for the management of gallstone dis-

ease. One of these was the use of lithotripsy, as had been applied to kidney stones. Initial results from Germany were promising, but that success could not be repeated in subsequent trials in which patient selection was not as stringent and in which general anesthesia and an immersion waterbath were not used. Subsequent trials also demonstrated that the efficacy of lithotripsy was highly dependent on the simultaneous administration of oral dissolution medications.

Two oral agents have been used, **chenodeoxycholic acid (CDCA)** and, more recently, **ursodeoxycholic acid (UDCA)**. Both of these exist in human bile as naturally occurring secondary bile acids. They act by expanding the bile salt pool and solubilizing cholesterol, as well as by other mechanisms that are less well understood. UDCA reduces cholesterol saturation by blocking HMG-CoA reductase. HMG-CoA reductase is an enzyme that is involved in cholesterol biosynthesis. It also forms highly soluble multilamellar vesicles and, in so doing, increases the nucleation time of the bile. The drug is used at 10–13 mg/kg/d and is about 50% successful. Dissolution of stones takes 6–12 months and the drug is generally only suited for cholesterol-rich, noncalcified stones. In addition, stones greater than 1.5 cm will rarely dissolve, and pigment stones are not susceptible.

All techniques that remove the stones without removing the gallbladder, including surgical procedures, are limited by the problem of recurrence of stones. In general, 50% of patients who are rendered stone-free without removing the gallbladder will have recurrence of their stones within 5 years of discontinuing therapy. This, plus the increased expense associated with serial imaging to determine progress, has all but eliminated interest in these therapies.

BENIGN & MALIGNANT BILIARY TRACT DISEASE

BILIARY COLIC & ACUTE CHOLECYSTITIS

Diagnosis

It is important to remember that the gallbladder and biliary tree have only autonomic innervation. In its early stages the pain of gallbladder disease, therefore, is visceral pain. It is often difficult to localize, but is commonly referred to the epigastrium or upper back. It is often, though not invariably, associated with nausea and vomiting, and may sometimes be described as a pressure sensation rather than pain. It is seldom if ever "fleeting." Instead, the pain of biliary colic rarely lasts fewer than several minutes. Actually, the term "colic" is an unfortunate misnomer, as biliary tract pain is never truly colicky in periodicity. It is sometimes impossible to distinguish biliary pain from that of cardiac angina, pyelonephritis, duodenal ulcer, gastroesophageal reflux (esophagitis), or pancreatitis, all of which may produce identical symptoms.

In the later stages of inflammation, physical findings and symptoms will localize more to the right upper quadrant. In this instance, bile salts, especially if they have been deconjugated by bile stasis or infection, produce transmural inflammation of the gallbladder. Physical findings secondary to peritoneal inflammation will ensue, and the omentum may migrate to the area of the inflammation and become adherent.

Obstruction of the cystic duct by a stone, or by acute or chronic cholecystitis, is the cause of biliary colic in the vast majority of cases. The role of bacteria in the presentation of symptoms is not at all well defined. An elevated white count may be present acutely, but does not necessarily imply that the patient is septic. Fever is more likely with sustained cystic duct obstruction and infection, but is not invariably present with acute cholecystitis. Obviously, some cases of acute cholecystitis will resolve without antibiotics or specific therapy.

Management

Prompt cholecystectomy is the treatment of choice for the majority of patients with acute cholecystitis, especially in the first 24–48 hours of onset of symptoms, and in most instances this can, and should, be performed laparoscopically. Broad-spectrum antibiotics are administered to decrease the risk of secondary infection. As stated earlier, there is a substantially increased risk of conversion to laparotomy in these cases, and in some patients the operation should clearly be performed by laparotomy, without an attempt at laparoscopy. If the diagnosis has been delayed and the patient is improving, it is best to make an effort to delay surgery for several weeks with the hope that the acute inflammatory process will resolve and make surgery less difficult and safer.

Rarely, percutaneous cholecystostomy may be the treatment of choice. The patient in the midst of a myocardial infarction, for example, can almost always be stabilized with a percutaneous cholecystostomy, with operation deferred until a later time when the patient's condition will better tolerate a general anesthetic and definitive surgical procedure. Although percutaneous cholecystostomy is only rarely necessary, it remains an important and effective means of deferring surgery in patients whose general medical condition or local conditions of inflammation would make a formal cholecystectomy technically difficult and dangerous. Percutaneous cholecystostomy should be performed under local anesthesia with CT or ultrasonographic guidance.

Symptoms and signs of acute cholecystitis occasionally present late and after significant complications of the early inflammatory process have progressed. These patients almost always require emergent surgery, however, in so doing it may be ill advised to remove the gallbladder. The decision to do so must be carefully weighed, and under these circumstances, a surgeon's experience is of great importance. Examples of these complications include free or localized perforation of the gallbladder with localized abscess, fistulization of the gallbladder to the duodenum or hepatic flexure of the colon, emphysematous (gas-gangrene) cholecystitis, and Mirizzi's syndrome, in which a large stone impacted in the neck of the gallbladder either erodes or otherwise obstructs the common duct. Often, these complications of acute cholecystitis must be treated appropriately during surgery, with a goal toward alleviating the inflammatory process; the patient would return at a later date for cholecystectomy under safer circumstances, when the anatomy of the biliary tract and blood supply to the liver can be clearly defined.

RETAINED COMMON DUCT STONES

Diagnosis & Management

A small number of patients following either open or laparoscopic cholecystectomy will present with retained common duct stones. The frequency of this problem is, of course, influenced by how aggressive the approach has been to clearing the common bile duct of stones, either prior to cholecystectomy or during the procedure. In recent years, improvements in ERCP have perhaps reduced the need to be overly aggressive at the time of surgery in patients with choledocholithiasis, reducing the risks of common duct injury and subsequent stricture.

The incidence of retained bile duct stones following laparoscopic cholecystectomy is estimated to be approximately 5%. Most patients present with biliary-type pain and mildly abnormal liver transaminases. They may or may not be jaundiced. Transabdominal ultrasonography may demonstrate duct stones or duct dilation. If these symptoms are not transient and if ultrasonography is confirmatory, an ERCP is performed with sphincterotomy and stone extraction. The success rate is 90–95% at experienced centers.

The complications are pancreatitis, bleeding, perforation, and infection and occur in 5–10% of cases. The mortality rate is approximately 0.5–1%. It is extremely rare today that patients cannot be managed successfully, either endoscopically or by a percutaneous transhepatic route, especially if they are willing to travel to specialized centers. As a result, open duct exploration has now become an exceedingly rare event in surgery. There is much less short-term and long-term risk for the patient and, obviously, significant cost savings.

ACALCULOUS CHOLECYSTITIS

Diagnosis

Rarely, patients may develop cholecystitis in the absence of stones. This occurs most commonly in patients who are critically ill in the intensive care unit, and particularly in patients who are not being fed enterally. Examples of patients at risk for acalculous cholecystitis include burn patients, trauma patients, and postsurgical patients with respiratory insufflation or multiorgan failure syndrome. Ischemia of the gallbladder is the responsible etiologic factor. The gallbladder wall itself may be frankly necrotic and contain bile that is thick and turbid. Infection, however, is not necessarily present. Fever and leukocytosis are commonly present, but may be attributable to other elements of the patient's underlying condition. Immunocompromised patients, especially patients with HIV infection, are also at risk. They develop a cytomegalovirus-related acalculous cholecystitis.

The diagnosis is often uncertain. Sedation, delirium, and previous abdominal operations may make interpretation of the abdominal examination difficult. Ultrasonography may demonstrate sludge without stones and gallbladder wall thickening, which are often nonspecific findings in seriously ill patients. The responsible physician must have a high index of suspicion in order to prevent a life-threatening complication. The HIDA scan will usually demonstrate nonvisualization of the gallbladder, but in this critically ill group of patients with prolonged fasting, its specificity is poor. This is a group of patients that benefit from CT scans—especially early in their course. The CT will generally document gallbladder-wall thickening and may demonstrate the presence of fluid around the gallbladder.

Management

Antibiotics are usually employed, though their role is not well defined. Cholecystectomy is the treatment of choice. When underlying critical illnesses preclude operative intervention, percutaneous cholecystostomy is an effective option and should be performed under CT or ultrasonographic guidance. Recently, endoscopic drainage of the gallbladder using a stent through the cystic duct has been reported. While somewhat difficult, such an approach could be useful in patients with ascites and coagulopathies.

GALLSTONE ILEUS

Diagnosis

Gallstone ileus refers to the condition in which a large gallstone has eroded through the gallbladder wall and the wall of the adjacent intestine, commonly the duodenum, causing a cholecystenteric fistula. These obstructions are usually incomplete, and the patients are often sufficiently ill that it may be difficult to elicit a history of gallbladder symptoms. The diagnosis may be suspected by abdominal radiographs demonstrating an intestinal obstruction and air in the biliary tree. The gallstone itself may be visible if it is sufficiently calcified. This condition is most often identified in elderly women and may carry a mortality rate as high as 20% because of the generally poor medical condition of the elderly patient. There is also substantial incidence of underlying or coincident gallbladder malignancy.

Management

Surgery is primarily directed at the intestinal obstruction. The stone may be removed by an enterotomy, or, occasionally, it may be milked into the colon, where it can be expected to pass. Primary treatment of the cholecystenteric fistula is most often unnecessary, as it usually closes spontaneously. Cholecystectomy should be performed at a later date when the patient's general condition has improved.

GALLSTONE PANCREATITIS

Diagnosis

Pancreatitis may be precipitated by the passage of stones through the ampulla of Vater. Approximately 10% of patients with a history of symptoms of acute cholecystitis have had an episode of gallstone pancreatitis. Gallstones and alcohol constitute the two most common causes of pancreatitis in this country.

The precise mechanism by which stones cause pancreatitis is not well understood. Sudden, abrupt obstruction of both the bile duct and the pancreatic duct is probably important, though the old notion that it is caused by reflux of bile into the pancreatic duct is probably not true. Why the majority of patients who pass stones or who have stents placed across the bile duct do not develop pancreatitis is not known.

Management

Most episodes of gallstone pancreatitis are characterized by a very high amylase (> 1000) that returns to normal within a few days, and for most patients the attacks are clinically mild. In such cases, early cholecystectomy—that is, during the initial hospitalization—is performed once the amylase has normalized and the patient appears recovered from the pancreatitis. Gallstone pancreatitis may be life-threatening, however, and patients who go on to develop extensive pancreatic necrosis may require urgent debridement. If left untreated, the risk of recurrence is 30–50% within 3–6 months; therefore, treatment is mandatory and, in general, is best done before discharging the patient.

Either cholecystectomy or endoscopic sphincterotomy will effectively eliminate the possibility of subsequent episodes of pancreatitis. The vast majority of patients will undergo cholecystectomy, but sphincterotomy alone may be appropriate in some patients who are too elderly or frail to tolerate a cholecystectomy, or if local inflammation from the pancreatitis makes a cholecystectomy unsafe. It is important to recall that the cholecystectomy itself does nothing to alter the outcome of a particular episode of pancreatitis; it only prevents subsequent episodes. There should be no urgency, therefore, to perform a cholecystectomy on a patient with gallstone pancreatitis because they are not recovering from the pancreatitis.

Recently, it has become apparent that in the small percentage of patients with severe pancreatitis, outcomes are improved by early ERCP, stone removal, and sphincterotomy. These patients are more likely than patients with mild pancreatitis to have a persistent stone impacted in the ampulla. Intervention to remove this has been shown to lessen the complications of gallstone pancreatitis (particularly septic complications) and to shorten hospital stay; with intervention, there is also a trend toward a lower mortality rate. Importantly, the utilization of ERCP during severe pancreatitis has not been shown to worsen the pancreatitis.

ACUTE CHOLANGITIS & OBSTRUCTIVE JAUNDICE

Diagnosis

Acute cholangitis is an infection of the bile ducts as a result of obstruction of the bile ducts. Biliary tract diseases associated with cholangitis include choledocholithiasis, bile duct or biliary anastomotic stricture, parasitic infections, and bile duct malignancies. Choledocholithiasis is the presence of gallstones within the common bile duct or hepatic ducts. This is a much more serious manifestation of calculus disease than cholelithiasis and should always be treated urgently. The vast majority of stones in the common duct form in the gallbladder and travel to the common duct through the cystic duct. Stones that are found in the common duct more than 2 years following cholecystectomy, however, are considered primary common duct stones. These stones are usually muddy brown stones and are invariably associated with chronic low-grade infections.

Stones in the common duct are often colonized with bacteria, and if they obstruct the ampulla, cholangitis is likely to occur. Normally, biliary pressures as low as 20 mm Hg may cause bile to spill over into the blood stream. If the bile is infected, the patient becomes cholangitic.

Patients with cholangitis are usually jaundiced and will typically have either high spiking fevers (occasionally > 40° C) or hypothermia and frank rigors. In fact, patients with cholangitis are more frequently hypothermic. If alert, the patient will have right upper quadrant pain and tenderness, but obtundation is common, especially in the elderly. Patients who have had a prior cholecystectomy often describe their pain as very similar to the pain they experienced during their "gallbladder attack." Either leukocytosis or leukopenia may occur, as well as thrombocytopenia. An abnormal prothrombin time is also common, probably as a consequence of sepsis as well as absence of bile within the gastrointestinal tract, producing a vitamin K deficiency. Most patients have elevated liver transaminases, often to a level of ten times above normal.

Management

Acute cholangitis is a true surgical emergency, even though its principle management is no longer surgical. Drainage of the biliary tree must be accomplished expeditiously. It is important to keep in mind that the immediate goal in a patient with cholangitis is *not* to achieve definitive cure of the obstructing lesion, but only to provide drainage of the biliary tree. Excessive manipulation of the biliary tree will exacerbate bacterial seeding and bacteremia. It is better to drain the biliary system and return when the patient is in better condition to try to eliminate the cause of the obstruction. Urgent drainage of the obstructed biliary tree is usually performed by ERCP, with placement of a biliary drain or a stent. An alternative is percutaneous transhepatic cholangiography and drainage. If the intrahepatic ducts are dilated this may be a reasonable approach, though it is not generally the first treatment approach.

Antibiotics must be given to patients with cholangitis and should be broad-spectrum and directed against the common organisms. The antibiotic of choice is piperacillin, which may be sufficient as a single agent for prophylaxis in a patient who is not septic. If the patient is septic, however, an aminoglycoside should be added; in severely septic patients, especially diabetics, transplant patients, immunodeficient patients, and the very elderly it may be appropriate to add Flagyl as well, because these patients are at risk to harbor anaerobes in their biliary tree.

Malignant obstruction of the biliary tree most commonly occurs from cancer of the head of the pancreas but may occur with cancer of the duodenum, ampulla, or common duct itself. Obstruction in these circumstances is usually painless unless the primary tumor is sufficiently advanced to cause pain. If the obstruction is below the cystic duct, the gallbladder may become considerably distended and be palpable (**Courvoisier's law**). Biliary ductal dilatation due to stone disease is usually mild or may even be absent. With malignant obstruction dilatation is usually pronounced, even before jaundice becomes clinically apparent. Cholangitis is very uncommon in malignant obstruction, except following instrumentation of the duct, in which case the obstructed biliary tree may become contaminated. Once the patient has recovered from the acute episode of cholangitis, the diagnostic evaluation is completed and a plan developed that provides the safest and surest opportunity to correct the underlying cause.

BILIARY DYSKINESIA

Diagnosis

This group of bile duct disease entities generally refers to benign non-calculous obstruction at the pancreaticobiliary duodenal junction, causing cholestasis, pancreatitis, occasionally cholangitis, and pain. The papilla will usually demonstrate inflammation, edema, and possibly fibrosis (scarring). At least one third of patients, however, will have no identifiable pathology on biopsy and the dysfunction may be secondary to a motor disorder of the sphincter.

Manometry has been described as a key tool in the evaluation of patients suspected of sphincter dysfunction, however, in reality, it is difficult to accurately perform, and most gastroenterologists rely on other findings. Manometry can generally be performed successfully at ERCP. It must, of course, be performed with only benzodiazepine sedation because narcotics, anticholinergics, and glucagon all affect the sphincter.

Dysfunctions are divided into three classes (all in postcholecystectomy patients). **Type I** include patients with pain, obstructive liver chemistries, an increase in bile duct diameter (12 mm in postcholecystectomy patients), and slow drainage of contrast from the bile duct (> 45 min) in the absence of stones. **Type II** include patients with pain but only one or two of the findings listed for Type I. Patients with **Type III** have suggestive pain but no other abnormalities. Manometry will be abnormal in 80% of Type I, 50% of Type II, and 25% of Type III patients. There is a slightly higher risk of pancreatitis when manometry is performed than with routine ERCP.

Management

Type I patients are treated generally quite successfully by sphincterotomy. It is probably best to offer Type II and III patients a trial of medical therapy, such as anticholinergics, calcium channel blockers, or nitrates, before proceeding to sphincterotomy. About 80% of Type II patients will benefit from this therapy as opposed to only about half of the Type III patients. The major risk, of course, is a leak at the site of the sphincterotomy. This can be a serious life-threatening complication. The complication rate is slightly higher than when sphincterotomy is done for stone disease. It is also important to recognize that our understanding of the causes of sphincter of Oddi dysfunction is still evolving and, therefore, refinements in the approach to therapy can be appreciated. Optimal patient care for these complex problems certainly requires an expert team of endoscopists, surgeons, and radiologists working for the patient.

BENIGN BILIARY STRICTURE

Diagnosis

Iatrogenic duct injury is estimated to occur at a rate of about one in 1000 open cholecystectomies and about seven or eight in 1000 laparoscopic cases. Injuries to the duct are classified in Table 29–5. When recognized at the time of surgery, such injuries should be repaired immediately. If it occurs during laparoscopic surgery, it may be best to convert to an open procedure for direct repair. Repair is accomplished over a T-tube of appropriate size using monofilament fine 5-0 or 6-0 interrupted sutures. If the injury is recognized later in the postoperative course, inflammation will be a considerable problem; efforts should consist of establishing internal and external (if needed) drainage. Once the inflammation has subsided (usually > 8 weeks), an open exploration is conducted to establish a biliary duct-to-intestine (Roux-en-Y) anastomosis over a temporary stent drain.

With iatrogenic duct injuries there is at least a 25%

Table 29–5. Classification of injuries to the bile duct.

I	Tangential partial opening
II	Clip injury
IIIa	Complete transection (or near-complete) without tissue loss
IIIb	Complete transection with tissue loss
IV	Injury to hepatic duct

stricture rate within 1 year and an associated 6% mortality. Thus, this is a serious complication. If a stricture is the presenting problem postcholecystectomy, the management is again an open exploration and construction of a bilidigestive anastomosis.

Although it is an uncommon problem, biliary stricture may have disastrous results if improperly managed. While benign biliary stricture may have a number of causes (Table 29–6), the majority of cases (≈ 90%) are the result of iatrogenic injury sustained during cholecystectomy. Patients with a biliary stricture will most often present with symptoms of obstructive jaundice, fever, and pruritus, which may include evidence of scratching marks on the patient's limbs. Hepatomegaly indicates long-standing obstruction. Leukocytosis is present in patients with associated cholangitis. The majority of patients will have an elevated serum bilirubin and serum alkaline phosphatase level.

The best means of identifying a biliary stricture are ultrasonography to confirm the presence of dilated ducts and percutaneous transhepatic cholangiography to identify the level and extent of the stricture and to help plan the subsequent repair.

Table 29–6. Causes of benign bile duct strictures.

Congenital strictures
    Biliary atresia
Bile duct injuries
    Postoperative strictures following
        Cholecystectomy and/or common bile duct exploration
        Biliary–enteric anastomosis
        Hepatic resection
        Portacaval shunt
        Pancreatic surgery
        Gastrectomy
        Miscellaneous procedures
    Strictures following blunt or penetrating trauma
Inflammatory strictures associated with
    Cholelithiasis or choledocholithiasis
    Chronic pancreatitis
    Chronic duodenal ulcer
    Abscess or inflammation in subhepatic region or in liver
    Parasitic infection
    Recurrent pyogenic cholangitis (oriental cholangiohepatitis)
Primary sclerosing cholangitis
Radiation-induced stricture
Papillary stenosis

Reprinted and modified, with permission, from Matthews JB, Blumgart LH: Benign biliary strictures. In: Blumgart LH (editor): *Surgery of the Liver and Biliary Tract,* 2nd ed. Churchill Livingstone, 1994, p. 865.

Management

Acute management of patients with a benign biliary stricture include administration of antibiotics and percutaneous biliary drainage with external or internal catheters to treat the obstruction. This is especially important for the patient with associated cholangitis. The best method of surgical repair of a biliary stricture is resection of the bile duct with an end-to-side Roux-en-Y hepaticojejunostomy. One of the main factors influencing a positive surgical outcome in these patients is the number of operations the patient has previously undergone. Therefore, initial satisfactory repair is of great importance. Approximately 90% of patients have successful operative repair of their biliary stricture, especially in the hands of an experienced surgeon. The operative mortality rate is reported as between 5% and 8%. The most common causes of death are uncontrolled hemorrhage, hepatic or renal failure, or a combination of both of these complications. In recent years, some benign strictures have been managed long-term by a series of percutaneous transhepatic balloon dilatations with or without internalized wall stents (30 French). A team approach with a surgeon and interventional radiologist is best positioned to select patients that might be successfully managed in this fashion and to know when to intervene surgically.

SCLEROSING CHOLANGITIS

Diagnosis

Sclerosing cholangitis is an inflammatory disease that causes chronic cholestasis, obliterative fibrosis, and multiple strictures of the bile ducts. The average age at presentation is 40–45 years, and males are more often affected than females. It has an incidence of between 10 and 40 per million population. The disease often progresses to cirrhosis with complications of portal hypertension. The cause of this disease remains unknown despite several proposed causes, including those arising from autoimmune, bacterial, congenital, viral, or drug- and toxin-induced disorders. The intra-arterial infusion of the chemotherapeutic agent floxuridine has been associated with features of sclerosing cholangitis. It is interesting that HLA haplotypes HLA-B2 and HLA-DX3 are more often present in patients with primary sclerosing cholangitis. These are the haplotypes most commonly found with autoimmune diseases. The common hepatitis viruses do not appear to play an etiologic role. Animal studies have suggested the possibility that toxins absorbed from the inflamed colon as well as bacterial peptides lead to a release of cytokines in the liver, causing ductal inflammation and injury. It is known, however, that approximately 70% of patients with sclerosing cholangitis have associated ulcerative colitis and, less commonly, Crohn's colitis. In most patients, the diagnosis of ulcerative colitis is established before symptoms of sclerosing cholangitis occur. The risk of patients with ulcerative colitis is estimated to be approximately 5%.

The signs and symptoms for sclerosing cholangitis are outlined in Table 29–7. The most common laboratory findings are elevated serum alkaline phosphatase and gamma glutamyl transferase levels. Radiographic diagnosis is best made using ERCP to access the ductal system for cholangiography. It is important to recognize that patients with primary sclerosing cholangitis have a unique increased risk of developing cholangiocarcinoma. Approximately 10% will develop this cancer.

Management

A liver biopsy is often indicated and is not only helpful in supporting the diagnosis but also in determining prognosis. However, liver biopsy in patients with ulcerative colitis has recently been reported to result in a pattern of small duct sclerosis in some patients; speculation exists as to whether this is a separate entity or simply an earlier stage of primary sclerosing cholangitis. Autoantibodies are often found, but their role in the actual disease process is unclear and, at least at this writing, they have not become an important diagnostic or prognostic tool.

Some patients progress rapidly to hepatic failure while others remain asymptomatic for years. Extrahepatic and hilar strictures can be managed using endoscopic procedures, such as balloon dilatation and stenting, and ursodeoxycholic acid has also proven effective in some patients. A dose regimen of 10–15 mg/kg/d in three to four divided doses has been used in most clinical studies, but determination of the exact benefit awaits completion of these trials. Some patients with strictures primarily located in the extrahepatic region may benefit from a Roux-en-Y hepaticojejunostomy. Patients with recurrent cholangitis or those with associated extensive cirrhosis may be effectively managed with liver transplantation. Prognosis varies but, on the average, the patient survives with progressive liver disease lasting approximately 10 years. The 5-year survival of patients managed with liver transplantation is essentially the same as that for patients with primary biliary cirrhosis, but these patients appear to require more retransplantation procedures.

Table 29–7. Symptoms and signs in primary sclerosing cholangitis.

Symptom or Sign	Percent at Presentation
Jaundice	45–55
Pruritus	40–50
Pain	45–50
Weight loss	25–30
Anorexia	35–40
Cholangitis	20–25
Asymptomatic	20–25
Hepatomegaly	50–60
Splenomegaly	30–35

Reprinted and modified, with permission, from Ahrendt SA, Pitt HA: Sclerosing cholangitis. In: Zinner MJ, Schwartz SI, Ellis H (editors): *Maingot's Abdominal Operations,* 10th ed. Appleton & Lange, 1997, p. 1794.

BILIARY TRACT CARCINOMA

Cancers of the biliary system are relatively uncommon and are often divided into intrahepatic cholangiocarcinoma, extrahepatic cholangiocarcinoma, gallbladder carcinoma, and tumors of the distal bile duct or ampullary cancer. In general, these tumors are difficult to manage successfully and have a high mortality-to-incidence ratio.

1. CHOLANGIOCARCINOMA

Diagnosis

Cholangiocarcinoma accounts for less than 10% of primary liver cancer. They have their origin from the epithelial cells in intrahepatic and extrahepatic bile ducts. More specifically, it is hypothesized that these cancers arise from a pluripotent stem cell of periductal glands. They are relatively rare, with a necropsy incidence variously reported between 0.089% and 0.46%, which is obviously higher in the jaundiced. Only a slight male predominance exists, and they tend to occur during the sixth and seventh decades of life.

Cholangiocarcinomas arising within the liver tend to become quite large before causing symptoms leading to diagnosis. The second group occurring at the bifurcation of the right and left bile ducts (Klatskin's tumor) are more likely to cause jaundice early in their growth. Similarly, tumors of the extrahepatic biliary tree, especially the distal common bile duct or papilla of Vater, have a more favorable prognosis because they produce signs of obstruction while the tumor is still quite small.

Several risk factors exist. For example, primary sclerosing cholangitis (7–9% will develop tumors), chronic ulcerative colitis (31-fold increase in relative risk), *Clonorchis sinensis* parasitic infection (liver flukes), as well as other biliary parasites induce hyperplasia and adenomatous proliferation within the ducts. Patients with choledochal cysts have a 3% risk of developing cholangiocarcinoma. Thirty percent have a history of stone disease. Other factors include polycystic liver disease, a history of thorotrast radiocontrast agent exposure, and α_1-antitrypsin deficiency.

Histologically, cholangiocarcinomas are mucin-secreting adenocarcinomas; this feature is often helpful in differentiating the tumor from hepatocellular cancer. Although greater than 90% of bile duct tumors are adenocarcinomas, occasionally a squamous cell tumor, a leiomyosarcoma, or very undifferentiated histological characteristics will be found.

Obstructive jaundice is the main feature of presentation. Alkaline phosphatase is elevated in greater than 90%. Serum carcinoembryonic antigen (CEA) is abnormal in less than 5%. Other important clinical findings include hepatomegaly (50–60%) and occult fecal blood (50%). In most patients, tumors are deemed unresectable at the time they present. CT scan is important in defining the extent of the tumor and whether metastases are suspected. MRI is considered helpful when the tumors are intrahepatic and often in this situation provides better definition of tumor borders.

Management

Percutaneous transhepatic cholangiography provides important information regarding the extent of the intraductal component and usually provides the most effective approach for decompression of the biliary ductal system. Frequently, tissue and cytological analysis can be obtained during this procedure. Interventional radiologists have routinely used angioplasty catheters to curette tumor and, occasionally, to direct choledochoscopy for visualization and biopsy. These are procedures generally available only in major treatment centers.

As noted, most patients with cholangiocarcinoma present at an advanced stage and are not candidates for resection. When this is the case, palliation consists of providing adequate decompression of the biliary ducts. Advances in stent design and manufacturing have significantly improved the ability to palliate these patients. New expandable metal stents can be placed through occluded ducts, either percutaneously for high lesions or endoscopically for distal duct lesions. They are expandable to 30 French and are a great improvement over the 10 or 12 French polyurethane stents used in the past. Tumor can grow through the interstices of the mesh, reoccluding the duct. This is managed by repeating the placement of a new stent inside of the old one. The expandable stents can be expected to remain patent at least 3 months in the vast majority of patients.

Further palliation may be achieved using newer techniques of conformal radiation, which specifically targets the tumor volume. This is usually done with protracted infusion of 5-fluorouracil (5-FU). In addition, responses have been reported using intraductal irradiation with ^{192}Ir wires. Chemotherapy consisting of mitomycin C, doxorubicin, and 5-FU has the greatest activity against cholangiocarcinoma, but the true response rates are relatively low ($\approx$ 29%), and median survivals are generally cited at, 6–12 months. Regional chemotherapy using floxuridine (FUDR) via the hepatic artery for proximal duct and intrahepatic tumors has some efficacy. A partial response rate of 43% with some prolongation of survival has been reported.

Of course, when possible, the treatment that offers the patient the best chance for prolonged survival is surgical resection. For Klatskin's (hilar) tumors, only about 30% will be resectable. The reported 5-year survival rates vary between 10% and 40% in the most optimistic reports. Some 62% can be expected to have localized regional recurrence. Recently, many have advocated resecting the caudate lobe, since this is a site of recurrence in almost all patients that fail. This undoubtedly occurs because bile ducts from the caudate lobe drain directly to the main left hepatic duct, and often to both left and right main ducts near the bifurcation. Such observations in recent years have led experienced liver surgeons to advocate en bloc liver resections as part of the resection of the extrahepatic duct system. Thus, either the surgeon performs an extended right hepatectomy with resection of caudate lobe and bile duct to the duodenum or, if the tumor is primarily left-sided, an extended left lobe resection. No 5-year survivors have been observed if margins of resection are microscopically positive, but there is some evidence that an aggressive resection does increase 5- and 10-year survival rates from 20% to 40% and 14%, respectively. Orthotopic liver transplantation has been reported in over 50 patients with hilar cholangiocarcinoma. At present, there is no evidence that transplantation offers any advantages over existing treatment.

Tumors arising in mid-common bile duct do not fare much better than the proximal tumors. Distal bile duct and papillary tumors are a different story; they have a more favorable prognosis. These tumors are managed by pancreaticoduodenectomy when deemed resectable (≈ 85% are resectable). The 5-year survival is at least 40% and appears to be improving, with at least one report as high as 62%. The prognosis is not as good if there is histological evidence of nodal spread. The majority of patients today receive additional 5-FU-based chemotherapy and radiation, even when surgical resection is potentially curative. What is truly needed are newer systemic agents with greater activity against these tumors. While they often appear indolent and slow-growing, they are rather relentless and, overall, fewer than 1% of patients with cholangiocarcinoma live 10 years.

2. GALLBLADDER CARCINOMA

Diagnosis

Adenocarcinoma of the gallbladder is more common than cholangiocarcinoma. It is the fifth most frequently diagnosed gastrointestinal malignancy. Currently, an estimated 6000–7000 cases are diagnosed each year in the United States. The autopsy incidence has been stated at 0.4–0.55%. Gallbladder cancer occurs most frequently in the sixth and seventh decades of life, with a 3:1 ratio of females to males. Over the last several decades, there has been evidence of a slight increase in this type of cancer.

Gallbladder cancer is found almost exclusively in patients with gallstones and, very interestingly, is six times more common among American Indians of the southwestern area of the United States. Mexican-Americans, Japanese-Americans, and Northeastern Europeans also have a higher incidence of both cholelithiasis and gallbladder cancer.

As with so many of the tumors of the gastrointestinal tract, the exact causes and risks remain to be elucidated. A number of risk factors are summarized in Table 29–8. Interestingly, there does not appear to be any direct relationship between any of the hepatitis viruses, the presence of

Table 29–8. Risk factors for gallbladder cancer.

Cholelithiasis
Choledochal cysts
Anomalous pancreatic-biliary duct junction (APBDJ)
Carcinogens (azotoluene, nitrosamines)
Estrogens
Typhoid carriers
Porcelain gallbladder
Adenomatous gallbladder polyps

Reprinted, with permission, from Yeo CJ, Cameron JL: Tumors of the gallbladder and bile ducts. In: Zinner MJ, Schwartz SI, Ellis H (editors): *Maingot's Abdominal Operations,* 10th ed. Appleton & Lange, 1997, p. 1837.

cirrhosis, or, for that matter, any of the mycotoxins or hepatic toxins. There are perhaps two carcinogens, 3-methylcholanthrene and nitrosamines, that are associated with a slightly higher incidence. In laboratory models, while hepatocarcinogens failed to induce or increase the incidence of gallbladder cancer, over 50% of the animals receiving hepatocarcinogens developed gallbladder cancer when they were also fed a gallstone-inducing diet. Another interesting association between stone disease and gallbladder cancer is the observation that the risk of developing cancer increases directly with enlarging stone diameter. For example, patients with stones 2.0–2.9 cm in diameter have a relative risk of 2.4. This increases to 10.1 when the stones are greater than 3.0 in diameter.

Another observation is the increased risk associated with calcification of the gallbladder wall—the so-called **porcelain gallbladder**. When this entity is discovered on radiography, the risk of the gallbladder having an adenocarcinoma present is at least 22%. It is also important to note that areas of mucosal dysplasia, atypical hyperplasia, discreet adenomas, as well as carcinoma-in-situ have been found in most gallbladders harboring invasive cancer. These findings raise the possibility that anything causing chronic inflammatory changes could induce transformation in a progressive fashion, beginning with the premalignant lesion. Finally, it has been observed that at least 17% of patients with gallbladder cancer have an anomalous confluence of the terminal bile duct and pancreatic duct. The incidence of this anomalous confluence is 3% in non-cancer populations. It has been postulated by various observers that this confluence results in a reflux of pancreatic secretions into the gallbladder, inducing mucosal inflammation. This has never been proven and this degree of reflux would seem to be physiologically difficult.

Histopathology. Greater than 90% of cancers of the gallbladder are adenocarcinomas, either scirrhous or papillary. The remaining 10% are comprised of anaplastic histologic types, such as adenoacanthoma, squamous cell carcinoma, and, very rarely, reported as a carcinoid tumor or embryonal rhabdomyosarcoma. Mucin production and signet ring cells are frequent findings. The cancer invades the muscle of the gallbladder wall and into the adventitial layers. Invasion into vascular spaces, lymphatic channels, and perineural sheaths is common and indicates aggressive behavior.

Only 10% are found incidentally with invasion confined to the gallbladder wall. Thus, most patients present with advanced disease, tumor extending into the liver and into regional structures. Extension into the liver indicates more widespread disease will be found in almost 90% of patients. The extrahepatic bile ducts are involved by direct extension of the tumor in 57% of cases and the duodenum, stomach, or colon in 40% when the liver is involved. Over half will have lymph node involvement. The American Joint Committee on Cancer staging system for gallbladder cancer is outlined in Table 29–9.

Symptoms are similar to those of patients with acute cholecystitis and include right upper quadrant pain (40–65%), jaundice (45%), and weight loss (37–77%), depending on the report. CEA levels for stage III or IV tumors is elevated in 80%. CT and high-resolution ultrasonography can identify early cancers, even as small as 5 mm in diameter, and are predictive in 88–95% of patients. Dynamic (dual-phase) CT is the most accurate way of defining the extent of tumor and determining resectability.

Management

Only 10–30% of patients are found to be candidates for curative resection. The extent of ideal resection is somewhat controversial but, in general, for early tumors found incidentally at the time of elective cholecystectomy and confined to the mucosa (T1aN0M0), cholecystectomy is felt to be adequate treatment. The incidence of positive lymph nodes has been reported as only 2.5% in such patients, thus making it difficult to justify the operative mortality (2%) and morbidity (30%) associated with aggressive nodal resections. On the other hand, T2 lesions have a much greater incidence of nodal metastases (> 50%) and even T1b lesions, in which the tumor invades the muscle layer, have a 15% incidence. For these stages, an aggressive "radical cholecystectomy" is the treatment most often employed.

For stage III, IV, and resected stage II tumors, most surgeons offer a more aggressive resection that includes the extrahepatic bile duct below the bifurcation (approximately 57% have invasion of the common bile duct). For stage V tumor that invades the liver, a resection of the lower segments of the right lobe of the liver is included. The Japanese have described hepatopancreaticoduodenectomy for locally advanced gallbladder cancer. The operative mortality rate of 15% and a 90% incidence of major morbidity would seem to preclude such approaches, since survival benefit cannot be demonstrated. Radical operations are rarely performed in this country, although occasional palliative procedures have included portal vein and hepatic artery resection with vascular reconstruction.

With 70,000 laparoscopic cholecystectomies performed per year in the Unites States for benign disease, the expected number of patients that will be found to have an unrecognized gallbladder cancer is approximately 1400 patients annually. Careful decisions will need to be made concerning accurate staging of their tumors and appropriate therapy.

The majority of patients with gallbladder cancer not found incidentally at laparoscopic cholecystectomy, unfortunately present with advanced tumor. Thus, taking all patients with carcinoma, the mean time of survival is 6–8 months and the 5-year survival is 5%. The obstructed bile ducts are palliated by percutaneous transhepatic stenting or, if it is determined that the tumor is unresectable at the time of laparotomy, a biliary-enteric bypass can be performed. Perhaps, as many as half of the patients with advanced gallbladder cancer will go on to develop gastric outlet obstruction from advancing tumor. These patients are managed by gastrojejunostomy or, if life expectancy is limited, by placement of a gastrostomy and feeding jejunostomy tube using, if possible, minimally invasive approaches.

Such patients are also offered chemotherapy initially with a combination of 5-FU and doxorubicin. Response rates are at best approximately 40%, but of limited duration. Radiation is given to a dose of at least 45 Gy, higher with conformal techniques. All of these approaches must be considered palliative, with most patients succumbing to their disease in 11 months or less. It is virtually impossible to evaluate therapies in a prospective fashion because of the low incidence of this tumor, but, to date, aggressive approaches have not provided any evidence for significant increases in the length of time patients can survive. A multidisciplinary approach to patients who unfortunately develop gallbladder cancer is essential.

Table 29–9. TNM staging for gallbladder cancer.

Stage	Tumor	Nodes	Metastases	5-year Survival Post-resection (%)
0	Tis	N0	M0	100
I	T1	N0	M0	85
II	T2	N0	M0	25–65
III	T1–2	N1	M0	10
	T3	N0–1	M0	
IV	T1–4	N2	M0	2
	T1–4	N0–2	M1	

Tis = Carcinoma in situ; T1 = Tumor limited to mucosa or muscularis; T2 = Tumor invades serosa; T3 = Tumor invades liver (< 2 cm) or one adjacent organ; T4 = Tumor extends > 2 cm into liver or two or more adjacent organs; N0 = No nodal involvement; N1 = Metastases in cystic duct, bile duct ,or hilar lymph nodes; N2 = Metastases in other lymph nodes; M0 = No distant metastases; M1 = Distant metastases.

Reprinted and modified, with permission, from Yeo CJ, Cameron JL: Tumors of the gallbladder and bile ducts. In: Zinner MJ, Schwartz SI, Ellis H (editors): *Maingot's Abdominal Operations*, 10th ed. Appleton & Lange, 1997, p. 1836.

SUGGESTED READING

Blumgart LH: *Surgery of the Liver and Biliary Tract*, 2nd ed. Churchill Livingstone, 1994.

Curly SA et al: Liver and bile ducts. In: Abeloff MD et al (editors): *Clinical Oncology*. Churchill Livingstone, 1995.

McFadden DW, Gadacz TR: Calculous diseases of the gallbladder and common bile duct. In: Miller TA (editor): *Physiologic Basis of Modern Surgical Care*. Mosby, 1988.

Warren KW et al: *Atlas of Surgery of the Liver, Pancreas, and Biliary Tract*. Appleton & Lange, 1991.

Zinner MJ et al: *Maingot's Abdominal Operations*, 10th ed. Appleton & Lange, 1997.

30

The Spleen & Lymphatics

Mark Vierra, MD

▶ Key Facts

- ▶ The adult spleen weighs approximately 100–175 g and measures approximately 14 cm in its greatest dimension.

- ▶ Accessory spleens occur in about 15–30% of patients and are usually found in close proximity to the splenic hilus.

- ▶ In adults, the spleen maintains certain immune functions, acts as a mechanical filter of the blood, and also plays an important role in antibody production, particularly in the production of IgM class immunoglobulins.

- ▶ Today, splenectomy is most commonly performed for certain hematologic illnesses, especially idiopathic thrombocytopenic purpura and hypersplenic states.

- ▶ The spleen is the most commonly injured intra-abdominal organ in blunt trauma. Nonoperative management may be used in selected circumstances.

- ▶ In selected patients, splenectomy may be performed laparoscopically. In general, this technique is best employed in cases in which the spleen is of normal size or only moderately enlarged.

- ▶ Complications of splenectomy include injury to the diaphragm, pancreas, stomach, and splenic flexure of the colon, pancreatic fistula, pleural effusion, hemorrhage (intraoperatively or postoperatively), and postsplenectomy sepsis.

- ▶ Postsplenectomy sepsis occurs rarely in patients who have undergone splenectomy. It is more common in young children and patients with underlying malignancies.

- ▶ Lymphedema is commonly described as primary lymphedema (uncommon idiopathic disorders that almost always involve the lower extremity) or secondary lymphedema (acquired as a consequence of some recognized trauma to the lymphatic drainage of an extremity or extremities).

THE SPLEEN

The spleen is an organ of the reticuloendothelial system. While not essential to life, it does participate in immune function, especially in the young. Splenectomy may be indicated when the spleen is damaged by trauma, for diagnostic purposes (eg, lymphoma), for symptoms of splenic enlargement or excess function (splenomegaly, hypersplenism), and for some hematologic illnesses.

ANATOMY & PHYSIOLOGY

The adult spleen weighs approximately 100–175 g and measures approximately 14 cm in its greatest dimension. In some disease states, however, the spleen may achieve massive proportions, weighing up to several kilos.

The spleen receives its blood supply from the splenic artery, which also gives off vessels to the greater curvature of the stomach via the short gastric arteries. Venous drainage is via the splenic vein, which is joined by the inferior mesenteric and superior mesenteric veins to become the portal vein. There is also venous drainage via short veins that drain to the greater curvature of the stomach. These veins are parallel to the short gastric arteries (Figure 30–1).

The spleen can usually survive even if the main splenic artery or vein is interrupted, relying on collaterals from the short gastric arteries and veins. Arterial or venous infarction may occur, however, and interruption of the splenic vein alone may be followed by the development of gastric varices or portal hypertensive gastropathy.

The spleen is attached to the diaphragm and posterior abdominal wall over the kidney and to the splenic flexure of the left colon by peritoneal reflections referred to as the **gastrosplenic**, **splenolienal**, and **splenocolic ligaments**. The short gastric arteries and veins run within the gastrosplenic ligament, while the other two ligaments are typically avascular.

An important point of surgical anatomy is that the spleen can be rotated toward the midline and delivered out of the recesses of the left upper quadrant without injuring or dividing any of its blood vessels. This is accomplished by dividing the posterior attachments of the spleen to the diaphragm, kidney, and colon. Once this is accomplished, the spleen can be elevated into the midline along with the tail of the pancreas and the greater curvature of the stomach. With the spleen elevated into the wound, it is easier and safer to control the vessels without injury to the tail of the pancreas or the stomach.

Accessory spleens occur in 15–30% of patients (Figure 30–2). **Accessory spleens** are generally found in close proximity to the splenic hilus, but may lie anywhere along the course of the splenic artery or vein, or in the greater omentum. Following splenectomy, these accessory spleens may retain some, although unpredictable, level of function, which is desirable if the splenectomy is performed for trauma but not if splenectomy has been performed for a hematologic illness, such as idiopathic thrombocytopenic purpura (ITP). The accessory splenic tissue left behind may hypertrophy, reproducing the problem. Thus, in performing splenectomy for diseases characterized by excessive splenic function, care is taken to look for accessory spleens.

During fetal development the spleen plays an important role in hematopoiesis, and though the spleen retains this potential throughout life, it generally ceases during about the fifth month of gestation. In the adult, it maintains certain immune functions and also acts to filter the blood, culling old cells, the nuclei of new red cells, and small impurities, such as Heinz bodies, Pappenheimer bodies, and spur cells that can be recognized in the circulation of patients who are asplenic. The spleen also filters bacteria, and is particularly important in the clearance of encapsulated bacteria, such as pneumococcus, hemophilus, and meningococcus. Its role in cancer surveillance is less clear. It is striking that despite its rich blood supply, intrasplenic metastases from tumors of the gastrointestinal tract are rare.

The spleen is also important in antibody production, particularly the production of IgM-class immunoglobulins. Larger antigens, in particular, are captured in the spleen, where they are transported to the germinal centers and presented to macrophages. There, the IgM response is thought to occur, and indeed, IgM antibody levels fall in asplenic individuals.

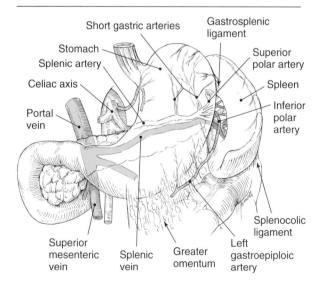

Figure 30–1. Anatomy of the spleen.

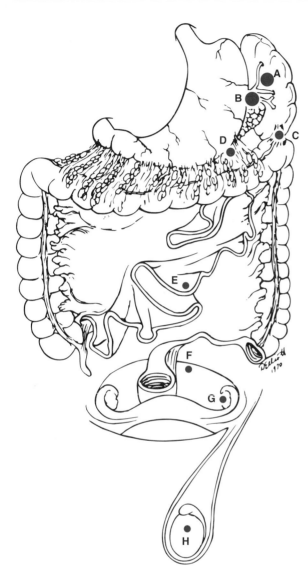

Figure 30–2. Location of accessory spleens. **A:** Splenic hilus. **B:** Along splenic vessels; tail of pancreas. **C:** Splenocolic ligament. **D:** Greater omentum; perirenal regions. **E:** Mesentery. **F:** Presacral region. **G:** Adnexal region. **H:** Peritesticular region. (Reprinted, with permission, from Schwartz SI, Adams JT, Bauman AW: Splenectomy for hematologic disorders. Curr Prob Surg, May 1971, p. 49.)

INDICATIONS FOR SPLENECTOMY

GENERAL INDICATIONS

Indications for splenectomy are changing. Trauma and the staging of Hodgkin's lymphoma have become increasingly uncommon reasons for the performance of a splenectomy. Today, splenectomy is most commonly per-

formed for hematologic illnesses, especially ITP and hypersplenic states. It is important to distinguish splenomegaly (splenic enlargement) from hypersplenism (excessive splenic function). Splenomegaly, per se, is not an indication for splenectomy, though early satiety, pain, or other local symptoms of splenic enlargement may be indications for splenectomy even in the absence of excessive splenic function.

More commonly, splenectomy may be indicated for symptoms of hypersplenism. It is important to recognize that while most patients with hypersplenism have at least mild splenomegaly, this is not always or necessarily the case. Hypersplenism produces cytopenias—anemia, neutropenia, or thrombocytopenia. These may be dangerous by themselves or may prohibit adequate chemotherapy necessary to treat the underlying illness.

TRAUMA

The spleen is the most commonly injured intra-abdominal organ in blunt trauma, and though the nonoperative management of splenic trauma has become increasingly common, laparotomy for both splenectomy and splenic repair continues to be necessary. In general, a trial of nonoperative management may be indicated in the hemodynamically stable patient who does not require a laparotomy for the repair of other injuries. Operation with splenic repair and salvage may be considered in patients with more severely injured spleens who do not respond to resuscitation using colloid or blood, or in patients with splenic injuries who require laparotomy for other reasons. Deep hilar injuries are not likely to be reparable, and heroic attempts at splenic repair, especially if this requires transfusion of additional blood products, is not indicated.

In children, much more severe splenic injuries may be tolerated and treated nonoperatively, in part because children seem to have a greater capacity to achieve spontaneous hemostasis than do adults, but also because the risk of postsplenectomy sepsis is far greater in children than in adults.

HEMOLYTIC DISORDERS

Among the Coomb's negative hemolytic disorders, hereditary spherocytosis, elliptocytosis, and the thalassemias generally respond well to splenectomy. Depending on the clinical course, splenectomy is usually deferred until after childhood to reduce the risks of postsplenectomy sepsis. Splenectomy is rarely indicated for sickle cell anemia and is not indicated for pyruvate kinase deficiency or G6PD deficiency.

Coomb's positive hemolytic anemias rarely demonstrate a durable response to steroids, though this is usually the initial treatment. Splenectomy, however, produces a durable response in about 60% of patients and may lessen steroid requirements, even in those patients who remain steroid-dependent.

ITP & TTP

Idiopathic thrombocytopenic purpura remains a common indication for splenectomy, producing a durable benefit in about three out of four patients. Interestingly, these patients may have surprisingly few bleeding complications, even with significant thrombocytopenia, presumably because their platelets maintain entirely normal function. Splenectomy is clearly indicated in patients who do not respond to steroids, but is generally indicated even in patients who are steroid-responsive but who remain steroid-dependent because of the significant side effects of prolonged steroid use. Patients who do not respond to steroids are also less likely to respond to splenectomy, but this is not invariably the case, and patients who fail steroids should be offered the option of splenectomy.

Thrombotic thrombocytopenic purpura (TTP) is much rarer than ITP and is most commonly treated with plasmapheresis, plasma exchange, steroids, and antiplatelet drugs. Splenectomy is rarely necessary but may be curative.

HYPERSPLENISM & SPLENOMEGALY

Hypersplenism and splenomegaly occur commonly in the setting of hepatic cirrhosis and portal hypertension. Splenectomy is rarely indicated under these circumstances. Splenorenal shunt usually produces sufficient improvement in counts that splenectomy is not necessary. More recently, liver transplantation has increasingly been used in this setting. With restoration of normal portal pressures after transplantation, splenectomy is rarely necessary. TIPS procedures (transhepatic, transjugular, interventionally placed intrahepatic portosystemic shunts) have all but replaced surgical shunt procedures, especially in patients for whom liver transplantation may be a future possibility.

Hypersplenism and splenomegaly occur commonly in agnogenic myeloid metaplasia and myelofibrosis, and splenectomy is sometimes indicated. Although it might seem that removal of an organ involved in extramedullary hematopoiesis might exacerbate anemia, this does not occur in practice. These patients are often hypermetabolic and have symptoms related to the size of the spleen, as well as cytopenias secondary to hypersplenism, and may benefit dramatically from splenectomy.

Chronic myelocytic leukemia, chronic lymphocytic leukemia, and, less commonly, hairy cell leukemia remain diseases in which splenectomy continues to play a role. Most commonly, splenectomy is indicated in patients who have difficulty tolerating chemotherapy due to their cytopenias. Occassionally, local symptoms (pain and satiety) from splenomegaly may be an indication for splenectomy.

Splenic vein thrombosis, most commonly related to pancreatitis or pancreatic neoplasm, may produce gastric and esophageal varices as well as hypersplenism. The treatment of choice is splenectomy, which is generally curative.

Lymphoma also remains an uncommon indication for splenectomy. At times, splenectomy may be indicated to achieve a diagnosis; more commonly, difficulty with cytopenias during chemotherapy may be an indication for splenectomy.

Splenectomy for staging of Hodgkin's lymphoma was once commonly performed in patients who were felt to be clinically stage 1 or 2, that is, with disease localized only above the diaphragm. Those patients could be treated with radiotherapy alone with excellent results, and staging laparotomy was commonly performed to rule out disease below the diaphragm in order to guide treatment. Approximately 30% of such patients were upstaged by splenectomy when they were found to have splenic involvement not suspected preoperatively. Currently, however, most patients are treated with chemotherapy, and radiation therapy alone for stage I or II disease is uncommon. With improvements in our imaging capabilities and greater confidence in our ability to stage patients radiographically, few patients now undergo staging laparotomy. Furthermore, salvage with chemotherapy for patients who relapse after radiotherapy alone has become sufficiently reliable to alleviate fears that a patient might be understaged and relapse. Staging laparotomy for Hodgkin's lymphoma, therefore, is now rarely performed.

MISCELLANEOUS CONDITIONS

Splenectomy may be performed for a number of more unusual conditions. Splenic abscesses are uncommon and are generally treated by splenectomy. Rarely, percutaneous drainage may be appropriate. Primary tumors of the spleen are uncommon apart from lymphomas; most of the remaining tumors have their origins in the blood vessel of the spleen, such as angiosarcomas.

Most splenic cysts are benign. Epithelial-lined (true) cysts may be congenital and multiple, rarely causing symptoms. Many cysts are actually pseudocysts, which lack an epithelial lining. These may arise following trauma, producing an intrasplenic blood clot or splenic fracture, or following pancreatitis.

Metabolic diseases, such as Gaucher's disease, may occasionally be an indication for splenectomy, but these diseases are extremely rare.

TECHNIQUE OF SPLENECTOMY

In an open splenectomy, either a midline or a left subcostal incision may be employed; rarely, a splenectomy may be performed through a left thoracotomy. In the classic open splenectomy, the lateral and posterior attachments of the spleen are divided, often by feel and without the aid of direct vision; the splenic flexure of the colon and greater omentum (splenocolic ligament) is separated from the lower pole of the spleen; and the spleen is delivered toward the midline. By bringing the spleen, along with the tail of the pancreas and the greater curvature of the stomach, into the midline, exposure is greatly facilitated (Figure 30–3A). This gives the operating surgeon easy access to the hilar structures and minimizes the risk of bleeding because the vessels are easily accessible.

Sometimes, due to size or adhesions, the spleen may not be easily rotated toward the midline. In this situation, the surgeon mobilizes the stomach away from the upper pole of the spleen by carefully dividing the short gastric arteries. The splenic artery and vein are ligated anteriorly in the splenic hilum.

Often, but not always, the splenic artery may be ligated first as it runs along the dorsal aspect of the pancreas (Figure 30–3B). This may allow some decompression of the spleen, making it easier to manipulate. Platelet adminis-

tration is usually deferred until after the spleen is removed, to prevent platelet sequestration.

Once the splenic artery and vein and the short gastric vessels are divided and ligated and the spleen is removed (Figure 30–3C), a careful search for accessory spleens should be carried out, depending on the indication for splenectomy (Figure 30–2).

When the hilar vessels are divided, care is taken to identify the pancreatic tail and to avoid pancreatic injury. If there is any possibility that the tail of the pancreas has been traumatized, it is appropriate to leave a drain for a few days in case there is a pancreatic leak. This is the only indication for which drainage is appropriate, and the drain should be a closed suction type to minimize the risk of infection. A considerable period of time should be devoted to the achievement of complete hemostasis, to assure that all peritoneal attachments that have been divided are dry.

In selected patients, splenectomy may be performed laparoscopically. In general, this technique is best employed in cases in which the spleen is of normal size or only moderately enlarged. It requires considerable technical expertise, but the technical details are very much like those for

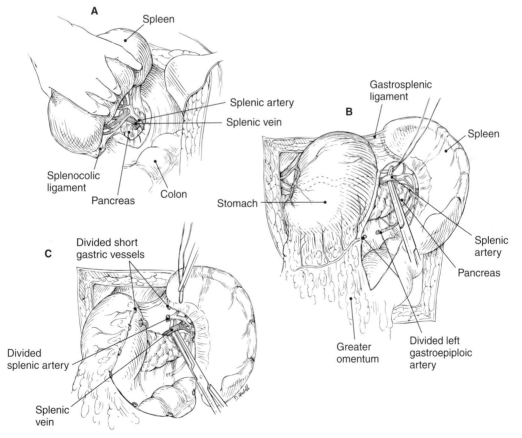

Figure 30–3. Technique of splenectomy. **A:** The spleen is elevated toward the midline to expose the splenic artery, splenic vein, and tail of the pancreas. **B:** The splenic artery may be ligated to allow for decompression of the spleen, making it easier to manipulate. **C:** The main splenic vein is carefully encircled with a 2-0 ligature. The splenic vein is then divided and the specimen removed

an open splenectomy. The patient is usually placed in the decubitus position with the left side elevated. This position helps to mimic the maneuver in open surgery in which the spleen is delivered into the midline. Once the splenic vessels and attachments are divided and the spleen is free, the spleen is placed into a bag, which is exteriorized through the umbilical port. The spleen may then be fractured and removed in pieces or morcellated if histological evaluation is not critical. Hospital stay is generally shortened and postoperative recovery is certainly easier for the patient, but operating times are at least twice that for an open splenectomy, and standards for patient selection are not yet well defined.

A nasogastric tube may be left in place after the procedure for a day or two, though increasingly this practice is being abandoned. It is important to be vigilant about the possibility of gastric distension, however, for all of the obvious reasons, and also because of fears that distension of the greater curvature of the stomach may cause ties or clips on the short gastric vessels to become dislodged, thereby producing postoperative hemorrhage.

COMPLICATIONS OF SPLENECTOMY

Splenectomy is almost always performed in patients with a serious underlying illness, upon which the risk and nature of complications is highly dependent. Anatomically, the diaphragm, pancreas, stomach, and splenic flexure of the colon are all at risk of injury during splenectomy. This risk may be increased in the presence of hilar adenopathy or previous splenic infarction, which may produce scarring to adjacent structures.

The pancreas is particularly at risk, as it may be so intimately associated with the hilum of the spleen that it is impossible to remove the spleen without transecting a small portion of the tail of the pancreas. Pancreatic fistula may occur in such instances, but this is usually not a problem if the splenic bed is well drained. The possibility of injury to the tail of the pancreas probably represents the only circumstance in which the placement of a drain into the splenic bed is indicated. The stomach may also be intimately associated with the spleen, and, rarely, a small portion of the greater curvature of the stomach may be removed with the spleen. This is most likely to be necessary in lymphoma, in which bulky hilar disease may make safe dissection of the spleen from the stomach impossible, or in which gastrosplenic fistula may have occurred.

Most patients undergoing splenectomy will suffer some degree of left lower lobe pulmonary atelectasis or small pleural effusion. This is seldom dangerous, but may predispose elderly and frail patients to pneumonia.

Hemorrhage, either intraoperatively or postoperatively, may be a serious risk, in part because of the rich blood supply to the spleen and also because of the illnesses for which splenectomy is indicated. Many patients may have

an associated coagulopathy not apparent on routine hematologic screening studies. While the risk of bleeding in a patient with ITP and a very low platelet count may be obvious, the patient with agnogenic myeloid metaplasia or chronic myelogenous leukemia is likely to have a far greater bleeding tendency, despite an apparently normal coagulation profile.

Postoperatively, most patients will have temporary thrombocytosis and leukocytosis—this is a normal phenomenon—and should be recognized without causing alarm. All patients will also thereafter have an abnormal peripheral blood smear, with such findings as Howell-Jolly bodies, Heinz bodies, and Pappenheimer bodies. This is probably of no real consequence.

Postsplenectomy thrombocytosis is common and has not been consistently demonstrated to correlate with an increased risk of thrombotic complications. On the other hand, some illnesses for which splenectomy is indicated—in particular, the agnogenic myeloid metaplasias and lymphomas—may predispose the patient to an increased risk of thrombotic complications; therefore, careful postoperative observation or specific therapy is warranted. Pneumatic compression boots should be used in all such patients during the operation, and in select patients, particularly those with a lupus anticoagulant, low-dose heparin may be indicated postoperatively. Splenic and portal vein thrombosis may occur and, on rare occasions, extend into the portal vein, resulting in death.

Postsplenectomy sepsis is an uncommon, but devastating, complication of splenectomy. As classically described, it is an overwhelming, rapidly progressive, and frequently fatal sepsis caused by an encapsulated gram-negative organism, usually pneumococcus or *Haemophilus influenzae*. The risk appears to be greatest in very young children and within the first 2 years following splenectomy. It is a far greater risk in patients with an underlying malignancy than in patients who have lost their spleens due to trauma, ITP, or hereditary spherocytosis. In young children without an underlying malignancy (eg, those undergoing splenectomy for trauma or spherocytosis), the lifetime risk of postsplenectomy sepsis is probably about 2%. In adults, the risk is substantially lower and may be negligible without an underlying immune suppressive disorder.

Vaccinations against pneumococcus and *H. influenzae* are routinely given to all patients who are expected to undergo splenectomy; vaccination against meningococcus may be added, particularly in children. There is some accumulating evidence that patients who have undergone splenectomy may have a slightly increased risk of other types of infections, such as pneumonias and wound infections. This has been less well demonstrated.

In addition to vaccination against encapsulated organisms, prophylactic antibiotic therapy is often indicated for young children who have undergone splenectomy. Penicillin is frequently given for an indeterminate period, usually 250 mg once or twice daily. There have been no good studies documenting the efficacy of this, and there are no firm guidelines about how long such prophylaxis should continue.

THE LYMPHATICS

LYMPH NODE DISEASE & LYMPH NODE BIOPSY

Lymph node biopsy may be indicated for diagnostic purposes or for staging of malignant disease. In adults, an isolated, significantly enlarged lymph node without an obvious infectious explanation may be an indication to perform a biopsy without a period of observation. In children, it is uncommon to do this without an initial trial of antibiotics and an observation period of up to 6 weeks.

Each lymph node is fed by vascular and lymphatic channels that enter on the undersurface of the lymph node, along both ends of the long axis of the node. It is important to ligate these channels when removing all but the smallest of lymph nodes to prevent a lymphatic leak. Such leaks may be substantial, especially if a large lymph node(s) is removed, but most will usually be asymptomatic in the free peritoneal space. Disruption of major lymphatic channels in the upper abdomen or thorax may result in chylous ascites or chylothorax. Treatment of this is usually with total parenteral nutrition or an elemental diet with medium-chain triglycerides. Chylous ascites and chylothorax are significant complications; if they do not resolve, they may require reoperation, either to perform a peritoneovenous shunt or to attempt to ligate the leaking lymphatics. A lymph fistula from a subcutaneous lymphadenectomy, as from a groin dissection or an axillary node dissection, predisposes the patient to cellulitis and lymphangitis, which significantly increases the risk of subsequent lymphedema of the involved extremity.

If a lymph node biopsy is being performed to establish a diagnosis, cultures should be sent based on clinical suspicion. Lymphoma is almost always in the differential diagnoses, and if this is a consideration, the specimen should be given fresh to the pathologist so that a portion may be frozen to allow for immunoperoxidase studies.

Lymph nodes may be the primary site of tumors such as lymphomas and are common sites of metastases for other malignancies such as colon or breast cancer. Some tumors, such as sarcomas, rarely metastasize to lymph nodes.

In some cases, lymph node metastasis is best thought of as a marker of disease severity, and the rationale for lymphadenectomy is for staging to determine the need for adjuvant therapy. In breast cancer, for example, removal of regional lymph nodes may be of benefit in preventing axillary recurrence (see Chapter 35), but does not demonstrably improve overall survival. In other malignancies, lymphadenectomy constitutes an important therapeutic part of the operation. For example, approximately 35% of patients with lymph nodes involved by colon cancer will be cured by surgery alone that includes regional lymphadenectomy. This survival benefit is far greater than can be achieved by any known adjuvant chemotherapy in patients with residual nodal disease.

LYMPHATIC MALFORMATIONS

Lymphatic malformations, or lymphangiomas, are usually apparent at birth or within the first 2 years of life. They are rarely life-threatening, and are generally slow growing but may produce profound cosmetic deformities. They often require surgical attention, which is the only known effective therapy.

The lymphangioma that most commonly requires surgical attention at presentation is cystic hygroma. These lymphangiomas contain large, complex cystic channels and usually occur in the axilla, cervical region, or both. Less common are lymphangioma simplex and cavernous lymphangioma, which may also require surgical treatment.

LYMPHEDEMA

Lymphedema is commonly described as primary or secondary lymphedema. The primary lymphedemas are uncommon disorders that almost exclusively involve the lower extremities. The most common type is lymphedema praecox, which occurs primarily in girls at about the age of puberty. Fortunately, less common is lymphedema congenita, which is a particularly severe form of lymphedema present at birth or appearing shortly thereafter.

Secondary lymphedema is acquired as a consequence of some recognized trauma to the lymphatic drainage of an extremity or extremities. The most common cause of secondary lymphedema worldwide is infection with *Wuchereria bancrofti*, a filarial organism that may produce massive lymphedema, most commonly of one or both lower extremities. In industrialized countries, the most common cause of lymphedema is iatrogenic, primarily following surgical lymphadenectomy. Though much less common now, lymphedema following mastectomy and axillary dissection for breast cancer was once a common and profound consequence of that procedure. Radiation therapy may also produce lymphedema, though it is rare for this to occur unless a surgical lymphadenectomy has also been performed or lymphatic drainage has been additionally compromised by tumor or trauma. Severe trauma to an extremity may cause lymphedema, often with an additional element of venous insufficiency. Tumor alone is a rare cause of lymphedema.

Infection occurring in an extremity with compromised lymphatic drainage significantly increases the risk of severity of lymphedema and must be avoided, if possible, and treated aggressively if it occurs. Postoperative infections after lymphadenectomy usually require aggressive intravenous antibiotics. Patients should be particularly careful to avoid even minor trauma to an extremity following lymphadenectomy.

Lymphangiosarcoma is a very rare tumor that occurs almost exclusively in patients with long-standing lymphedema. It is often not recognized until late because of the degree of abnormality of the extremity, and it is usually rapidly progressive and fatal.

A thorough discussion of the therapy of lymphedema is beyond the scope of this chapter. However, most cases can be managed with elastic compression garments, elevation, meticulous hygiene, and sometimes with the use of intermittent pneumatic compression. It is important that these measures be used aggressively before the subcutaneous tissues become fibrotic and the swelling irreversible.

Less commonly, surgical therapies may be employed. Microvascular lymphatic-venous anastomoses have been carried out, but these are largely described as case reports, and significant experience is lacking. Transfer of normal tissue with intact lymphatic drainage has also been attempted in the hope that lymphatic connections could be recruited from within the abnormal extremity. This has met with limited success, however, and is not commonly employed.

More commonly, a variety of procedures that involve excision of much or all of the subcutaneous tissues and the placement of either skin grafts or skin flaps directly on muscle fascia may be employed. These are generally of predictable, though limited, benefit.

SUGGESTED READING

Clarke PJ, Morris PJ: Surgery of the spleen. In: Morris PJ, Malt RA (editors): *Oxford Textbook of Surgery*. Oxford University Press, 1994.

Dupuy DE, Raptoupoulos V, Fink MP: Current concepts in splenic trauma. J Intensive Care Med 1995;10:76.

Perry JF: Anatomy of the spleen, splenectomy, and excision of acessory spleens. In: Nyhus LM, Baker JR (editors): *Mastery of Surgery*. Little, Brown, 1984.

Schwartz SI: Spleen. In: Schwartz SI (editor): *Principles of Surgery*, 6th ed. McGraw Hill, 1994.

Shaw JHF, Print CG: Postsplenectomy sepsis. Br J Surg 1989;76:1074.

Wilhelm MC, Jones RE, Mitchener JS: Splenectomy in hematologic disorders. Ann Surg 1989;207:581.

31

The Pancreas

J. Augusto Bastidas, MD, & John E. Niederhuber, MD

▶ Key Facts

- ▶ The pancreas is divided into five sections: the head, uncinate process, neck, body, and tail.

- ▶ The hormonal secretions of the pancreas, including insulin, glucagon, somatostatin, gastrin, and pancreatic polypeptide, originate from the cells of the islets of Langerhans.

- ▶ Congenital abnormalities of the pancreas include annular pancreas, a ring of tissue around the duodenum that may lead to duodenal obstruction, and pancreatic divisum, the term for dorsal (Santorini) ductal variants.

- ▶ The two most common risk factors for acute pancreatitis are gallstones and excessive alcohol consumption.

- ▶ Acute pancreatitis is usually a self-limiting process that resolves with bowel rest.

- ▶ Pancreatic pseudocysts (chronic peripancreatic fluid collections) are most often managed with parenteral nutrition, analgesics, and complete bowel rest.

- ▶ Patients with chronic pancreatitis usually suffer from chronic alcohol use, have an intrinsic defect in the pancreatic duct (ie, duct stenosis or stricture), or have an uncorrected metabolic defect.

- ▶ The treatment of chronic pancreatitis is most often focused on managing alcohol intake, abdominal pain, and replacement of pancreatic enzymes to reverse the symptoms of fat malabsorption.

- ▶ Pancreatic trauma is usually the result of significant external forces most often associated with multiple injuries. Therefore, overall mortality and morbidity are high.

- ▶ Pancreatic islet cell tumors may be benign or malignant and are classically described as functioning or nonfunctioning. Insulinomas are the most common functioning islet cell tumors.

- ▶ Pancreatic cancer is the fifth leading cause of cancer deaths in the United States, with approximately 6000 new cases diagnosed per year.

- ▶ The mortality of a pancreaticoduodenectomy (Whipple procedure) in the past has been significant. However, in centers where this procedure is commonly performed, the mortality is no higher than 1–2%.

ANATOMY & PHYSIOLOGY

GROSS ANATOMY & EMBRYOLOGY

The pancreas is both an endocrine and exocrine gland located within the retroperitoneum of the upper abdomen. Embryologically, it begins its development as two pancreatic buds from the foregut, which are seen by the fifth week of gestation. By the seventh week there is fusion of ventral and dorsal pancreatic buds. This fusion process explains the anatomy of the adult gland and also explains the variants when this process is altered (ie, pancreatic divisum, annular pancreas).

The developed pancreas is divided into five sections (Figure 31–1). These sections include the head of the pancreas and uncinate process (derived from the ventral bud), and the neck, body, and tail of the pancreas (derived from the dorsal bud). The duct of Santorini is derived from the embryologic duct of the dorsal bud, and the duct of Wirsung is derived from the ventral duct. In the adult gland, the duct of Wirsung and its opening to the duodenum are dominant. The luminal connection of the duct of Santorini is often obliterated, but can persist as a second point of drainage (minor papilla), or, in some cases, the two ductal systems remain distinct (Figure 31–2).

The head of the pancreas lies within the C-loop of the duodenum. The body and tail lie in the posterior aspect of the lesser sac behind the stomach, and the tail of the pancreas approaches the hilum of the spleen. There is an extensive blood supply to the pancreas, including arterial branches from both the celiac axis as well as the superior mesenteric artery (SMA). The gastroduodenal artery is the main branch to the head of the pancreas. Branches from the gastroduodenal artery and branches of the inferior pancreaticoduodenal artery from the SMA form an anterior and posterior arcade in the head of the pancreas. The splenic artery supplies several branches to the body and tail of the pancreas. The venous drainage is comprised of multiple branches into the superior mesenteric vein, portal vein, and splenic vein.

The pancreas has extensive lymphatic drainage consisting of the peripancreaticoduodenal, pyloric, and portal lymph nodes that drain the head of the pancreas. Nodes at the root of the mesentery and periaortic nodes contribute to the drainage of the uncinate process. The body and tail of the pancreas drain predominantly into two chains of nodes, the inferior pancreatic chain and the superior pancreatic chain. The pancreas receives both sympathetic and parasympathetic innervation. These nerves contain both afferent and efferent fibers to help modulate blood flow, as well as endocrine and exocrine function.

HISTOLOGY

The three major cell types in the pancreas include: **epithelial duct cells**, **acinar cells**, and **endocrine cells**. The acinar cells synthesize, store, and secrete pancreatic enzymes. The ductal cells begin as intercalated ducts leading from the acini. These join to form the intralobular ducts, which then form the interlobular ducts that drain into the main pancreatic duct. Compared to the acinar cells, the duct cells lack a developed secretory architecture (zymogen granules and rough endoplasmic reticulum) and instead are responsible for water and electrolyte secretion.

The acini comprise approximately 80% of the whole pancreas. These cells are organized in clusters located at the ends of the smallest ductules (Figure 31–3). These polar cells exhibit prominent zymogen granules and condensing vacuoles, supported by a well developed Golgi apparatus.

The **islets of Langerhans** are composed of the endocrine cells in the pancreas. These islets are interspersed throughout the pancreas and are composed of cells that secrete individual hormones (Table 31–1).

EXOCRINE PHYSIOLOGY

Composition of Pancreatic Juice

The two major components of pancreatic exocrine secretions are digestive enzymes, which are secreted by the acinar cells, and bicarbonate, other electrolytes, and water, which are secreted by the centrolobular and the intercalated duct cells. These secretions combine to create a total output of 1.5–2.5 L/d, with basal secretion ranging from 0.2–0.4 mL/m and maximal stimulated secretion reaching 3–4 mL/m.

The enzymes secreted are of various types and are present in all secretory granules. These enzymes include the predominant proteolytic, amylolytic, and lipolytic enzymes plus a small amount of nucleolytic enzymes (Table 31–2). Hydrolytic activation of the proteolytic enzymes occurs in the duodenum; the other enzymes are secreted in their active forms.

Water and electrolytes are secreted in the smallest ductules, with electrolyte concentrations being similar to serum. As flow increases, bicarbonate concentration increases in exchange for chloride ion. This exchange occurs predominately in the larger ductules and ducts and produces pancreatic juice with a pH of 8.0–8.4.

Regulation of Pancreatic Secretion

There is vagal modulation of pancreatic exocrine secretion during the cephalic and gastric phases of pancreatic exocrine secretion. However, the primary stimulation occurs from acid- and food-mediated release of gastrointestinal hormones during the "intestinal phase" of pancreatic secretion (Figure 31–4). Cholecystokinin (CCK) seems to be the predominant stimulus for enzyme secretion, whereas secretin is the predominant hormonal stimulus for bicarbonate secretion.

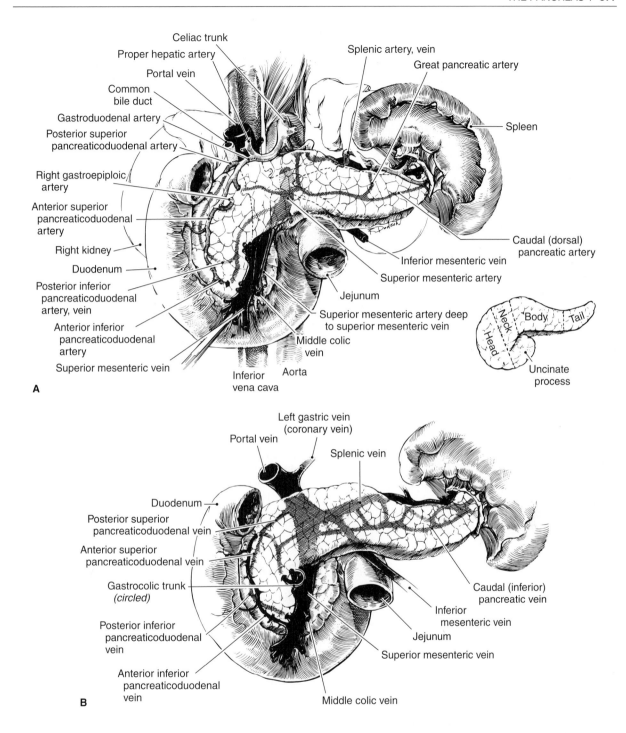

Figure 31–1. **A:** Gross anatomy and vascular anatomy of the pancreas. The pancreas is divided into five major regions. The head of the pancreas and uncinate process are derived from the ventral pancreatic bud. The neck, body, and tail of the pancreas are derived from the dorsal pancreatic bud. The arterial blood supply to the pancreas consists of the gastroduodenal artery and a branch of the celiac trunk, which divides into the posterior and anterior superior pancreatoduodenal arteries. These two vessels form an arcade and communicate with the anterior and posterior inferior pancreaticoduodenal arteries, which are branches of the proximal superior mesenteric artery. The body and tail of the pancreas are supplied by branches from the splenic artery. **B:** The venous drainage of the pancreas parallels the arterial supply with an anterior and posterior venous arcade around the head of the pancreas, draining into the superior mesenteric vein below and the portal vein above. The body and tail of the pancreas drain to the inferior pancreatic vein and to the branches of the splenic vein. (Reprinted, with permission, from Bastidas JA, Niederhuber JE: Pancreas. In: Abeloff MD et al (editors): *Clinical Oncology.* Churchill Livingstone, 1995, pp. 1374–1375.)

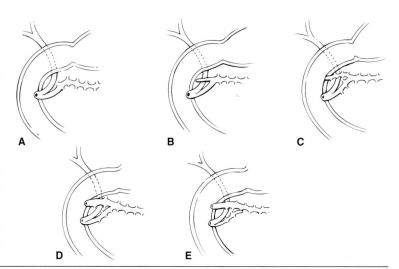

Figure 31–2. Pancreatic duct anatomy and variants. ***A:*** The main pancreatic duct (duct of Wirsung) is the usual drainage for the exocrine pancreatic secretions. ***B, C, D:*** The accessory pancreatic duct (duct of Santorini) usually communicates with the main pancreatic duct and has variable communication with the duodenum. ***E:*** In the extreme case, the two duct systems remain separated, and the predominant drainage is via the duct of Santorini. The separation of the two ducts is referred to as "pancreatic divisum." (Reprinted, with permission, from Bastidas JA, Niederhuber JN: Pancreas. In: Abeloff MD et al (editors): *Clinical Oncology.* Churchill Livingstone, 1995, p. 1376.)

ENDOCRINE PHYSIOLOGY

The hormonal secretions of the pancreas originate from the cells of the islets of Langerhans. The predominant cell type (75%) is the B (beta) cell, which produces insulin. The A (alpha) cell type comprises approximately 20% of the cells and produces glucagon. The D (delta) cells produce somatostatin, gastrin, and pancreatic polypeptide. Though these hormones are predominately involved in glucose homeostasis, they also influence pancreatic exocrine secretion, either directly or indirectly.

CONGENITAL & ACQUIRED BENIGN PANCREATIC DISEASES

ANNULAR PANCREAS

Diagnosis

Annular pancreas may present in the infant or adult as duodenal obstruction. Abnormal rotation of the pancreatic buds early in gestation creates a ring of pancreatic tissue around the duodenum. The severity of the duodenal constriction determines the age of presentation. Infants with severe duodenal obstruction present with an intrauterine history of polyhydramnios, early bilious vomiting, relatively undistended abdomen, and the classic "double bubble" sign of duodenal obstruction on plain x-ray. The differential diagnosis includes duodenal web or duodenal atresia.

In the adult, annular pancreas can present in a variety of ways, including pancreatic mass, pancreatitis, and peptic ulcer disease. Often the diagnosis is not made until laparotomy. Annular pancreas may also present as an incidental finding if there is relatively little obstruction. Treatment

may not be necessary if there are no signs or symptoms of duodenal obstruction.

Management

Initial treatment for patients presenting with duodenal obstruction includes nasogastric decompression, rehydration, and correction of electrolyte abnormalities. Once the patient is stabilized, laparotomy can be planned. Usually a duodenoduodenostomy or duodenojejunostomy can be performed to relieve the obstruction. Though gastrojejunostomy has been performed in the past, this treatment option is associated with a high late complication rate.

PANCREATIC DIVISUM

Diagnosis

Pancreatic divisum is a congenital abnormality that is defined by the persistence of the duct of Santorini (from the dorsal pancreatic bud) and its opening to the duodenum. In complete divisum the two duct systems remain separate (Figure 31–2). Pancreas divisum can be found in 5% of the population, however, its precise clinical significance remains controversial. Acute relapsing pancreatitis, chronic pancreatitis, and chronic abdominal pain syndrome have all been associated with pancreatic divisum. The diagnosis is made almost exclusively by endoscopic retrograde cholangiopancreatography (ERCP), although the newest generation computed tomographic (CT) scanners have sufficient resolution to sometimes suggest the diagnosis. When papillary stenosis is suspected, a secretin test measuring pancreatic duct output or an increase in pancreatic duct size by ultrasonography can be helpful in planning treatment.

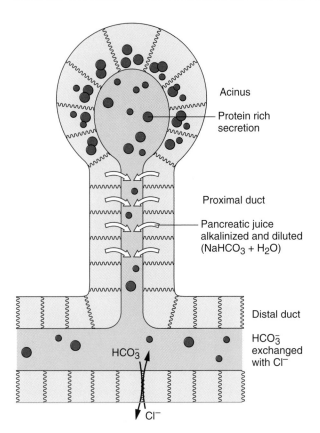

Table 31-1. Pancreatic cell types and function.

Exocrine Cells

Acinar cells
    Secrete multiple enzymes
Duct cells
    Secrete water and electrolytes, including bicarbonate

Endocrine Cells

Highly specialized cells organized as "islets of Langerhans" (2%
    of total pancreatic mass):
    A (alpha) cells produce glucagon
    B (beta) cells produce insulin
    D (delta) cells produce somatostatin, gastrin, and pancreatic
        polypeptide

Figure 31-3. Ductal origin of secretin-dependent pancreatic bicarbonate secretion. ***Open arrows*** indicate secretion of NaHCO₃ and water from the proximal duct cells. Some of the secreted HCO_3^- is exchanged with Cl^- in the distal ducts (***curved, solid arrows***). (Reprinted, with permission, from Raeder MG: The origin of and subcellular mechanism causing pancreatic bicarbonate secretion. Gastroenterology 1992;103: 1674.)

tion, myocardial infarction, and aortic dissection. A careful history may narrow the differential diagnosis by identifying risk factors for pancreatitis, including the two most common, gallstones and alcohol consumption. Other risk factors are outlined in Table 31-3.

Physical examination can usually narrow the differential diagnosis further. Fever and tachycardia are usually present. Marked epigastric tenderness with focal peritoneal irritation is common, though severe pancreatitis may cause tenderness in all quadrants of the abdomen. Patients may prefer to lie on their sides, sit up, or lie prone, since lying supine usually exacerbates their pain.

Hyperamylasemia is the hallmark of acute pancreatitis, though it is not essential for the diagnosis. Gallstone pancreatitis classically presents with amylase levels in excess of ten times normal (ie, greater than 1000 IU/mL). Alcoholic pancreatitis, as well as most other types of pancreatitis, usually exhibit lower levels of hyperamylasemia. In gallstone pancreatitis, it is also known that the high amylase can drop dramatically in the first 24–48 hours of symptoms. If the patient presents late, the serum amylase may

Management

Asymptomatic pancreatic divisum does not require treatment. However, patients with recurrent pancreatitis or chronic pain who also have stenosis of the minor papilla may benefit from operative sphincteroplasty. Endoscopic procedures, including sphincterotomy and stent placement across the minor papilla, may be of benefit in a small group of patients.

ACUTE PANCREATITIS

Diagnosis

Acute epigastric pain that usually radiates to the back, as well as nausea and vomiting, are the hallmarks of acute pancreatitis. This symptom complex has a wide differential diagnosis, including peptic ulcer disease, choledocholithiasis, cholecystitis, proximal small bowel obstruc-

Table 31-2. Pancreatic enzymes.

Proteolytic Enzymes (secreted as precursors requiring hydrolytic activation):

Endopeptidases
    Trypsin
    Chemotrypsin
    Elastase
Exopeptidases
    Carboxypeptidase A₁ and A₂
    Carboxypeptidase B₁ and B₂

Lipolytic Enzymes
Lipase (requires cofactor, colipase) Phospholipase A2 Nonspecific carboxylesterase
Amylolytic Enzymes
Amylase
Nucleolytic Enzymes
RNAse DNAse I

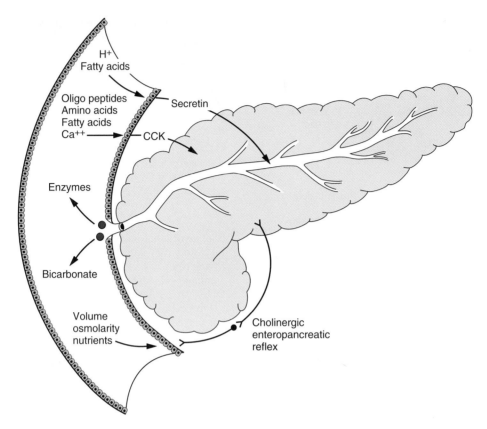

Figure 31–4. In the intestinal phase of pancreatic enzyme secretion, intestinal stimulants initiate enteropancreatic reflexes and release cholecystokinin (CCK), both of which act on pancreatic acinar cells to stimulate enzyme secretion. Hydrogen ions (H⁺) and fatty acids release secretin, which stimulates bicarbonate secretion. (Reprinted, with permission, from Owyang C, Williams JA: Pancreatic Secretion. In: Yamada T (editor): *Textbook of Gastroenterology,* 2nd ed. Lippincott, 1995, p. 376.)

have normalized. In these cases, it may be useful to obtain a lipase level, which tends to remain elevated longer. Lipase is also more specific for pancreatitis, since amylase is derived from a variety of tissues and can be elevated in parotitis, facial trauma, perforated gut, salpingitis, and ectopic pregnancy. To help in the resuscitation of the patient and to try to predict severe pancreatitis and estimate prognosis (Table 31–4), multiple other laboratory tests are often obtained: complete blood count (CBC), electrolytes (including calcium), arterial blood gas (ABG), liver panel, glucose, and blood urea nitrogen/creatinine (BUN/Cr). Occasionally, it is possible for a patient with a history of multiple episodes of pancreatitis, such as the chronic alcoholic, to present with a normal serum amylase. In these patients, one can consider measuring an amylase clearance from a 4- or 6-hour urine collection to confirm the diagnosis.

Occasionally, imaging studies are necessary to confirm the diagnosis of pancreatitis. A CT scan is best to outline inflammation of the pancreas. The addition of intravenous contrast is essential to identify areas of non-opacification, which represent pancreatic necrosis. Ultrasonography can also be used; while this modality is useful to image the

biliary tree and to identify gallstones, it is less reliable in providing adequate images of the pancreas. Plain films of the abdomen are usually nonspecific in pancreatitis, ranging from being essentially normal to showing a diffuse ileus pattern. Occasionally, one can identify a colon "cut-off sign," a sentinel loop of dilated small intestine or pancreatic calcifications.

Management

There is no specific therapy for acute pancreatitis. It is usually a self-limited process that resolves with bowel rest. Patients, therefore, usually only require supportive care, which includes hydration with intravenous fluids and analgesics as needed. The patient should be monitored closely. Generally, patients do not need nasogastric tubes for decompression unless they continue to vomit. Though usually febrile, patients with uncomplicated pancreatitis do not benefit from prophylactic use of systemic intravenous antibiotics. Although octreotide (an analogue of somatostatin) decreases pancreatic secretion, its use in acute pancreatitis has not been shown to improve the patient's clinical course.

Table 31–3. Causes of pancreatitis.

Drugs/Toxins

Alcohol
Thiazide diuretics
Estrogens
Salicylates
Anti-HIV medications
Sulfonamides
Immunosuppressives
Scorpion venom

Mechanical

Cholelithiasis
Duct obstruction
    Pancreatic and periampullary tumors
    Ascaris infestation
    Pancreatic duct strictures
    ? Pancreatic divisum
Trauma
ERCP

Metabolic

Hypertrigliceridemia
Hypercalcemia
Cystic fibrosis

Vascular

Postcardiopulmonary bypass
Ischemia
Collagen vascular diseases

Infectious

Viral (mumps, CMV, coxsackie, hepatitis, MMR vaccine)

Idiopathic

ERCP = endoscopic retrograde cholangiopancreatography; CMV = cytomegalovirus; HIV = human immunodeficiency virus; MMR = measles-mumps-rubella.

Table 31–4. Ranson's criteria and their relationship to prognosis in acute pancreatitis.

Initial Signs	Delayed Signs
Age > 55 years	↓Hct > 10%
WBC count > 16,000	↑BUN > 5 mg/dL
Blood glucose > 200 mg/dL	Calcium < 8 mg/dL
SGOT > 250 U/L	pO_2 < 60
LDH > 350 IU/L	Base deficit > 4 meq/L
	Fluid sequestration > 6 L

Mortality as a function of number of Ranson's signs

Number of signs	Mortality (%)
0–2	< 1
3–4	15
5–6	40
7–8	100

BUN = blood urea nitrogen; LDH = lactate dehydrogenase; SGOT = aspartate aminotransferase; WBC = white blood cells.

CHRONIC PANCREATITIS

Diagnosis

Patients with long-standing, recurring episodes of acute pancreatitis can develop chronic pancreatitis. This entity should be differentiated from patients who have recurrent acute pancreatitis, which can occur without apparent signs of chronic pancreatitis. Patients with chronic pancreatitis

Acute pancreatitis can be associated with pancreatic necrosis or persistent peripancreatic fluid collections (Figure 31–5). These two processes can remain sterile or become infected. The persistent peripancreatic fluid collections can organize into pancreatic pseudocysts, which by definition do not exist until after 6 weeks from the initial acute episode of pancreatitis.

Pancreatic necrosis is diagnosed by CT scanning and identification of hypoperfused segments of the pancreas. The presence of necrosis is associated with a more protracted and severe clinical course. With extensive necrosis, open debridement of the pancreas may be necessary in a patient who is not clinically stable or improving. Infected pancreatic necrosis, usually diagnosed by fine-needle aspiration or at laparotomy, mandates surgical debridement and drainage. Drainage can be achieved either open (ie, with open packing) or closed, with large drains in the pancreatic bed. Patients with severe pancreatitis associated with significant pancreatic necrosis may benefit from prophylactic antibiotics. Patients with severe pancreatitis and pancreatic necrosis often require prolonged care in the intensive care unit (ICU), including ventilatory support, nutritional support, and, sometimes, repeated operations for adequate debridement.

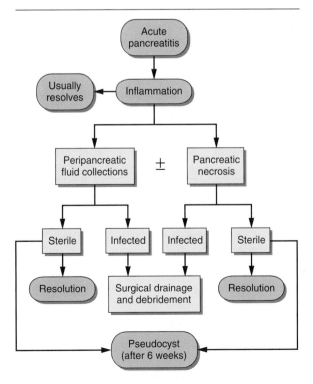

Figure 31–5. Clinical course of acute pancreatitis.

usually suffer from chronic alcohol use, have an intrinsic defect in the pancreatic duct (ie, duct stenosis or stricture), or have an uncorrected metabolic defect.

Chronic pancreatitis is characterized by fibrosis of the gland, often associated with pancreatic duct changes and pancreatic exocrine insufficiency. In severe cases, patients may develop a type of diabetes from altered endocrine function. This diabetes is a distinct entity from both type I (insulin deficiency) and type II (insulin resistance) diabetes mellitus. Islet architecture is often preserved, however, the insulin response to glucose is altered, as is the production of the counter-regulatory hormones, such as glucagon.

The most common symptom in patients with chronic pancreatitis is abdominal pain. Other prominent symptoms may include steatorrhea, weight loss, and malnutrition. The pain is usually epigastric, radiates to the back, and is usually exacerbated by eating. The etiology of the pain is thought to be related to duct obstruction, though it can be present in the absence of strictures and ductal dilatation. Confirmation of the diagnosis of chronic pancreatitis may be difficult. Plain radiographs may show calcifications in the pancreas. This finding would be a specific and distinguishing feature of chronic pancreatitis. However, in the absence of visible pancreatic calcifications on plain radiographs, the clinical suspicion of this diagnosis should lead to a CT scan. This imaging study will deliver information about the size and character of the pancreatic ducts and will also outline the status of the pancreatic parenchyma. ERCP is also an important adjunct in outlining ductal changes that may not be visible on the CT. Knowledge of the patient's ductal anatomy is vital in planning operative interventions.

Management

Treatment is focused on managing the three major symptoms and includes abstinence from alcohol and the judicious use of analgesics to manage the abdominal pain. Oral replacement of pancreatic enzymes can reverse the symptoms of fat malabsorption and sometimes improve pain management. Careful administration of insulin can be used to manage glucose intolerance. One must be aware that these patients can be very brittle in the management of their diabetes because of the lack of counter-regulatory hormones.

If pain persists after optimization of medical therapy, a variety of surgical procedures can be considered. These procedures can be classified as either "drainage" or "ablative" procedures and can achieve good pain control in the majority of patients. The drainage procedures (Table 31–5) can only be performed if there is significant ductal dilatation. These procedures have relatively low morbidity and have the advantage of preserving pancreatic parenchyma and salvaging some exocrine and endocrine function. The ablative procedures have the disadvantage of decreasing islet cell mass, and are associated with increased operative morbidity, but they generally offer better results with pain control.

Table 31–5. Surgical procedures for chronic pancreatitis.

Drainage Procedures
Transduodenal sphincteroplasty (for ampullary stenosis)
Puestow procedure (longitudinal pancreaticojejunostomy)

Ablative Procedures
Distal pancreatectomy
95% Pancreatectomy
Pancreaticoduodenectomy (Whipple procedure)
Total pancreatectomy

Miscellaneous Procedures
Autotransplantation of pancreas
Splanchnicectomy (operative or percutaneous)
Duodenal-preserving resection of the head of the pancreas

PANCREATIC PSEUDOCYSTS

Diagnosis

Following an episode of acute pancreatitis or duct disruption secondary to trauma, peripancreatic fluid collections may develop. If these collections persist, they can organize over a period of weeks into a defined collection that is walled off by the surrounding tissues. By definition, at 6 weeks these collections are referred to as pancreatic pseudocysts (Figure 31–6).

Patients with pseudocysts often have a protracted recovery from their episode of acute pancreatitis and have usually undergone imaging with either ultrasonography or CT scanning that has identified peripancreatic fluid collections. Occasionally, a patient will present with an abdominal mass, epigastric pain, nausea, vomiting, and, possibly, weight loss. These patients need to be evaluated carefully with a detailed history, physical examination, and laboratory evaluation (particularly amylase and lipase), followed by a high-resolution CT to try to differentiate a pseudocyst from a cystic neoplasm of the pancreas.

Pseudocysts may become complicated by infection, bleeding, or rupture, or they may cause obstruction of adjacent organs. Suspected infection can be confirmed at exploration or by percutaneous needle aspiration if the patient is stable. Bleeding can be identified by a gradual decrease in hemoglobin concentration, or, less commonly, as an acute bleed with altered hemodynamics. Bleeding into the cyst may arise from a pseudoaneurysm, often from the splenic artery. Cyst rupture usually presents as an acute abdomen or with pancreatic ascites. Lastly, a large cyst can cause partial gastric, duodenal, bile duct, or colonic obstruction.

Management

Supportive care and bowel rest is the usual treatment for symptomatic pseudocysts. This management usually entails parenteral nutrition, analgesics, and complete bowel rest. Occasionally, patients have asymptomatic pseudocysts. These patients can be followed closely on a low-fat diet and gastric acid suppression. The majority of

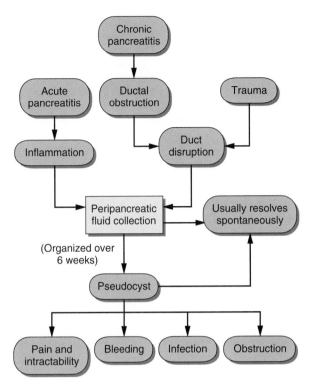

Figure 31–6. Pseudocyst formation and its complications.

small pseudocysts will resolve with this approach; additionally, a minority (20–30%) of larger pseudocysts (6 cm or greater) will also resolve without surgical intervention.

For persistent symptomatic pseudocysts, surgical decompression into the gastrointestinal tract is the standard treatment. Lesser sac collections can be drained into a Roux limb of small bowel or into the stomach through the posterior gastric wall. Cysts in the head of the pancreas can also be drained into the small bowel or, sometimes, directly into the duodenum. Recently, endoscopic cyst-gastrostomy and percutaneous drainage of cysts have been reported, but currently have limited application.

Infected pseudocysts require external drainage and systemic antibiotics. Acutely bleeding cysts are difficult to manage. Angiography with embolization is valuable to stabilize the patient and potentially control the bleeding. Control of pancreatic bed bleeding is often difficult to manage surgically. Occasionally, small pseudocysts are best managed with complete resection, particularly in the tail of the pancreas.

The outcome of surgical drainage of cysts is excellent. This surgery can be complicated by bleeding and infection. Urgent surgery for the complicated cysts, especially those that are infected or bleeding, carry significant perioperative morbidity.

PANCREATIC TRAUMA

Diagnosis

Penetrating injuries account for approximately two thirds of pancreatic trauma. The pre-hospital and postoperative mortality is high when these injuries are associated with major vascular injuries of the retroperitoneum or portal structures. The diagnosis is usually made at exploratory laparotomy for evaluation of a stab wound or gun shot wound. The important issue at exploration is to define all associated injuries, particularly to the duodenum, common bile duct, local vascular structures, and the main pancreatic duct.

Blunt trauma to the pancreas is usually the result of significant external forces, and, thus, is associated with multiple injuries. Injuries focused to the right of midline can include injury to the liver, bile duct, duodenum, and kidney. Midline trauma can lacerate the pancreas in the neck/midbody; this injury can also occur as an isolated injury when the pancreas is trapped between forces acting on the upper abdomen and the vertebral column. To the left of midline there is a high association with splenic injury.

The extent of injury ranges from simple contusion, to capsular and parenchymal rupture with or without duct injury, to combined injury with the duodenum. Patients who present in shock need to be resuscitated under standard trauma resuscitation protocols. Most patients then proceed to exploration. Some patients, however, present hemodynamically stable and pose significant difficulty in identifying a pancreatic injury. Symptoms can be vague and nonspecific. Early physical examinations can be fairly unrevealing. Laboratory tests, including serum amylase, have a relatively low predictive value. CT scanning is probably the most sensitive imaging study to identify pancreatic injury. However, even CT scans can be misleading early in the course of a pancreatic injury. ERCP can provide significant help in defining pancreatic duct injury in the stable patient. Intraoperative pancreatography is also used to define duct injury.

Management

Simple contusions and superficial lacerations usually only require external drainage using closed suction drains. Deeper lacerations and some duct injuries can be repaired and then drained. Body and tail duct injuries are sometimes best managed by distal pancreatectomy. Though this removes normal pancreatic parenchyma, the long-term consequences are really quite minimal, with virtually no exocrine or endocrine insufficiency. Complex injuries to the head of the pancreas and duodenum may require repair with extensive drainage, or, possibly, duodenal exclusion (oversewing of pylorus, gastrojejunostomy, biliary duct T-tube, duodenostomy tube, and feeding jejunostomy) or resection (Whipple procedure).

Overall postoperative mortality and morbidity is significant because of the commonly associated injuries and blood loss. Stab wounds have the best results, with a mortality of 10%; gunshot wounds are more lethal, as are blunt injuries with associated vascular injuries. These complex injuries may have a postoperative mortality as high as 50%.

BENIGN NEOPLASTIC DISEASE

SEROUS CYSTADENOMA

Diagnosis

Cystic neoplasms of the pancreas are rare entities. The older classification of these neoplasms emphasizes the microcystic versus macrocystic aspects of the gross histopathology. The current consensus is that these lesions are best classified as serous or mucinous. The serous lesions are benign in nature. Patients usually present with mild vague abdominal pain and, less commonly, a palpable abdominal mass. Serous lesions are now being discovered incidentally at the time of imaging the abdomen for other unrelated reasons. Ultrasonography and CT are the main imaging modalities to characterize cystic lesions of the pancreas. It is important to differentiate serous lesions from pancreatic pseudocysts, which are much more common and usually associated with a very clear history of acute pancreatitis. Serous cystadenomas are usually not in communication with the main pancreatic duct, so ERCP is not particularly helpful. In rare cases, percutaneous fine-needle aspiration of the cyst fluid may help in the differentiation between a pseudocyst and a cystic neoplasm.

Management

In general, the management of cystic neoplasms of the pancreas is by surgical resection. However, occasionally, when cysts are asymptomatic and found incidentally, the lesions can be followed closely, provided they satisfy all CT and ultrasonographic criteria of a serous cystadenoma. Since the serous nature of the cyst cannot be absolutely determined by imaging, it is preferable to excise these lesions to define their nature and to rule out a malignant process.

BENIGN ISLET CELL TUMORS

Diagnosis

Pancreatic islet cell tumors may be benign or malignant and are classically described as functioning (hormone-producing) or nonfunctioning. **Insulinomas** are the most common functioning islet cell neoplasm. Approximately 80% are solitary and benign. Some of these lesions may be discovered incidentally on CT scan. However, since many of the products of these lesions are functional, patients frequently present with a clinical syndrome related to the hormone being released by the tumor. Whipple's triad of central nervous system symptoms, hypoglycemia

(< 50 mg/dL), and reversal of symptoms with exogenous glucose is a classic description of the hyperinsulinemic state of an insulinoma. Confirmation of this syndrome usually involves fasting and documented severe hypoglycemia with inappropriate hyperinsulinemia. It is essential to exclude the possibility of exogenous insulin administration and oral hypoglycemics when evaluating these patients. A rare related disorder that needs to be considered in infants is nesidioblastosis (diffuse islet cell hyperplasia), which would present with clinical findings similar to insulinoma.

A **gastrinoma** (Zollinger-Ellison syndrome) may present in the pancreas or duodenum in what is often referred to as the gastrinoma triangle. These tumors are either of the sporadic type or associated with multiple endocrine neoplasia (MEN syndrome type I) and are characterized by complicated ulcer disease, diarrhea, and marked hypergastrinemia. The rarer syndromes are produced by vipomas, which are characterized by a profuse secretory diarrhea, and the glucagonomas, which present with diabetes as well as characteristic skin lesions.

Many islet cell tumors have been described as "nonfunctional," since there is no apparent clinical syndrome associated with the tumor. More recently, however, it has been discovered that many of these tumors actually produce excessive hormones, particularly pancreatic polypeptide. Only a small percentage of islet cell tumors are now considered "nonfunctional" (Table 31–6).

Management

The goal of therapy in managing islet cell tumors is control of symptoms. Disease that is limited to the pancreas is best treated with surgical resection. Simple resection (enucleation) of an adenoma is sometimes possible, especially for insulinoma. Depending on the location of the tumor, a Whipple procedure or distal pancreatectomy is required for larger or multiple lesions.

When there is extrapancreatic disease, such as liver metastasis, medical therapy of symptoms can be used. Metastatic gastrinoma can be managed with omeprazole to control the symptoms of excessive acid production. A somatostatin analogue, octreotide, can also be useful to control symptoms by inhibiting hormone release. This therapy is particularly useful in controlling diarrhea. Chemotherapy can be considered for symptomatic metastatic disease using streptozocin. This therapy will, however, induce diabetes, since it destroys all islet cells.

More traditional chemotherapeutic agents have been used, but generally have a poor response rate. However, to manage liver metastasis, chemoembolization through the hepatic artery has recently been reported to be a useful palliative approach.

Surgical resection is sometimes indicated for metastatic disease, since resection of the primary tumor and metastasis can offer significant palliation. Some patients have slow progression of their disease and can be offered repeated operations if medical management of their symptoms is inadequate.

Table 31-6. Overview of pancreatic endocrine tumors.

Syndrome	Hormone	Cell of Origin	Clinical Features	Frequency of Extra Pancreatic Tumor	Percent Malignant	Diagnostic Studies	Treatment
Insulinoma	Insulin (measure proinsulin and C peptide)	Beta	Whipple's triad / Hypoglycemia, altered mental status, syncope, dizziness, catecholamine surge / Most common islet cell tumor / 90% have single tumor / Equally distributed throughout pancreas / Must differentiate from paraneoplastic syndromes and other causes of hypoglycemia / Fewer than 10% have MEN-1	Rare	10–15	72-hour fast / Hyperinsulinemia / Elevated level C-peptide and proinsulin (also calcium and tolbutamide test) / Insulin/glucose ratio > 0.3	Enucleation / If close to duct or > 2 cm, best treated by distal pancreatectomy / Pancreaticoduodenectomy for head / Local resection of small number of hepatic metastases
Gastrinoma (Zollinger-Ellison syndrome)	Gastrin	G cell	Gastric acid hypersecretion, peptic ulceration, diarrhea (steatorrhea), weight loss, failure of medical treatment of peptic ulcer, post-bulbar ulcer, MEN-1 kindred / 25% associated with MEN-1 syndrome / Associated with prominent gastric rugal folds	Frequent	60–70	Secretin test / Calcium infusion	Omeprazole 20–200 mg/d / Patients with hepatic metastases not explored / Exploration with attention to "gastrinoma triangle" / Negative exploration rate is 5–20%
Glucagonoma	Glucagon	Alpha	Hyperglycemia, diabetes, skin rash (necrolytic migratory erythema), glossitis, thrombophlebitis, weight loss, anemia / 80% will have metastases	Rare	60	Hyperglucagonemia fasting > 150 pg/mL / Most located in body and tail / Hypoaminoacidemia	Octreotide for reducing symptoms / Resection—usually distal pancreas / Debulk metastatic lesions
Somatostatinoma	Somatostatin	Delta	Diabetes mellitus, gallstones, hypochlorhydria, steatorrhea, weight loss / Least common islet tumor (1 in 40 million population)	Rare	50	Fasting somatostatin > 150 pg/mL / Most located in head	Resection, debulking of metastases / Prophylactic cholecystectomy
WDHA, VIPoma (Verner-Morrison syndrome)	VIP (or prostaglandin E)	Delta	Watery diarrhea, hypokalemia, achlorhydria, dehydration (5 L/d), malabsorption, steatorrhea, psychosis / 20% have cutaneous flushing / 10% have extra-pancreatic tumors in retroperitoneum or thorax	10% of time	50	VIP / Single normal level does not rule out peptide histidine-isoleucine / Prostaglandins	Octreotide preoperatively / Resection, usually distal pancreatectomy / Debulking of metastatic tumor
Carcinoid	Serotonin (substance P)	EC	Flushing, diarrhea, tachycardia, abdominal pain / Rare islet cell tumors / Usually metastatic when diagnosed	Frequent	> 90	Calcium infusion, pentagastrin test / Elevated 5-HT (serotonin) / Elevated substance P / Elevated urinary 5-HIAA	Resection and debulking of metastases
PP-OMA	Pancreatic polypeptide	Delta	Weight loss, abdominal pain, diarrhea, jaundice / Possibly elevated PP in "non-functioning" tumors / "No functioning" tumors (lack of syndrome) produce symptoms by location and size, are most frequently located in head of pancreas	Rare	50–90	Evidence of MEN-1 / Elevated PP	Resection / 60% response rate with streptozocin plus doxorubicin

MEN = multiple endocrine neoplasia; PP = pancreatic polypeptide; VIP = vasoactive intestinal polypeptide; WDHA = watery diarrhea, hypokalemia, achlorhydria syndrome.

385

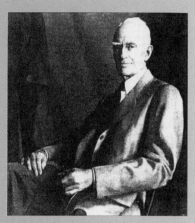

Allen O. Whipple, MD, in his seventies (1881–1963). (Courtesy of The New York Academy of Medicine Library, New York.)

Allen O. Whipple (1881–1963) is considered the father of modern pancreatic surgical treatment. He is eponymously remembered both for his contributions and modifications to the pancreaticoduodenectomy (Whipple's procedure) and for the classic triad for clinical diagnosis of insulinoma (Whipple's triad). Although the first successful pancreaticoduodenectomy was performed in 1912, it was not until 1935, when Whipple published his paper describing a unique two-stage en bloc resection of the head of the pancreas and the duodenum, that the procedure was popularized. Before that time, many surgeons considered the pancreas a dangerous and difficult organ, and the problems associated with pancreatic duct secretions were particularly troublesome as anastomoses of the pancreatic duct were apt to leak or break down. Whipple solved this problem by proving that maintenance of normal pancreatic duct flow was unnecessary. After several modifications, Whipple developed a one-stage procedure in 1940 that was further modified by I.R. Trimble in 1941.

The Whipple procedure still remained a formidable undertaking and was not widely performed until after Whipple's death in 1963. It was not until the 1980s that technical advances significantly lowered the operative mortality rate, which is now as low as 1–2% in centers where this procedure is performed on a regular basis.

Whipple's triad was first reported by Whipple and Frantz in 1935 and consists of three diagnostic indicators of the presence of an insulinoma: (1) symptoms caused by fasting or exercise; (2) hypoglycemia (< 45 mg/dL); and (3) relief of symptoms by administration of glucose.

In addition to these accomplishments, Whipple founded the Spleen Clinic in 1928 with Walter Palmer, from which emerged several remarkable advances in the surgical treatment of both the spleen and the liver (most notably the portacaval shunt for portal hypertension). Allen O. Whipple held the Valentine Chair of Surgery at Columbia Presbyterian Hospital in New York until his retirement in 1946. He was awarded all of the accolades due to a master surgeon, including election to several prestigious national and international surgical societies. He was recognized as a superb master of surgical technique, an excellent teacher and educator, as well as a great scientist and innovator.

MALIGNANT NEOPLASTIC DISEASE

PANCREATIC CARCINOMA

Pancreatic cancer is the fifth leading cause of cancer deaths, with approximately 6000 new cases diagnosed per year in the United States. The incidence of pancreatic cancer increases with age, but can present as early as the third decade of life. Known risks factors include smoking, high-fat diet, and inherited syndromes, including von Hippel-Lindau and familial atypical multiple mole melanoma syndrome. Other possible risk factors include previous gastric surgery, diabetes, and chronic pancreatitis. Most pancreatic cancers present in the head of the pancreas and have a resectability rate of approximately 15%. The lesions in the body and tail of the pancreas tend to present later and have a significantly lower resectability rate.

Diagnosis

The symptoms of pancreatic cancer are very vague and nonspecific, which may contribute to the fact that most patients present with advanced disease. The patient with lesions at the head of the pancreas will usually present with obstructive jaundice. Though these patients have classically been described as having "painless jaundice," on careful evaluation the majority of these patients usually present with epigastric or back pain. Usually patients who present with obstructive jaundice are best initially evaluated by ultrasonography to document biliary duct dilatation. In the absence of risk factors for gallstones, and in particular in the older patients, CT scan should be the next imaging study to assess the location of the obstruction and the potential of a periampullary mass.

It is preferable to perform the CT scan prior to ERCP, since many patients at ERCP have a stent placed to decompress the biliary system. The presence of this stent and the manipulation from ERCP sometimes contribute to artifact. Though a CT scan is extremely helpful in identifying the etiology of biliary obstruction, when the obstruction is due to gallstones the scan may not be diagnostic. Therefore, cholangiography (either endoscopic or percutaneous) is often an important adjunct, not only to visualize the biliary system but also to potentially decompress the obstructed biliary system.

The modern dynamic spiral CT is very effective in imaging the pancreas and periampullary area. These studies can delineate the pancreatic duct and bile duct anatomy, but can also assess vascular anatomy. In the absence of encasement of the celiac axis and mesenteric vessels, as well as in the absence of distant disease, the patient can be considered a surgical candidate. Some surgeons still obtain routine preoperative angiography, both to define anatomy and exclude vessel encasement; however, this imaging modality is becoming less and less important as CT scanning continues to improve.

Routine serum tumor markers, including CA 19-9 and carcinoembryonic antigen (CEA), should be assessed at presentation. These markers are nonspecific and do not contribute significantly to a precise diagnosis; rather, they help to identify a potential marker for disease that can be followed longitudinally throughout the course of therapy. Needle biopsy to confirm malignancy is not necessary in the majority of patients whose condition appears resectable. In patients with apparent metastatic disease, advanced local disease, or both, percutaneous biopsy may be useful to confirm a malignancy prior to consideration of nonsurgical therapy.

Management

Since the majority of patients are not candidates for surgical resection, the treatment for most patients with pancreatic carcinoma is palliative. The predominant symptoms at presentation are jaundice from bile duct obstruction and epigastric and back pain. Occasionally, there is also an element of duodenal obstruction that may require treatment.

Patients who present with metastases to the liver have a very short life expectancy. They generally are not candidates for exploration if the primary lesion is felt to be adenocarcinoma of the pancreas. If the patient has a lesion at the head of the pancreas and presents with jaundice, an endoprosthesis can be placed endoscopically to stent and relieve the distal bile duct obstruction.

The management of pain follows the general guidelines of pain management in oncologic patients, beginning with nonsteroidal agents and advancing to opiates. If the patient becomes difficult to manage with opiates, it is important to consider neurolytic splanchnicectomy. Percutaneous injections of alcohol into the celiac plexus usually provide excellent pain relief and allow patients to significantly decrease their narcotic use. If, however, the patient survives more than 6 months, a significant percentage will require repeat celiac blockade. Ordinarily, this would be as far as one would consider intervening for pain management in a patient with known metastatic disease.

Patients with diffuse liver metastasis, particularly those with ascites, have an extremely high morbidity from surgical intervention. However, patients with minimal liver disease may be considered for palliative surgical management of a primary tumor in conjunction with a possible liver resection, particularly young patients who wish to be aggressive with their treatment.

Another frequent presentation is that of a patient with locally advanced disease that is unresectable without evidence of metastatic disease. These patients are managed with biliary stent placement to control their obstructive jaundice and expectant management, depending on their symptoms. However, if the patient is young or if desires a very aggressive approach, one can consider combination chemoradiation therapy to try to slow progression of the disease locally. If there is extensive retroperitoneal involvement with encasement of the celiac axis, or extensive encasement of the mesenteric vessels, it is unlikely that chemoradiation will produce sufficient response to allow subsequent consideration of resection. Surgical intervention is not generally considered for these patients. The exceptions are those patients who develop duodenal obstruction. In these cases, a bypass procedure (gastrojejunostomy) is performed to allow the stomach to empty. A cholecystectomy and choledochojejunotsomy should also be considered at exploration. Intraoperative celiac chemical splanchnicectomy with alcohol injection is a proven therapy known to significantly decrease pain and the need for narcotics. This procedure should be performed whenever a patient is explored and not resected, whether or not the patient had pain preoperatively.

Patients who present with advanced disease, as described above, usually have significant cachexia and malnutrition. This alone often precludes any consideration for surgical intervention. On the other hand, if an aggressive approach is elected for these patients, appropriate nutritional support with either parenteral or enteral nutrition is indicated.

Another group of patients will present with questionable findings on the CT regarding resectability. This usually involves concerns regarding encasement of the superior mesenteric vein (SMV) or portal vein. Current CT scanning is usually sufficient to make these determinations and has essentially eliminated the use of angiography. For this group of patients, the two possible options include exploration and resection, including resection of the involved vein and vein graft substitution. If the patient is young, has not had significant weight loss, and has no other significant comorbidities, early exploration may be an option. On the other hand, if the patient is not an optimal candidate, there is a very good rationale to consider primary chemoradiation in the hopes that tumor shrinkage will allow subsequent resection. This period of primary therapy is usually with 5-fluorouracil (5-FU), given either as a continuous infusion or an intermittent bolus as a radiosensitizer for 45–55 cGy. This approach also allows a period of observation to see if an aggressive underlying biology can be declared for the patient's particular tumor. Specifically, there appears to be a group of patients who have very rapid progression to metastatic disease in the liver who, over a short period, will demonstrate these metastases in spite of therapy.

More important are those patients who respond well to chemoradiation and have significant shrinkage of tumor, such that vessel encasement is no longer seen and exploration for resection is appropriate. Again, once the patient is explored, a resection with a pancreaticoduodenectomy is completed (the details of this procedure will be discussed in the next section). On the other hand, if there is locally advanced disease, particularly invasion to the SMV or portal vein, surgical palliation with a choledochojejunostomy or duodenostomy can be achieved. Furthermore, a chemical splanchnicectomy with alcohol can be performed during the exploration. Most surgeons also perform a prophylactic gastrojejunostomy in the absence of evidence of gastric outlet obstruction. This issue is controversial, however, because only an estimated 15% of pa-

tients eventually develop significant gastric outlet obstruction that requires reoperation for gastric decompression. On the other hand, the rationale for prophylactic gastrojejunostomy is that the patient is already under anesthesia and is being explored. Morbidity from a gastrojejunostomy is infrequent.

Patients with masses at the head of the pancreas that do not appear to encase the celiac and SMA vessels and do not demonstrate impingement of the portal and SMV vessels, and who do not have metastatic disease involving other organs, can generally be considered candidates for surgical resection. At exploration a careful assessment of the entire abdomen and liver is made to rule out evidence of metastatic disease. If none is found, a stepwise evaluation to determine resectability is performed as follows.

A Kocher maneuver is used to mobilize the duodenum and head of pancreas off the retroperitoneum. This maneuver is performed to assure that the posterior aspect of the pancreas is free of the retroperitoneal vena cava and aorta. During the Kocher maneuver, the SMA is palpated and an assessment of nonencasement of the SMA by tumor of the uncinate process confirms potential resectability. Many surgeons then move to the celiac axis to determine if there is obvious adenopathy in this area, which ordinarily is not included in the resection. This issue remains controversial in that many surgeons feel that a complete node dissection, including the celiac nodes, should be a routine part of the pancreaticoduodenectomy. The next step in assessing resectability involves identifying the superior mesenteric vein and portal vein to make sure that they are free from the tumor. Ordinarily, a tunnel can be created behind the pancreas anterior to the SMV, all the way through to the anterior surface of the portal vein. Once the above issues have been clarified, the neck of the pancreas can be divided over the mesenteric vein and the proximal duodenum or stomach can be divided. At this point, the specimen can be dissected free of the SMV. The uncinate process is then released off of the SMA. The proximal jejunum is divided and its mesentery is taken down to allow en bloc removal of the duodenum and head of pancreas. This resection in general also encompasses the regional lymph node groups.

The reconstruction following the pancreaticoduodenectomy (Whipple's procedure) involves three major steps. First is the issue of management of the residual pancreas. Most surgeons have traditionally sewn the residual pancreas to a segment of proximal jejunum. More recently, an older technique of sewing the pancreas to the stomach has been resurrected and is reported to be technically easier, possibly with fewer complications. A hepatojejunostomy or choledochojejunostomy is performed to allow for adequate bile drainage. Lastly, a drainage procedure is established for the stomach. If a pylorus-saving procedure has been performed, the proximal duodenum is sewn in an end-to-side fashion into the jejunum. If, however, a partial gastrectomy was included in the resection, a gastrojejunostomy is created.

There continues to be the potential for significant morbidity from a pancreaticoduodenectomy. The two most common complications are delayed gastric emptying and pancreatic anastomotic leak. With modern care, the significance of these complications has diminished remarkably. Most surgeons place appropriate drains to assure adequate drainage if there is a pancreatic leak. The issue of delayed gastric emptying is more difficult, therefore, many surgeons routinely place feeding tubes at the original operation. This allows for enteral feeding to be initiated promptly and used to maintain the patient's nutrition if the stomach is slow to recover normal function. Occasionally, promotility agents are useful in the management of these patients.

Mortality from pancreaticoduodenectomy in the past has been significant. However, in centers where this procedure is commonly performed, the mortality rate should be no higher than 1–2%. The most devastating complication after pancreaticoduodenectomy is postoperative bleeding. This single complications may carry a mortality rate as high as 30–50%. Infection and abscess are often related to a pancreatic leak. This condition is often present prior to a significant hemorrhage. The management of postoperative bleeding may require urgent reexploration early in the postoperative period. However, if it occurs in a delayed fashion, angiography and consultation with an interventional radiologist for possible embolization should be considered in the hemodynamically stable patient.

Patients with lesions in the distal pancreas without evidence of metastatic disease can undergo distal pancreatectomy. Since this procedure usually includes splenectomy, preoperative vaccination for encapsulated bacteria should be considered to decrease the risk of postsplenectomy sepsis. The morbidity of distal pancreatectomy is significantly less than that of a pancreaticoduodenectomy.

After resection, adjuvant therapy with combined chemoradiation has been clearly shown to contribute to prolonged survival. The best prognosis is for patients with lesions less than 2 cm, no lymph node involvement, and negative surgical margins. This small group may have a 5-year survival that exceeds 50%. Node-positive tumors with a diameter greater than 2 cm have a 5-year survival of only approximately 10%. Some institutions have reported overall combined 5-year survival of 20–25%. These new results have provided renewed interest in the surgical management of this devastating disease.

CYSTIC NEOPLASM

Diagnosis

The presentation of cystic neoplasms can be similar to adenocarcinoma, particularly when they present in the head of the pancreas. Usually, they produce vague symptoms and an abdominal mass. Evaluation is as described above and depends primarily on CT scanning. These lesions, however, often have to be differentiated from pancreatic pseudocysts. This differentiation can be difficult and may require careful evaluation at surgical exploration.

Management

Mucinous cystic neoplasms present as frank metastatic malignancies or as mucinous tumors of the pancreas. These "benign-appearing" mucinous lesions have a high malignant potential and should be treated as malignancies. The treatment is surgical resection as described for adenocarcinoma, if there is no evidence of metastatic disease. Outcome is moderately improved over adenocarcinoma.

UNUSUAL TUMORS OF THE PANCREAS

Rare tumors of the pancreas include solid and papillary cystic neoplasms, acinar cell carcinomas, lymphoma, and sarcomas. The solid and papillary cystic neoplasms tend to present in young women and have a good prognosis when resected. Acinar cell tumors are treated like the more common adenocarcinomas. Pancreatic lymphoma may require laparotomy for diagnosis, however, its primary treatment is chemotherapy. Sarcomas are extremely rare and should be resected, if possible.

SUGGESTED READING

Bastidas JA, Niederhuber JE: Pancreas. In: Abeloff MD et al (editors): *Clinical Oncology.* Churchill Livingstone, 1995.

Niederhuber JE et al: The national cancer data base report on pancreatic cancer. Cancer 1995;76:1671.

Owyang C, Williams JA: Pancreatic secretion. In: Yamada T (editor): *Textbook of Gastroenterology,* 2nd ed. Lippincott, 1995.

Raeder MG: The origin of and subcellular mechanism causing pancreatic bicarbonate secretion. Gastroenterology 1992; 103:1674.

Udelsman R et al: Pancreaticoduodenectomy for selected pancreatic endocrine tumors. Surg Gyn Obstet 1993;177:269.

32

Hernias

David Oakes, MD

► Key Facts

► All abdominal hernias occur in one of three areas: (1) where the transversalis fascia has natural openings to permit the egress of normal structures; (2) where the fascia has been disturbed by surgical incisions or other penetrating trauma; (3) where there is a relative weakness of the fascial layer, related either to a failure of fusion of normal tissues or to an inherent weakness of a particular region of the fascial sac.

► Hernia strangulation develops when bowel trapped in the hernia no longer receives sufficient blood supply to prevent necrosis.

► Hernias will not heal spontaneously, the possible exception being small umbilical hernias in infants and children less than 2 or 3 years of age.

► General principles of the surgical repair of hernias are to define and reduce the herniated tissue, to define strong fascial margins in all directions, and to reapproximate those margins with strong sutures, tied without excessive tension.

► Hernias can be repaired under local, regional, or general anesthesia, or a combination of these techniques.

► The primary complications of hernia repairs are hematomas, infections, persistent postoperative pain, and recurrence.

► The most common abdominal hernias occur in the groin and include indirect inguinal, direct inguinal, and femoral hernias. Other types of abdominal hernias include umbilical, epigastric, and incisional.

OVERVIEW

It has been said that the history of hernia surgery is essentially the history of surgery. Indeed, many illustrious and skilled surgeons have added to our understanding of the anatomy of abdominal hernias and have contributed specific methods of repair. Unfortunately, they have frequently also contributed their names to various anatomic structures and surgical procedures, leading to what one author has referred to as a "ludicrous overuse of eponyms in this field" (Nyhus, 1992). This has often resulted in confusion and ambiguity rather than clarity and precision in the discussion of hernial anatomy and repair. With both acknowledgment of and apologies to the great hernial surgeons of the past, no eponyms will be utilized in this chapter.

DEFINITION

Hernia, the Latin word for "rupture," is used to describe the protrusion of any organ or tissue through the structure that normally confines it (Table 32–1). Thus, the brain stem can herniate through the tentorium secondary to increased intercranial pressure. A muscle can herniate through a tear or laceration of its investing fascia. An intervertebral disk can herniate and impinge upon adjacent spinal nerves. The heart can herniate through a pericardial defect, the lung through a disruption of the chest wall. The hernias of most common clinical significance are those involving the abdominal cavity, and specifically the anterior abdominal wall.

GENERAL ANATOMY

Normally, the abdominal contents are contained within a strong, nonyielding sac of fibrous tissue called the **transversalis fascia**. This tissue is interposed between the peritoneum and the musculature of the abdominal wall. All abdominal hernias occur in one of three areas: (1) where the transversalis fascia has natural openings to permit the egress of normal structures, (2) where the fascia has been disturbed by surgical incisions or other penetrating trauma, or (3) where there is a relative weakness of the fascial layer, related either to a failure of fusion of normal tissues or to an inherent weakness of a particular region of the fascial sac.

Examples of the first type, herniation through natural openings, include indirect hernias, umbilical hernias, and hiatal hernias. In these cases, the integrity of the transversalis fascia is of necessity violated to permit egress of the spermatic cord, the umbilical vessels, and the esophagus, respectively. Usually the fascia fuses completely to obliterate the umbilical defect, but an opening may persist and enlarge with time, secondary to normal or increased positive intra-abdominal pressure. The esophageal hiatus and the internal inguinal ring are normally defended by both fibrous rings and dynamic muscular slings, but both are capable of dilating and permitting herniation to occur.

Incisional hernias are examples of the second type. They arise from incomplete healing of fascial defects created by surgical incisions. This may occur because the patient's tissues are intrinsically weak, but more commonly are related to improper suture placement, tension on the wound edges, infection, or a combination of these factors.

Table 32–1. Hernia: definition.

Hernia (Latin: "rupture"): Protrusion of tissue through the structure normally confining it.

An abdominal hernia is the protrusion of extraperitoneal fat, peritoneum, omentum, bowel, or other viscera through a defect in the transversalis fascia.

Obesity is also a risk factor for incisional hernia formation.

Hernias of the third type, fascial weaknesses not related to defects for exiting structures, are not randomly distributed, but occur in predictable areas. The floor of the inguinal canal is one such site, giving rise to direct inguinal hernias. The area between the inguinal ligament and the pectineal ligament gives way to permit femoral hernias. Epigastric and anterior diaphragmatic hernias arise from the failure of fusion of midline structures. Posterolateral diaphragmatic hernias are also the result of incomplete joining of the embryological tissues.

INCIDENCE & PREVALENCE

Hernias are a common health problem in the United States. Although precise data are not available regarding the incidence and prevalence of this disorder, it is estimated that about 5% of males will develop inguinal hernias at some time during their lifetimes. Based upon a "Hospital Discharge Database," the National Center for Health Statistics reported 161,000 hernia repairs in the United States in 1993, of which 109,000 were inguinal, 44,000 umbilical, and 8000 femoral.

ETIOLOGY

Most hernias are acquired in the sense that they are not present at birth, but arise from areas of congenital weakness (see above). Anything that increases intra-abdominal pressure, either acutely or chronically, may convert an area of congenital weakness (eg, a patent processus vaginalis) into an actual hernia. Such factors include coughing, sneezing, straining to void or defecate, heavy lifting, pregnancy, ascites, peritoneal dialysis, and obesity.

COMPLICATIONS

Hernias produce discomfort and disability (a dragging sensation, inability to be physically active and to lift heavy loads) and may lead to the life-threatening complications of obstruction and strangulation. Serious complications occur only when the hernia is irreducible (incarcerated). Strangulation develops when bowel trapped in the hernia no longer receives sufficient blood supply to prevent necrosis. Strangulation does not occur without incarceration. On the other hand, hernias can be chronically incarcerated (irreducible) without being strangulated. This occurs when the incarcerated sac contains only preperitoneal fat or omentum—or when the bowel is held in the hernia sac by adhesive bands, rather than being trapped by a tight, constricting ring of fascia.

CLINICAL CONSIDERATIONS

HISTORY

The medical history is designed for two purposes: (1) to determine that a hernia is, in fact, present, and (2) to assess confounding factors that would influence the decision whether, and at what point, to advise surgical repair. Most patients will complain of pain, or a mass, or both in the inguinal, umbilical, or epigastric region. The mass may be intermittently or continuously present. If the mass is not reducible, the patient should be questioned about nausea, vomiting, distention, obstipation, fever, intense pain, or other symptoms of obstruction or strangulation. If present, these conditions require emergency operation.

More information is derived from observation and careful questioning, including:

- Is there a history of trauma?
- Have other masses been noted elsewhere in the body (eg, adenopathy)?
- Was there a precipitating event (eg, weightlifting)?
- How long have the symptoms been present?
- Is there frequent coughing secondary to asthma or chronic bronchitis?

- Does the patient strain to void or defecate?
- Is the patient overweight?
- Are there any skin lesions or other symptoms of infection, such as dysuria or sputum production?

Finally, the patient's cardiac, pulmonary, and overall health status needs to be assessed. If a hernia is present, does the patient desire elective surgery?

PHYSICAL EXAMINATION

The sine qua non of diagnosing an abdominal hernia is the demonstration of a mass. Acute groin pain does not always mean that a hernia is present, and muscular strains will heal spontaneously. When a patient is explored and no sac is found, extensive dissection must be undertaken to be sure that a hernia is not being missed. This surgical trauma may do considerable damage to the local tissues.

The physicial examination should begin with the patient standing. If a mass is palpable, see if it can be reduced—have the patient lie down if necessary. If a mass is not palpable, have the patient cough or strain while carefully palpating the area in question (Figure 32–1). For inguinal hernias in males, invaginate the scrotal skin to permit passage of a finger tip to and through the external ring

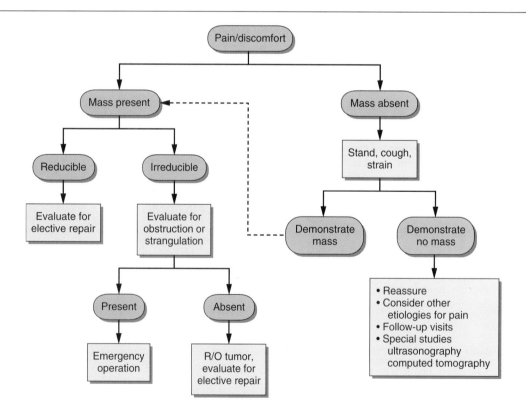

Figure 32–1. Management of a patient presenting with pain or discomfort in an area where hernias typically occur.

to feel for masses or impulses (a dilated external ring does not mean that a hernia is present—see below). Having the patient attempt to sit up without using his hands may help to demonstrate umbilical, epigastric, or incisional hernias. Even if a hernia is not present, all patients over 40 years of age should have a rectal examination in search of masses or occult blood.

If a mass cannot be demonstrated, reassure the patient (Table 32–2). If a hernia is too small to palpate, it will not likely cause obstruction or strangulation. If a hernia is in fact present, it will eventually enlarge and become palpable. If symptoms persist and if no mass can be palpated, consider imaging studies, such as ultrasonography or computed tomography. The latter is especially useful for obese patients when the differential diagnosis includes simple weakness of the abdominal wall, in addition to incisional or epigastric hernia (Figure 32–1).

PREOPERATIVE PREPARATION

Hernias will not heal spontaneously, the possible exception being small umbilical hernias in infants and children less than 2 or 3 years of age (see below). If a hernia can be unequivocally demonstrated, and if elective repair is desired, attention should be turned to identifying and correcting any reversible risk factors that may be present.

Coronary artery disease suggested by angina pectoris or a history of myocardial infarction should be assessed, at least by electrocardiography. More extensive cardiac workup, including stress tests, 24-hour monitoring, angiography, and even angioplasty or coronary artery bypass surgery, should be undertaken as indicated. These potentially life-threatening problems obviously should be dealt with before proceeding with elective hernia repair.

If the patient has chronic lung disease with a productive cough, a brief course of antibiotics may be indicated. Patients with alcoholic liver disease should be brought into optimal medical condition, with special attention to the prothrombin time and other clotting factors. Assistance of a hepatologist should be sought for those with cirrhosis, malnutrition, ascites, or stigmata of portal hypertension. Elective hernia repair may be inadvisable in patients with advanced liver disease.

Symptoms of prostatism should be investigated and significant prostatic obstruction corrected before elective

Table 32–2. Guidelines for management of patients with inguinal hernias.

1. Do not undertake an elective hernia repair unless a mass has been demonstrated.
2. Acute groin pain does not mean a hernia is present. Muscle strains will heal.
3. If a hernia is too small to palpate, it will not likely become obstructed or strangulated
4. Small, nonpalpable hernias will eventually enlarge and become papable. It is safe to wait.

hernia repair. Urinary tract or other infections should be treated before operation. Obese patients should be urged to lose weight—although the results are typically disappointing. Skin rashes or open lesions should be allowed to heal to minimize the risk of wound infection.

MANAGEMENT

ANESTHESIA

Hernias can be repaired under local, regional, or general anesthesia—or a combination of these techniques. Although local anesthesia may suffice in the hands of an experienced surgeon, it is not necessarily the safest technique for all patients. Patients may develop pain or discomfort just from being on the operating table—in areas remote from the surgical field. If a patient becomes agitated and hypertensive, the increased afterload may lead to myocardial ischemia. Local anesthesia has the theoretical advantage of avoiding excessive tension on the repair, because the patient's muscles are not relaxed. In practice, muscle relaxants do not contribute appreciably to problems of tension. General anesthesia can now be performed with short-acting agents, so prompt recovery and same-day surgery are still possible (see below). The choice of anesthetic agents and techniques is best left to the anesthesiologist, in consultation with both the surgeon and the patient.

GENERAL PRINCIPLES OF SURGICAL REPAIR

The general principles of surgical repair are, simply stated, to define and reduce the herniated tissue, to define strong fascial margins in all directions, and to reapproximate those margins with strong sutures, tied without excessive tension (Table 32–3). The hernia will usually be contained within a sac of peritoneum, but occasionally preperitoneal fat may present without a sac. In either case, the herniated tissue has forced itself into an anatomic site where it does not normally reside. For that reason, the tissue will not have a local blood supply, except perhaps for a few vascularized adhesive bands. Once the correct plane is entered, therefore, the hernia can be separated from the surrounding tissue by blunt dissection with minimal bleeding.

Table 32–3. Hernias: principles of repair.

Define, free, and reduce protruding tissue.
Define strong fascial margins.
Reapproximate with strong, nonabsorbable sutures.
Avoid excessive tension with relaxing incisions or prostheses.

Dissection is carried down until the fascial defect is defined circumferentially. At this point, it may be possible to reduce the herniated tissue through the fascial ring. If not, the sac is opened and the entrapped tissue freed of adhesive bands. Excess omentum or fat may be excised if it is not readily reducible. If all else fails, the fascial defect should be enlarged to permit reduction of the herniated tissue.

After the mass is reduced, it is important to clear the *underside* of the fascia for at least 2–3 cm beyond the edge of the defect in all directions to assure that the repair sutures can be placed into strong tissue without risk of damage to underlying viscera. The strength of the fascia should be tested by pulling against it with the needle holder as each suture is being placed. Midline defects can be closed either transversely or longitudinally, depending upon local factors, such as the quality of the fascia and the amount of tension generated by the alternative methods.

The choice of suture material (long-lasting absorbable, nonabsorbable, braided, monofilament) and the method of suture placement (interrupted, running, figure-of-eight) is a matter of surgeon's preference. Essentially all permutations and combinations have been successfully applied. If tension is thought to be excessive, it should be lessened by the use of relaxing incisions or some type of prosthetic mesh to bridge the fascial defect, allowing the opening to be closed without approximating fascial edge to fascial edge directly. Relaxing incisions involves dividing the tethering fascia at points remote from the area of closure, at sites where the integrity of the abdominal wall is maintained by multiple layers of muscle and fascia.

POSTOPERATIVE CARE

Postoperative care is simple and straightforward. Incisional pain must be controlled with appropriate oral or parenteral analgesics and, possibly, by injection of the operative area with long-acting local anesthetics (see below). The patient should be encouraged to walk as soon as possible after the operation, but to avoid strenuous activity for 6 weeks. Outpatients must demonstrate an ability to void and full recovery from their anesthetics prior to discharge. They should never drive on the day of operation and should be instructed in the signs of wound infection (redness, tenderness, swelling, warmth).

Patients should be seen in followup about 1 week after operation. It is traditional to have a final check up at 6 weeks, prior to returning to full activity. In the absence of obvious problems, this latter visit is primarily social, and may be omitted if the patient has no questions or concerns.

RESULTS

Recurrence

No method of hernia repair is perfect, and reherniation will occur in a certain percentage of cases. Precise data

are not available, but with modern surgical techniques the recurrence rate for primary repair of inguinal hernias should probably be less than 5%, with one specialized hospital reporting a rate of 0.61% in selected patients. The rate will obviously be higher for secondary repairs and for repair of incisional hernias.

Complications

The primary complications of hernia repairs are hematomas, infections, and persistent postoperative pain. Primary hernia repair is a class I ("clean") operation and should have an infection rate of less than 1%, too low to justify the use of prophylactic antibiotics. Recurrent hernias, however, are often associated with chronically infected suture material; prophylactic antibiotics are recommended in such cases.

Other general complications include urinary retention, atelectasis, pneumonia, deep vein thrombophlebitis, pulmonary emboli, injury to bowel or bladder, cerebral vascular accidents, myocardial infarctions, and even death. Major complications are rare, and elective hernia repair is generally advised in almost all symptomatic patients.

COMMON HERNIAS

THE INGUINAL ("GROIN") HERNIAS

REGIONAL ANATOMY

By far, the most common abdominal hernias occur in the groin. A basic understanding of the anatomy of this region is essential to the proper diagnosis and repair of groin hernias. Many texts provide diagrams of this area that illustrate the structures in elaborate, but often bewildering, detail. In fact, the basic anatomy of the region is really quite simple and straightforward.

Inguinal hernias are many times more common in men than in women because of the passage of the testis and spermatic cord through the abdominal wall and into the scrotum. The cord exits the abdomen through the **internal inguinal ring**, which is a defect in the transversalis fascia and transversus abdominus muscle just superior to the midportion of the inguinal ligament and just lateral to the deep inferior epigastric vessels (branches of the external iliac artery and vein). The cord contains the vas deferens, the spermatic vessels, and the processus vaginalis (usually obliterated but occasionally patent). The **processus vaginalis** is an outpouching of peritoneum, like the finger of a glove, which helps direct the testicle into the scrotum. The cord is covered by the cremaster muscle, attenuated fibers of the internal oblique muscle. The ilioinguinal nerve is usually adherent to the cremaster.

The anterior wall of the inguinal canal is formed by the

fascia of the external oblique muscle. The posterior wall (floor of the canal) is formed by the transversus abdominus muscle and the transversalis fascia. The superior portion of the floor is variously termed the conjoined tendon, the conjoined area, the falx inguinalis, or the arch of the transversus abdominus aponeurosis. The inferior portion of the floor, just above and parallel to the inguinal ligament, is called the iliopubic tract and is made up of a thickening of the inferior most portion of the transversalis fascia. The cord exits the canal through the external inguinal ring, a defect in the external oblique fascia lying just superior and lateral to the pubic tubercle.

The inguinal ligament is composed of the inferior most fibers of the external oblique fascia; its fibers extend from the anterior superior iliac spine to the pubic tubercle. The posterior portion of the inguinal ligament is referred to as the shelving edge. The inguinal ligament passes anterior to the femoral neurovascular bundle and encloses these structures between itself and the anterior pubic ramus posteriorly. The mnemonic **NAVEL** has been given to describe the arrangement of these structures from lateral to medial: Nerve, Artery, Vein, "Empty space" (for lymphatics), and Ligament. The anterior pubic ramus is covered on its anterior superior surface by dense fibrous tissue called the pectineal line or pectineal ligament (Figure 32–2).

INDIRECT INGUINAL HERNIAS

Indirect inguinal hernias occur when abdominal viscera pass through the internal ring within a patent processus vaginalis. The hernia sac lies within the spermatic cord; it can be confined to the inguinal canal or pass all the way into the scrotum. By definition, indirect inguinal hernias pass lateral to the deep inferior epigastric vessels.

On physical examination it may or may not be possible to distinguish an indirect from a direct inguinal hernia. It is not really important to do so, because the surgical approach is the same for both conditions. Most hernias that descend into the scrotum are indirect, although on rare occasions, a direct hernia also can do so. If a hernia can be reduced and held in place by pressure over the internal ring, it is probably indirect.

Surgical Repair: Anterior

Infants. The surgical approach is simpler in infants than in adults. A horizontal skinfold incision is made starting just above the pubic tubercle and carried laterally about 2 cm. The external ring is identified and enlarged. The cremasteric fibers are gently separated until the peritoneal sac (processus vaginalis) is identified. The sac is then carefully separated from the vas and vessels and transected. The proximal end is traced to the level of the inter-

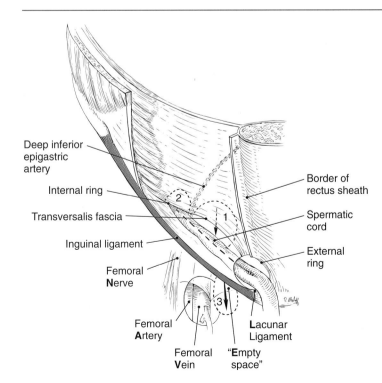

Figure 32–2. Anatomic location of groin hernias. *(1)* direct hernia, *(2)* indirect hernia, *(3)* femoral hernia. Also note the mnemonic NAVEL to denote the arrangement of the following structures from lateral to medial: Nerve, Artery, Vein, "Empty space" (for lymphatics), and Ligament.

nal ring, where it is suture-ligated and divided approximately 1 cm distal to the ligature. Because the internal ring has not been chronically dilated, repair of the floor of the inguinal canal is not necessary. High ligation and division of the peritoneal sac is all that is required. It is neither necessary nor desirable to remove the distal portion of the sac. Contrary to earlier teaching, hydroceles do not develop in the residual peritoneal tissue, and the cord structures can be easily damaged by extensive dissection.

Adults. Adult inguinal hernias differ from the infant variety primarily because the internal ring has become chronically dilated and the floor of the inguinal canal subsequently weakened. Repair of the latter structure is therefore indicated, in addition to high ligation and division of the peritoneal sac.

The operation can be performed from either an anterior or posterior approach. The anterior approach is more commonly used and begins with a transverse or oblique incision beginning about 2 cm above the pubic tubercle and carried laterally 2–3 cm superior to the inguinal ligament. (The location of the ligament is determined by palpation of its bony landmarks: anterior superior iliac spine and pubic tubercle). The external oblique fasica is exposed and cleared sufficiently to identify its inferior border and the external ring. The fascia is opened in the line of its fibers from the external ring laterally for 3–5 cm, with care taken not to injure the ilioinguinal nerve that typically courses along the anterior surface of the spermatic cord on the surface of the cremasteric muscle. If the nerve is visualized, it is carefully dissected free and retracted away from the areas of dissection. The canal contents are bluntly separated from the deep aspect of the lower flap of the external oblique fascia to reveal the shelving edge of the inguinal ligament. The dissection is carried medially to the level of the pubic tubercle, where a plane is developed between the bone and the cord structures. Similar blunt dissection is carried out superior to the cord, and the canal contents are completely encircled at the level of the pubic tubercle. A soft rubber drain is passed about the cord structures at this point for traction.

The fibers of the cremaster muscle are then gently teased apart by careful blunt dissection. This is usually accomplished using two surgical forceps to grasp the tissues, pulling them apart at right angles to the longitudinal axis of the cord. If a hernia is present, the surgeon will encounter the smooth, white surface of the peritoneal sac. This is then separated from the surrounding tissue by further blunt dissection, with care taken not to injure the vas or spermatic vessels.

If the sac extends only part way into the inguinal canal, it can be freed in its entirety. If it extends into the scrotum, it should be freed from the vas and vessels in the canal, transected, and traced proximally to the level of the internal ring—the distal portion being left undisturbed to avoid injury to the cord structures. At this point, the sac should be opened and the surgeon's index finger inserted into the peritoneal cavity. This will give some indication of the size of the internal ring and of the need for subsequent re-

pair. It will also allow palpation of the deep inferior epigastric vessels, thus confirming the indirect nature of the hernia. The floor of the canal medial to the epigastric vessels should also be palpated from within to assess the strength and integrity of the transversalis fascia in this area. Finally, the presence of a femoral hernia should be sought by palpating the area medial to the external iliac vein, posterior to the inguinal ligament, and anterior to the pectineal ligament (superior pubic ramus). The vein cannot actually be felt, but its position can be estimated by feeling the pulse of the external iliac artery as it passes under the ligament. The defect for a femoral hernia should occur 1.5–2.0 cm medial to the arterial pulsation.

The hernia is repaired by freeing the sac to a point just deep to the internal ring, and ligating and dividing it as high as possible, with care taken to avoid injury to intra-abdominal viscera. The proximal end of the sac should then retract well into the retroperitoneum (ligation, although always done, is probably not necessary, provided the sac is divided so that it no longer traverses the internal ring). The internal ring is tightened around the cord to prevent recurrent herniation through this space. If the ring is only slightly dilated, and if the surrounding tranversalis fascia is strong, repair can be accomplished through simple placement of a few interrupted sutures to tighten the fascia medial to the cord (Figure 32–3A). Usually, however, the entire posterior wall of the canal is compromised, and it is therefore tightened by sewing the transversalis fascia (conjoined tendon, conjoined area, falx inguinalis, arch of the transversalis abdominus aponeurosis) to the shelving edge of the inguinal ligament, starting at the pubic tubercle and proceeding laterally to the internal ring (Figure 32–3B).

Prior to this maneuver, the cord is carefully defined by resecting the posterior bands of cremasteric muscle to permit full visualization of the shelving edge of the inguinal ligament. In this repair, the inguinal ligament is the only structure that is actually *visualized*. The superior edge of the repair (the presumed transversalis fascia) is simply *palpated* by invaginating the posterior wall of the canal and feeling for a firm band of tissue superiorly. Once felt, this tissue is grasped with atraumatic clamps and drawn inferiorly toward the inguinal ligament.

The tissue should feel sturdy when traction is applied and should produce an easily palpable fibrous ridge. Multiple interrupted sutures of strong, nonabsorbable material are then placed at intervals of about 1 cm, starting at the pubic tubercle and continuing laterally until the internal ring has been closed snugly around the spermatic cord. The internal ring must be closed tightly enough to avoid recurrent herniation, but not so tightly as to interfere with the venous drainage of the testicle. Each time the needle is passed into the superior band of tissue, the strength of the fascia should be tested by gentle traction on the needle holder. If the tissue seems to give way, stronger fascia must be sought. Some surgeons say the internal ring should be closed to the point where it will admit the tip of the index finger "snugly"; others insert a closed hemostat

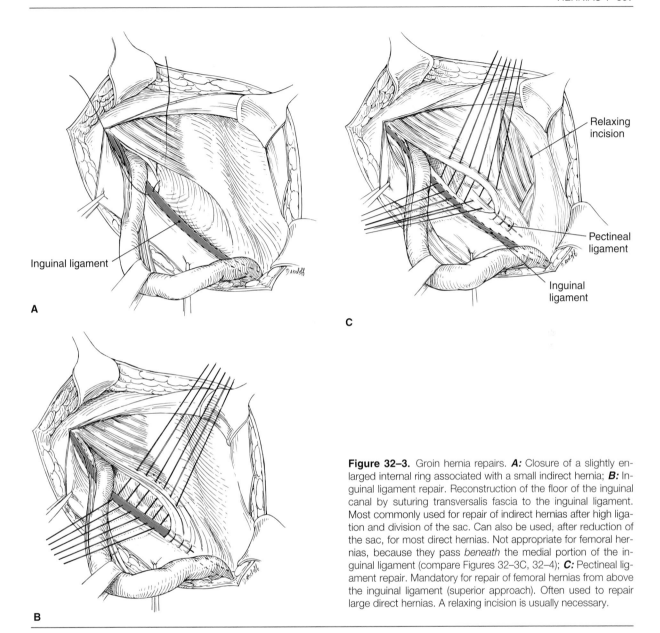

Inguinal ligament

A

B

Relaxing incision

Pectineal ligament

Inguinal ligament

C

Figure 32–3. Groin hernia repairs. ***A:*** Closure of a slightly enlarged internal ring associated with a small indirect hernia; ***B:*** Inguinal ligament repair. Reconstruction of the floor of the inguinal canal by suturing transversalis fascia to the inguinal ligament. Most commonly used for repair of indirect hernias after high ligation and division of the sac. Can also be used, after reduction of the sac, for most direct hernias. Not appropriate for femoral hernias, because they pass *beneath* the medial portion of the inguinal ligament (compare Figures 32–3C, 32–4); ***C:*** Pectineal ligament repair. Mandatory for repair of femoral hernias from above the inguinal ligament (superior approach). Often used to repair large direct hernias. A relaxing incision is usually necessary.

alongside the cord to gauge the appropriate degree of tightness. There are, as yet, no objective guidelines for how tightly to close the internal ring, and this maneuver remains a matter of surgical judgment. Technical improvements are indicated, because about 5% of males will develop testicular atrophy, presumably secondary to cord ischemia, after inguinal hernia repair. (In women, the round ligament is divided and the internal ring closed completely.)

Some surgeons argue that, because the transversalis fascia normally inserts into the pectineal ligament, all repairs of the posterior wall of the inguinal canal should be done

by reapproximating the transversalis fascia to the latter structure. This requires the floor of the canal to be opened to permit exposure of the pectineal ligament (Figure 32–3C). Note that the femoral vessels pass anterior to the pectineal ligament and limit the lateral extent to which this structure can be used in the repair. At the level of the femoral vein, a "transition" stitch must be placed to permit the lateral portion of the repair to be done to the shelving edge of the inguinal ligament anterior to the femoral vessels. The more posterior location of the pectineal ligament (relative to the inguinal ligament) usually means that there is greater tension on the transversalis fascia, and a "relaxing incision" is always recommended. This is done by dissecting under the superior flap of the external oblique fascia to its junction with the rectus sheath medially. A curvilinear incision is then made in the latter structure, with the transversalis fascia allowed to slide laterally and inferiorly, thus relieving tension on the repair. (Although the pectineal ligament repair is theoretically "more anatomic" than the inguinal ligament repair, reported results are similar. The author, therefore, favors the inguinal ligament procedure, because of its relative simplicity.)

After repair to the posterior wall of the canal, the cord and ilioinguinal nerve are returned to their anatomic positions, and the external oblique fascia reapproximated over them. Note that the external oblique fascia is not really part of the repair, because the hernia occurred *underneath* it. If the transversalis fascia is felt to be weak and the integrity of the repair of the posterior wall of the canal is suspect, the upper flap of the external oblique fascia can be passed *beneath* the cord and sutured to the inguinal ligament from the pubic tubercle to the internal ring. The cord is, thus, transposed from a subfascial to a subcutaneous position, and the external ring directly overlies the internal ring. The external oblique fascia now contributes to the integrity of the repair.

DIRECT INGUINAL HERNIAS

Direct inguinal hernias do not occur in infants. In adults they may be diffuse or discrete (pedunculated, diverticular), the diffuse form being vastly more common. Direct hernias present through a defect in the floor of the inguinal canal medial to the deep inferior epigastric vessels. Unlike indirect hernias, they are not related to a natural defect in the transversalis fascia, but rather arise from an acquired weakness of the latter structure.

Surgical repair is essentially identical to that described above for indirect inguinal hernias. After the cord is isolated with a rubber drain, it should be carefully dissected to expose its individual components ("skeletonized") in order to rule out the presence of an indirect sac. (Simultaneous indirect and direct hernias are termed "pantaloon" hernias, the crotch of the pantaloon being formed where the two sacs are draped over the deep inferior epigastric vessels.)

Direct hernial sacs need not—and probably *should not*—be excised because of potential injury to underlying bowel or bladder (see below). As described above under General Principles of Surgical Repair, the herniated mass is dissected free from surrounding tissue, reduced, and held in place by closing the fascial defect with strong sutures. A discrete (pedunculated, diverticular) direct hernia can be repaired by simple closure of the ring of the fascial defect. Diffuse direct hernias should be repaired by sewing the transversalis fascia to the inguinal or pectineal ligaments, exactly as described above for indirect hernias (Figure 32–3B, 3C).

SLIDING HERNIAS

A **sliding hernia** is a special type of inguinal hernia, either direct or indirect, in which a viscus (cecum, sigmoid colon, or bladder) forms an integral part of the wall of the herniated mass, rather than being simply contained within it. In the past, elaborate operations involving multiple concentrically placed pursestring sutures were devised to reduce and repair sliding hernias. In fact, the general principles of repair apply: define and reduce the mass and close the fascial defect. It is necessary neither to open the sac nor to excise redundant peritoneum. Occasionally, sliding hernias may be incarcerated and refractory to reduction through the fascial defect. In such cases a laparotomy may be needed to reduce the sigmoid colon or cecum from above. Fascial repair then proceeds as for other indirect or direct inguinal hernias (see above).

FEMORAL HERNIAS

A femoral hernia protrudes through an acquired fascial defect and passes posterior to the inguinal ligament and medial to the femoral vein. It is further bounded medially by the arch of fibrous tissue that joins the medial end of the shelving edge of the inguinal ligament to the more posteriorly situated pectineal ligament. This is termed the **lacunar ligament** (lacuna, Latin "a pit"). Because, unlike indirect and direct hernias, femoral hernias pass *beneath* the inguinal ligament, they cannot be repaired by approximating the transversalis fascia to the latter structure. If approached superior to the inguinal ligament (through the external oblique fascia as described above), femoral hernias *must* be repaired using the pectineal ligament so as to obliterate the causative fascial defect (Figure 32–3C).

Femoral hernias, however, can also be approached from below (inferior to) the inguinal ligament. Here the general principles of hernia repair still apply: define and reduce the herniated tissues and close the fascial defect without tension (Table 32–3). Frequently, this can be done simply by suturing the medial portion of the inguinal ligament directly to the adjacent, more posteriorly situated pectineal ligament (Figure 32–4). If this cannot be done without tension, some surgeons recommend placing a patch or plug of prosthetic mesh into the defect and securing it to the inguinal ligament anteriorly and to the pectineal ligament posteriorly.

Surgical Repairs: Posterior

All three types of groin hernias can also be repaired from a posterior approach. Midline, transverse, or oblique incisions are used to enter the peritoneal cavity or—more frequently—the preperitoneal space. The general principles of repair then apply. The herniated tissues are freed and reduced, this time by *pulling* rather than *pushing* them into the abdomen. The fascial edges and securing ligaments are defined and closed in a fashion analogous to that described above, but with the sutures placed from

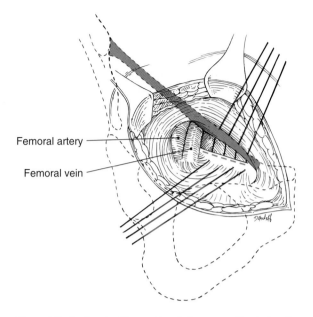

Figure 32–4. Repair of femoral hernia from a position below the inguinal ligament (inferior approach). The inguinal ligament is approximated to the pectineal ligament (pectineal line). A plug of prosthetic mesh is often inserted to fill the space between the two ligaments, thus relieving tension on the sutures.

their deep rather than their superficial aspects. Relaxing incisions are not possible from this approach. Many surgeons advocate the insertion of prosthetic mesh to reinforce these repairs. The mesh is usually sutured loosely in place, but is sometimes simply interposed between the peritoneal sac and the fascial defects, relying upon the positive intraperitoneal pressure to hold it in place until scarring occurs (Figure 32–5).

The posterior approach is particularly recommended for repair of multiply recurrent hernias, especially if they are bilateral. Excellent results are reported by advocates of this technique, although it is rarely used by most general surgeons. The advent of laparoscopic herniorrhaphy is producing renewed interest in this approach (see below and Chapter 12).

UMBILICAL HERNIAS

A defect in the transversalis fascia is necessary to permit the umbilical vessels to reach the placenta during fetal life. This defect contracts after birth and normally is completely obliterated within a few weeks. In some individuals, the defect persists or reopens during adult life as a result of chronically increased intra-abdominal pressure (eg, pregnancy, ascites, obesity, peritoneal dialysis).

Hernias in this area present as masses directly underlying the umbilicus. The mass may be large or small, reducible or irreducible. Small, irreducible, tender masses (1–2 cm in diameter) typically contain only preperitoneal fat. They are repaired to alleviate pain or discomfort.

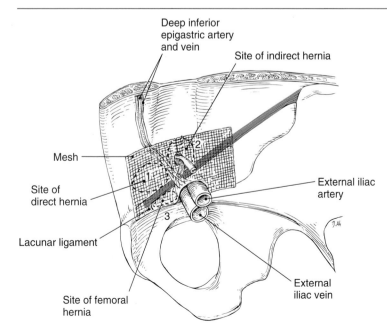

Figure 32–5. Right groin anatomy, posterior view. Closure of *(1)* direct hernia; *(2)* indirect hernia; *(3)* femoral hernia, utilizing a prosthetic mesh patch over the defects via a posterior (preperitoneal) approach. Note that all of the illustrations in this chapter show the anatomy of the right groin. In this figure, the structures appear reversed, because they are viewed from behind (from their deep surfaces). By way of orientation, the right pubic tubercle is to the left of the drawing and the right anterior superior iliac spine is to the right.

Larger hernias may contain omentum, small intestine, or even transverse or sigmoid colon. These should be repaired to prevent obstruction or strangulation, as well as to ameliorate symptoms and decrease disability.

Unless the defect is greater than 3 cm, operation in children is generally delayed until age 5 or 6 years to allow for possible spontaneous closure. It is stated that 95% of umbilical fascial defects less than 1 cm will close by 6 years of age but that those greater than 1.5 cm "seldom" will. There are, however, no accurate data relating the size of the defect to the chance of spontaneous closure.

Repair of these hernias follows the general principles discussed above (Table 32–3). The herniated mass is freed from the surrounding tissues, reduced below the fascia, and the fascia reapproximated over it. In the past, a transverse closure, in which the superior flap of fascia was drawn down over the inferior flap ("vest over pants" technique) was advocated. This has been largely abandoned in favor of simple closure using widely spaced nonabsorbable sutures. The closure may be transverse or longitudinal, depending on the individual anatomy. If the fascial defect is large and rigid, and the edges are not easily approximated without tension, it may be necessary to use prosthetic mesh to bridge the defect. This is done with some trepidation, because of the increased risk of infection in umbilical hernia repairs. Infection of a large piece of prosthetic mesh can become a surgical nightmare—frequently requiring removal of the mesh and alternative complex methods of repair. Prophylactic antibiotics are indicated if prosthetic mesh is to be placed. Mesh can be sewn to the underside of the fascia, the superficial aspect, or both. In all cases, care should be taken to interpose omentum or peritoneum between the mesh and the underlying bowel to minimize adhesive bands and possible fistula formation. The reduction of large umbilical hernias will leave a considerable potential space in the subcutaneous fat, predisposing to hematoma or seroma formation. Closed suction drainage catheters are left in such cases.

EPIGASTRIC HERNIAS

Epigastric hernias occur through midline defects in the fascia of the upper abdomen (between the umbilicus and the xiphoid). They probably arise from a failure of complete fusion of the midline fascia. They are usually small and become symptomatic only when preperitoneal fat becomes incarcerated. Their management is identical to that of umbilical hernias.

INCISIONAL HERNIAS

By definition, all incisional hernias can be considered "recurrent" in that they represent failure of healing of a previous surgically created fascial defect. Many of the factors that led to the original failure of wound healing may still be present (obesity, intrinsically weak tissues, large areas of fascial loss, persistent infection), thus predisposing to further recurrences. Recurrence rates of 15–20% are not unusual in such cases, regardless of the operative technique.

Hernias in midline incisions are often larger and more complicated than they initially appear. If fascial healing has failed in one place, it frequently has failed in other parts of the incision. The incision must, therefore, be explored in its entirety, clearing the undersurface of the scar well beyond the obvious area of herniation to check for other small occult defects. Left unrepaired, these smaller defects will likely enlarge and produce clinically apparent hernias in the future.

The general principles of repair are described above (Table 32–3). It is important to free the fascia widely in all directions to assure placement of sutures into strong fascial structures. If the wound edges cannot be reapproximated without undue tension, relaxing incisions or prosthetic mesh must be used to bridge the defect. The latter technique has largely replaced the former in modern surgical practice. The potential hazards of prosthetic mesh are described above (see Umbilical Hernias). Closed suctioned drains will frequently be required, especially in obese patients.

AREAS OF CURRENT INTEREST/CONTROVERSY

INPATIENT/OUTPATIENT SURGERY

The past 20 years has seen a complete shift from inpatient to outpatient management of routine hernia repair in all but the most high-risk patients. Health care costs have been significantly lowered with no adverse effect upon outcome (recurrence rate, morbidity, mortality). Admission is still indicated for patients of advanced age, with multiple medical problems, or with large incisional hernias.

ANESTHESIA

As discussed above, routine inguinal hernias can be repaired under local, regional, or general anesthesia. Factors to be considered are the overall medical condition of the patient, the skill and experience of the surgeon, and the need to utilize short-acting agents if surgery is being performed in the outpatient setting. Satisfactory results can be obtained with all of the techniques. Choice of anesthesia should be individualized, with patient, surgeon, and anesthesiologist all involved in the final decision. Local anesthesia presents difficulty if the surgeon and the patient cannot communicate easily during the procedure—if, for example, they do not share a common language.

Some surgeons routinely inject a long-acting local anesthetic into the wound following inguinal hernia repair. The usual agent used is bupivacaine, which can have effects for as long as 24 hours. Use of this agent may lessen, but rarely replace, the need for systemic analgesics. Double-blind, prospective, randomized, controlled clinical trials have not established a clinically important role for this technique in most patients—at least not to the satisfaction of this author.

ONLAY PROSTHETIC MESH

The use of prosthetic mesh is sometimes unavoidable, for example, when fascial defects simply cannot be brought together because of loss or contraction of tissue in the abdominal wall. In that setting, mesh is used to *bridge* the gap—acting as an artificial fascia and allowing the wound to be closed without tension. More recently, some surgeons have advocated the routine use of mesh as an **onlay patch** on top of the completed repair to encourage scarring and fibrosis and to provide a stronger repair. Used in this fashion, mesh will not adhere to or damage the bowel, but it is still subject to infection and subsequent chronic problems. The use of mesh is important in certain techniques of laparoscopic hernia repair (see below) (Figure 32–5).

It remains to be proven that the routine use of mesh as an onlay patch will appreciably reduce the risk of recurrence for uncomplicated inguinal hernias. Because literally millions of hernias have been successfully repaired without mesh, it clearly is not an essential part of the operation in all cases.

LAPAROSCOPIC HERNIA REPAIR

In recent years, techniques have been developed to repair inguinal hernias laparoscopically. The anatomic concept is identical to that of the posterior approach described above. The laparoscope is used to visualize and define the hernia sac and the fascial defect from the deep aspect of the abdominal wall. The dissection is performed either intraperitoneally or in the preperitoneal space. The herniated mass is identified and reduced by pulling it back into the abdomen. The fascial defect is defined and closed with sutures or special staples, or by covering it from the inside with a patch of prosthetic mesh (Figure 32–5).

Laparoscopic hernia repair has been shown to be feasible, but it remains to be established whether or not it has any meaningful advantage over conventional techniques in terms of morbidity, mortality, cost, time of disability, or durability of repair. A number of cases of bowel obstruction have been reported following laparoscopic hernia repair, a complication rarely seen with traditional techniques (see Chapter 12).

SUGGESTED READING

Bendavid R: The Shouldice method of inguinal herniorrhaphy. In: Nyhus LM, Baker RJ (editors): *Mastery of Surgery*, 2nd ed. Little, Brown, 1992.

Condon RE: Iliopubic tract repair of inguinal hernia: The anterior (inguinal canal) approach. In: Nyhus LM, Baker RJ (editors): *Mastery of Surgery*, 2nd ed. Little, Brown, 1992.

De Lorimier AA, Harrison MR: Pediatric surgery. In: Way LW (editor): *Current Surgical Diagnosis & Treatment*, 8th ed. Appleton & Lange, 1988.

Deveney KE: Hernias and other lesions of the abdominal wall. In: Way LW (editor): *Current Surgical Diagnosis & Treatment*, 8th ed. Appleton & Lange, 1988.

Heydorn WH: Abdominal hernia. In: James EC, Corry RD, Perry JF, Jr (editors): *Principles of Basic Surgical Practice*. Hanley and Belfus, 1987.

Knol JA, Eckhauser FE: Inguinal anatomy and abdominal wall hernias. In: Greenfield LJ (editor): *Surgery: Scientific Principles and Practice*. Lippincott, 1993.

McGregor DB et al: The abdominal wall, including hernia. In: Lawrence PF (editor): *Essentials of General Surgery*, 2nd ed. Williams & Wilkins, 1992.

Nyhus LM: Iliopubic tract repair of inguinal and femoral hernia: The posterior (preperitoneal) approach. In: Nyhus LM, Baker RJ (editors): *Mastery of Surgery*, 2nd ed. Little, Brown, 1992.

Nyhus LM, Bombeck CT, Klein MS: Hernias. In: Sabiston DC, Jr (editor): *The Textbook of Surgery: The Biological Basis of Modern Surgical Practice*, 14th ed. WB Saunders, 1991.

Ponka JL: The Ponka approach to the repair of groin hernias. In: Nyhus LM, Baker RJ (editors): *Mastery of Surgery*, 2nd ed. Little, Brown, 1992.

Rutledge RH: Cooper ligament repair of groin hernias. In: Nyhus LM, Baker RJ (editors): *Mastery of Surgery*, 2nd ed. Little, Brown, 1992.

Stoppa RE, Warlaumont CR: The midline preperitoneal approach to and prosthetic repair of groin hernias. In: Nyhus LM, Baker RJ (editors): *Mastery of Surgery*, 2nd ed. Little, Brown, 1992.

Wantz GE: Abdominal wall hernias. In: Schwartz SI, Shires GT, Spencer FC (editors): *Principles of Surgery*, 6th ed. McGraw-Hill, 1994.

33

The Head & Neck

Jimmy J. Brown, DDS, MD, Hee Wan Park, MD, PhD, & Willard E. Fee, Jr, MD

► Key Facts

► A thorough head and neck examination includes adequate exposure by means of a headlight or mirror, application of topical anesthesia to decrease patient discomfort, and the administration of a nasal decongestant, such as Neo-Synephrine or oxymetazoline.

► The most common site of facial trauma is the nose. Complicated fractures, such as nasoethmoid, orbital, "blow out", and zygomatic complex fractures, may require ophthalmologic or neurosurgical consultations.

► Maxillary fractures are classified into three groups (LeFort I, II, and III) based on the course of fracture lines through the facial and skull bones.

► Congenital lesions of the nose include nasal dermoids, nasal gliomas, and encephaloceles.

► Although nasal neoplasms are uncommon, clinical signs may include nasal obstruction, blood-tinged mucus, and frank epistaxis.

► For acute sinusitis, surgical management may be considered when there are impending complications of intraorbital or intracranial spread.

► Pleomorphic adenomas are the most common benign salivary neoplasm in the adult population, while mucoepidermoid carcinomas are the most common malignant neoplasms. Both are man-

aged with surgical excision and in cases adjuvent radiotherapy.

► Removal of the tonsils or adenoids for an infectious process is usually preceded by clinical documentation of at least five episodes per year or absence from school or work for 2 weeks per year.

► Laryngeal papilloma is the most common benign neoplasm of the larynx and may occur in both juveniles and adults. Most cases require serial endoscopies with resection. The CO_2 laser is also useful for debulking or removing the lesion.

► Approximately 11,000 new cases of laryngeal cancer are diagnosed annually. Risk factors associated with the disease include tobacco use, alcohol consumption, occupational or industrial exposure, and radiation.

► The differential diagnosis of a neck mass includes four broad categories: congenital, inflammatory, neoplastic, and acquired.

► The primary site for most cancers that metastasize to the neck is the upper aerodigestive tract, but cancers from the lungs, prostate, kidney, breast, testicle, and gastrointestinal tract may also metastasize here.

The head and neck region represents a compact zone of muscles, nerves, and blood vessels supported by a bony architecture covered by specialized epithelial surfaces that functions to maintain the homeostasis of this region. Epithelial surfaces of the aerodigestive tract also form part of this unit. These various epithelial surfaces are prone to the formation of disease. A high level of suspicion must be maintained when evaluating patients with complaints in this region. Far too often, there is a delay in diagnosis of conditions requiring timely attention.

A detailed history and physical examination cannot be overemphasized. Specifically, etiologic agents such as tobacco, alcohol, exposure to industrial agents, radiation, and dietary factors should be explored. A thorough head and neck examination begins with adequate exposure, which includes the use of a head light or mirror. The mucosa should be anesthetized topically to suppress a cough or gag reflex, and the nose should be decongested with Neo-Synephrine or oxymetazoline (Table 33–1).

ANATOMY & PHYSIOLOGY

FACE

The bony architecture of the face is actually a conglomerate of several individual bones fused at various suture lines (eg, frontal, nasal, lacrimal, zygomatic, maxilla, and mandibular bones). Certain points of union between individual bony units, called **buttresses**, are particularly reinforced. These buttresses are akin to the pillars of a temple and can withstand a great deal of force. Understanding

Table 33–1. Approach to the head and neck.

- Develop a system by which the regions of the head and neck are evaluated and a presumptive diagnosis is reached.
- Perform a detailed, comprehensive history and physical examination.
- Maintain a high level of suspicion for malignancies in the head and neck.
- Appreciate the difficulty posed in examining some regions of the head and neck, such as the nasopharynx, hypopharynx, and larynx.
- Have the appropriate instruments available during examination.
- Think of the acronym V.I.N.D.I.C.A.T.E.S., a system of differential diagnosis that groups related conditions or systems: V = vascular, I = infections, N = nutrition, D = drugs, C = cancer, A = allergies, T = trauma, E = endocrine conditions, S = systemic illnesses.
- Do not minimize the examination of any region of the head and neck based on the patient's complaints. A complaint-directed examination is performed only for "established" patients.
- Consider imaging studies only after obtaining a complete history and performing a physical examination.

these buttresses is a key to the repair of facial fractures as well as congenital and acquired cosmetic deformities.

The anatomic region of the nasoethmoid complex includes the nasal bones, ethmoid sinus labyrinth, lacrimal bone, lacrimal sac, and medial canthal tendon. The configuration of the ethmoid sinus is similar to that of a piece of cardboard with two bony plates separated by interbridging thin plates of bones. Its roof is the anterior cranial fossa. The lateral wall of this labyrinth is the medial wall of the orbit, with the lacrimal bone anteriorly contributing to part of this wall. The lacrimal bone has two crests, one anteriorly and one posteriorly. Each serves as an attachment for one slip of medial canthal tendon (tendon of orbicularis oculi muscle) (Figure 33–1). The lacrimal sac is cradled within the fossa of the lacrimal bone, with the anterior and posterior slips of medial canthal tendon on each side.

The facial muscles are a study in contrast to the usual concept of muscles acting as joint movers in the rest of the skeleton. In the face, the muscles have bony origin and soft tissue (skin) insertion. This arrangement creates various permanent topographical features, such as brow lines, crow's feet, nasolabial folds, and mentolabial folds that become more pronounced with age. All muscles of facial expression are innervated by branches of the seventh cranial nerve (CNVII). Sensory innervation is mediated via branches of the fifth cranial nerve (CNV). The muscles and their investing fascia form a unit structure referred to as the **superficial muscular aponeurotic system**. This system is the key to the surgical planes of the face. Specifically, a successful rhytidectomy (face-lift) is predicated on having a sound knowledge of the superficial muscular aponeurotic system.

Vascular supply to the face is derived from both the internal and external carotid systems. The internal system contributes to the **ophthalmic artery**. This artery passes through the optic canal along with the optic nerve, providing nutrients to the intraorbital contents and entering the nose as the anterior and posterior ethmoidal arteries. It exits the orbit onto the forehead via the supratrochlear and supraorbital foramina, bearing the name of each foramen respectively. Veins of the face follow a course similar to that of arteries. Tributaries of the scalp and deeper structures of the head coalesce to form main channels. For example, angular veins coursing at the nasofacial angle receive tributaries from the scalp and cavernous sinus via the inferior ophthalmic vein. These vessels are valveless, hence, flow of blood may be bidirectional. Therefore, bacteria from facial infectious foci can embolize centrally.

NOSE

The nose is a pyramidal structure comprised of paired bones that are fused to the nasal process of the frontal bone and frontal process of the maxilla. Distal to the nasal bony structure is a mobile unit comprised of paired upper and lower lateral cartilages. Muscles and strong ligaments attach this cartilaginous framework to a "pear-shaped"

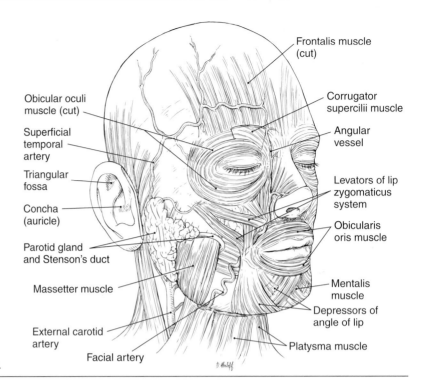

Figure 33–1. Anatomy of facial soft tissues.

opening of the facial skeleton called the **piriform aperture**.

Intranasally, the lateral wall is formed by the **turbinates**. The space beneath each turbinate is called the **meatus**. The inferior meatus lies beneath the inferior turbinate and is the site for the opening of the nasolacrimal duct. The middle meatus, the site of opening for the maxillary, ethmoid, and frontal sinuses, boasts the ethmoid bulla, a conglomerate of anterior and middle ethmoid air cells. The anterior and middle ethmoid chambers open into the ethmoid bulla. Inferior to the ethmoid bulla is a slit-like structure, the hiatus semilunaris. The sphenoid sinus opens near the superior meatus in the area of the sphenoethmoid recess. Traveling anteriorly to posteriorly along the floor of the nose, one would encounter the paired choanae, representing the posterior aperture of the nose. The intricate nature of the intranasal anatomy serves to process the air we breathe by filtering, warming, moistening, and streamlining its flow.

Vascular supply to the nose is derived from both internal and external carotid systems. The **ophthalmic artery**, a branch of the internal carotid artery, gives off the anterior and posterior ethmoidal arteries via their respective ethmoidal foramina at the frontoethmoidal suture line. The location of the anterior and posterior ethmoidal foramina from a fixed point anteriorly (**maxillolacrimal suture line**) is a crucial surgical landmark to avoid injury to the optic nerve when the ethmoidal arteries must be ligated, for example, in intractable epistaxis. These arteries, after supplying the air cells of the ethmoid sinus, give off main branches to the attic of the nasal cavity and septum.

The **sphenopalatine artery**, which is the main blood supply to the nose, is the terminal branch of the internal maxillary artery, itself a branch of the external carotid artery. The sphenopalatine artery ramifies most of the nasal vault, giving off lateral and septal branches. It enters the nasal cavity via the sphenopalatine foramen on the posterior superior aspect of the septum. Venous drainage follows in the same basic pattern as arterial supply. Knowledge of the vascular anatomy of the internal nose is crucial to successful management of epistaxis.

Innervation of the nasal cavity is via the **maxillary nerve** (V2), carrying somatic sensory, special sensory, and secretomotor (parasympathetic) information.

PARANASAL SINUSES

There are four pairs of paranasal sinuses named after the bone in which they are housed: **maxillary**, **ethmoid**, **frontal**, and **sphenoid**; they develop as outgrowths of nasal mucosa (Figure 33–2). These sinuses are air-filled chambers lined by typical respiratory epithelium (mucosa). The blood supply and nervous innervation are derived from branches of the carotid and trigeminal systems, respectively.

Lymphatic channels of the nose and paranasal sinuses pass posteriorly and coalesce into larger channels in the region of the eustachian tube. Subsequently, they pick up other channels from the nasopharynx and then empty into retropharyngeal lymph nodes. Secondary lymph channels

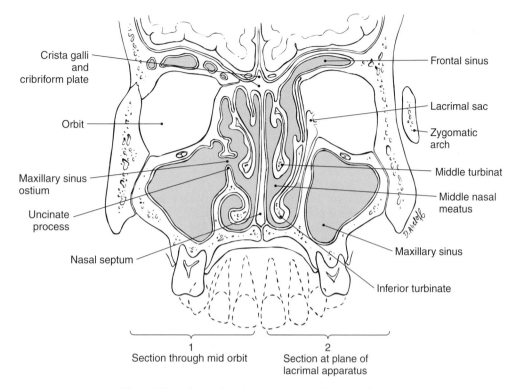

Crista galli and cribriform plate

Orbit

Maxillary sinus ostium

Uncinate process

Nasal septum

Frontal sinus

Lacrimal sac

Zygomatic arch

Middle turbinat

Middle nasal meatus

Maxillary sinus

Inferior turbinate

1
Section through mid orbit

2
Section at plane of lacrimal apparatus

Figure 33–2. Coronal anatomy, paranasal sinuses, and nose.

leave the retropharyngeal nodal station (primary nodal station) and empty into the deep jugular chain.

SALIVARY GLANDS

There are three pairs of major salivary glands in the head and neck and between 750 and 1000 minor salivary glands throughout the upper aerodigestive tract. The first of the major salivary glands is the **parotid gland**. It is the largest of the salivary glands, paired, and located on either side of the face, between the mastoid and posterior aspect of the ramus of mandible (parotid fossa). Superficially, the skin and dermis cover the gland. Medially, the gland is buttressed by the styloid process and its muscles: the styloglossus, stylohyoid, and stylopharyngeus. The carotid sheath is also medial to the gland. Superiorly, the zygomatic arch marks its limit and, inferiorly, the anterior border of the sternocleidomastoid muscle. Embryologically, the parotid gland is the earliest to be seen developmentally, and the last to complete its encapsulation. For this reason, adjacent lymph nodes become entrapped within the substance of the gland during this final stage of development. The gland is artificially divided into a superficial and a deep lobe, demarcated by the plane of the CNVII as it ramifies through the gland.

The parotid duct (Stenson's duct) is a coalescence of several ductules emanating from the substance of gland. It travels anteriorly over the masseter muscle, turning suddenly medially, piercing the buccinator muscle and mucosa of the cheek, and opening at the level of the second maxillary molar.

The **submandibular gland** fills the major portion of the digastric or submandibular triangles on each side. The duct of the submandibular gland (Wharton's duct) emerges from its deep portion and courses anteriorly between the two muscles of the floor of the submandibular triangle, the mylohyoid and the hyoglossus. It opens into the floor of the mouth near the lingual frenulum on either side of the midline. The duct has an important anatomic relationship with the lingual nerve. Posteriorly, the nerve crosses the duct laterally, while anteriorly the nerve lies medial to the duct.

The **sublingual gland**, also paired, lies superficially in the floor of the mouth, deep to mucosa only. The gland can be easily palpated bilaterally in the floor of the mouth. It does not develop a single draining duct, but has several ductules that may open separately into the floor of the mouth or into the submandibular gland duct.

The parotid gland receives secretomotor fibers from the inferior salivary nucleus of the brain stem, which travels with the ninth cranial nerve (CNIX). The CNIX then sends fibers via the tympanic plexus to the otic ganglion as the lesser petrosal nerve. The otic ganglion, which resides in the infratemporal fossa, sends post-ganglionic fibers via auriculotemporal nerve to the parotid gland. This system regulates the production of saliva.

The submandibular and sublingual glands are regulated by secretomotor tracts that originate in the superior salivatory nucleus. These fibers leave the brain stem as the intermediary fibers of CNVII, which course through the temporal bone. The fibers leave the main trunk of CNVII at the posterior wall of the middle ear as the chorda tympani nerve. This nerve travels through the middle ear space between the malleus and the incus, exiting anteriorly and entering the infratemporal fossa to join the lingual nerve. The fibers then travel with the lingual nerve to synapse with the submandibular ganglion in the submandibular space. From here, post-ganglionic fibers are given off to the submandibular gland and sublingual gland for their secretory functions.

Minor salivary glands are present throughout the upper aerodigestive tract and are particularly numerous in the soft palate. They contribute to the total homeostasis of the overlying mucosa of the upper aerodigestive system. The minor salivary glands can also be the source of neoplastic disease processes.

EAR

The external ear comprises the auricle, cartilaginous ear canal, and lateral tympanic membrane surface (Figure 33–3). The **auricle** is a fibroelastic structure with an undulating lateral surface having a perichondrium and skin firmly attached to it. The major undulations are the concha, scaphoid fossa, triangular fossa, antihelix, and helix. On the posterior surface, the covering is thicker and more loosely attached. This framework is firmly attached to the tympanic part of the temporal bone by a continuation of the cartilaginous ear canal (anterior, superior and posterior ligaments) and corresponding intrinsic muscles. Innervation is by the CNV, CNVII, CNIX, CNX, and the cervical plexus (greater auricular). All contribute sensory innervation to the ear canal and auricle. The blood supply is via the branches of the external carotid artery. The posterior auricular and the superficial temporal artery are the main branches.

The external auditory canal is cartilaginous in its lateral one third and bony in its medial two thirds, culminating at the tympanic membrane. It has an area of incomplete union. The "fissure of Santorini" traverse its anterior walls. This fissure can transmit infection or tumor from the ear canal to the parotid fossa.

The middle ear anatomy consists of the tympanic cavity and the bony part of the eustachian tube. The **tympanic cavity** contains the sound-pressure transformer mechanism. The posterior wall contains structures such as the pyramidal process, facial nerve, and chorda tympani. The anterior wall is common, with a thin plate of bone covering the carotid artery (carotid canal). Medially, the middle ear shares a common wall (the basal turn of cochlea) with the inner ear, called the promontory. The inner ear has a complex system of channels responsible for converting sound energy into electrical energy. This system is the labyrinth of the cochlea and vestibular apparatus. The vascular supply to the middle ear is vast, originating from internal and external carotids. The anterior

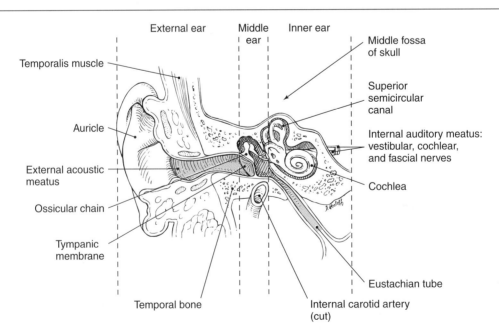

Figure 33–3. Relationship of external, middle, and inner ear.

tympanic, superior tympanic, deep auricular, and inferior tympanic arteries are various branches of the carotid system supplying the middle ear. Nerves of the middle ear include the chorda tympani, which has no real function in the middle ear, but carries taste fibers to the anterior two thirds of the tongue along with secretory motor fibers to the submaxillary and sublingual glands. The tympanic nerve, or Jacobson's nerve, runs submucosally over the promontory and provides sensation to the middle ear mucosa.

ORAL CAVITY

The anatomic boundaries of the oral cavity begin with the vermilion borders of upper and lower lips anteriorly and extend posteriorly to the junction of the hard and soft palate superiorly, and to the circumvallate papillae of the tongue inferiorly. Contained in this area are the lips, buccal region, alveolar ridges (with teeth and gingiva), retromolar trigone, floor of the mouth, anterior two thirds of tongue (oral tongue), and hard palate. The **lips** begin at the junction of vermilion border and skin and include only that portion or surface that comes into contact with each other. They are joined laterally at the commissures of the mouth. The **buccal region** includes all the mucosa lining the inner aspect of the cheeks, deep to which is the buccinator muscle. The **alveolar ridges** are the alveolar processes of both the maxilla and mandible. On the mandible, this extends posteriorly to the retromolar area and ramus. On the maxilla, the posterior extent is the maxillary tuberosity. The **retromolar trigone area** is the mucosally covered anterior ramus of mandible bilaterally, starting immediately posterior to the third molars on either side. The **floor of the mouth** is the semilunar-shaped space extending from the inner aspect of the alveolar ridge of the mandible to the under surface of the tongue. Its posterior limit is the base of the anterior tonsillar fossa. The ostia of both the submandibular and sublingual glands open into the anterior floor of the mouth on either side of the frenulum; a mucosal band extends from the median raphe of the tongue to attach to the alveolar ridge of the mandible. The **hard palate** is the semilunar area between the upper alveolar ridge and the mucus membrane covering the palatine process of maxillary bone and palatine bone. Its posterior termination begins with the soft palate, an oropharyngeal structure. The **oral tongue** is the anterior most two thirds occupying the oral cavity. Its posterior limit is the circumvallate papillae. Its surfaces are dorsal, lateral, ventral, and tip.

The oral cavity has a rich supply of blood vessels, including arteries that originate from the external carotid artery. The innervation is via the trigeminal nerve (CNV) for pain, pressure, and temperature sensation. Sensation for taste is via the chorda tympani to the anterior two thirds of the tongue. All the structures comprising the oral cavity act in concert to masticate and prepare food for deglutition and digestion.

OROPHARYNX

The anatomic boundaries of the oropharynx extend from the plane of the hard palate superiorly to the plane of the hyoid bone inferiorly. In this defined area, posterior to the oral cavity, are the **faucial arches**, including the soft palate, tonsils, and the anterior and posterior tonsillar pillar. The base of the tongue extends posteriorly from the circumvallate papillae. The median and lateral glossoepiglottic folds are all part of the oropharynx. When one views the oropharynx from the oral cavity, the posterior pharyngeal wall is in full view and is the limit posteriorly. Blood supply to this region is via branches of the external carotid, while innervation is via the ninth cranial nerve for somatic sensation and taste to the posterior one third of the tongue. The phase of swallowing occurring at the level of the oropharynx is considered involuntary. The tongue presses the food against the soft palate, and with contraction of the oropharyngeal musculature the food is propelled into the introitus of the esophagus.

NASOPHARYNX

The anatomic boundaries of the nasopharynx are the skull base and sphenoid sinus, the paired tori of the eustachian tubes bilaterally, as well as the recesses between the posterior lateral walls and the elevation of the tori (fossa of Rosenmüller) (Figure 33–4). Anteriorly, the limit of this space is the posterior opening into the nose (the choanae). This space is also separated from the oropharynx by an imaginary line drawn from the level of the hard plate anteriorly to the posterior pharyngeal wall. Branches of the external carotid artery supply this area, while innervation is via the pharyngeal plexus. The nasopharynx is involved in the important functions of smell, taste, and speech, and passively facilitates the act of swallowing, as well.

NECK

The neck is divided into **triangles** by muscle bellies, bones, and fascial layers (Figure 33–5). The posterior triangle on each side of the neck is bounded by the sternomastoid, trapezius, and middle third of clavicle. It is further divided into the occipital triangle superiorly and the subclavian triangle inferiorly by the lower belly of the omohyoid muscle. The anterior triangle is bound by the sternomastoid, body of the mandible, and midline of the neck. It is subdivided into the digastric triangle by both bellies of the digastric muscles and by the inferior border of mandible. The submental triangle is bound by both the anterior bellies of the digastric muscles and the hyoid bone inferiorly. The carotid triangle is bound by the sternomastoid muscle, posterior belly of the digastric, and upper belly of the omohyoid.

The **deep fascial system** of the neck has three layers:

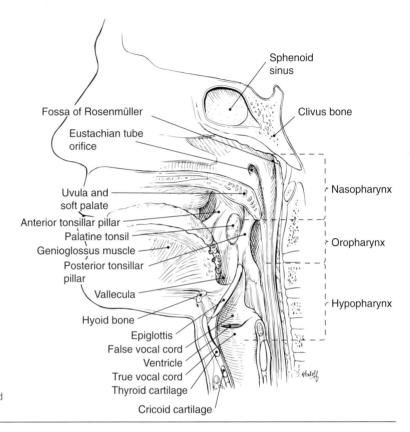

Figure 33–4. Nasopharynx, oropharynx, and hypopharynx (laryngopharynx).

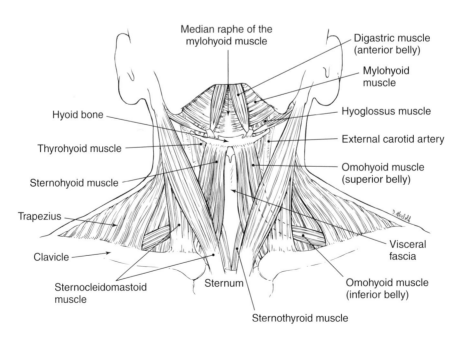

Figure 33–5. General anatomic scheme of neck.

superficial, middle, and deep. The superficial layer of this system invests the triangles of the neck and each individual muscle of the triangles. The middle layer, or visceral layer, invests the visceral structures of the neck (trachea, larynx, esophagus, and thyroid). The deep layer invests the scalenus and levator muscles. The brachial plexus and phrenic nerve lie deep to this fascia. The **carotid sheath** (another complex fascial system) is comprised of layers from all three divisions of the deep fascial system. The carotid sheath contains the internal jugular vein, common and internal carotid arteries, and vagus nerve.

The **strap muscles** are the sternohyoid, sternothyroid, thyrohyoid, and omohyoid. They are innervated by C1 and C2 of the nerve loop formed with the hypoglossal nerve (ansa hypoglossi). The strap muscles overlie the thyroid and parathyroid glands as well as the larynx and trachea, which are contents of the anterior compartment of the neck. The superficial layer of the deep fascial system invests the strap muscles.

TRAUMA

FACE & NOSE

Facial trauma is a common occurrence in any major medical center around the United States. The major causes include motor vehicle accidents, industrial accidents, sporting events, and interpersonal altercations. The most common site of facial trauma is the nose.

NASAL FRACTURES

Diagnosis & Management. Nasal fractures may be associated with the formation of nasoseptal hematoma. A nasoseptal hematoma may progress to the formation of an abscess, which can destroy the nasal support mechanism and result in nasal dorsal collapse (saddle nose deformity). Therefore, a careful assessment of any patient who suffers facial trauma should include ruling out a septal hematoma. The treatment of a hematoma is incision and drainage.

Nasoethmoid complex fractures, as the name implies, are complicated fractures of the nasal and ethmoid bony labyrinth with medial canthal tendon disruption. This injury will frequently demand the expertise of an ophthalmologist to manage any associated eye injuries. Neurosurgery consultation may also be needed if a cribriform plate fracture is present. Some nasal fractures can be repaired immediately by closed reduction of the bony fragments. The nasoethmoid complex fractures may require an open procedure for access to the medial canthal tendon attachments. In orbital fractures, blunt trauma to the globe with a fist or baseball may transmit the forces to the or-

bital floor, which has a natural weakness created by the passage of the infraorbital nerve. Selective fracture here will produce a blow-out fracture. With a blow-out fracture, the contents of the orbit may herniate into the maxillary sinus.

MANDIBULAR FRACTURES

Diagnosis & Management. Mandibular fractures are the second most common type of facial fracture, second only to nasal fractures. Anatomic areas of the mandible include the arch, symphysis, body, angle, ramus, coronoid process, and the condylar neck and head (Figure 33–6).

Clinical diagnosis includes assessment of dental occlusion, palpation of irregularities and distracted bony segments, bleeding, mucosal ecchymosis, and point tenderness. A panorex imaging study should be done to confirm and document these fractures.

The management of mandibular fractures has several objectives (Table 33–2). The status of the dentition plays an important role. For example, if the fracture line passes through and also fractures a tooth root, it is prudent to extract that tooth. If the tooth is not fractured and indeed helps in the stabilization of the reduced fracture, the tooth should be saved and attention paid to possible endodontic therapy (root canal). When a tooth is saved in a fracture line, a watchful eye for early infection is prudent.

Various techniques and devices have been used for reduction and stabilization of mandibular fractures. Technique selection may be influenced by the surgeon's preference, age of the patient, site of fracture, and whether the patient is edentulous or not. Some methods include closed reduction with arch bars and intermaxillary fixation. Other methods include open reduction using wire fixation, followed by arch bars and intermaxillary fixation, with similar results. Compression plates, a technique in which the

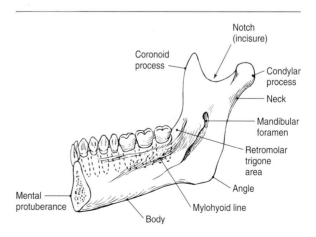

Figure 33–6. Anatomy of the mandible.

Table 33–2. Objectives in the management of mandibular fractures.

Reestablishment of premorbid occlusion
Reduction and fixation of fracture segments
Establishment of infection-free bony union
Full functional mobilization of the mandible

fracture segments are pressed against each other to achieve primary bone healing, is another useful technique that may avoid intermaxillary fixation.

ZYGOMATIC FRACTURES

Diagnosis & Management. Zygomatic fractures are referred to as "tripod fractures." This is a misnomer, however, as the zygoma has four articulation points and not three (frontal, maxillary, temporal, and sphenoid). This fracture can often be assessed without the use of radiographic studies. There is usually a loss of prominence to the zygoma, as the fracture is displaced posteriorly and medially. There may be attendant hypesthesia over the distribution of V2 and a palpable step-off at the fracture lines.

Repair of this fracture usually entails surgical access adjacent to the anticipated fracture lines. An intraoral approach is sometimes included in the repair, especially if the zygoma cannot be reduced by the external approach alone. The zygomatic arch, which is an extension of the zygoma posteriorly, articulates with the temporal bone and may present as an isolated fracture. This may be accompanied by trismus, or inability to open one's mouth.

Maxillary fractures are classified into three groups (**LeFort I, II, and III**) based on the course of fracture lines through the facial and skull bones. Radiologic assessment using plain films or computed tomography (CT) scans prove to be extremely useful in this subset of patients. LeFort I fractures involve the entire maxilla in a horizontal plane from anterior to posterior, just above the apices of the maxillary teeth and into the pterygoid plate. LeFort II fractures, also called "pyramidal" fractures, extend across the nasofrontal suture line down the lamina papyracea and across the floor of the orbit (near the intraorbital grove). It then extends laterally below the zygoma to separate the zygomaticomaxillary buttress and posteriorly to the pterygoid plate at a higher level than the LeFort I fractures. LeFort III fractures are referred to as "craniofacial dislocation" fractures because all bony buttresses attaching the maxilla to the cranium are disrupted, hence, an elongated facial appearance results. The fracture line begins across the nasofrontal suture line and travels across the frontoethmoid suture line and the superior orbit. It then extends across the frontozygomatic suture, crosses the temporal fossa to the pterygomaxillary space, and continues across the root of the pterygoid plates. The cribriform plate, ethmoidal arteries, optic nerve, and internal maxillary artery are all at risk for injury.

LeFort fractures are most often repaired with open reduction and internal fixation. Facial fracture repair can usually be delayed for up to 7–10 days until more pressing patient needs, such as cranial, abdominal or thoracic injuries, are addressed.

SALIVARY GLANDS

Diagnosis & Management. Acute injuries, such as lacerations or glandular avulsion, along with ductal disruption, are frequently addressed in the emergency room setting. First, wounds should be cleansed with "tissue-kind" antimicrobial solutions. If there is only a laceration into the gland parenchyma, it can be repaired when skin injury is repaired. If, in the case of the parotid and submandibular glands, the duct is lacerated, it must be reanastomosed or reimplanted. A silastic tubing is sometimes needed to stent open the duct during the healing phase.

For facial nerve injury, the ends are sought with a microscope, and a tensionless repair (using 9-0 suture) is performed. If this is not possible, then an auricular nerve graft may be interposed to add length and decrease tension.

Salivary fistula, which may occur as a result of injury to gland parenchyma, can be treated conservatively with pressure, anticholinergic agents, or resection of the gland if uncontrolled by conservative means.

EAR

Diagnosis & Management. Traumatic injury to the ear and temporal bone include auricular or external canal laceration or avulsion, hematoma, tympanic membrane perforation, ossicular disruption, and temporal bone fracture.

Each category provides its own management challenges. However, for auricular lacerations, the wound is cleaned, possibly debrided, and reapproximated with monofilament sutures. Partial or total avulsion is treated by primary repair, replacing the avulsed part, followed by intravenous antibiotics and possible steroid therapy. Serially puncturing the edematous repaired areas with an 18-gauge needle decreases pressure and venous stasis. Aspirin, Trental, and small-molecular-weight dextran can also be used to increase blood flow and decrease venous stasis. Medicinal leeches are also valuable adjuncts in this situation.

Hematomas are drained with placement of a small drain and pressure dressing for 3–5 days to decrease recurrence, which is fairly common. Extensive ear canal lacerations frequently have to be stented with packing to avoid scarring and stenosis, which are difficult to correct, once they have occurred.

Ossicular disruption may be repaired in a delayed fashion after all evidence of acute injury has cleared. Frequently, the ossicular injury is an incudostapedial joint separation or fracture dislocation of the stapes.

Temporal bone fractures may occur after blunt trauma to the skull. There are essentially three types of fractures: longitudinal fractures (70–90%), transverse fractures (10–20%), and mixed fractures (a combination of both types). Longitudinal fractures follow the long axis of the temporal bone, while transverse fractures run transversely through the otic capsule, causing nerve deafness, and through the fallopian canal, causing facial nerve paralysis.

Management strategies are based on whether the facial nerve was paralyzed acutely or in a delayed fashion, presence of cerebrospinal fluid otorrhea, and hearing loss. Surgical intervention largely addresses the status of the facial nerve acutely if it is thought to have been severed on impact.

LARYNX, HYPOPHARYNX, & NECK

Diagnosis & Management. The major cause of trauma to the aerodigestive tract is automobile accidents. The extent of the injury is determined by the speed of the vehicle and the use of seat belts. Other blunt or penetrating traumatic events can cause upper aerodigestive injuries, such as those produced by the fist, knife, bullet, and baseball bat. The neck is usually divided into three zones based on certain fixed landmarks. Zone I lies below the sternal notch, zone II lies between the sternal notch and the angle of the mandible, and zone III is above the angle of the mandible. Each zone has specific requirements for assessment.

Initial evaluation includes assessment of the airway, control of bleeding, and evaluation of cardiovascular and neurologic status. Some diagnostic tools used in this setting include plain films of the neck for soft tissue detail, cervical spine radiographs, barium swallow, CT scan, magnetic resonance imaging (MRI), and arteriography. Zones I and III may require angiographic studies before any surgical intervention is planned.

After a full assessment, the decision for endoscopy under general anesthesia and neck exploration may be guided by several factors: site of injury (ie, zone of neck), type of injury (blunt versus penetrating), depth of penetration, crepitus in the neck, airway compromise, expanding mass, active bleeding, or any signs of cerebrovascular insufficiency. Some authorities believe any penetrating trauma deep to the platysma may require mandatory exploration. Specific signs and symptoms of blunt or penetrating neck trauma depend on the structures that are damaged. For example, laryngeal fractures may present with dysphagia, odynophagia, hoarseness or aphonia, dyspnea, hemoptysis, point tenderness, and neck crepitus.

A cardiovascular surgical consultation may be warranted for expansile hematomas. A ruptured hollow viscus may be repaired primarily with strategic drains placed to avoid collection of fluid and infection.

Some larynx fractures are managed conservatively with steroids and antibiotics. This group of patients has minimal symptomatology and physical findings and are observed in the hospital setting. If the airway is compromised and an artificial airway is required, the patient should receive a tracheostomy under local anesthesia rather than be intubated, which will avoid further injury that may compromise laryngeal function later.

If fracture sites are determined to be displaced on examination or imaging studies, the neck is opened for exploration of the larynx, and fractures are reduced and fixed with sutures, wires, or microplates.

Mucosal tears are repaired with absorbable sutures and exposed cartilage covered with mucosa or split thickness skin graft. Hospitalization on intravenous antibiotics, steroids, and tracheostomy tube management may last from 3–5 days, in most cases. The tracheotomy tube is removed when an endoscopy shows a patent airway.

BENIGN & MALIGNANT DISEASE PROCESSES

NOSE

CONGENITAL LESIONS

Nasal Dermoid
Diagnosis & Management. The dermoid sinus lesion is located between nasal cartilages and/or the bone of the dorsum. This may raise or widen the nasal dorsum. Clinically, a lesion can be readily discerned by its location over the nasal dorsum at the bony cartilaginous junction. Radiologic evaluation is by CT scan. Management strategies center around total surgical excision. Surgical access can be made by a horizontal ellipse, "Y"-shaped or "H"-shaped incision over the dorsum and root of the nose.

Nasal Glioma
Diagnosis & Management. These lesions represent deposition of glial tissue extradurally, although 15% may maintain a connection with the subarachnoid space. Clinically, these lesions can present intranasally or extranasally. They are usually noticed at birth or during early childhood. Intranasally, there may be nasal obstruction manifested by difficulty in feeding. Lesions appear as firm, pink, noncompressible, polypoid masses that do not distend when the child cries or when the jugular vein is compressed (Furstenberg's sign).

Management of extranasal and intranasal gliomas is surgical. The extranasal gliomas can be excised with an approach similar to that of a dermoid. Some gliomas may

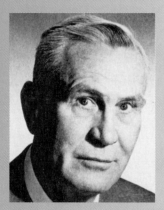

Hayes Martin, MD (1892–1977). (Reprinted, with permission, from Am J Surg 1989;158:279.)

Hayes Martin (1892–1977) made considerable contributions to head and neck surgery in the United States and throughout the world. He was not only responsible for major advances in the field, he was also a key figure in establishing head and neck cancer surgery as a unique specialty. After attending medical school at the University of Iowa, he served in the Navy during World War I. Upon his return to the United States in 1919, he began his internship at Poly Clinic Hospital in New York City and also rotated to Bellevue. He then received an internship at Memorial Hospital beginning in the summer of 1922 and stayed on until 1923. After an additional 2-year residency at Bellevue, Martin returned to Memorial as a clinical assistant surgeon. He was appointed chief of the head and neck service at Memorial Hospital in 1934, and it was here that he established the field of head and neck cancer surgery as a separate entity that required special training, specific experience, and unique qualifications.

One of the first contributions he made to the field of head and neck cancer, and to cancer management in general, was the discovery of the aspiration biopsy while he was still a resident at Bellevue. He performed the first aspiration biopsy on a deceased patient (who was still on the ward) using a needle with a large syringe and the patient's last radiograph as a guide. The specimen was sent to the laboratory and successfully read as cancer by the chief of pathology. Despite the success of the procedure, he was told he would be fired if he continued "doing autopsies on the ward." It was not until he returned to Memorial Hospital as a clinical assistant surgeon that Martin was once again allowed to perform the aspiration biopsy. The procedure was soon adopted as a standard practice on all solid tumors. The first paper to describe it was published in 1930. Aspiration biopsy is now performed worldwide.

require a craniotomy procedure if there is a connection centrally. Therefore, a thorough preoperative evaluation is mandatory, which includes an MRI of the lesion and its relation to the central nervous system.

Encephalocele

Diagnosis & Management. An encephalocele is an extracranial herniation of the meninges and brain through a cranial defect. Only if the meninges alone herniate can the term meningocele be used. Encephaloceles can present in the nose, nasopharynx, or orbit. Clinical presentation of an anterior encephalocele may be associated with rhino-

rhea and feeding difficulty. On examination, a pulsatile mass that is expansile with crying or jugular venous compression may be noted. Widening of the nasal vault may also be seen. An MRI will fully delineate the lesion. Surgical management employs a staged or combined head and neck/neurosurgical approach.

BENIGN NEOPLASMS

Diagnosis & Management. In general, nasal cavity neoplasms are uncommon. Occupational exposure may

In Martin's early days at Memorial Hospital, head and neck cancer was most often treated using radium and radon seeds. Martin wrote numerous articles on radiation therapy and was president of the American Radium Society. In fact, he was one of the rare people who had board membership in three different areas, including the American Board of Radiology, the American Board of Surgery, and the American Board of Plastic Surgery.

During and after World War II, remarkable advances in anesthesia and the advent of antibiotics allowed surgical treatment to dominate much of head and neck cancer management. In 1954, together with Grant Ward, Martin founded the Society of Head and Neck Surgeons and became its first president. He was also a founding member of the James Ewing Society, now known as the Society of Surgical Oncology.

He contributed numerous publications to the field of head and neck surgery, including his remarkable book, *Surgery of Head and Neck Tumors* (Hoeber Harper, 1957). This book represented a major step in the advancement of the surgical management of head and neck cancer. Two of his earlier papers—"Cancer of the Head and Neck" (JAMA 1948;137:1306) and "Neck Dissection" (Cancer 1951;4:441)—were so popular that the American Cancer Society had to order reprints by the thousands to keep up with requests.

Hayes Martin was a dedicated educator, a skilled surgeon, and a creative influence that transformed the field of head and neck surgery. He suffered a stroke in 1971 and died in Memorial Hospital on Christmas Day in 1977 as a result of respiratory complications.

play a causative role, as in the case of woodworkers, leather workers, and workers in nickel or chromium refining plants, who are at increased risk.

Clinical assessment requires a high degree of suspicion, as the symptoms of nasal tumors are not striking. Nasal obstruction, blood-tinged mucus, and sometimes frank epistaxis are the most common signs. Epiphora or tearing unilaterally along with facial numbness may be late signs. Physical examination includes meticulous inspection and palpation. Eye position, visual problems, tooth instability, nasal obstruction, and trismus are important signs to look for. An MRI to determine extent of tumor is important to surgical planning.

The **inverting papilloma** is so named because of its characteristic epithelial growth pattern of finger-like inversions into underlying stroma. It is thought to arise from the "schneiderian epithelium" lining the sinonasal tract. This epithelium is derived from the nasal placodes during embryogenesis and is ectodermal, unlike the rest of the endodermally derived upper aerodigestive tract. Three critical points of emphasis are (1) inverting papillomas are treated by total surgical excision; (2) they have a high rate of recurrence when inadequately excised; and (3) approxi-

mately 10% of inverting papillomas may show squamous cell carcinoma within the specimen. Surgical management techniques include lateral rhinotomy and medial maxillectomy with en bloc ethmoidectomy.

The **juvenile nasopharyngeal angiofibroma** (JNA) is a benign tumor that occurs only in adolescent males and usually presents with a long history of nasal obstruction and recurrent epistaxis. The site of origin is postulated as posterior to the nasal cavity in the area of the sphenopalatine foramen. These lesions can obliterate the maxillary sinus by pushing an intact posterior wall anteriorly. Lateral extension into the pterygomaxillary space and superiorly into the sphenoid sinus or CNS also occurs.

Treatment of JNA should always be preceded by imaging studies to delineate the extent of the tumor. MRI scanning to determine intracranial extension is of vital importance. Angiography with embolization of the main feeding vessels to decrease intraoperative bleeding is indicated for larger tumors. Biopsy of this lesion in a clinic setting is dangerous because of the potential for intractable bleeding.

Surgical approaches to JNA include a lateral rhinotomy or sublabial or transpalatal degloving. Occasionally, a lateral infratemporal fossa approach or a combination of approaches is necessary. While several other approaches are described in the literature, these seem to be the most common. Low-dose radiation for recurrent JNA or intracranial extension is occasionally required.

MALIGNANT NEOPLASM

Diagnosis & Management. The physical and radiologic examination should proceed similar to that for benign neoplasms. Squamous cell carcinoma (SCCA) is the most common malignant neoplasm of the nasal cavity and can originate from any site within the nasal cavity. Nasal vestibule and lateral wall lesions are uncommon while septal lesions are extremely rare. Other malignant lesions of the nasal cavity include adenocarcinomas, adenoid cystic carcinomas, malignant melanoma, esthesioneuroblastoma, hemangiopericytoma, and various sarcomas.

Surgery is the treatment of choice for intranasal SCCA, the surgical approach being alar rhinotomy. Larger lesions may require more extensive procedures, such as a rhinectomy. Lateral wall tumors may be difficult to separate from maxillary sinus tumors, however, management may ultimately be the same. The current accepted mode of therapy is surgery, followed by radiation therapy for large tumors. Surgery may also include an approach via a Weber-Fergusson incision with medial or total maxillectomy.

PARANASAL SINUSES

INFECTIONS

Diagnosis & Management. The most important signs and symptoms of sinus disease are outlined in Table 33–3. Acute sinus infections with impending spread to contiguous structures, such as the orbit or cranium, may necessitate immediate surgical intervention. Before surgery is performed, the appropriate antibiotic coverage must be instituted. Empiric antibiotic therapy is directed toward microbes known to cause acute sinus infection: *Streptococcus pneumoniae*, *Haemophilus influenzae*, and *Moraxella catarrhalis* are the primary pathogens.

For chronic disease, the microbial picture may be different and may include staphylococci and gram-negative species. Fungal infections, such as aspergillus may present a challenge, requiring surgery in combination with antifungal drug therapy.

For acute sinusitis, surgical management may be considered when there are impending complications of intraorbital or intracranial spread. Approaches may include frontal trephination, ethmoidectomy, or sphenoidotomy. For chronic sinusitis, surgical approaches are essentially the same, with emphasis on widening the natural ostia and removing diseased mucosa via endoscopic or open techniques.

In certain situations of chronic sinusitis, allergic sinus disease, or previous trauma, **mucoceles** may develop. These are mucus-filled cystic structures that are slow-growing and reside within the sinus cavity. The appropriate management for mucoceles is surgical excision. The approach may vary, depending upon which sinus is involved. For the frontal sinus, a frontal osteoplastic flap is employed to gain access to the sinus, followed frequently by obliteration of the sinus to prevent recurrence.

NEOPLASMS

Risk factors for paranasal sinus neoplasms are similar to those of the nasal cavity. Neoplasms of the paranasal sinuses are uncommon in the general population. The maxillary sinus is the most common site for sinus neoplasm. Squamous cell carcinoma is the most common malignancy of the paranasal sinuses, occurring in the maxillary sinus 80% of the time.

Diagnosis & Management. The most common symptoms associated with paranasal sinus carcinoma are nasal obstruction and epistaxis (bloody nasal discharge). As the disease progresses it extends into other regions, giving rise to diplopia from compression or invasion of the orbit. Epiphora (excess tearing) occurs when there is obstruction of the nasolacrimal duct. Facial swelling, malocclusion, and trismus occur when there is extension into soft tissues overlying the face and pterygomaxillary space. Hearing loss and facial numbness occur when the tumor extends into the nasopharynx, causing serous otitis media and trigeminal nerve hypesthesia. After adequate evaluation, including MRI imaging, a biopsy may be performed for definitive diagnosis. Cervical lymph node involvement is uncommon at the time of presentation and is an ominous sign when present.

Caldwell-Luc, a popular procedure in which the anterior face of the maxillary sinus is removed and its contents exenterated, is inappropriate for malignant neoplasms.

Table 33–3. Signs and symptoms of sinus disease.

Signs and Symptoms	Infection	Neoplasm
Headaches	+++	+
Rhinorrhea—pus vs blood	+++ pus	+++ blood
Nasal obstruction	++	++
Post-nasal discharge	++	++
Tooth pain	++	++
Tooth laxity	+	+++
Eye pain	++	+
Epiphora	+	+++
Visual disturbance	+	++
Facial hypesthesia	+	+++
Skin lymphedema	–	++
Decreased sense of smell	+	+++

(–) absent; (+) somewhat likely; (++) likely; (+++) very likely.

Also, an external ethmoidectomy, which utilizes an incision just medial to the brow in the shadow of the nasofrontal angle, is inappropriate. Surgical exposure is limited significantly by these approaches that compromise total removal of a malignant tumor. They may be useful, however, for resection of benign neoplasms, for drainage, and, sometimes, for enhancing exposure during biopsy. Medial maxillectomy via a lateral rhinotomy or a sublabial approach may be used for smaller malignant tumors limited to the medial wall, but there may be limitation of access to the posterior and superior margins of resection.

Maxillectomy is the standard operation for advanced carcinoma of the maxillary sinus. It may incorporate the orbital contents above or the pterygoid space contents posteriorly. A **Weber-Fergusson** incision is used for surgical exposure. This incorporates an incision on one side of the face, midway between the nasal dorsum and medial canthus, extending inferiorly to split the upper lip. This exposes the entire maxilla and nasal bones and provides access to the ethmoid labyrinth and, sometimes, the pterygoid plates. Regions inaccessible by a Weber-Fergusson approach are the ethmoid roof and posterior orbit. When tumor involves the ethmoid roof, cribriform plate, or frontal region, a combined craniofacial frontoethmoidectomy is indicated.

SALIVARY GLANDS

INFECTIONS

Diagnosis & Management. Acute suppurative bacterial infections most often occur in the parotid gland and are more common in elderly and diabetic patients. The infecting organism is usually *Staphylococcus aureus*, but *Haemophilus influenzae*, *Streptococcus pyogenes*, *Escherichia coli*, and *Pseudomonas aeruginosa* have also been isolated. Treatment includes antimicrobial therapy with incision and drainage of any abscess formation. A safe approach to incision and drainage for parotid abscess is to use the standard parotid incision or the modified Blair incision, bluntly dissecting along the direction of the facial nerve, looking for loculations of pus. Obstructive inflammatory processes with stone formation may require excision of the gland. The submandibular gland is usually the more common site for stone.

BENIGN NEOPLASMS

Diagnosis & Management. The salivary glands can develop a wide range of tumors. Eighty percent occur in the parotid gland. Of these, 80% are benign. Pleomorphic adenomas are the most common benign salivary neoplasm in the adult population (Table 33–4). It is second to hemangiomas in the pediatric age group. The majority of be-

Table 33–4. Benign neoplasms of the salivary glands.

Adenomas
  Pleomorphic adenoma (mixed tumor)
  Adenolymphoma (Warthin's tumor)
  Monomorphic adenoma
  Sebaceous lymphadenoma

Oncocytoma

Myoepithelioma

Vascular Tumors
  Hemangiomas
  Lymphangiomas

nign tumors present as painless, slow-growing, mobile masses without facial nerve dysfunction. Submandibular gland benign tumors essentially behave in the same fashion. Benign minor salivary gland tumors usually present intraorally on the palate as painless, mucosally covered, rubbery masses.

A thorough history and detailed physical examination will most often point to a benign neoplasm (especially in the parotid gland). The other salivary glands may present more of a diagnostic challenge. Fine-needle aspiration for cytology and imaging studies may further delineate and narrow the scope of the differential diagnosis, however, they are seldom necessary because surgical excision is the treatment of choice, regardless of the pathology.

Surgery is the mainstay of treatment for benign salivary gland tumors. All other factors being equal, the minimum surgery for a parotid neoplasm is a superficial parotidectomy. For other major salivary gland neoplasms, excision of the entire gland is a sound oncologic practice. In the case of minor salivary gland neoplasms, a wide local excision is acceptable. The pleomorphic adenoma has a propensity to recur when the surgical resection is compromised by a conservative approach, such as enucleation.

MALIGNANT NEOPLASMS

Diagnosis & Management. The most common malignant salivary gland neoplasm in both the adult and pediatric populations is the **mucoepidermoid carcinoma** (Table 33–5). While some patients may present with a lesion found on routine clinical examination, a large percentage of patients would have noticed an enlarging mass of the parotid space, submandibular space, or palate. Associated hypesthesia, nerve paralysis, ulceration, pain, firmness, and fixation are some signs of malignancy and represent a poor prognosis. Imaging studies, such as MRI or CT scans, may offer some help in evaluation, especially for those parotid tumors encroaching into the parapharyngeal space or skull base.

Histopathologic characteristics and biologic behavior are strongly correlated in these tumors. Tumors are divided into two main groups: low-grade and high-grade.

Table 33–5. Malignant salivary gland tumors.

Mucoepidermoid carcinoma
Malignant mixed tumor (pleomorphic)
Adenoid cystic carcinoma
Acinic cell carcinoma
Adenocarcinoma
Malignant oncocytoma
Squamous cell carcinoma
Undifferentiated or anaplastic carcinoma

The low-grade tumors include acinic cell carcinoma, low-grade mucoepidermoid carcinoma, and adenoid cystic carcinoma. The high-grade group consists of high-grade mucoepidermoid carcinoma, adenocarcinomas, malignant mixed tumor, and squamous cell carcinomas. The separation of mucoepidermoid carcinoma into low and high grades is based on the ratio of epidermoid to mucinous cell population, mitotic index, and clinical invasiveness. Patients with low-grade tumors clearly have better long-term survival rates.

Management options are based on histopathologic factors and the extent of involvement of contiguous structures. Low-grade tumors of the parotid gland limited to the superficial lobe without facial nerve involvement are treated with superficial parotidectomy with facial nerve preservation. For the submandibular gland, the entire gland is removed. Wide local excision is employed for minor salivary gland malignancies.

When the facial nerve is involved, it is resected with the tumor specimen. The nerve is grafted with a suitable donor, such as the greater auricular or sural nerve. This will likely encompass a total parotidectomy. More extensive tumors may require resection of the mandible, masticatory muscles, facial muscles, and skin. Postoperative radiation therapy usually follows.

EAR

INFECTIONS

Diagnosis & Management. Infectious disease processes requiring surgical intervention may include acute otitis media, recurrent otitis media, chronic otitis media, or chronic suppurative otitis media with cholesteatoma. Complication of ear infections, such as mastoiditis with or without neck abscess formation (Bezold abscess), petrositis, facial nerve paralysis, or temporal lobe abscess, may all require surgical intervention as primary treatment along with intravenous antibiotics. **Cholesteatoma** is an epidermal inclusion cyst of the middle ear, mastoid, or petrous bone. **Petrositis** is an infectious process of the petrous part of the temporal bone.

Some surgical treatment modalities include placement of ventilation tubes to vent the middle ear and mastoid cavity. Since chronic otitis media portends a perforated

tympanic membrane, reconstruction of the tympanic membrane is usually needed (tympanoplasty). If cholesteatoma is present, it is painstakingly removed and the ossicular chain reestablished with various ossicular prostheses, if needed. The mastoid usually has to be exenterated in this situation.

NEOPLASMS

Diagnosis & Management. Neoplasms occur at the auricle and external auditory canal much the way they do in other cutaneous areas of the body (Table 33–6). Clinically benign neoplasms may present as raised, smooth, corrugated, pigmented, flat, or ulcerated lesions, which may on occasion simulate malignancy. This, however, poses no treatment dilemma, since an excisional biopsy adequately treats these lesions.

Malignant neoplasm of the auricle and external auditory canal account for approximately 6% of all skin malignancies. Clinically, they may present with pain, otorrhea, cranial nerve palsy, and lymphadenopathy. Imaging studies may show temporal bone lytic lesions. Squamous cell is the most common histopathologic finding in the adult. Rhabdomyosarcoma is the most common aural malignancy of childhood. The ear is the third most common site of head and neck rhabdomyosarcoma behind the orbit and nasopharynx.

Treatment for malignant tumors of the external ear varies. For auricular lesions, excision with wide margins with reconstruction is usually adequate. For external auditory canal lesions, surgery may include modified temporal bone resection and parotidectomy, followed by radiation therapy. The leading therapeutic modalities for rhabdomyosarcoma are irradiation and chemotherapy involving a variety of drugs, such as vincristine, dactinomycin, and cyclophosphamide.

The most common middle ear neoplasm is the glomus tumor, but facial nerve schwannoma, adenoma, menin-

Table 33–6. Tumors of the external ear (auricle and external auditory canal).

Malignant

Squamous cell carcinoma
Basal cell carcinoma
Malignant melanoma
Rhabdomyosarcoma

Benign

Hidradenoma
Sebaceous adenoma
Neurofibroma
Keloid
Eosinophilic granuloma
Fibrous dysplasia
Keratoacanthoma
Actinic keratosis

gioma, hemangioma, and glioma (all benign) are also seen (Table 33–7). Malignant lesions primarily arising within the middle ear cleft include squamous cell carcinoma, rhabdomyosarcoma, adenocarcinomas, and mesenchymal tumors, such as chondrosarcoma. Metastatic neoplasms should also be kept in mind. Clinically, these lesions may be noticed early because of hearing loss, fullness, and pain, which may be present early in the course of the disease.

Benign tumors limited to the middle ear space may be extricated via the ear canal, with minimal morbidity. However, some benign tumors extending outside the middle ear cleft can pose a significant surgical challenge, since preservation of vital structures of hearing, facial nerve function, and so forth are of critical importance.

Malignant lesions, on the other hand, require more radical resection. Thanks to the collaboration of surgical subspecialists, the techniques have evolved to such a degree that vital aural structures and cranial nerves can be preserved while better access, decreased mortality, and improved long-term survival can also be achieved.

ORAL CAVITY, OROPHARYNX, & NASOPHARYNX

INFECTIONS

Diagnosis & Management. Odontogenic infections are one of the most common infections inflicting humans. Most resolve without complications. However, some will progress beyond the site of the offending tooth source. When this occurs, an abscess may form. If an abscess forms, its location is usually determined by the site of the offending tooth, type of bone surrounding the tooth, and the muscle attachments. For example, a second or third mandibular molar with its root tip extending past the mylohyoid ridge, where the mylohyoid muscle is attached, will most always present an abscess into the submandibular space rather than sublingually or in the buccal space (space between the buccinator muscle and subcutaneous fat of the cheek).

A particularly serious infection occurring within the submental, sublingual, and submandibular space is called **Ludwig's angina.** This infection spreads rapidly and may lead to airway obstruction. It is akin to a necrotizing cellulitis and not strictly an abscess. The microbiological picture of oral infections is that of normal flora, by all accounts. These include streptococcus species (anaerobic or facultative varieties), bacteroides, and fusobacterium. Staphylococcus species originating from an odontogenic source are uncommon.

Oral cavity infections with abscess formation require directed antibiotic therapy to cover the microbes previously described. Penicillin continues to be a useful antibiotic for this therapy as well as clindamycin, cephalosporins, and Flagyl.

Surgical intervention in the form of incision and drainage is almost always required. A passive drain is usually left in place for 2–5 days to effect prolonged drainage of pus. Ludwig's angina requires that the submental and submandibular space be opened widely. The airway is usually secured with tracheotomy or intubation.

The most common oropharyngeal infection is tonsillitis. While "routine" tonsillitis may be amenable to medicinal therapy with antibiotics, the complication of a peritonsillar abscess or a lateral pharyngeal space abscess can present treatment challenges. A peritonsillar abscess may occur in the setting of a tonsillitis that has been inadequately treated with oral antibiotics that later suppurates within the soft tissue surrounding the offending tonsil.

Another important infectious process of the oropharynx is that of the retropharyngeal space abscess. This is usually seen in the age group between 2 and 6 years. It is thought to result from suppurative lymphadenitis of retropharyngeal lymph glands, which have usually involuted by age 6 or so. The potential space between the buccopharyngeal and the prevertebral fascia represents the site of pus collection. Treatment of these infectious states may require incision and drainage in the operating room along with systemic antibiotic therapy. Artificial airway support in the form of a tracheostomy or endotracheal tube is almost always required. A peritonsillar abscess can be managed in the emergency room setting via needle aspiration or incision and drainage. If the airway is compromised, the patient should be hospitalized with airway precautions.

Nasopharyngitis and adenoiditis are the two significant infections of the nasopharynx. Removal of the tonsils or adenoids is usually preceded by clinical documentation of at least five episodes per year or 2 weeks absence from school or work per year.

BENIGN NEOPLASMS

Diagnosis & Management. A variety of cystic and solid lesions may occur within the bony structures or soft

Table 33–7. Tumors of the middle ear.

Malignant
Squamous cell carcinoma
Rhabdomyosarcoma
Adenocarcinomas
Mesenchymal tumors (chondrosarcoma, etc)

Benign
Glomus tympanum
Facial nerve schwannoma
Adenoma
Meningioma
Hemangioma
Glioma
Osteoma
Cholesteatoma

tissues of the oral cavity or oropharynx. Cystic lesions include fissural, odontogenic, mucus retention phenomenon, and dermoid cysts. Their treatment requires total excision. Solid lesions include fibromas, papillomas, granular cell tumors, rhabdomyomas, bony exostoses, and various other mesenchymal tumors. Most will require surgical excision, however, bony exostoses, such as torus palatinus and mandibularis, are only removed if they prevent proper seating of dentures.

Hemangiomas are frequently observed and sometimes treated with systemic steroids, especially in children. Laser therapy has also become a useful method of treatment, especially those lasers with wavelengths that are absorbed by the hemoglobin of blood (KTP-532 laser).

Differential diagnosis of benign lesions arising in the nasopharynx includes fibromas, vascular polyps, teratomas, and JNA. Fibromas are rare and occur from local injury, and teratomas are usually noticed at birth. Vascular polyps are also rare and occur from neovascularization. Clinically, the most common complaint is nasal obstruction, followed by epistaxis. Facial deformity may also be a part of the clinical picture.

Benign lesions of the nasopharynx are treated surgically. The nasopharynx can be accessed surgically by removing a portion of the hard palate (**transpalatine approach**), opening the anterior face of the maxillary, ethmoid, and sphenoid sinuses (**transmaxillary approach**), or placing an incision over the parotid region and traversing the parotid fossa (**infratemporal fossa approach**). Other surgical approaches are described in the literature but are beyond the scope of this text (Thawley, 1987).

MALIGNANT NEOPLASMS

Oral Cavity & Oropharynx

Diagnosis & Management. The differential diagnosis of malignant neoplasm in this region include tumors of epithelial as well as mesenchymal origin. These include squamous cell carcinoma (by far the most common), melanoma, and minor salivary gland tumors. Mesenchymal tumors may include the variety of sarcomas. Lymphomas and extramedullary plasmacytoma may also occur.

Squamous cell carcinoma is the most common malignant neoplasm in both the oral cavity and oropharynx. Several variant forms of SCCA occur. For example, the spindle cell variety has a population of cells resembling mesenchymal cells present in varying numbers. There is a verrucous variety, considered a histologic variant of a well-differentiated SCCA with a particular histologic picture of papillomatous epithelium. Verrucous carcinoma is locally aggressive with limited tendency to metastasize. Adenoid squamous cell carcinoma is another rare variant. These may be confused, histologically, with minor salivary gland adenoid cystic carcinoma.

There are several etiologic factors, some carrying greater significance in the oral cavity as compared to the oropharynx. Some etiologic factors have geographic predilection. For example, in India, where the oral cancer incidence may approach 50% (as compared to 5% in the United States), the main causes are thought to be the chewing of betel nuts and the custom of reverse smoking (placing the lighted end of the cigarette into the oral cavity). Ethanol consumption is also an important risk factor, thought to compound the problem when combined with cigarette smoking. Actinic exposure is the most important risk factor for lip SCCA. Dietary deficiencies, poor oral hygiene, syphilis, herpes simplex, and occupational exposures have also been implicated.

Lesions of SCCA can mimic several other lesions of this region. A high degree of suspicion is, therefore, required to diagnose incipient lesions. The smaller the lesion at diagnosis, the better the prognosis. When lymph nodes of the neck are involved, the chance of survival is diminished by 25% or more. Diagnosis may be achieved by biopsy, which is warranted for an oral or oropharyngeal lesion that does not heal after 2 weeks of antibiotic therapy.

A small but important percentage of patients (1–3%) with oral and oropharyngeal SCCA will have a second concurrent SCCA in the upper aerodigestive tract. Twenty-five percent of patients treated successfully for their initially diagnosed cancer (the index tumor) will eventually develop a second primary tumor. The most common site for this second cancer is the esophagus.

Clinical examination is by far the most important tool in diagnosing oral and oropharyngeal cancers. Imaging studies serve only as adjuncts in assessing these lesions. A biopsy is the hallmark of diagnosis after clinical suspicion.

The treatment selection includes surgery, radiation therapy, chemotherapy, or a combination of these modalities. The selection of treatment may be complex but is largely guided by the tumor's extent and location, patient's physical and social status, and physician's experience. For early disease, surgery or radiation therapy has proved to be essentially equal in efficacy. Chemotherapy, sadly, has not shown efficacy for primary therapy. For surgery, as a sole modality or in combined therapy, the goal is to excise the lesion with a margin of normal tissue. Resection of vital structures, such as the tongue base, may result in problems of aspiration, mastication, and speech. Once the cancer has been extirpated, reconstruction may be done by primary closure or regional or distant transfer of tissue flaps. Various designs of flaps have been used to close defects of the head and neck (Table 33–8).

Resection of the mandible is required when it is involved grossly with cancer. However, when the mandible is not clinically involved, one must depend on preoperative imaging studies to plan the surgical approach. For oropharyngeal carcinomas, such as base of tongue and tonsil lesions, external beam radiotherapy combined with interstitial implants, such as iridium[192], have proved to be efficacious.

Table 33–8. Commonly used flaps in head and neck surgery.

Flap Type	Nutrient Vessels	Some Sites of Use
Pectoralis major myocutaneous flap	Thoracoacomial artery	Pharynx/oral cavity
Trapezius flap	Transverse cervical artery	Cheek/oral cavity
Latissimus dorsi flap	Thoracodorsal artery	Anywhere in head and neck where bulk is needed
Deltopectoral flap	Perforators from internal mammary artery	Pharynx/esophagus
Forehead flap	Superficial temporal artery	Cheek/floor of mouth
Microvascular free flap (eg, radial forearm)	Branch of radial artery	Floor of mouth Composite mandibular reconstruction

Nasopharynx

Diagnosis & Management. The nasopharynx is a difficult area to examine, even by physicians trained in the diagnosis of lesions of this region. Consequently, malignant lesions in this region often go undiagnosed until late in their course. By far the most common histopathologic type of lesion is squamous cell carcinoma. Squamous cell carcinoma of the nasopharynx is divided into three groups, based on histopathologic typing. World Health Organization (WHO) type I lesions show features of a high degree of differentiation with keratin production. WHO type II is a nonkeratinizing lesion that shows more pleomorphism than WHO type I. WHO type III is undifferentiated carcinoma.

Nasopharyngeal carcinoma is rare in the United States, yet common in southern China, Malaysia, Singapore, and Tunisia. Etiologically, a genetic predisposition exists and relationships to the herpes virus and Epstein-Barr virus have also been confirmed. Other risk factors have also been established, such as consumption of salted fish in childhood (nitrosamines) and inadequate fresh fruit and vegetable consumption.

Diagnosis is established by biopsy. The disease can easily be missed, because of its submucosal nature. Serologic testing for IGA titers against viral capsid antigen and early antigen have proven to be useful. MRI scan of the nasopharynx with gadolinium contrast and fat suppression is the diagnostic imaging study of choice. Treatment is standardized to external beam radiation therapy with surgery reserved for those who have failed this therapy. Five-year disease-free survival ranges from 37 to 57%.

LARYNX & HYPOPHARYNX (LARYNGOPHARYNX)

INFECTIONS

Several infectious processes of the larynx and hypopharynx require surgical intervention, especially if there is an obvious abscess or swelling with impending airway compromise. Any infectious process can compromise the larynx and hypopharyngeal airway, but the two most significant entities are laryngotracheitis (croup) and epiglottitis. Both diseases were once considered to be emergencies requiring tracheostomy. However, advances in nonsurgical airway management have obviated the need for tracheostomy in most cases. Chronic infections pose less of an immediate threat and rarely need surgical airway management. Examples are syphilis, tuberculosis, and various fungi.

Laryngotracheitis

Diagnosis & Management. Laryngotracheitis (croup) is an acute or subacute viral illness characterized by fever, "barking" cough, and stridor developing over 1–3 days. Its main causative agents are parainfluenza viruses I and II along with influenza virus type A. This condition is seen predominately among children ages 1–3 years.

The crucial factor with croup is the amount of airway swelling in the subglottic area. This can be assessed using a plain film posterior/anterior view of the neck, looking for the so-called "steeple sign," a narrowing of the subglottic area, creating a shadow on x-ray akin to a church steeple. In the differential diagnosis, foreign-body aspiration, epiglottitis, and bacterial tracheitis must all be considered.

The mainstay of management is humidification. Other modalities of treatment are racemic epinephrine, systemic steroids, and, rarely, artificial airway management. There is still controversy regarding the efficacy of systemic steroid therapy.

Epiglottitis

Diagnosis & Management. This condition is better called supraglottitis, since the infection is not limited to the epiglottis but involves most or all the supraglottic structures. It is usually caused by *Haemophilus influenzae* type B in the pediatric age group and *Staphylococcus aureus* or streptococcal species in the adult population. This condition is more likely to require artificial airway management. The hallmark of epiglottitis is a severe sore throat developing over a matter of hours.

Clinically, the child may appear "toxic," with elevated temperature, drooling, and severe odynophagia. The child usually assumes the most comfortable posture with neck extended. There is controversy whether a child suspected of having epiglottitis should be examined or manipulated before preparation for artificial airway management, as this may precipitate further airway compromise. A soft tissue lateral film of the neck will make this diagnosis in close to 80% of patients where the "thumbprint sign," characteristic of a swollen epiglottis, is considered pathognomonic. Several authorities believe, however, that the patient should be taken to the operating room for diagnosis, followed by intubation and intravenous antibiotics. Most frequently, a tracheostomy is avoided. The duration of intubation ranges from 48–72 hours. With the patient intubated, laryngoscopy can be performed every 24 hours to determine the optimal time of extubation.

Medical management may include a variety of antibiotics directed at the known causative agents. Chloramphenicol in combination with ampicillin are the two drugs most recommended. However, cephalosporins have been shown to be efficacious, for example, cefuroxime and cefotaxime. The use of steroids is controversial, and racemic epinephrine has no value.

BENIGN NEOPLASMS

Diagnosis & Management. The benign lesions are separated into two groups. The first group is caused by mucosal reaction to abnormal stresses and irritants. These are not true neoplasms. They include nodules, polyps, cysts, laryngoceles, granulomas, glottic sulci, and stenosis. In Table 33–9, group 2 lesions are true neoplasms.

Nodules and polyps primarily affect the true vocal cords and are related to inflammation and vocal abuse. These lesions affect the phonatory characteristics of the vocal cords and are treated by a combination of conservative measures, including voice rest, antiinflammatory

Table 33–9. Benign lesions of the larynx and hypopharynx.

Group 1

Nodules
Polyps
Cysts/laryngoceles
Contact granulomas
Glottic sulci
Subglottic stenosis

Group 2

Squamous papillomatosis
Hemangiomas
Rhabdomyoma
Lipoma
Benign minor salivary gland neoplasm
Chondroma
Neurofibroma
Neurilemoma
Granular cell myoblastoma

medications such as steroids, and speech therapy. Surgical treatment is rarely necessary and follows failure of conservative measures. Surgical strategies include microlaryngeal procedures aimed at removing the lesion and conserving the mucosal coverings (**phonosurgery**).

Cysts and laryngoceles are disorders of the saccule of the larynx. The saccule is that blind pouch that is a continuation of the laryngeal ventricle. It is lined with mucus-producing glands responsible for lubrication. The cyst is a collection of this mucus causing expansion of the saccule, while a laryngocele is air-filled. Both may present with mild airway symptoms to significant airway obstruction. Treatment of either lesion involves surgical excision or marsupialization. The CO_2 laser has been found to be useful in this endeavor.

Laryngeal papillomas are the most common benign neoplasm of the larynx and may occur in either a juvenile or an adult. In children, this may be a relentless disease refractory to all modes of therapy. Some occasional cases have been known to regress spontaneously at puberty, but most require serial endoscopies with resection. The CO_2 laser is useful for their debulking or removal.

Adult forms usually do not present with the same level of respiratory distress as the juvenile type. Tracheostomy in these patients is to be avoided if at all possible, since this is associated with seeding of the tracheobronchial tree, a condition that can lead to serious consequences, including death.

Hemangiomas are another group of lesions that present with different features in infants and adults. In adults, the lesion is usually supraglottic with larger caliber vessels, while in the infant, the lesion is usually subglottic with smaller vessels. In infants, the lesion may be associated with another lesion elsewhere on the body, sometimes on the skin. Treatment in the infant group is achieved with the use of a CO_2 laser to ablate the lesion. Adult hemangiomas are not as amenable to laser treatment and are better left alone unless there is airway compromise. All other benign lesions of the larynx or hypopharynx are treated with resection, mostly via endoscopy or by a laryngofissure approach. A laryngofissure involves opening of the larynx anteriorly, in the midline, to gain access to endolaryngeal structures.

Subglottic stenosis is a congenital or acquired narrowing of the space immediately below the true vocal cords (subglottis). The acquired form is much more prevalent, especially since the advent of the neonatal intensive care unit, where immature infants may remain intubated for an extended period. A developmental defect or infection in utero is implicated for the congenital form. Treatment is surgical to widen the airway (laryngotracheoplasty).

MALIGNANT NEOPLASMS

Larynx

Diagnosis & Management. Cancer of the larynx accounts for about one fifth of all head and neck cancers

(Table 33–10). Approximately 11,000 new cases are diagnosed annually, according to the National Cancer Institute. In general, this cancer has a favorable prognosis, with a 5-year survival approaching 70%. It is likely to be a preventable malignancy, in the majority of cases.

The incidence of laryngeal cancer peaks at about the seventh decade of life, with a male to female ratio of 5 to 1. Risk factors associated with the disease include tobacco use, alcohol consumption, occupational exposure, and radiation exposure. Viral infections and dietary deficiencies are linked to a lesser extent.

Laryngeal cancers often produce early symptoms that may lead to early diagnosis and treatment with excellent preservation of function. Symptomatology includes voice change or hoarseness in tumors of the true vocal cords, or muffled voice as in tumors of the supraglottic region. Tumors of the subglottic region are rare, and airway obstruction may be the prominent clinical presentation. Odynophagia, dysphagia, and even otalgia may be present. A neck mass and constitutional sign of weight loss may be a sign of advanced laryngeal cancer.

Clinical examination should follow the previously outlined steps. Facility with the use of a laryngeal mirror and headlight or fiberoptic laryngoscope greatly increases the diagnostic yield (Figure 33–7). Imaging studies, such as barium contrast films, CT scan and MRI, may augment the clinical examination. These may be particularly helpful in determining cartilage invasion, a sign of late stage disease. Since chronic infectious states, such as fungi, syphilis, and microbacteria, may simulate malignancy in the larynx, a tissue biopsy is always needed for diagnosis.

Glottic carcinomas constitute the majority of primary laryngeal tumors (60%). Symptoms usually present early in the form of voice change. Though involvement on the anterior commissure is not included in the official staging system, it portends a poor prognosis. The most important prognostic factor for the vocal cord lesion is cord mobility. A fixed vocal cord is a negative prognostic factor.

Subglottic tumors are rare and constitute approximately 1% of laryngeal primary malignancies. Tumors here carry a poor prognosis in general, because symptoms do not occur until tumors are advanced. Subglottic tumors also have a high propensity to spread extralaryngeally.

There are several factors guiding treatment of laryngeal tumors. Notably, the patient's age, sex, general health, personal preferences, and social circumstances, the location of tumor and stage, availability of a facility for treat-

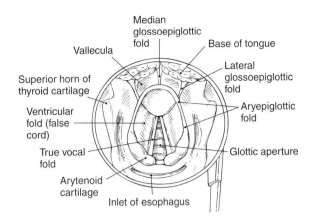

Figure 33–7. Larynx as viewed from above with an examination mirror.

ment, and the experience of the treating physician. The standard choices are surgery or radiation therapy as a single modality, a combination of both, or in combination with chemotherapy.

For early laryngeal carcinomas, radiation therapy has the best functional outcome, with treatment cures comparable to surgery. For late stage diseases, however, radiation therapy as a single modality has not proved to be as successful in terms of long-term survival or local control of disease. Radiation therapy may also cause mucositis, dry mouth, dermatitis, scarring, and chondroradionecrosis. Surgical options include conservation procedures, such as endoscopic removal of the lesion, laryngofissure with cordectomy, horizontal and vertical laryngectomy, and near-total laryngectomy. Nonconservative measures include total laryngectomy.

Hypopharynx

Diagnosis & Management. Squamous cell carcinoma is the predominant malignant neoplasm of this region. It may arise from any subsite of the hypopharynx, including the posterior pharyngeal wall, postcricoid region, or pyriform sinus.

The same risk factors for laryngeal carcinoma apply for hypopharyngeal tumors. However, one unique condition, the Plumber-Vinson syndrome (glossitis, splenomegaly, esophageal stenosis, achlorhydria, and iron-deficiency anemia), has a predisposition for postcricoid carcinoma.

There are fewer barriers to the spread of hypopharyngeal cancer as compared to the compartmentalization seen in the larynx. Therefore, a pyriform sinus tumor can readily extend to the larynx. Also significant is the high degree of spread to the neck. In fact, at presentation, 60–70% of primary hypopharyngeal tumors have already metastasized to the neck. This may also be related to the silent nature of this tumor, affording late diagnosis. Symptoms may include pain on swallowing, dysphagia, ear pain, or

Table 33–10. Malignant tumors of the larynx.

Squamous cell carcinoma
Verrucous squamous cell
Carcinosarcoma
Adenocarcinoma
Adenoid cystic and mucoepidermoid carcinoma
Lymphomas
Sarcomas
Metastatic malignancies

neck mass. The evaluation includes a thorough history and physical, triple endoscopy with biopsies, and an MRI.

A large percentage of patients with hypopharyngeal carcinoma may have other serious illnesses, such as cirrhosis, chronic obstructive pulmonary disease, or cardiovascular disease, and are also usually in a negative nitrogen balance. The treatment may include hypopharyngectomy, which usually consists of a total or near-total laryngectomy, and neck dissection followed by postoperative radiation therapy.

NECK

THE NECK MASS

Diagnosis & Management. Unearthing the diagnosis of a neck mass can be a challenging endeavor. Although most neck masses are benign, it may be the presenting symptom in 12% of patients with head and neck cancer (especially in patients over 40 years of age). Eighty-five percent of the metastatic carcinoma to cervical lymph nodes arises from an upper aerodigestive tract primary tumor, and 10% arise from tumors below the clavicle. In 5% of cases, the primary site of cancer is never found.

The differential diagnosis of a neck mass usually includes four broad categories: congenital, inflammatory, neoplastic, and acquired (Table 33–11). Congenital lesions are usually first seen in early childhood, but can sometimes be seen in adulthood. An example is the branchial cleft cyst, which is usually located in the upper neck along the anterior border of the sternocleidomastoid muscle. The most common branchial cleft cyst is derived from the second branchial arch. Another example is the thyroglossal duct cyst, which usually appears in the midline of the neck below the level of the hyoid bone. This lesion will move upwards during the act of swallowing. Cystic hygroma (or lymphangioma) are multiple large lymph-filled spaces that transilluminate and can occur anywhere in the face or neck.

Inflammatory causes of neck masses usually present with erythema, induration, and tenderness. Lymphadenitis is by far the most common inflammatory neck mass. This is usually secondary to a pyogenic organism, such as staphylococcus or streptococcus. A common cause of an inflammatory neck mass in the Third World is *Mycobacterium tuberculosis*. In the United States, this remains uncommon, except in the case of cervical lymphadenitis in children, which is frequently caused by atypical mycobacteria. The cervical lymphadenitis associated with cat scratch disease is not always caused by the scratch of a cat but may be caused by the scratch of other animals. Toxoplasmosis, which is spread via the feces of cats, rare pork, or raw beef, occurs in children or adults, resulting in lymphadenitis.

Neoplastic lesions presenting as neck masses can either

Table 33–11. Differential diagnosis of a neck mass.

Neoplasm

Primary neoplasm
  Fibroma
  Lipoma
  Angioma
  Paraganglioma
  Schwannoma and neurilemoma
  Salivary gland tumor
  Thyroid gland tumor
Metastatic neoplasm
  Head and neck primary tumor
  Distant primary tumor
Constitutional neoplasm
  Leukemia, lymphoma, Hodgkin's disease

Congenital and Developmental

Sebaceous and epidermal cysts
Branchial cleft cyst
Thyroglossal duct cyst
Dermoid cyst
Ectopic thyroid tissue
Laryngocele
Zenker's diverticulum
Thymic cyst
Lymphangioma
Cystic hygroma

Inflammatory

Infectious
  Bacterial—*Staphylococcus aureus*, group A beta-hemolytic streptococci
  Viral—Epstein-Barr virus, cytomegalovirus, human immunodeficiency virus
  Granulomatous—tuberculosis, sarcoid, actinomycosis, lymphogranuloma venereum
  Syphilis
Noninfectious
  Mucocutaneous lymph node syndrome
  Necrotizing lymphadenitis
  Sinus histiocytosis with massive lymphadenopathy
  Angioimmunoblastic lymphadenitis
  Systemic lupus erythematosis lymphadenitis
  Rheumatoid arthritis lymphadenopathy
  Dilantin hypersensitivity

Acquired

Arteriovenous fistula
Fat necrosis
Hematoma

be primary or metastatic. Lymphomas are usually primary and should be suspected in a rubbery neck mass or multiple similar nodes at other body sites. Primary cancers may occur more commonly in the thyroid or salivary gland, but metastatic disease to these glands should not be overlooked. Vascular tumors have a characteristic feature of compressibility or the presence of a bruit. Imaging studies, such as an MRI scan, may show a "flow void" or a "blush" as seen on a contrast CT scan.

As already mentioned, the primary site for most cancers that metastasize to cervical lymph nodes is the upper aerodigestive tract, but cancers from the lungs, prostate, breast, testicle, and gastrointestinal tract may also metastasize here. It is the left side of the neck that characteristically gets metastasis from infraclavicular primaries. This is thought to be due to the presence of the thoracic duct.

Investigating the causes of a neck mass should proceed in a logical, cost-effective manner. Most head and neck physicians believe that premature biopsy of a cervical lymph node that contains metastatic cancer from a head and neck primary is unnecessary and results in undue delay. The diagnostic evaluation should begin with a thorough history and physical examination. A slow, continuously enlarging neck mass is likely to be cancer, while a mass that appears acutely with associated pain and fluctuates in size is likely an inflammatory process.

A history of trauma, such as insect bites or animal scratches, may point to lymphadenitis, which may suggest cat scratch disease. Other blunt or penetrating trauma may suggest fat necrosis, hematoma, or pseudoaneurysm. A history of tuberculosis exposure may point to the causes of the mass.

Hoarseness or a muffled voice may signal malignancy at the glottis, epiglottis, tonsillar region, or tongue base. Patients presenting with a history of throat pain may be harboring cancer in the larynx or pharynx. Pain in the ear may be referred from any of the aforementioned sites. Hearing loss may be the result of serous otitis media, which could indicate nasopharyngeal carcinoma.

Dysphagia or odynophagia may suggest a hypopharyngeal or esophageal cancer, especially if there is associated weight loss. Any history of cough should be characterized, since this may represent a pulmonary primary, especially if there is associated hemoptysis.

Familial tendency for most head and neck cancers is uncommon, but of note is medullary thyroid carcinoma, which occurs as part of the multiple endocrine neoplastic syndrome. Also, carotid body tumors may have familial tendencies in up to 10% of cases.

The physical examination should involve all body systems to encompass a wide differential diagnosis. The obvious neck mass is examined, coupled with a general examination that includes the breasts, prostate, rectum, and lymphatic structures in other regions. All epithelial surfaces of the head and neck should be examined in a detailed fashion. The tympanic membrane should be examined closely to rule out serous otitis media, which is frequently seen with nasopharyngeal carcinomas. A pulsatile mass in the middle ear associated with a neck mass may suggest a glomus tumor. The nasal cavity and sinuses should be examined grossly and with the use of telescopes. However, by the time a sinonasal tumor has caused cervical adenopathy, it has likely grown to an obstructing and sometimes disfiguring size. The oral cavity and oropharynx should be inspected and then bimanually palpated. As compared to the sinonasal region, tumors of the oral cavity and oropharynx may present with a neck mass (60% in some series). The larynx and hypopharynx are examined with the aid of a laryngeal mirror or fiberoptic flexible scope. Attention is paid to the pyriform sinus, since small, inconspicuous lesions may present with cervi-

cal lymphadenopathy quite early in their course. Supraglottic and subglottis cancer also have a propensity for spread to cervical lymph nodes—54% and 60%, respectively. The thyroid gland should be inspected while the patient is instructed to swallow. Frequently, an obscured mass may be made prominent by this maneuver. One should not trivialize the examination of the scalp. The scalp is a frequent site for squamous carcinoma as well as melanoma, which may present with a neck mass or parotid mass. The use of a comb may facilitate this examination.

On examination of the neck mass in question, if metastatic cancer is suspected the location of the mass may give some clue to its primary source. For example, the more cephalad the mass, the more likely it is a head and neck primary cancer. Consistency of the mass can sometimes give a clue as to its cause. A mass that is hard and fixed to adjacent structures most likely represents a malignancy. Multiple, rubbery, matted masses may represent lymphoma. Fluctuance in a mass may represent infectious processes, especially if other signs of inflammation are present. However, this may also represent necrosis in a tumor that has outgrown its blood supply.

Assuming you are the first physician to see a patient for a workup of a neck mass, and your history and physical are not enlightening as to its cause, it is appropriate to give the patient a 10-day course of antibiotics (penicillin or cephalexin) and have the patient return in 2 weeks. In about 10% of cases, the neck mass will have disappeared and no further workup is necessary. If the neck mass is still present, a complete examination should be performed to locate the primary site (Figure 33–8). Fine-needle aspiration of the mass can be performed in the clinical setting without anesthesia; with a highly trained cytopathologist, this study carries a high degree of sensitivity (95%). Although seldom needed by an experienced head and neck surgeon, it can be a useful test for the inexperienced clinician.

Laboratory tests may be useful, but must be tailored to the history and physical examination. A complete blood count with slide differential may be helpful, especially if an infectious or lymphoproliferative cause is suspected. Serologic testing for infectious mononucleosis should be done in teenagers or young adults, especially if their classmates have any history of the disease. Although syphilis is an uncommon explanation for lymph node hyperplasia, this diagnosis can remain elusive without a Venereal Disease Research Laboratory (VDRL) test. A test for human immunodeficiency virus should be performed for any patient at risk. A toxoplasma titer is warranted when an individual consumes rare steak or pork, or if they clean cat litter boxes. Epstein-Barr virus antibodies are indicated if the patient is of southern Chinese descent, or is from Malaysia, Tunisia, Singapore, or is an American Eskimo. IgA (not IgG or IgM) antibodies to viral capsid antigen and early antigen diffuse are the proper tests to rule out nasopharyngeal carcinoma. If there is a strong likelihood that the mass represents carcinoma, liver function tests

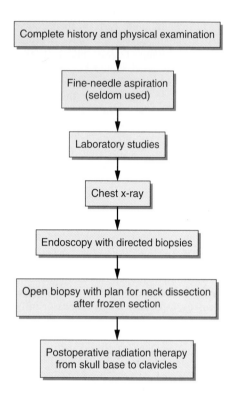

Figure 33–8. Diagnostic approach to the neck mass with primary site unknown.

should be obtained to rule out hepatic metastasis. If the patient has a prostate nodule on physical examination, a prostate-specific antigen (PSA) test is indicated. For a patient with a thyroid mass and a positive family history of thyroid carcinoma, a serum thyrocalcitonin is indicated. Similarly, if the patient has had multiple neurofibromas, or symptoms of hypercalcemia, the serum calcium and parathormone level should be obtained.

Radiologic imaging studies should be tailored to the history and physical examination. A chest radiograph is routinely obtained to rule out other metastatic foci. An MRI with gadolinium from the skull base to the clavicles

may be helpful to find the primary site of malignancy, but in our experience this has been positive only in approximately 10% of patients. Although we have not had extensive experience with its use, positron emission tomography (PET) has been helpful in locating primary disease. Plain films of the neck, thyroid scans, bone scans, contrast study of the gastrointestinal tract, and CT scans are seldom worthwhile and rarely obtained in the initial workup.

If the neck mass is indeed SCCA, then it is necessary to locate the primary tumor and any additional primary tumor sites. Panendoscopy, which is sequential laryngoscopy, bronchoscopy, nasopharyngoscopy, and esophagoscopy, is used to determine this. During these procedures, if the primary lesion is found, it is biopsied. If the primary lesion is not found, then selected biopsies are performed at the areas known to harbor occult primaries, including the nasopharynx, tonsils, base of tongue, and pyriform sinus. Bronchial washings are obtained from both lungs but have a low yield in most series reviewed. A second primary tumor is then sought, since this can occur in up to 3% of patients. In fact, a second primary is usually the cause of death in a sizeable percentage of patients whose index tumor (the first to be diagnosed) was appropriately treated. A common site for a second primary is the esophagus.

Management strategies at this stage vary depending upon the philosophy of the head and neck surgeon and the wishes of the patient. Some surgeons will perform an open biopsy with frozen section and proceed with a formal neck dissection under general anesthesia; this is followed by postoperative irradiation to the known primary sites and neck when there is no apparent primary site for the cancer. Others may await the permanent results of the biopsies to the known primary sites before performing an open biopsy to the suspected neck cancer. The neck mass, however, should never be subjected to an open biopsy in the clinical setting before a thorough workup is completed.

The primary site of the cancer is identified in only 10% of patients who present with a neck mass arising from an unknown primary. Five-year survival statistics for these patients ranges from 50–70%. If the primary becomes evident after treatment is completed during the follow-up period, the survival is reduced by 20%.

SUGGESTED READING

Collins SL et al: Head and neck. In: Abeloff MD et al (editors): *Clinical Oncology*. Churchill Livingstone, 1995.

Cummings CW et al: *Otolaryngology–Head & Neck Surgery*, 2nd ed. Mosby, 1993.

Hollinshead WH: *Anatomy for Surgeons*, Vol. 1, 3rd ed. Harper and Row, 1982.

Jacobs CD, Goffinet DR, Fee WE: Head and neck squamous cancers. *Current Problems in Cancer*. Year Book Medical Publishers, January/February 1990, Vol XIV(1).

Kaur A, Fee WE: Head and neck cancers. In: Niederhuber JE (editor): *Current Therapy in Oncology*. Mosby Year Book, 1993.

Krespi, YP, Ossoff RH: *Complications in Head and Neck Surgery*. Saunders, 1993.

Netter FH: *Atlas of Human Anatomy*. Ciba-Geigy, 1989.

Thawley SE, Panje WR: *Comprehensive Management of Head and Neck Tumors*. Saunders, 1987.

34

The Endocrine System

Ronald J. Weigel, MD, PhD

▶ Key Facts

- ▶ Thyroidectomy is the most common operation performed by endocrine surgeons and is the standard treatment for thyroid carcinoma.

- ▶ The main function of the thyroid is production of thyroid hormones, thyroxine (T_4), and triiodothyronine (T_3).

- ▶ There are approximately 14,000 new cases of thyroid carcinoma in the United States annually.

- ▶ The majority of thyroid nodules are benign and evaluation is aimed at determining which nodules are benign, but laboratory values as well as careful clinical examination are required to determine which nodules might be malignant and require operation.

- ▶ Most patients with thyroid carcinoma have an excellent prognosis, with 10-year disease-free survival of 80–90%.

- ▶ The parathyroid gland is normally composed of chief cells and water-clear cells that both secrete parathyroid hormone (PTH).

- ▶ Approximately 80% of patients with primary hyperparathyroidism (HPT) have a solitary parathyroid adenoma. Surgery is indicated for patients with symptomatic HPT.

- ▶ Patients with adrenal carcinoma often will have large tumors that are locally invasive or metastatic at presentation. These patients should undergo a debulking procedure to remove as much tumor as possible.

- ▶ Pheochromocytoma is a rare tumor of the chromaffin cells of the adrenal gland that secrete catecholamines.

THYROID

Thyroidectomy is the most common operation performed by endocrine surgeons. Indications for thyroidectomy include abnormal thyroid function, suspicion of malignancy, or local symptoms of airway compromise or dysphagia. To make decisions concerning the treatment of thyroid diseases requires a thorough understanding of the normal physiologic and pathologic processes affecting the thyroid gland.

ANATOMY & PHYSIOLOGY

The thyroid is derived from the first and second pharyngeal pouches. It is located in the central neck just inferior to the cricoid cartilage. The gland is composed of two lobes connected by a central part called the isthmus. The thyroid is highly vascular and derives its blood supply from two paired arteries. The **superior thyroid artery** is a branch of the external carotid artery and enters the gland as branched vessels supplying the superior pole. The **inferior thyroid artery** is a branch from the thyrocervical trunk, and its branches enter the gland near the central part of the lobe. Vessels called **thyroid ima vessels** are derived from the aortic arch and can provide additional blood supply to the inferior aspects of the gland.

The main function of the thyroid is production of thyroid hormones, thyroxine (T_4), and triiodothyronine (T_3). Thyroid hormone is synthesized from tyrosine by oxidation and iodination. Hormone is stored as colloid within the acinar of the thyroid follicle. Synthesis of thyroid hormone is precisely regulated through the hypothalamus–pituitary–thyroid axis (Figure 34–1). The hypothalamus synthesizes **thyrotropin-releasing factor** (TRF), which is a tripeptide. TRF is secreted into the portal circulation and is carried to the pituitary gland. Within the anterior pituitary, TRF stimulates release of **thyroid stimulating hormone** (TSH), which is a peptide hormone carried by the circulation to the thyroid gland. TSH stimulates the thyroid to grow and synthesize the thyroid hormones T_4 and T_3. Thyroid hormone exerts a negative regulation upon the hypothalamus and pituitary to balance the production of hormone. The blood levels of these various hormones can be measured and provide information about the homeostasis of the thyroid axis.

Thyroid function tests are routinely employed in the evaluation of patients with thyroid problems. The commonly employed thyroid function tests are shown in Table 34–1. In patients with hyperthyroidism, T_4, T_3, and free T_4 (FT_4) are elevated and TSH is suppressed. In hypothyroid states, T_4, FT_4, and T_3 are low and TSH is elevated. TSH is valuable in that it is the single most sensitive indi-

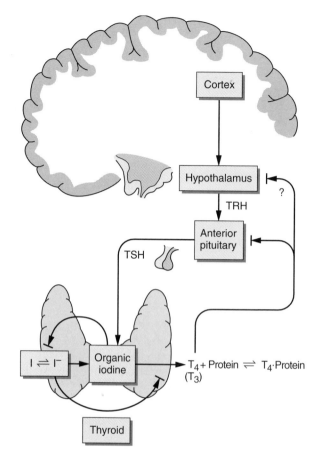

Figure 34–1. Schema of the homeostatic regulation of thyroid function. Thyroid-stimulating hormone (TSH) stimulates release of thyroid hormone. Secretion of TSH is regulated by a negative feedback mechanism acting directly on the pituitary gland and is normally inversely related to the concentration of unbound hormone in the blood. Release of TSH is induced by thyrotropin-releasing hormone (TRH). Factors regulating secretion of TRH are uncertain but may include the free hormone in the blood and stimuli from higher centers. (Reprinted, with permission, from Ingbar SH, Woeber KA: The thyroid gland. In: Williams RH (ed): *Textbook of Endocrinology,* 6th ed, Saunders, 1981, p. 134.)

Table 34–1. Laboratory evaluation of the thyroid patient.

Test	Normal Values
Free T_4	0.73–2.01 ng/dL
TSH	0.4–4.0 µIU/mL
T_3, total	100–190 ng/dL
T_4, total	6.1–11.8 µg/dL
Thyroglobulin	With thyroid gland: < 20 ng/mL
	Athyreotic on T_4: < 2 ng/mL
	Athyreotic off T_4: < 5 ng/mL
Anti-thyroid microsomal	Negative: < 0.3 U/mL
24-hour ^{131}I uptake	5–30%

TSH = thyroid-stimulating hormone.

cator of thyroid function. The thyroid scan is often helpful in determining the etiology of abnormal thyroid function and can help with decisions for further treatment. For example, thyrotoxicosis may be due to a toxic nodule that can be imaged using a thyroid scan. Each of these tests must be considered in light of an overall clinical picture.

BENIGN DISEASE

GOITER

Goiter is a term usually indicating any one of a number of benign enlargements of the thyroid gland. A goiter may develop as a result of iodine deficiency or exposure to goitrogens. **Endemic goiter** is a term that applies to the increased incidence of goiter within a defined geographic region. Although iodine deficiency and goitrogens are the likely etiology of endemic goiter, genetic influences may also be involved.

In most instances, patients with goiters will have normal T_4, T_3, and TSH. Treatment with thyroxine to suppress the gland is rarely effective unless TSH is elevated. Although thyroxine therapy may halt thyroid enlargement, large symptomatic goiters will not shrink significantly and surgery is usually indicated due to local symptoms of compression. Surgery is also indicated in multinodular goiters when malignancy is suspected.

HYPOTHYROIDISM

Hypothyroidism is usually the result of chronic thyroiditis or of surgical resection or radioiodine ablation. Symptoms of hypothyroidism include fatigue, cold intolerance, weight gain, impaired intellectual function, dry skin and hair, enlarged tongue, hoarse voice, congestive heart failure (CHF), and constipation. Thyroid function tests usually reveal a low T_4, FT_4, and elevated TSH. Treatment is supplementation with thyroid hormone (Synthroid), starting with a low dose and increasing the dose to achieve a euthyroid state confirmed by a normal TSH. Hypothyroidism rarely presents as a surgical problem. Patients with thyroiditis can sometimes develop a hard fibrotic gland that can cause airway compromise or that can be concerning for carcinoma. In these instances, thyroidectomy may be indicated.

HYPERTHYROIDISM

Hyperthyroidism is characterized by excess thyroid hormone, which results in a hypermetabolic state. Hyperthyroidism is usually the result of Graves' disease, toxic multinodular goiter, toxic adenoma, acute thyroiditis, or iatrogenic hyperthyroidism resulting from excess thyroid

hormone replacement. Symptoms of hyperthyroidism include heat intolerance, excitability, tremulousness, emotional instability, weight loss, diarrhea, palpitations, tachycardia, atrial fibrillation, muscle weakness, and restlessness. **Thyroid storm** is a particularly impressive presentation of severe hyperthyroidism that can occur as a complication of surgery or of trauma or sepsis in a patient not treated or partially treated for Graves' diseases. Manifestations include fever, CHF, hypotension, and circulatory collapse. Treatment includes fluid resuscitation and cooling blankets. Patients are given potassium iodine intravenously to inhibit thyroid hormone synthesis and cortisol to treat associated adrenal insufficiency. Propranolol is effective in controlling cardiac manifestations.

Graves' disease presents with hyperthyroidism in association with a diffuse goiter and exophthalmos. Thyroid scan reveals a diffusely enlarged gland with elevated uptake. The eye findings are due to an autoimmune process involving the eye muscles and retro-orbital tissue and may not be present at the time of initial presentation. **Toxic multinodular goiter** presents with several palpable nodules that are hot on thyroid scan. A solitary toxic nodule may also cause hyperthyroidism and generally occurs at a younger age than toxic multinodular goiter.

The initial treatment is aimed at establishing a euthyroid state by treatment with propylthiouracil (PTU) or methimazole (Tapazole). These drugs decrease the synthesis of thyroid hormone by interfering with the organification of iodine in the thyroid. Serious side effects include agranulocytosis and aplastic anemia. Some patients with hyperthyroidism are also treated with beta-blockers, such as propranolol, to control cardiac arrhythmias.

Once patients have achieved a euthyroid state, definitive therapy is based on surgical resection or ^{131}I ablation. Surgical treatment is indicated in patients with a suspicion of malignancy, such as in Graves' disease with an associated cold nodule, or in patients who are pregnant. Surgery is also preferred in several situations where ^{131}I is contraindicated or is predicted to be ineffective due to the extent of radioiodine uptake on thyroid scan.

THYROID CARCINOMA

There are approximately 14,000 new cases of thyroid carcinoma in the United States annually. Table 34–2 lists the common types of thyroid malignancies. This section deals with the well-differentiated thyroid carcinomas that are the most common of the thyroid malignancies.

ETIOLOGY

A number of studies have reported an association between external ionizing radiation and the development of well-differentiated thyroid cancer. The relationship be-

Table 34–2. Classification of thyroid cancers.

Papillary adenocarcinoma
    Classic papillary
    Follicular variant
Follicular adenocarcinoma
    Follicular micro- or macro-invasive
    Hürthle cell carcinoma
Medullary carcinoma
Undifferentiated (anaplastic) carcinoma
Lymphoma
Sarcoma
Metastatic

Table 34–3. Causes of solitary nonfunctional thyroid nodules.

Type of Nodule	Note
Adenoma	Subtypes are macrofollicular (simple colloid), microfollicular (fetal), embryonal (trabecular), Hürthle-cell (oxyphil, oncocytic) adenomas, atypical adenomas, adenomas with papillae, and signet-ring adenomas.
Carcinoma	Subtypes are papillary (70%), follicular (15%), medullary (5–10%), anaplastic carcinomas (5%) and thyroid lymphoma (5%).
Cyst	Simple cysts and other cystic thyroid lesions (see text) may present as thyroid cysts.
Nodule of an unrecognized multinodular colloid goiter	Small multinodular colloid goiters may contain a dominant nodule that is clinically indistinguishable from a macronudular follicular adenoma.
Other	Includes inflammatory thyroid diseases (subacute thyroiditis, chronic lymphocytic thyroiditis, granulomatous disease) and developmental abnormalities (unilateral lobe agenesis, cystic hygroma, dermoid, teratoma). All are very rare causes of solitary nodules.

Reprinted and modified, with permission, from Mazzaferi L: N Engl J Med 1993;328(8):557.

tween radiation exposure and carcinoma appears to be linear, with even small doses associated with increased risk. There is also an effect with age at exposure, indicating that younger patients seem more susceptible to the effect of radiation. Although most studies have indicated a long lag time between exposure and development of carcinoma, recent studies of radiation exposure from the Chernobyl nuclear disaster have indicated an increased incidence of thyroid carcinoma occurring within 3 years of exposure.

Some studies describe a familial association for the predisposition to papillary thyroid carcinoma. This association has not been as extensively studied as for familial predisposition to medullary thyroid carcinoma. Family inheritance for development of medullary thyroid cancer has been shown to be due to mutations of the ret proto-oncogene. Ret mutations have also been described in papillary carcinomas.

Several studies have reported an incidence of occult papillary carcinoma of approximately 20% in the general population. Although these small lesions are histologically identical to clinically apparent papillary carcinomas, these occult papillary cancers rarely become large enough to detect as a thyroid nodule. Since there are only 14,000 new cases of papillary thyroid carcinoma annually, the vast majority of occult papillary carcinomas are clinically insignificant.

EVALUATION OF THE THYROID NODULE

Most patients with a thyroid carcinoma present with a thyroid nodule. Thyroid nodules are quite common, and incidence increases with age. The majority of the nodules are benign; evaluation is aimed at determining which nodules are benign and can be followed, and which are malignant and require operation. Table 34–3 presents a list of causes of thyroid nodules. Clinical features and selected tests are helpful in distinguishing benign and malignant thyroid nodules.

The patient history can provide important information in the evaluation of thyroid nodules. A previous history of thyroid carcinoma, a history of radiation exposure in childhood, rapid growth of the nodule, or development of

a hoarse voice would raise a suspicion of thyroid carcinoma. A family history of medullary thyroid carcinoma (MTC) would increase the likelihood that a thyroid nodule is MTC. On physical examination, suspicion of malignancy is increased for nodules that are hard, solitary, locally fixed, or associated with lymphadenopathy. Larger nodules are also more likely to be malignant.

Ultrasonography of the thyroid is useful for discriminating between cystic and solid lesions. Cancer is more likely to be solid, but some papillary carcinomas can have a major cystic component. Nodules that are hot on radioisotope scan are unlikely to be malignant. Since only 20% of cold nodules are malignant, thyroid scan is unlikely to provide useful information to discriminate between benign and malignant lesions.

Thyroid fine-needle aspiration (FNA) cytology is the most useful test in determining the likelihood of malignancy of thyroid nodules. FNA for thyroid nodules has a false-negative rate of only 4–6%, with an overall accuracy of 95%. For small nodules, ultrasound-guided FNA can be used to increase sampling accuracy. Figure 34–2 provides a useful guide to the evaluation of thyroid nodules. A benign thyroid FNA is characterized by abundant colloid and scant cellularity, with few follicles containing benign-appearing cells. Cytological characteristics of papillary thyroid carcinoma include papillary architecture, nuclear grooves, pseudonuclear inclusions, and clumped "bubble gum" colloid. Within these diagnostic groups, FNA is accurate in distinguishing benign from malignant.

The FNA evaluation of microfollicular lesions remains a diagnostic problem. The differentiation between a be-

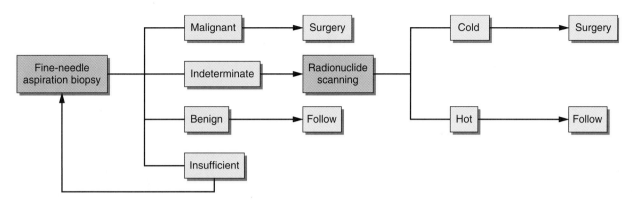

Figure 34–2. Sequence for the evaluation of patients with a thyroid nodule. The results of radionuclide scanning are expressed as "hot" or "cold" to indicate function of the nodule in relation to the normal thyroid tissue in the patient. (Reprinted, with permission, from Mazzaferri EL: Management of a solitary thyroid nodule. N Engl J Med 1993;328:553.)

nign microfollicular adenoma and a malignant follicular carcinoma is based upon capsular or angiolymphatic invasion. These features cannot be determined by FNA cytology. Since the incidence of follicular carcinoma is 20–30% in microfollicular lesions, thyroidectomy is indicated for the "indeterminate" FNA.

No single test can be relied upon for the evaluation of thyroid nodules. The overall clinical presentation must be considered when evaluating a patient with a thyroid nodule. Table 34–4 presents a list of clinical features and a relative score related to the suspicion of malignancy. In general, surgery is advisable in any patient with a score of five in any category.

TREATMENT OF WELL-DIFFERENTIATED THYROID CANCER

Total thyroidectomy is the standard treatment for any patient with thyroid carcinoma. Figure 34–3 provides a description for performing a thyroidectomy. On occasion, resection of a thyroid lobe involved with carcinoma necessitates disruption of the blood supply to the parathyroid glands. In these instances, a contralateral near-total thyroidectomy may decrease the severity of postoperative hypocalcemia. Operation for papillary thyroid carcinoma also includes dissection of mid-neck lymph nodes. In cases where lymph node metastases are clinically apparent, a modified neck dissection to include involved nodes is also indicated. Postoperatively, patients should be monitored for hypocalcemia and for development of neck hematoma, which can cause airway compromise.

Mortality from a total thyroidectomy is extremely low. Morbidity from recurrent laryngeal nerve paralysis is 1–2%, and permanent hypocalcemia has been reported to be 6–9%. The incidence of complications is low for individuals who devote the majority of their practice to endocrine surgery. Although lesser operations (eg, lobectomy) have been advocated by some, total thyroidectomy

has a lower recurrence rate and improved cancer-related mortality. Total thyroidectomy also has the advantage that patients can be monitored for thyroglobulin postoperatively as an indicator for recurrence. Treatment with ^{131}I ablation is also facilitated in patients who have undergone total thyroidectomy.

Treatment with radioactive ^{131}I has been used for many years as an adjunct to surgical resection. Metastases to

Table 34–4. Risk factors for malignancy in nodular thyroid.

		Low Risk ⟵⟶ High Risk				
		1	2	3	4	5
Age	Elderly				●	
	Child				●	
Sex	Male				●	
	Female		●			
Low-dose radiation in childhood						●
Family history			●			
Cystic mass		●				
Solid mass					●	
Multiple masses			●			
Solitary mass				●		
Growing mass						●
Stable mass				●		
Hot scan		●				
Cold scan				●		
Warm scan			●			
Fine-needle aspiration (–)			●			
Fine-needle aspiration (+)						●
Associated cervical adenopathy						●
Complete resolution to thyroid suppression		●				
Partial resolution to thyroid suppression				●		
No response to suppression					●	

Reprinted and modified, with permission, from Myers E, Suen J (editors): *Cancer of the Head and Neck,* 2nd ed. Churchill Livingstone, 1989, p. 766.

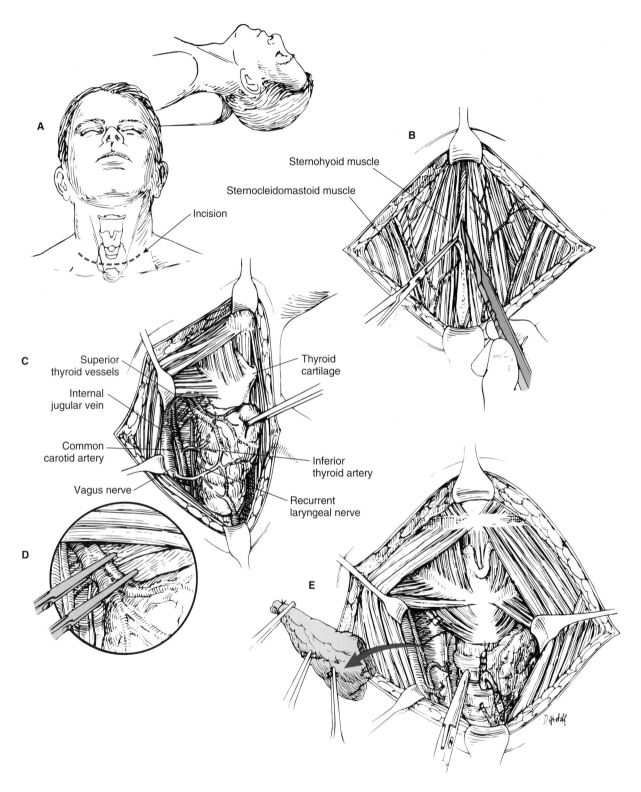

Figure 34–3. Thyroidectomy. **A:** The patient is placed with the neck in extension. The thyroid is approached through a Kocher collar incision, which is commonly made approximately 2.0 cm superior to the sternal notch. **B:** The strap muscles are divided in the midline to expose the thyroid gland. **C:** The strap muscles are retracted laterally and the thyroid is retracted medially, exposing the structures of the mid-neck. The recurrent laryngeal nerve can be seen lying within the tracheoesophageal groove. **D:** The superior pole vessels are individually clamped and ligated as they enter the thyroid gland. Inferior thyroid vessels, as well as the vessels of the thyroid (ima), are individually suture-ligated. **E:** The dissection is completed by dissection of the thyroid gland off the trachea. The isthmus is then transected and can be oversewn with a suture for hemostasis. (Reprinted, with permission, from Macdonald J, Haller D, Weigel R: Endocrine System. In: Abeloff MD (ed): *Clinical Oncology.* Churchill Livingstone, 1995, p. 1051.)

lymph nodes that are not clinically apparent are effectively treated by [131]I. Although ^{131}I ablation is contraindicated during pregnancy, there do not appear to be any long-term side effects from treatment. Prior to treatment with ^{131}I, thyroid hormone replacement is withheld and patients are allowed to become hypothyroid. The elevation in TSH stimulates any remaining thyroid tissue or carcinoma, which increases the effectiveness of the radioiodine. New studies are investigating the use of recombinant human TSH, which will alleviate the need to make patients hypothyroid prior to treatment.

OUTCOME

Most patients with thyroid carcinoma have an excellent prognosis, with 10-year disease-free survival of 80–90%. Prognosis after treatment of well-differentiated thyroid cancer is influenced by the tumor stage. One commonly used staging classification is as follows:

Class I: Intrathyroidal disease
Class II: Positive cervical nodes
Class III: Extrathyroidal invasion
Class IV: Distant metastases

Patients with class I and II disease have a longer time to recurrence and lower cancer-related mortality than patients with class III and IV disease. Early studies indicated that locoregional lymph node involvement did not ad-

versely affect prognosis. However, more recent series have demonstrated that the 30-year cancer-related mortality approaches 0% for class I disease, compared with 6% for class II disease. The 30-year recurrence rate is 8% for class I, compared with 30% for class II disease.

Age of the patient at presentation is also an important determinant for mortality related to thyroid cancer. Interestingly, there is a bimodal distribution of recurrence rate with age, but cancer mortality is low for young patients. There is a nearly linear increase in cancer mortality with age for patients over the age of 45 years (Figure 34–4).

Size of the tumor has a significant influence upon prognosis. Tumors smaller than 1.5 cm have 0.4% 30-year cancer-related mortality rate, compared with a 7% mortality rate for tumors 1.5–2.5 cm. For tumors larger than 3.0 cm, 30-year mortality approaches 50%. It has also been reported that papillary tumors have a more favorable prognosis when compared to follicular carcinomas. However, recent studies that compare tumors by size, age, and stage have failed to note a significant difference in the prognosis of papillary versus follicular carcinomas.

Extent of surgery strongly influences outcome for thyroid cancer. The 30-year recurrence rate is 26% for total thyroidectomy as compared to 40% for patients treated with lesser operations (Figure 34–5). There is also a higher mortality among patients who have had a delay in diagnosis. In a recent series, patients who were cured of thyroid carcinoma had a mean delay of 4 months, compared to 18 months in patients who died of thyroid carcinoma.

There is a highly significant reduction in recurrence

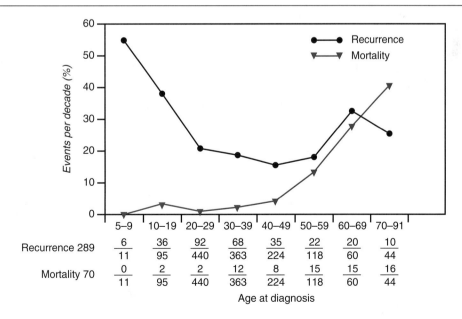

Figure 34–4. Tumor recurrence and cancer deaths according to the patient's age at the time of diagnosis. Numerators are the number of events during each time interval, and denominators are the number of patients at the beginning of each time interval. (Reprinted by permission of the publisher from Mazzaferri EL, Jhiang SM: Long-term impact of initial surgical and medical therapy on papillary and follicular thyroid cancer. Am J Med 97:422, Copyright 1994 by Excerpta Medica, Inc.)

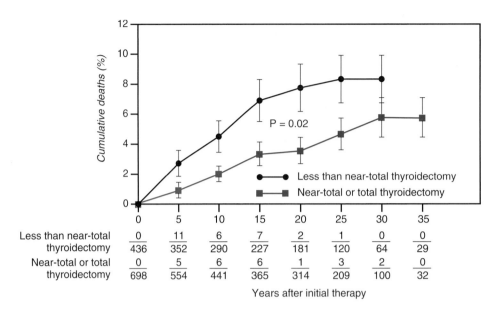

Figure 34–5. Cancer mortality in 698 patients with stage 2 or 3 tumors treated with near-total or total thyroidectomy compared with 436 who underwent less extensive surgery. Those treated more conservatively were slightly older (mean age, 37.1 years), but fewer had cervical lymph node metastases (37% versus 54%). (Reprinted by permission of the publisher from Mazzaferri EL, Jhiang SM: Long-term impact of initial surgical and medical therapy on papillary and follicular thyroid cancer. Am J Med 97:424, Copyright 1994 by Excerpta Medica, Inc.)

rate and mortality for patients treated with ^{131}I ablation as an adjunct to initial surgical therapy. The 30-year recurrence rate for patients treated with ^{131}I ablation is 15%, compared to 30% for patients treated with thyroid hormone replacement alone. This fact is even more impressive when one considers that patients treated with ^{131}I ablation tend to have tumors with a worse prognosis. Radioiodine ablation also plays an important role in treating patients with locoregional recurrence of thyroid carcinoma and patients who develop distant metastases. Papillary thyroid carcinoma most often metastasizes to the lung. Follicular thyroid carcinoma most often metastasizes to lung and bone. These metastases can be effectively treated, in most instances, with radioactive iodine.

PARATHYROID GLANDS

ANATOMY & PHYSIOLOGY

Four parathyroid glands are normally found adjacent to the thyroid. The upper glands arise from the fourth brachial pouch and descend slightly in association with the thyroid. The upper gland is usually located within a small area near the upper pole of the thyroid (Figure 34–6). The lower parathyroid glands are derived from the third brachial pouch and migrate inferiorly with the thymus. Consequently, their location is more variable but the majority of lower glands are found near the inferior pole of the thyroid. Occasionally, the inferior gland may be located within the mediastinum or the carotid sheath.

The average weight of a normal parathyroid gland is 30–35 mg. During pathologic states, a parathyroid can enlarge to as much as 1.0–3.0 g. The parathyroid glands derive their blood supply from the branches of the superior and inferior thyroid arteries. On occasion, an aberrant artery may provide a clue to the location of a parathyroid adenoma.

The parathyroid gland is normally composed of chief cells and water-clear cells that both secrete parathyroid hormone (PTH). Oxyphil cells are also present and can represent the dominant cell type in some adenomas. Normal parathyroid glands have fat dispersed throughout the gland, and the proportion of fat increases with age. Parathyroid adenomas normally demonstrate a sheet of chief cells, but water-clear cells can be intermixed. Little or no fat is found within adenomas.

The parathyroid glands synthesize PTH, which is involved in calcium homeostasis. Serum calcium is regulated primarily through the actions of PTH and vitamin D. Calcitonin is synthesized by the C cells of the thyroid and can inhibit bone resorption. However, calcitonin appears not to have a major role in calcium homeostasis in humans.

PTH acts on bone and kidney through interaction with a

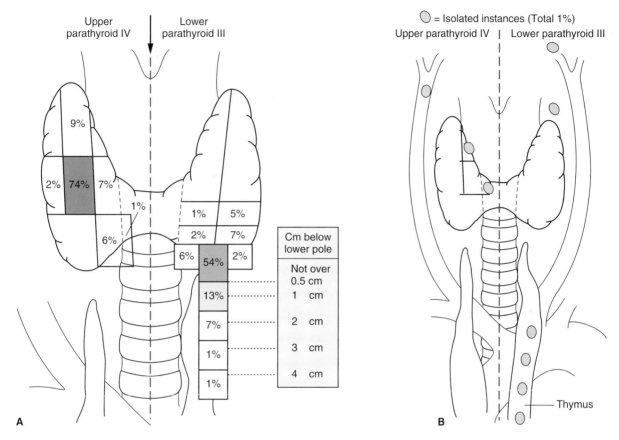

Figure 34–6. **A:** Frontal view of common anatomical locations of upper and lower parathyroid glands. **B:** Location of uncommon aberrant upper and lower parathyroid glands. (Reprinted, with permission, from Gilmour JR: J Pathol 1937:45:507.)

PTH receptor that utilizes cyclic AMP as a second messenger. In bone, PTH stimulates activity of osteocytes and results in an increase in calcium release. Within the kidney, PTH stimulates the reabsorption of calcium and also stimulates the synthesis of 1,25-dihydroxy-vitamin D_3 [$1,25(OH)_2D_3$]. This metabolite is the active form of vitamin D; it stimulates the mobilization of calcium and phosphorous from bone and augments absorption of calcium in the small bowel.

PRIMARY HYPERPARATHYROIDISM

Approximately 80% of patients with primary hyperparathyroidism (HPT) have a solitary parathyroid adenoma. Hyperplasia involving more than one gland can occur in 20% of patients and can be asymmetric, making the distinction between hyperplasia and multiple adenomas somewhat academic. HPT occurs twice as often in women as in men. Patients can present with a number of symptoms caused by hypercalcemia, kidney stones being the most common. Patients can also develop osteoporosis, pathologic fractures, bone pain, joint pain, fatigue, muscle weakness, mental disturbances, pancreatitis, polyuria, and polydipsia. Prolonged HPT can also result in renal dysfunction. In recent series, the majority of patients with HPT are asymptomatic, with no physical findings, and are identified by an elevated calcium on routine screening blood work. The presence of a neck mass in a patient with HPT is most often attributed to an associated thyroid nodule; however, the rare occurrence of parathyroid cancer can result in a palpable neck mass.

Laboratory tests are used to confirm a diagnosis of HPT. Serum calcium is elevated, as is ionized calcium, and phosphorous is usually low. Alkaline phosphatase may be elevated and is an indication of bone demineralization. Creatinine should be normal in most patients and should be checked to exclude secondary HPT. PTH levels are evaluated using a radioimmunoassay. A number of peptide fragments can be found in blood, and different antibodies can independently measure the N-terminal, mid-molecule, and C-terminal peptides. A double antibody test to measure intact PTH is most specific for HPT. An elevated calcium in the presence of an elevated intact PTH is pathognomonic for HPT.

Bone resorption in HPT is most prominent in the radial side of the middle and distal phalanges and the outer end of the clavicles. Bone density measurement is also now employed to document changes of generalized osteoporosis. Skull films, bone scan, and chest x-ray may be helpful in cases where hypercalcemia is considered to be secondary to malignancy.

SECONDARY HYPERPARATHYROIDISM

Hypocalcemia occurring as a result of chronic renal failure will result in a compensatory hyperplasia of the parathyroid glands. Hyperphosphatemia is also usually present and is a dominant feature of secondary HPT. The use of phosphate binding agents, calcium, and vitamin D supplementation will control bone and mineral metabolism in most patients. In some patients, a severe bone disease called **renal osteodystrophy** can result from chronic HPT that is due to parathyroid hyperplasia. These patients are characterized by bone pain, severe bone demineralization, and elevated alkaline phosphatase. Parathyroidectomy is indicated in this condition.

Chronic stimulation of the parathyroid glands can result in autonomous parathyroid hyperplasia, which is not responsive to correction of serum calcium. If a patient with chronic renal failure receives a kidney transplant, the autonomous parathyroid gland can continue to produce HPT. This condition is known as **tertiary hyperparathyroidism** and may result in nephrolithiasis in the transplanted kidney. Parathyroidectomy is indicated in these patients.

LOCALIZATION OF PARATHYROID GLANDS

Many surgeons do not perform localization studies prior to operating on patients with HPT. In recent years, there has been a renewed interest in localizing parathyroid glands prior to surgery to decrease operative time and extent of surgery. Clearly, localization is indicated in the setting of recurrent HPT or in cases of previous neck exploration. New modalities of ultrasound have increased the ability to localize parathyroid adenomas preoperatively using this technique. Most series have found ultrasonography will correctly localize an adenoma in 60–80% of cases. The results for ultrasonography are clearly affected by experience of the radiologist. Technetium-99 sestamibi is a new agent that has also been successful in localizing adenomas. In some series, sestamibi scans have been able to localize 80–90% of all adenomas. MRI scan is also use-

ful in parathyroid localization, especially in reoperative surgery. Newer modalities of intraoperative MRI may be used in the future. On occasion, it may be necessary to use venous PTH sampling to localize an abnormal gland for a patient in whom other imaging techniques have failed. Definitive localization can be achieved in most patients and is necessary prior to surgery for recurrent disease.

SURGERY FOR HYPERPARATHYROIDISM

Surgery is indicated for patients with symptomatic HPT. Many endocrine surgeons also advocate parathyroidectomy for "asymptomatic" patients with HPT, since subtle symptoms, such as fatigue or emotional instability, often may not be evident preoperatively. In addition, prolonged HPT may result in acceleration of osteoporosis. There is debate as to whether older patients with mild hypercalcemia should undergo parathyroidectomy.

The operation for HPT begins the same as for thyroidectomy, as described in Figure 34–3. The procedure involves identification of all four parathyroid glands. A parathyroid adenoma is identified as a large gland with a classic brick-red color. Enlarged glands should be removed and the normal glands should be biopsied to confirm their identity as parathyroid glands. The location of the normal glands should be marked with nonabsorbable suture to facilitate their identification in case future neck explorations are required.

Preoperative localization allows a directed operation to be performed. In cases where an enlarged gland is identified that corresponds to the localization studies and a normal gland is identified on the same side, a contralateral neck exploration can be avoided. The incidence of a second adenoma that is not imaged and would result in postoperative hypercalcemia is 2–5%. The intraoperative rapid PTH test can be used to confirm that an adequate resection has been performed.

Postoperatively, patients should be followed for hypocalcemia. The common symptoms of hypocalcemia include tingling of the fingertips and around the lips or nose. Patients may also develop a **Chvostek's sign**, which is a contraction of the facial muscles when tapping over the facial nerve. Severe hypocalcemia may be manifested by tetany or convulsions. Postoperative hypocalcemia is treated with calcium supplementation. Symptomatic patients should have a calcium level drawn and be given intravenous calcium, which should alleviate symptoms. If hypocalcemia is confirmed by laboratory studies, patients should be treated with oral calcium supplementation.

Postoperative hypocalcemia is often attributed to "bone hunger" as the result of chronic elevated PTH. However, postoperative hypocalcemia is usually the result of disruption of the vascular supply to the normal parathyroid glands. This conclusion is supported by a decreased incidence of postoperative hypocalcemia in patients who do not have the normal parathyroid glands biopsied. Most patients have a normal calcium off supplementation within 4–6 weeks. Severe postoperative hypocalcemia may also require vitamin D supplementation. Permanent hypoparathyroidism can occur in 2% of patients postoperatively.

Patients should be followed by periodically checking serum calcium. Parathyroidectomy cures 95–98% of patients with primary HPT after the first operation. Patients with parathyroid hyperplasia are at an increased risk for recurrent HPT. To avoid the need for a second neck exploration, a total parathyroidectomy can be performed in patients with hyperplasia (eg, renal failure or multiple endocrine neoplasia). A small amount of parathyroid tissue can be reimplanted into the muscles of the forearm. This tissue will be revascularized and will provide PTH to establish normal calcium homeostasis. If recurrent HPT occurs in this situation, some parathyroid tissue can be removed from the forearm under local anesthesia.

ADRENAL

ANATOMY & PHYSIOLOGY

The **adrenal glands** are paired organs located in the retroperitoneum lying superior and medial to the kidney on each side. The arterial supply is variable and is composed of multiple branches from the aorta, phrenic artery, and renal artery. On the left, the main adrenal vein drains into the left renal vein. On the right, a variable number of adrenal veins drain directly into the inferior vena cava.

A normal adrenal gland weighs 3.5–5.0 g and displays a chrome yellow-brown color. There are three layers of the adrenal cortex—**zona glomerulosa, zona fasciculata**, and **zona reticularis**. These three layers synthesize the three steroid hormones—aldosterone, cortisol, and adrenal androgens. Each of these steroid hormones are synthesized from cholesterol. The **adrenal medulla** is the central part of the adrenal gland and synthesizes the catecholamines—epinephrine, norepinephrine, and dopamine. The catecholamines are synthesized from the amino acid phenylalanine. Epinephrine and norepinephrine are metabolized by monoamine oxidase (MAO) and catecholamine methyltransferase (CMT) to the metanephrines and vanillylmandelic acid. These metabolites are excreted in the urine and can be measured as a screening test for pheochromocytoma.

ADRENAL CORTEX

PRIMARY HYPERALDOSTERONISM

Primary hyperaldosteronism occurs in one in 200 patients with hypertension. Patients present with hypertension, hypokalemia with inappropriate kaliuresis, and elevated plasma and urinary aldosterone. Plasma renin levels are suppressed and the ratio of plasma aldosterone to renin is elevated. Primary hyperaldosteronism may be due to either an aldosterone-producing adenoma (APA) or idiopathic hyperaldosteronism (IHA) stemming from bilateral cortical hyperplasia. Patients with APA are likely to benefit from surgery, whereas patients with IHA generally do not improve with adrenalectomy.

Patients with clinical and biochemical evidence of primary hyperaldosteronism should be evaluated with abdominal computed tomography (CT) with fine cuts through the adrenal glands. Patients with APA should have a solitary adrenal cortical adenoma, and the remaining adrenal cortex of both adrenal glands should be thin. Adenomas greater than 1.0 cm are usually imaged by CT. Adrenal vein catheterization has also been used with success to localize adenomas; however, this technique is more accurate for left-sided adenomas because of the variability of venous drainage of the right adrenal gland. Postural studies have also been helpful in distinguishing between APA and IHA, since aldosterone secretion in patients with IHA is sensitive to small fluctuations in renin concentration induced by postural changes.

Unilateral adrenalectomy is advised for patients with APA. Hypokalemia is correctable in 90–95% of patients following adrenalectomy. Correction of hypertension is less uniform, with only 60% of patients being cured by adrenalectomy. However, blood pressure control is improved in most patients. There is also some evidence that the response of hypertension to surgery is influenced by duration of symptoms; patients who have had hypertension for less than 5 years may be more likely to be cured than patients with long-standing hypertension.

HYPERADRENOCORTICISM

Cushing's syndrome is characterized by cortisol excess. Cortisol hypersecretion can be caused by pituitary tumors that produce adrenocorticotrophic hormone (ACTH), ectopic ACTH-producing tumors, or adrenal tumors. Patients with Cushing's syndrome present with truncal obesity, hirsutism, moon facies, acne, buffalo hump, purple abdominal striae, hypertension, and diabetes. In states of ACTH excess, increased skin pigmentation is also a feature.

Evaluation of a patient suspected of having Cushing's syndrome should begin with a 24-hour urinary free cortisol measurement. As shown in Figure 34–7, a low-dose

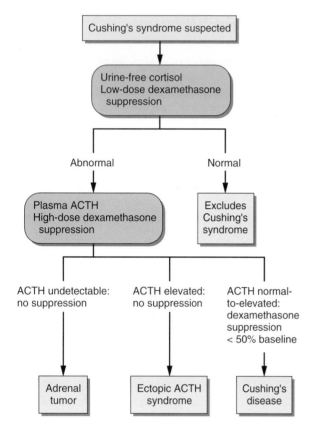

Figure 34–7. Flow diagram for the evaluation of Cushing's syndrome. Boxes enclose clinical decisions and circles enclose diagnostic tests. (Reprinted, with permission, from Baxter JD, Tyrell JB: In: Felig P et al (editors): *Endocrinology and Metabolism.* McGraw-Hill, 1981, p. 475.)

treatment with corticosteroids to avoid addisonian crisis. Steroids can be tapered, and the manifestations of cortisol excess will subside within 3–4 months.

ADRENAL MEDULLA

PHEOCHROMOCYTOMA

A **pheochromocytoma** is a tumor of the chromaffin cells of the adrenal gland that secretes catecholamines. Extra-adrenal pheochromocytomas also occur and are referred to as **paragangliomas**. Chromaffin tissue is embryologically related to a group of endocrine tissues that secrete polypeptide hormones. These cells are termed **amino precursor uptake and decarboxylation (APUD) cells**. Pheochromocytomas can develop in any location where chromaffin tissue migrates during embryogenesis.

Patients with pheochromocytoma present with a plethora of symptoms. Hypertension is present in most patients and can be sustained or paroxysmal. Hypertensive crisis during general anesthesia necessitates evaluation for pheochromocytoma. Headache, palpitations, diaphoresis, anxiety, tachycardia, and flushing are prominent features of the disease. Patients will often describe "spells" characterized by a number of these symptoms attributed to catecholamine excess.

Patients suspected of having pheochromocytoma should undergo biochemical screening. Plasma levels of epinephrine and norepinephrine are useful if severely elevated but may be normal because of the transient nature of hypersecretion. The most reliable test is a 24-hour urine for catecholamines and metabolites. Urine should be evaluated for epinephrine, norepinephrine, and the metabolites metanephrines and vanillylmandelic acid. When all of these substances are examined, 98% of patients with a pheochromocytoma will have at least one abnormality.

One useful test to distinguish pheochromocytoma from essential hypertension is the clonidine suppression test. Clonidine will lower blood pressure in patients with essential hypertension and pheochromocytomas, but will only lower plasma levels in patients with essential hypertension. Clonidine acts centrally to inhibit neurally mediated catecholamine release at axon terminals of sympathetic postganglionic neurons. In essential hypertension, this is the main source of plasma catecholamines, therefore, a reduction in the low levels of normal plasma catecholamines is observed. In pheochromocytomas, the normal sympathetic regulation occurs, and only a small fraction of the high plasma levels of catecholamines is active at the synaptic level. Therefore, clonidine will lower blood pressure in patients with pheochromocytoma but will have little effect on the high plasma levels from the tumor.

Once the diagnosis of pheochromocytoma is established, the tumor must be localized before resection can

dexamethasone suppression test is helpful in confirming the diagnosis of Cushing's syndrome. In patients identified with Cushing's syndrome, plasma ACTH levels are used to distinguish between adrenal and extra-adrenal etiologies. Following high-dose dexamethasone suppression, undetectable ACTH with no cortisol suppression indicates the presence of an adrenal adenoma, adrenal carcinoma, or, rarely, nodular adrenal dysplasia. Ectopic ACTH syndrome is most often the result of small cell carcinoma of the lung. Elevated ACTH with suppression of 17-hydroxycorticosteroids is likely to be due to a pituitary adenoma (Cushing's disease). Pituitary exploration is indicated in patients with Cushing's disease.

Unilateral adrenalectomy is curative for patients with an adrenal adenoma. Patients with adrenal carcinoma will often have large tumors that are locally invasive or metastatic at presentation. These patients should undergo a debulking procedure to remove as much tumor as possible. Patients with nodular hyperplasia can be treated with bilateral adrenalectomy. Postoperatively, patients require be considered. CT scan of the abdomen with special attention to the adrenal glands provides the best anatomic localization of pheochromocytoma. MRI scan is being used more frequently since pheochromocytomas have a characteristic bright appearance on T-2 weighted images. ^{131}I-metaiodobenzylguanidine (MBIG) scans are also helpful in localizing tumors, particularly in cases where CT scan or MRI have failed to identify a tumor.

Prior to surgery, patients are treated with phenoxybenzamine, which is an α-adrenergic blocking agent. Treatment is titrated to maximize blood pressure control while limiting orthostatic hypotension. In patients whose tumors secrete epinephrine, the cardiac dysrhythmias can be controlled with beta-adrenergic blockers but only after sufficient alpha blockade has been established. Adequate fluid resuscitation is an important aspect of preoperative and intraoperative management. During adrenalectomy, hypertension can still be a problem despite adequate blockade, especially during manipulation of the tumor. Short-acting agents such as intravenous nitroprusside are useful in controlling hypertension intraoperatively. Intraoperative transesophageal echocardiography is routinely employed to evaluate mitral valve function, which can provide additional information concerning the fluid status of the patient, as well as other hemodynamic parameters.

ADRENAL SURGERY

The surgical approach to the adrenal gland is through an abdominal incision or through a posterior incision as outlined in Figure 34–8. The posterior approach is preferable for well-localized, small adrenal tumors where risk of malignancy is low. Large tumors are best approached through the abdomen. New techniques of laparoscopic adrenalectomy have received considerable interest over the last few years.

MULTIPLE ENDOCRINE NEOPLASIA

Multiple endocrine neoplasia (MEN) is an inherited cancer syndrome characterized by the development of multiple tumors within distinct endocrine tissues. Both syndromes are inherited as an autosomal dominant trait with a high degree of penetrance. The features of MEN1 and MEN2A and 2B are outlined in Table 34–5.

MEN1

Linkage analysis has established that the gene for MEN1 is located at 11q13. Affected individuals develop parathyroid hyperplasia, pancreatic islet cell tumors, and pituitary adenomas. Parathyroid hyperplasia is usually the first manifestation of the disease, which is normally clinically manifest by the third to fourth decade of life. Treatment of parathyroid hyperplasia involves neck exploration with resection of abnormal glands. Pancreatic islet cell tumors are often multiple, and curative resection is not achieved in most cases.

MEN2

MEN2 is characterized by medullary thyroid carcinoma (MTC), pheochromocytoma, and the development of parathyroid hyperplasia (2A), or multiple mucosal neuromas with a marfanoid habitus (2B). Expressivity of the trait is dependent upon the kindred. There is also a familial MTC not associated with other tumors. All of these syndromes have been linked to mutations of the ret proto-oncogene located at the centromeric region of chromosome 10. Genetic screening now allows identification of affected individuals from birth.

MTC is treated by total thyroidectomy. In MEN2A, total parathyroidectomy with reimplantation to the forearm is performed at the same time as thyroidectomy. Patients with MTC should be screened for pheochromocytoma. In patients with pheochromocytoma, adrenalectomy is performed first. Several studies have reported a combined operation of adrenalectomy and thyroidectomy with good results. Genetic screening has also allowed thyroidectomy to be performed prior to the development of overt MTC. This approach will likely improve survival in these patients.

Table 34–5. Syndromes of multiple endocrine neoplasia.

MEN1	MEN2

Pituitary tumors
    Eosinophilic adenoma
        (acromegaly)
    Prolactinoma
    Nonfunctional tumors
    ACTH-secreting tumors
	MEN2A and 2B
	    Medullary carcinoma
	        of the thyroid
	    Pheochromocytoma

Hyperparathyroidism	MEN2A Hyperparathyroidism

Pancreatic tumors
    Most common
        Pancreatic polypeptide-
            secreting tumor
        Gastrinoma
        Insulinoma
    Uncommon
        Glucagonoma
        VIPoma
        Grfoma
	MEN2B
	    Mucosal neuromas
	    Marfanoid habitus
	    Typical facies
	    Bowel abnormalities

ACTH = adrenocorticotropic hormone; MEN2A, 2B = multiple endocrine neoplasia types 2A, 2B.
Reprinted and modified, with permission, from Abeloff MD et al: *Clinical Oncology,* Churchill Livingstone, 1995, p. 1064.

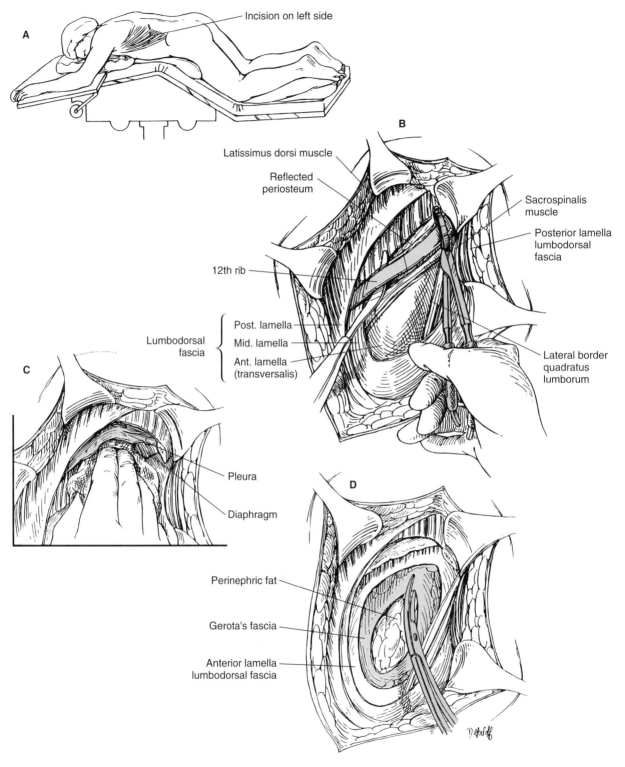

Figure 34–8. Posterior approach to the adrenal gland. **A:** The patient is placed in jackknife prone position and a curvilinear incision is made in the flank. **B:** The 12th rib is removed subperiosteally, exposing the lumbodorsal fascia. **C:** The pleura is swept superiorly with a gauze-covered finger. **D:** The diaphragm is transected, exposing Gerota's fascia, which is then opened. **E:** The adrenal gland is exposed, and **F:** vessels of the gland are ligated with hemoclips and then transected. (Reprinted, with permission, from Macdonald J, Haller D, Weigel R: Endocrine System. In: Abeloff MD (editor): *Clinical Oncology.* Churchill Livingstone, 1995, pp. 1058–1059.)

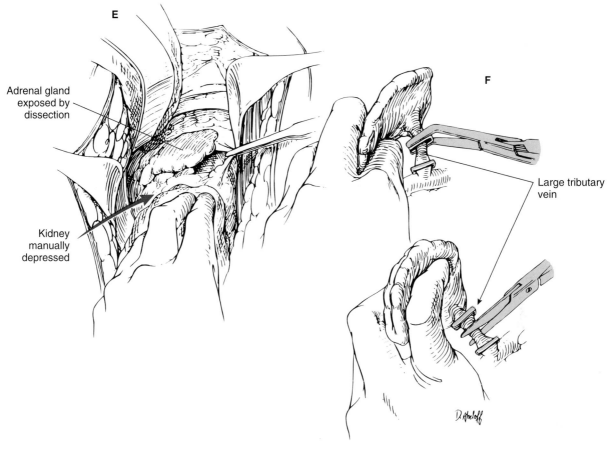

E

Adrenal gland
exposed by
dissection

Kidney
manually
depressed

F

Large tributary
vein

D. Abeloff

Figure 34–8.   Continued

SUGGESTED READING

Macdonald J, Haller D, Weigel R: Endocrine system. In: Abeloff MD et al (editors): *Clinical Oncology*. Churchill Livingstone, 1995.

Myers E, Suen J: *Cancer of the Head and Neck*, 2nd ed. Churchill Livingstone, 1989.

Wilson JD, Foster DW: *Williams' Textbook of Endocrinology*, 8th ed. Saunders, 1992.

35

The Breast

Stefanie S. Jeffrey, MD, Frank E. Stockdale, MD, PhD, & Robyn L. Birdwell, MD

► Key Facts

- ► Physical examination of the breasts includes inspection for nipple and skin changes, physical deformities, such as bulges or dimpling in the skin, and overall symmetry.

- ► The breast normally has a varied architecture that may feel lumpy or nodular in most patients, but this should not be confused with a dominant mass, which requires diagnostic evaluation.

- ► A screening mammogram is the radiologic evaluation of breasts with no known abnormalities, while diagnostic mammography is recommended for patients with abnormal screening mammograms or complaints of a palpable lump, pain, or nipple discharge.

- ► Palpable masses may be biopsied by several different methods, including fine-needle aspiration, needle core biopsy, or incisional or excisional open biopsy.

- ► Mammographic abnormalities can be classified as masses, microcalcifications, architectural distortions, or areas of asymmetric densities.

- ► Hookwire surgical biopsy or stereotactic needle biopsy is used to biopsy nonpalpable mammographic lesions.

- ► Breast cancer falls into three general categories: the ductal carcinomas, the lobular carcinomas, and the special types, such as tubular, medullary, colloid/mucinous, and papillary carcinomas.

- ► Once the diagnosis of primary breast cancer has been established, therapeutic decisions must be made in two major areas: (1) local-regional treatment (the removal of tumor and determination of lymph node involvement); (2) systemic treatment (adjuvant therapy to stop the growth of any tumor cells that may have traveled to distant sites).

- ► With few exceptions, patients who have a relapse of breast cancer will die of their disease.

ANATOMY & PHYSIOLOGY

The breast is composed of skin, adipose tissue, a ligamentous framework (Cooper's ligaments), ducts, and alveoli-containing lobules (Figure 35–1). Embryologically, breast development extends as an ectodermal band known as the milk streak from the base of the forelimb bud, or primitive axilla, to the base of the hindlimb bud, or primitive inguinal region. Normal development results in single bilateral organs, but with failure of involution during fetal development, accessory breast tissue may be

440

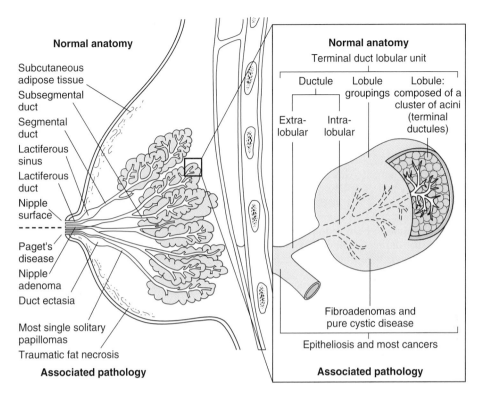

Figure 35–1. The anatomy of the breast, demonstrating the organization of the elements comprising the terminal duct lobular unit and their relationship to specific pathologic abnormalities. (Reprinted, with permission, from Hayes D: Breast cancer. In: Skarin AT (editor): *Atlas of Diagnostic Oncology.* Lippincott, 1991, p. 6.4.)

found anywhere along the line from the axilla (most common site) to the inguinal region. Supernumerary nipples may occur along this line in both sexes and may be mistaken for dermal nevi.

At birth, the breast has only a rudimentary network of branching ducts. Fluid known as colostral milk, or "witch's milk," may be secreted by the neonate in the first postpartum week due to residual maternal hormones. During adolescence the female breast responds to hormonal stimulation, resulting in lobular development and ductal and stromal enlargement. Physical examination of the peripubertal breast may reveal firm and sometimes asymmetric areas beneath the nipples. This is a normal physical finding and excisional biopsy of the prepubertal and peripubertal breast is never recommended, as breast bud removal or injury will result in failure of breast development.

As development proceeds, all components of the breast grow, including the ductal-alveolar system. Fifteen to 20 ducts open onto the nipple. These ducts arborize from their largest diameter under the nipple to their smallest branches at the terminal duct-lobular units (TDLU). The ducts drain segmental areas of the breast without predictable pattern and without histologically defined boundaries separating one lobe from another. The vast majority of breast cancers begin in the TDLU; investigation has focused on many aspects of anatomic developmental, and environmental factors leading to pathologic abnormalities in this region. Exposure to ionizing radiation during puberty and deleterious environmental influences occurring prior to mature breast development may subsequently lead to breast cancer. More recent studies are focusing on molecular changes that occur within the TDLU.

The ductal and lobular systems demonstrate histologic and functional changes based on hormonal influences. During pregnancy there is a proliferation of lobules that ultimately lead to the postpartum secretion of milk during lactation. Following lactation and even more profoundly as menopause is achieved, the ductal-lobular tissues involute and are replaced by fatty tissue. In general, by mammography, a young woman's breast tends to appear more dense due to increased fibroglandular tissue, while the older breast is more radiolucent secondary to fatty replacement. This is, however, not a predictable pattern and can be affected and even reversed by hormonal replacement therapy.

The breast is supplied by arterial flow from branches of the axillary, intercostal, and internal mammary arteries.

Venous drainage predominantly follows the same routes. Lymphatics primarily drain to the axilla; a minor drainage pathway is to the internal mammary lymph nodes.

PHYSICAL EXAMINATION OF THE BREAST

Prior to examination of the breasts, a focused history should be elicited from the patient. This should include any recent breast symptoms and recording of family history, menopausal status or date of last menstrual period, parity and age at birth of first child, lactation history, history of hormone use, exposure to head and neck or chest wall radiation (especially during childhood or adolescence), and results of previous breast biopsies/surgery, if applicable.

Physical examination of the breasts includes inspection for overall symmetry, nipple and skin changes, and physical deformities such as bulges or dimpling of the skin. Keep in mind that many women have asymmetrical breasts. If this is not a recent change, it is considered normal. Skin edema (postsurgical or from lymphatic obstruction by tumor) can produce a skin texture change known as **peau d'orange** because the prominent skin pores cause it to look like the skin of an orange. On physical examination, arm movements may reveal areas of abnormal breast contour. The patient should be asked to: (1) raise her arms (in order to visualize lesions fixed to ligaments that pull on the overlying skin, causing skin dimpling); (2) place her arms on her hips and squeeze elbows forward (in order to visualize lesions that may be adherent to the pectoral fascia); (3) lean forward (in order to visualize lesions in the lower half of ptotic breasts).

The supraclavicular region, infraclavicular region, and axilla may be palpated with the patient in the upright position and the breast examined in all quadrants. The breast tissue is also examined with the patient in the supine position. All portions of the breast must be palpated from the sternum medially to the clavicle superiorly to the midaxillary line laterally to below the inframammary fold inferiorly. This may be done with light and firm pressure using rotary motions of the index and middle fingers held together, or by making alternating motions of the index and middle fingers (like playing the piano). The use of these motions in progressive vertical strips efficiently examines the breast (Figure 35–2). The patient may then turn to a lateral decubitus position for the breast to be reexamined (with the patient on her side, it is easier to feel the lateral, posterior, and axillary portions of the breast). The breast may also be repalpated with the patient upright, using a hand or firm surface to support the underlying breast tissue.

The breast normally has a varied architecture, which may feel lumpy or nodular in some patients. Fibrofatty nodules or glandular tissue in the upper outer portions of

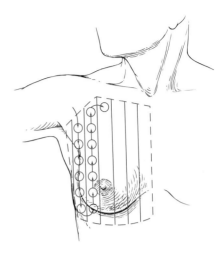

Figure 35–2. The breast is examined in a vertical manner with small palpating motions, using the sensitive pads of the fingers.

the breast or along the inframammary fold may be confused with a breast lump but actually represent normal findings. A **dominant mass** is a nodule or lump that is different than the surrounding tissue. The dominant mass remains constant in texture with change in patient position. It is not important to decide whether a mass is cancer, but only if a mass is dominant and requires diagnostic workup. Since most cancers are found by the woman herself, special attention should be given to any abnormalities noticed by the patient.

It is helpful to record the breast examination using a diagram that visually specifies the location of lumps or thickenings and records the presence or absence of clinically abnormal lymph nodes (Figure 35–3). When the location of a breast lump is verbally discussed, the breast is usually divided into four quadrants: the upper outer, lower outer, upper inner, and lower inner, to specify the location of the lump. Often, the position is indicated using clock face terminology (eg, 10 o'clock position).

BREAST IMAGING

The American Cancer Society recommends that women 40 years of age and older should have an annual physical examination and an annual mammography to detect breast cancer. The addition of mammography to the standard clinical examination began in the 1960s. Randomized clinical trials performed in Europe, Canada, and the United States have demonstrated that smaller, and in many cases lower grade, cancers can be imaged before they can be felt. In general, the smaller the cancer the less chance for invasion or metastases.

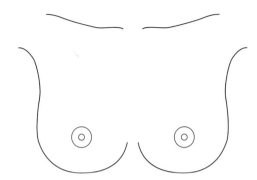

Figure 35–3. Site-specific visual diagram to record the presence of lumps or thickenings in the breast during physical examination.

The term **screening mammogram** is used to describe the radiologic evaluation of breasts in which no abnormalities are reported by the patient or the examining health care professional. The examination requires a dedicated mammography machine and includes two standard views of each breast. Each breast is examined in the medial lateral oblique (the side view) and the craniocaudal (the up and down view) position, with compression using an automated transparent plate applied similarly in both projections. Screening examinations may be performed in an office by a qualified technologist and read at a later time, and sometimes in a different location, by a radiologist. The focus of this approach is to minimize cost and maximize volume, resulting in a decrease in cost to the patient.

Diagnostic mammography is recommended for patients with complaints, which may include a palpable lump, pain, or nipple discharge. The interpretation of mammograms, whether screening or diagnostic, is performed by a radiologist with special training in mammography. The radiologist will take into account the overall composition of the breast tissue as well as any perceived abnormalities. Breasts vary in size and density. In general, the premenopausal breast is composed of fibroglandular tissue alternating with varying amounts of fat. With age, the breast tissue involutes with the deposition of additional fat. In some women on hormone replacement therapy, this pattern of fatty predominance can revert to a more premenopausal glandular appearance. On x-ray, fat is dark and abnormalities that are light or "white" may be more evident. Fibroglandular patterns tend to be more radiographically dense ("white") and abnormalities may not be so easily visualized.

Mammography is a method of *detection* rather than *diagnosis* of breast cancer in that many abnormalities may appear to be cancer but are, in fact, benign. Mammographically detected abnormalities in the breast include masses, calcifications, architectural tissue pattern distortion, and asymmetry of tissue (Figure 35–4). Additional abnormalities that may suggest breast cancer include skin thickening, an overall increase in breast density, and axillary lymphadenopathy.

Although mammography is the only imaging method shown to be beneficial as a screening examination of the breasts, other modalities can be very helpful in further characterizing focused areas of abnormality. In some cases of mammographically detected masses, breast sonography is used to further evaluate the nature of the mass. Cysts may be diagnosed by their sonographic characteristics, including a round or elliptical shape with smooth borders, no internal echoes within the mass, and increased transmission of the echo beam. This latter finding is a result of the refocusing of the sonographic beam by the fluid within the cyst. Although some sonographic characteristics of solid masses are highly suggestive of malignancy, the findings of a solid mass by sonography are nonspecific and may warrant biopsy.

Mammography of silicone breast implants to substantiate clinical suspicion for rupture is fairly insensitive, particularly if the silicone is not free within the breast. These women may benefit from sonography, but magnetic resonance imaging (MRI) has been shown to be more sensitive in diagnosing intracapsular rupture. The use of MRI for breast cancer is still in the experimental stages, but early results suggest that breast MRI will play an important role, especially when mammography is not clearly diagnostic (Figure 35–5).

THE SYMPTOMATIC PATIENT

BREAST PAIN

Diagnosis & Management

The most common breast complaint is breast pain, which is estimated to occur at some time in almost half the female population. Occasionally, breast pain is due to pressure from an enlarging and usually palpable breast cyst. Less frequently, an area of focal mastitis may present as a tender breast mass with or without overlying skin erythema. Advanced inflammatory breast cancer may be a rare cause of breast tenderness, but the physical signs of skin erythema with a firm mass or overall distortion of the involved breast usually makes this diagnosis obvious. The cause of most breast pain is not well understood. Upon questioning, women commonly describe an area of diffuse tenderness that may radiate to the axilla or upper arm (distribution of the intercostobrachial sensory nerve). The pain is commonly cyclic, occurring most often at the time of ovulation or in the week before the onset of menses. Although most breast pain is not due to malignant disease, focal, persistent, noncyclic pain in an area that the patient can point to with one finger must be suspect, since 10–17% of breast cancers are preceded by or associated with focal pain.

Workup of breast pain includes a thorough physical ex-

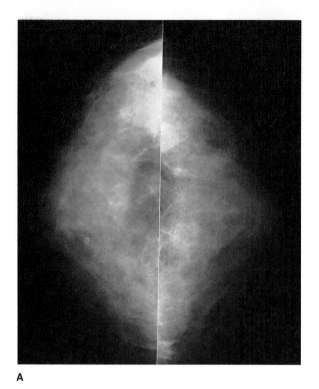

A

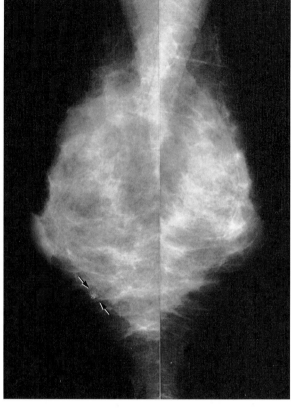

B

C

Figure 35–4. Depicted in this figure is a bilateral mammogram (an X-ray) characrterized as "dense" because of the dominant fibroglandular tissue (white material) with very little accompanying fat (seen as black on mammography). This examination is almost totally normal with the exception of a small focus of calcifications in the left breast (arrows). **A.** This is the craniocaudal view of the breasts which is produced when the X-ray beam is directed from the patient's head to her feet. **B.** This view is the medio-lateral projection where the woman is placed into the dedicated mammography machine at an oblique angle, compression applied, and the X-ray beam captured on specialized X-ray film after traveling in the medial to lateral direction. The arrows point to a very small group of microcalcifications in the left breast. This area of the breast was normal on physical examination. **C.** Magnification of the very small microcalcifications within the left breast demonstrates to better advantage the variation in calcification sizes and shapes which is an indicator of concern for malignancy warranting a biopsy recommendation. Pathology showed intraductal carcinoma.

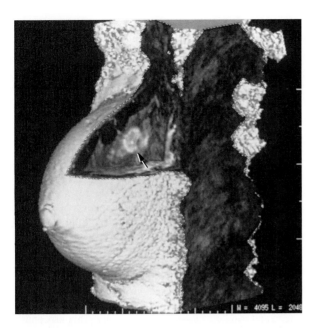

Figure 35–5. This 3-dimensional image is a computer rendering of information from a magnetic resonance image (MRI) of a breast following the injection of gadolinium contrast material which enhances the moderate sized, rim enhancing, irregularly shaped carcinoma (arrow).

amination in all women and mammography in women over 35 years of age. When the pain is focal, breast sonography at the specific site of pain may be used to identify (or show lack of presence of) a solid or cystic mass. Any mass, area of architectural distortion, or mammographic or sonographic abnormality at the site of breast pain should be biopsied, either by needle biopsy (fine-needle aspiration [FNA] or core biopsy) or surgical biopsy. Symptomatic cysts can be aspirated. When no mass is identified by physical examination or breast imaging, the patient should have a follow-up physical examination within 2–3 months and be questioned to see if any of the treatment modalities discussed below have been helpful.

Since the majority of women believe the reason for breast pain is a cancer growing in their breast, the most important part of treatment is reassurance that the pain is not related to breast cancer. For breast pain that is not related to disease, a 3-month trial of caffeine restriction and/or vitamin E 800 IU/d has been helpful in individual women, although randomized series in large populations of women do not show a difference over placebo. The effect of caffeine on breast pain may be related to cyclic-AMP stimulation. Also unproven in randomized clinical trials, but often helpful in individual cases of cyclic breast swelling and tenderness, is vitamin B_6 150–200 mg/d for 1 week prior to the onset of her menstrual period. Vitamin

B_6 may act like a natural diuretic and diminish fluid retention. The woman should be warned that chronic large doses of vitamin B_6 can lead to a reversible peripheral neuropathy, so it should not be abused. Of proven benefit in randomized clinical series is Oil of Evening Primrose. A common dosage is 6 capsules per day for 1 month, then 4 tablets per day for 2 more months. Adjustments of estrogen and progesterone if the woman is on postmenopausal hormone supplementation may also be of benefit. Very severe breast pain interfering with a woman's daily life may be treated with bromocriptine, a pituitary antagonist; danazol, an androgen; or luteinizing hormone/releasing hormone (LH/RH) agonists. All of these drugs have been shown to be helpful in clinical trials, but they carry significant side effects and are rarely used in the treatment of breast pain.

NIPPLE DISCHARGE

Diagnosis & Management

Physiologic nipple discharge can be expressed from about 10–60% of breasts of nonlactating women. It is usually bilateral and can be elicited from multiple ducts. A woman may note a discharge when she squeezes her nipples during breast self-examination or while washing. The color can range from golden brown to dark green to milky. Women should be reassured that this is very common and not caused by breast cancer. No workup is required other than routine breast examination and screening mammography if she is eligible by age and has not had this done within the previous 6 months. Mammography is performed not for the nipple discharge, but to make sure that the patient does not have synchronous pathology.

Pathologic nipple discharge is usually unilateral, spontaneous, and comes from a single duct. The patient often complains of finding a wet spot on her bra or nightgown without any antecedent event. All bloody nipple discharges must be evaluated. The most common cause (35–50%) for a pathologic nipple discharge is an intraductal papilloma. Malignant neoplasm may account for 15–20% of pathologic nipple discharges, although a bloody nipple discharge in a postmenopausal woman is malignant 30% of the time. The older the patient, the greater the chance that the discharge is a sign of underlying cancer. Mammary duct ectasia or fibrocystic change accounts for the remainder of cases of pathologic nipple discharge.

In women with pathologic discharge the breast is palpated, especially in the periareolar region, to determine if there are any associated masses. The nipple is sequentially compressed in a clockwise fashion to determine if the discharge is associated with a periareolar duct opening on the nipple. Mammography is performed but is often negative, since the process causing the discharge is usually intraductal. A galactogram may demonstrate intraductal filling defects and may help to identify lesions in the more distal ductal system.

To diagnose a pathologic nipple discharge, a nipple duct surgical exploration is done, beginning at the nipple and extending the dissection distally for about 5 cm into the breast tissue. Injection of methylene blue dye into the involved duct is helpful in identifying the subareolar duct system to be followed.

PALPABLE BREAST MASSES

Diagnosis & Management

When evaluating breast masses or thickenings, the clinician must first decide whether a true dominant abnormality is present or whether the "lump" is part of the normal breast architecture. It is not unusual for a fibrofatty nodule or an area of glandular tissue to feel like a lump, especially along the inframammary fold or in the upper outer quadrant of the breast. If other similar-feeling tissue is palpable elsewhere in the same or opposite breast, or if the abnormality is no longer palpable with a change of position, then a true dominant mass is unlikely. Normal architectural "lumpiness" may change with the menstrual cycle. These areas may enlarge or feel indurated the week prior to onset of menstruation and regress in the 7–10 days following the first day of menstruation (the optimal time for routine breast palpation or routine mammography). When an abnormality is felt by the patient or her physician, it is not necessary to decide by palpation alone whether an abnormality is malignant; it is only necessary to decide whether an abnormality exists and requires imaging or biopsy.

After physical examination demonstrates that a mass indeed exists, the next step depends on the likelihood that the mass is a simple cyst that can be diagnosed and treated by aspiration alone. If there has not been a recent mammogram, the next part of the workup is breast imaging. Mammography is important, not only in the characterization of a mass but also to look for multifocal (same quadrant) or multicentric (different quadrant) cancer as well as any abnormality in the opposite breast (synchronous contralateral disease). Breast sonography may identify whether the mass is cystic or solid and, if cystic, whether there are findings suggestive of neoplastic growth within the cyst wall. It is important to perform the breast imaging prior to any needle aspiration, since bleeding after the needle stick may change the mammogram or breast sonogram image and it may take about 3 weeks for the changes to resolve. Mammography is not usually performed for breast masses in women less than 35 years old unless there is a high clinical likelihood that the mass is malignant.

Palpable masses may be biopsied by a number of methods. The choice of method may depends on patient age, experience of the clinician, and availability of a skilled cytologist.

Needle aspiration alone refers to the aspiration of a mass to determine whether it is cystic (fluid-filled) or solid. Cyst fluid is aspirated into a syringe and the site of the cyst is then palpated to determine if there is any residual mass that may be present in cases of cystic carcinomas.

A **fine-needle aspiration** (FNA) biopsy is a technique that provides a cytologic sample from a solid mass(es) or area of mammographic abnormality. Multiple to-and-fro passes are made with an 22- to 23-gauge needle using syringe suction. Cell clusters and individual cells are cut and aspirated into the hub of the needle. The cells are then pushed out and smeared onto a slide that can be air-dried or fixed and then stained. Because the breast epithelial cells that are sampled are not seen in relation to ducts or lobules, it is important to consult an experienced cytologist, since usual histologic structural features are absent. FNA biopsies, for example, cannot distinguish between in situ and invasive carcinoma. Due to the subtle cytologic differences between some atypical hyperplasias and ductal carcinoma in situ, any atypia in an FNA biopsy requires open surgical biopsy.

Core needle biopsy refers to the use of a specialized needle (such as a Tru-cut 14-gauge needle) that cuts a core of tissue. The core of tissue provides a sample that is sectioned and can be evaluated histologically. This procedure can be more painful than FNA biopsy. Similar to FNA biopsy, accuracy of core biopsy depends on the experience of the person performing the biopsy but is not dependent on the cytologic reading, as actual tissue is available for evaluation.

Open surgical biopsy may be **excisional** or **incisional**. Excisional biopsy, the preferred technique, refers to removing the entire mass, whereas incisional biopsy means cutting into the mass and only taking a portion of it, such as in the case of a very large mass. **Hookwire localization** surgical biopsy will be discussed in the section under management of mammographic abnormalities.

The majority of breast masses are benign and can be cystic or solid. Breast cysts are normally benign (more than 99% of the time). They may be aspirated in the office for diagnosis or to relieve pressure symptoms. Breast sonography is also a helpful technique for following patients with multiple bilateral breast cysts (benign cystic mastopathy) and in guiding aspiration of multiple cysts.

Solid breast masses may be fibrocystic lesions, fibroadenomas, or breast malignancies. **Fibrocystic change** refers to a pathologic entity, not just palpably lumpy breasts. In the spectrum of histologic fibrocystic change is one or more of the following: micro or macro cyst formation, apocrine metaplasia, fibrous change, and epithelial (ductal or lobular) hyperplasia.

Atypical hyperplasia may be diagnosed by the development and proliferation of a single cell population within a breast duct or lobule, with varying severity of nuclear cytologic changes. A "borderline lesion" refers to severe atypical ductal hyperplasia that has an appearance very similar to the cells of ductal carcinoma in situ. Atypical hyperplasia, especially in conjunction with a family history of breast cancer, is associated with a marked increase in risk for the future development of breast cancer.

Fibroadenomas are a proliferation of ductal (epithelial) elements and fibrous tissue. They may be diagnosed by FNA or core needle biopsy and treated conservatively once the cytologic or histologic diagnosis has been established. About one third will completely resolve within 2 years. It is important not to assume that a mass is a fibroadenoma without cytologic or histologic confirmation and such patients should be followed closely. About 2 or 3 of 1000 fibroadenomas may contain an associated malignancy inside or at the edge of the mass. Usually the association of cancer with a fibroadenoma occurs in patients older than 40; therefore, any clinical change in size or mammographic appearance of a fibroadenoma necessitates excisional biopsy. Low axillary lymph nodes may also present as a mass in the axillary tail of the breast. These are easily diagnosed by FNA biopsy.

Most palpable cancers can be diagnosed with FNA biopsy preoperatively. In experienced hands, the accuracy approaches 95–98%. Any mass that is diagnosed cytologically as atypical, suspicious, or frankly malignant should be surgically removed. Fine needle aspiration biopsies reported as an indeterminate diagnosis or nondiagnostic because of hypocellularity should be repeated, unless the mass clinically feels like a lipoma or fibrofatty nodule. It is important to be aware that with FNA cytology, it is sometimes difficult to detect an infiltrating lobular carcinoma because single-file infiltration of normal tissue by malignant cells may not be easily aspirated. Diffuse infiltrating lobular carcinoma may also be associated with false negative mammograms because they may cast a nonspecific image on mammography.

THE ABNORMAL MAMMOGRAM

Diagnosis & Management

In 1992, Congress passed the Mammography Quality Standards Act, mandating the standardization of both the production and the interpretation of mammograms. As of October 1, 1994, all mammography facilities were required by law to be certified by the Food and Drug Administration (FDA). Included in this document is the requirement of strict adherence to quality assurance and follow-up of all abnormal mammograms with a system established for reviewing outcome data, including disposition and correlation of surgical biopsy results with mammogram reports. Abnormal mammograms often describe benign findings; an appropriate follow-up may be a short interval 6-month mammogram examination. However, indeterminate or suspicious masses, calcifications, and areas of architectural distortion not associated with a history of prior biopsy or trauma usually warrant biopsy.

Mammographic abnormalities can be classified as masses, microcalcifications, architectural distortions, and areas of asymmetric densities. Very-low-suspicion abnormalities (termed "probably benign") can be mammographically followed at 6 months, 12 months, and annually thereafter. Masses and microcalcifications that remain stable for a period of 3 years are considered benign. Indeterminate lesions may be mammographically or sonographically followed or undergo tissue biopsy. All suspicious lesions should be biopsied.

Newer, less invasive percutaneous techniques for diagnosing mammographic abnormalities include sonographically guided FNA or core needle biopsy and stereotactic needle biopsy. Stereotactic biopsy uses specialized computer and x-ray equipment to guide a 14- or 11-gauge needle to a mammographically detected lesion. As stated previously, FNA cannot distinguish between in situ and invasive ductal carcinoma, and it is less accurate for microcalcifications alone. Core needle biopsy is more accurate for diagnosing microcalcifications because the tissue core can be radiographed to verify the presence of microcalcifications at the time of the procedure. When determining which patient to follow mammographically, which patient to stereotactically biopsy, and which patient to surgically biopsy, the clinical history, the number of lesions, the location of the lesions, and other risk factors (such as history of previous breast cancer or atypical breast lesions or a history of radiation as a child or adolescent) should be taken into account.

Hookwire localization biopsies are performed under local anesthetic for mammographic lesions that cannot be palpated. A hookwire is placed under mammographic or sonographic guidance and the nonpalpable lesion is then surgically excised. Mammographic masses may or may not be palpable from within the breast tissue at surgery, and microcalcifications are not visible to the naked eye. Thus, the surgical specimen must be oriented three-dimensionally by tagging margins and sent for specimen radiography. If the lesion appears close to a margin, it is usually easier to re-excise the involved margin at the time of biopsy than to return later to re-excise the entire biopsy cavity. After specimen radiography, a biopsy specimen should be sent to pathology for inking of margins. The surgeon should refrain from cutting into breast biopsy specimens prior to inking, as this will affect the evaluation of surgical margins for malignant cells.

BREAST CANCER

According to the American Cancer Society, more than 185,000 new breast cancers and over 44,000 deaths from breast cancer occurred in the United States alone in 1996. Breast cancer is the most common malignancy in women in the United States and the second leading cause of cancer death. Although the incidence of breast cancer has increased in the last few decades, the mortality has remained fairly constant, suggesting that improved treatment regimens have been increasingly successful.

RISK FACTORS

There are a number of factors associated with the risk of developing breast cancer (Table 35–1). Understanding

Table 35–1. Risk factors for breast cancer.

Family history of breast cancer
High-fat diet/postmenopausal obesity
Alcohol consumption
Use of oral contraceptives
Use of postmenopausal estrogen replacement therapy
Early age of menarche
Older age at menopause
Previous benign breast biopsy, especially if atypical hyperplasia present
Previous breast cancer
Irradiation of breast

Reprinted and modified, with permission, from Abeloff MD et al: Breast. In: Abeloff MD et al (editors): *Clinical Oncology.* Churchill Livingstone, 1995, p. 1624.

these factors and how they interact with one another allows for the construction of better screening and prevention approaches. It should be noted, however, that approximately 70% of women who develop breast cancer have no major risk factor that can be identified other than increasing age and being female.

PATHOLOGY

Breast cancer falls into three general categories: the ductal carcinomas, the lobular carcinomas, and special types. Ductal or lobular carcinomas are the most common and can be either invasive, meaning that the neoplastic cells invade the substance of the breast (its supporting stromal tissue), or noninvasive (usually called **carcinoma in situ**), where the neoplastic cells remain confined to the ducts or lobules of the breast and do not invade through the basement membrane.

Ductal Carcinoma In Situ

Ductal carcinoma in situ (DCIS) is composed of neoplastic cells confined to the ducts of the breast. They can be as small as two millimeters or can reach several centimeters in size without invasion occurring. Within the category of ductal carcinoma in situ are several subtypes that were previously described by architecture (ie, comedo, cribriform, solid, micropapillary, and papillary), but more recently classified by nuclear grade and the presence or absence of necrosis (Table 35–2). The clinical significance of the subtypes is under investigation. The comedo ductal carcinoma in situ is composed of cells that have cytologic features often associated with a poor prognosis when found in invasive ductal carcinomas. DCIS is associated with a heightened risk of subsequent development of invasive breast cancer in the ipsilateral breast.

Lobular Carcinoma In Situ

Lobular carcinoma in situ (LCIS) is a noninvasive neoplasm of the glandular tissue of the breast in which the lobules are distended with neoplastic cells. Also known as lobular neoplasia, LCIS is not considered a true carcinoma, but

Table 35–2. Classification of ductal carcinoma in situ.

High grade
High nuclear grade, necrosis
Comedo
Intermediate grade
Intermediate nuclear grade
Commonly solid architectural type
Low grade
Low nuclear grade, no necrosis
Commonly cribriform/micropapillary architectural type

rather may be an indicator marker for future development of breast cancer in either breast. The probability of developing subsequent infiltrating cancer is seven to nine times greater in patients with foci of LCIS than in the general population, and the risk of death from breast cancer is approximately 11 times greater. LCIS is usually multifocal (many locations within a single quadrant of the breast) and often multicentric (involvement of more than a single quadrant of the breast). More often than with DCIS, LCIS can be a process that is bilateral at presentation. LCIS is often an incidental finding at biopsy for another lesion.

Invasive Ductal Carcinomas

Most breast cancers (70–80%), either invasive or in situ, are of the ductal type. Infiltrating ductal carcinomas are subtyped by tumor grade as described by the Scarff-Bloom-Richardson method. **Tumor grade** is determined by tubule formation (structural grouping of cancer cells which mimic breast ductal architecture), nuclear pleomorphism, and mitotic rate of the malignant cells. Increasing grade (I–III) is associated with less defined tubule formation, increasingly atypical cytologic appearance, and more numerous mitotic cells. Grade I infiltrating ductal carcinomas are well-differentiated, grade II are moderately differentiated, and grade III are poorly differentiated. Prognosis varies with the tumor grade, but prognosis in general is dictated by a combination of the stage of the cancer and the biologic properties of the tumor.

Invasive Lobular Carcinoma

Invasive lobular carcinomas constitute about 5–10% of invasive breast cancers. They differ from invasive ductal carcinomas in several ways: they usually have very uniform nuclei; the cells of the tumor frequently infiltrate into the stroma of the breast in a linear fashion; and they are more likely to have positive steroid receptors. There are subtypes based on cytologic features that may identify those with a poorer prognosis, but this is less developed than with ductal carcinomas, where grading is important in prognosis.

Special Types

Other types of invasive carcinomas include tubular carcinoma (which can be considered a very well differentiated type of ductal carcinoma), medullary carcinoma, colloid/mucinous carcinoma, and papillary carcinoma. These special types of breast cancer generally carry a better prognosis per stage than infiltrating ductal carcinoma.

STAGING

Staging in breast cancer is based upon the anatomic distribution of the tumor at the time of presentation. The **TNM system** of classification is used to stage all primary breast cancer patients (Table 35–3). The key considerations are the size of the tumor (T); the involvement of lymph nodes with metastatic breast cancer cells (N); and whether or not the tumor has metastasized to distant sites or the supraclavicular or cervical lymph nodes (M). The staging system is used to predict patient survival. Stage I patients have a higher rate of being cured of their cancer than stage II or III patients. Stage IV patients have less than a 1% chance of surviving their disease. Staging should be based upon pathologic findings rather than clinical findings alone, because the measurement of tumor size and detection of nodes by palpation is inaccurate.

Prognosis is also be determined by **biologic features** of the tumor. These consist of tumor grade (index of the extent to which the tumor lacks tubule formation, has atypical nuclei, and has a large number of mitotic figures), presence and amount of estrogen or progesterone receptors, diploid or aneuploid DNA index, percentage or fraction of tumor cells in S phase, and over-expression of some oncogenes and other factors. These biologic measures can identify patients at higher risk of relapse than the stage of tumor may indicate.

MANAGEMENT OF PRIMARY BREAST CANCER

Primary breast cancer refers to the original tumor that is diagnosed, in contradistinction to a tumor recurrence. Once the diagnosis of primary breast cancer has been established, therapeutic decisions must be made in two major areas: (1) local-regional treatment (removal of the breast tumor [local] and determination of any spread into axillary lymph nodes [regional]); (2) systemic treatment (determining whether and what kind of adjuvant chemotherapy or hormonal therapy is indicated to stop the growth of any systemic micrometastases that are not yet clinically detectable). The choice of local-regional treatment does not affect whether systemic treatment is indicated (see section on systemic adjuvant therapy). Because of the complexity of the disease process, the availability of multiple treatment options, and the need to individualize each woman's care, a multidisciplinary approach to breast cancer treatment is essential.

Local-Regional Treatment

The local treatment of breast cancer (Figure 35–6) involves the surgical removal of the entire tumor with a surrounding rim of *tumor-free* breast tissue. There are two methods of doing this: (1) mastectomy or (2) lumpectomy,

Table 35–3. TNM staging system for breast cancer.

Primary Tumor (T)

TX		Primary tumor cannot be assessed.
T0		No evidence of primary tumor.
Tis		Carcinoma in situ: Intraductal carcinoma, lobular carcinoma in situ, or Paget's disease of the nipple with no tumor.
T1		Tumor 2 cm or less in greatest dimension.
	T1a	0.5 cm or less in greatest dimension.
	T1b	More than 0.5 cm but not more than 1 cm in greatest dimension.
	T1c	More than 1 cm but not more than 2 cm in greatest dimension.
T2		Tumor more than 2 cm but not more than 5 cm in greatest dimension.
T3		Tumor more than 5 cm in greatest dimension.
T4		Tumor of any size with direct extension to chest wall or skin.
	T4a	Extension to chest wall.
	T4b	Edema (including peau d'orange) or ulceration of the skin of breast or satellite skin nodules confined to same breast.
	T4c	Both T4a and T4b.
	T4d	Inflammatory carcinoma.

Lymph Nodes (N)

NX	Regional lymph nodes cannot be assessed (eg, previously removed).
N0	No regional lymph node metastasis.
N1	Metastasis to movable ipsilateral axillary lymph node(s).
N2	Metastasis to ipsilateral axillary lymph node(s) fixed to one another or to other structures.
N3	Metastasis to ipsilateral internal mammary lymph node(s).

Distant Metastasis (M)

MX	Presence of distant metastasis cannot be assessed.
M0	No distant metastasis.
M1	Distant metastasis (includes metastasis to ipsilateral supraclavicular lymph node[s]).

Stage Grouping

0	Tis	N0	M0
I	T1	N0	M0
IIA	T0	N1	M0
	T1	N1[1]	M0
	T2	N0	M0
IIB	T2	N1	M0
	T3	N0	M0
IIIA	T0	N2	M0
	T1	N2	M0
	T2	N2	M0
	T3	N1	M0
	T3	N2	M0
IIIB	T4	Any N	M0
	Any T	N3	M0
IV	Any T	Any N	M1

[1]Note: The prognosis of patients with N1a is similar to that of patients with pN0.
Reprinted and modified, with permission, from Beahrs OH et al (editors): *Manual for Staging of Cancer,* 4th ed. Chicago. American Joint Committee on Cancer, 1992.

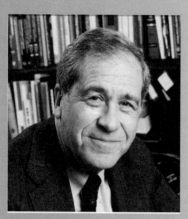

Bernard Fisher, MD. (Courtesy of the University of Pittsburgh School of Medicine.)

During the past 30 years, surgical management of primary operable breast cancer evolved from the use of radical mastectomy in all women to breast conservation followed by radiation therapy in appropriate patients. Almost simultaneously, it was recognized that an improvement in survival could result only through the use of postoperative systemic adjuvant therapy. The evolution of these conceptual changes in therapy has largely been a result of the pioneering work of Dr Bernard Fisher in the clinical biology of breast cancer and to his leadership in organizing over 6000 medical professionals at 600 medical centers in North America into a group known as the National Surgical Adjuvant Breast and Bowel Project (NSABP). The NSABP is one of the largest cooperative groups supported by the National Cancer Institute to conduct research in the treatment of breast cancer.

Dr Fisher was a founding member of the NSABP, which was established in 1958. He served on its board of directors, was chairman of the group from 1967 to 1994, and is currently the NSABP scientific director. As chairman, he moved the headquarters from Roswell Park Cancer Institute in Buffalo, New York, to the University of Pittsburgh in 1971. Since that time, nearly 50,000 patients have entered more than 25 major prospective randomized clinical breast cancer trials conducted by the NSABP.

Many of these studies have provided seminal information regarding the natural history of breast cancer and have contributed to a reassessment of the principles of cancer management, particularly as they relate to surgery and systemic adjuvant chemotherapy. These trials were, for the most part, conceived, designed, and implemented as a result of Dr Fisher's nearly 2 decades of laboratory and clinical investigation into the phenomenon of tumor metastasis. In 1968, Dr Fisher formulated a hypothesis of tumor biology different from the anatomic one proposed by William Halsted that had served as the basis for cancer treatment for 100 years. Two important studies conducted by Dr Fisher and his associates since 1970 support his alternative hypothesis. Findings from these randomized clinical trials have justified breast-preserving surgery and replacement of the Halstedian paradigm for cancer management with one that is biologic in concept. The first trial demonstrated that, after 20 years, there was no significant difference in the rates of disease-free survival (DFS), distant disease-free survival (DDFS), or survival (S) of patients treated by conventional radical mastectomy or less extensive breast-removal procedures (ie, total (simple) mastectomy without axillary dissection and with or without postoperative breast irradiation). The second trial, conducted as a result of preliminary observations from the *continued* **HISTORICAL FACTS**

first, has shown, after 12 years of follow-up, that lumpectomy and axillary dissection with or without breast irradiation, when compared with modified radical mastectomy, results in no significant difference in DDFS or S among the three groups. This is despite the fact that, following lumpectomy alone, almost 40% of patients developed an ipsilateral breast tumor recurrence (IBTR) whereas, following lumpectomy and radiation therapy, only about 10% had an IBTR. As a result of these findings, a National Cancer Institute consensus panel in 1990 concluded that breast preservation is the recommended treatment for women with stage I and II breast cancer.

Early in his investigations, Dr Fisher postulated that major improvement in the outcome of breast cancer patients would result only from the use of systemic adjuvant therapy following surgery. This led to clinical trials using adjuvant chemotherapeutic regimens or hormonal therapy. Dr Fisher was the first to report from randomized clinical trials in 1968 and 1973 that adjuvant chemotherapy resulted in a benefit in DFS and S. His subsequent studies demonstrated the advantage from such therapy for the treatment of patients with positive as well as negative nodes.

Dr Fisher's 1989 publications in the New England Journal of Medicine indicating the value of chemotherapy for women with estrogen receptor (ER)-negative tumors and of tamoxifen for women with ER-positive tumors were responsible for altering the management of node-negative breast cancer patients. In 1990, he demonstrated that tamoxifen plus chemotherapy is better than tamoxifen alone for the treatment of node-positive patients. He is now evaluating the worth of preoperative therapy in a study that could alter the current approach to breast cancer therapy. He has also recently published findings from a major NSABP trial indicating the value of lumpectomy and radiation therapy for the treatment of mammographically detected ductal carcinoma in situ.

In 1992, under Dr Fisher's leadership, the NSABP began its largest trial, the Breast Cancer Prevention Trial, the first women's health trial to evaluate the use of a preventive agent (tamoxifen) for breast cancer. A major justification for that study related to his findings indicating that tamoxifen not only enhanced the DFS of node-negative, ER-positive patients but also decreased the incidence of contralateral breast cancer. Nearly 13,000 women at high risk for the disease have entered the trial and will be followed for life. The study is viewed as the culmination of Dr Fisher's 30 years of research in the biology and treatment of breast cancer.

followed by radiation therapy (XRT) (also known as breast-conserving treatment).

The decision for mastectomy versus breast-conserving treatment depends on multiple factors. These include:

(1) the size and location of the tumor in relation to the size of the woman's breast (ie, the ability to achieve tumor-free margins and still leave a cosmetically acceptable breast)
(2) the presence of multifocal (multiple sites in same quadrant) or multicentric (multiple sites in different quadrants) disease, which would necessitate too much breast removal for lumpectomy
(3) ease in ability to follow the postoperative breast mammographically and by physical examination for evidence of recurrent cancer
(4) patient preference

Collagen-vascular diseases are also a relative contraindication to breast-conserving treatment because of skin complications related to radiation. A prior history of

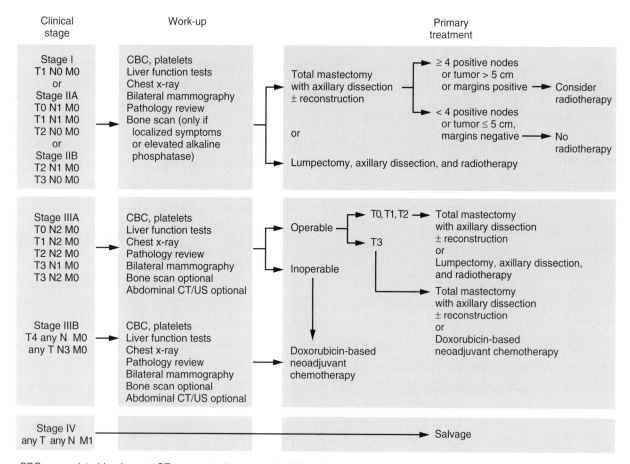

CBC = complete blood count; CT = computed tomography; US = ultrasonography

Figure 35–6. National Comprehensive Cancer Network Practice Guidelines for Invasive Breast Cancer. (Reprinted and modified, with permission, from Oncology 1996;120(Suppl), pp. 56–57.)

radiation to the chest wall (since the total amount of radiation required for lumpectomy and XRT may exceed lifetime limits) is also a contraindication to breast conservation.

The local recurrence rate following lumpectomy and XRT is highly dependent on the ability to achieve tumor-free margins. The surgical margins should be inked and, if possible, the specimen should be oriented in a three-dimensional manner for the pathologist. If the tumor microscopically approaches the surgical margins, it should be re-excised.

An axillary dissection is usually performed as part of the mastectomy or breast-conserving treatment for invasive cancers. Axillary lymph nodes are generally classified as levels I, II, or III (Figure 35–7). Examination of the axillary lymph nodes for metastatic disease is principally done for prognostic purposes, although there is still debate

as to the therapeutic value of axillary lymph node dissection. The more lymph nodes that are removed, the higher the incidence of postoperative lymphedema of the arm. Generally, a level I and II axillary lymph node dissection is performed. The morbidity of a standard lymph node dissection is usually low, but the procedure can be associated with limitations in shoulder mobility (especially in older patients with pre-existing conditions), cutaneous nerve numbness, rare motor nerve injury, and recommendations to avoid blood draws or intravenous lines in the ipsilateral arm.

When a lumpectomy is performed, the axillary dissection is usually done through a separate transverse incision at the lower edge of the axillary hair line (Figure 35–8). When a modified radical mastectomy is performed, the axillary dissection is done through the mastectomy incision.

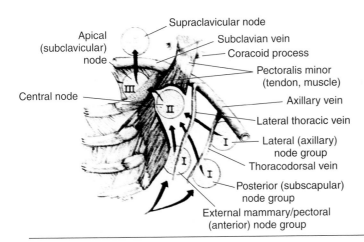

Supraclavicular node

Apical
(subclavicular)
node

Subclavian vein

Coracoid process

Pectoralis minor
(tendon, muscle)

Central node

Axillary vein

Lateral thoracic vein

Lateral (axillary)
node group

Thoracodorsal vein

Posterior (subscapular)
node group

External mammary/pectoral
(anterior) node group

Figure 35–7. Schematic drawing illustrating the major lymph node groups associated with the lymphatic drainage of the breast. The Roman numerals indicate three levels or groups of lymph nodes that are defined by their location relative to the pectoralis minor. Level I includes lymph nodes located lateral to the pectoralis minor; level II, lymph nodes located deep to the muscle; and level III, lymph nodes located medial to the muscle. The arrows indicate the general direction of lymph flow. The axillary vein and its major tributaries associated with the pectoralis minor are included. (Reprinted, with permission, from Romrell LJ, Bland KI: Anatomy of the breast, axilla, chest wall, and related metastatic sites. In: Bland KI, Copeland EM (editors): *The Breast: Comprehensive Management of Benign and Malignant Diseases.* Saunders, 1991, p. 30.)

Although most women with small invasive breast cancers do not have axillary lymph node metastases, they still must undergo axillary lymph node dissection to know for sure. Sentinel lymph node (SLN) biopsy is a new technique to determine whether axillary lymph nodes harbor tumor cells. SLN is the first lymph node along the afferent lymphatic pathway from the breast. It may be located in the axilla or in the internal mammary chain. SLN biopsy removes only one to four axillary lymph nodes, thereby preserving most lymphatics and cutaneous nerves that traverse the axilla. The SLN is identified by injection of blue vital dye or radiolabeled colloid around the breast tumor or by biopsy cavity. The dye or radioisotope is taken up by afferent lymphatics in the breast and travels to the SLN. The blue lymphatic tract and SLN is visually identified; the radioactive SLN is located using a handheld gamma detection probe (similar to a small Geiger counter).

Initial studies have suggested that if an axillary SLN is negative for tumor cells when analyzed by serial sectioning and immunohistochemical stains, this is highly predictive of no other axillary metastases from the breast cancer. However, as tumors grow larger (> 2 cm), multiple afferent lymphatic drainage pathways may develop, and we have observed two or three anatomically separate SLN clusters containing metastatic tumor, as well as false-negative SLN biopsies in some of these patients. Larger clinical trials are under way to better define the accuracy of this procedure and patient selection criteria. It is nonetheless likely that SLN biopsy, which can be performed with minimal morbidity under local anesthesia or conscious sedation, will replace standard axillary lymph node dissection in the surgical treatment of women with small invasive breast cancers.

Following lumpectomy, radiation therapy is usually given 5 days a week for 5–6 weeks until a total dose of 4000–5000 cGy is achieved. This may include an additional 1500 cGy boost of radiation therapy directed at the primary site. Radiation therapy is not usually given to the chest wall following mastectomy *except in special circumstances*: tumors greater than 5 cm, evidence of dermal lymphatic invasion, evidence of tumor invasion through the pectoralis major muscle fascia, or large number of axillary lymph node metastases (four or greater). These factors are all associated with high rates of local chest wall recurrence following mastectomy, and XRT reduces this risk.

For noninvasive breast cancer (DCIS), therapeutic options include total mastectomy, lumpectomy and XRT, or lumpectomy alone. The treatment choice must be individualized and should take into account tumor size, histologic subtype, mammographic findings, and patient preference. Axillary lymph node dissections are generally not performed for DCIS, unless the DCIS is large or diffuse, is of a high nuclear grade (comedo subtype), or there is microinvasion. In such cases, a low level I axillary dissection may be performed.

For invasive breast cancers, breast-conserving treatment gives equivalent overall survival and disease-free survival results as mastectomy in properly selected patients with invasive tumors less than 4 cm (stages I and II). The remaining breast tissue must be radiated following lumpectomy to prevent local recurrence. If the breast is radiated after lumpectomy, the rate of recurrence of cancer in the same breast is under 5–10% percent; if the breast is not radiated, the local recurrence rate approaches 40–50% in long-term follow-up. These numbers must be compared to chest wall local recurrence rates following mastectomy, which are about 2–4%. A level I and II axillary lymph node dissection is usually performed as mentioned earlier.

Locally advanced breast cancer (stage III) is usually treated with a multimodality approach beginning with chemotherapy and will be discussed later in this chapter.

Breast Reconstruction. If a woman decides to undergo mastectomy, the breast can be reconstructed at the same time as the mastectomy (immediate reconstruction) or can be performed some time in the future (delayed reconstruction). The period of delay can be as short as 6 weeks to 3 months, or delayed, in some cases, for many years after mastectomy. The choice of immediate versus delayed reconstruction is usually individualized to the pa-

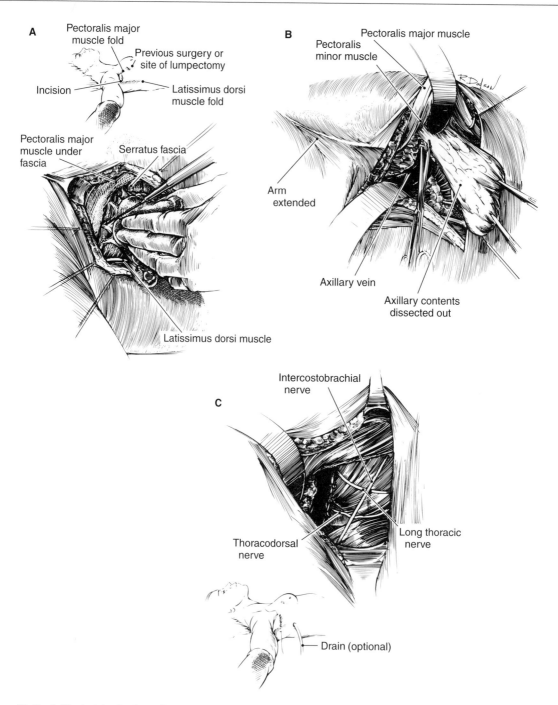

Figure 35–8. *A:* The incision for the axillary node dissection is placed at the inferior aspect of the axillary hairline and extends from the lateral border of the pectoralis major muscle to the anterior border of the latissimus dorsi muscle. Nylon traction sutures are placed in the dermis. Flaps are raised superiorly and inferiorly. *B:* The pectoralis major and minor muscles are retracted to facilitate dissection of the lymph node-bearing fatty tissue from beneath the muscles and away from the axillary vein and chest wall. *C:* The completed dissection showing the isolated nerves to the serratus muscles, the latissimus dorsi muscle, the pectoral muscles, and the sensory nerve to the inner aspect of the upper arm. (Reprinted, with permission, from Abeloff MD et al: Breast. In: Abeloff MD et al (editors): *Clinical Oncology.* Churchill Livingstone, 1995, p. 1660.)

tient and may be influenced by need for postoperative chest wall radiation. Most women who undergo lumpectomy do not require breast reconstruction.

There are generally three types of postmastectomy breast reconstructions: (1) the use of a subpectoral breast implant or tissue expander; (2) a latissimus dorsi myocutaneous flap; and (3) a transverse rectus abdominis myocutaneous (TRAM) flap. When a tissue expander is used, the expander is placed under the pectoralis and serratus muscles and expanded with saline during postoperative office visits over time so that the overlying skin and muscles are slowly stretched. It may be left in place or later replaced with a different or permanent saline-filled breast implant. A myocutaneous flap is used to bring in more skin (vascularized by the underlying muscle) so that the ptosis ("droop") of the opposite breast may be better imitated. The flap can be rotated from the back or abdomen, using existing blood supply, or it can be a free flap in which its blood vessels are anastomosed to branches of axillary blood supply. If a latissimus dorsi flap from the back is used, then a saline-filled breast implant must be placed under the flap to give the breast its shape. If a TRAM flap from the abdomen is used, there is usually enough associated fat under the abdominal skin to mold a new breast without the need of a breast implant. Research continues concerning the possibility of using other sites to reconstruct the absent breast.

Systemic Adjuvant Treatment

All patients with a diagnosis of breast cancer who have undergone their initial local treatment should be considered for adjuvant systemic chemotherapy or hormone therapy. The patient needs to understand that surgery or radiation treat the local (breast) and regional (lymph node) disease, but do not address the risk of developing systemic metastases from tumor cells that were shed prior to tumor excision. The risk of developing distant metastases directly relates to the anatomic distribution of the primary breast cancer within the breast (size and extension to chest wall, skin, or nipple), the involvement of axillary lymph nodes, and biologic properties of the breast cancer, such as tumor grade, estrogen receptors, ploidy, percentage of tumor cells actively dividing, and the over-expression of some oncogenes. Based on the anatomic and biologic characteristics of their tumor, patients with primary breast cancer can be subgrouped by risk parameters to determine eligibility for systemic therapy regimens (Figure 35–6).

There are two goals of adjuvant systemic therapy: to cure the patient or to lengthen the time until distant relapse. Once a patient develops distant metastases (distant relapse), she generally will die of breast cancer. There is evidence, both in women under 50 years and over 50 years, that adjuvant therapy improves overall survival. A general rule is that adjuvant therapies will *reduce* the risk of relapse by about 20–25%; it does not eliminate relapses in all patients. Should the patient relapse after systemic

therapy, a very important benefit is the lengthening of time to relapse.

For *premenopausal* women, the most commonly used combination chemotherapy is either six cycles of Cytoxan, methotrexate, and 5-fluorouracil (CMF), which takes 24 weeks, or four cycles of Adriamycin and Cytoxan (AC), which takes 12 weeks. Loss of ovarian function is the most important irreversible toxicity of these treatments, most likely to be experienced by patients in the age group of 45–50. The consequence of this toxicity is the inability to bear children and the advent of the physiologic changes associated with menopause.

Postmenopausal women are generally most benefited by adjuvant tamoxifen or adjuvant chemotherapy plus tamoxifen. There are probably subsets within this group who will only benefit from adjuvant chemotherapy. Loss of ovarian function is not a consequence of treatment for this group because they usually do not have functional ovaries. If patients have been taking hormone replacement therapy, it is recommended that this be stopped; the patient will then experience menopausal symptoms from hormone withdrawal. Patients in this age group with estrogen-positive tumors of low grade are most likely to benefit from tamoxifen alone or chemotherapy and tamoxifen. In patients with receptor-negative cancers, chemotherapy is usually indicated. The major complaint of patients receiving tamoxifen is an increase in hot flashes and vaginal secretions. For those receiving chemotherapy, there is hair loss, fatigue, nausea, and weight gain.

Patients with locally advanced primary breast cancer (stage III) usually have a large breast cancer (> 5 cm) involving the skin of the breast or attachment to the chest wall. They are best treated with a combination of chemotherapy and radiation therapy to achieve local control of the breast cancer. In some patients, mastectomy may be part of the treatment program. These patients frequently have large numbers of palpable axillary nodes that may be attached to one another or the chest wall. The tumor is best assessed by needle biopsy to establish diagnosis. This is followed by combination chemotherapy that includes doxorubicin, and treatment is continued until there is no further reduction in the size of the palpable cancer in the breast and axilla (usually four, but no more than six, cycles). These patients are then irradiated, usually to higher doses (6000–7000 cGy to the whole breast) than doses used for the stage I or II patient who has undergone breast preservation (4500–5000 cGy). If it is documented by physical examination or breast imaging (mammography or sonography) that considerable tumor volume remains after four to six cycles of chemotherapy, a mastectomy or lumpectomy may be indicated prior to radiation therapy. In either case, the local treatment is followed by additional combination chemotherapy lacking Adriamycin for up to six cycles. Thus, the entire treatment period is 10–12 months. At the completion of therapy all patients are placed on tamoxifen for 5 years, irrespective of their steroid receptor status. With these combined modality approaches, 85% of patients have local control and 50% are free of distant disease at 5 years. However, there is continued relapse over time in this group of patients, to a long-term survival rate of about 25–30%.

MANAGEMENT AT RELAPSE

Principles of Treatment

Confirmation of a clinical impression of first recurrence of breast cancer with a tissue or cytologic diagnosis is important. With few exceptions, all patients who relapse will ultimately die of their disease. Thus, a relapse has profound implications for the patient, and it changes the goals of therapy for the physician. For these reasons, it is important that presumption of relapse be demonstrated pathologically. Concurrent with confirmation of relapse is an assessment of the extent of the relapse, in particular, whether the relapse is confined to "favorable" sites, such as skin, bone, lymph node, and pleura, or is predominately within the liver, lung, or brain. The distribution of the relapse is determined by physical examination and imaging.

Therapy for breast cancer in relapse consists of local modalities, such as radiation therapy and surgery, and systemic therapy, such as hormonal therapy or chemotherapy. The principles of treatment of first and subsequent relapses are to manage local problems with surgery or radiation therapy and treat generalized problems associated with relapse with systemic therapies.

When relapses present simultaneously in multiple sites or as multiple lesions within a single site or organ, treatment focuses on the systemic use of hormones or chemotherapy. Some patients may have a threatening local problem, such as a lytic bone metastasis in a femur where there is danger of fracture. Such a patient will require integrated irradiation and systemic treatment. The goal of therapy after relapse is palliation rather than cure. Thus, the toxicities, ease of treatment, and other medical problems of the patient must be considered in all judgments about which local and which systemic treatment will be used.

First Relapse of Breast Cancer

After there is pathologic confirmation of recurrence of breast cancer and the extent of the process is defined, a general treatment plan should be outlined for the patient. Radiation therapy is most commonly delivered by high-energy radiation equipment (usually linear accelerators). In most instances therapy is given once a day, 5 days per week, in what are called **fractions**. Most fractions are in the range of 150–200 cGy, with a total duration of treatment of 3–4 weeks and total doses in the range of 3000–5000 cGy. Some organs (such as the spinal cord, lung, and liver) tolerate maximal dosages that are less than the ranges outlined. By proper planning and defining of areas to be irradiated (radiation fields), and considera-

tion of which organs will be irradiated, toxicities are minimized.

Hormonal therapy should be considered for all patients at first relapse. Those patients who are most likely to benefit from hormonal treatment have the following clinical characteristics: age greater than 55 years; long intervals from diagnosis to relapse (> 2 years); relapses predominately in bone, skin, lymph node, or pleura; tumors that are positive for estrogen or progesterone receptors; and single site of relapse.

A second group that is likely to respond to hormones are those who have had a favorable response to one hormonal agent or manipulation and then have had progression. Those who are least likely to benefit from hormonal therapy are those with relapses in the brain, liver (with impaired liver function), or lung (with impaired respiratory function), and meninges. The latter groups of patients should receive radiation therapy followed by chemotherapy alone, or chemotherapy in addition to hormones if they are steroid hormone receptor-positive. Radiation treatment and either chemotherapy or hormonal therapy at relapse can be integrated by paying careful attention to overlapping toxicities of these modalities. The timing of treatment depends upon which problem dominates, the systemic or the local problem.

Chemotherapy is used first, particularly when there is clear physiologic derangement of major organs, especially in the liver or lung. Involvement of the liver or lung is not an absolute contraindication to the use of hormones when a patient has otherwise favorable clinical characteristics and little physiologic derangement. Chemotherapy is indicated when there is lymphangitic spread of cancer in the lung or hepatic involvement with compromised hepatic function, particularly in individuals who have short disease-free intervals (the time from diagnosis to first relapse) of less than a year or those with tumors that contain no estrogen or progesterone receptors.

Systemic Forms of Treatment

The most commonly used group of agents are estrogen receptor antagonist/agonists, such as tamoxifen. Tamoxifen (20 mg/d) is the agent to be used first in patients with clinical characteristics associated with a high likelihood of benefit, with the expectation that as many as 50–60% will have an objective response or stabilization of metastases. The best indicators that there will be a favorable response are a long disease-free interval, steroid hormone receptor positivity, and bony sites of involvement. Patients with one or more of these should be given a trial of tamoxifen. The side effects are an increase in hot flashes if the patient is having hot flashes prior to initiation of treatment, an increase in vaginal secretions, an increase in the thickness of the endometrium, and, very rarely, endometrial cancer or damage to the retina. Patients should be told that tamoxifen may cause endometrial cancer, and any vaginal bleeding needs to be evaluated with an endometrial biopsy. These patients taking tamoxifen should have a careful gynecologic examination and vaginal ultrasonography annually for assessment of the thickness of the endometrium (endometrial stripe). If there is vaginal bleeding or irregularities of the endometrial stripe, the endometrium should be biopsied.

Progestational agents, such as Megace, are usually used after a patient has been treated with tamoxifen and had a favorable response but develops progressive disease again. As long as such patients retain favorable characteristics, Megace or other hormonal agents should be considered. Megace has the principle side effect of appetite stimulation. If the patient responds to the increase in appetite by an increase in caloric intake, they may gain over 10 kg of weight in a matter of months.

There are also a number of agents that prevent the conversion of steroids into estrogen. The aramidase inhibitors, in particular, prevent the conversion of androgenic precursor in peripheral fat into estrogen. These agents should be used in women who no longer have ovarian production of estrogens—following oophorectomy, natural menopause, or chemotherapy-induced menopause. Commonly used agents are aminoglutethimide and fadrozole. Agents that bind to the receptors in the pituitary for gonadotropin-releasing factors can result in a depletion of gonadotrophin in premenopausal women and affect a drug-induced suppression of the release of estrogen, sometimes called a "medical oophorectomy." Following withdrawal of the agent, estrogen production resumes. These agents are useful in patients who are premenopausal and have characteristics favorable for hormonal response.

In selected patients, evidence supports the efficacy of high-dose chemotherapy and autologous bone marrow or stem cell rescue. This may be an important therapeutic option for young women with advanced cancer in the high-risk category (stage III breast cancer or 10 or more positive nodes). Women with hormone-unresponsive metastatic breast cancer have been shown to have overall response rates of greater than 80% and complete responses two to three times that observed with conventional-dose polydrug therapy. As would be expected, the morbidity associated with such therapy is considerable, and the treatment-related mortality may range from 5% to 10%. However, ongoing improvements are decreasing the potential risks as well as evidence for prolonged remissions of disease that often exceed 2 years.

Ablative Hormonal Treatment

Premenopausal women that are over 45 with favorable characteristics may have as high as a 40% chance of response to removal of the ovaries. This, of course, introduces premature menopause, which is not symptomatically treated with estrogen replacement. For patients 45–50 years old, this procedure should be considered as part of treatment planning, as this group may have prolonged periods of disease control.

FOLLOW-UP OF PATIENT WITH BREAST CANCER

When the breast cancer patient has completed her local-regional and adjuvant therapy, there is a need for continued follow-up. There are two reasons for this: There is a risk of relapse from the cancer that has just been treated, and there is a heightened risk of a new breast cancer in the opposite breast of women who have had previous breast cancer. Therefore, one focuses on detection of relapse and new breast cancers.

The usual number of visits in the first 2 years is three to four per year, and then twice a year for many years. The frequency can be tempered by the individual patient's risk of relapse. These visits will include a complete history and physical examination with attention to the most common sites of relapse: the chest wall if a mastectomy has been performed; the treated breast if conservation has been performed; the lymph node areas draining the involved region; the lungs; and the liver. Historical items of importance are persistent pain in the back, hips, or ribs, as the most common sites of relapse of breast cancer are the large bones.

The usual studies performed on these visits are a general serum laboratory screening panel that includes liver function studies. All patients need the uninvolved breast carefully examined for evidence of a new primary cancer. The opposite breast is rarely a site of metastasis. This will include physical examination of the breast on each visit and an annual mammogram. It is not clear that outcome is changed by obtaining chest x-rays or bone scans, imaging the liver, or following serum markers for recurrence. Studies show no difference in survival in patients followed by careful history and physical examination alone versus those followed by these studies in addition to history and physical examination. The important element in follow-up is to listen carefully to the patient and pursue persistent complaints.

PSYCHOLOGIC ASPECTS OF BREAST CANCER

It goes without saying that a woman who has been told she has breast cancer is very frightened. This is the case even when the findings are favorable, such as for women with ductal carcinoma in situ or those with low-grade cancers and negative axillary lymph nodes. The important elements in wholesome interactions at this time are:

- Have a well-thought-out plan before you inform the patient.
- Be supportive, reassuring, and understanding of the patient's fears.
- Provide adequate information to make the most immediate decisions.

- Do not dwell on derivative decisions that can only be made after assessment is complete.

Thus, from the first interaction, it is important to be supportive, concerned, and prepared to tell patients how you can help.

When informing a patient of a positive biopsy, it is important that one be prepared to know exactly how to proceed. Patients are reassured if a definite plan for the initial evaluation and treatment can be outlined at the time they are told their diagnosis. Sometimes there is more than one option, therefore, be prepared to weigh these options and explain them. It is important to be deliberate in the process of assessment of their problems. Do not be hurried, as this reassures the patient that all factors are being considered and someone is in control of what is a seemingly uncontrolled process. Many patients will not remember what they were told; therefore, one must be patient in repeating findings and plans on subsequent visits. Suggesting that the patient bring another person or a tape recorder to the visit may be helpful. All interactions should end with reassuring comments, even when there are ominous findings.

Most patients benefit from participating in support groups where they can talk and listen to other women with similar problems. It is important to include their spouse and other family members in discussions, as they are likely to remember details of your advice. Rarely will patients need professional psychologic care unless they were under treatment prior to diagnosis. But all women take many months before they can begin to function without recurring thoughts and fears about their diagnosis.

SUGGESTED READING

Abeloff MD et al: Abeloff MD et al (editors): Breast. In: *Clinical Oncology*. Churchill Livingstone, 1995.

Baker RR, Niederhuber JE: *The Operative Management of Breast Disease*. Saunders, 1992.

Bland KI, Copeland EM: *The Breast: Comprehensive Management of Benign and Malignant Diseases*. Saunders, 1991.

Bland KI et al: Surgery for benign and malignant disease of the breast: Indications and techniques. In: Bland KI et al (editors): *Atlas of Surgical Oncology*. Saunders, 1995.

Giuliano AE et al: Sentinel lymphadenectomy in breast cancer. J Clin Oncol 1997;15:2345.

Harris JR et al: *Diseases of the Breast*. Lippincott-Raven, 1996.

National Comprehensive Cancer Network: Breast cancer practice guidelines. Oncology 1996;10(Suppl):47.

36

Soft Tissue Sarcomas

John E. Niederhuber, MD

► Key Facts

- ► An estimated 6000 new cases of soft tissue sarcomas are diagnosed annually in the United States, for an incidence of approximately two per 100,000 population.

- ► Predisposing factors to sarcoma formation include radiation exposure, chemotherapy exposure, chemical exposure, and chronic lymphedema.

- ► Extremity sarcomas usually present as a painless mass of sudden onset and increasing size.

- ► Retroperitoneal tumors or visceral sarcomas present either as an abdominal mass or with vague abdominal symptoms related to the gastrointestinal tract.

- ► The physical examination should document the location and size of the mass, character of the overlying tissues, neurologic findings, and regional node status.

- ► MRI is the optimal imaging modality for truncal and extremity lesions because it provides better contrast of the tumor margins with surrounding muscle and other (especially vascular) structures.

- ► Sarcoma is staged primarily based on tumor size, tumor grade, and presence or absence of regional or distant disease.

- ► Current therapy of sarcomas combines several modalities. Almost 90% of extremity sarcomas are managed with limb-sparing treatment.

- ► Over 50% of retroperitoneal sarcomas will have microscopically positive tumor resection margins; at least half of the patients demonstrate intra-abdominal recurrent tumor, usually within 2 years.

- ► The lung is the most common site of first failure from metastatic sarcoma. Patients with pulmonary metastasis may be candidates for resection.

While relatively rare tumors, an estimated 6000 soft tissue sarcomas are newly diagnosed yearly in the United States, for an incidence of approximately 2 per 100,000 population. Slightly more than half these patients ($\approx$ 3600) die each year from the metastatic spread of their tumor, underscoring the difficulty of providing curative treatment. There is a slightly higher male incidence, with a 1.1:1.0 male-to-female ratio. There do not appear to be any specific race or geographic "hot spots" for the development of sarcomas in the United States. They comprise approximately 6.5% of pediatric cancers and less than 1% of all adult tumors. They occur in all age groups, but half are diagnosed after the age of 60 years. Although they can be found in every tissue of the body, the majority arise from cells derived from a common mesodermal origin. The exceptions are neurosarcomas and primitive neuroectodermal tumors.

The ability to evaluate therapy in a prospective fashion is extremely difficult because of the huge diversity of histologically distinct tumors and the relative rarity of each histologic subtype. Their relative rarity has also caused surgeons to feel uncertain regarding the management of these tumors. Thus, it is extremely important to understand the approach to diagnosis, biopsy techniques, staging of tumors, and multimodality treatments. The multimodality approach to treatment of sarcomas has achieved a place in the history of surgery, for it represents one of the initial advances in organ preservation (limb-sparing) and, thus, a very real contribution to quality of life.

ETIOLOGIC FACTORS

The specific genetic mechanisms and induction factors for sarcomas remain to be determined. There are, however, several apparent predisposing factors, such as radiation exposure, chemotherapy exposure, chemical exposure, and chronic lymphedema. For example, sarcomas have developed in prior therapeutic radiation fields used for treating lymphoma, head and neck cancer, pelvic malignancies, benign skin, and thymic disorders. The most common radiation-induced sarcoma is osteosarcoma, but fibrosarcoma, malignant fibrous histiocytoma, and angiosarcoma are also common subtypes. There is a documented dose effect with a relative risk of 0.6 in patients receiving 10 Gy or less, and a 38.3 relative risk when the radiation dose exceeds 60 Gy. Almost all radiation-induced sarcomas ($\approx$ 90%) are high-grade tumors, and almost all occur more than 10 years after the radiation treatment regimen.

A variety of chemicals are also known to increase the risk of developing a sarcoma. Examples are the phenoxyacetic acids (forestry and agriculture workers), chlorophenols, Thorotrast (a radiologic contrast agent no longer in use), vinyl chloride, and arsenic. Alkylating chemotherapeutic agents (cyclophosphamide, melphalan, procar-

bazine, etc) have been suspected of causing sarcomas. The most common relationship is in children previously treated for acute lymphoid leukemia. Another classic example is the patient who develops chronic severe lymphedema of her arm as a complication of her breast cancer therapy, and subsequently a lymphangiosarcoma arises in the swollen arm. Sites of heavy scarring (such as old burn scars), chronic tissue trauma, and foreign body invasion (such as old shrapnel wounds) have been reported as areas where sarcomas may develop.

Several genetic conditions also predispose to formation of soft tissue sarcomas. For example, neurofibromatosis (von Recklinghausen's disease), Li-Fraumeni syndrome, and familial polyposis coli are inherited syndromes associated with an increased lifetime risk of developing sarcomas. The risk for patients with neurofibromatosis is variously reported to be 7–10% and the *NF1* gene, located on chromosome 17q, has been implicated in the development of benign fibromas. Recently, evidence has suggested that a subsequent deletion or mutation on 17p involving the *p53* tumor suppressor gene may be related to the transition of a benign neurofibroma to a malignant peripheral nerve tumor. Fibrosarcomas are also seen in patients with neurofibromatosis. Enlarging tumors in neurofibromatosis patients must be excised, if technically possible.

An abnormal or deleted *Rb1* gene is thought to be part of the genetic explanation of why retinoblastoma patients have an increased risk of developing osteosarcoma and other soft tissue sarcomas. The *p53* gene has also been implicated in the Li-Fraumeni syndrome, but other genes are also certainly involved. Patients with Gardner's variant of familial polyposis coli have an 8–12% chance of developing low-grade fibrosarcoma (desmoid tumor).

CLINICAL PRESENTATION

The ability of these sarcomas to form in virtually any site in the body where connective tissue resides, and the resultant variability in histological features, often complicates discovery and diagnosis. The various connective tissues present in all organs of the body can, of course, give rise to a sarcomatous tumor that is either benign or malignant. Such tumors are much more rare than similar tumors developing in the somatic tissues. Of the somatic tissue sarcomas, roughly 60% occur in the extremities, with a 3:1 ratio of lower to upper extremity tumors. Approximately 75% of the lower extremity sarcomas are found proximal to the knee. The head and neck region accounts for 9%, and 31% of sarcomas are truncal. Within the truncal group, approximately 40% are retroperitoneal. These are general percentages and vary slightly from one large center to another.

Extremity sarcomas usually present as a painless mass the patient suddenly becomes aware of and notes is increasing in size (Figure 36–1). Often, local trauma to the

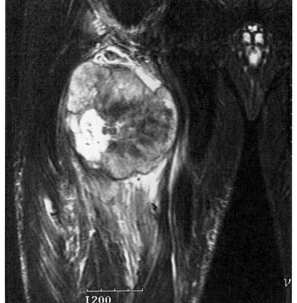

A

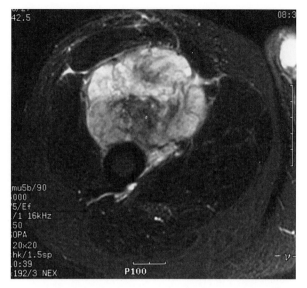

B

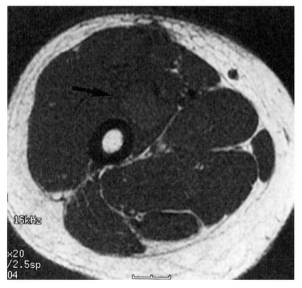

C

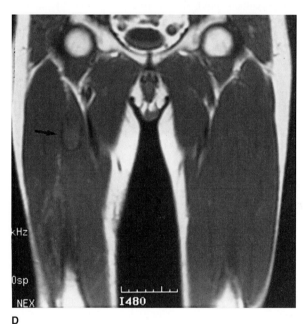

D

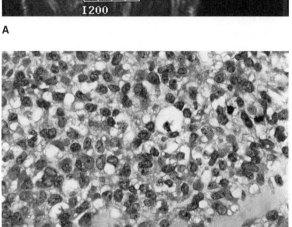

E

Figure 36–1. *A, B:* Preoperative MRI (anterior view *[A]* and cross-section *[B]*) of a 49-year-old male who presented with a soft tissue mass in the anterior right thigh measuring 10 x 12 cm. Patient initially complained of slight pain and muscle aches in anterior right mid-thigh when working out at the gym. ***C:*** A surgical biopsy was performed. Pathologic diagnosis was consistent with primitive neuroectodermal tumor, a malignant tumor more common in children (H & E × 160). ***D, E:*** Preoperative (primary) chemotherapy using three cycles of high-dose Cytoxan/Adriamycin/vincristine and radiation therapy totaling 5000 cGy in 25 fractions over 5 weeks prompted almost total regression of tumor as seen on MRI (anterior view *[D]* and cross-section *[E]*). The resected tumor measured 2.6 × 4.2 × 2 cm.

area is what catches the patient's attention. The traumatic event causes pain and may produce some hemorrhage. Pain, when present, may be the result of progressive tumor growth that causes pressure or stretching of adjacent structures and sensory nerves. Muscle weakness and distal extremity swelling secondary to venous and lymphatic compression are generally late symptoms.

Retroperitoneal tumors or **visceral sarcomas** present as an abdominal mass or with vague abdominal symptoms related to the gastrointestinal tract. Pain is a feature in half the patients. Retroperitoneal sarcomas often reach rather large dimensions before causing symptoms. Visceral sarcomas, of course, must be distinguished from the much more common adenocarcinomas of the gastrointestinal tract. The evaluation of a retroperitoneal mass should include serum tumor markers for beta-human chorionic gonadotropin (β-HCG) and alpha-fetoprotein.

The physical examination is important and needs to accurately document the location and size of the mass, character of the overlying tissues, neurologic findings, and regional node status. The most important step in the evaluation is the performance of a biopsy. Unless the lesion is quite small (< 3 cm) one should perform an incisional biopsy. Small lesions may be totally excised. The incision should be made directly over the center of the tumor and should be placed in a longitudinal direction on the extremity to facilitate placement of the definitive resection incision (see Chapter 9). Biopsy incisions for head and neck and truncal lesions should be kept small and positioned to facilitate subsequent surgical resection and, perhaps, flap reconstruction.

It is important to ask the pathologist to examine the fresh biopsy specimen to determine if there is adequate viable tumor for histopathologic and immunohistochemical studies. The surgeon should avoid raising tissue flaps during the biopsy and make every effort to leave the site with absolute hemostasis.

Fine-needle aspirations are not indicated. They are unnecessarily invasive and provide no useful information. Whether core needle biopsies under computed tomographic (CT) or ultrasonographic direction can provide adequate tissue samples for complete histologic staging is currently being studied.

Retroperitoneal tumors and visceral tumors do not need to be biopsied. They are, by their very presence, an indication for surgical exploration, and the less they are disturbed or invaded the better chance the patient will have of avoiding further tumor seeding of the abdominal cavity. The exceptions to this rule are when the tumor is deemed unresectable, or if the diagnosis is not clear from imaging studies and the tumor could represent lymphoma, a germ cell tumor, or a metastasis from another tumor.

Prior to biopsy, it is best to complete the imaging evaluation. Both CT and magnetic resonance imaging (MRI) are useful. MRI is optimal for truncal and extremity lesions because it provides better contrast of the tumor margins with surrounding muscle and other (especially vascular) structures. MRI also provides both sagittal and coronal planes. Within the abdomen, new-generation helical CT scanning with thin slices provides the best assessment. It is important to include a chest CT or MRI as well. At this time, there does not appear to be any particular advantage to using other imaging techniques, such as gallium scans or positron emission scanning.

HISTOPATHOLOGY & STAGING

Sarcomas are classified according to the determined cell of origin. This determination becomes more difficult as the tumor becomes less well differentiated, and often pathologists will disagree on the exact pathologic diagnosis. Establishing the histologic subtype is important in providing insight into the anticipated natural history of the tumor, tumor grade, and the potential for response to different therapies.

The most commonly diagnosed sarcomas are those derived from primitive mesenchymal cells that are pluripotent and develop as fibroblasts, fibrocytes, myocytes, and so forth. Today, tumors arising from these connective tissues are grouped as malignant fibrous histiocytomas. Occasionally, pathologists will further define these tumors as fibroblastic, histiocytic, or pleomorphic.

Other sarcomas arising in adipose tissue are termed **liposarcomas**. They may be very low grade and lipoma-like or very high grade with extensive spindle cell components and a marked pleomorphic cellular histology. Smooth muscle and striated muscle tumors are termed **leiomyosarcomas** and **rhabdomyosarcomas**. **Angiosarcomas** are malignant tumors of blood vessel origin and **lymphangiosarcomas** are from lymphatic vessels. Malignant schwannoma, neurofibrosarcoma, neurogenic sarcoma, and malignant neurilemoma are terms used for **peripheral nerve tumors**. **Chondrosarcomas** arise from cartilage. **Osteosarcoma** is quite rare, generally occurring in the sixth decade or greater, usually in the thigh or buttock regions, and they almost always present as high-grade tumors.

For each tumor, the pathologist must report a histologic diagnosis (often best accomplished by a review of several pathologists), an accurate assessment of tumor size, and a careful evaluation of the inked gross and microscopic margins. Anything less than 1 mm from the ink is considered a positive margin. Finally, an assessment of tumor grade and reactivity with specific antibody markers is critical (Table 36–1). Tumor grade has been clearly established as a major factor in determining prognosis.

The sarcoma is staged primarily based on tumor size, tumor grade, and whether there is regional or distant disease. Two systems for staging are used, the American Joint Committee on Cancer (AJCC) (Table 36–2) and the Memorial Sloan-Kettering Cancer Center (MSKCC) system (Table 36–3). Unfavorable prognostic factors are listed in Table 36–4.

Table 36–1. Guideline to histologic grading of sarcomas.

Low-Grade Sarcomas	High-Grade Sarcomas
Good differentiation	Poor differentiation
Hypocellular	Hypercellular
Hypovascular	Hypervascular
Much stroma	Minimal stroma
Minimal necrosis	Much necrosis
Fewer than 5 mitoses per 10 high-power fields	More than 5 mitoses per 10 high-power fields

Reprinted, with permission, from Hajdu SI: *Pathology of Soft Tissue Tumors.* Philadelphia, Lea & Febiger, 1979, p. 45.

MULTIDISCIPLINARY THERAPY

EXTREMITY SARCOMAS

Therapy of sarcomas, especially those involving the extremities, has undergone significant change. Just 2 decades ago, essentially all extremity sarcomas of any significant size were managed by amputation because of the high local recurrence rate when treated by excision alone (variously reported as 33–63%). Five-year survival rates with amputation were variously cited as 30–50%.

Table 36–2. American Joint Committee on Cancer sarcoma staging system.

Stage		Description		
G	Tumor grade			
	GX	Grade cannot be assessed		
	G1	Well differentiated		
	G2	Moderately differentiated		
	G3	Poorly differentiated		
	G4	Undifferentiated		
T	Primary tumor site			
	TX	Primary size cannot be assessed		
	T0	No evidence of tumor		
	T1	Tumor size ≤ 5 cm		
	T2	Tumor size > 5 cm		
N	Regional lymph node status			
	NX	Regional nodes cannot be assessed		
	N0	No regional lymph node metastasis		
	N1	Regional lymph node metastasis		
M	Distant metastasis			
	MX	Presence of distant metastasis cannot be assessed		
	M0	No distant metastasis		
	M1	Distant metastasis		
Stage	G	T	N	M
IA	G1	T1	N0	M0
IB	G1	T2	N0	M0
IIA	G2	T1	N0	M0
IIB	G2	T2	N0	M0
IIIA	G3, G4	T1	N0	M0
IIIB	G3, G4	T2	N0	M0
IVA	Any G	Any T	N1	M0
IVB	Any G	Any T	Any N	M1

Reprinted, with permission, from Beahrs OH et al: Soft tissues. In: *American Joint Committee on Cancer Manual for Staging of Cancer.* Lippincott, 1992, p. 31.

Table 36–3. MSKCC staging scheme.

Stage	Grade	Size (cm)	Depth
0	Low	< 5	Superficial
1	Low	< 5	Deep
	Low	> 5	Superficial
	High	< 5	Superficial
2	Low	> 5	Deep
	High	< 5	Deep
	High	< 5	Deep
3	High	> 5	Deep

MSKCC = Memorial Sloan-Kettering Cancer Center.
Reprinted, with permission, from Hajdu SI: *Pathology of Soft Tissue Tumors.* Philadelphia, Lea & Febiger, 1979, p. 45.

It was then recognized that soft tissue sarcomas are not encapsulated but have only a pseudocapsule composed of compressed tissue surrounding the tumor. The pseudocapsule develops as the sarcoma expands. It was also recognized that projections of tumor cells extend beyond the pseudocapsule and, in fact, nests of tumor cells can frequently be found some distance from the primary growth among tumor bundles and other structures of the extremity compartment.

Currently, therapy combines several modalities, and almost 90% of extremity sarcomas are managed with limb-sparing treatment. This results in a marked improvement in quality of life by maintaining a functioning extremity. In addition, the 5-year survival rate now approaches 60–90%, depending on the tumor grade and location.

The question of limb-sparing surgery as an acceptable approach to extremity sarcomas was initially addressed in a now-classic clinical trial at the National Cancer Institute (NCI). In the NCI trial, patients were prospectively randomized to receive limb-sparing surgery and postoperative radiotherapy or amputation. Both study arms also received postoperative chemotherapy consisting of cyclophosphamide, doxorubicin, and methotrexate. Five of 27 patients in the limb-sparing group developed local recurrence while one of 17 patients undergoing amputation had local failure ($p = 0.22$). The overall survival was 70% and 71%, respectively ($p = 0.97$), with over a decade of follow-up. This important trial established the efficacy of limb preservation using a multimodality approach to treat-

Table 36–4. Unfavorable prognostic factors.

High grade
Deep location
Size ≥ 5 cm
Extracompartmental
Invasion of bone or a neurovascular structure
Inadequate surgical margin
Age ≥ 50 years
Proximal size
Lower extremity
Female sex
Presentation with recurrent disease

ment. The key to the success of this approach is the size and location of the tumor. If a functional extremity cannot be obtained, then amputation may provide the best chance for rapid rehabilitation.

The decision of whether or not to employ adjuvant chemotherapy is very much dependent upon the size of the primary tumors and the histologic grade. Patients with tumors less than 5 cm in diameter and whose tumors are low grade are generally not offered adjuvant chemotherapy. This decision is supported by a meta-analysis of 11 prospective randomized trials using adjuvant therapy for extremity sarcomas. This type of statistical analysis is not without its critics, and the advantage for chemotherapy was quite modest at best. These chemotherapeutic regimens cannot be undertaken lightly, since all are doxorubicin-based and carry a 10–15% risk of subsequent congestive heart failure.

In recent years there has been an interest in treating patients with tumors greater than 5 cm (high grade) with primary chemotherapy (Figure 36–1). There are several rationales for this approach. The obvious advantage is that of providing systemic treatment early in an effort to significantly impact on micrometastases elsewhere in the body. Chemotherapy provided up front also gives an indication of whether or not the tumor is sensitive to the drugs used. A significant response may facilitate a later surgical resection.

While irradiation alone is not ideal therapy, there is increasing interest in sequencing radiation therapy immediately following the primary chemotherapy. In so doing, treatment fields are smaller (when used following surgery, the field must encompass all of the flap dissection area). The risk of intravascular and wound seeding with viable tumor cells during surgical manipulation is decreased, and a further reduction in tumor volume facilitates surgical resection. The negative side to this approach is an increase in postoperative complications, especially in relation to normal healing, and a need for second operations in approximately 25% of patients to deal with wound complications. These approaches, therefore, must be regarded as investigational, and patients are best managed on a suitable clinical trial.

INTRA-ABDOMINAL SARCOMAS

Pelvic tumors often provide the greatest challenge to the surgeon. The goal for tumors in this region must be adequate resection. The most common histologic types are liposarcoma, leiomyosarcoma, and fibrosarcoma. Margins of surgical resection should have at least 3 cm of normal tissue. Frequently, this margin may need to be compromised because of the close proximity of major vascular structures (aorta, vena cava), critical organs, and the spine. Resection of adjacent organs may need to be performed in 50–80% of cases in order to gain adequate margins.

This aggressive approach is needed because over 50%

of retroperitoneal sarcomas will have microscopically positive tumor resection margins, and at least half of the patients demonstrate intra-abdominal recurrent tumor, usually within 2 years. Patients with low-grade lesions have a higher median survival than those with high-grade tumors (80 months versus 20 months) as well as a greater 5-year survival rate (70% versus 20%) (Figure 36–2).

While the use of postoperative adjuvant chemotherapy has not yet been shown to be of significant benefit, the difficulty in irradiating retroperitoneal sarcomas has been reason enough to employ all modalities, including intraperitoneal installation of chemotherapy in the immediate postoperative period. The most common chemotherapeutic agents employed include doxorubicin, cyclophosphamide, and methotrexate. Unfortunately, these regimens have failed to demonstrate any significant change in survival outcome.

Patients who develop local recurrence in general should have another surgical attempt to eliminate their tumor. The results of what is known as "salvage surgery" for recurrent tumor are promising, with over two thirds of patients experiencing long-term survival. If radiation therapy was not used at the time the primary tumor was removed, it should be used in this setting of recurrence. If full-dose irradiation was already given, intraoperative radiation therapy (IORT) or external beam radiation should be considered.

TREATMENT OF DISTANT RECURRENCE

The lung is the most common site of first failure from metastatic sarcoma. Patients with pulmonary metastases may be candidates for resection if they meet the following

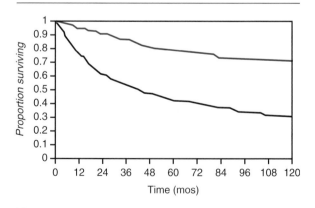

Figure 36–2. Proportion of patients with retroperitoneal sarcoma surviving from the date of first operation for high-grade tumor **(black line)** and low-grade tumor **(blue line)** in MSKCC trial. (Reprinted, and modified, with permission from Jacques DP et al: Management of primary and recurrent soft-tissue sarcoma of the retroperitoneum. Ann Surg 1990;212:51.)

criteria: (1) there is control of the primary tumor; (2) the lung is the only site of metastatic disease; (3) the patient is an acceptable operative risk; and (4) all metastatic disease appears resectable. In at least one report, local tumor control using 50 Gy was better with preoperative than postoperative radiotherapy (97% versus 91%), especially when tumors were greater than 15 cm. Postoperative doses are generally higher in the 60–65 Gy range. Clearly, radiation is an important part of the treatment program. Surgery alone can only be expected to achieve a 65% local control rate.

On an experimental basis, there is an interest in using limb perfusion to treat extremity sarcoma. Patients may receive doxorubicin intravenously and cisplatin by isolated limb perfusion. This may prove to be of special benefit to the subgroup of patients that, because of tumor size and location, would not be candidates for limb preservation.

Retroperitoneal sarcomas deserve special attention. As noted earlier, they tend to occur late, when the tumor is quite large. Their location and relationship to vital organs often pose significant problems to the surgeon trying to obtain an adequate margin. Their location also precludes preoperative radiation. Surgical exploration is the initial therapy. Often it will be necessary to resect portions of adjacent organs in an effort to obtain clear margins. There is an important role for intraoperative radiotherapy and brachytherapy to deliver adjuvant radiation to the tumor bed and high-risk margins. Intraoperative treatment is followed by external beam treatment. The author has frequently used tissue expanders filled with saline to displace radiation-sensitive organs, such as the small bowel, away from the target of radiation. Chemotherapy of distant metastases has not shown great benefit. Current interest is in polydrug regimens and in dose intensification using autologous marrow cells for growth factor stimulation. While these regimens show a higher response rate ($\approx 40\%$), there is considerable toxicity and, to date, no evidence for a significant survival benefit. As a result, aggressive surgical approaches are indicated, often even in the face of metastatic tumor.

SUGGESTED READING

Antman K et al: An Intergroup phase III randomized study of doxorubicin and dacarbazine with or without ifosfamide and mesna in advanced soft-tissue sarcomas. J Clin Oncol 1993;11:1276.

Conlon KC, Brennan MF: Soft tissue sarcomas. In: Murphy GP et al (editors): *American Cancer Society Textbook of Clinical Oncology*, 2nd ed. American Cancer Society, 1995.

Dooley WC: Soft tissue sarcoma of the extremity. In: Cameron JL (editor): *Current Surgical Therapy*. Mosby-Year Book, 1992.

Geer Rj et al: Management of small soft-tissue sarcoma of the extremity in adults. Arch Surg 1992;127:1285.

Karakousis CP: Principles of surgical resection for soft tissue sarcomas of the extremities. Surg Clin N Am 1993;2:547.

Pisters PW, Brennan MF: Soft tissue sarcomas. In: Abeloff MD et al (editors): *Clinical Oncology*. Churchill Livingstone, 1995.

37

The Heart

37.1 Acquired Disease of the Heart

Kwok L. Yun, MD, & Thomas A. Burdon, MD

► Key Facts

- ► Cardiovascular disease is the number one cause of death in America and accounts for nearly 44% of all deaths.

- ► The basic components of the cardiopulmonary bypass circuit are a venous drainage line and reservoir, an oxygenator/heat exchanger, a pump, and an arterial inflow line.

- ► Currently, more than 30,000 heart valves are replaced annually in the United States.

- ► Aortic dissection is the most frequent catastrophe involving the aorta, being twice as common as ruptured abdominal aortic aneurysm.

- ► The major risk factors for development of coronary atherosclerosis include hypercholesterolemia, habitual tobacco use, and hypertension.

- ► Ischemic heart disease typically presents as precordial chest pain radiating to the arm, neck, or jaw. It may also manifest as dyspnea, epigastric pain, or fatigue.

- ► Coronary artery bypass grafting is the most commonly performed operation in cardiac surgery today.

- ► Complications of myocardial infarction include postinfarction ventricular septal defect, postinfarction acute mitral insufficiency, and left ventricular aneurysm.

- ► Complications of pericarditis requiring surgical intervention include cardiac tamponade, chronic pericardial effusion, and chronic constrictive pericarditis.

- ► Cardiac neoplasms are relatively uncommon, with metastatic disease involving the heart 20–40 times more frequently than primary cardiac tumors.

Cardiovascular disease is the number one cause of death in America and accounts for nearly 44% of all deaths. Two out of every five Americans die of cardiovascular disease, resulting in approximately 2500 deaths per day. Of those with heart disease, 52.2% are male, 47.8% are female, 88.2% are white, 9.5% are black, and 2.4% are of other races. As many as 50 million Americans suffer from hypertension, the leading contributor to heart disease, yet approximately 70% are not receiving therapy. Clearly, heart disease is a national concern, and awareness of its prevalence, prevention, and management are of the utmost importance to the surgeon. It is vital to be aware of the signs and symptoms of underlying cardiac disease in order to take appropriate preventive measures.

This chapter begins with a detailed discussion of the techniques currently used for extracorporeal circulation, or **cardiopulmonary bypass (CPB)**. A thorough understanding of the principles outlined in this section is essential for the student or resident who will be exposed to cardiothoracic cases in his or her career. CPB is used to prevent blood loss and reduce arterial flow through the heart to allow the surgeon to operate in a motionless, bloodless field. Following the section on CPB, we then proceed into discussions of the diagnosis, evaluation, treatment, and results of the most common acquired heart disorders, which include valvular and ischemic heart disease as well as cardiac tumors.

EXTRACORPOREAL CIRCULATION

GENERAL CONSIDERATIONS

The basic components of CPB circuit consist of a venous drainage line and reservoir, a pump, an oxygenator-heat exchanger, an arterial filter, and an arterial inflow line (Figure 37.1–1). Additionally, drainage of pooled blood and, when appropriate, blood from cardiac chambers are provided for by cardiotomy suckers and "vent" lines, respectively. Other adjuncts include a cardioplegia delivery system, blood gas analyzer, and in-line monitors.

CONDUCT OF CPB

The extracorporeal bypass circuit is usually primed with a balanced salt solution to dilute the red cell mass to a hematocrit of 20–25%. If the patient is severely anemic and the expected dilutional hematocrit is less than 20%, then blood is added to the pump prime. Hemodilution lowers blood transfusion requirement, reduces trauma to blood cells and proteins, and augments urine flow and clearance of creatinine. It does, however, decrease intravascular oncotic pressure, leading to greater interstitial edema.

Prior to cannulation for CPB, anticoagulation is achieved with approximately 300 units/kg of intravenous heparin. Adequacy of anticoagulation is measured by the **activated clotting time** (ACT), with a level greater than 400 seconds required for initiation of CPB. A range of 800–1000 seconds is recommended when aprotinin is utilized to reduce postoperative bleeding. The ACT is reassessed every 20–30 minutes to ensure adequate anticoagulation. Heparin resistance is noted in patients with antithrombin III deficiency and those with heparin-induced thrombocytopenia. In these cases, safe anticoagula-

tion can be achieved with pretreatment using fresh frozen plasma and aspirin/dipyridamole, respectively.

Venous drainage is accomplished by gravity into a reservoir placed below the level of the right atrium. One two-stage or two one-stage cannulae are used, dependent on the type of procedure and the preference of the surgeon. These are placed via the right atrium, or directly into the superior and inferior venae cavae. Access can also be achieved via the femoral veins for partial CPB during thoracic aortic procedures, difficult reoperations, and emergency situations.

For most cardiac procedures, arterial access can be accomplished via the distal ascending aorta. Femoral artery cannulation is often used in cases of acute aortic dissection, severe aortic calcification, reoperation, and when rapid cannulation is necessary to establish partial CPB. The arterial cannula selected should be of a caliber adequate to provide sufficient systemic flow rates without generating a large gradient across the cannula tip in order to avoid cavitation, gaseous emboli, and hemolysis.

Commencement of CPB is usually associated with a transient decrease in arterial pressure resulting from a fall in systemic vascular resistance. Systemic flow rates of 2.2–2.5 L/min/m^2 are required at normothermia to maintain adequate peripheral perfusion and oxygen delivery. The flow rate may be lowered with the onset of hypothermia (approximately 1.8 L/min/m^2 at 28°C) because of the decrease in metabolic rate. Unnecessarily high flow rates can cause blood element trauma, gaseous emboli, and increased noncoronary collateral and systemic venous return to the heart, resulting in premature cardiac rewarming. Mean arterial pressure during normothermic CPB is maintained between 50 and 70 mm Hg. Pressures less than 45 mm Hg are associated with increased risk of neurologic complications. With moderate hypothermia (28°C), pressures as low as 35 mm Hg are considered safe. Blood pressure is controlled by adjusting the flow rate, using vasoactive agents, and varying the level of anesthesia.

The oxygenator system is equipped with a heat exchanger that can cool and warm the blood. Systemic rewarming usually occurs much more slowly than cooling because the temperature gradient between the blood leaving and entering the patient is more difficult to maintain. Temperature differences between the patient and the perfusate are limited to 10–14°C in order to prevent gaseous emboli. Because metabolic activity decreases with body temperature, hypothermia reduces oxygen requirement and allows lower flow rates without producing lactic acidosis. The extent of hypothermia is guided by the type, complexity, and anticipated length of the procedure. Moderate hypothermia (28–32°C) is frequently utilized for routine operations. However, profound hypothermia with temperatures below 20°C may be necessary or advantageous during corrective congenital heart surgery in neonates and infants, or in aortic arch reconstruction, when circulatory arrest is required to optimize exposure.

CPB may be weaned when the patient is fully rewarmed and resuscitated, with all monitored parameters within the

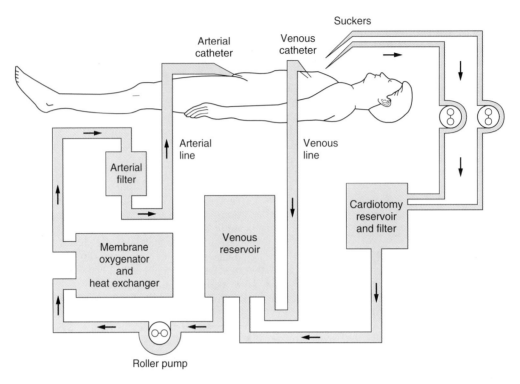

Figure 37.1–1. Diagram of a typical cardiopulmonary bypass setup with a membrane oxygenator. (Reprinted, with permission, from Baue AE et al: *Glenn's Thoracic and Cardiovascular Surgery,* 5th ed. Appleton & Lange, 1991, p. 1402.)

normal range. These include cardiac hemodynamics, peripheral perfusion, electrolytes, glucose, acid-base balance, gas exchange, glucose, temperature, and hematocrit. When CPB is terminated, the heart is decannulated and anticoagulation is reversed with protamine. ACT may occasionally remain elevated in the absence of heparin activity because of platelet dysfunction or depletion of coagulation factors. Furthermore, protamine is cleared from the circulation faster than heparin. This may result in residual rebound heparin effect after the initial protamine dosing. In these circumstances, direct measurement of heparin levels may be useful in determining the need for additional protamine administration. On rare occasions, protamine may cause anaphylactic reactions due to preexisting antibodies to protamine, thereby producing severe pulmonary vasoconstriction. Treatment includes nitroglycerin, epinephrine, calcium chloride, phenylephrine, and, not infrequently, emergent reinstitution of CPB.

MYOCARDIAL PROTECTION

To facilitate surgical exposure during operations for acquired heart disease, cessation of cardiac activity is usually desirable. While the patient is on CPB, this is readily accomplished by cross-clamping the ascending aorta with interruption of coronary blood flow. With the nonperfused myocardium in a flaccid state, the heart can be manipulated to provide adequate visualization in a bloodless field. However, ischemic arrest may lead to irreversible myocardial injury. Although many techniques have been developed over the years to preserve myocardial cellular function, pharmacologic cardioplegia and hypothermia have emerged as the most commonly employed methods to lower the metabolic demand of the heart during arrest.

The principles of chemical cardioplegia are: to stop the heart, create a milieu for continued energy production, and mitigate the deleterious effects of ischemia. Arrest can be achieved with a cardioplegic solution containing potassium, magnesium, or procaine. To further reduce metabolic rate, myocardial temperature should be lowered with a cardioplegia solution that is cold. The additional need for continuous topical hypothermia with cold saline solution or commercially available cooling jacket remains controversial. Substrates such as glucose are provided for continued energy production as well as to act as an osmotic agent to minimize myocardial edema. To maximize aerobic metabolism, blood is preferentially utilized as the cardioplegic vehicle, since it is a physiologic source of oxygen and minimizes hemodilution. Additionally, blood has an excellent intrinsic buffering capacity and is an abundant source of endogenous oxygen free radical scavengers in the form of superoxide dismutase, catalase, and glutathione, which may reduce oxygen-mediated reperfusion injury. To obtain an ideal pH solution, an appropriate buffer, such as tromethamine, bicarbonate, or phosphate, is usually added. Finally, some degree of membrane stabilization is obtained with low concentration of exogenous calcium.

After aortic cross-clamping, rapid diastolic arrest with cold blood cardioplegia lowers myocardial metabolic requirements and preserves energy stores. However, in severely ischemic hearts with depleted energy reserves, some have advocated the use of a period of warm blood cardioplegia induction enriched with Krebs cycle intermediates, such as glutamate and aspartate. It has been proposed that under this normothermic condition, the heart is able to utilize oxygen optimally for cellular repair and replenishment of energy stores. Similarly, controlled reperfusion with glutamate/aspartate-enriched warm blood cardioplegia prior to release of the aortic crossclamp has been demonstrated to result in improved metabolic recovery, enhanced preservation of high-energy phosphates, and improved post-reperfusion ventricular performance.

During the course of the operation, noncoronary blood flow to the heart tends to wash away all cardioplegic solutions and elevate the myocardial temperature. To counteract this collateral washout, multidose cardioplegia at 20-minute intervals is necessary to maintain arrest, restore sufficient hypothermia, buffer acidosis, replenish the supply of oxygen and substrate for aerobic metabolism and production of high-energy phosphates, and minimize edema with hyperosmolarity. Although continuous administration of blood cardioplegia may provide superior myocardial protection, its major disadvantage is obscuring of the operative field. Also, large volume may lead to hyperkalemia, hemodilution, and myocardial edema.

While antegrade administration via the aortic root is the commonly employed route of cardioplegia delivery, retrograde cardioplegia via the coronary sinus has been shown to be as effective in providing myocardial preservation in many clinical circumstances. It can produce more uniform cooling distal to coronary obstruction, distribute cardioplegia without removing the retractors during mitral valve surgery, and obviate the need for direct coronary ostia cannulation in cases of mild aortic insufficiency as well as during operations on the ascending aorta or aortic valve. Commercially available self-inflating retrograde cardioplegic cannula has made possible successful transatrial cannulation of the coronary sinus in over 95% of patients without a right atriotomy. Isolated retrograde cardioplegia, however, does not provide consistent right ventricular cooling and preservation, as nutritive right ventricular retroperfusion is only 20% of that to the left ventricle. Furthermore, a larger volume of cardioplegia is required, and the interval before arrest is achieved is longer, because 30% of retroperfusion is nonnutritive. This can be offset by combining antegrade and retrograde cardioplegia to ensure rapid diastolic arrest and uniform cardioplegic distribution.

POSTOPERATIVE MANAGEMENT

The goal of the early postoperative period after CPB is optimization of cardiac output to maintain adequate end-organ perfusion. This stage is characterized by capillary leak syndrome with fluid shift and potential hemodynamic instability. The duration and severity of this phase are influenced by the degree of preoperative cardiac dysfunction, the duration of CPB, the type of operation performed, the extent to which the pathology has been corrected, and coexisting medical illnesses. Heart rate, arterial blood pressure, central venous blood pressure, temperature, mediastinal tube output, and urine output are monitored continuously, while potassium, hemoglobin, coagulation parameters, and arterial blood gas are measured at frequent intervals. For high-risk patients and those with labile hemodynamics, a Swan-Ganz catheter is used to guide fluid management and determine the degree of cardiac dysfunction.

The most important predictor of hospital survival and clinical outcome is cardiac output, which is determined by heart rate and stroke volume. Stroke volume, in turn, depends on preload, afterload, and cardiac contractility. Bradycardia can be treated with chronotropic agents or electrical pacing. Conversely, atrial tachyarrhythmias are treated with digoxin, beta-blockers, calcium channel antagonists, or electrical cardioversion. Preload is optimized to maintain hemodynamic stability and adequate urine output. A filling pressure higher than preoperative level is generally required, due to myocardial edema and decreased ventricular compliance after CPB. In response to extracorporeal circulation, hypothermia, pain, hypoperfusion, and surgical stimulation, circulating catecholamine levels are generally elevated, causing greater impedance to left ventricular pump function. This leads to an increase in intramyocardial systolic wall tension and, consequently, higher myocardial oxygen consumption and possible cardiac ischemia. Vasodilatation may be accomplished with afterload reducing agents, such as sodium nitroprusside, once intravascular volume has been replenished. Finally, cardiac output can be increased with inotropic agents, such as dopamine, dobutamine, or adrenaline. However, these drugs must be used with caution, as they all increase myocardial oxygen utilization and may exacerbate myocardial ischemia.

Despite the above interventions, approximately 2–6% of patients undergoing myocardial revascularization or valvular surgery cannot maintain adequate cardiac output in the absence of cardiac tamponade. In these cases, the use of intra-aortic balloon counterpulsation may be preferred over administration of inotropic agents in nonphysiologic ranges. Diastolic blood pressure augmentation with balloon inflation increases myocardial perfusion, while balloon deflation prior to systolic ejection lowers resistance to flow, thereby, reducing myocardial oxygen consumption. Rarely, temporary left ventricular assist with the aid of a centrifugal pump may be considered in

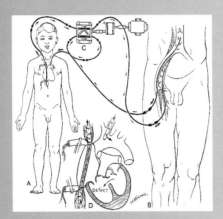

A depiction of the method of direct-vision intracardiac surgery utilizing extracorporeal circulation by means of controlled cross-circulation. *A:* The patient, showing sites of arterial and venous cannulations. *B:* The donor, showing sites of arterial and venous (superficial femoral and great saphenous) cannulations. *C:* The single Sigmamotor pump precisely controlling the reciprocal exchange of blood between the patient and donor. *D:* Close-up of the patient's heart, showing the vena caval catheter positioned to draw venous blood from both the superior and inferior venae cavae during the cardiac bypass interval. The arterial blood from the donor was circulated to the patient's body through the catheter that was inserted into the left subclavian artery. (Reprinted, with permission, from Gravlee GP, Davis RF, Utley JR: *Cardiopulmonary Bypass: Principles and Practice.* Williams & Wilkins, 1993, p. 10.)

It is difficult to imagine that less than 50 years ago, open heart surgery was not the commonplace event it is today. As recently as 1952, a surgeon whose patient was dying of an intracardiac malformation was at a loss to do anything but pray for a recovery. There is no doubt that open heart surgery is one of the most important medical advances to have occurred in the latter part of this century.

After years of laboratory and clinical study, Dr John Gibbon developed a heart-lung apparatus to the point where 12 of 20 dogs survived the closure of a surgically created ventricular septal defect. With these results as justification, Gibbon performed the first successful open heart surgery with the aid of a heart-lung machine for the repair of an atrial septal defect on May 6, 1953. Unfortunately, this initial success was followed by several unsuccessful efforts, both by Dr Gibbon and others.

Because of the limited early success of cardiopulmonary bypass (CPB) using the heart-lung machine, Dr C. Walton Lillehei and his team at the University of Minnesota performed open heart surgery for the repair of congenital heart defects in the mid-1950s. They used selected patients in whom intra-aortic counterpulsation proved to be inadequate.

Less than 5% of patients undergoing cardiac surgery manifest excessive bleeding postoperatively. Initial workup includes evaluation for heparin excess, thrombocytopenia or platelet dysfunction, disseminated intravascular coagulation (DIC), and clotting factor deficiency due to massive transfusion or hepatic dysfunction. Heparin excess, as indicated by prolonged activated coagulation time, is treated with additional protamine. Thrombocytopenia or platelet dysfunction as a result of CPB and/or aspirin intake is managed with transfusion of fresh platelets. DIC is usually self-limited once the patient is off CPB, but may require fresh frozen plasma and cryoprecipitate. Persistent chest tube drainage of more than 100 mL/h for several hours in the presence of relatively normal coagulation parameters mandates immediate mediastinal exploration for surgically correctable causes. Exploration should also be considered for possible cardiac tamponade in those with low cardiac output in association with elevated pulmonary capillary wedge and central venous pressures.

All patients, with a few exceptions, require mechanical ventilatory support in the immediate postoperative period. With emergence from the effects of anesthesia and surgery and in the absence of hemodynamic instability, insufficient end-organ perfusion, mediastinal bleeding, and arrhythmias, weaning from the ventilator is initiated. Once fully awake, cooperative, and able to maintain adequate gas exchange with minimal respiratory support, the

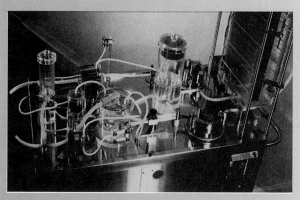

The Mayo Clinic-Gibbon Screen Oxygenator. This model was used in 1955 during the first series of open heart operations performed by Dr John Kirklin and associates at the Mayo Clinic, Rochester, Minnesota. (Photo courtesy of JW Kirklin.) (Reprinted, with permission, from Gravlee GP, Davis RF, Utley JR: *Cardiopulmonary Bypass: Principles and Practice.* Williams & Wilkins, 1993, p. 14.)

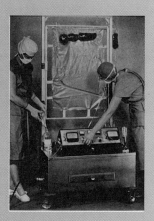

A DeWall-Lillehei unitized plastic, sheet oxygenator, commercially manufactured and shipped sterile ready to hang up, prime, and use as shown here. (Photo courtesy of DA Cooley.) (Reprinted, with permission, from Gravlee GP, Davis RF, Utley JR: *Cardiopulmonary Bypass: Principles and Practice.* Williams & Wilkins, 1993, p. 17.)

controlled cross-circulation, in which the patient is connected to a donor's circulation (usually the parent) for oxygenation and perfusion during the procedure (Historical Figure, p. 470). The overwhelming success of clinical cross-circulation operations stimulated intensive laboratory work on alternative methods of CPB without the need of a living donor.

In 1955, Dr John Kirklin and associates at the Mayo Clinic performed the first successful series of operations using the Mayo Clinic-Gibbon Screen Oxygenator (Historical Figure, p. 471, upper) for CPB. Despite the early success of the cross-circulation technique, in that same year the DeWall-Lillehei bubble oxygenator became the sole method of oxygenation for cardiopulmonary bypass at the University of Minnesota (Historical Figure, p. 471, lower). Today, 2000 surgeries every 24 hours are performed using this technique.

patient is extubated from the ventilator. Thereafter, cough, deep breathing, and incentive spirometry are encouraged, along with ambulation. Aerosol treatment with bronchodilators may be indicated for those with active bronchospasm.

Approximately 12 hours after CPB, there is usually cessation of capillary leakage. This is followed by mobilization of excess interstitial fluid into the intravascular space, which may exacerbate pulmonary congestion. Therapy includes fluid restriction and gentle diuresis with small doses of furosemide. Once the patient is transferred from the intensive care unit, there is gradual resumption of normal daily activity. The main goals during the second to fifth postoperative day are prevention of pulmonary complications and prophylaxis or treatment of supraventricu-

lar arrhythmias. Patients with prosthetic valves are placed on warfarin therapy, with achievement of adequate anticoagulation prior to discharge from the hospital.

VALVULAR HEART DISEASE

Acquired valvular heart disease can be manifested as either stenosis, insufficiency, or a combination of both. Before the discovery of penicillin, rheumatic fever was the most common etiology of valvular dysfunction in the

United States. Since that time, degenerative changes, infectious endocarditis, congenital valvular malformations, and ischemic heart disease have accounted for an increasing proportion of cases.

Currently, more than 30,000 heart valves are replaced annually in the United States. Despite the numerous valve substitutes introduced, no single design has fulfilled all the criteria for an ideal valve substitute. These include physiologic flow dynamics without hemolysis, durability, biocompatibility, resistance to thrombosis and infection, easy implantability, and lack of noise. Generally, prosthetic valves available today can be divided into either mechanical or tissue valves (Figure 37.1–2). While mechanical valves are more durable and have lower reoperation rates, bioprosthetic valves offer the distinct advantage of not requiring indefinite anticoagulation, with an attendant lower risk of thromboembolism and anticoagulant-related hemorrhage. The type of valve used is determined by age, gender, occupation, lifestyle, coexisting medical conditions, access to medical care, compliance, psychological attitude, personal preference, valvular pathology, annular size and geometry, and size of the left ventricle or aortic root.

AORTIC STENOSIS

GENERAL CONSIDERATIONS

The most common etiology of aortic stenosis in patients younger than the age of 70 years is the thickening and calcification of the congenitally bicuspid aortic valve. In older patients, degenerative changes result in extensive calcification of a trileaflet valve, often with involvement of the anterior leaflet of the mitral valve. Rheumatic etiology can be invoked in 35% of cases, which is characterized by fibrosis and retraction of the aortic cusps with varying degrees of commissural fusion.

Regardless of the etiology, obstruction of left ventricular outflow causes a pressure overload of the left ventricle. As an adaptation to the increased afterload, the heart undergoes concentric left ventricular hypertrophy in order to maintain adequate systemic cardiac output. Eventually, the ventricle decompensates and becomes dilated, producing signs and symptoms of congestive heart failure. Since atrial contraction can augment cardiac output by 25–35% in patients with hypertrophied hearts, the development of atrial fibrillation can herald the onset of rapid clinical deterioration. The increases in left ventricular mass and systolic pressure cause a proportionally higher oxygen demand and reduced subendocardial blood flow, thereby producing angina pectoris without significant coronary artery disease. Fixed obstruction to left ventricular ejection can also lead to cerebral hypoperfusion and syncope, especially during exercise-induced systemic vasodilatation. Finally, sudden death is responsible for 20% of deaths in patients with aortic stenosis. Whether the mech-

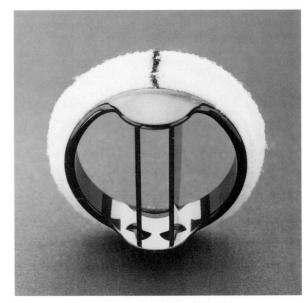

A

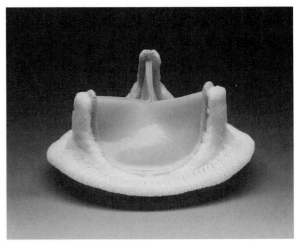

B

Figure 37.1–2. Prosthetic valves are categorized into **A:** mechanical (Courtesy of St. Jude Medical, St. Paul, Minn), and **B:** bioprosthetic types (Carpentier-Edwards porcine valve, courtesy of Baxter Healthcare Corporation, Edwards CVS Division).

anism is related to ventricular arrhythmias or other causes is unknown.

CLINICAL EVALUATION

Physical examination reveals a loud, harsh, crescendo-decrescendo systolic murmur with radiation to the neck. In advanced disease, however, the murmur may be attenuated because of a diminished gradient generated by the failing ventricle. With the development of left ventricular hypertrophy, an S4 is commonly heard at the apex of the heart. Peripheral pulses are delayed with a diminished upstroke. Electrocardiogram demonstrates left ventricular hypertrophy with a strain pattern.

Chest x-ray typically shows normal or mild enlargement of the cardiac silhouette. Significant cardiomegaly with pulmonary venous hypertension may develop during the late stages of aortic stenosis. Calcification of the aortic valve is often present, and poststenotic dilatation of the ascending aorta may occasionally be seen.

Two-dimensional echocardiography, either transthoracic or transesophageal, is used to demonstrate the thickening and calcification of the leaflets and to evaluate the degree of aortic valve narrowing. Doppler measurements can noninvasively quantify the aortic valve gradient and determine the aortic valve area, which correlate well with angiographic findings. Echocardiographic mean aortic valve gradients greater than 50 mm Hg or aortic valve areas less than 0.75 cm^2 (normal = 2.5–3.5 cm^2) suggest the presence of severe aortic stenosis. Since the transvalvular gradient and calculation of aortic valve area are dependent on cardiac output, a low gradient does not necessarily exclude critical aortic stenosis in patients with severely impaired left ventricular function.

Routine cardiac catheterization must be used with caution in patients with a failing left ventricle and elevated pulmonary arterial wedge pressure. It is generally reserved for patients over 40 years of age or younger patients with symptoms of angina, for whom coronary arteriography is warranted. Occasionally, cardiac catheterization is indicated in those with discordant clinical symptoms and echocardiographic findings (Table 37.1–1).

TREATMENT

The indications for surgical treatment of aortic stenosis are the presence of symptoms, including angina, congestive heart failure, syncope, or episode of sudden death. These symptoms are usually accompanied by findings of severe aortic stenosis by echocardiographic or angiographic assessment. Management of asymptomatic patients with evidence of critical aortic stenosis (mean gradient > 50 mm Hg or valve area < 0.75 cm^2) remains controversial. However, most of these patients will develop symptoms within a short period of time, thereby requiring surgical intervention.

Table 37.1–1. Aortic stenosis: Essentials of diagnosis.

Harsh basal crescendo-decrescendo systolic murmur in the right second intercostal space with transmission to the neck
Diminished and delayed peripheral pulse (pulsus parvus et tardus)
Evidence of significant aortic valve obstruction with left ventricular hypertrophy by Doppler echocardiography or cardiac catheterization

The surgical procedure of choice is aortic valve replacement with either a mechanical or a bioprosthetic substitute. As a result of the potential prosthetic-related complications, including structural valve deterioration, thromboembolism, and anticoagulant-related hemorrhage, alternatives to conventional aortic valve replacement have been proposed. In children and young adults, women of childbearing age, and patients with valvular endocarditis, the use of cryopreserved homografts has been advocated. To improve long-term durability, the Ross procedure was designed, which involves the translocation of the patient's own pulmonary valve to the aortic position and reconstruction of the pulmonary valve with a homograft. Freedom from degeneration has been reported as high as 80% at 20 years. Mechanical debridement and decalcification have been used in selected patients with moderate degenerative aortic stenosis, small aortic root, or contraindication to anticoagulation. Percutaneous balloon aortic valvuloplasty may be considered in those who are not surgical candidates or as a temporizing measure to stabilize a patient for subsequent aortic valve replacement. Complications include cardiac tamponade, myocardial infarction, aortic regurgitation, and stroke. Although most patients will experience moderate clinical improvement, the restenosis rate can be as high as 75% within 9 months.

RESULTS

The operative mortality has been reduced to less than 5% in recent years. The incidence of stroke following aortic valve replacement is 3–5% in the older population. Maintenance of normal sinus rhythm is important for filling of the noncompliant, hypertrophied left ventricle in the postoperative period. Inotropic agents must be used with caution for treatment of hypotension in those with inadequate preload and near obliteration of the left ventricular cavity. With the relief of outflow obstruction, left ventricular performance is improved, with regression of concentric hypertrophy and reduction in end-diastolic pressure. Long-term survival is increased compared to medical management. Actuarial survival estimate at 10 years is approximately 60%. Factors that adversely affect long-term survival include advanced age, significant coronary artery disease, and left ventricular dysfunction.

HYPERTROPHIC OBSTRUCTIVE CARDIOMYOPATHY

GENERAL CONSIDERATIONS

Despite the fact that hypertrophic obstructive cardiomyopathy (HOCM) is a primary disorder of the heart muscle, it is discussed in this section because it is a form of subaortic stenosis (hence the old term of "idiopathic hypertrophic subaortic stenosis"). It may occur sporadically or it can be transmitted in an autosomal dominant pattern. Classically, it is characterized by asymmetric hypertrophy of the interventricular septum, causing left ventricular outflow tract obstruction. Histologically, the myocytes are disorganized, with fibrosis and thickened intramural coronary arteries. This process may extend to the anterolateral or posterior wall or the right ventricle.

Symptoms of HOCM result from a triad of diastolic dysfunction, left ventricular outflow tract obstruction, and myocardial ischemia. Decreased left ventricular compliance and prolongation of isovolumic relaxation lead to elevated pulmonary venous hypertension, which can produce symptoms of congestive heart failure. Further impairment of left ventricular filling due to the onset of atrial fibrillation is usually accompanied by clinical deterioration. Left ventricular outflow tract obstruction is caused by the anterior systolic motion of the anterior leaflet of the mitral valve toward the thickened interventricular septum. This dynamic intraventricular obstruction is exacerbated by maneuvers that reduce chamber volume, such as a Valsalva maneuver, vasodilatation, or the use of amyl nitrate or isoproterenol. The combination of increased oxygen demand due to increases in work load and muscle mass and decreased oxygen supply secondary to reduced coronary blood flow, narrow intramural vessels, and systolic compression of large intramyocardial vessels may result in exertional angina in the absence of coronary artery disease.

CLINICAL EVALUATION

Physical findings typically include a systolic crescendo-decrescendo murmur, an S_4 gallop, and a bisferious pulse. Although electrocardiogram usually reveals normal sinus rhythm with a left ventricular hypertrophy pattern, holter monitoring demonstrates premature ventricular contractions in the majority of patients and, not infrequently, nonsustained ventricular or supraventricular tachyarrhythmias. Chest x-ray is often unremarkable except for evidence of left ventricular hypertrophy.

The diagnosis of HOCM is usually made on the basis of echocardiographic findings. In the M-mode, systolic anterior motion of the mitral valve can be illustrated. Asymmetric septal hypertrophy is confirmed by demonstrating a ratio of end-diastolic septal thickness to posterior free wall thickness greater than 1.3. With Doppler measurement, an estimate of the left ventricular outflow tract gradient is calculated. Cardiac catheterization is no longer indicated except to exclude to presence of coronary artery atherosclerotic disease.

TREATMENT

Symptoms are usually treated with a combination of beta-blockers, calcium channel antagonists, and antiar-

rhythmic agents. Beta-blockers decrease oxygen demand and prolong diastolic filling. The most extensively utilized calcium channel blocker is verapamil, which acts by decreasing contractility, reducing heart rate, and augmenting diastolic relaxation. Disopyramide and amiodarone are the most frequently used agents for prevention and control of supraventricular and ventricular tachyarrhythmias. More recently, the use of dual-chamber pacing has also been shown to decrease the outflow gradient by altering the electrical activation sequence of the left ventricle and prolonging ventricular relaxation rate.

Surgery is reserved for patients with persistent symptoms despite maximal medical therapy. Operation is also indicated in those who survived sudden death and have significant (> 50 mm Hg) resting or provocable gradients. Although controversial, there is evidence that surgical intervention can improve long-term survival in younger asymptomatic patients with intraventricular gradients exceeding 80 mm Hg. Conversely, surgery is contraindicated for patients with left ventricular dysfunction and small outflow gradients and for symptoms related to atrial or ventricular arrhythmias.

In most centers, the procedure of choice for HOCM is **septal myotomy and myectomy**. This technique involves resection of septal muscle between the nadir of the right coronary cusp and the commissure between the right and left coronary sinuses. By enlarging the outflow tract and the mitral-septal separation, the left ventricular outflow tract gradient is reduced. Complications of septal myotomy and myectomy include ventricular septal defect, complete or left bundle branch block, and new or progressive aortic regurgitation.

As a result, a few surgeons still advocate mitral valve replacement as the surgical treatment for HOCM. However, it is generally reserved for intraventricular septal dimension less than 18 mm, atypical septal morphology in which the hypertrophied muscle lies outside the field of resection, persistent symptoms after septal myectomy, and concurrent mitral regurgitation due to organic valvular disease.

RESULTS

Without treatment, HOCM is associated with an annual sudden death rate between 2.5% and 4% in adults and 4% and 6% in children. The etiology of sudden death is thought to be most likely an arrhythmia. In contrast to medical treatment, which has not been demonstrated to prevent sudden death or improve long-term survival, septal myectomy has resulted in a lower sudden death rate (2% per year). The reported operative mortality rates range from 3% to 7%, with sustained symptomatic improvement in 80–90% of patients. The overall 10-year survival estimate is approximately 85% and is adversely influenced by advanced age.

AORTIC INSUFFICIENCY

GENERAL CONSIDERATIONS

The most common cause of aortic regurgitation is rheumatic fever, with fibrous thickening and retraction of one or more cusps causing abnormal coaptation. This is followed by infective endocarditis, producing destruction of valve leaflets or annulus. Other less common causes include aortic root dilatation in patients with Marfan's syndrome or annuloaortic ectasia and loss of commissural support and cusp prolapse in patients with ascending aortic dissection.

The regurgitant volume in aortic insufficiency may be as high as 70% of the stroke volume. To maintain an adequate output, stroke volume is increased. As a result, the aortic systolic pressure is elevated while the diastolic pressure is lowered because of the regurgitation.

In the acute setting, usually resulting from endocarditis or aortic dissection, the heart is unable to compensate by dilatation to accommodate the volume overload. This leads to an acute elevation in left ventricular end-diastolic pressure, and consequently, congestive heart failure and acute pulmonary edema. Furthermore, coronary perfusion is also compromised as a result of lower aortic diastolic pressure. Acute aortic regurgitation is generally poorly tolerated, and urgent aortic valve replacement is required.

In chronic aortic regurgitation, the left ventricle undergoes both eccentric hypertrophy and dilatation in response to the pressure and volume overload, respectively. As a result, systolic wall stress is minimized and left ventricular diastolic compliance is increased to maintain a normal end-diastolic pressure. Without surgical intervention, the heart eventually reaches a size beyond which it can no longer maintain cardiac output by the Frank-Starling mechanism. At this point, patients begin to develop symptoms of congestive heart failure.

CLINICAL EVALUATION

Patients with moderate, even severe, aortic insufficiency may remain asymptomatic for many years. Early symptoms include decreased exercise tolerance, fatigue, and exertional dyspnea. Occasionally, there may be a mid-diastolic murmur due to fluttering of the anterior leaflet of the mitral valve, known as the **Austin Flint** murmur. Physical examination reveals a short, high-pitched, blowing diastolic murmur along the left sternal border. Peripheral pulse pressure is widened with a water hammer pulse (Corrigan's sign). Arterial diastolic pressure may paradoxically rise, with worsening congestive heart failure and elevated left ventricular end-diastolic pressure. Other signs related to widened pulse pressure may include pulsating nail beds (Quincke's pulse), bobbing of the head

(de Musset's sign), pistol shot–like sounds heard over large arteries (Traube's sign), and murmur along the femoral arteries (Duroziez's sign).

Chest film demonstrates cardiomegaly, and a prominent ascending aorta and root may also be seen. Doppler echocardiography is used to measure the degree of aortic insufficiency and left ventricular function, as well as to delineate the etiology of the regurgitation. Serial studies can evaluate the rate of left ventricular dilatation and provide an appropriate timing for surgical intervention. Cardiac catheterization is performed to measure right and left heart pressures and to assess coronary anatomy in patients over 40 years of age and those presenting with angina or risk factors for coronary artery disease (Table 37.1–2).

TREATMENT

Patients with acute aortic regurgitation should undergo aortic valve surgery as soon as possible. Since the survival rate for those with symptomatic chronic aortic insufficiency is markedly decreased (median survival rate approximately 2 years), early aortic valve replacement is also recommended for this cohort of patients. The indications for surgery for asymptomatic patients with moderate-to-severe aortic insufficiency, however, remain controversial. Classically, ejection fraction less than 45%, fractional shortening less than 25%, end-diastolic dimension greater than 70 mm (40 mm/m^2), or end-systolic dimension greater than 55 mm (30 mm/m^2) are associated with poor long-term outcome. More recently, a preoperative end-systolic stress/end-systolic volume ratio (a relatively load-insensitive measure of left ventricular performance) of less than 2.9 has been demonstrated to predict persistent left ventricular dysfunction after aortic valve replacement.

As with patients with aortic stenosis, the treatment of choice for patients with aortic regurgitation is aortic valve replacement with either a mechanical or bioprosthetic valve substitute, homograft, or pulmonary autograft. Recently, reconstructive techniques have been developed in an attempt to restore aortic valve competence. In patients with aortic regurgitation due to acute aortic dissection involving the ascending aorta, the aortic valve can usually be preserved by resuspension of the aortic commissures. Other maneuvers include commissurotomy, cusp resuspension, resection of redundant prolapsing leaflet, commissural annuloplasty, or cusp plasty using

Table 37.1–2. Aortic insufficiency: Essentials of diagnosis.

Left ventricular heave
Decrescendo diastolic blowing murmur along the left sternal border
Bounding peripheral pulse (water-hammer pulse) with widened pulse pressure
Echocardiographic or angiographic evidence of aortic valvular insufficiency

glutaraldehyde-treated pericardium. Although short-term results are encouraging, long-term follow-up is necessary before the durability of these procedures is known.

RESULTS

The operative risk of aortic valve replacement for aortic insufficiency is less than 5%, but slightly higher than in patients with aortic stenosis. The most important predictor of operative mortality and long-term survival is the preoperative left ventricular function. After aortic valve replacement, those with relatively normal preoperative cardiac function can expect improved long-term survival as well as symptomatic improvement, with gradual reduction in chamber dilatation and left ventricular hypertrophy. Although patients with markedly depressed left ventricular function may experience symptomatic relief following surgery, response to exercise usually remains abnormal. The 5-year survival estimate is significantly reduced compared to those with normal left ventricular performance (65% versus 90–95%). Extended use of diuretics and afterload reducing agents may be necessary. Therefore, it is prudent to provide closed serial echocardiographic follow-up of patients with asymptomatic aortic insufficiency in order to prevent irreversible left ventricular dysfunction.

MITRAL STENOSIS

GENERAL CONSIDERATIONS

Mitral stenosis is almost exclusively due to chronic rheumatic disease. The initial event is fibrous thickening of the leaflets and fusion of the commissures. This is followed by fibrosis and shortening of the subvalvular apparatus, thereby causing progressive functional obstruction to diastolic left ventricular inflow. The resultant elevated left atrial pressure leads to pulmonary venous hypertension and symptoms of congestive heart failure. Exercise tolerance is poor, due to inadequate cardiac output caused by the limited left ventricular filling. Left atrial enlargement is common and predisposes the patient to the development of atrial fibrillation and thrombus formation. Not infrequently, hemoptysis may be noted in association with the development of pulmonary hypertension.

CLINICAL EVALUATION

Auscultation may reveal an opening snap after the second heart sound due to immobility of the chordae tendineae. This is followed by an apical diastolic rumble with presystolic accentuation if the patient is in sinus rhythm. The onset of atrial fibrillation may herald the onset of congestive heart failure symptoms, including dyspnea, orthopnea, paroxysmal nocturnal dyspnea, and wheezing.

Chest x-ray typically shows left atrial enlargement with a "double density" on the right side of the cardiac silhouette. Calcification of the mitral valve and annulus may also be noted. In advanced cases, pulmonary congestion, redistribution of the pulmonary vasculature, and basal interstitial edema with engorgement of lymphatics (Kerley B lines) are commonly present.

Echocardiography is a useful noninvasive technique to assess the size of the left atrium, the extent of involvement by the disease process, left ventricular function, and the presence of left atrial thrombus. With Doppler measurements, the transvalvular gradient and mitral valve area can be determined with reasonable accuracy. A mitral valve area is considered mild if it is 1.5–2.0 cm^2 (normal being 4–6 cm^2), moderate if it is 1.0–1.5 cm^2, and critical if it is less than 1.0 cm^2.

Cardiac catheterization typically demonstrates elevated pulmonary artery and capillary wedge pressures. Together with left ventricular pressures, the transvalvular gradient can be determined and the mitral valve area computed using the Gorlin formula. Coronary arteriography is also necessary in patients over 40 years of age or those suspected of having coronary artery disease (Table 37.1–3).

TREATMENT

Surgical intervention is indicated for symptomatic patients in order to improve the quality of life, prolong survival, prevent the development of atrial fibrillation, and reduce the risk of thromboembolism. However, the optimal timing for mitral valve replacement in those with an unfavorable valve quality for repair is unclear. Closed mitral commissurotomy for the treatment of mitral stenosis was introduced in 1923 and popularized in the late 1940s. However, with the advent of cardiopulmonary bypass in 1953, open mitral commissurotomy became the preferred procedure because it allowed for direct visualization and repair of valvular and subvalvular obstruction, with a 90% success rate. Operative techniques include splitting of commissures, separation of fused chordae and papillary muscles, and debridement of calcium. Compared to the closed technique, the incidence of reoperation is lower with open commissurotomy (10–20% versus 50% at 10 years).

Table 37.1–3. Mitral stenosis: Essentials of diagnosis.

Dyspnea, orthopnea, paroxysmal nocturnal dyspnea, and cough
Opening snap and apical crescendo diastolic rumble on auscultation
Echocardiographic evidence of left atrial enlargement, elevated diastolic mitral valve gradient, and significantly reduced mitral valve area (< 1 cm^2)

The concept of closed commissurotomy, however, has not been totally abandoned, as it led to the development of percutaneous balloon mitral valvotomy in 1984. Via the femoral vein, a balloon catheter system is introduced across the interatrial septum into the left atrium. The fused commissures are fractured by controlled balloon inflations. The best results are obtained with younger patients in sinus rhythm with pliable leaflets, minimal subvalvular calcification, and trivial mitral regurgitation. Complications include left atrial or ventricular rupture, persistent atrial septal defect, thromboembolism, and conduction abnormalities.

Commissurotomy is preferable to mitral valve replacement whenever possible, since significant functional improvement can be derived from a small increase in effective mitral valve area to 2 cm². However, when the extent of valvular or subvalvular disease involvement precludes a satisfactory mitral commissurotomy, mitral valve replacement should be performed.

RESULTS

In the early postoperative period, prolonged ventilatory support may be necessary, since patients with advanced mitral stenosis frequently have an element of pulmonary arterial and venous hypertension. Pulmonary arterial blood pressures usually decrease after correction of mitral stenosis. However, residual pulmonary hypertension may require the use of pulmonary vasodilators. Although the left ventricle is protected from both pressure and volume overload in this disease entity, cardiac performance may be compromised from right ventricular failure as a result of the long-standing pulmonary hypertension and poor right ventricular protection during CPB. The combination of inotropic agents and pulmonary vasodilators is often required in improving right ventricular performance.

With modern techniques and current advances in postoperative management, the operative mortality rate for uncomplicated mitral valve replacement is less than 5%. Important determinants of operative risk are advanced age, higher New York Heart Association (NYHA) functional class, degree of irreversible pulmonary hypertension, and extent of right ventricular failure. In patients with preoperative atrial fibrillation, return of normal sinus rhythm occurs in less than 30%. It is usually irreversible in those with significant left atrial enlargement (> 50 mm) and prolonged atrial fibrillation (> 1 year duration).

The majority of patients (85–90%) return to NYHA functional class I–II following surgical relief of mitral stenosis. About 20% of patients undergoing open commissurotomy will require mitral valve replacement within 10 years, and 50% in 20 years. Long-term survival rates following mitral commissurotomy and mitral valve replacement are approximately 85% and 60%, respectively. Significant incremental risk factors for late deaths include older age and higher NYHA functional class.

MITRAL REGURGITATION

GENERAL CONSIDERATIONS

In the United States, myxomatous degeneration of the mitral valve leaflets with elongation of chordae tendineae is the most common cause of mitral insufficiency. Rheumatic disease may result in fibrotic thickening and retraction of the mitral valve, resulting in noncoaptation of the leaflets. This is further exacerbated by annular calcification with immobilization of the base of the leaflets. Myocardial ischemia or infarction may produce chordal rupture, or, more commonly, papillary muscle dysfunction. Less frequent causes of mitral regurgitation include endocarditis, dilated cardiomyopathy, congenital defects, and trauma.

Acute mitral regurgitation results from chordal rupture or endocarditis with leaflet perforation. Due to the low compliance of the left atrium, this produces an abrupt elevation in left atrial and pulmonary venous pressures, leading to acute pulmonary edema. The loss of effective forward flow usually causes significant hemodynamic compromise. Although the use of inotropic and afterload-reducing agents can temporize the situation, emergent mitral valve repair or replacement is frequently warranted.

In contrast, chronic mitral regurgitation is usually well tolerated for many years without symptoms. The left ventricle compensates by eccentric hypertrophy and dilatation, thereby accommodating the volume overload with an increase in end-diastolic volume without significant elevation in end-diastolic pressure. Furthermore, the left atrium also dilates and becomes more compliant. This increases its ability to accept a larger regurgitant volume. Although the total ejection fraction frequently remains unchanged or even increased, forward stroke volume may not be adequate, particularly during exercise. The initial complaint is often fatigue, followed by symptoms of congestive heart failure with progressive decompensation of the left ventricle. The onset of atrial fibrillation reduces left ventricular filling and leads to worsening of symptoms.

CLINICAL EVALUATION

In patients with long-standing mitral regurgitation, physical examination often demonstrates a prominent apical impulse and parasternal lift. Auscultation typically reveals a holosystolic murmur best heard at the apex, with radiation to the axilla. In those with severe congestive heart failure, an S_3 gallop is often present. There is usually evidence of left atrial enlargement on electrocardiogram and chest x-ray.

The most useful modality of assessing mitral regurgitation is transthoracic or transesophageal echocardiography with color Doppler. The amount of mitral regurgitation, the extent of left atrial enlargement, and degree of left ventricular dysfunction can be quantified. Importantly, the structural abnormality responsible for the mitral regurgitation is often identified, which may be useful in terms of determining the likelihood of successful mitral valve repair. In general, the direction of the mitral regurgitant jet is opposite the leaflet involved.

On cardiac catheterization, a V wave may be seen on the pulmonary artery capillary wedge pressure tracing. Regurgitant fraction can be calculated from the angiographic stroke volume and Swan-Ganz thermodilution cardiac output. Coronary anatomy is also assessed in elderly patients and those with significant risk factors or symptoms for coronary artery disease (Table 37.1–4).

TREATMENT

Acute mitral insufficiency with hemodynamic compromise, due to ruptured chordae (idiopathic or ischemic) or endocarditis, mandates urgent mitral valve repair or replacement. Patients with class III or IV symptoms due to chronic mitral regurgitation usually have depressed left ventricular function. Surgery is indicated except in cases of advanced disease where ejection fraction is decreased, suggesting irreversible left ventricular dysfunction. For those with minimal or no symptoms, mitral valve surgery is warranted when there is evidence of progressive left ventricular dilatation or dysfunction. Echocardiographic indicators include fractional shortening less than 30% or end-diastolic dimension greater than 75 mm.

Because of its ease of implantation and reliability, mitral valve replacement had been the procedure of choice for mitral insufficiency until the mid-1980s. Because of the problems of thromboembolism and anticoagulant-related hemorrhage with mechanical prostheses and the limited durability of bioprosthetic substitutes, a variety of mitral valve reconstructive techniques were developed in Europe in the 1970s. The most widely accepted are those described by Carpentier, which include annuloplasty for annular dilatation, quadrangular resection for posterior leaflet prolapse, chordal shortening for elongated chordae, and chordal transfer for ruptured chordae of the anterior leaflet.

When mitral valve reconstruction is not possible, mitral valve replacement using chordal sparing techniques is recommended. Conventional mitral valve replacement with excision of the entire subvalvular apparatus has been associated with higher mortality rates and depressed left ventricular function postoperatively. It is thought that the elimination of systolic unloading into the low impedance left atrium after mitral valve replacement creates an after-load mismatch, thereby increasing left ventricular wall stress. Preservation of papillary-annular continuity has been demonstrated in clinical and experimental studies to improve left ventricular performance. Chordal excision is associated with significant increases in postoperative left ventricular end-systolic volume and stress, along with a decline in ejection fraction. When these techniques are utilized for implantation of mechanical valves, it is important that the subvalvular structures do not interfere with disc motion. The posterior leaflet can simply be plicated into the suture line, but special techniques are required for preservation of the anterior leaflet in order to prevent left ventricular outflow tract obstruction. The integrity of the subvalvular apparatus is also thought to minimize the potential postoperative left ventricular rupture.

RESULTS

Postoperative care regarding ventilatory support and pulmonary dilatation to manage right ventricular failure is similar to that following mitral valve surgery for critical mitral stenosis. In contrast to mitral stenosis, however, correction of mitral regurgitation with elimination of systolic unloading may unmask significant left ventricular dysfunction. Therefore, prolonged inotropic support with adrenaline or noradrenaline may be necessary to treat early left ventricular failure.

Compared to conventional mitral valve replacement, the operative mortality rate is lower for patients undergoing mitral valve repair (2–4% versus 5–8%). Long-term survival also appears to be superior with mitral reconstruction (85% versus 55% at 10 years). Preoperative risk factors that are found to adversely influence long-term survival include left ventricular dysfunction, higher NYHA functional class, concomitant coronary artery disease, ischemic etiology for mitral regurgitation, and advanced age. In terms of durability, mitral repair is comparable to mitral valve replacement except in cases of rheumatic valve disease.

However, not all causes of mitral insufficiency are amendable to satisfactory reconstruction. The best candidates are those with degenerative disease with a single prolapsed scallop of the posterior leaflet. In cases where mitral valve replacement is necessary, preservation of the mitral subvalvular apparatus may be important in optimizing left ventricular performance postoperatively.

TRICUSPID STENOSIS

GENERAL CONSIDERATIONS

Tricuspid stenosis is most often of rheumatic origin. It is rarely an isolated lesion without involvement of other valves. There are fusion of the commissures, leaflet thick-

Table 37.1–4. Mitral regurgitation: Essentials of diagnosis.

Apical holosystolic murmur radiating into the axilla
Left atrial and left ventricular enlargement with pulmonary
  congestion
Echocardiographic or angiographic evidence of mitral
  insufficiency

ening, and coexistent valvular regurgitation. In contrast to rheumatic mitral valve disease, there is less involvement of the subvalvular apparatus, and calcification is rarely present. Other less common causes of tricuspid stenosis include carcinoid syndrome, fibroelastosis, endomyocardial fibrosis, and lupus erythematosus.

Tricuspid stenosis results in inflow obstruction to the right ventricle, producing right atrial enlargement and hypertension. Transvalvular gradient is exacerbated by exercise, due to increased venous return. Early symptoms include fatigue and exercise intolerance. Evidence of systemic congestion (hepatomegaly, ascites, and peripheral edema) is noted with advanced disease and when transvalvular gradient exceeds 5 mm Hg. Symptoms are worsened with the onset of atrial fibrillation.

CLINICAL EVALUATION

Physical examination is remarkable for a diastolic jugular venous A wave in patients with sinus rhythm. Approximately one half of patients have atrial fibrillation and demonstrate slow venous emptying. A diastolic murmur can be heard along the left lower sternal border, which is accentuated with inspiration and attenuated with expiration. Pathognomonic radiographic findings are right atrial enlargement with clear lung fields and normal-sized pulmonary arteries. However, right ventricular and pulmonary arterial enlargement are frequently noted, as a result of the presence of severe mitral valve disease. Echocardiography is significant for right atrial enlargement with restricted diastolic tricuspid leaflet excursion. Stenosis is considered severe when the transvalvular gradient is 5 mm Hg or more, as estimated by echocardiography or measured by cardiac catheterization (Table 37.1–5).

TREATMENT

Early symptoms are usually amenable to control with diuretics and salt restriction. The development of class III–IV symptoms and the onset of signs of systemic congestion refractory to medical treatment are indications for surgical intervention. Tricuspid commissurotomy is the procedure of choice unless there is extensive disease or significant regurgitation, in which case tricuspid valve replacement is necessary. Commissurotomy is usually carried out at the an-

Table 37.1–5. Tricuspid stenosis: Essentials of diagnosis.

Prominent diastolic jugular venous pulsation with diastolic murmur at the lower left sternal border
Peripheral edema, ascites, and hepatomegaly
Right atrial enlargement without right ventricular or pulmonary artery dilatation
Right atrial pressure > 12 mm Hg and effective valve area < 1.5 cm^2

---

teroseptal and the posteroseptal commissures, because of the higher incidence of tricuspid regurgitation with incision of the anteroposterior commissure. Tricuspid annuloplasty is often required to avoid residual regurgitation.

TRICUSPID REGURGITATION

GENERAL CONSIDERATIONS

Isolated tricuspid regurgitation is rare. It commonly occurs on a functional basis as a result of pulmonary hypertension secondary to mitral valve disease. Tricuspid insufficiency can occur as a part of multivalvular rheumatic involvement. It is seen with increasing frequency because of endocarditis in intravenous drug users. Other organic causes include trauma, carcinoid, and congenital heart disease. Symptoms resulting from tricuspic regurgitation develop gradually and usually are severe only with concomitant pulmonary hypertension. Right ventricular output can be maintained with slight elevation of systemic venous pressure in the presence of normal pulmonary artery pressures. Signs of systemic venous hypertension are the same as those for tricuspid stenosis (eg, peripheral edema, hepatomegaly, and ascites).

CLINICAL EVALUATION

The most common physical finding is hepatomegaly, followed by distended neck veins. The incidence of systolic pulsation of the liver and peripheral veins is variable. A systolic murmur may be heard at the lower left or right sternal border, which may be confused with those of left-sided lesions.

Chest x-ray demonstrates right atrial and ventricular enlargement. The most useful diagnostic test for documenting tricuspid regurgitation is two-dimensional echocardiography with color Doppler. The severity of tricuspid insufficiency can be quantified by the ratio of the regurgitant jet area to right atrial area. Typically, a high right atrial systolic V wave is noted on the pressure tracing obtained during cardiac catheterization. Functional tricuspid regurgitation is suggested by pulmonary hypertension with systolic pulmonary arterial pressure greater than 60 mm Hg, where it is usually less than 40 mm Hg for organic tricuspid regurgitation. The extent of valvular insufficiency and annular dilatation is estimated by right ventriculography (Table 37.1–6).

TREATMENT

Surgery is indicated for severe, symptomatic, tricuspid regurgitation and moderate, functional, tricuspid insufficiency in the presence of elevated pulmonary artery pres-

Table 37.1–6. Tricuspid regurgitation: Essentials of diagnosis.

Prominent systolic jugular venous pulsation with a holosystolic
  murmur along the left sternal border
Right atrial and ventricular enlargement with regurgitant V wave
  on right atrial pressure tracing

sure and resistance. Functional tricuspid regurgitation that is mild or moderate in the absence of pulmonary hypertension usually resolves after correction of the mitral valve lesion, and therefore, does not require intervention. In contrast, organic tricuspid insufficiency generally requires either annuloplasty or replacement.

Tricuspid regurgitation can be corrected with either annuloplasty or replacement. Several annuloplasty techniques and their modifications have been developed over the years. The Kay annuloplasty procedure essentially converts the tricuspid valve into a bicuspid valve by plication of the annulus over the posterior leaflet with figure-of-eight sutures. Another accepted technique is the De-Vaga semicircular annuloplasty, which involves the plication of the dilated portion of annulus between the anteroseptal and posteroseptal commissures, with two rows of plicating sutures along the annulus. The most frequently employed method is ring annuloplasty with either a rigid Carpentier-Edwards or flexible Duran ring.

Tricuspid valve replacement, when necessary, can be performed with the aorta unclamped. Mechanical valves have a greater incidence of postoperative thrombosis because of the low pressure of the right side of the heart. The newer generation of bileaflet mechanical valves appears to have lower thrombosis rates. Despite the low incidence of postoperative complete heart block (2–7%), placement of permanent epicardial ventricular pacing leads should also be considered, since a transvenous pacing lead will interfere with valve leaflet excursion. Given these limitations of mechanical prostheses in the tricuspid position, bioprostheses have been advocated by some surgeons because of their greater durability compared to those implanted in the mitral or aortic positions. Another advantage of bioprosthetic valves is that a Swan-Ganz catheter can be placed across them, if necessary, for postoperative hemodynamic management.

RESULTS

Since tricuspid annuloplasty is rarely performed as an isolated procedure, its effect on operative mortality and long-term survival is difficult to assess directly. Generally, excellent results in terms of durability have been reported. All annuloplasty techniques are associated with mild diastolic gradients in 40% of patients and variable degrees of residual insufficiency in 30–50%. Because annular geometry is preserved with ring annuloplasty, the incidence of residual regurgitation tends to be less. Despite

its limitation, clinical improvement is observed in 90% of patients when coexisting left-sided lesions are corrected, with resolution of their attendant pulmonary hypertension and elevated pulmonary resistance.

The operative mortality rate for isolated tricuspid replacement is approximately 5%. This figure is substantially higher with concomitant mitral and/or aortic valve replacement. Actuarial survival estimate is about 50–55% at 10 years. Both operative risk and long-term survival are adversely influenced by higher preoperative NYHA functional class and ventricular dysfunction.

THORACIC AORTIC ANEURYSM

GENERAL CONSIDERATIONS

Aneurysms of the thoracic aorta may involve the sinus of Valsalva, ascending aorta, transverse arch, descending aorta (with or without extension into the abdominal aorta), or their combinations (Figure 37.1–3). Approximately 50% of thoracic aneurysms are located in the descending aorta, 25% in the ascending aorta, and 10% in the aortic arch. Another 10% involve both the ascending aorta and the transverse arch. Rarely, aneurysms of the thoracic aorta are limited to the sinuses of Valsalva.

Aneurysms of the ascending aorta and arch usually re-

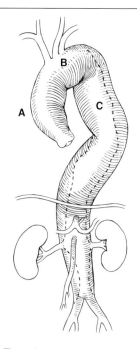

Figure 37.1–3. Thoracic aneurysms may involve the ascending aorta **(A)**, transverse arch **(B)**, or descending aorta **(C)**.

sult from myxomatous degeneration of the medial layer of the aortic wall or cystic medial necrosis, which is often associated with Marfan or Ehlers-Danlos syndromes. In contrast, those involving the distal arch and descending aorta are most commonly due to atherosclerosis. Other causes include chronic dissections, trauma, and infection. Occasionally, poststenotic dilatation of the ascending aorta can occur, with significant aortic valvular stenosis. Conversely, aneurysms of the ascending aorta may extend to the aortic annulus, resulting in annuloaortic ectasia. Sinus of Valsalva aneurysms are either congenital, owing to the absence of normal elastic and muscular tissue in the sinus (most commonly involving the right coronary sinus), or acquired as a result of endocarditis, cystic medial necrosis, trauma, or syphilis.

CLINICAL EVALUATION

Most patients with thoracic aortic aneurysms are asymptomatic until there is rapid expansion of the aneurysm, with compression and invasion of adjacent intrathoracic structures. Symptoms, therefore, are related to the size and location of the aneurysm. Congestive heart failure symptoms may result from progressive aortic insufficiency associated with dilatation of the aortic root or annuloaortic ectasia. Bony erosion of the sternum, ribs, or vertebral bodies can produce chest pain or back pain. Stretching of the vagus or recurrent laryngeal nerve may result in hoarseness. Compression of the airway may cause cough and hemoptysis. Dysphagia and hematemesis may occur, with erosion into the esophagus. Rarely, involvement of the cervical ganglia may produce Horner's syndrome. Those with congenital sinus of Valsalva aneurysms commonly present with dyspnea on exertion, palpitations, fatigue, and chest pain due to rupture into the cardiac chambers that results in a significant left to right shunt. These patients typically have a hyperdynamic heart, a wide pulse pressure, and a machinery-like murmur. In contrast, the acquired form of sinus of Valsalva aneurysm usually ruptures into the pericardial space, causing cardiac tamponade.

The diagnosis of a thoracic aortic aneurysm is suggested by a widened mediastinum on chest radiograph. Echocardiography is most useful for evaluating size of the aneurysm, degree of aortic root dilatation and aortic regurgitation, presence of intimal flap, and left ventricular function. Contrast computed tomography (CT) scanning is an excellent imaging modality for quantifying the precise size and extent of aneurysm as well as identifying intimal flap and intraluminal thrombus. In comparison, magnetic resonance imaging (MRI) has the additional advantage of providing images in the sagittal and coronal planes, as well as in the transverse plane, without the need for radiation or contrast. Aortography is most important for assessing the proximal and distal extent of the aneurysm and delineating the anatomy of significant intercostal or spinal

Table 37.1–7. Thoracic aortic aneurysm: Essentials of diagnosis.

Chest pain, back pain, hoarseness, cough, dysphagia, or Horner's syndrome (variable)
Enlarged mediastinal silhouette on chest x-ray
Radiologic evidence of aortic abnormality by aortography, computed axial tomography, or magnetic resonance imaging

arteries. Cardiac catheterization is performed, when necessary, to evaluate aortic valvular competency and presence of coronary disease (Table 37.1–7).

TREATMENT

Once a diagnosis of thoracic aortic aneurysm is made, over 50% of patients die within 2 years. Rupture is responsible for nearly half of these deaths, with the remainder from associated cardiovascular diseases. Therefore, elective rather than emergency repair is recommended for aneurysms that are infectious in origin, symptomatic, progressively expanding on serial imaging studies, or greater than 6 cm in diameter or twice the diameter of the uninvolved aorta if asymptomatic. Surgical intervention should also be considered for ascending aortic aneurysms greater than 4 cm in association with significant aortic regurgitation.

The fistula of a ruptured congenital sinus of Valsalva aneurysm may be approached through the aorta, the chamber into which it ruptured, or both. All aneurysmal and fistulous tract tissue should be excised and the aortic defect closed primarily or with a patch. Concomitant aortic valve replacement may be necessary for coexisting aortic regurgitation.

Aneurysms of the ascending aorta are resected and replaced with a woven double velour Dacron graft. Large aneurysms displacing the heart and mediastinal structures, thereby preventing access to cannulation, may require perfusion through the femoral vessels. Associated aortic regurgitation with dilated aortic root will require replacement using a composite valve graft conduit and reimplantation of the coronary arteries. If the aneurysm extends into the proximal arch, a hemi-arch repair is performed whereby the graft is beveled to replace the lesser curve of the transverse arch.

Repair of the transverse arch aneurysm is more complicated, involving the use of profound hypothermic circulatory arrest to provide exposure and minimize neurological complications. Using this technique, the patient is cooled systemically to 18°C, the head is packed in ice, and methylprednisolone is administered. The distal anastomosis to the descending aorta distal to the left subclavian artery is performed, followed by the reimplantation of the cerebral vessels as an island. The graft is clamped and the perfusion is reinstituted via the femoral artery while the proximal anastomosis is completed. Concomitant involvement of the descending aorta may require a stage re-pair using the "elephant trunk" technique, where the distal anastomosis is performed with an infolded graft, thereby leaving a portion of the graft dangling in the descending aorta beyond the anastomosis. In this fashion, proximal control during repair of the descending aortic aneurysm involves only opening the aneurysm and quickly clamping the elephant trunk graft.

Aneurysms of the descending aorta are approached via a left thoracotomy. Distal perfusion after aortic cross-clamping is provided by left atrial-to-femoral artery by-pass or partial femorofemoral bypass with systemic cooling. When the aneurysm involves the distal aortic arch, or is so large as to preclude safe proximal aortic clamping, a period of profound hypothermia and circulatory arrest may be necessary to perform the proximal anastomosis. For high-risk patients, repair with the deployment of an endovascular stent via the femoral artery has been successful, if anatomy is favorable.

RESULTS

The operative mortality for the repair of ruptured sinus of Valsalva aneurysms is less than 10%. The long-term prognosis is excellent, with an 80% 25-year survival rate. Similarly, the operative mortality rate for tube graft replacement of ascending aortic aneurysms ranges from 5% to 10%, being the same for those requiring a composite valve-graft conduit. Risk factors include advanced age, diabetes, reoperative aortic surgery, and emergency operation for rupture. The 5-year survival estimate is 65–75% and is adversely influenced by the presence of aortic dissection, transverse arch involvement, coexisting coronary disease, and Marfan's syndrome.

Operation for transverse arch aneurysms is technically more complex and is associated with higher mortality and morbidity rates. With the development of profound hypothermia and circulatory arrest, improved graft material, and refined postoperative management, the operative mortality has significantly decreased from 50% to 10–20%. The most serious complication is stroke, which accounts for approximately 20–25% of deaths.

The operative risk for resection of descending aortic aneurysms is about 15%. Predictors for operative death include advanced age, emergency operation, and presence of congestive heart failure. Both paraplegic and renal failure rates range between 5–10%. Factors that have been demonstrated to be determinants of spinal cord injury include duration of ischemia, interruption of critical intercostal arteries, extent of aneurysm, level of involvement, adequacy of distal perfusion, perioperative hypotension, and systemic temperature. Adjuncts such as somatosensory evoked potential monitoring, spinal fluid drainage, and pharmacologic agents to increase spinal cord tolerance to ischemia have not been demonstrated to reduce the risk of paraplegia. Long-term survival is variable. The

5-year survival rate is 40–60%, with rupture of associated abdominal aortic aneurysms and complications of cardiovascular disease accounting for one quarter and one third of late deaths, respectively.

AORTIC DISSECTION

GENERAL CONSIDERATIONS

Aortic dissection is the most frequent catastrophe involving the aorta, being twice as common as ruptured abdominal aortic aneurysm. If untreated, acute aortic dissection involving the ascending aorta is associated with a mortality rate of about 1% per hour during the first 48 hours. Causes of death include intrapericardial rupture resulting in cardiac tamponade, acute aortic valvular regurgitation, or compromised cerebral or coronary perfusion. For patients with aortic dissection limited to the descending aorta, the leading causes of death are rupture and compromised blood flow to vital organs.

Aortic dissection is most frequently seen in middle-aged men with a history of hypertension. Patients with connective tissue disorders, such as Marfan's syndrome or Ehlers-Danlos syndrome, have a predisposition for dissection due to degeneration of the elastic element within the aortic wall. In young women, dissections not uncommonly occur during the third trimester of pregnancy, during labor, or in the postpartum period, often causing the death of either the mother, fetus, or both.

The primary event is a tear in the aortic intima with secondary extension into the media, thereby creating a true and false lumen. Along its path, the dissection can affect the origin of important arterial branches by extrinsic compression by the false lumen, leading to end-organ ischemia. The false lumen can enlarge over time to give rise to false aneurysms that may require late reoperation. An intramural hematoma may form, with primary hemorrhage in the aortic media without a true dissection process. Clinically, reports of intramural hematoma evolving into acute aortic dissection suggest that it may be a precursor of dissection in some patients.

Based on the Stanford classification scheme, dissections involving the ascending aorta, irrespective of the site of primary intimal tear and regardless of the distal extent of propagation, are termed **type A dissections**. If the ascending aorta is not involved, it is called a **type B dissection** (Figure 37.1–4). Arbitrarily defined, the dissection is considered acute if symptoms occurred less than 14 days earlier and chronic if longer than 14 days. Approximately two thirds of dissections are type A dissections, typically with the intimal tear located just distal to the sinotubular ridge. In patients with type B dissections, the tear is usually just distal to the left subclavian artery (25%). The remainder of intimal tears are located

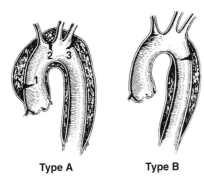

Type A   **Type B**

Figure 37.1–4. Aortic dissections involving the ascending aorta are termed **type A,** irrespective of the site of intimal tear or the extent of propagation. If the ascending aorta is not involved, then it is called a **type B dissection.** (Reprinted, with permission, from Mcgoon DC: *Cardiac Surgery.* FA Davis Company, 1982, p. 246.)

in the aortic arch (10%), or on rare occasions, in the abdominal aorta (2%).

CLINICAL EVALUATION

The clinical manifestations of acute aortic dissection are protean, as a result of the unpredictable disturbances of end-organ perfusion as the dissecting process propagates. Therefore, a high index of suspicion is imperative when a patient presents with signs and symptoms involving seemingly unrelated, multiple organ systems. The most common symptom is excruciating chest or interscapular pain, with subsequent migration. The blood pressure is often elevated, and aortic rupture or cardiac tamponade should be suspected if hypotension is present. Ascending aortic dissection can cause aortic valvular incompetence, thereby leading to congestive heart failure symptoms. Rupture into the pericardium or accumulation of transudate from the inflamed, dissected ascending aorta may result in cardiac tamponade. Coronary occlusion and acute myocardial ischemia may be the dominant features, as suggested by a pericardial rub and electrocardiographic changes. Approximately one third to one half of all patients develop one or more central or peripheral vascular complications. These include neurologic deficits, paraplegia, limb ischemia, renal insufficiency, and mesenteric ischemia.

Because of the lethal nature of the disease, the best initial diagnostic test is the one that can be performed most rapidly and accurately. The preferred screening test is transesophageal echocardiography. It can confirm the diagnosis of aortic dissection and reliably determine the involvement of the ascending aorta. The presence of aortic insufficiency, pericardial effusion or tamponade, and left

ventricular function can also be assessed. Magnetic resonance imaging is an excellent technique to provide comprehensive mapping and flow within the entire aorta. While it is more accurate than transesophageal echocardiography, it is time-consuming and may be impractical in critically ill patients. In centers where MRI is not available or logistically difficult to obtain, contrast-enhanced CT is a relatively accurate method in diagnosing aortic dissection. Although aortography has been previously considered the diagnostic gold standard, this procedure is invasive, time-consuming, and not infallible. The only indication today for angiography is in stable patients with known or suspected coronary artery disease (Table 37.1–8).

TREATMENT

While confirmatory diagnostic procedures are performed, the initial goal is to control the mean arterial blood pressure between 60 and 70 mm Hg with the use of beta-blockers and short-acting vasodilators, while maintaining adequate coronary, cerebral, and renal perfusion. Whether the patient is managed medically or surgically, oral antihypertensive medications are continued indefinitely.

For patients with acute type A aortic dissections, emergency surgical repair is the treatment of choice. The operation involves replacement of the ascending aorta, resection of the primary intimal tear if possible, obliteration of the false lumen with restoration of flow into the true lumen, and repair of concomitant injuries to the aortic arch, coronary arteries, or aortic valve. Extension of aortic replacement to include the transverse arch is indicated for patients with rupture or impending rupture of the arch, or those with cerebral flow compromise, or to resect a tear located in the arch in young, low-risk patients. In most cases, an open distal aortic anastomosis using a brief period of profound hypothermia and circulatory arrest is recommended. This method ensures a more technically secure and reliable distal anastomosis and avoids further aortic injury from the crossclamp. Finally, the aortic valve can be preserved in the majority of cases by resuspending the aortic commissures. Aortic valve replacement is advocated only in patients with connective tissue disorders or gross annuloaortic ectasia.

Because of the high operative mortality rate, patients with acute type B dissections are usually managed with

Table 37.1–8. Aortic dissection: Essentials of diagnosis.

Excruciating chest pain with migration
Multitude of seemingly unrelated cardiovascular end-organ
    dysfunctions
Shock-like state with poor peripheral perfusion during late stages
Evidence of dissection on echocardiography, computed
    tomography, magnetic resonance imaging, or angiography

antihypertensive and negative inotropic agents to control blood pressure. Surgery is recommended for rupture, acute expansion, intractable pain, uncontrollable hypertension, and distal organ ischemia. The role of early operative intervention for low-risk patients with uncomplicated acute type B dissections remains controversial, since it may confer some protection against late development of false aneurysms in the distal aorta, acute redissection, or ischemic compromise of major aortic tributaries. For patients with Marfan's syndrome, early surgical graft replacement is advocated in experienced centers. In most cases, only a limited resection of the most severely diseased segment of the descending aorta is recommended in order to minimize the risk of spinal cord injury.

Recently, endovascular techniques using intravascular ultrasonographic guidance have been developed to manage the subset of high-risk patients presenting with major dissection-related complications. Using this approach, fenestrations can be created to decompress the false lumen when antegrade flow in the distal true lumen is compromised by extrinsic compression by the false lumen. Furthermore, balloon-expandable stents can be used to revascularize important end-organs which are compromised when the true lumen is extrinsically obstructed by the dissected false lumen.

Indications for operation in patients with chronic type A dissections are restricted to congestive heart failure due to aortic insufficiency, pain due to aneurysmal degeneration of the ascending aorta, and asymptomatic aneurysmal enlargement to greater than twice the diameter of contiguous normal aorta. Similarly, for patients with chronic type B dissections, surgery is recommended when the aortic false aneurysm reaches 5–6 cm, especially if it is confined to a relatively short segment. Because of the higher risk of paraplegia, more extensive resections are indicated only for aneurysms greater than 7–8 cm.

RESULTS

As a result of earlier diagnosis, more advanced surgical techniques, and improved postoperative care, the operative mortality rate for acute aortic dissection, type A or B, has improved over the years to less than 25%. For those with chronic dissections, the operative risk is approximately 15%. Predictors of operative death include hypertension, cardiac tamponade, coronary artery disease, renal dysfunction, stroke, and advanced age.

The overall long-term survival is about 50% at 10 years for hospital survivors, independent of the acuity or the type of dissection. Freedom from late reoperation related to the dissection process is 65% at 10 years, with an operative mortality rate of 35%. These late procedures include treatment failures in which the initial operation was either incomplete or failed prematurely, and late sequelae, representing progression of the underlying dissection process. This underscores the need for closed aortic imaging sur-

veillance and earlier surgical intervention before the development of complications.

ISCHEMIC HEART DISEASE

ANGINA PECTORIS

GENERAL CONSIDERATIONS

Coronary artery disease results from significant hemodynamic obstruction of coronary vessels due to development of atherosclerosis. Although coronary autoregulation compensates for a decrease in perfusion beyond a coronary stenosis by vasodilatation, distal blood flow is reduced during exercise and at rest when vessel luminal diameter is decreased, respectively, by 50% and 85%. When myocardial perfusion is inadequate to meet metabolic demands, the resulting ischemia can lead to angina, myocardial infarction, congestive heart failure, ventricular arrhythmias, or sudden death. Early mortality following acute myocardial infarction is usually related to left ventricular failure and cardiogenic shock. Other mechanical complications of myocardial infarction, such as severe mitral regurgitation, ventricular septal perforation, and left ventricular aneurysm, are associated with a poor outcome.

The major risk factors for development of coronary atherosclerosis include hypercholesterolemia, habitual tobacco use, and hypertension. The risk of coronary artery disease increases in a nonlinear fashion with elevation of total serum cholesterol beyond 180 mg/dL. It also correlates directly with low-density lipoprotein and inversely with high-density lipoprotein. Cigarette smoking increases the risk of nonfatal myocardial infarction by threefold, which returns toward baseline 2 years after cessation of smoking. Both systolic (> 140 mm Hg) and diastolic (> 90 mm Hg) blood pressures are independent determinants of coronary atherosclerosis, with an increase in risk by 30% for each 10-mm Hg rise in systolic pressure. Other less important risk factors that have been identified as independent predictors of coronary artery disease include diabetes mellitus, strong family history of coronary atherosclerosis, obesity, stress, and hyperuricemia.

CLINICAL EVALUATION

Signs & Symptoms

Ischemic heart disease typically presents as precordial chest pain radiating to the arm, neck, or jaw. It may also manifest as dyspnea, epigastric pain, or fatigue. Angina usually occurs with exertion, stress, or exposure to cold.

Symptoms are relieved with rest and sublingual nitroglycerin. Chronic stable angina refers to chest pain that has been stable for 4–6 weeks without significant changes in pattern or severity. In contrast, unstable angina has been defined as new onset of severe angina, crescendo angina, or angina at rest. Physical examination is generally unrevealing. Occasionally, an S_3 gallop or rales may be auscultated, suggesting ischemic left ventricular dysfunction.

Laboratory & Imaging Studies

Routine laboratory studies are usually normal except for an elevated serum cholesterol. Electrocardiogram may show evidence of previous myocardial infarction and ST segment depression. Treadmill testing using a graded protocol will demonstrate electrocardiographic changes in 85% of patients with coronary artery disease. Sensitivity and specificity are improved with thallium scanning. Significant coronary disease is suggested by the development of ST segment depression persisting into the recovery phase, angina, fall in systolic blood pressure, and reversible perfusion defects or increased lung uptake by thallium scan. For patients unable to exercise, Persantine administration mimics the redistribution of blood flow during exercise. Metabolic studies utilizing positron emission tomography (PET) have high predictive value in distinguishing viable, hibernating myocardium from scar tissue. Stress and dobutamine echocardiography have been demonstrated to be sensitive methods of detecting segmental wall motion abnormalities due to myocardial ischemia.

Coronary arteriography is indicated when a patient with suspected coronary artery disease based on clinical findings and/or stress testing is considered for either balloon angioplasty or bypass surgery. Angiography is used to evaluate and delineate the extent of coronary disease. A stenosis is considered significant when it results in 70% decrease or more in the luminal diameter. This criteria is reduced to 50% for the left main coronary artery. Left ventriculography can also be performed at the time of coronary angiography to assess left ventricular function and to detect the presence of segmental wall motion abnormalities, mitral regurgitation, and left ventricular aneurysm (Table 37.1–9).

TREATMENT

Medical Treatment

Myocardial oxygen consumption is determined primarily by the interplay of preload, afterload, contractility, and heart rate. Since most ischemic syndromes are related to increases in oxygen demand, the main goal of medical therapy is directed towards modification of these factors. The most commonly used anti-angina regimen includes nitrates, beta-blockers, and calcium channel antagonists. Nitrates produce a decrease in preload and reduce coronary vascular resistance. Beta-blockers slow the heart rate and have a negative inotropic effect, but must be used cautiously in patients with congestive heart failure or significant reactive airway disease. Calcium channel antagonists lower systemic resistance and produce coronary vasodilatation. Additionally, contractility is decreased and heart rate is reduced by certain calcium channel blockers, such as verapamil and diltiazem. Cholesterol- and lipid-reducing agents have been shown to be effective in secondary and, possibly, primary prevention of fatal and nonfatal myocardial infarctions. Modification of other risk factors includes cessation of smoking, treatment of hypertension, and dietary and exercise programs to attain ideal weight and to control hypercholesterolemia and hyperglycemia.

Surgical Treatment

Coronary artery bypass grafting is the most common operation in cardiac surgery today, performed on approximately 1 in every 1000 persons in the United States. It involves revascularization of the myocardium by means of grafts bypassing the coronary obstruction (Figure 37.1–5). The most frequently used and available conduit is the patient's own greater saphenous vein, which routes blood from the ascending aorta to the distal epicardial coronary arteries. When the greater saphenous vein is significantly diseased with varicosity and thrombophlebitis, the lesser

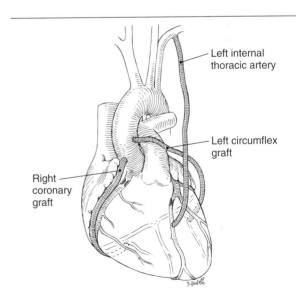

Figure 37.1–5. Schematic demonstrating aortocoronary bypass vein grafts and bypass grafting using the left internal thoracic artery as an arterial conduit.

Table 37.1–9. Angina pectoris: Essentials of diagnosis.

Substernal chest pain
Electrocardiographic evidence of ischemia during chest pain
Demonstration of ischemia by treadmill testing, radionuclide scan, or stress echocardiography
Significant angiographic obstruction of major coronary arteries

saphenous vein can serve as a satisfactory alternative. Since arterial conduits have higher patency rates, internal mammary arteries are often utilized to bypass obstructed coronary vessels directly from the subclavian arteries. Other available arterial grafts include the pedicled right gastroepiploic artery, the free inferior epigastric artery, and the free radial artery. Because of their poor patency rates, arm veins, cryopreserved homologous veins, and synthetic polytetrafluoroethylene grafts have limited usage.

The goals of coronary artery bypass are to relieve ischemia and the symptoms of angina, prolong survival, prevent myocardial infarction, preserve left ventricular function, and improve exercise tolerance. Indications for surgery include the following: (1) disabling angina refractory to medical management; (2) unstable angina; (3) postinfarction angina; (4) ischemic pulmonary edema; (5) failed balloon angioplasty and catheter-related complications; (6) acute myocardial infarction resulting in cardiogenic shock, severe mitral regurgitation, ventricular septal perforation, or left ventricular rupture; (7) significant left main coronary artery obstruction; (8) three-vessel coronary artery disease with left ventricular dysfunction; (9) three-vessel coronary artery disease with inducible ischemia on physiologic testing; (10) two-vessel coronary disease with proximal left anterior descending artery stenosis; and (11) adjunct to concomitant cardiac procedures.

More recently, transmyocardial laser revascularization techniques have been developed in an attempt to improve myocardial perfusion in those with nonbypassable coronary disease. Thus far, this procedure has been associated with significant palliation of angina symptoms without definitive objective evidence of improved myocardial perfusion by radionuclide scans. Longer follow-up is needed to assess the utility of this method for the treatment of coronary artery disease.

Nonsurgical Revascularization

Percutaneous transluminal coronary angioplasty (PTCA) is a viable alternative to coronary artery bypass surgery and is most suitable for patients with intractable stable angina and significant stenosis of one coronary artery accessible to balloon angioplasty. The procedure has been extended successfully to those with multivessel disease, acute myocardial infarction, or contraindication to surgery. The encouraging results of PTCA have led to the development of other devices designed to relieve obstructed coronary arteries by various methods. **Directional atherectomy** removes atherosclerotic plaques by means of a cylindrical cutting piston and entraps the material into a side chamber. **Rotary ablation** utilizes a high-speed rotating diamond-covered burr, which pulverizes the plaque into microparticles to be removed by the reticuloendothelial system. It is most widely used for hard, calcific lesions. The **transluminal extraction atherectomy catheter** (TEC) technique involves removing a portion of the plaque with a rotating conical cutting head and aspirat-

ing it through the catheter by suction. It has been used primarily in thrombosed vein grafts and vessels with bulky irregular plaques. Laser optics, developed to remove plaques by photoablation and mechanical disruption, have been used largely for long lesions and ostial lesions. More recently, various types of **endovascular stents** have been popularized to improve restenosis rates after PTCA by exerting radial force on the artery and creating a smoother lumen by covering fractures and intimal flaps. Current indications for the use of stents include abrupt closure or dissection following PTCA and unfavorable lesions with high restenosis rates after balloon angioplasty.

RESULTS

Elective coronary bypass surgery for stable angina with good left ventricular function yields an operative mortality rate of 1% or less. For patients with unstable angina, postinfarction angina, moderate left ventricular dysfunction, and failed PTCA, the operative risk is about 3–5% and increases to 10–20% in those with severely depressed left ventricular function requiring urgent operation. Postinfarction cardiogenic shock complicated by mitral regurgitation or ventricular septal defect is associated with poor outcome, with reported operative mortality rates exceeding 40%. Important determinants of operative risk include left ventricular dysfunction, reoperation, emergency operation, advanced age, and female gender.

Over 90% of patients obtain good relief of angina symptoms after myocardial revascularization, with objective improvement in exercise tolerance. About 10–15% of vein grafts occlude within the first year, and 2–5% per year occlude thereafter, with a 10-year patency rate of about 50%. In contrast, the internal mammary artery has a patency rate of 90–95% at 10 years and improves event-free survival by 10%. Despite the superior long-term patency rates of internal mammary arteries, recurrent angina still occurs in 35% of patients, primarily because of vein graft occlusion and progression of disease in nonbypassed vessels or in bypassed vessels beyond the site of the distal anastomosis. However, angina symptoms can usually be controlled with medical therapy, with only 10% of patients requiring reoperation at 10 years. The operative mortality rate of reoperation is generally two to three times higher because of the risks of catastrophic bleeding during mediastinal reentry, injury to patent grafts, and atheroembolism from manipulation of patent grafts. Revascularization is usually less satisfactory because coronary arteries are frequently obscured as a result of epicardial scarring.

The incidence of perioperative myocardial infarction is approximately 2–3% for stable angina, 5–10% for unstable angina, and 30–50% for emergency revascularization following failed PTCA. Thereafter, the late myocardial infarction rate is about 1–3% per year. Compared to medical management, coronary bypass surgery is associated with a lower incidence of fatal infarction and sudden death.

There is also evidence to suggest that late infarctions tend to be smaller with better preserved left ventricular function. If only saphenous vein grafts are used, the long-term survival after surgery is approximately 80% and 65% at 5 and 10 years, respectively. These figures are improved to 90% and 75%, respectively, if internal mammary arterial conduits are utilized as well. The most important predictor adversely influencing long-term prognosis is left ventricular dysfunction.

The long-term follow-up of patients undergoing single-vessel PTCA is favorable, with a 10-year survival rate of approximately 90%. However, additional angioplasty is required in 30% and bypass surgery in another 25%. Results of angioplasty of vein graft stenoses are favorable for lesions located at the distal anastomotic site, but poor for those in the mid-graft and proximal anastomotic positions. In the setting of acute myocardial infarction, primary angioplasty can be performed with a high level of success. Compared to thrombolytic therapy, PTCA appears to be superior in older patients and in those with anterior infarctions. The use of endovascular stents has reduced the need for emergency bypass surgery and reintervention. It has also resulted in larger luminal size at 6 months follow-up angiography. However, due to the vigorous anticoagulation regimen, there is a higher incidence of bleeding complications, resulting in a significantly longer hospital stay. These results may improve with better antiplatelet agents and lower targeted levels of anticoagulation.

The indications for PTCA versus bypass surgery are not clearly defined. In the setting of single-vessel disease producing ischemia, angioplasty is a good alternative to coronary bypass grafting in alleviating angina symptoms. It is associated with lower costs and morbidity, but has a recurrent stenosis rate of 25–30%, depending on the size of the vessel as well as the location and severity of the lesion. In patients with two- or three-vessel disease and good left ventricular function, there are no differences between the two methods of revascularization in terms of death, myocardial infarction, or the amount of ischemia on follow-up radionuclide scans. However, freedom from subsequent bypass grafting or repeat angioplasty is significantly higher for those undergoing operation.

COMPLICATIONS OF MYOCARDIAL INFARCTION

Postinfarction Ventricular Septal Defect

The incidence of postinfarction ventricular septal defect (VSD) is about 1–2%. It is most common following first myocardial infarctions in patients with one-vessel coronary artery disease and poorly developed collaterals. Two thirds of postinfarction VSDs involve the anteroapical septum, and one third are located in the posterior septum. The infarct is transmural, with perforation through a zone of necrotic myocardial tissue usually within 2 weeks. The resulting left-to-right shunt causes pulmonary edema and cardiogenic shock. Without surgical treatment, the prognosis is poor, with mortality rates of 25% within the first 24 hours and 50% at 1 week.

Diagnosis. The diagnosis is suggested by the development of recurrent chest pain and abrupt hemodynamic deterioration several days after an acute myocardial infarction. A harsh, pansystolic murmur is often present along the left lower sternal border. To differentiate postinfarction VSD from mitral regurgitation stemming from papillary muscle rupture (which can produce a similar clinical scenario), right heart catheterization can be performed to confirm an oxygen saturation step-up between the right atrium and pulmonary artery. More commonly, echocardiography with color-flow Doppler mapping is used to accurately demonstrate the presence and location of septal rupture. Coronary angiography is necessary to provide information concerning the extent of coronary artery disease.

Treatment. Initial therapy is directed toward stabilization of hemodynamics to ensure sufficient peripheral organ perfusion. This is best accomplished by unloading the left ventricle while augmenting coronary blood flow with an intra-aortic balloon pump, as well as by using inotropic and afterload-reducing agents. While delayed surgical repair after 6 weeks has been recommended in the past to allow for scar maturation, immediate operation is currently advised to prevent irreversible end-organ failure and to lower operative mortality. Classically, the operative approach involved extensive debridement of the necrotic septum and ventricular free wall and closure with a double patch technique. More recently, an endocardial repair has been developed in which a patch of Dacron or bovine pericardium is secured to the normal left ventricular endocardium around the infarct via a transinfarct left ventriculotomy, using a continuous polypropylene suture. This is followed by primary closure of the left ventriculotomy without resecting myocardium. In this fashion, the VSD and infarcted myocardium are excluded from the high-pressure left ventricle, tension on friable muscle is avoided, and ventricular geometry is preserved. Concomitant coronary revascularization is also recommended, as it has been demonstrated to significantly improve long-term survival.

Results. With prompt surgical intervention, postinfarction VSD can be repaired with an operative mortality as low as 15%. Posterior infarctions are associated with a higher operative risk due to right ventricular infarction and dysfunction. Other factors adversely affecting outcome include cardiogenic shock, emergency operation, and multiorgan system failure. Long-term results are favorable with respect to survival and functional rehabilitation. Approximately 70% of hospital survivors are expected to be alive at 5 years, with over 75% in NYHA functional class I or II. Recurrent or residual septal defects occur in 10–25% of patients. If symptomatic or the left-to-right shunt is greater than 2 to 1, these defects should be closed, either surgically or in the catheterization laboratory using a clam-shell device.

Postinfarction Acute Mitral Insufficiency

Postinfarction acute mitral insufficiency complicates myocardial infarction in 1–5% of cases and generally develops within the first week. Mitral incompetence can result from papillary muscle rupture or, more commonly, from papillary muscle dysfunction due to extensive myocardial injury. The posteromedial papillary muscle is most frequently involved, in association with an extensive inferior wall infarction and right coronary artery occlusion. Occasionally, occlusion of the left anterior descending artery results in rupture of the anterolateral papillary muscle. Due to a normally small and, therefore, noncompliant left atrium, acute mitral regurgitation results in pulmonary venous hypertension and congestion as well as cardiogenic shock. If untreated, the death rate is approximately 50% within 24 hours and 80% at 1 week.

Diagnosis. Acute mitral regurgitation following myocardial infarction is suggested by sudden deterioration of hemodynamics and the presence of a new holosystolic apical murmur. A V wave is often seen on the pulmonary arterial wedge pressure tracing. In contrast to postinfarction VSD, there is no oxygen saturation step-up from the right atrium to the pulmonary artery. Two-dimensional echocardiography, particularly via the transesophageal approach, is performed to determine the presence and the extent of mitral insufficiency. The extent of coronary artery disease is assessed by selective coronary angiography.

Treatment & Results. As with postinfarction VSD, patients in cardiogenic shock are managed initially with inotropic agents, vasodilators (if not hypotensive), and intra-aortic counterpulsation to allow temporary hemodynamic improvement while preparations are made for emergency operation. Frequently, intubation with mechanical ventilation is required for hypoxemia and pulmonary failure. Coronary revascularization and mitral valve replacement is the procedure usually performed. Because of the presence of left ventricular dysfunction, recent infarction, and cardiogenic shock, the operative mortality has been reported to be as high as 50%. In this respect, mitral valve repair may prove to be superior to valve replacement. Technically, exposure of the mitral valve can be difficult because of the small size of the left atrium. Some have advocated mitral valve repair through the infarcted left ventricle. Most patients are in NYHA functional class I and II postoperatively.

Left Ventricular Aneurysm

Left ventricular aneurysm is a thin-walled transmural scar that results from progressive expansion of infarcted myocardium over several months following an acute myocardial infarction. The reported incidence varies from 10–30%, depending on the definition of the aneurysm and the diagnostic modality utilized. However, clinically significant aneurysms occur in only 2–4% of patients. With increasing use of interventional catheter techniques and thrombolytic therapy, the number of patients referred for aneurysm resection has decreased. The majority of the aneurysms are located in the anteroapical region because of proximal left anterior descending coronary artery occlusion with poor distal collateral perfusion. About 10% result from occlusion of the right or circumflex vessels and involve the posteroinferior wall.

The paradoxical motion of a left ventricular aneurysm during systole and diastole results in significant left ventricular dysfunction. With time, the left ventricle becomes dilated and noncompliant. This, in turn, causes increased wall stress and higher oxygen consumption in the remaining normal myocardium, with decreased oxygen delivery. These changes can precipitate or aggravate symptoms of angina or congestive heart failure. Malignant ventricular arrhythmias originating at the junction of normal and scarred tissue are the major causes of death in the first year after infarction. Although organized thrombus on the endocardial surface of the aneurysm forms in about 50%, the incidence of systemic embolization is relatively low.

Diagnosis. The most common symptom of left ventricular aneurysm is congestive heart failure, followed by angina pectoris. The incidence of ventricular arrhythmias varies between 5% and 20% and correlates with the size of the aneurysm. Examination reveals a diffuse sustained apical impulse with a "rocking" precordium. Electrocardiogram usually shows Q waves in the anterior precordial leads and persistent ST segment elevation. Two-dimensional echocardiography is excellent for evaluating global and regional wall motion abnormalities and for detecting mural thrombus. Although CT and MRI can accurately delineate the anatomy of the aneurysm, contrast ventriculography remains the gold standard in defining cardiac function and coronary anatomy.

Treatment. Small asymptomatic aneurysms without left ventricular dysfunction are treated medically unless significant ventricular arrhythmias develop. Symptomatic patients with congestive heart failure or angina or those with asymptomatic large aneurysms are considered for operation. Traditionally, coronary artery bypass combined with aneurysmectomy and linear closure reinforced with Teflon felt strips was the procedure most commonly employed. Although this approach may be adequate for small aneurysms, it can lead to significant distortion of ventricular geometry and impairment of left ventricular function in those with large aneurysms. This has led to the development of a Dacron or bovine pericardium endoventricular patch technique in an attempt to maintain left ventricular geometry. In patients with ventricular arrhythmias, intraoperative mapping, endocardial resection, or cryoablation of arrhythmogenic tissue may be indicated.

Results. Recently reported operative mortality rates range between 4% and 20%, being the lowest for those repaired by the endoventricular patch plasty method. Increased operative risk is associated with extensive coronary artery disease and advanced NYHA functional class, due to depressed function of the remaining nonaneurysmal myocardium. The overall 5-year survival following left ventricular aneurysm resection is about 65%, which compares favorably to 47% for those treated medically. Again, left ventricular dysfunction is the most important predictor of decreased long-term survival.

PERICARDITIS

GENERAL CONSIDERATIONS

Acute pericarditis is an inflammation of the parietal and visceral layers of the pericardium. The majority of cases are idiopathic, with generally a benign course. Other etiologies include infectious processes (viral or bacterial infection, tuberculosis, or rheumatic fever), uremia, neoplasm, trauma, myocardial infarction, and postcardiotomy syndrome. Most patients with pericarditis can be treated conservatively with medical therapy. Complications of pericarditis requiring surgical intervention include cardiac tamponade, chronic pericardial effusion, and chronic constrictive pericarditis.

CLINICAL EVALUATION

Typically, patients with acute pericarditis experience chest pain that is exacerbated in a supine position. Dyspnea may result from chest wall splinting. On physical examination, a pericardial rub is usually present. Although fever is variable, leukocytosis is a common finding. The ECG characteristically demonstrates diffuse ST segment elevation. Chest x-ray is normally unremarkable except in cases of chronic effusion or calcific constriction. Echocardiography is most useful for detection of a pericardial effusion. Diagnosis can be made by either pericardiocentesis and, if necessary, by open or thoracoscopic pericardial biopsy.

COMPLICATIONS

Acute Cardiac Tamponade
Cardiac tamponade can result from rapid accumulation of pericardial fluid or addition of a small amount of fluid to a large chronic effusion. This leads to an elevation of intrapericardial pressure, which interferes with diastolic filling and reduces stroke volume. If untreated, cardiac output continues to fall, with ensuing hypotension and circulatory compromise.

The patient may appear agitated and confused. The classic findings of Beck's triad, which include distant heart sounds, distended neck veins, and hypotension, are variable. Pulse pressure is narrow, and **pulsus paradoxus**, defined as an inspiratory decrease in arterial systolic blood pressure of more than 10 mm Hg, may also be present. Echocardiography characteristically demonstrates

right atrial and right ventricular diastolic collapse. Hemodynamic measurement on cardiac catheterization reveals elevation and equilibration of intrapericardial and intracardiac pressures.

Chronic Pericardial Effusion
Chronic pericardial effusion is a nonspecific response to inflammation of the pericardium, most commonly from neoplastic, uremic, and idiopathic causes. The amount of fluid that can accumulate without cardiac tamponade depends upon the compliance and distensibility of the pericardium. When the effusion becomes hemodynamically significant, the patient may develop fatigue, dyspnea, and anorexia. Examination demonstrates Beck's triad, ascites, hepatomegaly, and peripheral edema.

A widened cardiac silhouette is usually seen on chest x-ray. Electrocardiogram is remarkable for diffuse decreased voltage. Echocardiography is commonly used to confirm the diagnosis and demonstrate any right atrial and right ventricular compression suggestive of cardiac tamponade. Right heart catheterization can also be performed to establish the hemodynamic significance of the effusion.

Chronic Constrictive Pericarditis
Constrictive pericarditis is caused by chronic inflammation of the pericardium, resulting in marked thickening with or without calcification of the pericardium. The process involves both parietal and visceral pericardium with encasement of the heart. The main physiologic consequence is impairment of ventricular filling. In the past, tuberculous pericarditis was the most common cause of chronic constrictive pericarditis. Today, most cases in the United States are idiopathic.

Typically, the patient presents with gradual onset of fatigue and dyspnea on exertion, followed by signs and symptoms of systemic venous hypertension. Eventually, hepatomegaly and ascites develop, with or without peripheral edema. Physical examination demonstrates distended neck veins and pulsus paradoxus only in the presence of sinus rhythm. Auscultation of the heart is remarkable for inspiratory splitting of the first heart sound, a loud third heart sound, or a pericardial knock due to rapid ventricular filling in early diastole.

Chest x-ray is only useful if it demonstrates calcification of the pericardium. Echocardiography, CT, or MRI is helpful in confirming the presence of a thickened pericardium. The diagnosis of constrictive pericarditis is made definitively by cardiac catheterization. The classic finding is the characteristic early right ventricular dip and plateau or the square root pattern in the right ventricular pressure tracing. The reflects a prominent descent of rapid ventricular filling, followed by an elevated diastolic plateau. There are also elevation and equalization of mean right atrial, pulmonary artery wedge, right ventricular, and left ventricular end-diastolic pressures.

TREATMENT & RESULTS

Most cases of acute pericarditis are self-limited and respond well to conservative management with bed rest and nonsteroidal anti-inflammatory agents for pain. When a specific cause is identified, direct therapy, such as dialysis or antibiotics, is undertaken. Occasionally, corticosteroids may be used for idiopathic acute pericarditis, but with high relapse rates.

Pericardiocentesis is employed to obtain fluid for diagnosis or treatment of a hemodynamically significant chronic pericardial effusion. Recurrent effusions can be treated with repeat pericardiocentesis or a pericardial window draining into either the pleural space or peritoneal cavity. Occasionally, sclerosing agents can be instilled into the pericardial space with a drainage catheter for malignant pericardial effusions.

Acute cardiac tamponade or chronic pericardial effusions manifesting tamponade physiology mandate immediate decompression of the pericardial space. Pericardiocentesis may be performed to improve hemodynamics until any necessary definitive surgical measures can be taken. These include immediate bedside sternotomy in postoperative cardiac surgery patients, left thoracotomy for trauma patients with suspected cardiac tamponade, or subxiphoid pericardial drainage in those with chronic pericardial effusions.

In general, pericardiectomy is indicated for patients diagnosed with chronic constrictive pericarditis. Because of the underlying myocardial dysfunction in patients with radiation-induced constrictive pericarditis, operation is delayed until symptoms are advanced, and it is certain that the symptoms are attributable to pericardial constriction. The procedure entails complete removal of the pericardium over the cardiac chambers and great vessels, extending from pulmonary veins on the right side to those on the left via a sternotomy or an anterior left thoracotomy. Pericardiectomy is usually followed by brisk diuresis and symptomatic improvement. Incomplete response is usually due to inadequate decortication of the ventricles, failure to remove the layer of constrictive epicardium, or underlying myocardial dysfunction or atrophy.

Pericardiectomy carries an operative mortality rate of 5–15%. The majority of postoperative deaths are due to low cardiac output syndrome. Significant predictors of higher operative risk include more advanced NYHA functional class symptoms, elevated right ventricular end-diastolic pressure (> 30 mm Hg), and radiation-induced pericardial constriction. The time-related survival estimates, including hospital deaths at 5 and 10 years, are approximately 75% and 65%, respectively. In favorable cases, these figures approach those of an age-, race-, and gender-matched population. Advanced preoperative NYHA functional class has also been identified as a risk factor for late death after operation. Thus, early pericardiectomy is recommended before dense fibrosis and myocardial atrophy develop.

CARDIAC TUMORS

GENERAL CONSIDERATIONS

Cardiac neoplasms are relatively uncommon, with metastatic disease 20–40 times more frequent than primary cardiac tumors. Tumors of the heart can produce a variety of clinical symptoms or may remain asymptomatic until they become large. If pedunculated, a tumor may cause valvular dysfunction or ventricular outflow tract obstruction, resulting in signs of either left or right heart failure. If friable, it can embolize to either the systemic or pulmonary circulation. If the tumor is invasive, it can produce a cardiomyopathy or it may involve the conduction system, leading to arrhythmias or heart block. Extension to the epicardial surface can result in hemopericardium and cardiac tamponade as well as pericardial constriction. Finally, cardiac tumors can be manifested primarily by constitutional symptoms of fever, malaise, fatigue, and weight loss.

BENIGN TUMORS

Of the primary cardiac tumors, 75% are benign, with myxomas comprising approximately 50%. In the pediatric age group, rhabdomyoma predominates and is frequently associated with tuberous sclerosis. Other less frequent benign tumors include lipoma, papillary fibroelastoma, hemangioma, fibroma, AV node mesothelioma, teratoma, and granular cell tumor.

MYXOMAS

Myxomas are the most common benign cardiac tumors. Grossly, they are usually pedunculated, gelatinous masses with a short fibrovascular attachment. Approximately 75% arise from the fossa ovalis of the left atrium and another 20% from the right atrium. Sporadic cases of myxomas are usually seen in young women while familial myxomas tend to occur in younger men and are frequently multicentric. The most common presentation is obstruction of the mitral valve, causing congestive heart failure symptoms that mimic mitral stenosis. Systemic embolization has been reported to occur in 25–40% of patients, most commonly to the brain and kidneys. The majority of patients also manifest various constitutional symptoms with nonspecific laboratory findings.

Auscultatory examination frequently reveals an accentuated first heart sound and a diastolic murmur. Occasionally, an early diastolic "tumor plop" may be present. Change in the murmur with time and position is suggestive of a myxoma. The most commonly employed noninvasive modality for the diagnosis of myxoma is echocardiography, with sensitivity approaching 100%. Although CT and MRI can provide additional information regarding extent of tumor involvement, the diagnosis is made by echocardiography in the majority of cases.

Treatment of choice for myxomas is surgical en bloc resection without fragmentation. The overall operative mortality is less than 5%. The early postoperative course is frequently complicated by supraventricular tachyarrhythmias, occasionally requiring long-term antiarrhythmic medications. After resection, most patients are cured, with an actuarial 20-year survival of greater than 90%. The recurrence rate is 1–3% and is higher for the familial form of myxomas. It is thought that tumor recurrence is most likely to be related to multicentric growth rather than tumor implantation or inadequate resection.

MALIGNANT TUMORS

Primary cardiac malignancies comprise 25% of all primary cardiac tumors. Of these, sarcomas account for 80% with angiosarcoma being the most frequent, followed by rhabdomyosarcoma. They are rapidly invasive and usually in an advanced metastatic stage when diagnosed. Although echocardiography is the preferred screening test, contrast-enhanced CT or MRI can more accurately delineate the extent of intramyocardial or mediastinal invasion. Prognosis is dismal, with poor clinical response to chemotherapy and radiotherapy. However, symptomatic relief can occasionally be obtained surgically, despite incomplete resection.

ANGIOSARCOMA

Angiosarcoma is the most common primary malignant cardiac tumor and occurs with the highest frequency in middle-aged men. Approximately 75% arise from the right atrium and invade the venae cavae, tricuspid valve, and pericardium, causing symptoms of right heart failure. Metastases to the lung, liver, or brain are not uncommon. Although chemotherapy and irradiation may be of some benefit, most patients die of local invasion within a year of diagnosis. Cardiac transplantation has not been associated with prolonged survival.

METASTATIC TUMORS

Although metastatic involvement of the heart is infrequently encountered clinically, cardiac metastases are noted in approximately 10–20% of patients dying of disseminated cancer. Metastatic spread to the heart can occur hematogeneously, via the lymphatics or by direct invasion, or extend into the right atrium via the inferior vena cava. The most common types of neoplasm that secondarily involve the heart are bronchogenic carcinoma, breast carcinoma, leukemia, lymphoma, and melanoma. The epicardium and pericardium are most frequently affected and may lead to hemorrhagic pericardial effusion and hemodynamic compromise. Extensive infiltration can produce congestive heart failure and cardiac arrhythmias.

Surgical treatment of metastatic cardiac tumors is generally palliative. In those patients with significant pericardial effusion, creation of a pericardial window is frequently effective. Debulking procedures are indicated for those with valvular or outflow tract obstruction. Renal cell carcinomas that extend up the inferior vena cava into the right atrium can often be extracted under CPB and profound hypothermic circulatory arrest, with excellent reported survival rates. While lymphoproliferative metastases may respond to radiotherapy and chemotherapy, solid tumors rarely respond for a substantial period of time. In general, the prognosis for a metastatic cardiac tumor is extremely poor.

SUGGESTED READING

Ameli A, Shah PK: Cardiac tamponade: Pathophysiology, diagnosis, and management. Cardiol Clin 1991;9:665.

Baue AE et al: *Glenn's Thoracic and Cardiovascular Surgery*, 5th ed. Appleton & Lange, 1991.

Bonow RO: Asymptomatic aortic regurgitation: Indications for operation. J Cardiac Surg 1994;9(suppl):170.

Buckberg GD et al: Integrated myocardial management in valvular heart disease. J Heart Valve Dis 1995;4(suppl II):S198.

Carabello BA: Management of valvular regurgitation. Curr Opin Cardiol 1995;10:124.

CASS Principal Investigators and Their Associates: Coronary artery surgery study (CASS): A randomized trial and coronary artery bypass surgery. Survival data. Circulation 1983;68:939.

Dake MD et al: Transluminal placement of endovascular stent-grafts for the treatment of descending thoracic aortic aneurysms. N Engl J Med 1994;331:1729.

Dion R: Ischemic mitral regurgitation: When and how should it be corrected? J Heart Valve Dis 1993;2:536.

European Coronary Surgery Study Group: Long-term results of prospective randomized study of coronary artery bypass surgery in stable angina pectoris. Lancet 1982;2:1173.

Fananapazir L et al: Long-term results of dual-chamber (DDD) pacing in obstructive hypertrophic cardiomyopathy. Evidence for progressive symptomatic and hemodynamic improvement and reduction of left ventricular hypertrophy. Circulation 1994;90:2731.

Fann JI et al: Surgical management of aortic dissection during a 30-year period. Circulation 1995;92(suppl II):II-113.

Fowler NO: Constrictive pericarditis: Its history and current status. Clin Cardiol 1995;18:341.

Fraser CD Jr et al: Repair of insufficient bicuspid aortic valves. Ann Thorac Surg 1994;58:386.

Grossi EA et al: Endoventricular remodeling of left ventricular aneurysm. Functional, clinical, and electrophysiological results. Circulation 1995;92(suppl II):II-98.

Jamieson WR: Modern cardiac valve devices—bioprostheses and mechanical prostheses: State of the art. J Cardiac Surg 1993;8:89.

Kratz J: Evaluation and management of tricuspid valve disease. Cardiol Clin 1991;9:397.

Odell JA, Orszulak TA: Surgical repair and reconstruction of valvular lesions. Curr Opin Cardiol 1995;10:135.

Palacios IF: Percutaneous mitral balloon valvotomy for patients with mitral stenosis. Curr Opin Cariol 1994;9:164.

Reynen K: Cardiac myxomas. N Engl J Med 1995;333:1610.

Robbins RC, Stinson EB: Long-term results of left ventricular myotomy and myectomy for obstructive hypertrophic cardiomyopathy. J Thorac Cardiovasc Surg 1996;111:586.

Safian RD, Kuntz RE, Berman AD: Aortic valvuloplasty. Cardiol Clin 1991;9:289.

Stone PH: Management of the patient with asymptomatic aortic stenosis. J Cardiac Surg 1994;9(suppl):139.

Svensson LG, Crawford ES: Aortic dissection and aortic aneurysm surgery: Clinical observations, experimental investigations, and statistical analyses—Part III. Curr Prob Surg 1993;30:1.

Vaitkus PT et al: Treatment of malignant pericardial effusion. JAMA 1994;272:59.

Yacoub M et al: Fourteen-year experience with homovital homografts for aortic valve replacement. J Thorac Cardiovasc Surg 1995;110:186.

37.2 Congenital Disease of the Heart

Robert C. Robbins, MD, David D. Yuh, MD, & Bruce A. Reitz, MD

▶ Key Facts

▶ Congenital heart disease is estimated to occur in 40,000 (1%) of new babies annually. Approximately 50% of these children will require treatment in the first year of life.

▶ Congestive heart failure in infants is manifested by poor weight gain, tachypnea, irritability, and slow feeding associated with diaphoresis.

▶ Exertion dyspnea, chest pain, syncope, and palpitations are common symptoms of older children with congenital heart disease.

▶ In neonates with congenital heart disease, cyanosis can be episodic and associated with feeding and crying.

▶ The most common obstructive lesions include valvular pulmonary stenosis (10%), coarctation of the aorta (6.5%), valvular aortic stenosis (5%), and pulmonary atresia with intact ventricular septum (1–1.5%).

▶ The most common left-to-right shunts or acyanotic defects include ventricular septal defects (20%), patent ductus arteriosus (12–15%), and atrial septal defects (10–15%).

▶ Rare malformations generally comprise fewer than 1% of congenital heart defects and include cor triatriatum, congenital mitral valve disease, aortic-pulmonary window, aneurysm of the sinus of Valsalva, double-inlet single ventricle, Ebstein's anomaly, anomalies of the coronary arteries, double outlet right ventricle, hypoplastic left heart syndrome, and congenitally corrected transposition of the great arteries.

There are approximately 4 million live births per year in the United States. Congenital heart disease is estimated to occur in 40,000 new babies (1%) annually. Approximately one half of these children will require treatment in the first year of life. The frequency is about ten times greater among members of the same family than in the general population. Virtually all fetal cardiac structures are formed between the third and eighth week of pregnancy; however, in most cases of congenital heart disease, a specific etiologic factor cannot be determined. Although the large number of congenital cardiac anomalies that have been described can be somewhat daunting, a relatively small number of defects comprise the majority of abnormalities seen. These include ventricular septal defect, atrial septal defect, pulmonic valvular stenosis, aortic valvular stenosis, patent ductus arteriosus, coarctation of the aorta, and *d*-transposition of the great arteries. This section describes the pathophysiology, diagnosis, and treatment of the majority of congenital heart defects encountered in an active pediatric cardiac clinical setting.

THE PEDIATRIC CARDIAC PATIENT: GENERAL CONSIDERATIONS

SIGNS & SYMPTOMS

Most neonates with congenital heart disease are initially referred for evaluation because of cyanosis, congestive heart failure (CHF), or detection of a precordial murmur. CHF in infants is manifested by poor weight gain, tachypnea, irritability, and slow feeding associated with diaphoresis. Cyanosis can be episodic and associated with feeding and crying. Exertion dyspnea, chest pain, syncope, and palpitations are common symptoms of older children with congenital heart disease.

Clinical signs of congenital heart disease are generally apparent with a concentrated physical examination. A complete set of vital signs, including four extremity blood pressure measurements, should be obtained. A pulse oximeter can provide accurate assessment of the systemic oxygen saturations and is particularly useful in cyanotic patients. Careful precordial auscultation can detect characteristic murmurs, gallops, or rales suggestive of cardiac abnormalities. Hepatomegaly is a sensitive sign of CHF in young children and underscores the need for a complete abdominal examination. The quality and strength of peripheral pulses can be particularly helpful in the diagnosis of obstructive aortic anomalies.

DIAGNOSTIC STUDIES

Routine Studies

A routine chest radiograph should be obtained in patients with suspected congenital heart disease. Cardiac size and contour, aortic position, and patterns of pulmonary vasculature are important points of assessment. Many of the most frequently observed congenital cardiac abnormalities can be classified into lesions with normal, increased (left-to-right shunt), or decreased pulmonary flow (right-to-left shunt). Electrocardiograms can assess rhythm, ischemic changes, axis, and chamber hypertrophy and should be obtained in children with a history and physical findings suggestive of cardiac pathology.

Specialized Studies

Echocardiography should be performed in all suspected cases of congenital heart disease. Technologic advancements combined with increased clinical experience with echocardiography has resulted in a high degree of diagnostic specificity for the majority of congenital cardiac lesions. Most cases can be referred for operative intervention based on solid echocardiographic data combined with the other routine evaluations. This is especially true for most neonatal anomalies where cardiac catheterization may be detrimental in these critically ill babies.

Although most congenital cardiac lesions can be reliably diagnosed by echocardiography, cardiac catheterization is essential for the evaluation of many specific aspects of congenital heart disease. Cardiac catheterization is required for measurement of intracardiac pressures, calculation of intracardiac shunts, and assessment of pulmonary vascular resistance. In addition, definition of coronary and pulmonary artery anatomy is best achieved with angiographic contrast studies. Catheterization is often necessary in cases where the echocardiographic diagnosis is uncertain. Magnetic resonance imaging (MRI) is emerging as an important adjunct to catheterization and may play an important role in the future.

PREOPERATIVE MANAGEMENT

The medical management of congenital heart disease is primarily focused on the treatment of CHF. Decongestive therapy with digoxin, diuretics, and afterload reduction is generally effective for the treatment of most left-to-right shunting lesions. The use of indomethacin for the closure of patent ductus arteriosus in newborns has utility in selected cases. The intravenous infusion of prostaglandin E_1 (PGE_1) has had a dramatic effect on the management of infants with ductal-dependent circulation. PGE_1 is specifically useful in aortic obstructive lesions for the maintenance of distal perfusion and to assure adequate pulmonary perfusion in lesions that limit pulmonary flow. This permits stabilization and preoperative optimization of patients. The use of inotropic support and endotracheal intubation for critical ill patients can be beneficial in preparation for operative intervention and as primary therapy for certain anomalies. The use of pulmonary vasodilatation with oxygen, hyperventilation, nitrates, PGE_1, and inhaled nitric oxide can be useful in the management of pulmonary hypertension.

The timing of operative repair for congenital heart disease is related to the efficacy of medical therapy. Obstructed total anomalous pulmonary venous connection and critical aortic stenosis are indications for emergent operative intervention because of the lack of any effective medical therapy. The inability to restore or maintain patency of the ductus arteriosus in ductal-dependent lesions additionally constitutes the need for immediate operative treatment. Ductal-dependent lesions that can be stabilized with PGE_1 need intervention on a semi-elective basis. Hypercyanotic episodes in patients with tetralogy of Fallot represent an indication for urgent operation.

Patients with *d*-transposition of the great arteries and truncus arteriosus should generally undergo elective operation soon after the diagnosis is made. Patients with significant left-to-right shunts are usually effectively managed with decongestive therapy and brought to operation if medical management fails. Overall, there is an evolving strategy for the early operative intervention of most congenital heart defects.

INTRAOPERATIVE MANAGEMENT

Intraoperative management of congenital heart disease involves the coordination of the surgical team, anesthesiologists, and perfusionists. Careful induction of general anesthesia and placement of arterial and venous monitoring lines are imperative prior to commencement of the operation. It is important, particularly in children with right-to-left intracardiac shunting, that air bubbles are not inadvertently introduced into any intravenous lines since systemic embolization could result from this; specially designed filters can be used to prevent this. All intracardiac repairs require cardiopulmonary bypass (CPB). Venous drainage cannulae are placed in the right atrium or directly into the vena cavae. Blood flows into the heart-lung machine by gravity drainage. An oxygenator removes carbon dioxide and adds oxygen to the blood prior to infusion into the ascending aorta via an arterial cannula. The heart-lung machine, therefore, takes over cardiopulmonary function to facilitate the operative repair.

Systemic hypothermia is accomplished with a cooling unit integrated into the bypass apparatus. This lowers the metabolic demands of the patient and allows for reduced arterial flow, which decreases the amount of blood returning to the operative field. In addition to providing better visibility to perform the operation, systemic hypothermia is an adjunct to myocardial protection. The majority of cases require a motionless, bloodless operative field, which is achieved by clamping the aorta proximal to the arterial perfusion cannula. Myocardial protection is accomplished by the instillation of a cold hyperkalemic cardioplegia solution into the aortic root proximal to the aortic cross-clamp. This produces diastolic arrest of the heart and maintains the myocardial temperature at about 10–15°C during the repair.

Aortic arch reconstruction, repair of total anomalous pulmonary venous connection, and intracardiac repairs performed in patients weighing less than 3 kg are facilitated with a period of profound hypothermia, exsanguination, and total circulatory arrest. The generally accepted safe period for circulatory arrest is approximately 45 minutes at core temperatures of 15–18°C. This is usually well tolerated but may result in early postoperative seizures or other neurologic complications.

The use of epidural anesthesia for non-CPB pediatric cardiac operations is helpful, especially with thoracotomy incisions. It provides excellent intraoperative and postoperative pain control and facilitates early extubation. We have extended the use of supplemental regional anesthesia to all routine CPB cases, including Fontan procedures, with satisfactory results.

Transesophageal echocardiography is an invaluable tool for the intraoperative evaluation of operative repairs. Assessment of ventricular function, residual septal defects, valvular regurgitation, and residual obstructive lesions should be performed routinely.

POSTOPERATIVE MANAGEMENT

Use of supplemental regional anesthesia to facilitate intraoperative or early postoperative extubation requires careful patient selection. Excellent communication and cooperation between surgeon, anesthesiologist, and intensivist is mandatory. This patient management strategy can simplify postoperative management and decrease hospital stays in selected routine cases. Even without regional anesthesia, most routine cases are extubated within 24 hours postoperatively. Early extubation is especially beneficial with cavopulmonary connection procedures (eg, bidirectional Glenn shunts and Fontan procedures) because of improved pulmonary flow in the absence of positive pressure ventilation. Neonates and more complex procedures usually require longer periods of ventilatory support, especially in the presence of reactive pulmonary hypertension or persistent pulmonary congestion.

Most patients will return to the intensive care unit with arterial and central venous monitoring lines. Transthoracic left atrial and pulmonary artery lines can be useful in the postoperative management of patients with left ventricular dysfunction or pulmonary hypertension. The presence of hypotension and a low left atrial pressure (< 3–5 mm Hg) indicates hypovolemia. A combination of hypotension and a high left atrial pressure generally is indicative of left ventricular dysfunction requiring inotropic support. The majority of routine cases require minimal inotropic support. More complex repairs will generally need some degree of inotropic support with dopamine, dobutamine, epinephrine, a phosphodiesterase inhibitor, or a combination of these drugs, depending on institutional preferences.

Frequent detailed assessment of cardiac output is essential in the management of critically ill children following cardiac operations. Persistent metabolic acidosis, poor peripheral perfusion, and diminished urine output (< 1 cc/kg/h) are signs of inadequate cardiac output. Hypovolemia, poor ventricular function, increased pulmonary resistance, cardiac tamponade, and residual cardiac defects should all be considered as potential causes. Central venous, pulmonary artery, left atrial, and systemic arterial pressures are helpful in making the correct diagnosis and guiding therapy. Echocardiography should be utilized for the evaluation of persistently low cardiac output. Prolonged unexplained requirements of inotropic and ventilatory support should be investigated with cardiac catheterization.

Profound ventricular failure, persistent hypoxia, or supersystemic pulmonary hypertension unresponsive to inhaled nitric oxide may be an indication for a period of extracorporeal membrane oxygenation (ECMO) support. Survival following postcardiotomy ECMO support is approximately 50%, with recovery usually seen within 5–7 days.

Significant postoperative hemorrhage is unusual following most pediatric cardiac surgical procedures but may be problematic in cyanotic patients. Bleeding in excess of 3–5 cc/kg/h over 3–4 hours following operation or any sudden episode of significant chest tube drainage should be treated with reexploration. The coagulation profile should be normalized and platelet infusion administered during the immediate postoperative period, however, prolonged periods of bleeding are not well tolerated, especially in critically ill neonates.

OBSTRUCTIVE LESIONS

The most common obstructive lesions include valvular pulmonary stenosis, pulmonary atresia with intact ventricular septum, valvular aortic stenosis, and coarctation of the aorta. These malformations impede systolic ventricular emptying, which generally results in hypertrophy of the affected ventricle. Although cardiac enlargement is usually not readily apparent with chest radiography, ventricular hypertrophy can be assessed with electrocardiography and echocardiography (Table 37.2–1).

PULMONIC VALVULAR STENOSIS

General Considerations

Congenital maldevelopment of the pulmonary valve can result in stenosis. It is a common defect, constituting about 10% of congenital heart defects. No known developmental cause has been identified, however, rubella infection during pregnancy has been implicated. There is a wide spectrum of pulmonary valvular stenoses, ranging from a mild degree of leaflet adhesion to a completely imperforate valve observed in pulmonary atresia. The severity of stenosis varies considerably and is most simply de-

fined by determining the systolic pressure gradient between the right ventricle and pulmonary artery. Mild, clinically insignificant stenosis is associated with a peak systolic gradient less than 50 mm Hg. The obstruction to blood flow produces elevated right ventricular pressures and hypertrophy. Critical stenosis may be present in the newborn period and requires immediate intervention.

Diagnosis

The clinical presentation of patients varies widely according to the degree of stenosis. In mild stenosis, the right ventricle is enlarged but functions adequately, resulting in an asymptomatic patient. Overall, 30–40% of patients with severe pulmonary stenosis beyond the neonatal period are asymptomatic when first examined. With moderate stenosis, the right ventricle gradually hypertrophies, resulting in symptoms of dyspnea and easy fatigability because of inadequate pulmonary flow, especially with physical exertion. Neonates with severe pulmonary stenosis are critically ill, irritable, tachypneic, and cyanotic as the result of right-to-left shunting at the atrial level. Patients with long-standing stenosis may experience angina and arrhythmias.

A left parasternal systolic flow murmur with a substernal right ventricular lift are characteristic physical findings of pulmonary stenosis. Right ventricular hypertrophy (RVH) with right axis deviation and occasionally right atrial enlargement are typical electrocardiographic findings. Enlargement of the main pulmonary artery from poststenotic dilatation and right ventricular enlargement on the lateral projection may be observed with chest radiography. Echocardiography is usually diagnostic, with demonstration of pulmonary valve abnormalities and increased valvular gradients. Cardiac catheterization is performed when intervention is indicated from echocardiographic data and history.

Treatment

Intervention is generally not recommended in asymptomatic patients with mild pulmonary stenosis. Pulmonary valvotomy is indicated in symptomatic patients or in patients with severe pulmonary stenosis (transvalvular gradient > 50 mm Hg). In cases of critical pulmonary stenosis in neonates, valvotomy must be performed in the first few days or weeks of life.

Percutaneous balloon valvuloplasty is extremely effective in relieving the valvular gradient and is the treatment of choice. Open valvotomy is reserved for percutaneous failures. In open pulmonary valvotomy, the stenotic pulmonary valve is approached through a vertical pulmonary arteriotomy and its fused leaflets opened with a knife blade. Adequate opening of the valve is of paramount importance; portions of the valve may be excised if other methods fail to achieve a wide opening. The procedure is performed with CPB support and without aortic crossclamping.

Table 37.2–1. Obstructive lesions.

Defect	Incidence (%)	Pathophysiology	Signs & Symptoms	Diagnostic Tests	Treatment	Operative Results
Pulmonic valvular stenosis	10	Stenotic pulmonary valve obstructs RV emptying and pulmonary blood flow, producing RVH	Initially asymptomatic followed by dyspnea and fatigue, systolic left parasternal murmur, substernal lift	ECG: RVH Echo: Abnormal pulmonary valve, RVH, transvalvular gradient Cath: RV->pulmonary artery gradient	Percutaneous balloon valvuloplasty; open pulmonary valvotomy for percutaneous failures	Mortality < 1%; good long-term results
Pulmonary atresia with intact ventricular septum	1–1.5	Atretic pulmonary valve and RV and tricuspid valve hypoplasia leads to inadequate pulmonary blood flow and hypoxia	Severe cyanosis	CXR: "Boot-shaped" heart ECG: RA enlargement, RVH Echo: Absent pulmonary valve, hypoplastic RV or PA (rare), abnormal tricuspid valve	Stage 1: Systemic-PA shunt (eg, Blalock-Taussig) w/ or w/o transannular patching Stage 2: Bidirectional Glenn shunt or biventricular repair (adequate RV) Stage 3: Fontan procedure or biventricular repair	Perioperative mortality 20%
Left ventricular outflow tract obstruction	5	Obstruction of left ventricular outflow tract produces LVH	Pulmonary congestion, diminished peripheral pulses, right parasternal systolic murmur	CXR: Pulmonic congestion ECG: LVH w/ strain pattern Echo: Bicuspid or abnormal Ao valve, subaortic membrane or septal hypertrophy, LVH Cath: LV->Ao gradient	Aortic valvotomy; AVR; resection of subaortic membrane or septal hypertrophy; patch enlargement of ascending Ao	Perioperative mortality 2–5% (> 1 yr old), 10–35% (neonates esp. w/ associated defects)
Coarctation of the aorta	6.5	Narrowed Ao produces obstruction to blood flow and LVH	Upper extremity hypertension w/ diminished lower extremity pulses, fatigue, diminished growth, CHF	CXR: LVH, "3" sign, rib notching ECG: RVH (infants), LVH (older children) Echo: Ao narrowing w/ ↑ gradient; bicuspid Ao valve, LVH Cath: Gradient across coarctation	Resection with end-to-end anastomosis; subclavian flap augmentation	Mortality 1–3% (older children), 5–10% (w/ associated defects); recurrence 5–20%
Vascular rings and slings	< 1	Maldevelopment of embryonic Ao arches, producing vascular ring/sling around esophagus and/or trachea	Tracheal and esophageal compression leading to respiratory distress, recurrent infections, and dysphagia	CXR: Tracheal compression, right Ao arch or ill-defined arch w/ double arch vascular ring Barium swallow: Diagnostic; posterior esophageal compression (ring), anterior esophageal compression (sling) CT/MRI: Diagnostic confirmation	Division of vascular ring/sling	Mortality 1–2%; good long-term results

Ao = aorta/aortic; AVR = aortic valve replacement; CHF = congestive heart failure; CXR = chest x-ray; ECG = electrocardiogram; LA = left atrium; LV = left ventricle; PA = pulmonary artery; RA = right atrium; RV = right ventricle; RVH/LVH = right/left ventricular hypertrophy.

Results

Mortality after percutaneous or open valvotomy for pulmonary stenosis approaches zero. Immediate and durable relief of the gradient is usually obtained. Most patients with a normally developed right ventricle experience excellent late functional results with normal exercise capacity.

PULMONARY ATRESIA WITH INTACT VENTRICULAR SEPTUM

General Considerations

Pulmonary atresia with intact ventricular septum is a rare congenital malformation, comprising 1–1.5% of all defects, and represents the most extreme lesion in the spectrum of pulmonary stenosis. The pulmonary valve is atretic, with no flow from the right ventricle to the main pulmonary artery. This results in varying degrees of right ventricular and tricuspid valve hypoplasia.

Associated cardiac malformations include a tricuspid valve with thickened, incompletely separated leaflets, abnormal chordae, and a small annular diameter. The right ventricular cavity is usually diminished in size secondary to massive ventricular wall hypertrophy. Approximately 50% of patients with pulmonary atresia and intact ventricular septum display coronary sinusoids with right ventricular-coronary artery fistulae on cineangiography, and 10% possess a right ventricular-dependent coronary circulation. Cumulatively, these malformations markedly compromise pulmonary blood flow. Pulmonary atresia with intact ventricular septum is associated with a high early mortality, with 2-week and 6-month survival rates of 50% and 15%, respectively. Death is caused by severe hypoxia and metabolic acidosis that usually results from spontaneous closure of the ductus arteriosus. Continuous infusion of PGE_1 is instituted in affected neonates to maintain ductus patency.

Diagnosis

Infants with pulmonary atresia and intact ventricular septum initially appear normal except for cyanosis. Cyanosis is usually obvious on the first day of life and, as the ductus closes, rapidly becomes more severe with resultant respiratory distress and metabolic acidosis. Classically, chest radiography reveals clear lung fields with a flat or concave pulmonary artery segment producing a "boot-shaped" heart. Electrocardiographic evidence of right atrial enlargement is common, with occasional signs of RVH. Two-dimensional echocardiography is diagnostic and can be used to measure the dimensions of the tricuspid valve. Furthermore, right ventricular-coronary artery fistulae may be identified. Once a diagnosis of pulmonary atresia with intact ventricular septum is made, cardiac catheterization and angiography are used to find coronary arterial stenoses, coronary sinusoids, and right ventricular-coronary artery fistulae. Furthermore, the size, configuration, and function of the right ventricle are also determined.

Treatment

Without treatment, pulmonary atresia with intact ventricular septum is uniformly fatal. The initial operation is based on evaluation of the likelihood of a subsequent biventricular repair which is, in turn, determined by tricuspid valve annular size, right ventricular size, and whether or not there is a well formed infundibular component to the right ventricle. Concomitant pulmonary transannular patching and systemic-pulmonary artery shunting are performed in patients thought to have some chance of eventual right ventricular growth leading to a two-ventricle circulation. Patients with severe hypoplasia of the tricuspid valve and right ventricle initially receive a systemic-pulmonary artery shunt without decompression of the hypertensive right ventricle. The modified **Blalock-Taussig shunt** is constructed with a Gore-Tex tube graft placed between the innominate-subclavian artery junction and right pulmonary artery. Cardiac catheterization and echocardiography are subsequently performed at 3–6 months to assess right ventricular growth and pulmonary artery anatomy. Patients with poor right ventricular growth should have a superior vena cava-pulmonary artery bidirectional Glenn shunt performed at 4–6 months, followed by a completion Fontan operation at 18–24 months.

The **Fontan operation** consists of directing systemic venous return to the pulmonary artery, effectively bypassing the right heart. Several variations of the original operation described by Fontan in 1971 employ anastomoses from the right atrium or venae cavae to the right pulmonary artery. The preference at Stanford is an extracardiac inferior vena cava-to-pulmonary artery connection in the Fontan operation (Figure 37.2–1). The inferior vena cava is transected at the junction of the right atrium. A Gore-Tex tube graft is then interposed end-to-end between the inferior vena cava and the inferior surface of the right pulmonary artery. The operation is conducted with CPB support and has the advantage of not requiring aortic cross-clamping.

Patients in whom the right ventricle is deemed adequate to support a biventricular circulation should undergo trial occlusion of the shunt and interatrial communication. If the systemic blood pressure and arterial oxygen saturation are maintained and the right atrial pressure does not significantly rise, then plans should be made for a biventricular repair consisting of permanent closure of the shunt and interatrial communication.

A small subset of patients may potentially be converted to "one-and-a-half ventricle repair." These are patients who have some growth of the right ventricle but not enough to support total systemic venous return. In this repair, a superior vena cava-pulmonary artery bidirectional connection is performed and the interatrial communication is closed so that the right ventricle supports only inferior vena caval return to the pulmonary circulation.

Patients with right ventricular-dependent coronary circulation are at risk of myocardial ischemia and death. Some centers have recommended cardiac transplantation

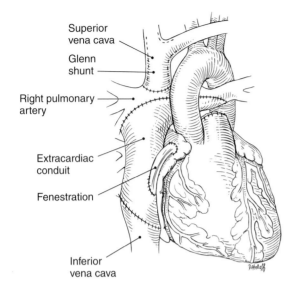

Superior
vena cava

Glenn
shunt

Right pulmonary
artery

Extracardiac
conduit

Fenestration

Inferior
vena cava

Figure 37.2–1. The extracardiac Fontan operation with placement of an extracardiac conduit between the inferior vena cava and the inferior aspect of the right pulmonary artery. A previously constructed bidirectional Glenn shunt between the superior vena cava and right pulmonary artery is also illustrated. A fenestration placed between the conduit and the right atrium serves to reduce systemic venous pressure in the early postoperative period.

for this subset of patients. Satisfactory results have been achieved with initial shunting and tracking toward an eventual modified Fontan procedure. This seems to be a reasonable approach to this high-risk cohort of patients in view of the critical shortage of donors.

Results

The overall perioperative mortality among neonates treated for pulmonary atresia with intact ventricular septum is about 20%. The 1-, 2-, and 4-year survival rates among a heterogeneous group of treated patients are 70%, 65%, and 60%, respectively.

LEFT VENTRICULAR OUTFLOW TRACT OBSTRUCTION

General Considerations

Congenital aortic stenosis represents a group of malformations that obstruct blood flow from the left ventricle to the aorta. These malformations are classified as supravalvular, valvular, discrete subvalvular, and hypertrophic muscular subaortic stenosis. These defects comprise approximately 5% of congenital heart defects. Approximately 25% of patients diagnosed with congenital aortic stenosis have other cardiovascular defects, includ-

ing coarctation of the aorta, patent ductus arteriosus, ventricular septal defect, and pulmonary stenosis.

In **congenital aortic stenosis**, the left ventricle experiences an increase in pressure and wall tension, leading to left ventricular hypertrophy (LVH). An associated increase in the systolic ejection period necessitates a diminished diastolic interval and, hence, reduction in coronary perfusion. The combined effects of LVH and diminished coronary perfusion lead to left ventricular ischemia and dysfunction.

Diagnosis

Neonates and infants presenting with severe aortic stenosis usually present with pallor, diminished peripheral pulses, dyspnea, and pulmonary congestion. These patients typically develop rapidly progressive CHF and die within a few days or weeks of birth, if no intervention is attempted. Children and young adults may be asymptomatic in cases of mild to moderate stenosis, however, severe stenosis usually manifests as some combination of dyspnea on exertion, angina, and syncope. When symptoms are delayed until the patient is older than 1 year of age, heart failure is rare and survival without treatment is generally prolonged.

Auscultation typically reveals a harsh systolic right parasternal murmur radiating into the carotids with a systolic ejection click. The electrocardiogram and chest film may display characteristics of LVH, however, it is not uncommon for these tests to appear normal. Echocardiography is an excellent means to assess the morphology and severity of the stenotic aortic valve as well as the size, contractility, and wall thickness of the left ventricle. The flow velocity across the stenotic valve and, hence, transvalvular pressure gradient can be estimated. Cardiac catheterization is used to determine the valve area and pressure gradient. A valve area less than $0.5 \text{ cm}^2/\text{m}^2$ or a peak systolic gradient greater than 50–75 mm Hg represents severe stenosis. An elevated left ventricular end-diastolic pressure suggests a left ventricle that is either noncompliant or in failure. These diagnostic data are combined to classify the degree of aortic stenosis as mild, moderate, or severe.

Treatment

The type of operative intervention for congenital aortic stenosis depends upon the type of obstruction present and the patient's age. Neonates with critical aortic valvular stenosis require immediate intervention. Careful echocardiographic examination of left ventricular size is imperative, especially when a large patent ductus arteriosus is present. Patients with small left ventricles may be more effectively treated with the Norwood procedure if there is a predominance of right-to-left shunting at the ductal level. Critical aortic stenosis of the newborn is usually treated with open valvotomy. However, in many centers percutaneous balloon valvuloplasty via the umbilical artery or from the carotid artery has been as effective as the open procedure and is emerging as the treatment of choice. **Open valvotomy** is performed with CPB support, moderated systemic hypothermia, and cardioplegic arrest. This approach involves division of the fused valve commissures exposed through an ascending aortotomy. An alternative approach to open valvotomy is dilation of the valve antegrade through the left ventricular apex with the heart beating during CPB.

Supravalvular aortic stenosis is treated by enlarging the aorta just superior to the aortic annulus with an autologous pericardial patch. Discrete subvalvular stenosis is treated with resection of the obstructing subvalvular membrane. Aortic valve replacement with a mechanical prosthetic valve is a therapeutic option in older children but requires lifelong anticoagulation. Aortic valve replacement by translocation of a pulmonary autograft and replacement of the pulmonary artery root with a cryopreserved homograft, the **Ross procedure**, is an attractive alternative to mechanical valve replacement because anticoagulation is not required and there is the potential for autograft growth. Tunnel subaortic obstruction has traditionally been treated by enlarging the left ventricular outflow tract with the **Konno procedure**, which entails a mechanical aortic valve replacement. The modified Ross-Konno procedure augments the left ventricular outflow tract and uses the pulmonary autograft for aortic valve replacement.

Results

Neonates presenting with critical aortic stenosis have an operative mortality of 10–35% following aortic valvotomy. Percutaneous balloon valvuloplasty may achieve palliation with lower mortality in this group of critically ill patients. Surgical interventions performed beyond the first year of life have a perioperative mortality ranging from 2% to 5%. Patients undergoing aortic valvotomy at an early age may experience recurrent stenosis or aortic insufficiency later in life. Consequently, many of these patients may eventually require aortic valve replacement.

COARCTATION OF THE AORTA

General Considerations

Coarctation of the aorta is a congenital narrowing of the upper descending thoracic aorta, adjacent to the site of attachment of the ductus arteriosus. Rarely, coarctation occurs between the left common carotid and subclavian arteries. The aorta is usually dilated distal to the coarctation. These relatively common defects comprise approximately 6.5% of all congenital heart defects. Approximately 11% of individuals born with coarctation have a coexisting ventricular septal defect (VSD) and about 7% have other significant coexisting intracardiac defects. Coarctation of the aorta is associated with Turner syndrome and Von Recklinghausen's disease. The pathogenesis of coarctation is not clear, however, the prevalent theories have associated the localized narrowing with closure of the ductus arteriosus and patterns of fetal blood flow.

A pressure gradient exists across the length of aortic narrowing that can be quite severe. The luminal cross-sectional area must be reduced by more than 50% before a hemodynamically significant gradient exists, although longer coarctations may result in significant gradients with lesser narrowing. A collateral circulation develops to circumvent significant coarctation and is comprised of enlarged internal mammary, intercostal, subscapular, and other arteries. These vessels become dilated and sometimes aneurysmal and may be a significant source of hemorrhage if not respected during surgical repair.

In 5–10% of infants, left ventricular failure may be severe and even fatal during the first month of life without correction. After the first year of life, CHF rarely occurs before the age of 20. Without treatment, the average life expectancy among these patients is 30–40 years. The most common causes of death include aortic rupture, cardiac failure, intracranial hemorrhage, and bacterial endocarditis.

Diagnosis

Classically, the combination of upper extremity hypertension with absent or diminished lower extremity pulses suggests aortic coarctation. A systolic murmur is usually audible over the left hemithorax. The signs and symptoms of coarctation presenting in the neonate are those of heart failure. In infants, manifestations of severe CHF—including tachypnea, failure to thrive, and frequent respiratory infections—are accompanied by marked cardiomegaly and pulmonary congestion on chest radiography. Electrocardiography reveals signs of RVH as the result of right ventricular-dependent lower body perfusion. Older children and adolescents complain of headaches, lower extremity weakness, dyspnea on exertion, and fatigue.

Electrocardiography and chest films typically reveal signs of LVH from long-standing hypertension. Chest films also may display signs of rib notching and the classic "3" sign produced by the hourglass configuration of the aorta in the region of coarctation. Echocardiography is usually diagnostic, with anatomical definition of the coarctation associated with accelerated pulse Doppler flow. VSD, bicuspid aortic valve, and LVH may be observed. The transverse aortic arch should be carefully assessed. Hypoplasia of the arch requiring arch reconstruction should be considered in neonates if the arch measures (in millimeters) less than 1 plus the infant's weight (in kilograms). Cardiac catheterization is reserved for equivocal echocardiographic findings.

Treatment

Severe CHF in neonates with coarctation warrants immediate operative correction. An extended **end-to-end anastomosis** of the descending aorta to the distal aortic arch with excision of all ductal tissue is the procedure of choice. The graft interposition and subclavian flap aortoplasty techniques are alternative techniques used by some centers. All procedures are performed through a posterolateral thoracotomy in the fourth intercostal space. Some centers have experience with percutaneous balloon dilatation of native coarctation, but, presently, percutaneous procedures are generally limited to the treatment of postoperative recurrence of the coarctation, which is usually related to scarring of residual ductal tissue left at the anastomotic site.

Patients with severe juxtaductal coarctation of the aorta and a large VSD should be treated with repair of both lesions via median sternotomy, with circulatory arrest for the aortic reconstruction. A similar approach should be employed for the repair of coarctation associated with aortic arch hypoplasia.

Results

The overall operative risk is less than 5%. Corrections performed in infants in CHF and with associated cardiac anomalies may incur an operative risk as high as 5–10%. In general, long-term results are satisfactory following surgical correction, however, persistent hypertension requiring medical management and restenosis does occur and may be related to the technique of repair and age at which it was performed. Recurrent coarctation of the aorta occurs in 5–20% of cases and can be effectively managed with percutaneous balloon dilatation.

VASCULAR RINGS & SLINGS

General Considerations

Abnormal regression or persistence among the six primitive aortic arches connecting the dorsal and ventral aortic roots during embryonic development give rise to vascular rings that compress the trachea and/or esophagus. This anomaly comprises less than 1% of congenital heart defects. The most common types of vascular rings are the (1) double aortic arch and (2) right aortic arch with a left-sided ligamentum arteriosus. A pulmonary artery sling is produced by posterior compression of the trachea by the anomalous origin of the left pulmonary artery from the right pulmonary artery. The left pulmonary artery courses between the trachea and esophagus.

Diagnosis

This diagnosis should be suspected in all newborns displaying symptoms of airway obstruction or dysphagia without an obvious cause. Severe respiratory distress and dysphagia may present shortly after birth. In older children and young adults, dysphagia is usually a more prominent symptom. Physical examination reveals sequelae of respiratory distress, including tachypnea, stridor, wheezing, cyanosis, and intercostal retractions. Aspiration pneumonia is another associated finding. The electrocardiogram is usually normal, however, chest radiography may reveal signs of tracheal compression or pneumonia. A barium swallow is extremely useful in detecting both tracheal and esophageal compression. Demonstration of posterior compression of the esophagus is diagnostic of a vascular ring. Anterior compression of the esophagus with posterior encroachment of the trachea is associated with a

pulmonary artery sling. MRI scanning is extremely accurate in demonstrating the anatomical configuration of the ring or sling. Fiberoptic bronchoscopy should be used to look for tracheomalacia, especially in cases of pulmonary artery slings. Echocardiography can identify abnormal arch anatomy and associated intracardiac defects but has limited utility in clearly defining the anatomy of these lesions. Cardiac catheterization is rarely indicated.

Treatment

Patients diagnosed with vascular rings who experience signs and symptoms of tracheal or esophageal compression should undergo operative treatment. The majority of vascular ring anomalies are approached through a left thoracotomy in the fourth intercostal space. In general, the offending vascular ring must be divided to completely relieve any esophageal or tracheal compression and, at the same time, maintain normal perfusion. In most cases, the ligamentum arteriosus (or ductus arteriosus) must be divided to completely free the constricting ring.

In the case of the double aortic arch, the ring is divided at an atretic point usually located distal to the origin of the left subclavian artery on the anterior arch. If no such point exists, the smaller of the anterior or posterior arches is divided. This serves to relieve the compression while maintaining adequate perfusion. Repair of a pulmonary artery sling may be accomplished with division of the left pulmonary artery at the origin from the right pulmonary artery and translocation anterior to the trachea with anastomosis to the main pulmonary artery. Because of the high incidence of tracheomalacia at the site of the sling, an alternative approach is to perform tracheal resection with primary anastomosis of the trachea posterior to the left pulmonary artery. Meticulous attention to postoperative respiratory care, including pulmonary toilet, is essential. The effects of tracheal edema and tracheomalacia due to prolonged tracheal compression warrants cautious extubation.

Results

Correction of vascular rings is associated with a low operative mortality (< 3%) and good long-term relief of obstructive symptoms. Most morbidity and mortality is associated with the degree of tracheal maldevelopment.

LEFT-TO-RIGHT SHUNTS (ACYANOTIC DEFECTS)

Since pressures in the left heart chambers are normally higher than those in the right heart chambers, defects in either the atrial or ventricular septa result in shunting of oxygenated blood from the left to right side of the heart. This generally increases pulmonary blood flow and leads to pulmonary congestion and a tendency to develop pulmonary hypertension. The most common types of defects in this category are ventricular septal defects, atrial septal defects, and patent ductus arteriosus (Table 37.2–2).

ATRIAL SEPTAL DEFECTS

General Considerations

Atrial septal defects (ASDs) are among the most common congenital cardiac defects, constituting 10–15% of all cases. ASDs vary widely in size and location and are broadly classified as ostium secundum, sinus venosus, and ostium primum type defects.

Ostium secundum (or fossa ovalis) defects, the most common type of ASD, results from a failure of the septum secundum to develop completely and cover the ostium secundum (Figure 37.2–2). Most secundum defects are located in the midportion of the atrial septum, lying within an area defined by the limbus anteriorly, superiorly, and posteriorly. **Sinus venosus defects** occur high in the atrial septum near the superior vena caval orifice and are usually associated with anomalous entry of one or more superior pulmonary veins into the vena cava. The net physiologic effect of both of these ASD types is a left-to-right shunting of blood at the atrial level leading to increased pulmonary blood flow. The degree of shunting is dependent upon the size of the defect and relative compliances of the left and right ventricles. **Shunting** is reported as the ratio of pulmonary (Q_P) to systemic (Q_S) flow from cardiac catheterization measurements. During the first few months of life, the similar structures of the left and right ventricles result in a relatively low shunt. After several months, as pulmonary vascular resistance falls, right ventricular compliance increases along with the left-to-right shunt. Eventually, as pulmonary hypertension develops from abnormally increased pulmonary blood flow, right ventricular compliance decreases, often leading to a reversal of the shunt, cyanosis, and right ventricular failure.

Ostium primum ASDs occur low in the atrial septum, just above the atrioventricular (A-V) valves and result from failure of the septum primum to fuse with the endocardial cushions. These defects are more properly classified as part of the spectrum of atrioventricular canal defects and are discussed later.

Diagnosis

Isolated ASDs rarely produce symptoms in infancy or early childhood. Symptoms of CHF, including dyspnea on exertion, tachypnea, and frequent respiratory infections, occur as a result of increased pulmonary blood flow. Approximately 1% of patients with large ASDs are symptomatic during the first year of life. Paroxysmal atrial tachycardia or atrial fibrillation usually present after the age of 30. On physical examination, a soft midsystolic pulmonary flow murmur, fixed splitting of the second heart sound, and a diastolic tricuspid flow murmur are frequently observed in patients with significant left-to-right shunting (Q_P:Q_S > 1.5:1) at the atrial level. Prolonged increased pulmonary flow may result in significant pulmonary hypertension in some patients. This leads to an accentuated second heart sound and a marked right ventricular lift. Chest radiography often reveals an enlarged right ventricle, right atrium, and pulmonary artery. Electrocardiography demonstrates right atrial enlargement and RVH. Echocardiography is diagnostic and will demonstrate right atrial, right ventricular, and pulmonary artery enlargement in association with defects in the atrial septum. Contrast echocardiography will reveal the left-to-right shunt across the atrial septum. The diagnosis of sinus venous defects by transthoracic echocardiography is frequently difficult, and transesophageal echocardiography or cardiac catheterization should be used to confirm this diagnosis. Cardiac catheterization is otherwise seldom indicated for the diagnosis of ASDs. It can be helpful in the measurement of pulmonary artery pressure and pulmonary vascular resistance as well as in shunt calculations in older patients prior to intervention.

Treatment

In general, ASDs with left-to-right shunts (Q_P:Q_S) greater than 1.5:1 or 2.0:1 require closure. Since most patients are diagnosed by history, physical findings, and echocardiographic data, the magnitude of the shunt is not generally calculated. The physical findings of a diastolic tricuspid flow murmur and a fixed split of the second heart sound indicating a delayed closure of the pulmonary valve as the result of increased flow across the valve generally correlates well with Q_P:Q_S ratios greater than 1.5:1. Patients with severe pulmonary hypertension and significantly elevated pulmonary vascular resistance (greater than 6 Wood units) should be considered carefully for closure if the pulmonary resistance can be lowered with aggressive pulmonary vasodilatation.

Repair is usually performed via a median sternotomy on CPB. A right anterolateral thoracotomy approach is also satisfactory and provides female patients with superior cosmetic results. Once on CPB, the defect is accessed via an atriotomy. Secundum defects can usually be closed directly with suture, however, for large defects, an autologous pericardial patch is used. Sinus venosus defects usually require a patch to close the defect and direct the anomalous pulmonary venous flow to the left atrium.

Results

In uncomplicated ASD repairs performed during early childhood, the operative risk is less than 1%, however, this figure rises considerably in adults with pulmonary hypertension and increased pulmonary vascular resistance. Patients who undergo repair early in life usually recover rapidly, with a long-term prognosis equivalent to that of the normal population. Most often, pulmonary hypertension will regress following closure except in cases of extremely high pulmonary vascular resistance.

Table 37.2-2. Left-to-right shunts (acyanotic defects).

Defect	Incidence (%)	Pathophysiology	Signs & Symptoms	Diagnostic Tests	Treatment	Operative Results
Atrial septal defect	10–15	Septal defect permits left-to-right atrial shunting and ↑ pulmonary blood flow	Sometimes asymptomatic, CHF symptoms, systolic murmur	CXR: Enlarged RA, RV, and PA; pulmonary congestion ECG: RA enlargement, RVH Echo: Septal defect, RV enlargement Cath: Left-to-right atrial shunt	Closure	Mortality < 1% for early repair, ↑ for repair in adulthood and w/ pulmonary hypertension and ↑ pulmonary vascular resistance
Atrioventricular septal defects	5	Failure of endocardial cushions to meet septum primum produces a defect low in atrial septum (incomplete A-V canal); incomplete development of endocardial cushions produces common A-V valve, VSD, and low ASD (complete A-V canal); left-to-right shunting; mitral/tricuspid regurgitation; pulmonary hypertension	CHF symptoms, systolic murmur, hepatomegaly	CXR: Cardiomegaly, pulmonary congestion ECG: RVH, LVH Echo: Defect low in atrial septum, abnormal A-V valves (incomplete A-V canal); single A-V valve, ASD, VSD (complete A-V canal) Cath: Left-to-right shunt, mitral regurgitation, "goose-neck" deformity of left ventricular outflow tract, ↑ RV and PA pressures, ↑ pulmonary vascular resistance (complete A-V canal)	Patch repair of A-V septal defects	Mortality < 2% (partial A-V canal), 5–13% (complete A-V canal); long-term results dependent on degree of mitral regurgitation
Ventricular septal defect	20	Septal defect permits left-to-right ventricular shunting in proportion to defect size; can produce heart failure in infancy and irreversible pulmonary hypertension later	CHF	CXR: Cardiomegaly, ↑ pulmonary vascularity and "pruning" ECG: LVH, RVH Echo: Enlarged LA and LV, septal defect Cath: Left-to-right ventricular shunt	Patch closure	Mortality 1–2% (isolated VSD), 5–10% (multiple VSDs)
Patent ductus arteriosus	12–15	Blood flow from thoracic Ao to the PA leads to pulmonary overcirculation and CHF	Sometimes asymptomatic, CHF symptoms in newborns, characteristic continuous precordial murmur, wide pulse pressure w/ bounding peripheral pulses	CXR: Enlarged heart and PA, ↑ pulmonary vascularity ECG: LVH Echo: LA enlargement, Ao->PA flow Cath: Left-to-right shunt +/- pulmonary hypertension	Indomethacin, percutaneous embolization, or surgical ligation/division	Mortality < 1%, ↑ in adults; excellent long-term results

Ao = aorta/aortic; A-V = atrioventricular; ASD = atrial septal defect; AVR = aortic valve replacement; CHF = congestive heart failure; CXR = chest x-ray; ECG = electrocardiogram; LA = left atrium; LV = left ventricle; PA = pulmonary artery; RA = right atrium; RV = right ventricle; RVH/LVH = right/left ventricular hypertrophy; VSD = ventricular septal defect.

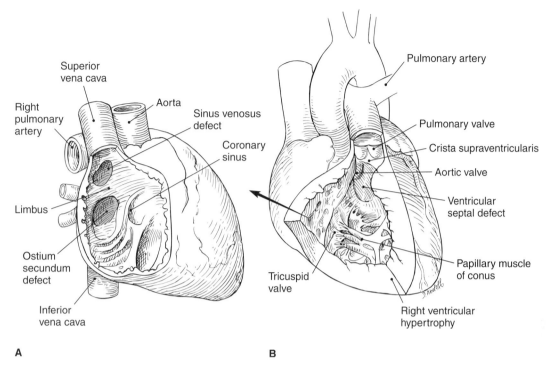

Figure 37.2–2. Atrial and ventricular septal defects. **A:** Anatomical locations of ostium secundum and sinus venosus type atrial septal defects. **B:** The four morphologic features of the tetralogy of Fallot are (1) the aorta overrides the ventricular septum, (2) hypoplastic infundibulum and hypertrophied parietal and septal muscle bands obstruct the right ventricular outflow tract, resulting in (3) right ventricular hypertrophy; and (4) a ventricular septal defect permits right-to-left shunting.

ATRIOVENTRICULAR SEPTAL DEFECTS

General Considerations

Atrioventricular septal (canal) defects represent a wide spectrum of anomalies caused by the maldevelopment of the endocardial cushions. This results in defects above and below the A-V valves. A-V septal defects are classified as partial or complete. Partial A-V septal defects (ostium primum ASDs) occur because the superior aspect of the endocardial cushion fails to develop and close the ostium primum portion of the atrial septum. This defect is frequently associated with incomplete development of the left A-V valve, resulting in a "cleft" in the mitral valve. Complete A-V septal defects have deficiencies in both the atrial and ventricular septum, the latter of which is produced by a failure of the inferior extension of the endocardial cushion to close the ventricular septum. These defects are associated with abnormalities of the right and left sides of the resultant common A-V valve.

A-V septal defects comprise approximately 5% of congenital cardiac lesions and account for 30–40% of the cardiac defects observed in Down's syndrome patients. The most commonly associated cardiac anomalies include tetralogy of Fallot, transposition of the great arteries, double outlet right ventricle, and anomalous pulmonary venous connection. The pathophysiology of A-V septal defects is related to left-to-right shunting at the atrial and/or ventricular levels, producing pulmonary overcirculation and CHF, particularly during infancy. The degree of A-V valve regurgitation is an additional factor involved in the hemodynamic pattern of these defects. Rapidly progressive pulmonary vascular disease can be associated with complete A-V septal defects, especially in the patients with trisomy 21.

Diagnosis

The symptoms associated with A-V septal defects are dependent on the magnitude of left-to-right shunting and A-V valve regurgitation. CHF symptoms of failure to thrive, tachypnea, and recurrent pulmonary infections appear in the first few months of life in patients with complete A-V septal defects. Patients with partial A-V septal defects usually have less severe heart failure symptoms that tend to be manifested beyond the first year of life. Significant A-V valve regurgitation can accentuate symptoms in both forms of the defect. Flow murmurs and fixed splitting of the second heart sound are typically detected with partial defects. A loud systolic precordial murmur, loud second heart sound, right ventricular lift, and hepatomegaly are consistent physical findings in complete A-V septal defects.

Radiographic findings of cardiomegaly and increased

pulmonary vascular markings are observed with these defects and are directly related to the degree of left-to-right shunting. Electrocardiographic patterns of RVH, prolongation of the P-R interval, and the characteristic pattern of leftward and superior axis changes are observed in patients with A-V septal defects. Specific echocardiographic findings are diagnostic of A-V septal defects. Cardiac catheterization is utilized to quantify pulmonary artery pressure, pulmonary vascular resistance, and the degree of shunting in selected patients.

Treatment

Cardiopulmonary bypass with bicaval venous cannulation and cardioplegic arrest is employed for repair of both partial and complete A-V septal defects. Patients with partial A-V septal defects can generally be repaired electively in the first few years of life. Earlier repair may be indicated if refractory heart failure results from significant A-V valve regurgitation. Repair is performed with an autologous pericardial patch closure of the atrial defect, with suture closure of the associated left A-V valve cleft in most cases.

Complete A-V septal defects should have primary repair at 4–6 months of age. These patients typically develop significant CHF and can rapidly develop pulmonary vascular disease, especially those patients with associated trisomy 21. The principles of repair include closure of both the ventricular and atrial components of the defect, dividing the common A-V valve into the left-sided "mitral" and right-sided "tricuspid" valves with attachment of these new valves to the top of the VSD patch, and closure of the septal commissure or "cleft" in the left-sided valve. The repair may be achieved with either a **single-patch** or a **two-patch technique**. We prefer the two-patch technique, which involves closure of the ventricular component with a Dacron patch and use of an autologous pericardial patch for closure of the atrial component.

Transesophageal echocardiography is an invaluable tool for intraoperative evaluation of A-V septal defects prior to and following repair. Careful assessment of A-V valve regurgitation or stenosis, intraventricular or atrial shunting, left ventricular outflow, and ventricular function should be made immediately following repair. Pulmonary artery banding has a very limited role in the management of patients with complete A-V septal defects and should be reserved for selected complex cases.

Results

Operative mortality for partial A-V septal defects is less than 2% and for complete A-V septal defects 5–13%. Significant preoperative A-V valve regurgitation and elevated pulmonary vascular resistance are both associated with increased operative risk. Postoperative complications include complete heart block (1–2%), residual interventricular shunt (5–7%), and left A-V valve regurgitation (5–10%) requiring subsequent repair or replacement.

VENTRICULAR SEPTAL DEFECT

General Considerations

Ventricular septal defects (VSDs) are the most common congenital heart defects, accounting for about 20% of all defects. Four major anatomical types of VSDs have been characterized, depending upon the location in the ventricular septum. These include supracristal, perimembranous, septal leaflet (inlet), and muscular defects (Figure 37–7). The most common defect is the perimembranous VSD, which comprises 80% of VSDs and is related to the aortic and tricuspid valves. The bundle of His passes along the posterior and inferior portions of the defect before branching into the left and right bundle branches.

The two major consequences of VSDs are cardiac failure and pulmonary hypertension. The differential pressures between the left and right ventricles results in a left-to-right shunt across the VSD, leading to increased pulmonary blood flow. The magnitude of the shunt is a function of the defect size and pulmonary vascular resistance. Defects are termed "nonrestrictive" if the defect is larger than the aortic annulus. This results in nonrestrictive blood flow from the high-pressure left ventricle across the defect. Nonrestrictive defects are less likely to spontaneously close and generally result in CHF early in life. While small increases in pulmonary blood flow are generally well tolerated, large increases to more than twice the systemic flow may produce cardiac failure, severe pulmonary congestion, and poor growth during infancy. Elevated pulmonary blood flow leads to pulmonary hypertension produced by changes in the media and intima of pulmonary arterioles. As pulmonary vascular resistance rises, flow reversal leading to right-to-left shunting occurs, producing arterial hypoxemia. This phenomenon is referred to as the **Eisenmenger's syndrome** and occurs in 10% of untreated nonrestrictive VSDs.

Diagnosis

Small VSDs are usually asymptomatic while larger defects result in congestive symptoms, including dyspnea on exertion, hepatomegaly, rales, and frequent pulmonary infections. Patients who develop Eisenmenger's syndrome generally present later in life when cyanosis evolves. Auscultation reveals a loud harsh pansystolic ejection murmur along the left sternal border in the third and fourth interspaces. The pulmonic second sound is increased in cases of significant pulmonary hypertension. Radiographic findings are usually associated with larger defects and include enlargement of the heart and pulmonary arteries with signs of pulmonary congestion. Electrocardiography shows signs of left and right ventricular hypertrophy. Echocardiographic imaging is diagnostic, with reproducible localization and measurement of the defect. Cardiac catheterization is rarely indicated for the diagnosis of an isolated VSD. Catheterization may be necessary, however, for the measurement of pulmonary artery pressure, pulmonary vascular resistance, and calculation of shunt size in patients suspected of fixed pulmonary resistance or to provide this data in complex cases.

Treatment

Since 60–70% of small VSDs close spontaneously in early life, these generally should be observed. Infants with large nonrestrictive defects are treated with decongestive therapy consisting of digoxin and diuretics. CHF unresponsive to medical therapy is an indication for VSD closure. Supracristal defects are located just below the pulmonary and aortic valves. Aortic regurgitation is common with these defects due to the Venturi effect from flow across the VSD, causing the aortic leaflet to be pulled inferiorly. Therefore, all supracristal VSDs should be closed.

Most VSDs can be repaired through a right atriotomy with retraction of the tricuspid valve. Supracristal defects are accessed more easily through the pulmonary valve. A right ventriculotomy may be required for closure of some inferiorly located muscular VSDs. A Dacron patch is placed over the VSD, with care taken not to place sutures through the adjacent conduction fiber bundles.

Results

The overall mortality for isolated VSD repair is about 1–2%. Operative risk increases to 5–10% with preexisting pulmonary vascular disease and multiple VSDs. Permanent heart block requiring pacemaker placement is most frequently a complication of perimembranous VSD closure and occurs in 2–5% of cases. A significant residual VSD requiring reoperation can occur in up to 5% of cases. The routine use of intraoperative transesophageal echocardiography can identify any residual VSDs. Early repair generally results in dramatic improvement of CHF, prevents the development of pulmonary vascular disease, and is associated with excellent long-term outcome.

PATENT DUCTUS ARTERIOSUS

General Considerations

Patent ductus arteriosus (PDA) is an open communication that is usually between the upper descending thoracic aorta and the main pulmonary artery, resulting from persistent patency of the fetal ductus arteriosus. In fetal life, the ductus arteriosus shunts blood from the pulmonary artery to the aorta because pulmonary circulation is not necessary in utero. Shortly after birth, the muscular contraction in the wall of the ductus results in closure as the pulmonary vascular resistance falls with lung expansion. In some cases, the ductus remains open for several weeks or even longer, resulting in left-to-right shunts of varying degrees, depending on the size of the ductus and the pulmonary vascular resistance. This anomaly, comprising 12–15% of congenital heart defects, may be well tolerated for years in some patients, however, a persistent shunt can produce heart failure early in life as well as progressive pulmonary hypertension later on.

Diagnosis

Many patients with isolated PDA are asymptomatic, however, CHF may present early in life. Physical examination reveals a characteristic continuous harsh flow murmur in the left second intercostal space. A wide pulse pressure results in bounding peripheral pulses. Electrocardiography may be normal in cases of small shunts, but will reveal some degree of LVH in large shunts. Similarly, chest radiography may be normal in small shunts, however, if the shunt is large, mild cardiomegaly with a prominent pulmonary artery may present. Increased pulmonary vascularity and LVH may also be evident on chest film. Echocardiography is diagnostic, demonstrating blood flow from the aorta to the pulmonary artery with associated LVH and left atrial enlargement. Cardiac catheterization is usually not required.

Treatment

Early administration of indomethacin may cause ductal closure in many premature infants, obviating surgical treatment. Indomethacin therapy, however, is generally contraindicated if renal insufficiency or intracranial bleeding is present. Surgical closure of the ductus is recommended when a significant left-to-right shunt is present. Ductal closure for bacterial endocarditis prophylaxis is generally indicated for smaller PDAs, but this is controversial. In most cases, adequate exposure of the ductus is achieved through a small left posterolateral thoracotomy in the fourth intercostal space. The ductus is interrupted with a surgical clip in neonates or divided between appropriate vascular clamps, with oversewing of the ends in older children.

Percutaneous coil embolization has produced satisfactory results in selected cases and may emerge as the treatment of choice in the future. Some centers have achieved good results with clip ligation of PDAs using a thoracoscopic approach.

Results

For isolated PDA ligation, the operative mortality is well below 1%. The risk is greater in the older patient with preexisting pulmonary hypertension. Rare complications include bleeding and damage to the recurrent laryngeal and phrenic nerves. Immediate improvement in pulmonary vascularity and heart size is often seen after PDA ligation in infants with CHF. Long-term results are excellent.

RIGHT-TO-LEFT SHUNTS (CYANOTIC DEFECTS)

This category of anomalies is characterized by the shunting of venous blood into the systemic circulation, resulting in arterial hypoxemia and cyanosis. In general, pulmonary blood flow is diminished (Table 37.2–3).

Table 37.2–3. Right-to-left shunts (cyanotic defects).

Defect	Incidence (%)	Pathophysiology	Signs & Symptoms	Diagnostic Tests	Treatment	Operative Results
Tetralogy of Fallot	12	Tetralogy consisting of VSD, RV outflow tract obstruction, overriding Ao, and RVH, leading to obstruction of pulmonary blood flow, right-to-left shunting, and cyanosis	Cyanosis, harsh systolic pre-cordial murmur	CXR: RVH w/ small PA ("boot-shaped" heart), diminished pulmonary vascularity, right Ao arch (25%) ECG: RVH Echo: Large overriding Ao, small PA, large malalignment VSD Cath: ↑ RV pressure, RV->PA gradient, right-to-left shunt, VSD, coronary artery anomalies	Total correction in cases w/ favorable anatomy; palliative systemic-PA shunt (eg, Blalock–Taussig) in cases w/ unfavorable anatomy	Mortality 3–5%; good long-term results
Tricuspid atresia	1–3	Atretic tricuspid valve, hypoplastic RV, and ASD resulting in right-to-left shunting and cyanosis	Cyanosis, CHF, holosystolic murmur, hepatomegaly	CXR: Pulmonary congestion and plethora ECG: RA hypertrophy, LVH Echo: Absent right A-V valve, great artery relationship, VSD, pulmonary stenosis	Stage 1: Palliative Blalock-Taussig shunt or PA band in infancy Stage 2: Glenn shunt Stage 3: Fontan operation	Mortality < 10%; satisfactory long-term results

Ao = aorta/aortic; ASD = atrial septal defect; A-V = atrioventricular; CXR = chest x-ray; ECG = electrocardiogram; LA = left atrium; LV = left ventricle; PA = pulmonary artery; RA = right atrium; RV = right ventricle; RVH/LVH = right/left ventricular hypertrophy; VSD = ventricular septal defect.

TETRALOGY OF FALLOT

General Considerations

The tetralogy of Fallot is one of the most common cyanotic defects, constituting over half of all cases of cyanotic heart disease and approximately 12% of all congenital heart defects. The four related defects comprising the tetralogy are (1) a large VSD, (2) obstruction of the right ventricular outflow tract, (3) an overriding aorta, and (4) RVH (Figure 37.2–3). This constellation of defects can be explained by the abnormal anterior and leftward rotation (malalignment) of the infundibular ventricular septum during cardiac development. Associated defects commonly include an ASD or patent foramen ovale, resulting in the **pentalogy** of Fallot. A right aortic arch occurs in about 25% of these patients. Maldevelopment of the right or left pulmonary artery (stenosis) and pulmonary valve (atresia) is also associated with the tetralogy. Five percent of patients have coronary artery anomalies, the most important of which is a left anterior descending artery arising from the right coronary artery, which, in turn, courses across the right ventricular outflow tract to reach the left ventricle.

The defects comprising the tetralogy of Fallot act to obstruct pulmonary blood flow with an associated right-to-left shunting of blood across the VSD into the aorta. The net pathophysiologic effect is cyanosis. The degree of cyanosis is largely dependent upon the degree of right ventricular outflow tract obstruction. Cyanosis is usually ameliorated at birth due to supplemental pulmonary blood flow across a patent ductus arteriosus. If the right ventricular outflow tract obstruction is severe enough, however, closure of the ductus over the ensuing days or weeks after birth results in significant cyanosis. If the pulmonary valve is atretic, cyanosis is severe at birth. If left to progress untreated, RVH increases, leading to progressive right ventricular outflow tract obstruction and worsening cyanosis. The main causes of death in the first year of life are cerebral infarction and cardiac arrest from thrombosis or anoxia.

Diagnosis

Although some patients with mild outflow tract obstruction remain asymptomatic for quite some time, less than 10% of untreated patients with the tetralogy survive to the age of 20. Dyspnea and cyanosis, worsened by exertion, are the most striking symptoms in tetralogy patients. Cyanotic spells, or sudden episodes of intense cyanosis followed by unconsciousness, are prevalent between 2 and 6 months of age. Relief of dyspnea by squatting is another aspect of this syndrome observed in older children and represents an adapted maneuver to increase systemic vascular resistance, thereby forcing more blood across the VSD and the obstructed right ventricular outflow tract. Squatting is seldom seen in this country because most cases are diagnosed and treated early in life, but it continues to be part of the natural history of the disease in developing countries. Besides cyanosis, physical examination reveals digital clubbing and a systolic murmur along the left sternal border in the third and fourth intercostal spaces. The second pulmonic sound is weak or absent while the aortic second sound is enhanced.

Chest films reveal the so-called "boot-shaped" heart that results from a concave pulmonary artery segment, concentric RVH, and a small left ventricle. Decreased pulmonary vascularity is also often noted. Electrocardiography typically reveals RVH. Echocardiography is diagnostic and usually highlights the anatomic characteristics of the tetralogy. Cardiac catheterization is not mandatory and is reserved for patients in whom there is some echocardiographic uncertainty.

Treatment

There is a trend toward early total correction in all cases of tetralogy of Fallot, with palliation by a systemic-to-pulmonary artery shunt reserved for cases with extremely small pulmonary arteries, an anomalous coronary artery crossing the right ventricular outflow tract, or associated complex cardiac lesions. Some centers have established excellent results with palliative shunting followed by complete repair at 1 year of age for patients presenting with hypercyanotic spells early in life.

In patients with adequate pulmonary annular size, the repair may be performed through the tricuspid valve and pulmonary artery to resect the infundibular obstruction and repair the VSD. Patients with a small pulmonary annulus are generally repaired through a right ventriculotomy. Hypertrophied septal and parietal bands are resected and the VSD is closed with a prosthetic patch. An

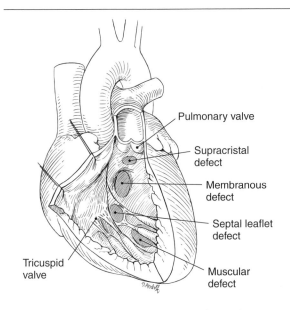

Figure 37.2–3. Anatomical locations of the four major types of ventricular septal defects, including supracristal, perimembranous, septal leaflet (inlet), and muscular defects.

autologous pericardial patch is used to close the right ventricle and is extended across the pulmonary annulus, widening it. In patients with pulmonary atresia or an anomalous origin of the left anterior descending coronary artery from the right coronary artery, reconstruction of the right ventricular outflow tract with placement of a cryopreserved homograft between the right ventricle and pulmonary artery may be necessary.

Results

In patients with favorable anatomy, the operative mortality ranges from 3–5% with generally good long-term results and an actuarial survival of approximately 85% at 20 years. Varying degrees of right ventricular failure in the early postoperative period and mild, well-tolerated pulmonary insufficiency are not uncommon. Residual right ventricular outflow tract obstruction requiring reoperation occurs in approximately 5% of cases. Long-term ventricular tachyarrhythmias can occur in 3–5% of cases.

TRICUSPID ATRESIA

General Considerations

Tricuspid atresia results from developmental failure of the A-V valve between the right atrium and right ventricle. It is the third most common form of cyanotic congenital heart disease after the tetralogy of Fallot and *d*-TGA and comprises 1–3% of congenital heart defects. The classification of tricuspid atresia is based on the relationship of the great vessels and the degree of obstruction to pulmonary blood flow. The most common form of tricuspid atresia has normally related great arteries, a restrictive VSD, and pulmonary stenosis. All forms of tricuspid atresia have an ASD and a hypoplastic right ventricle. There is a right-to-left atrial level shunt resulting in cyanosis. The degree of cyanosis is related to the extent of pulmonary blood flow obstruction. Approximately 70% of patients have restricted pulmonary flow and 30% have pulmonary overcirculation with mild oxygen desaturation.

Diagnosis

Most patients with tricuspid atresia will present with some degree of cyanosis. Patients with tricuspid atresia and normally related great arteries tend to become cyanotic in the first month of life and may have a history of hypercyanotic spells. Patients with tricuspid atresia and *d*-TGA are less cyanotic and present later in life with signs and symptoms of CHF. A holosystolic VSD murmur may be detected with tricuspid atresia, and hepatomegaly is observed in patients with pulmonary overcirculation and CHF.

Electrocardiography demonstrates right atrial hypertrophy, LVH, and left axis deviation. These findings observed in a cyanotic patient strongly suggest tricuspid atresia. The chest radiograph may demonstrate pulmonary overcirculation or pulmonary plethora, depending on the degree of pulmonary obstruction. Echocardiographic demonstration of absence of the right A-V valve is diagnostic of tricuspid atresia. Additional information concerning the relationship of the great arteries, VSD, and the degree of pulmonary stenosis is readily obtained by echocardiography. Cardiac catheterization is not needed for the initial assessment of tricuspid atresia, but is helpful in planning subsequent staging toward eventual construction of a total cavopulmonary connection.

Treatment

The initial treatment of tricuspid atresia is related to the balance between pulmonary and systemic flow. Patients with pulmonary obstruction and cyanosis will require a modified Blalock-Taussig systemic-pulmonary artery shunt in the newborn period. Patients with unrestricted pulmonary flow will require pulmonary artery banding. All patients with tricuspid atresia are tracked toward an eventual modified Fontan procedure. This process begins with a superior vena cava-pulmonary artery anastomosis (bidirectional Glenn shunt) with takedown of the systemic-to-pulmonary artery shunt, if present, at 4–6 months of age. The **Damus-Kaye-Stansel procedure** may be combined with the bidirectional Glenn shunt in patients with *d*-TGA and subaortic stenosis. In this procedure, the proximal cut end of the main pulmonary artery is anastomosed end-to-side to the proximal ascending aorta, bypassing the subaortic obstruction and providing ventricular outflow.

The modified Fontan procedure performed at approximately 2 years of age is the definitive repair for patients with tricuspid atresia and establishes a total cavopulmonary connection. Fenestration of the Fontan circuit may be used in high-risk patients but is generally not required in patients with tricuspid atresia and good left ventricular function.

Results

The overall operative mortality for patients with tricuspid atresia through all stages to total cavopulmonary connection is less than 10%. Long-term results have been satisfactory, with complications related to those previously outlined for the Fontan procedure.

COMMON MIXING LESIONS (CYANOTIC DEFECTS)

These cyanotic lesions are based on the total intracardiac mixing of blood from the right and left sides of the heart. Balanced or increased pulmonary blood flow is present in these lesions (Table 37.2–4).

Table 37.2-4. Common mixing lesions (cyanotic defects).

Defect	Incidence (%)	Pathophysiology	Signs & Symptoms	Diagnostic Tests	Treatment	Operative Results
Total anomalous pulmonary venous connection	1–2	Pulmonary veins drain into RA; obstruction of anomalous connection leads to pulmonary hypertension and congestion	Respiratory distress, cyanosis (obstructed), CHF (unobstructed)	CXR: Pulmonary congestion ECG: RA enlargement, RVH Echo: Anomalous pulmonary venous flow Cath: anomalous pulmonary venous connections	Redirection of pulmonary venous return to RA	Mortality 10%; excellent long-term results
d-Transposition of the great arteries	7–8	Ao arises from RV; PA arises from LV; can occur w/ IVS or w/ VSD; systemic and pulmonary circulations placed in parallel; intracardiac shunt required to allow oxygenated blood to enter systemic circulation; ↑ pulmonary blood flow leads to pulmonary hypertension	Cyanosis in infancy w/ IVS; CHF w/ VSD	ECG: RVH w/ IVS; LVH w/ VSD CXR: "Egg-shaped" heart w/ narrowing of superior mediastinum +/– pulmonary congestion Echo: Abnormal great vessel relationship +/– VSD Cath: Ventriculoarterial discordance, intracardiac shunting +/– ↑ pulmonary vascular resistance	Atrial or arterial switch operation	Mortality < 5%; good long-term results
Truncus arteriosus	1–3	Single common artery overlying ventricular septum and VSD gives rise to both systemic and pulmonary circulations; mixing of blood from both ventricles leads to arterial hypoxemia; excessive pulmonary blood flow leads to CHF and pulmonary hypertension	CHF followed by cyanosis; systolic thrill, apical impulse	ECG: Biventricular enlargement CXR: Cardiomegaly, pulmonary congestion and vascular changes Echo: Truncus overlying ventricular septum w/ large semilunar valve, VSD Cath: Biventricular pressure equalization, left-to-right shunting, truncal anatomy	Remove PA from truncus and reestablish continuity w/ RV via valved conduit; VSD closure	Mortality 10–20%; increased when performed later in life w/ ↑ pulmonary vascular resistance

Ao = aorta/aortic; CHF = congestive heart failure; CXR = chest x-ray; ECG = electrocardiogram; IVS = intact ventricular septum; LV = left ventricle; PA = pulmonary artery; RA = right atrium; RV = right ventricle; RVH/LVH = right/left ventricular hypertrophy; VSD = ventricular septal defect.

TOTAL ANOMALOUS PULMONARY VENOUS CONNECTION

General Considerations

Total anomalous pulmonary venous connection (TAPVC) is a rare anomaly, comprising 1–2% of congenital cardiac cases. TAPVC comprises a wide spectrum of lesions in which the entire pulmonary venous return to the heart drains into the right atrium. Classification of TAPVC is based on the anatomical connection to the right atrium and includes supracardiac (45%), cardiac (25%), infracardiac (25%), and mixed (5%) patterns of drainage. In the **supracardiac** configuration a pulmonary venous confluence drains into the right atrium via a vertical vein leading into the innominate vein or directly into the superior vena cava. The **cardiac** pattern has pulmonary venous return to the coronary sinus or directly into the right atrium. The **pulmonary venous** confluence drains via a vertical vein below the diaphragm into the portal vein or directly into the inferior vena cava in the infracardiac variety of TAPVC. The **mixed** pattern consists of combinations of the other patterns.

The pathway of pulmonary venous return to the right atrium may be obstructed or unobstructed. The infracardiac type is most commonly obstructed and the cardiac type is rarely obstructed. Since pulmonary blood flow empties into the right atrium, an interatrial right-to-left shunt is needed to maintain systemic output and survival. This shunting leads to pulmonary congestion and cyanosis. The degree of cyanosis is related to the size of the right-to-left shunt which is, in turn, determined by the degree of obstruction to pulmonary venous return. Pulmonary venous obstruction effectively increases pulmonary vascular resistance, increasing right-to-left atrial shunting and systemic arterial desaturation.

Diagnosis

Neonates with obstructive TAPVC present with respiratory distress and profound cyanosis in the first few hours of life. Arterial blood gas analysis demonstrates severe hypoxia and metabolic acidosis. Severe pulmonary edema and a normal cardiac silhouette are consistently observed on chest radiography. Right atrial enlargement and right ventricular hypertrophy are frequently noted on the electrocardiogram. Echocardiography is usually diagnostic, with findings of a pulmonary venous confluence without connection to the left atrium and Doppler venous flow patterns away from the heart. Cardiac catheterization may be detrimental in a critically ill acidotic infant and should be reserved for cases of the mixed variety or when the echocardiographic information is not clearly diagnostic.

Infants with unobstructed TAPVC generally present with CHF symptoms in the first few months of life. Older children with the cardiac type of TAPVC may have a more indolent course with mild symptoms. Catheterization may be indicated in these patients to better define the anatomical pattern.

Treatment

The treatment for all cases of TAPVC is operative repair. The timing of the repair is related to the degree of obstruction to pulmonary venous return. Neonates with obstructive TAPVC are critically ill and require emergent repair. Patients with nonobstructive TAPVC should have an elective repair soon after diagnosis to diminish the adverse affects of cyanosis, pulmonary hypertension, and right heart volume overload.

The goal of operative repair is to direct the entire pulmonary venous return to the left atrium. The technique used for repair of supra- and infracardiac TAPVC involves the direct anastomosis of the left atrium and the posteriorly located pulmonary venous confluence, ligation of the vertical vein, and autologous pericardial patch closure of the ASD. The cardiac type of TAPVC is repaired with an autologous pericardial patch placed over the ASD and the coronary sinus ostium such that the pulmonary venous return is baffled into the left atrium.

Placement of a transthoracic pulmonary artery monitoring catheter is frequently helpful for the postoperative management of patients with obstructed TAPVC. Pulmonary artery pressures of systemic magnitude are not unusual in this subset of patients. Hyperventilation, heavy sedation, and inhaled nitric oxide therapy is generally effective in lowering pulmonary vascular resistance in the perioperative period.

Results

The overall operative mortality for TAPVC repair is approximately 10%. Preoperative acidosis, obstruction to pulmonary venous return, and the infracardiac type of TAPVC are all associated with increased operative mortality. The most common cause of postoperative death is persistent pulmonary hypertension. Inhaled nitric oxide should significantly decrease the morbidity and mortality in these patients. Pulmonary venous obstruction occurs in 5–10% of patients following repair of TAPVC and usually develops within the first 6 months after repair; it is associated with an extremely poor prognosis. Overall, repair of TAPVC is associated with excellent long-term results.

d-TRANSPOSITION OF THE GREAT ARTERIES

General Considerations

d-transposition of the great arteries (*d*-TGA) is a congenital cardiac defect in which the aorta arises from the right ventricle and the pulmonary artery arises from the left ventricle. It accounts for 7–8% of all congenital heart disease. There is a 2:1 male-to-female ratio. Approximately 75% of patients with *d*-TGA will have an intact ventricular septum (IVS) with no other significant cardiac malformations other than a PDA. This is referred to as **"simple" TGA**. About 20% of TGA cases have a VSD and are termed **"complex"**; these are associated with a 20% incidence of left ventricular outflow tract obstruction

(LVOTO). Aortic arch obstruction is associated with 7–10% of d-TGA/VSD cases.

Transposition of the great arteries results in several physiologic and anatomical derangements. First, the pulmonary and systemic circulations are in parallel with each other instead of in series. In other words, oxygenated blood circulates through the lungs and the left side of the heart while deoxygenated blood circulates through the systemic circulation and the right side of the heart. Without an intracardiac shunt between the two circuits to allow oxygenated blood to enter the systemic circulation, this derangement is incompatible with life. Typically, this shunt is in the form of an ASD, VSD, or PDA.

Second, since this anomaly requires pulmonary blood flow to be greater than systemic blood flow for effective systemic oxygenation to occur, obstructive pulmonary vascular disease rapidly develops in untreated patients. Finally, the right ventricle is typically hypertrophied and large, because it must work against systemic vascular resistance.

Diagnosis

Infants with d-TGA commonly present with varying degrees of cyanosis or CHF. The severity of these symptoms depends largely upon the extent of communication and mixing between the two parallel circulations. Patients with d-TGA/IVS usually have poor mixing through a patent foramen ovale or ASD and develop a rapidly progressive cyanosis beginning in the first hours of life. Without treatment, early death usually occurs. On the other hand, patients with d-TGA/VSD generally have good mixing and do not present with CHF until the end of the first month of life when the pulmonary resistance begins to fall. Tachycardia, tachypnea, hepatomegaly, and pulmonary congestion are other common signs.

Electrocardiographic changes consistent with RVH are usually observed with d-TGA/IVS. Changes associated with LVH also tend to occur in cases of d-TGA/VSD. Characteristic changes on chest radiography include an oval, "egg-shaped" cardiac silhouette on the end of a narrow vascular pedicle constituting the superior mediastinum. This is sometimes associated with signs of pulmonary congestion due to increased pulmonary blood flow. Echocardiography can be diagnostic for TGA by revealing inversion of ventricular systolic time intervals and the abnormal relationship of the great vessels. Moreover, associated malformations, including valvular malformations, VSD/ASD, LVOTO, aortic arch obstruction, and coronary artery anomalies, are consistently well-detailed with echocardiography. Catheterization is not routinely performed to diagnose TGA, however, useful information can be obtained from such studies, including calculation of pulmonary vascular resistance, the locations of intracardiac shunts and great vessels, the size and function of the A-V valves, the condition of both ventricles, and the presence of other cardiac anomalies.

Left untreated, the overall long-term life expectancy of patients with d-TGA is poor. Taking all varieties of TGA into account, the 1-month, 6-month, and 1-year survival rates are approximately 55%, 15%, and 10%, respectively. The prognosis is particularly poor in untreated patients with d-TGA/IVS, with survival rates of 17% and 4% at 2 months and 1 year, respectively.

Treatment

Operative repair of d-TGA falls into two major categories: **atrial switch** and **arterial switch** operations. Atrial switch operations are designed to (1) redirect systemic venous return to the mitral valve, left ventricle, and pulmonary artery and (2) transpose pulmonary venous return to the tricuspid valve, right ventricle, and aorta. The **Mustard operation** utilizes a pericardial baffle to achieve this transposition of venous return. The **Senning operation** uses flaps of atrial tissue as baffles to redirect systemic and pulmonary venous inflow. Although these operations achieve good results, they have the disadvantage of committing the right A-V valve and ventricle to support the systemic circulation. Poor right ventricular function is often seen on follow-up catheterizations after atrial switch operations, prompting concerns about premature right ventricular failure. Additionally, long-term atrial arrhythmias and baffle obstruction and leaks have resulted from excessive realignment in the atria. These problems led to the development of a more "anatomical" correction, namely the arterial switch operation.

During recent years, the arterial switch operation has become the preferred technique for treatment of d-TGA. This type of correction has the benefit of placing the systemic circulatory work load on the more powerful left ventricle. Performed under CPB, the ascending aorta, pulmonary trunk, and coronary artery ostia are transposed.

Results

Results with the Mustard and Senning atrial switch operations are good, with an operative mortality rate less than 5%. However, these procedures are associated with the long-term complications of systemic right ventricular failure, atrial arrhythmias, baffle obstruction of superior vena caval inflow, baffle leaks, tricuspid regurgitation, and LVOTO. In institutions with adequate experience, mortality rates for the arterial switch operation are 2–5%. Mortality is most often due to ventricular failure secondary to imperfect coronary artery transfers or right ventricular dysfunction in the presence of severe pulmonary vascular disease. The most common complication following arterial switch operations is supravalvular pulmonary artery stenosis. Excellent ventricular function can be expected following arterial switches, and long-term survival rates have been estimated to be around 90%.

TRUNCUS ARTERIOSUS

General Considerations

Truncus arteriosus is a defect in which one large arterial trunk arising from the base of the heart and overlying the interventricular septum gives rise to the coronary, systemic, and one or both pulmonary arteries. At the origin of this artery is a semilunar valve composed of two to six cusps; beneath it lies a VSD. This defect results from a lack of partitioning of the conus during embryogenesis. Four type of truncus defects have been identified by the Collett-Edwards classification, however, most clinical cases consist of type I or type II defects or an intermediate variant. In **type I defects**, a single arterial trunk gives rise to the aorta and main pulmonary artery, while in **type II defects**, the right and left pulmonary arteries arise immediately adjacent to one another from the dorsal wall of the truncus. Physiologically, the truncus receives blood from both ventricles, resulting in mixing of systemic and pulmonary venous blood leading to systemic arterial desaturation. In most infants with this lesion, pulmonary blood flow is excessive, leading to CHF and pulmonary vascular hypertension if left untreated.

Diagnosis

Infants with truncus defects typically present in some degree of heart failure with tachypnea, dyspnea, tachycardia, and failure to thrive. Cyanosis becomes evident after the development of significant pulmonary vascular obstructive disease. Physical examination reveals a systolic thrill over the left third and fourth intercostal spaces and a prominent apical impulse. Electrocardiography and chest radiography demonstrate biventricular enlargement and cardiomegaly. Radiographic evidence of augmented pulmonary blood flow is usually present. Echocardiographic findings include a characteristically large truncal root overlying the ventricular septum, an absent pulmonary valve, and VSD. Cardiac catheterization with cineangiography is helpful in selected cases of truncus arteriosus to further define the pulmonary artery anatomy, pulmonary vascular resistance, and aortic arch anatomy.

Treatment

All diagnosed cases of truncus arteriosus should be repaired as early in life as possible, since about 50% of truncus patients managed medically die during the first month of life. Operative repair may be contraindicated in older patients with prohibitively high pulmonary vascular resistances.

Complete repair begins with excision of the pulmonary trunk from the main truncus and pericardial patch closure of the resultant aortic defect. A right vertical ventriculotomy is then performed and the VSD is identified and closed with a Dacron patch. A cryopreserved homograft is then anastomosed between the ventriculotomy and the distal pulmonary trunk, thereby directing right ventricular outflow into the pulmonary arteries (Figure 37.2–4).

Results

Early mortality following truncus repair ranges between 10–20% and is dependent upon the anatomical anomalies, pulmonary vascular resistance, and preoperative condition of the infant. Patients undergoing repair at an early age usually require reoperation for conduit replacement as the child grows.

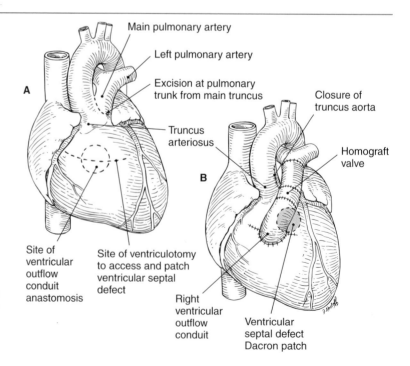

Figure 37.2–4. Truncus arteriosus. **A:** In type I truncus, a single arterial trunk gives rise to the aorta and main pulmonary artery. A ventricular septal defect (VSD) is always present. **B:** Repair involving resection of the main pulmonary artery from the truncus and reestablishing continuity with the right ventricle using a valved conduit. The VSD is closed.

RARE MALFORMATIONS

Most of the following congenital cardiac malformations generally comprise less than 1% of all congenital heart defects, but warrant brief discussion since they all require surgical correction and display interesting pathophysiology (Table 37.2–5).

COR TRIATRIATUM

General Considerations

Cor triatriatum is a rare congenital heart defect in which the pulmonary veins enter a proximal "accessory" left atrial chamber (common pulmonary venous sinus), which is separated from the more distal "true" left atrium by a thick-walled muscular diaphragm containing one or more restrictive ostia. The restricted pulmonary venous flow results in pulmonary hypertension, with significant pressure gradients noted between the venous sinus and true left atrium. The size of the ostia draining the common pulmonary venous chamber into the true left atrium determines the clinical course of patients with cor triatriatum. If the aperture is small and severely restrictive, as it is in about 75% of patients born with classical cor triatriatum, the infant becomes critically ill during the first few months of life and, without surgical treatment, dies at an early age. Conversely, if the hole is larger, or when the common pulmonary venous chamber communicates with the right atrium through a fossa ovalis ASD, the patient presents later in childhood or young adulthood with a clinical picture resembling mitral stenosis. Isolated cor triatriatum occurs in 30% of cases. The most common associated cardiac anomalies include PDA, TAPVC, unroofed coronary sinus with left superior vena cava, VSD, coarctation of the aorta, and tetralogy of Fallot.

Diagnosis

Infants with restrictive cor triatriatum typically present in a low cardiac output state with pallor, tachypnea, poor peripheral perfusion, and failure to thrive. If there is an associated left-to-right shunt, signs and symptoms of pulmonary congestion may also be present. Children and young adults with cor triatriatum who present later in life typically display the signs and symptoms of pulmonary venous hypertension and right heart failure. Electrocardiography and chest radiography may show evidence of RVH if a significant left-to-right shunt exists. Two-dimensional echocardiography is diagnostic with demonstration of the bipartite left atrium and obstructing membrane. Transesophageal echocardiography can further define the anatomical pattern of cor triatriatum. Cardiac catheterization is rarely needed for diagnosis but may be useful for more complex cases.

Treatment

Correction of classical cor triatriatum with a restrictive diaphragmatic communication is indicated in the first year of life. Under moderately hypothermic CPB, the common pulmonary venous chamber is opened through a vertical incision made anterior to the right pulmonary veins. The partitioning diaphragm is identified, exposed, and excised. If present, the ASD is closed.

Results

Mortality after surgical correction of isolated cor triatriatum is extremely low except in cases when the infant is critically ill prior to repair. Operative mortality is related to the severity of associated anomalies. The life expectancy after repair, especially when performed in infancy, approaches that of the general population.

CONGENITAL MITRAL VALVE DISEASE

General Considerations

Congenital mitral valve disease (CMVD) comprises a spectrum of rare malformations of one or more components of the mitral valve, including portions of the left atrial wall adjacent to the mitral valve annulus. These malformations generally result in congenital mitral valve stenosis, incompetence, or degrees of both. **Congenital mitral stenosis** is caused by narrowing at the valve or points above or below the valve. **Congenital mitral incompetence** may be caused by prolapse or dysplasia of one or both of the valve leaflets. Significant flow obstruction or regurgitation of the mitral valve results in elevated pulmonary venous pressures and pulmonary congestion. Pulmonary vascular changes secondary to pulmonary hypertension lead to RVH and failure. CMVD is commonly associated with other cardiac anomalies, including ASD, VSD, aortic stenosis, and coarctation of the aorta.

Diagnosis

The clinical signs and symptoms of isolated CMVD are identical to those present in acquired mitral valve disease (eg, pulmonary hypertension and congestion), with the natural history dependent on the severity of mitral stenosis or incompetence and any coexisting lesions. Signs include flow murmurs and a right ventricular lift.

Isolated congenital mitral stenosis is usually severe and presents in the first months to years of life, whereas isolated mitral incompetence is usually acquired, presenting somewhat later in life with moderately severe symptoms. In both cases, symptoms and the need for correction comes earlier when other cardiac anomalies exist. Electrocardiographic evidence of left atrial enlargement and RVH typically present with CMVD. Overall cardiac enlargement, particularly left atrial enlargement, is the foremost radiographic sign. Signs of pulmonary venous hypertension may also present. Echocardiography and catheterization studies with cineangiography are diagnos-

Table 37.2-5. Rare malformations.

Defect	Incidence (%)	Pathophysiology	Signs & Symptoms	Diagnostic Tests	Treatment	Operative Results
Cor triatriatum	< 1	Persistence of common pulmonary vein forming an accessory chamber that communicates w/ LA; varying degrees of flow restriction into LA by fibromuscular diaphragm leading to pulmonary venous obstruction	Dyspnea, pulmonary infections, failure to thrive; severity dependent upon degree of pulmonary venous obstruction; older patients may present w/ right heart failure	ECG: RVH CXR: Pulmonary venous congestion Echo: Diagnostic; septation of LA; ASD	Excision of partitioning diaphragm	Mortality low; excellent long-term results
Congenital mitral valve disease	< 1	Malformation of mitral valve leading to mitral stenosis, insufficiency, or both	CHF symptoms, flow murmur, RV lift	ECG: LA enlargement CXR: Cardiomegaly Echo: Malformed mitral valve apparatus Cath: ↑ pulmonary wedge pressures	Mitral valve repair or replacement	Variable; generally ↑ mortality in infants < 1 yr; reoperation often required later for valve revision
Aortic-pulmonary window	< 0.5	Large communication between Ao and PA leading to high-flow left-to-right shunt, rapidly progressive CHF, and pulmonary hypertension	CHF symptoms in infancy, systolic flow murmur, wide pulse pressure	ECG: LA and biventricular enlargement CXR: Cardiomegaly, pulmonary congestion Echo: Aortopulmonary communication Cath: Aortopulmonary shunt	Closure of aortopulmonary window	Mortality low; excellent long-term results
Double-inlet single ventricle	2–3	Single functional ventricle receiving both systemic and pulmonary venous return, leading to arterial hypoxemia; associated pulmonary overcirculation or decreased pulmonary blood flow dependent upon degree of pulmonary obstruction	Varying degrees of heart failure, pulmonary congestion, and cyanosis	ECG: Nondiagnostic CXR: Pulmonary congestion or patterns of decreased pulmonary blood flow Echo: Absent intraventricular septum, augmented/diminished pulmonary blood flow +/– atretic/stenotic pulmonary outflow tract Cath: Single functional ventricular anatomy, augmented/diminished pulmonary blood flow	Modified Fontan operation	Mortality 5–10% w/ results similar to other defects treated w/ Fontan
Ebstein's anomaly	< 1	Downward displacement of posterior and septal tricuspid valve leaflets; "atrialization" of RV leading to diminished RV output from tricuspid insufficiency and/or ventricular dysfunction; usually associated with patent foramen ovale/secundum ASD	Varying degrees of CHF and cyanosis; older patients may have arrhythmias	ECG: RA enlargement, Wolff-Parkinson-White syndrome (10–20%) CXR: Cardiomegaly, decreased pulmonary vascularity Echo: Enlarged RA, displaced tricuspid valve, atrialized RV Cath: ↑ RA pressures, right-to-left shunt across ASD, tricuspid displacement and insufficiency; RV dysfunction	Tricuspid valve replacement or repair, ASD closure	Mortality 5–8%; good long-term results

Condition	%	Pathophysiology	Signs/symptoms	Diagnosis	Treatment	Prognosis
Aneurysm of the sinus of Valsalva	< 1	Aneurysmal dilatation of sinus of Valsalva (usu. right coronary sinus); rupture leads to dysfunction of affected chamber and heart failure	Sudden or gradual onset of chest pain, dyspnea, and/or palpitations, continuous parasternal murmur +/– thrill	ECG: Cardiac hypertrophy CXR: Cardiomegaly, pulmonary congestion Echo: Aneurysmal origin, dysfunctional cardiac chamber Cath: Aneurysmal origin, affected chamber	Excision of aneurysmal sac to aortic origin, patch defect closure	Mortality low; excellent long-term results
Coronary artery anomalies: ALCAPA CAVF	< 1	Creation of coronary steal and myocardial ischemia	Often mild to absent in infancy; includes angina, dyspnea, failure to thrive, cyanosis; occasional flow murmurs	ECG: LVH (ALCAPA); ventricular overload (CAVF) CXR: Cardiomegaly, pulmonary congestion Echo: Ventricular dilatation; hypokinesis (ALCAPA); arteriovenous fistula connection (CAVF) Cath: Abnormal left coronary ostial origin (ALCAPA); arteriovenous fistula, left-to-right shunts (CAVF)	Establish continuity between ascending Ao and left main coronary ostium (Takeuchi procedure) (ALCAPA); Ligate fistulae (CAVF)	Mortality highly variable w/ ALCAPA, very low w/ CAVF; excellent long-term results for operative survivors (ALCAPA, CAVF)
Double-outlet right ventricle (DORV)	1–2	Both great vessels arise from RV; left-to-right shunt across VSD leads to increased pulmonary blood flow and congestion; associated w/ pulmonary stenosis, which leads to decreased pulmonary blood flow and cyanosis	CHF symptoms w/ increased pulmonary blood flow; cyanosis w/ decreased pulmonary blood flow, d-TGA, or inverted ventricles	ECG: RVH CXR: Cardiomegaly, pulmonary congestion Echo: Relationships between VSD, A-V valves, and great vessels Cath: Origins of great vessels w/ respect to ventricles and VSD	Intraventricular tunnel repair for simple DORV w/ subaortic VSD and no pulmonary stenosis; Repair similar to tetralogy of Fallot for simple DORV w/ subaortic VSD and pulmonary stenosis	Mortality 5–10%; variable long-term results
Hypoplastic left heart syndrome	7–10[1]	Marked hypoplastic, nonfunctional LV; RV supports pulmonary and systemic circulations w/ PDA-dependent parallel flow; CHF and systemic hypoperfusion result as pulmonary:systemic blood flow ↑	Tachypnea, cyanosis, CHF, left parasternal systolic murmur, right ventricular lift	ECG: RA and RV enlargement CXR: Cardiomegaly, pulmonary congestion Echo: Hypoplastic LV and Ao; PDA, ASD, tricuspid insufficiency	Norwood procedure or cardiac transplantation	Mortality 20–50% for Norwood stage 1, lower for stages 2 and 3; early mortality 20% for transplantation
Congenitally corrected transposition of the great arteries	< 1	Combined discordant ventriculoarterial and atrioventricular connections resulting in "corrected" transposition of systemic and pulmonary circulations; pathophysiology stems from high incidence of associated intracardiac anomalies: VSD, pulmonary outflow tract obstruction, A-V conduction defects, "tricuspid" regurgitation	Related to associated congenital cardiac anomalies	ECG: A-V conduction abnormalities CXR: Anterior and leftward position of Ao Echo: Associated cardiac anomalies Cath: Pulmonary artery anatomy, intracardiac pressures, pulmonary vascular resistance	Based upon associated cardiac anomalies	Mortality 10–20%; 25% require reoperation, usually for progressive left-sided A-V valve incompetence

[1]7–10% of defects in neonates diagnosed with congenital heart disease.

ALCAPA = anomalous left coronary artery from the pulmonary artery; Ao = aorta/aortic; ASD = atrial septal defect; A-V = atrioventricular; CAVF = coronary arteriovenous fistula; CHF = congestive heart failure; CXR = chest x-ray; d-TGA = d-transposition of the great arteries; ECG = electrocardiogram; LA = left atrium; LV = left ventricle; PA = pulmonary artery; RA = right atrium; RV = right ventricle; RVH/LVH = right/left ventricular hypertrophy; VSD = ventricular septal defect.

tic of CMVD, defining the malformed mitral valve and quantifying elevated left atrial (wedge) pressures.

Treatment

Only about 20% of patients with CMVD survive to 3 years of age without surgical correction. Significant pulmonary venous hypertension leading to severe signs and symptoms indicate early operation in patients with CMVD. Furthermore, significant pulmonary hypertension, even in the absence of symptoms, is also a strong indication for operation. Surgical techniques of repair and replacement for the many types of mitral valve disease closely resemble those used for acquired valvular disease in adults. Valve repair should be attempted, since valve replacement in the pediatric population requires a mechanical prosthesis; tissue valves can rapidly deteriorate in children. Commissurotomy and papillary muscle splitting are useful techniques for patients with parachute mitral valves and a single papillary muscle.

Results

Hospital mortality is highly variable considering the wide spectrum of clinical presentations and valve anomalies, but satisfactory results can usually be achieved with valve repair when feasible. High early mortality frequently results from the technical difficulties associated with mitral valve replacement in children under 1 year of age. Many patients who undergo early correction of CMVD require future reoperation for valve replacement or correction of residual mitral valve incompetence.

AORTIC-PULMONARY WINDOW

General Considerations

Aortic-pulmonary (A-P) window represents a rare congenital anomaly in which a large communication exists between the proximal ascending aorta and the main pulmonary trunk (type I) or the more distal aorta and origin of the right pulmonary artery (type II). Physiologically, this results in a high-flow left-to-right shunt leading to rapidly progressive CHF if left untreated. The augmented pulmonary artery flow also results in obstructive pulmonary vascular changes. There is no tendency for spontaneous closure of this defect. From 30% to 50% of all patients with A-P window have a coexisting cardiac anomaly, including VSD, tetralogy of Fallot, subaortic stenosis, ASD, right aortic arch, and PDA.

Diagnosis

Infants with isolated A-P window typically present early in life with signs and symptoms of CHF, including tachypnea, failure to thrive, and frequent respiratory infections. Physical examination reveals a systolic flow murmur of varying intensity and wide pulse pressures. Electrocardiography and chest films typically present signs of left and right ventricular enlargement as well as left atrial enlargement due to pulmonary overcirculation. Echocardiography effectively demonstrates A-P window, however, cardiac catheterization with cineangiography may be required for better anatomical definition.

Treatment

Symptomatic infants with A-P window should be operated on early after the diagnosis is made, preferably before 3 months of age. Since CHF and pulmonary vascular changes are usually severe with this anomaly, corrective surgery is recommended for all patients with A-P window, except in advanced cases with very high pulmonary vascular resistances. On CPB, the defect is accessed through a transverse opening made in the aorta (or pulmonary trunk if necessary). Small windows may be closed with sutures alone while larger defects are patched from within the aorta with prosthetic material or autologous pericardium.

Results

Mortality after early A-P window repair is low, with excellent long-term results. Later repairs are often subject to the effects of high pulmonary vascular resistances.

DOUBLE-INLET SINGLE VENTRICLE

General Considerations

Double-inlet single ventricle (DISV) is a very rare congenital syndrome characterized by a single functional ventricle into which both A-V valves empty; the interventricular septum at the inlet is absent. It presents in several forms, with variation in the types of functioning and hypoplastic ventricles (right or left), malformations of the A-V valves, and great vessel origins. The most common anatomical pattern is double-inlet left ventricle, consisting of a rudimentary right ventricle and discordant ventriculoarterial connection. In this pattern, both atria drain into a dominant right-sided left ventricle that empties into the pulmonary artery. This chamber communicates with the rudimentary right ventricle from which the aorta arises. The two most common physiologic manifestations of this syndrome are (1) hypoxemia from mixing of oxygenated and deoxygenated blood prior to ejection into the aorta and (2) increased pulmonary blood flow resulting in pulmonary hypertension and CHF.

Diagnosis

The clinical presentation of DISV varies with the degree of pulmonary obstruction. Infants with increased pulmonary blood flow are not severely cyanotic, but suffer from pulmonary congestion and cardiac failure. On the other hand, infants with decreased pulmonary blood flow secondary to pulmonary atresia or stenosis suffer from significant cyanosis. Electrocardiography and chest radiography may reveal signs of DISV, particularly cardiomegaly and pulmonary congestion, however, echocardiography is usually diagnostic. The hallmark echocardiographic sign of DISV is the absence of the interventricular septum.

Treatment

The majority of patients with DISV morphology are tracked toward a modified Fontan procedure. Patients with unrestricted pulmonary flow may require pulmonary artery banding prior to the Fontan procedure. Many patients with pulmonary outflow obstruction require a palliative systemic-pulmonary artery shunt (bidirectional Glenn shunt) at 4–6 months of age as the initial procedure prior to the Fontan operation.

Subaortic obstruction and discordant ventriculoarterial connection develops in most patients with DISV, resulting from restriction of the bulboventricular foramen. This can be managed with the Damus-Kaye-Stansel procedure at the time of the bidirectional Glenn shunt. The extracardiac modification of the Fontan procedure is then performed at about 2 years of age.

Results

The results of the Fontan operation for single ventricle are similar to those achieved when this operation is performed for pulmonary atresia. The operative mortality is 5–10% with satisfactory long-term results, especially for patients who have a morphologic left ventricle as the dominant ventricle.

EBSTEIN'S ANOMALY

General Considerations

Ebstein's anomaly is a rare congenital cardiac lesion defined by malformation of the posterior and septal leaflets of the tricuspid valve. The anterior septal leaflet is usually normal or enlarged to some degree. The malformed leaflet origins are inferiorly displaced into the right ventricle, creating a thin-walled "atrialized" portion of the right ventricle. A patent foramen ovale or secundum defect is usually associated with this anomaly. Moderate cyanosis is found in about 50% of these patients because of right-to-left shunting across the ASD. Ebstein's anomaly varies widely in severity. The main physiologic disturbance associated with this defect is inadequate right ventricular output stemming from tricuspid insufficiency and right ventricular dysfunction. The natural progression of disability from this anomaly is generally gradual, however, approximately 50% of severely symptomatic patients die in infancy.

Diagnosis

Signs and symptoms of Ebstein's anomaly depend upon the degree of tricuspid insufficiency, the size of the ASD, and the degree of right ventricular dysfunction. Consequently, many infants present with cyanosis and severe CHF. Older patients with this anomaly usually present with dyspnea and cyanosis. Arrhythmias are associated with this anomaly; 10–20% of these patients have Wolff-Parkinson-White (WPW) syndrome. Physical examination generally reveals a systolic flow murmur from tricuspid insufficiency, cyanosis, and clubbing. Electrocardiography and chest radiography usually reveal cardiomegaly, due to a markedly dilated right atrium, and decreased pulmonary vascularity. Characteristic echocardiographic findings include delayed closure of the tricuspid valve compared to the mitral valve, a downwardly displaced tricuspid valve, a small atrialized right ventricle, and an enlarged right atrium. Definitive diagnosis of Ebstein's anomaly is usually made with echocardiography.

Treatment

Indications for surgical correction include New York Heart Association class III or IV functional status, moderate to severe cyanosis, paradoxic emboli, right ventricular outflow tract obstruction, and intractable arrhythmias. As a result of the wide anatomical variability of Ebstein's anomaly, a variety of techniques for surgical correction are available. The most common approach involves repair or replacement of the tricuspid valve and ASD closure. Valvular repair is preferred to replacement, especially in young children. Neonates with severe heart failure and cyanosis may be treated by oversewing the tricuspid valve and performing a systemic-pulmonary artery shunt. These patients are hence converted to a single ventricle configuration and are tracked toward an eventual modified Fontan procedure. In cases of WPW, accessory pathways are sectioned.

Results

Overall early mortality after surgical correction of Ebstein's anomaly is about 5%, usually from acute cardiac failure. Late deaths are uncommon after tricuspid repair or replacement and ASD closure, with most surviving patients achieving a significantly improved functional status.

ANEURYSM OF THE SINUS OF VALSALVA

General Considerations

Aneurysm of the sinus of Valsalva is defined by a thinning of the aortic media layer in the wall of the sinus of Valsalva, usually involving the right coronary sinus (67%). Right coronary sinus aneurysms rupture into the right ventricle. The noncoronary sinus is involved less frequently (25%) and usually ruptures into the right atrium. Involvement of the left coronary sinus is infrequent (8%). Morphologically, these aneurysms resemble a windsock, with a wide base at the aortic origin and tapered tip extending into the chamber where it may rupture. This lesion is also associated with VSD and aortic valve prolapse.

Diagnosis

There are usually no physical manifestations of this anomaly prior to rupture unless the aneurysm distorts the aortic leaflets to such an extent that aortic insufficiency results. Once rupture occurs, on average at around 30 years of age, about one third of afflicted patients experience a sudden onset of chest pain followed by dyspnea and palpitations. A characteristic parasternal continuous murmur often associated with a thrill also presents. In nearly one half of these patients, however, aneurysmal rupture is associated with a more gradual onset of symptoms. Over the ensuing weeks and months after rupture, cardiac failure progresses, becoming intolerable within 1–2 years. Electrocardiography and chest radiography reveal cardiac hypertrophy and pulmonary congestion. Echocardiography is often diagnostic. Catheterization and cineangiography are useful in localizing the aneurysm's site of origin, identifying the cardiac chamber involved, and defining any associated defects.

Treatment & Results

A ruptured sinus aneurysm should be repaired promptly. The aneurysmal sac is excised back to its aortic origin and the defect is closed, usually with a prosthetic patch. Postoperative mortality after surgical repair of this anomaly is very low. Results and long-term prognosis after repair are generally excellent.

CORONARY ARTERY ANOMALIES

1. ANOMALOUS LEFT CORONARY ARTERY FROM THE PULMONARY ARTERY

General Considerations

Anomalous left coronary artery from the pulmonary artery (ALCAPA) is a rare congenital cardiac defect in which the left main coronary ostium originates from the proximal main pulmonary artery or, less frequently, from the proximal right main pulmonary artery. The branching pattern of the left coronary artery and the right coronary artery ostia are normal. Physiologically, the right coronary artery supplies the entire myocardium and intracoronary collaterals which, in turn, feed the left coronary artery. Therefore, left coronary artery flow is reversed and drains into the pulmonary artery. A significant coronary steal results, leading to myocardial ischemia, left ventricular dilatation, and heart failure in infancy.

Diagnosis

Symptoms of myocardial ischemia can present within 1–2 weeks of birth. These symptoms include circumoral pallor and cyanosis, poor feeding, sweating, dyspnea, tachycardia, and discomfort, many of which probably stem from angina. When symptoms do not present in infancy, CHF and ischemia may not become obvious until 20 years of age. Physical examination commonly reveals a precordial lift, hepatomegaly, and pulmonary rales. Electrocardiographic signs consistent with anterolateral infarction and LVH suggest this diagnosis; cardiac enzymes may be elevated. Chest radiography reveals cardiomegaly and interstitial pulmonary edema. Echocardiography usu-

ally shows a dilated, hypokinetic left ventricle. Definitive diagnosis requires cardiac catheterization and cineangiography to demonstrate the anomalous left coronary ostium and retrograde left coronary artery blood flow.

Treatment & Results

The diagnosis of ALCAPA in infancy or adulthood is an indication for early surgical correction to prevent sequelae of myocardial ischemia. The optimal operation is the construction of a two-coronary system, which entails the creation of direct continuity between the left coronary ostium and the ascending aorta. This is achieved with coronary translocation and a direct anastomosis or the creation of a tunnel from the aorta to the anomalous origin of the left coronary artery (**Takeuchi procedure**). The mortality associated with correction of ALCAPA varies widely, and follow-up data is somewhat lacking; however, it is assumed that most patients who recover from this operation have a good long-term prognosis.

2. CORONARY ARTERIOVENOUS FISTULA

General Considerations

Coronary arteriovenous fistula is defined as the presence of one or more communication(s) between a coronary artery and any one of the four cardiac chambers, coronary sinus, and tributaries thereof, superior vena cava, pulmonary artery, or pulmonary veins. Most commonly, isolated coronary arteriovenous fistulae (CAVF) from the left or right coronary arteries terminate in the right heart chambers or pulmonary artery. Such fistulae lead to myocardial ischemia by creating a coronary steal and imposing an additional volume load on the left ventricle.

Diagnosis

Signs and symptoms of CAVF depend upon the volume of fistula flow and are usually absent-to-mild in infancy. Most patients are diagnosed and treated late in life, after 20 years of age. In fact, detection of this anomaly often results from a continuous murmur found on routine physical examination or mild signs of cardiomegaly and pulmonary congestion on chest films. Symptoms are generally nonspecific and include effort dyspnea and fatigue and CHF signs; angina and myocardial infarction are rare. Electrocardiography and chest films are often normal but may occasionally suggest right or left ventricular overload, cardiomegaly, and pulmonary congestion. Cardiac catheterization with selected coronary cineangiography is required for definitive diagnosis and planning of surgical repair.

Treatment & Results

Since some congenital arteriovenous fistulae enlarge with age and predispose to heart failure, accelerated atherosclerotic changes, coronary aneurysmal dilatation, and bacterial endocarditis, surgical closure of all but the smallest of fistulae is recommended. Mortality associated with closure of congenital CAVF approaches zero. Complications are rare and the long-term prognoses are generally excellent.

DOUBLE-OUTLET RIGHT VENTRICLE

General Considerations

Double-outlet right ventricle (DORV) is a rare congenital cardiac defect in which both great arteries arise from the right ventricle. It is usually associated with a VSD located beneath the aorta or pulmonary artery. Pulmonary stenosis is often associated with DORV. Discussion of the many DORV variants is beyond the scope of this chapter, however, classification is based upon the presence or absence of pulmonary stenosis, the relationship of the great arteries to the ventricles, and the presence or absence of ventricular inversion. DORV with a subpulmonic VSD is termed a **Taussig-Bing anomaly**.

The pathophysiology of DORV depends upon the anatomical variant. In the absence of pulmonary stenosis, left-to-right flow across the VSD results in pulmonary hypertension, obstructive pulmonary vascular disease, and CHF. If the great arteries are transposed or if the ventricles are inverted (without pulmonary stenosis), the pathophysiology resembles that of *d*-TGA with a VSD, specifically hypoxemia and high pulmonary blood flow. If pulmonary stenosis is present, significant cyanosis and polycythemia result from inadequate pulmonary blood flow.

Diagnosis

Signs and symptoms associated with DORV include those of CHF. Cyanosis is particularly prominent with pulmonary stenosis. Physical examination often reveals a parasternal murmur. Electrocardiography may show evidence of RVH. Chest radiography typically reveals a cardiomegaly with pulmonary congestion in the absence of pulmonary stenosis. Echocardiography and cineangiography define important anatomical relationships between the VSD, great vessels, A-V valves, and ventricles.

Treatment & Results

DORV anatomical variability has resulted in different approaches to treatment. In general, simple DORV with subaortic VSD and without pulmonary stenosis should be repaired early (before 6 months) to avoid complications from chronic pulmonary overcirculation. The indications for DORV with significant pulmonary stenosis resemble those for the tetralogy of Fallot; the repair can be deferred until 6–24 months of age or until significant symptoms develop.

Simple DORV with a subaortic VSD and no pulmonary stenosis is repaired by creating a tunnel within the right ventricle that conducts left ventricular blood from the VSD to the aorta (**intraventricular tunnel repair**). DORV with a subaortic VSD and pulmonary stenosis is repaired in a manner similar to the tetralogy of Fallot, substituting construction of an intraventricular tunnel for the simple VSD repair. The Taussig-Bing anomaly is best treated with an arterial switch and VSD closure, since an intraventricular tunnel repair is not feasible. The overall operative risk associated with repair of DORV ranges between 5–10%, with variable long-term prognoses.

HYPOPLASTIC LEFT HEART SYNDROME

General Considerations

Hypoplastic left heart syndrome (HLHS) represents left-sided cardiac maldevelopment, with most cases displaying left ventricular hypoplasia, atresia of the ascending aorta, and an intact ventricular septum. HLHS occurs in 7–10% of newborns diagnosed with congenital heart disease and accounts for 25% of cardiac deaths within the first week of life. Since the left ventricle is nonfunctional, the right ventricle supports the pulmonary and systemic circulations with parallel flow. Blood is pumped into the main pulmonary artery with systemic flow provided via a typically large PDA. Retrograde flow from the PDA into the aortic arch and ascending aorta delivers coronary and cerebral perfusion. Antegrade flow from the PDA into the descending aorta provides lower body systemic perfusion. Pulmonary venous return to the left atrium is shunted across a patent foramen ovale or ASD into the right atrium and ventricle. The balance between systemic and pulmonary blood flow is related to the difference in systemic and pulmonary resistances. Pulmonary vascular resistance is high in the newborn period, generally providing a proper balance between pulmonary and systemic perfusion. CHF, renal insufficiency, and acidosis develop as the pulmonary resistance drops and pulmonary flow increases. ASD size is an important determinant of pulmonary blood flow as the pulmonary vascular resistance falls.

Diagnosis

Neonates with HLHS typically display tachypnea and mild cyanosis in the first 24–48 hours of life. A single heart sound, a left sternal systolic murmur, and right ventricular lift are usually apparent on physical examination. Right atrial and ventricular enlargement are suggested on electrocardiography. Chest radiography indicates cardiomegaly and pulmonary overcirculation. A pattern of obstructive pulmonary venous return may be observed if intra-atrial shunting is excessively restrictive. Echocardiography is diagnostic of HLHS and defines the sizes of the ascending aorta, PDA, and ASD, in addition to the degree of tricuspid regurgitation.

Treatment

The preoperative management of HLHS is important. The two major goals are the maintenance of (1) ductal patency and (2) the balance between pulmonary and systemic flow ($Q_P:Q_S = 1$). Ductal patency can be maintained with an infusion of PGE_1. Most neonates with HLHS diagnosed in the first few days of life have a $Q_P:Q_S$ of approximately 1 and do not require mechanical ventilation. Some patients have a nonrestrictive ASD and require mechanical ventilation to increase pulmonary vascular resistance and reduce pulmonary flow. Ventilation with CO_2 (1–3%) added to the room air inspired gas mixture is effective in treating systemic hypoperfusion and pulmonary overcirculation in these patients. Some patients are effectively managed without mechanical ventilation using a hood ventilated with room air and supplemental CO_2.

Surgical treatment of HLHS is directed toward cardiac transplantation or the staged **Norwood procedure**. The mortality for neonates with HLHS is approximately 40% during the waiting period for a donor heart. Improvements in the operative mortality for the Norwood procedure have prompted most centers to recommend the first stage of the operation, since the operative mortality is generally less than the combined mortality associated with waiting for and performing cardiac replacement. This decision does not preclude cross-over to transplantation.

There are three stages to the Norwood procedure. The first stage, performed in the neonate, replaces the PDA as the systemic outflow conduit with construction of a "neoaorta" comprised of the proximal portion of the transected main pulmonary artery anastomosed to the ascending aorta and arch. After an atrial septectomy is done, a systemic-pulmonary artery (modified Blalock-Taussig) shunt is constructed to supply pulmonary blood flow.

As the pulmonary vascular resistance falls in the weeks after completion of the first stage, the systemic-pulmonary artery shunt would become excessive and lead to congestive failure. Therefore, the second stage of the Norwood reconstruction involves conversion of the systemic-pulmonary artery shunt to a bidirectional cavopulmonary (Glenn) shunt, usually at 6 months. The third and final stage of the Norwood reconstruction is a modified Fontan operation performed between 18 months and 2 years of age.

Results

In the Norwood staged reconstruction, operative mortality is 20–50% for the first stage and lower mortalities for each of the second and third stages. Cardiac transplantation is associated with a lower operative mortality (20%); however, 20–40% of neonates on waiting lists do not receive donor hearts. Moreover, transplantation requires lifelong immunosuppression.

CONGENITALLY CORRECTED TRANSPOSITION OF THE GREAT ARTERIES

General Considerations

Congenitally corrected transposition of the great arteries (CC-TGA) is also referred to as *l*-transposition of the great arteries (*l*-TGA) to distinguish this anomaly from *d*-TGA. In patients with CC-TGA, systemic venous blood returns to the right atrium and crosses a right-sided mitral A-V valve into a morphologic left ventricle. The right-sided "left" ventricle pumps blood into the pulmonary artery. Blood returning from the lungs into the left atrium crosses a left-sided tricuspid A-V valve into a morphologic right ventricle. The left-sided "right" ventricle pumps blood into the aorta, thereby completing the normal intracardiac flow of blood. The coronary circulation and A-V valves follow the ventricular morphology. The left-sided "right" ventricle is supplied by a morphologic right coronary artery, and the right-sided "left" ventricle is supplied by a morphologic left coronary system.

Associated cardiac anomalies are common with CC-TGA and influence the clinical course. A VSD is present in about 70% of patients with CC-TGA. Pulmonary outflow tract obstruction, A-V conduction defects, and left A-V valve "tricuspid" regurgitation are also observed.

Diagnosis

Patients with no associated cardiac anomaly may be asymptomatic for years. Most symptoms are related to the presence of an associated cardiac abnormality. Patients with tricuspid regurgitation or a VSD will have a characteristic precordial murmur. The association of pulmonary outflow stenosis and VSD may result in cyanosis. Roentgenographic evidence of pulmonary overcirculation may be seen in patients with VSD and pulmonary congestion in patients with tricuspid regurgitation. The anterior and leftward position of the aorta produces a characteristic radiographic silhouette. Varying patterns of A-V conduction abnormalities may be observed with electrocardiography. Echocardiography is diagnostic and reliably identifies associated cardiac malformations. Cardiac catheterization may be needed to more clearly define pulmonary artery anatomy or for the measurement of intracardiac pressures and pulmonary resistance.

Treatment

The treatment of CC-TGA is based on the associated cardiac anomaly. The timing of VSD closure is the same as for other patients. There is an increased incidence of complete heart block after VSD repair in these patients due to the unusual course of the conduction tissue. Relief of pulmonary outflow tract stenosis generally requires a ventricular-to-pulmonary artery conduit because a transannular patch with resection of subvalvular tissue is associated with heart block. Tricuspid valve regurgitation in these patients generally requires valve replacement or repair.

Left-sided "right" ventricular failure occurs in some of these patients as a result of long-term pumping against systemic vascular resistance. Aggressive afterload reduction may be beneficial with cardiac transplantation reserved for medical failures. The use of the arterial switch operation in conjunction with an atrial switch procedure has been used to treat patients with CC-TGA. This "double switch" operation is only useful in patients with nonobstructed ventriculoarterial connections and when the right-sided left ventricle has maintained conditioning by functioning at systemic pressures, usually as the result of pulmonary outflow tract obstruction.

Results

The overall operative mortality for intracardiac repair in patients with CC-TGA is about 10–20%. The incidence of perioperative heart block is also 10–20%. Approximately 25% of patients will require reoperation, usually for progressive left-sided A-V valve regurgitation.

SUGGESTED READING

Castaneda AR et al: *Cardiac Surgery of the Neonate and Infant.* Saunders, 1994.

Kirklin JW, Barratt-Boyes BG: *Cardiac Surgery.* Churchill Livingstone, 1993.

Mavroudis C, Backer CL: *Pediatric Cardiac Surgery,* 2nd ed. Mosby-Year Book, 1994.

Nichols DG et al: *Critical Heart Disease in Infants and Children.* Mosby-Year Book, 1995.

Stark J, de Leval M: *Surgery for Congenital Heart Defects,* 2nd ed. Saunders, 1994.

38

The Lung, Chest Wall, & Pleura

38.1 Pulmonary Diseases

Stephen C. Yang, MD, & Richard F. Heitmiller, MD

> ## ► Key Facts

- ► Anomalies of the lung are uncommon, but include bronchogenic cysts, pulmonary sequestration, congenital cystic adenomatoid malformations, and congenital lobar emphysema.

- ► Vascular anomalies that directly influence pulmonary functions include congenital absence of the pulmonary artery, pulmonary arteriovenous malformations, and the scimitar syndrome.

- ► Noninfectious interstitial lung disorders that would be diagnosed surgically (via mediastinoscopy, anterior mediastinotomy, or lung biopsy) include sarcoidosis, interstitial pneumonitis, interstitial pulmonary fibrosis, allergic pulmonary hypersensitivity, and bronchiolitis obliterans with organizing pneumonia.

- ► More than 14 million Americans suffer from various stages of chronic obstructive pulmonary disease (COPD), with smoking as the most common cause.

- ► Fewer than 1% of patients with COPD have indications for palliative surgery that would include bullectomy, lung transplantation, and lung volume reduction surgery.

- ► Indications for palliative surery for COPD include end-stage disease, maximized medical therapy, good rehabilitation potential, and demonstrated compliance to medical therapy.

- ► Approximately 25% of lung transplantation procedures are performed for COPD.

ANATOMY

Surgical anatomy of the lungs, airway, and pulmonary vasculature is of prime importance to the thoracic surgeon. Knowledge of the anatomic relationships and possible anomalies is critical in the diagnosis and surgical management of patients with pulmonary diseases. Pulmonary vasculature, lobar, and segmental anatomy is reviewed in Figures 38.1–1 and 38.1–2.

CONGENITAL LESIONS OF THE LUNG

Anomalies of the lung are uncommon. They usually become apparent in children and young adults but can present at any age. These anomalies occur as a consequence of abnormalities in development of the lungs and trachea from the ventral bud of the primitive foregut.

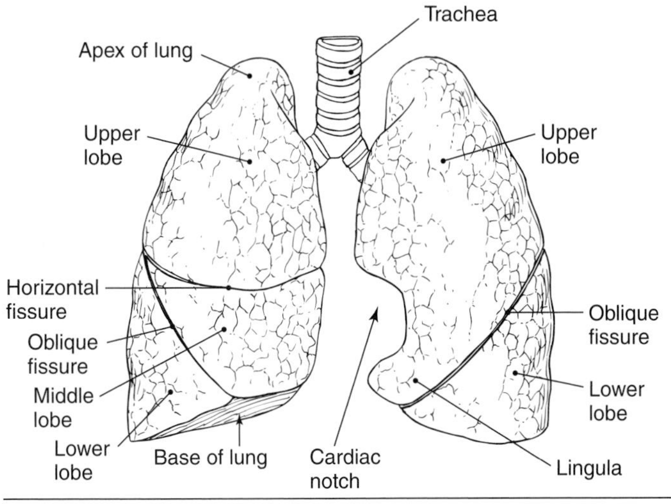

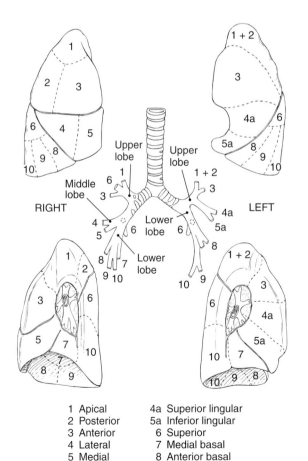

Figure 38.1–1. Topical anatomy of the lungs (anterior view).

1 Apical
2 Posterior
3 Anterior
4 Lateral
5 Medial
4a Superior lingular
5a Inferior lingular
6 Superior
7 Medial basal
8 Anterior basal
9 Lateral basal
10 Posterior basal

Figure 38.1–2. Segmental anatomy of the bronchopulmonary system.

BRONCHOGENIC CYST

A bronchogenic cyst is a spherical cyst of bronchial origin, formed by abnormal budding of the respiratory tract anlage during embryogenesis, which is lined with bronchial epithelium. Paratracheal, subcarinal, parahilar, and intraparenchymal cyst locations have been reported. Although rare, malignancies have been reported originating from these cysts. Symptoms depend on the size and location of the cyst, and whether it has a bronchial connection. Most patients, however, are asymptomatic. The diagnosis is suggested by identification of a round, cystic intrathoracic mass on chest film or computed tomography (CT). Treatment is resection to confirm the diagnosis and to prevent complications.

SEQUESTRATION

A sequestration (Figure 38.1–3) is a segment or lobe of lung that has no airway communication with the native lung, and which has a systemic blood supply. There are two types. Eighty-five percent of sequestrations are intralobar, in which the abnormal lung tissue is surrounded by adjoining normal lung tissue, and 15% are extralobar, in which the sequestrated segment is completely separate from the normal lung tissue and invested in its own pleural lining. A sequestration is often identified as an asymptomatic mass on chest film. Symptoms, when present, include recurrent respiratory infections due to pneumonia within the sequestration, and less frequently, hemoptysis. The diagnosis is best made by contrast chest CT, which demonstrates both the sequestration and its systemic blood supply. Prior to the advent of CT, angiography was used to identify the aberrant arterial blood supply. Surgery is recommended to prevent recurrent respiratory infections.

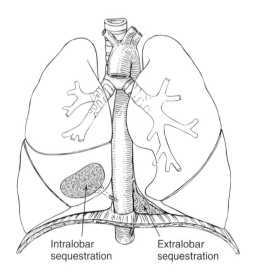

Intralobar
sequestration

Extralobar
sequestration

Figure 38.1–3. Pulmonary sequestration.

CONGENITAL CYSTIC ADENOMATOID MALFORMATIONS

Congenital cystic adenomatoid malformations result from an overgrowth of bronchial tubular structures and a lack of mature alveoli. Three variants are described: cystic, intermediate, and solid. The abnormality causes air trapping and progressive distention of the abnormal lung leading to respiratory distress. The degree of symptoms vary from milder degrees of respiratory distress in patients with cystic lesions, to solid lesions that are fatal. Older children and adults may present with an asymptomatic radiographic finding on chest film, or with recurrent respiratory infections. A multicystic lung lesion, best seen by chest CT, suggests the diagnosis. Surgical resection is indicated, sometimes emergently, to treat or prevent respiratory compromise of the compressed noninvolved lung.

CONGENITAL LOBAR EMPHYSEMA

Congenital lobar emphysema is a condition in which there is isolated lobar hyperinflation without extrinsic bronchial obstruction. Focal agenesis of bronchial wall support resulting in a segment of bronchomalacia is responsible for this air-trapping condition. The left upper lobe is most commonly affected. Symptoms usually present in infancy and include tachypnea, wheezing, chest wall retractions, and repeated respiratory infections. On examination, symptomatic patients have tracheal deviation away from the affected side, and decreased breath sounds and hyperresonance on the affected side. On chest film, the hyperexpanded lung is identified. Sometimes it may be mistaken for a pneumothorax. Treatment is lobectomy.

VASCULAR ANOMALIES

Congenital absence of the pulmonary artery, pulmonary arteriovenous malformations, and the scimitar syndrome are considered vascular anomalies.

Agenesis of the pulmonary artery is rare. Most patients die early of severe pulmonary hypertension and right heart failure. In patients who survive, there is often anomalous systemic blood supply to the affected lung as well as enlarged ipsilateral bronchial arteries. Patients present with recurrent respiratory infections and hemoptysis. The diagnosis is made by right heart catheterization. The treatment is pneumonectomy.

Pulmonary arteriovenous fistula (AVF) may occur with either a pulmonary arterial or systemic arterial blood supply. The former is more common. Patients with AVF are divided into those with multiple hereditary telangiectasias (Osler-Weber-Rendu syndrome) and those without it. There is a prognostic significance to this classification in that those patients with Osler-Weber-Rendu syndrome more often have multiple AVF, progressive symptoms, and more complications. Half the patients with AVF are symptomatic with dyspnea, palpitations, and easy fatigability. Only one in five patients present with the classic triad of cyanosis, polycythemia, and clubbing. Onset of symptoms is usually the third or fourth decade. Patients may have documented decrease in PO_2 or oxygen saturation. A lobulated mass with a density connecting it to the hilum, usually solitary and involving the lower lung fields, is seen on chest film. Chest CT shows the AVF anatomy in greater detail, however, pulmonary arteriography, to determine the vascular anatomy of the fistula, hemodynamic measurements, and number of AVF, is still indicated. Only those AVF that are small and asymptomatic should be followed. Surgical resection is indicated for good-risk patients with symptomatic or large, solitary fistula. Patients with multiple AVF, or who are not surgical candidates, are considered for angiographic embolization of the fistulas.

SCIMITAR SYNDROME

Abnormal pulmonary venous drainage of the right lung to the inferior vena cava produces a characteristic curve-shaped radiographic density that resembles a scimitar and is therefore known as the scimitar syndrome. There is a high incidence of associated abnormalities of the right lung, pulmonary artery, bronchus, and heart. Reported symptoms include dyspnea, fatigue, cough, and respiratory infections. On chest film there is a small right hemithorax, shift of the heart to the right, and the characteristic scimitar shadow. There is right ventricular hypertrophy on electrocardiography. The diagnosis may be made by echocardiography or cardiac catheterization. For large shunts, both resection and surgical correction of the defect have been described.

INFLAMMATORY DISEASES
OF THE LUNG

LUNG ABSCESS

Lung abscess (Figure 38.1–4) is a suppurative, necrotizing process within the pulmonary parenchyma. Aspiration is the most common etiology; other causes include secondary infection of a lung bulla, trauma, lung infarction, or pulmonary extension of an intra-abdominal infection. Differential diagnosis must exclude cavitary tuberculosis and cavitary lung carcinoma. Patients characteristically present with fever and cough productive of copious and foul-smelling sputum. A round or oval parenchymal density with an air-fluid level is commonly noted on chest film. Early in the clinical course, however, the chest film may not show an air-fluid level.

Early flexible bronchoscopy is indicated in most cases to obtain cultures and to rule out bronchial obstruction (as with a bronchogenic carcinoma). Medical therapy with systemic antibiotics and chest physiotherapy is effective in over 90% of cases. Surgical intervention is warranted for persistent symptoms, large (or enlarging) size (> 6 cm), inability to differentiate from carcinoma, or spontaneous pleural drainage. There are two surgical options: (1) direct tube drainage of the abscess and (2) resection. Because of the inflammation and the often debilitated state of patients with lung abscess, surgery continues to have a mortality of 10% or greater.

BRONCHIECTASIS

Bronchiectasis, or dilatation of the bronchus, results from severe or recurrent respiratory infections (eg, immune-compromised patients and pertussis) and in association with congenital abnormalities, such as alpha$_1$ antitrypsin deficiency, cystic fibrosis, and Kartagener's syndrome (pansinusitis, situs inversus, bronchiectasis), or following external beam radiation therapy. Patients present with cough productive of large amounts of infected sputum, recurrent respiratory infections, and hemoptysis. Most cases are located in the lower lobes, and half are bilateral. Radiologic diagnosis in the past relied upon characteristic bronchial dilatation on bronchography (Figure 38.1–5). Today, chest CT is the recommended diagnostic test.

In the pre-antibiotic era, mortality reached 85%. With appropriate antibiotics, the rate is down to 25% in the late stages, and can be as low as 5% in the appropriately selected surgical candidate. Surgical resection may be indicated in patients who have localized resectable disease that fails medical therapy.

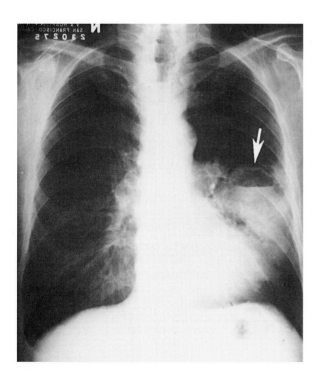

Figure 38.1–4. Posterior-anterior chest film showing left mid-lung abscess *(arrow)* with air-fluid level.

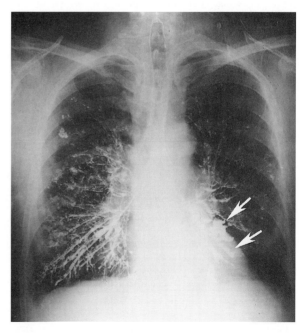

Figure 38.1–5. Bronchiectasis of the left lower lobe. Contrast bronchography demonstrates saccular dilatation of the bronchi *(arrows)* and normal caliper airways on the right.

MIDDLE LOBE SYNDROME & BRONCHOLITHIASIS

Extrinsic compression by bronchial lymph nodes or obstruction of the middle lobe orifice causes the middle lobe syndrome. Surgical resection, typically lobectomy, is required for recurrent intractable or recurrent pneumonia, abscess, bronchial stenosis, and exclusion of cancer.

Erosion of calcified lymph nodes into the bronchial lumen is known as broncholithiasis and is rare. It is usually a late complication of histoplasmosis (most common), tuberculosis, or coccidiomycosis (least common). Patients may present with a cough productive of gritty particles, respiratory infection, or hemoptysis. The diagnosis is made by identifying stones in the sputum or visualizing stones bronchoscopically. Surgery is infrequently indicated (25% of patients) for persistent airway obstruction or massive hemoptysis.

TUBERCULOSIS

Once a common cause of death in the United States, the incidence of tuberculosis has markedly declined over the past 5 decades. It remains the number one infectious-related cause of death worldwide. The species most often obtained is *Mycobacterium tuberculosis*, but may include *M bovis, M avium* and other "atypical" types. Less than 20% of the US population is tuberculin-positive; pulmonary symptoms present only when the disease is quite advanced. Medical treatment consists of multidrug therapy, including rifampin, streptomycin, isoniazid, and ethambutol. Surgery is indicated for empyema (see Chapter 38.2), bronchopulmonary fistula, hemoptysis, lung abscess, or in patients who remain persistently culture-positive despite antitubercular therapy.

MYCOTIC INFECTIONS

Surgery is often indicated in patients with mycotic infections (Figure 38.1–6). Procedures include lung biopsy

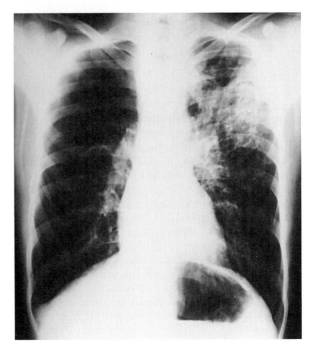

Figure 38.1–6. Aspergilloma of the left upper lobe. "Fungus ball" is seen inside a well-circumscribed cavity.

for diagnosis, resection to rule out cancer, surgical treatment of complications, such as hemoptysis, and surgical treatment of localized disease in suitable patients who are resistant to medical therapy. The clinical and radiographic characteristics and treatment of specific mycotic infections are listed in Table 38.1–1.

Table 38.1–1. Mycotic lung infections.

Infectious Process	Endemic Region/Source	Clinical Features	Radiologic Findings
Histoplasmosis	Mississippi River Valley/ contaminated soil	Acute URI symptoms, late mediastinal fibrosis	Acute pneumonitis, late calcified granuloma, nodes
Coccidiomycosis	Southwest US/spore-laden dust	Mild URI symptoms, arthritis; often asymptomatic	Acute pneumonitis, late coin lesion
Blastomycosis	Southeastern US/ contaminated soil	Mild URI symptoms, skin lesions	Acute pneumonitis, late fibronodular lesions
Cryptococcosis	No specific region/ contaminated soil	Mild URI symptoms, meningismus	Variable and not diagnostic
Aspergillosis	No specific region/ contaminated soil, airborne spores	Three forms: aspergillar bronchitis, "fungus ball," disseminated	Depends on form; "fungus ball" shown in Figure 38.1–6

URI = upper respiratory infection.

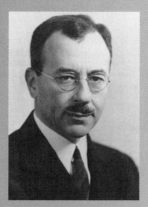

John Alexander, MD (1891–1954). (Courtesy of the University of Michigan.)

The name of John Alexander, MD, is held in high regard in thoracic surgery circles. He is particularly well known for his interest in the surgery of pulmonary tuberculosis. He graduated from the University of Pennsylvania in 1916 and served in France during World War I. Before returning home, he spent a short period in Lyons in the clinic of Leon Bérard, where they began implementing surgery in the treatment of tuberculosis. This experience played a large role in deciding John Alexander's future interests.

In 1920, Alexander joined the faculty at the University of Michigan, where he became the Head of Thoracic Surgery in 1928 at the first residency training program of its kind in the United States. Unfortunately, shortly after his arrival at the university, he developed spinal tuberculosis. It is widely believed that this setback actually unleashed hidden reserves of courage. During his enforced sojourns at Saranac Lake, he not only became a prolific writer, he also designed a special support structure that held a book in place for the bedridden reader. The two classic texts for which John Alexander is best known are *The Surgery of Pulmonary Tuberculosis* (Lea & Febiger, 1925) and *The Collapse Therapy of Pulmonary Tuberculosis* (Lea & Febiger, 1937).

John Alexander was not only a skillful surgeon and an inspiring teacher, he also possessed a charming and caring manner that earned him the respect and admiration of all who knew him. He trained more thoracic surgeons than any other teacher of his era. After his death, his trainees were responsible for writing and publishing the *John Alexander Monograph Series* on various aspects of thoracic surgery, which they dedicated to his memory "with affection, admiration and gratitude of the thoracic surgeons whom he trained."

INTERSTITIAL LUNG DISEASE

A detailed description of interstitial lung disease is beyond the scope of this surgical text. There are, however, a number of noninfectious, interstitial lung disorders in which the surgeon is involved in making the diagnosis, either by mediastinoscopy, anterior mediastinotomy, or lung biopsy (open versus thoracoscopic). These include sarcoidosis, interstitial pneumonitis, interstitial pulmonary fibrosis, allergic pulmonary hypersensitivity, and bronchiolitis obliterans with organizing pneumonia (BOOP).

CHRONIC OBSTRUCTIVE PULMONARY DISEASE

More than 14 million Americans suffer from various stages of chronic obstructive pulmonary disease (COPD). Smoking is the most common cause of this disease. Many advances have been made over the past 15 years to provide surgical options for patients with advanced disease. However, fewer than 1% of patients with COPD have indications for surgery. It should be stressed that these procedures are only palliative and not curative, with

Table 38.1–2. Surgical therapy for emphysema.

Surgical Technique	Indication
Bullectomy	Large bulla (> 1/2 hemithorax) FEV_1 > 40% predicted Compressed normal lung
Transplantation	Survival < 24 months FEV_1 < 20% predicted
Volume reduction	Heterogeneous disease FEV_1 20–30% predicted Lung hyperexpansion Flat hemidiaphragms

Table 38.1–3. Indications for lung transplantation.

Single-Lung Transplantation	Double-Lung Transplantation
Emphysema Primary pulmonary hypertension Idiopathic pulmonary fibrosis Sarcoidosis Alpha$_1$ antitrypsin deficiency Secondary pulmonary hypertension with corrected cardiac defect	Primary pulmonary hypertension Cystic fibrosis Alpha$_1$ antitrypsin deficiency Secondary pulmonary hypertension with corrected cardiac defect

the main goals of improving quality of life, exercise tolerance, and pulmonary function. These techniques include bullectomy, lung transplantation, and a new procedure called lung volume reduction surgery. The latter option was developed initially as a bridge to transplantation but is now indicated for patients not sick enough or too old for transplant. A summary of the indications and approaches for these options are listed in Table 38.1–2. Absolute indications for each procedure are the requirements that these patients have end-stage disease, maximized medical therapy, good rehabilitation potential, and demonstrated compliance to medical therapy.

Following bullectomy, early results are excellent, but at best 20% remain symptomatically improved at 10 years. Since the beginning of modern-day lung transplantation in 1983, actuarial 4-year survival has been 50%. Though a relatively new procedure, early results with lung volume reduction surgery show a plateau of improvement in the above-mentioned goals at 3 years. Follow-up reveals relative improvement in chest wall mechanics and diaphragmatic excursion. Long-term results will be required to determine efficacy and cost benefit with this procedure.

LUNG TRANSPLANTATION

The first successful human lung transplantation occurred in 1963 by Hardy and associates. The modern era began in 1983 and is credited to the Toronto experience, which coincided with the advent of cyclosporin. Since then, more than 3100 single-lung, double-lung, and bilateral sequential lung transplantation procedures have been performed worldwide (see Chapter 40.11). The current indications are summarized in Table 38.1–3. More than 25% of these procedures are performed for COPD.

The average waiting time for a single lung is 300 days; for two lungs, 400 days. Sepsis is the primary cause of postoperative death during the first year while bronchiolitis obliterans is the leading cause of late mortality.

The overall 1- and 4-year survival for lung transplantation patients is 70% and 50%, respectively. Patients with COPD do the best, while those with pulmonary hypertension have a 10% lower survival. Patients with single-lung and bilateral lung transplants have an actuarial survival rate of 53% and 62%, respectively. Nevertheless, lung transplantation is now an effective surgical option for select patients with end-stage lung disease.

SUGGESTED READING

Battistell F, Benfield JR: Blunt and penetrating injuries of the chest wall, pleura, and lungs. In: Shields TW (editor): *General Thoracic Surgery*, 4th ed. Lea & Febiger, 1994.

Bryan-Brown CW: Physiology of respiration. In: Miller TA (editor): *Physiologic Basis of Modern Surgical Care*. Mosby, 1988.

Campbell DB: Trauma to the chest wall, lung and major airways. Semin Thorac Cardiovasc Surg 1992;4:234.

Connolly JE, Wilson A: The current status of surgery for bullous emphysema. J Thorac Cardiovasc Surg 1989;97:351.

Cooper JD et al: Bilateral pneumectomy (volume reduction) for chronic obstructive pulmonary disease. J Thorac Cardiovasc Surg 1995;109:106.

Davis RD, Passkey M: Pulmonary transplantation. Ann Surg 1994;221:14.

Flynn A, Thomas AN, Schecter WP: Acute tracheobronchial injury. J Trauma 1989;29:1326.

Jurkovich GJ, Moore EE: Thoracic trauma. Trauma Q 1984;1:37.

Kaye MP: The registry of the international society for heart and lung transplantation: Tenth official report—1993. J Heart Lung Transplant 1993;12:541.

LoCicero J, Mattox KL: Epidemiology of chest trauma. Surg Clin North Am 1989;69:15.

Luck SR, Reynolds M, Raffensperger JG: Congenital bronchopulmonary malformations. Curr Prob Surg 1986;23:251.

Pohlsan EC et al: Lung abscess: A changing pattern of disease. Am J Surg 1985;150:97.

Richardson JD, McElvein RB, Trinkle JK: First rib fracture: A hallmark of severe trauma. Ann Surg 1975;181:251.

Trulock EP: Recipient selection. Chest Surg Clin North Am 1993;3:1.

38.2 Chest Wall & Pleural Disease

Stephen C. Yang, MD, & Richard F. Heitmiller, MD

▶ Key Facts

- ▶ Congenital anomalies of the chest wall include absence of ribs, cervical ribs, pectus excavatum, and pectus carinatum.

- ▶ Inflammatory chest wall infections include subpectoral and subscapular infections, osteomyelitis, and costochondritis.

- ▶ Chest wall tumors comprise 1% of all tumors and are malignant in 60% of cases.

- ▶ Metastases to the chest wall most commonly originate from soft tissue sarcomas, and breast, genitourinary, lung, and thyroid primary tumors.

- ▶ Traumatic injuries of the chest wall include sternal fractures, rib fractures, and flail chest. In most cases, treatment is rest and pain control.

- ▶ Blood in the pleural space, or hemothorax, is a common occurrence after chest trauma and is managed in 90% of patients by tube thoracostomy.

- ▶ Pneumothorax, defined as air in the pleural space, has the potential (called tension pneumothorax) to deviate the mediastinum, impair venous return to the heart, and severely decrease cardiac output.

- ▶ Indications for chest tube placement for pneumothorax include (1) a large pneumothorax; (2) a

pneumothorax in an unstable or ventilated patient; (3) bilateral pneumothorax; and (4) tension pneumothorax. Surgery is indicated in patients with persistent airleaks or recurrent disease.

- ▶ Pleural empyema is defined as pus in the pleural space and should be considered a surgical disease because of the need for surgical intervention for management. Therapeutic options vary, depending on the presenting phase (acute/exudative, transitional/fibrinopurulent, and chronic/organizing).

- ▶ Chylothorax is injury to the thoracic duct or its branches, with leakage of fluid into the pleural space. In 50% of patients, it can be managed nonoperatively, and surgical management is successful in 90% of cases.

- ▶ Pleural mesothelioma is subclassified into three groups: benign (11%), localized malignant (23%), and diffuse malignant (66%). Treatment and prognosis are based on subclassification.

- ▶ Pleural metastases are most commonly produced from breast and lung cancer, as well as lymphoma, and are significant for disabling pain and shortness of breath.

The chest wall is a conical-shaped cage that has the capacity to expand during lung ventilation. The shape of the lung is largely determined by the bony structures surrounding it (the ribs and sternum) and by the inferior muscular boundary, the diaphragm. The sternum is approximately 18 inches long in the adult and consists of the manubrium, the body of the sternum, and the xiphoid connected via three cartilaginous joints.

The sides of the chest wall include the upper ten ribs, which are attached to the sternum, and ribs 11 and 12, which are only attached posteriorly to their corresponding thoracic vertebra. As a result of this, ribs 11 and 12 are sometimes referred to as the "floating ribs."

Each lung is invested by two layers of pleural membranes. The **parietal pleura** is the outermost lining of the two layers and is divided into four parts—the cupula (cervical pleura), costal pleura, mediastinal pleura, and diaphragmatic pleura. The visceral pleura is the innermost layer and closely adheres to the surfaces of the lungs. The potential pleural space between the two layers normally contains only a few drops of serous fluid. However, this space may become enlarged with fluid, pus, or blood in pathologic conditions (Figures 38.2–1, 38.2–2, 38.2–3).

CHEST WALL

CONGENITAL ANOMALIES

Congenital chest wall anomalies produce a spectrum of symptoms that range from asymptomatic to those that are cosmetically, structurally, and physiologically detrimental. This section will discuss some of these clinical entities that require surgical intervention.

Rib Abnormalities

Most rib anomalies are asymptomatic and are usually identified as incidental findings on chest film. Congenital absence of rib(s) may result in herniation of lung through the chest wall defect. Most defects that result in paradoxical chest wall motion are small and usually asymptomatic. Symptoms, when present, include chest pain and dyspnea. Plain chest films may be normal, but chest computed tomography (CT) will demonstrate the defect and determine its extent. If the defect is symptomatic, the treatment of choice is surgical repair as described above.

Cervical ribs occur in approximately 1% of the population, and, when present, are bilateral in 80% of patients.

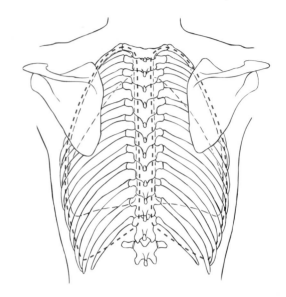

Figure 38.2–2. Posterior view of the pleural reflections.

From a surgical standpoint they are significant for their association with the **thoracic outlet syndrome** (TOS), in which the subclavian vessels and lower portion of the brachial plexus become stretched out as they pass over these ribs before entering the arm. Bony abnormalities, including cervical ribs, bifid first rib, fusion of the upper ribs, or clavicular deformities, are present in 30% of patients with TOS. Either neurologic or, less commonly, vascular compression symptoms may result.

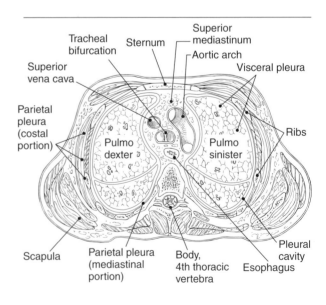

Figure 38.2–3. Cross-section of the thorax at the level of the tracheal bifurcation and the fourth thoracic vertebra.

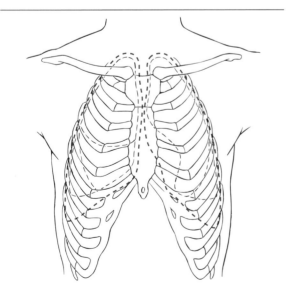

Figure 38.2–1. Anterior view of the pleural reflections.

The diagnosis of TOS is made primarily on the basis of history and physical examination. Primary management is nonoperative, however, surgical removal of the cervical rib may be indicated for suspected vascular occlusion and for neurologic symptoms that are unresponsive to nonoperative therapy.

Sternal Anomalies

Pectus excavatum, posterior displacement of the sternum as a result of abnormal costal cartilage development, is the most common congenital deformity of the sternum. Symptoms that have been attributed to pectus excavatum include frequent respiratory infections and impaired exercise tolerance. The diagnosis is made clinically. Some have argued that the deformity is of cosmetic interest only, while others have documented associated respiratory and cardiac compromise. It is generally agreed that pectus excavatum results in some degree of compromise in cardiac and respiratory function, especially with exertion. Surgical repair, which involves removal of the deformed cartilages and fixing the sternum in a more normal position, should be done before the age of 7.

Pectus carinatum ("pigeon breast"), in which there is forward protrusion of the sternum due to costochondral overgrowth, occurs ten times less frequently than pectus excavatum. Two forms are recognized in which either the upper or lower sternum protrudes. The defect increases the anterior-posterior diameter of the chest, in effect, fixing it in full inspiration and, therefore, increasing the work of breathing. Symptoms include dyspnea, wheezing, and respiratory infection. Surgical repair, by removing the abnormal cartilage and reducing the sternum posteriorly, is indicated if the defect is severe.

INFLAMMATORY CHEST WALL DISEASE

Spontaneous chest wall infections are infrequent and usually occur in immunosuppressed patients or after trauma or surgery.

Subpectoral & Subscapular Infections

These infections may be difficult to recognize, as they lie under the chest wall muscle fascia. The etiology includes previous chest, breast, or pacemaker surgery, trauma, prior radiation therapy, and empyema. Symptoms include erythema, induration, and local pain, sometimes with arm motion. The diagnosis is confirmed by chest CT. Treatment involves surgical drainage and appropriate antibiotic coverage. Tuberculosis, fungus, or actinomycosis should be entertained if the infection remains unresponsive to antibiotic therapy.

Osteomyelitis

Prior to antibiotics, primary osteomyelitis of the ribs was caused by typhoid fever and tuberculosis. Now it is seen as a complication of surgery, immunosuppression, and drug addiction. Sternal osteomyelitis most commonly occurs as a complication of median sternotomy for open heart surgery. The diagnosis is suspected postoperatively in a patient with an unstable sternum, sternotomy wound infection, or signs of mediastinitis. Therapy requires intravenous antibiotics and aggressive mediastinal and sternal debridement often with mediastinal muscle or omental flap coverage.

Costochondritis

Infection of the costal cartilage may be difficult to treat, since the anterior costal cartilage is relatively avascular. It can present as nonspecific chest wall tenderness and may progress to induration, abscess formation, and even chronic draining sinuses. For those patients who fail medical therapy, wide resection of both the involved cartilage and contiguous bony structures with soft tissue coverage is indicated.

CHEST WALL TRAUMA

Sternal Fractures

Sternal fractures usually result from motor vehicle steering wheel injuries. Patients complain of pain and the sensation that the sternum moves or "clicks." The diagnosis is made on lateral sternal films. The treatment is rest and pain control. Open reduction with fixation is required if displacement and separation of the fragment occurs. Observation for occult myocardial contusion is necessary in all instances of significant sternal trauma, with serial cardiac enzyme levels and electrocardiograms.

Rib Fractures

Rib fractures are significant for their potential complications, including hemothorax, pneumothorax, and flail chest, all of which are life-threatening problems. In addition, fractures of the upper three ribs and scapula are associated with a 10% incidence of high-speed deceleration major vascular injuries, therefore, studies to evaluate the aorta and its arch vessels should be considered. Patients complain of focal pain that is worse with cough or deep breathing. Rib fractures may not be evident on chest film. Oblique rib views will demonstrate the fracture. For uncomplicated rib fracture, treatment is rest and pain control. Flail chest and hemothorax are discussed in this section; pneumothorax is discussed in the section on pleural disease.

Fracture of more than one rib in more than one place results in a flail chest. The resultant chest wall instability results in paradoxical motion of the chest wall, markedly increasing the work of breathing, and impairing lung ventilation. Flail chest is frequently associated with lung contusion, which compounds the degree of respiratory compromise. Therapy is directed at pain control and pulmonary toilet. For severe cases, ventilatory support is needed. Surgical reduction and fixation is rarely indicated.

Blood in the pleural space, or hemothorax, is a common occurrence after chest trauma. At least 250 mL must be present before it is visible on erect chest film. Hemothorax is potentially a life-threatening emergency with both volume loss, and a tension component (see tension pneumothorax). The diagnosis is made radiographically. Ninety percent of patients are managed successfully by tube thoracostomy. Thoracotomy is indicated for excessive bleeding, which is defined as an initial loss of 1500 mL, or an ongoing loss estimated by the "800 rule": 800 mL over 1 hour, 400 mL/hr for 2 hours, or 200 mL/hr for 4 hours.

CHEST WALL TUMORS

Chest wall tumors comprise 1% of all tumors. Incidence and treatment outcome statistics for these tumors vary, sometimes widely, depending on the series cited. In general, chest wall tumors are malignant in 60% of cases; of these, just over half are primary tumors, and the remainder are metastatic to the chest wall. For benign tumors, wide local resection is curative. For the majority of malignant tumors, despite advances in chemotherapy and radiation therapy, surgical resection remains an important part of the treatment plan.

The principles of chest wall resection and reconstruction involve resection of involved ribs or sternum with associated soft tissue, followed by rigid prosthetic replacement of the chest wall and soft tissue coverage. Further details of the procedure can be obtained from the suggested reading list.

Benign Chest Wall Tumors

The characteristics of benign chest wall tumors are listed in Table 38.2–1. Most present as a painless mass, and complete excision is curative. Desmoid tumors, also known as fibromatosis, are listed as a benign tumor, however, some consider them to be low-grade sarcomas.

Malignant Chest Wall Tumors

The presenting age, symptoms, location, radiographic features, treatment, and outcome for selected malignant chest wall tumors are shown in Table 38.2–2. The tumors are listed in order of frequency.

Metastases to the chest wall most commonly originate from soft tissue sarcoma, breast, genitourinary, lung, and thyroid primaries. Usually, surgery is involved for diagnosis; however, in select patients, wide local excision may be indicated.

PLEURAL SPACE

PNEUMOTHORAX

Pneumothorax is defined as air in the pleural space, and its significance is in the potential to develop air under pressure (**tension pneumothorax**) which deviates the mediastinum, impairs venous return to the heart, acutely drops cardiac output, and is a life-threatening emergency. A pneumothorax is classified on the basis of etiology (primary or spontaneous and secondary to underlying disease) or the mode of presentation (open, tension, or stable).

The most common symptom is ipsilateral chest pain. Shortness of breath (SOB) and cough are less common. Physical examination may reveal diminished breath sounds, with increased tympany to percussion on the affected side. With a tension pneumothorax, there are also signs of developing shock and shift of the trachea away from the affected side. A chest radiograph, with an expiratory phase film, will confirm the diagnosis. Most describe the pneumothorax size as a percent of the total hemithorax volume. A more reproducible approach (with less reader variability) describes the chest radiographic findings quantitatively in terms of the distance of the lung apex to the apical chest wall and how far down the side of the chest wall the pneumothorax extends (Figure 38.2–4).

Treatment is based on pneumothorax size, type (open, stable, or tension), and patient stability. Air is spontaneously resorbed from the pleural space, therefore, patients with small, stable pneumothorax may be managed by observation alone. Hospitalization is recommended in order to rule out a tension component. Once it is established by serial radiographs that the pneumothorax is stable, patients are followed as outpatients until the pneumothorax is resolved. No further work-up is needed unless underlying lung disease is diagnosed or there is a recurrence. Needle aspiration of pleural space air, by means of a technique similar to that used in thoracentesis, will hasten resolution of larger, stable pneumothoraces. Anterior second or third interspace needle aspiration may also be used emergently to stabilize a patient with a tension pneumothorax until chest tube drainage can be established.

The indications for chest tube placement include (1) a large pneumothorax; (2) a pneumothorax in an unstable, or ventilated patient; (3) bilateral pneumothorax; and

Table 38.2–1. Characteristics of benign chest wall tumors.

	Chondroma	Fibrous Dysplasia	Osteochondroma	Fibromatosis (Desmoid)
Age	Teens–20s	Young adults	Young adults	Teens–40s
Symptoms	Painless mass	Painless mass	Painless mass	Painless mass
Location	Costochondral junction	Posterior ribs	Costochondral junction	Intercostal
Radiologic features	Medullary mass, thin cortex	Osteolytic mass, intact cortex	Bony protuberance with calcified cap	Soft tissue mass
Treatment	Excision	Excision	Excision	Excision

Table 38.2–2. Characteristics of malignant chest wall tumors.

	Chondrosarcoma	Osteogenic Sarcoma	Ewing's Sarcoma	Plasmacytoma (Myeloma)
Age	40s	Teens–40s	Adolescent	50s
Symptoms	Painful mass	Painful mass	Fever, malaise, mass	Fever, malaise, mass
Location	Costochondral junction	Chest wall	Ribs	Ribs
Radiologic features	Invasive, osteolytic mass	"Sunburst" appearance	"Onionskin" appearance	Osteolytic mass pathologic fracture
Treatment	Excision	Excision, chemotherapy	Radiation therapy/ chemotherapy/excision	Radiation therapy/chemotherapy
5-year survival	14–96%	10–20%	5–40%	20–45%

(4) tension pneumothorax. Surgery is indicated in patients with persistent airleaks or recurrent disease. The standard open technique used a transaxillary approach with ligation or stapling of emphysematous blebs or other airleak site and pleurodesis or pleurectomy. Currently, videothoracoscopy has largely replaced the open approach.

EMPYEMA

Pleural empyema is defined as pus in the pleural space and should be considered a surgical disease because of the need for surgical intervention for diagnosis and management. Empyema is classified into three types: acute/exudative, transitional/fibrinopurulent, and chronic/organizing, based on its presentation. The characteristics of these phases are listed in Table 38.2–3. Empyema most commonly occurs as a complication of pneumonia (50% of

cases). Parapneumonic, post-thoracic surgical, and traumatic empyema together account for 75–80% of cases.

The symptoms are not specific but reflect the underlying disease process responsible for the empyema, however, pleuritic chest pain, cough, fever, and shortness of breath are often observed.

The diagnosis is made by thoracentesis. Approximately 20–50 mL are required and should be sent for specific gravity, white blood cell (WBC) count, pH, lactate dehydrogenase (LDH), glucose, and culture. Both aerobic and anaerobic cultures should be obtained, as anaerobic organisms are involved in over 75% of empyemas. The typical laboratory findings in empyema include a specific gravity of 1.018, WBC count 500–1500 cells/mm^3, glucose less than 40–50 mg/dL, pH less than 7.0, and LDH greater than 1000 U/L.

Therapeutic options vary, depending on the presenting phase of the empyema. In all cases, treatment of any associated disease (eg, pneumonia) must occur concomitantly, and pneumonitis must be controlled *before* procedures are performed that require general anesthesia. For acute phase empyema treatment includes complete evacuation (by chest tube or thoracentesis) of the free-flowing infection and appropriate antibiotic coverage. For transitional phase empyema, chest tube drainage is adequate for most patients, however, for those with early fibrinous loculations, thoracoscopic-assisted drainage provides more effective pleural space drainage. For chronic phase empyema, treatment options are tube drainage, local rib resection and drainage, or thoracotomy, debridement, and lung decortication.

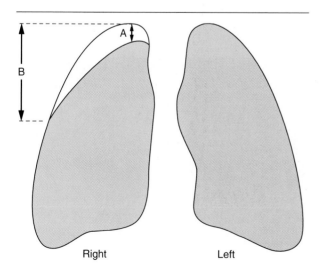

Figure 38.2–4. Recommended method to describe the size of a pneumothorax in terms of how far (in centimeters) from the apex the lung has fallen **(A)**, and how far down the side of the chest wall it extends **(B)**.

Table 38.2–3. Empyema classification.

Fluid Composition	Acute	Transitional	Chronic
Fluidity	Free flowing	Free flowing/ turbid	Loculated
WBC	Low	Rising	High
LDH	Low	Rising	High
Glucose	Normal	Decreasing	Low
pH	Normal	Decreasing	Low

LDH = lactate dehydrogenase; WBC = white blood cell count.

CHYLOTHORAX

An injury to the thoracic duct or its branches with leakage of chylous fluid into the pleural space is termed a chylothorax. Although it is infrequent, lengthy hospitalization and high mortality make it a significant complication. Blunt, penetrating, or surgical trauma to the thoracic duct is the most common cause. Congenital ductal anomalies and neoplastic obstruction and invasion of the thoracic duct are less common etiologies. The symptoms are those of a pleural effusion, with pleuritic pain or pressure and shortness of breath.

The diagnosis should be suspected in patients with large, rapidly occurring (or recurring) pleural effusion following surgery near the thoracic duct. Evaluation of the effusion by thoracentesis or chest tube drainage will show non-clotting, milky fluid with a fat content which exceeds that of plasma, a triglyceride level greater than 110 mg/100 mL, and a cholesterol/triglyceride ratio less than 1.0. On microscopic evaluation, lymphocytes are the predominant cellular component.

Initially, patients may be treated by cessation of oral feedings, pleural drainage (by repeated thoracentesis or chest tube drainage), and intravenous hyperalimentation. If the chylous leak resolves, oral intake is resumed before discontinuing chest tube drainage. If the chylous leak persists for 2 weeks without signs of resolution, then surgery should be considered. The preferred technique involves a right thoracotomy with ligation of the thoracic duct proximally. Alternatively, the leak site may be plugged with fibrin glue and mechanical pleurodesis or pleurectomy added. Currently, videothoracoscopy is often selected as the surgical approach over open thoracotomy.

Nonoperative therapy results in closure of the chylous leak in 50% of cases. Surgery is successful in controlling 90% of chylous leaks, with a low operative mortality.

PLEURAL NEOPLASTIC DISEASE

Mesothelioma

Pleural mesothelioma is subclassified into three groups: benign, localized malignant, and diffuse malignant. Benign mesothelioma, also referred to as pleural fibroma, accounts for 11% of all pleural mesotheliomas. Often, the tumors are attached to the adjacent pleura by a stalk. No known risk factors have been reported. Symptoms are not specific and include cough and chest pain; however, more than half of patients with benign tumors are asymptomatic. A localized, smooth-walled, pleural-based or peripheral intrathoracic tumor is noted on chest CT. Treatment is complete surgical resection, which is curative.

Localized malignant tumors account for 23% of pleural mesotheliomas. Only 10% of patients report a previous asbestos history. Extensive local tumor invasion is common, as are the presenting symptoms of chest pain, dyspnea, and fever. A locally invasive pleural-based mass is seen on chest CT. Percutaneous needle biopsy is cytologically diagnostic in the majority of cases. The treatment consists of thoracotomy with wide local excision, including pulmonary and chest wall resections if necessary. Complete resection should result in a cure. Patients whose tumors are incompletely resected have a median survival of 7 months and are candidates for postoperative radiation therapy. Diffuse malignant tumors account for 66% of all pleural mesotheliomas. Most patients present in the fifth to seventh decade, with a strong male predominance, and asbestos exposure history is noted in 20–85% of cases. Histologically, the tumor presents in three forms: epithelial (40%), fibrosarcomatous (20%), and mixed (40%). Epithelial tumors produce pleural effusions early, whereas fibrosarcomatous tumors are dry with marked pleural thickening. Symptoms vary, depending on the propensity of the tumor to produce a symptomatic pleural effusion. Chest CT findings include pleural effusion, contracted hemithorax, diffuse, irregular pleural thickening, and a nonshifted mediastinum despite a pleural effusion (Figure 38.2–5). A preoperative tissue diagnosis by thoracentesis or percutaneous needle biopsy is often difficult to make. On the other hand, thoracoscopy has proved to be reliable in diagnosing these tumors.

Diffuse malignant disease is invariably fatal, and surgical treatment, chest tube placement, or pleurectomy and decortication are directed at palliating symptoms, including chest pain from pleural invasion and shortness of breath from effusion and entrapped lung. Pleuropneumonectomy, an extensive operative procedure designed to attempt surgical cure, has an operative mortality of 6–15% and no documented survival advantage over palliative therapy.

Radiation therapy is reserved to palliate limited-region symptoms. Chemotherapy is considered experimental for these patients.

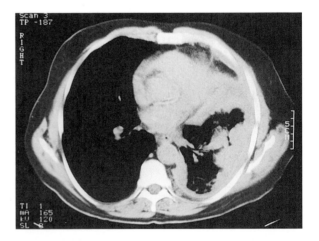

Figure 38.2–5. Computed tomography of the chest through the level of the inferior pulmonary vein, demonstrating the characteristic radiographic findings of diffuse mesothelioma (see text).

Pleural Metastatic Disease

Pleural metastases are significant for the often disabling symptoms of pleuritic pain and shortness of breath, which limits patients' quality of life. Lung cancer, breast cancer, and lymphoma are most notable for producing pleural metastases. Symptoms include pleuritic chest pain, shortness of breath, and a cough. There may be additional symptoms related to the primary tumor. The diagnosis may be suspected radiographically by demonstrating diffuse, pleural nodularity and a pleural effusion in a patient with a known malignancy. A bloody pleural exudative effusion by thoracentesis is very suggestive and may be confirmed by cytopathology. Thoracoscopy is also effective at diagnosis, but if performed in a patient suspected of having a malignant effusion, the surgeon should be prepared to both diagnose and treat the effusion.

For treatment, the primary malignancy should be managed as per routine. Treatment of the malignant effusion is palliative. Treatment options include repeated thoracentesis, chest tube drainage with sclerotherapy, or pleurodesis/pleurectomy using an open or thoracoscopic approach.

SUGGESTED READING

Arnold PG, Pairolero PC: Chest wall reconstruction: Experience with 100 consecutive patients. Ann Surg 1984;199:725.

Daniel TM: Diagnostic thoracoscopy for pleural disease. Ann Thorac Surg 1993;56:639.

Ferguson MK: Thoracoscopy for empyema, bronchopleural fistula, and chylothorax. Ann Thorac Surg 1993;56:644.

Greene PS, Heitmiller RF: Thoracoscopy for pleural space disease. Surg Laparosc Endosc 1994;4:100.

Heitmiller RF: Pneumothorax. In: Cameron JL (editor): *Current Surgical Therapy*. BC Decker, 1992.

Heitmiller RF: Pleural mesothelioma. In: Niederhuber JE (editor): *Current Therapy in Oncology*. BC Decker, 1993.

LoCicero J III: Thoracoscopic management of malignant pleural effusion. Ann Thorac Surg 1993;56:641.

Sabiston D (editor): *Textbook of Surgery*, 14th ed. Saunders, 1992.

Shamberger RC et al: Anterior chest wall deformities and congenital heart disease. J Thorac Cardiovasc Surg 1988;96:427.

Shields TW (editor): *General Thoracic Surgery*, 4th ed. Lea & Febiger, 1994.

Urschel Jr HC, Paulson DL, McNamara JJ: Thoracic outlet syndrome. Ann Thorac Surg 1968;61:1.

Weissberg D, Ben-Zeev I: Talc pleurodesis. J Thorac Cardiovasc Surg 1993;106:689.

Welch KJ: Chest wall deformities. In: Holder TM, Ashcraft KW (editors): *Pediatric Surgery*. Saunders, 1980.

38.3 Lung Cancer

Stephen C. Yang, MD, & Richard F. Heitmiller, MD

▶ Key Facts

- ▶ Lung cancer is currently the number one cause of cancer-related deaths for both men and women in the United States, and the number is rising.

- ▶ Lung cancer is divided into two histologic groups: non-small cell (NSC) (82%) and small cell (18%).

- ▶ Accurate staging of NSC lung cancer is vital, as therapy and prognosis are directly based on it.

- ▶ Surgical therapy for NSC lung cancer includes pneumonectomy, lobectomy, segmental lung resection, and wedge resection. However, lobectomy continues to be the standard lung resection for patients with adequate pulmonary function.

- ▶ Radiation therapy for NSC lung cancer is indicated for patients who are not candidates for surgery because of poor pulmonary function, comorbid medical disease, or by patient choice.

- ▶ Small cell lung cancer often presents as a systemic disease requiring systemic chemotherapy as the primary therapy.

Lung cancer is currently the number one cause of death for both men and women in the United States, and the incidence is rising. Therefore, for any new abnormal chest radiographic finding, regardless of age, gender, or smoking history, the diagnosis of lung cancer must be strongly considered. Lung cancer is subdivided into two histologic groups: non-small cell (NSC) cancers (82%), and small cell (SC) cancers (18%). The pretreatment evaluation, treatment options, and prognosis are different for the two groups, and these will be discussed separately in this chapter. Primary lung cancer, regardless of cell type, is most common in patients aged 55–85, with a peak in the early seventh decade, however, the diagnosis of lung cancer must always be considered, even in younger age patients. Whenever a lung cancer is identified, the possibility that it represents a pulmonary metastasis (see Chapter 38.1 on pulmonary diseases) must also be considered.

CLASSIFICATION

The current understanding of lung neoplasia is that tumors arise from a single cell type, which then differentiates into specific cell lines, such as squamous cell, adenocarcinoma, or small cell cancer. The fact that tumors arise from a single pluripotential cell type readily explains the observed phenomena of mixed cell type cancers. A classification of lung tumors based on tumor histology is shown in Table 38.3–1, and the frequency of lung tumors by cell type is shown in Table 38.3–2. Adenocarcinoma has only recently surpassed squamous cell tumors as the most common lung cancer.

NON-SMALL CELL LUNG CARCINOMA

DIAGNOSIS

Clinical Symptoms

The presenting symptoms in patients with lung cancer vary considerably according to tumor size, location, and stage. Frequently, with early-stage tumors, patients are totally asymptomatic. Tumors that involve the airway may present with shortness of breath, cough, wheezing, he-

Table 38.3–1. Histologic classification of malignant lung carcinoma.

Squamous cell variant
Small cell carcinoma
Adenocarcinoma
Large cell carcinoma
Adenosquamous carcinoma
Carcinoid tumors
Mucoepidermoid/adenoid cystic tumors

Table 38.3–2. Frequency of malignant lung carcinoma by cell type.

Cell Type	Frequency (%)
Squamous cell carcinoma	29
Small cell carcinoma	18
Adenocarcinoma	32
Large cell carcinoma	9
Carcinoid	1
Other	11

Reprinted and modified, with permission, from Travis WD, Travis LB, Devesa SS: Lung cancer. Cancer (Suppl) 1995; 75:191.

moptysis, or postobstructive pneumonia. Tumors that invade the parietal pleura or chest wall produce intense, persistent, localized chest pain. Depending on the specific site of involvement, metastatic disease can result in a spectrum of symptoms. There are, as well, paraneoplastic syndromes associated with some lung cancers.

Radiologic Findings

Lung cancer may present with a variety of radiographic findings. Old chest films are helpful in determining whether a lesion is chronic and may be followed, or whether it is new and needs further evaluation. In general, lung cancer radiographically presents in two forms: (1) as

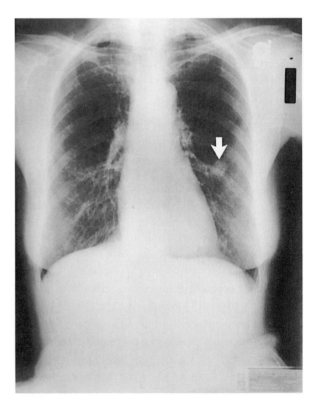

Figure 38.3–1. Posterior-anterior chest film showing left lung non-small cell carcinoma *(arrow)*.

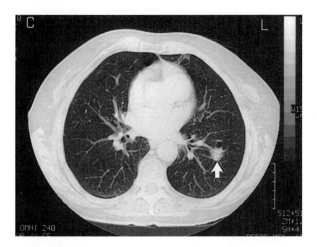

Figure 38.3–2. Chest computed tomographic section through the tumor demonstrates the radiographic features of the lesion in greater detail.

a pneumonia with or without airway obstruction and (2) as a primary tumor (Figure 38.3–1) or nodal mass. Regardless, all new chest radiographic findings may represent lung cancer and should be managed accordingly. A chest computed tomography (CT) scan is the best way to further evaluate the radiographic features of a lung lesion (Figure 38.3–2), to screen intrathoracic lymph nodal status, and to triage diagnostic testing.

Pathologic Diagnosis

The decision regarding preoperative tissue diagnosis of a suspected lung cancer is individualized. A documented new lung lesion in a patient who is a smoker, with radiographic features highly suspicious for a cancer, may reasonably justify surgery without a tissue diagnosis. On the other hand, if the patient is a poor candidate for surgery, or the lesion is radiographically indeterminant for cancer, it may be more prudent to pursue a tissue diagnosis. If this is the case, sputum cytology is the easiest approach. The accuracy of this technique varies, depending on the size and location of the tumor. A series of three early morning specimens optimizes the diagnostic yield (approximately 80%). More recently, monoclonal antibody staining techniques are being used to increase the accuracy of early diagnosis of lung cancer.

Percutaneous needle biopsy (PcNBx) is a safe, accurate technique to diagnose peripheral lung lesions greater than 1.0 cm. PcNBx may also be used to diagnose possible metastatic foci. Endobronchial or hilar lesions, which are often inaccessible by PcNBx, may be diagnosed by flexible (or sometimes rigid) bronchoscopy. Transtracheal and transbronchial biopsy using the Wang needle technique has further extended the bronchoscopic diagnostic options. Mediastinoscopy and anterior parasternal medi-

astinotomy require general anesthesia but permit direct biopsy of the primary tumor or adenopathy in the paratracheal and anterior hilar regions, respectively. Videothoracoscopy has not replaced mediastinoscopy in assessing mediastinal adenopathy, but does allow excisional wedge biopsy of small peripheral lung lesions in a fashion less invasive than with an open thoracotomy. Despite the wide array of diagnostic procedures, there are patients in whom a tissue diagnosis cannot be made. For these patients, the management options are: (1) to proceed with thoracotomy and resection and (2) to follow the lesion with serial chest CT scans (usually at 3-month intervals) with the plan to repeat diagnostic procedures or to resect the lesion if it enlarges.

STAGING

Tumor staging in non-small cell lung cancer is of more than academic interest in that decisions regarding therapy and prognosis are directly based on clinical and pathologic tumor staging. The TNM (tumor, node, metastasis) criteria and staging system is shown in Table 38.3–3.

Table 38.3–3. TNM staging for lung cancer.

Stage	T	N	M
0	CIS		
Ia	1	0	0
Ib	2	0	0
IIa	1	1	0
IIb	2	1	0
	3	0	0
IIIa	3	1	0
	1–3	2	0
IIIb	4	0–2	0
	1–4	3	0
IV	Any	Any	1

Primary Tumor (T)

CIS = carcinoma in situ.

T1   Tumor < 3 cm without evidence of invasion proximal to lobar bronchus
T2   Tumor > 3 cm, visceral pleural invasion, or with atelectasis/pneumonia extending proximally to hilum
T3   Tumor invading chest wall, diaphragm, mediastinal pleura, pericardium, or within 2 cm of carina
T4   Tumor involving mediastinum, heart, great vessels, trachea, esophagus, vertebral bodies, carina; malignant effusion

Nodal Involvement (N)

N0   No nodal metastasis
N1   Metastasis to peribronchial or ipsilateral hilar nodes
N2   Metastasis to ipsilateral mediastinal and/or subcarinal nodes
N3   Metastasis to contralateral mediastinal nodes or any scalene or supraclavicular nodes

Distant Metastasis (M)

M0   No distant metastasis
M1   Distant metastasis

THERAPY

Surgery

Indications. To determine if a patient is a candidate for surgery, the patient must have a general medical condition adequate to permit safe general anesthesia, sufficient pulmonary reserve, and localized disease. Evaluation of medical condition prior to general anesthesia for thoracotomy is no different than for nonthoracotomy cases. Although advancing age is associated with increased surgical risks, thoracotomy has been shown to be safe, even in the octogenarian.

In evaluating pulmonary reserve, the goal is to predict what the patient's pulmonary function will be *following* lung resection. Briefly, in order to do this, three assumptions are made: (1) forced expiratory volume at 1 second (FEV_1) in liters is a number that reflects pulmonary reserve, much like ejection fraction (EF) reflects cardiac function; (2) the volume of expired air at 1 second (FEV_1) comes from the lung equally; and (3) the measured lung volume represents normally functioning lung. Spirometry generates data on lung volumes such as FEV_1 and forced vital capacity (FVC). Pulmonary ventilation and perfusion ($\dot{V}/\dot{Q}$) scanning quantitates the distribution of lung function, and single-breath diffusing capacity for carbon monoxide (DLCO) reflects lung function. As always, pulmonary function test results should be interpreted in conjunction with the clinical assessment of pulmonary function.

Whereas a wide array of TNM combinations fall within the category of localized disease, there are only three TNM criteria—T4 tumors, N3 nodal metastatic disease, and M1 metastases—that absolutely render the patient unresectable. Therefore, if preoperative staging with physical examination, chest and abdominal CT scanning, assessment of mediastinal lymph nodes, bone scans, and brain CT or MRI, fail to show T4, N3, or M1 disease, the disease is technically resectable.

Technique. There are two options for pulmonary resection: anatomic or nonanatomic techniques. Anatomic techniques all involve dissection, ligation, and division of the pulmonary vessels and airway to the portion of lung to be removed. Lung anatomy is reviewed in Chapter 38.1. Segmental lung resection is the smallest anatomic unit of lung that can be removed and, therefore, has the advantage of being lung-sparing. Lobectomy, on the basis of its wide parenchymal and lymphatic margin, has been the gold standard technique for lung cancer since its introduction in the early 1940s. Involvement of the proximal pulmonary artery or airway may sometimes require pneumonectomy. Nonanatomic resection involves resection of the lung tumor without regard to pulmonary anatomy, such as with a wedge resection or lumpectomy using electrocautery or laser.

The importance of tumor staging has already been alluded to. In order to accurately pathologically stage lung cancer, nodal staging or "mapping" should be performed at surgery, using the nodal staging classification shown in Figure 38.3–3. Of particular importance with regard to staging, prognosis, and qualification into multitherapy protocols are nodal stations 4, 7, and 10 on the right, and 4, 5, and 7 on the left.

A wide range of thoracic incisions can be used to perform the resections listed above. In general, when dealing with carcinoma, it is the resection, not the incisional approach, that is most important.

Videothoracoscopy is an established thoracic surgical technique, however, its role in the routine surgical management of patients with lung cancer is unresolved. It has yet to be shown that survival with equivalent open and thoracoscopic resections is the same, and lobectomy, the standard open resection technique, is difficult to perform thoracoscopically in the majority of patients.

Results. The overall surgical mortality in patients with NSC lung cancer is approximately 3–4%. The individual mortality varies according to extent of resection (wedge/segmentectomy < 1%, lobectomy < 3%, pneumonectomy < 6%), age, pulmonary function, and comorbidities. Morbidity is primarily cardiorespiratory, with cardiac arrhythmias, atelectasis, tracheobronchitis, and pneumonia leading the list. The survival by stage is: stage Ia, 67%; stage Ib, 57%; stage IIa, 55%; stage IIb, 39%; stage IIIa, 24%; stage IIIb, 3–7%; stage IV, 1%. On the basis of its operative safety, low local recurrence rates, and survival, lobectomy continues to be the standard lung resection for patients with adequate pulmonary function.

RADIATION THERAPY

Radiation therapy for NSC lung cancer is indicated for patients who are not candidates for surgery because of poor pulmonary function, comorbid medical diseases, unresectable disease, or by patient choice. Like surgery, radiation therapy is local therapy with its effects limited only to the region treated. The usual radiation dose administered is 5000–6000 cGy in daily doses of 180–200 cGy, 5 days per week. Radiation therapy may result in cure for patients with localized disease, however, the local and metastatic recurrence rates remain high with this form of therapy.

CHEMOTHERAPY

The role of chemotherapy in the management of patients with NSC lung cancer is controversial. There are no data demonstrating a survival advantage using chemotherapy alone. Currently, chemotherapy is most commonly used to palliate patients with metastatic disease or as combination therapy with either surgery or radiation therapy (usually in a protocol setting). Effective single-agent chemotherapy includes cisplatinum, ifosfamide, vindesine, and mitomycin C.

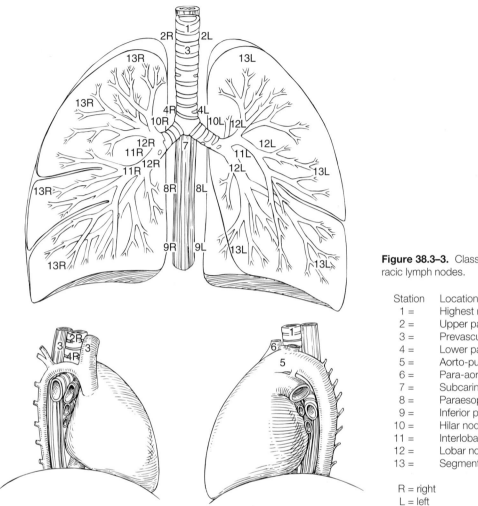

Figure 38.3–3. Classification of regional intrathoracic lymph nodes.

Station	Location
1 =	Highest mediastinal node
2 =	Upper paratracheal node
3 =	Prevascular and retrotracheal nodes
4 =	Lower paratracheal node
5 =	Aorto-pulmonary node
6 =	Para-aortic node
7 =	Subcarinal node
8 =	Paraesophageal node
9 =	Inferior pulmonary ligament node
10 =	Hilar node
11 =	Interlobar node
12 =	Lobar node
13 =	Segmental node

R = right
L = left

SMALL CELL LUNG CARCINOMA

Small cell lung cancer invariably presents as a systemic disease requiring systemic chemotherapy as the primary therapy. Small cell lung tumors are staged as **localized disease**, defined as intrathoracic disease that can be included within a single radiation therapy port, or as **extensive disease**, having tumor extending beyond the single radiation port or metastasizing to distant sites or organs. More recently, subclassification of localized disease using the standard TNM system has proven useful in defining therapeutic options and predicting outcome.

For localized disease, therapy includes multi-agent chemotherapy and radiation therapy. The most common chemotherapeutic regimens include cyclophosphamide, Adriamycin, and vincristine (CAV); cyclophosphamide, Adriamycin, and etoposide (CAE); etoposide, ifosfa-

mide, and cisplatinum (ICE); etoposide with cisplatinum (EP); and cyclophosphamide, lomustine, and methotrexate (CCM). Prophylactic cranial irradiation (PCI), whose benefit is controversial, is sometimes considered. For extensive disease, recommended therapy is chemotherapy alone.

The role of surgery in the management of patients with small cell lung cancer is limited and includes (1) establishing the diagnosis (eg, mediastinoscopy, mediastinotomy, open biopsy); (2) resecting T1 or T2, N0, M0 lesions in conjunction with pre- or postoperative chemotherapy; (3) resecting the non-small cell component of mixed small and non-small cell lung tumors (10–15% occurrence) in patients in whom the small cell component is controlled with systemic therapy.

Two-year survival in patients with limited disease who receive combination chemoradiation therapy varies from 71–53%, depending on the series and specific treatment regimen.

SUGGESTED READING

Eagan RT: Management of regionally advanced (stage III) non-small cell lung cancer. LCSG 831. Chest 1994;106(6 Suppl): 340S.

Ettinger DS: Small cell lung cancer. In: Niederhuber JE (editor): *Current Therapy in Oncology*. BC Decker, 1993.

Faber LP: Current status of neoadjuvant therapy for non-small cell lung cancer. Chest 1994;106(6 Suppl):355S.

Feld R et al: Lung. In: Abeloff MD et al (editors): *Clinical Oncology*. Churchill Livingstone, 1995.

Holmes EC, Ruckdeschel JC: Preoperative chemotherapy for locally advanced non-small cell lung cancer. Semin Oncol 1994;21(3 Suppl 6):97.

Martini N: The role of surgery in N1 and N2 lung cancer. Front Radiat Ther Oncol 1994;28:92.

Mountain CF: Value of the new TNM staging system for lung cancer. Chest 1989;97:935.

Mountain CF: Revisions in the international system for staging lung cancer. Chest 1997;111:1710.

Mountain CF: Surgery for stage IIIa–N2 non-small cell lung cancer. Cancer 1994;73:2589.

Pearson FG: Current status of surgical resection for lung cancer. Chest 1994;106(6 Suppl):337S.

Rendina EA et al: Comparative merits of thoracoscopy, mediastinoscopy, and mediastinotomy for mediastinal biopsy. Ann Thorac Surg 1994;57:992.

Travis WD, et al: Lung cancer. Cancer (Suppl) 1995;75:191.

39

Vascular Surgery

39.1 Evaluation of Patients With Vascular Disease

Ronald L. Dalman, MD

► Key Facts

- ► Evaluation of the patient with vascular disease requires a working knowledge of vascular anatomy, pathology, and pathophysiology.

- ► A busy vascular surgeon may see 2000 or more patients a year with various end-organ manifestations of atherosclerotic vascular disease.

- ► Risk factors for atherosclerotic disease include a family history of peripheral vascular occlusive disease, use of tobacco in any form, history of diabetes mellitus, and hypertension.

- ► Arterial abnormalities tend to manifest in one of two categories: (1) insufficient end-organ arterial perfusion, causing clinical symptoms; (2) progressive arterial degeneration, with loss of arterial integrity and aneurysmal enlargement.

- ► The objective measurement of the degree of distal flow in the lower extremity is most commonly accomplished by the assessment of the ankle-brachial index.

- ► Aneurysm is a progressive, degenerative condition of the arterial wall that results in vessel enlargement.

- ► Sudden onset of discolored feet or toes, especially when pedal pulses are present or even normal, suggests embolization from a more proximal source, most commonly an aneurysm.

- ► The patient with acute unilateral lower extremity edema must be evaluated for the presence of deep venous thrombosis.

- ► The signs and symptoms associated with acute limb ischemia are referred to as the "seven *P*'s" (aka, "the five *P*'s"): pulselessness, pallor, polar (cold), paresthesias, paralysis, pain, and past midnight (in reference to when these conditions usually occur).

- ► The most versatile, sensitive, and specific imaging instrument currently used in the vascular laboratory is the duplex scanner.

- ► More than any other single component in vascular surgery, precise preoperative arterial imaging is paramount to the expectation of success.

HISTORICAL FACTS

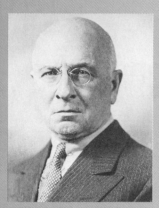

Alexis Carrel (1873–1944). (Courtesy of the Rockefeller University Archives.)

Alexis Carrel (1873–1944) is considered by many to be the "father of vascular surgery." His extraordinary imagination and foresight led to unparalleled accomplishments, both in vascular surgery and in organ transplantation.

Born in Lyon in 1873, his father died when he was just 5 years old. It is believed that the responsibility of helping to raise a younger brother and sister had an early maturing effect. After 3 years at the medical school at the University of Lyon, he became an extern at the Red Cross Hospital and the Hospital Antiguaille. In 1895, he fulfilled 1 year of military service with the French mountain troops. The next 5 years were spent completing his internship in several hospitals in Lyon.

In 1904, Carrel left France for Montreal, having failed to gain a surgical faculty position in Lyon. In that same year, he presented a paper on vascular surgery to the Second Medical Congress of the French Language of North America, which was very well received. A member of the audience, Karl Beck, a respected Chicago surgeon, approached Carrel with the possibility of working in the United States. Carrel accepted a position at the University of Chicago under the chairmanship of Dr George Stuart.

ESSENTIAL ASPECTS OF A CAREFUL VASCULAR ASSESSMENT

UNDERSTANDING ARTERIAL DISEASES

Diseases of the blood vessels are appropriately grouped into arterial and venous disorders. Arterial disease is dominated by atherosclerosis and its related complications. Other congenital or acquired pathological conditions exist, but their incidence varies from infrequent (heterozygous deficiency of cystathionine B-synthase, 1/70–1/200) to rare (Marfan's syndrome 4/100,000–6/100,000), to extremely unusual (pseudoxanthoma elasticum 1/200,000). By contrast, atherosclerotic plaque formation starts as early as the fourth or fifth decade of life and is universally present in select locations within the arterial vasculature after the sixth decade. A busy vascular surgeon or internist may see 2000 or more patients a year with various end-organ manifestations of atherosclerotic vascular disease. During that same time, perhaps one or two patients will be seen for thromboangiitis obliterans or one of the other more common arteritides. Thus, while keeping the possibility of more exotic arterial disease processes in mind, the clinician taking a patient history should direct questions towards the presence and significance of atherosclerosis.

Atherosclerosis is an age-related, progressive, degenerative disease that occurs in a distinct population of men and women with appropriate age (mean, 68 years) and coexistent risk factors. These risk factors include a family history of peripheral vascular occlusive disease, use of tobacco in any form, and presence of diabetes mellitus and hypertension. Risk factors more commonly associated with the risk of coronary artery occlusive disease, such as hypercholesterolemia, are apparently less relevant to peripheral vascu-

It was here that Carrel formed his legendary partnership with Claude Guthrie, a young physiologist. Between November 1904 and August 1906, they wrote 28 papers together. Their experimental work included perfection of vascular anastomoses and the use of vein grafts, development of tissue preservation methods, reimplantation of limbs, and the transplantation of kidneys, ovaries, thyroids, and hearts. This collaboration ended in 1906 when Carrel moved on to the Rockefeller Institute in New York. Once in New York, Carrel continued his experimental efforts in vascular, cardiothoracic, and transplantation surgery and also devoted much of his time to improving techniques of tissue preservation.

In 1912, Carrel was awarded the Nobel Prize for Physiology and Medicine, and in 1913 he was made a Knight of the Legion of Honor by the French government. In 1915, Carrel became a Commander in the French Army's Legion of Honor, and in 1917 he established the first mobile army hospital.

After the war, Carrel gained worldwide fame for his collaboration with the great aviator, Charles Lindbergh. Working together, they created the first organ perfusion pump, the Lindbergh pump, which sustained a cat thyroid gland for 18 days. This extraordinary invention laid the groundwork for the development of modern pump oxygenators.

Unfortunately, Carrel was forced into retirement at the age of 65 by the Rockefeller Institute. He was very bitter over this decision and left for France in the early 1940s. Later, amid unfounded accusations of Nazi collaboration, Carrel suffered his first heart attack in 1943, and a second one that took his life in 1944. History has exonerated him of all wrongdoing and has recognized him as one of the most ingenious and innovative figures in the history of surgery.

---

lar occlusive disease (Table 39.1–1). In addition, age, sex, and coexistent disease factors are also very important. Typical age of onset can vary from the fourth through the tenth decade of life. In women, the age of symptomatic presentation tends to lag behind men by 10 years or more.

In the absence of recognized risk factors, or if age of onset is before the fourth decade, or if other disease processes are coexistent, alternative arterial conditions should be considered. If a young women complains of arm fatigue with exercise, or symptoms of a transient ischemic attack (TIA), and also notes a history of a febrile illness with rash and or other connective tissue disease symptoms, the possibility of Takayasu's arteritis should be considered. If an older woman complains of similar systemic symptoms in conjunction with temporary or permanent loss of vision and severe headache, giant cell arteritis will be more likely. In women and men, Raynaud's phenomenon may develop as a distinct, mild, primary condition, or may portend the development of more serious systemic connective tissue diseases, such as scleroderma or lupus erythematosus. Early distal obliterative arterial disease, often associated with venous thrombosis, sometimes involving the upper extremities, suggests thromboangiitis obliterans, especially if the patient is a young man (fourth or fifth decade) with prodigious tobacco consumption. When evaluating a new patient, it is useful to establish a working diagnosis of either atherosclerosis or an alternative arterial disease. This initial distinction (based largely on the historical factors listed above) serves as a useful guide to further diagnostic and management decisions.

ARTERIAL OCCLUSIVE DISEASES

Arterial abnormalities tend to manifest themselves in one of two categories: either (1) insufficient end-organ arterial perfusion causing clinical symptoms or (2) progressive arterial degeneration with loss of arterial integrity and aneurysmal enlargement. Peripheral arterial involvement

Table 39.1–1. Risk factors associated with the development of lower extremity arterial disease, disease progression, and mortality.

Risk factor	Development of disease	Progression	Mortality
Smoking	Yes	Yes	Yes
Diabetes	Yes	Yes/No	Yes
Hyperlipidemia	Conflicting results for triglyceride, cholesterol, and lipoprotein	Conflicting results	Conflicting results
Systolic blood pressure	Yes (blood pressure a strong predictor in most, but not all, studies)	Yes/No	Yes/No
Physical activity	NAI	Yes/No	No
Hemorheologic factors	Unclear	NAI	NAI
Obesity	No (however, may be a weak risk factor in men)	NAI	NAI
Genetic factors	NAI	NAI	NAI

NAI = not adequately investigated.

occurs most commonly at arterial bifurcations (common carotid, aortic, iliac, femoral) or specific regions of unbranched arteries (infrarenal aorta, superficial femoral artery). Patients with aneurysmal degeneration of the aorta may have significant occlusive disease in the other predictable locations in the peripheral vasculature, and vice versa. The specific pathological processes associated with occlusive versus aneurysmal disease will be reviewed in later chapters. However, the careful clinician will be alert for the coexistence of occlusive and aneurysmal arterial abnormalities when examining any vascular patient, regardless of his or her preexisting diagnosis or presenting complaint.

Occlusive diseases tend to present and be distinguished by ischemia of the end organ. **Vasculogenic claudication** is a term specific to the lower extremities. It describes leg pain with walking secondary to inadequate limb blood flow, relieved by rest. Ischemic rest pain, or **metatarsalgia**, refers to generally more severe lower extremity ischemia. Metatarsalgia represents the most severe manifestation of limb ischemia, with limb perfusion compromised to such a degree that pain is continuous. Such pain is usually only improved by dependent positioning of the involved limb. This position supposedly optimizes oxygen extraction from pooling and stasis of the arterial and venous blood that is present. Claudication is also present, but walking itself may not be possible, precluding the recognition of claudication symptoms.

The severely ischemic lower limb is prone to develop non-healing ulcerations. This is especially true in the forefoot. These can remain open and indolent or can progress to wet or dry gangrene. Plantar fasciitis can result from seemingly innocuous lesions, especially in diabetic patients. The painful, ischemic, ulcerated lower extremity often becomes the fulcrum upon which the elderly patient's life turns. Failure to heal the wound or salvage the limb severely exacerbates the patient's immobility and isolation. Amputation often is the first step in a relentless decline that includes full-time nursing care, debility, institutionalization, depression, and death. In the review of a patient's social history, attention to the activities of daily living and home support provide essential perspective on the suitability of various care options for each patient.

The severity and location of lower extremity ischemic symptoms are closely related to the location of the stenosis/occlusions. In general, symptoms of claudication tend to manifest themselves one level below the level of the occlusion. Thus, patients with aortoiliac disease usually complain of thigh or buttock pain with ambulation. When combined with symptoms of impotence and physical examination findings of absent femoral pulses in men, this symptom complex is known as **Leriche syndrome** (in deference to the early 20th century French vascular surgeon René Leriche). Further distally, superficial femoral artery stenosis or occlusion is consistently associated with calf pain, and popliteal or tibial disease usually is not related to claudication but rather to severe foot and ankle ischemia, as classically noted in diabetic patients. A careful history and physical examination can accurately localize areas of obstruction without any additional imaging studies under these circumstances. In general, the severity of ischemia is closely related to the degree of luminal reduction present in any one location. Serial stenoses are usually present in the setting of profound ischemia. Thus, patients with absent femoral pulses indicating iliac stenoses or occlusion (a term referred to as **inflow disease**) frequently walk one or more blocks before the onset of symptoms. However, if additional stenoses are also present in the vessels at or distal to the inguinal ligament (**outflow disease**), the patient is probably experiencing pain at rest, or worse. Collateral flow may be so well developed as to allow palpable pedal pulses to still be present in the setting of single-level (iliac/femoral or popliteal) disease, but in general, occlusion at any level usually obliterates the distal pulse.

In the setting of the absent pedal pulse, estimates of pedal perfusion can be deceptive, based on capillary refill time or skin temperature. Thus, objective measurement of the degree of distal flow and obstruction becomes necessary. This is most commonly accomplished by the assessment of the ankle-brachial index (ABI). This bedside procedure should be considered part of the physical examination of patients with clinical signs of ischemia and absent pedal pulses. The examiner places blood pressure cuffs around both ankles (Figure 39.1–1). A hand-held, continuous wave Doppler instrument is used to identify the dorsal pedal and posterior tibial arteries on the foot. The cuffs are then inflated until the signals are obliterated. Usually, this procedure needs to be repeated several times to determine the highest pressure/best signal on either

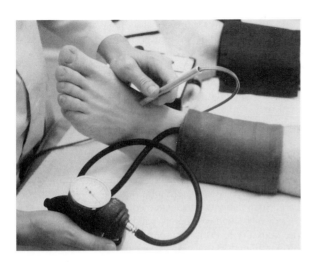

Figure 39.1–1. Measurement of ankle-brachial index. Blood pressure cuffs are placed around each ankle while a hand-held continuous wave Doppler instrument identifies the dorsal pedal and posterior tibial arterial flow through the foot.

foot. Then, the higher of the two brachial pressures is determined and used as the denominator to calculate the index. The scale from 1.0 to 0.0 is a useful method of determining the severity of limb ischemia. In general, an ABI of greater than 0.5 is more consistent with viable limbs that experience some degree of claudication, and an ABI of less than or equal to 0.5 is indicative of more severe, limb-threatening ischemia (Figure 39.1–2).

Vasculogenic upper extremity pain with exercise is much less common than claudication. Atherosclerosis rarely involves the upper extremity arteries, despite advanced involvement in other arterial beds. When present, significant lesions usually are an extension of aortic arch disease involving the great vessels. The range of differential diagnoses is much broader for symptoms of upper extremity ischemia than for lower. Conditions such as arterial impingement at the thoracic outlet, primary vasospastic processes, autoimmune-related connective tissue diseases, thromboangiitis obliterans, diabetes-associated vasculopathy, and embolic phenomenon are much more likely etiologic considerations in this setting. Close attention should be paid to comorbid disease processes, underlying health issues, family history, and frequency, severity, and dura-

tion of symptomatic episodes. As is true in the lower extremities, careful segmental pulse examination can reliably identify the location and extent of occlusion or stenosis in many patients. Severe ischemia is usually more proximal, inaccessible, and, thus, more reliant on objective evaluation in the laboratory to assess degree and location of obstruction.

Visceral ischemic syndromes remain poorly defined almost a century after their description. Unlike the extremities, the end organs of the renal or mesenteric vessels are not available for direct examination. Reliance on the patient's history and clinical status becomes paramount to the diagnostician. Newer examination methods, such as duplex ultrasonographic scanning or magnetic resonance imaging, may play a more significant role in identifying these patients in the future.

ANEURYSMAL ARTERIAL DEGENERATION

In addition to occlusion, the infrarenal aorta and distal vessels may also be prone to aneurysmal degeneration. These processes also tend to occur at predictable locations. These include the infrarenal aorta and common iliac arteries, the femoral arteries, the popliteal arteries, and, less frequently, the internal iliac (hypogastric) and superficial femoral arteries. **Aneurysm formation** is a progressive, degenerative condition of the arterial wall that results in vessel enlargement. Over the course of years (for "atherosclerotic aneurysms") or days (for mycotic aneurysms), the wall loses integrity and begins to enlarge. Subsequent symptoms may be the result of enlargement and external impingement of surrounding structures, leak or rupture, or distal embolization of aneurysm contents or aneurysm thrombosis.

Risk factors and the average age of onset for aneurysm formation are very similar to those of occlusive disease. Family history may play a very significant role. For our purposes in this chapter, the diagnosis of aneurysm disease relies on the skill and knowledge of the examiner. When presented with a patient with an appropriate risk profile (age, risk factors, comorbidity, tobacco use, and so forth), the possibility of aneurysmal disease must be considered, even if symptoms seem unrelated on the initial evaluation. For example, flank or back pain and lower extremity weakness or pain suggestive of sciatica may mask

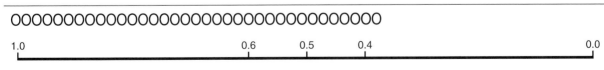

Figure 39.1–2. Ankle-brachial index. Used to determine severity of lower extremity ischemia. O's denote range consistent with claudication; X's denote area of limb-threatening ischemia. Note area of considerable overlap around 0.5.

a contained rupture of an aortic or iliac aneurysm. Sudden onset of discolored feet or toes, especially when pedal pulses are present or even normal, suggests embolization from a more proximal source, most commonly an aneurysm. If present on both feet, the aorta is more likely; unilateral foot involvement suggests a more distal lesion.

Peripheral aneurysm disease is notoriously multifocal. Five percent of patients with aortic aneurysms may develop popliteal aneurysms. However, half of patients with popliteal aneurysms may also have aortic aneurysms. Many patients may also develop femoral or superficial femoral aneurysms years later. Aneurysm disease should be considered a work in progress, lasting the life of the patient.

Naturally occurring aneurysms, either atherosclerotic or mycotic, generally involve the entire vessel wall (intima, media, and adventitia). Degenerative aneurysms arising from infected or injured arteries are more commonly "false" in the sense that all three layers are not present. These false aneurysms, or "pseudoaneurysms," frequently complicate previous vascular procedures, such as aortic surgery or arterial catheterization. Thus, patients with a history of previous arterial surgery or serious injury warrant regular review and examination of their vascular status, focused not only on the possibility of new aneurysms, should such have previously been repaired, but also on the potential failure of previous repairs or unrepaired, injured arteries as well.

VENOUS DIAGNOSTIC CONSIDERATIONS

Low pressure in the venous system, and the requirement of active muscle function necessary for venous return from the lower extremities, distinguish venous disease and its sequelae. Venous disease includes (1) congenital abnormalities of the venous circulation; (2) thrombotic occlusion and subsequent impaired limb drainage; (3) pulmonary embolization following thrombotic occlusion; (4) impaired venous hemodynamics following thrombosis and venous valvular incompetence. Evaluation of the patient with complaints referable to the extremities or the pulmonary circulation must include consideration of venous abnormalities.

Extremity swelling, either at rest or during exercise, is the sine qua non of venous dysfunction. The patient with acute unilateral lower extremity edema must be evaluated for the presence of deep venous thrombosis (DVT). This is especially true if calf pain or tenderness is also present. Pain, however, may not be prominent. The solicitation of "Homans's sign," as distinguished by palpation of a "cord" with the calf itself, is not sensitive enough to be used with confidence during clinical evaluation. Important historical information includes prolonged inactivity, ipsilateral limb injury, recent orthopedic surgery or fixation, past history of DVT, or other causes of hypercoagulability. Bilateral acute limb edema may or may not represent central or iliocaval thrombosis. If caval thrombosis is present, edema and swelling are usually severe, and venous compartmental hypertension may become an issue.

Acute DVT is a common occurrence in ambulatory care units and emergency rooms. More perplexing are the various limb sequelae associated with chronic venous occlusion or valvular insufficiency. These patients often complain of progressive limb swelling during the day, relieved by elevation in the evening. Skin changes, such as pigmentation or frank ulceration, may occur in the perimalleolar area or the distal one third of the calf. In advanced cases, chronic edema and ulceration create indurated limbs and persistent ulceration, requiring intensive wound care. Such patients either have congenitally deficient vein valves or secondary venous valvular insufficiency due to previous DVT. Prominent superficial veins and perforating veins may suggest abnormal or occluded deep veins. History taking in patients with chronic venous diseases should focus on family history; previous trauma, thrombosis, or surgery; functional limitations; and potential coexisting systemic or dermatologic diseases.

VASCULAR EMERGENCIES

Arteries can occlude, rupture, or dissect. If chronic stenosis is present, progressive stenosis/occlusion may be well tolerated, but when otherwise normal vessels occlude due to cardiogenic embolization, external pressure, or penetrating injury, then limb loss, stroke, or death may ensue. Acute arterial limb ischemia usually becomes symptomatic shortly after the event and progresses over the next several hours. The signs and symptoms associated with acute limb ischemia are frequently referred to as the "seven P's" (also abbreviated as the "five P's"): pulselessness, pallor, polar (cold), paresthesias, paralysis, pain, and past midnight (in reference to when these conditions usually occur). When present, these signs and symptoms need to be pursued aggressively, as delay in revascularization can lead to tissue necrosis, reperfusion injury, nerve palsy, compartment syndrome, and, ultimately, limb loss.

Arterial rupture is most commonly associated with aneurysmal degeneration of the aorta, but can occur with profound clinical consequences at any location in the body. Femoral and popliteal aneurysms, though commonly associated with aortic aneurysms, rupture only infrequently. Abdominal aortic aneurysms (AAA) are best treated by elective repair after identification of asymptomatic aneurysms, but this protocol is not always possible. Typically, patients with ruptured AAA present to the emergency room with severe abdominal pain of recent onset, hypotension, and a prominent aortic pulse or absent pedal pulses. Prompt operative repair of the aneurysm is the only hope of survival in this situation, requiring clear thinking and goal-driven diagnostic analysis in the emergency room.

If aneurysm rupture is considered a likely diagnosis, the preoperative assessment should be limited to obtaining a clot tube for the blood bank, a 12-lead ECG, and, possibly, emergency ultrasonography or computed tomographic (CT) scanning. Imaging tests are obviously not appropriate for hypotensive, unstable patients. If myocardial ischemia is not thought to be the cause of the patient's problems, and profound or worsening pain, abdominal girth, hypotension, and anemia are present, then any further evaluation or imaging study is not appropriate and operative repair is paramount. Musculoskeletal back pain (acute or chronic), indigestion, and renal or biliary colic can all mimic the symptoms of AAA, and, conversely, the diagnosis of AAA should be strongly considered in the evaluation of patients with these symptoms.

Arteries can also rupture if they have been previously subjected to instrumentation (intentionally or inadvertently) or have been weakened through infection (mycotic aneurysm), previous arterial reconstructive surgery (pseudoaneurysm), or penetrating injury. The possibility of arterial injury and catastrophic operative bleeding or exsanguination should always be considered when one contemplates surgery on patients with these conditions or assesses patients with penetrating injuries that appear to be in close proximity to major arteries.

Arterial dissection may mimic occlusion or rupture. Primary aortic dissection is classically associated with severe back, chest, and abdominal pain. During dissection, blood flow creates a new channel within the arterial wall, known as the **false lumen**. The false lumen may provide flow to some or all of the visceral arteries or one or both extremities. Aortic dissection, thus, is associated with acute mesenteric, renal, spinal, or lower extremity ischemia. If the false lumen decompresses back into the true lumen without compromising other arteries, there may be no sequela. Dissection may also occur near the aortic root, compromising coronary flow or aortic valvular integrity.

When hypertensive patients present with unusual symptoms of limb or organ ischemia, the diagnosis of dissection should be considered. In collagen vascular disorders, such as Ehlers-Danlos or Marfan's syndrome, spontaneous dissection and primary arterial rupture become much more likely.

UNDERSTANDING THE VASCULAR LABORATORY

TESTING MODALITIES

Modern vascular surgery and medicine rely heavily on the objective assessment of blood pressure, flow, and direct vessel imaging to confirm or establish the clinical diagnosis. These examinations are usually performed in a dedicated vascular laboratory. Such a facility should be accredited by the Intersocietal Commission for the Voluntary Accreditation of Vascular Laboratories. The Registered Vascular Technologist (RVT) credential of the American Registry of Diagnostic Medical Sonographers distinguishes a professional technologist who is knowledgeable in the natural history and assessment of patients with all manner of vascular diseases. Achievement of the credential is by examination. Private as well as junior college-based training programs exist to prepare candidates for examination.

The *Journal of Vascular Technology*, formerly *Bruit*, is the official journal of the Society of Vascular Technologists. This journal publishes original research related to vascular patient assessment, as well as timely and comprehensive reviews of current testing strategies. The name change effected by this journal several years ago was made in recognition of the fact that a bruit, appreciated on physical examination by auscultation or palpation, is only a marker of turbulence and, as such, is not a reliable indicator of stenosis or occlusion. This change reflects the increasing objective focus of vascular technology.

The development of noninvasive vascular testing has been closely associated with the development of vascular surgery as a distinct specialty. Original reliance on indirect methods of flow and pressure assessment (such as plethysmography) has given way to direct vascular imaging and estimation of flow using Doppler-derived frequency shifts of reflected ultrasonographic beams. Today, laboratory testing is focused on lower extremity pressure and flow studies, serial postbypass graft surveillance, vein mapping prior to graft harvest, extracranial and intracranial cerebrovascular flow and imaging studies, aortic and mesenteric imaging and flow studies, and venous imaging and valve function studies. Testing indications and results appropriate to specific disease processes will be reviewed in the appropriate following chapters. This section will focus on methods of vascular imaging and flow assessment and their application to vascular patient evaluation.

The most versatile, sensitive, and specific imaging instrument currently used in the vascular laboratory is the duplex scanner. This device combines the imaging strength of B-mode ultrasonography with Doppler spectral frequency analysis. The Doppler equation can be used to determine the speed of moving blood, based on the premise that the frequency of a transmitted ultrasonographic beam is shifted by its reflection by the blood, and the degree of that shift is proportional to the speed. The Doppler shift (f) can be expressed as:

$$f = 2 \times F \times V \times \cos. \text{theta}/C,$$ where F = frequency, V = velocity, theta = the angle between the ultrasound beam and the direction of moving blood, and C = the speed of ultrasound transmitted through tissue.

Solving for velocity,

$$V = f \times C/F \times 2 \times \cos. \text{theta}$$

This equation determines the frequency shift generated by moving red blood cells through a given region under consideration. This information, along with the angle of insonation, is computed to provide the flow velocity of blood in cm/s. Color is applied to the image to distinguish flow toward the probe (red) or away (blue), as well as the velocity profile of the cross-sectional image.

By combining the image with the flow velocity data, areas of stenosis or occlusion can be assessed with extreme accuracy. In general, scanning accuracy is inversely related to depth of penetration. Although the relationship between flow velocity and arterial stenosis can vary depending on the distal resistance, in general, flow velocity increases after a 50% reduction in diameter, continues to increase until diameter reduction reaches 95%, and then rapidly diminishes as diameter reduction approaches total occlusion. Knowledge of the relationship between velocity and stenosis in a given circulation can be and has been used to develop criteria for predicting the location and severity of stenotic lesions in the arterial system in a noninvasive fashion. The scope of this text is not appropriate for a more detailed discussion of the duplex scanner and its related technologies; the reader is referred to the references at the end of this chapter for further information.

DISEASE-SPECIFIC TESTS & RESULTS REPORTING

EXTRACRANIAL CEREBRAL ARTERIAL EXAMINATION

Patients who have suffered a transient ischemic attack (TIA), episode of amaurosis fugax, or stroke are frequently the victims of embolic events that have originated at the carotid bifurcation. These patients should be examined to rule out a source for embolization, especially when these patients have audible bruits present in the neck or other symptoms of peripheral vascular occlusive disease. The role of such testing in asymptomatic patients with bruits or appropriate risk factors remains less certain.

Examinations are usually performed with the patient in a supine position. The technologist identifies the common carotid artery and the carotid bifurcation with the duplex scanner and uses the color flow to confirm location and suggest areas of possible stenosis. Precise determination of degree of stenosis is accomplished by the determination of flow velocity in the areas of interest as described above. Criteria for stenosis are based on peak systolic and end-diastolic velocity and the ratio of internal to common carotid artery velocities (Table 39.1–2). The risk of subsequent cerebrovascular events has been determined in retrospective and large, prospective, multicenter, randomized trials in patients with increasing degrees of stenosis present in these arteries. Similar flow determinations can also be made in the vertebral and subclavian arteries, although the angle of insonation is often not known with certainty; therefore, precise determinations of stenosis are not possible.

Currently, patients in our practice are examined if their history or physical examination suggests that a flow-limiting lesion may be present. If carotid lesions are present, but do not warrant surgery, patients are followed every 3, 6, or 12 months, depending on the severity and instability of the stenosis.

ARTERIAL LUMINAL DIAMETER

The presence, diameter, and extent of peripheral artery aneurysms can easily be appreciated by B-mode (two-dimensional) ultrasonographic imaging. Clear criteria exist for intervention in aortic aneurysms. Indications for surgery are less well defined for other peripheral

Table 39.1–2. Relationship of stenosis to Doppler findings.[1]

Diameter Stenosis	Peak Systolic Velocity (m/s)	End Diastolic Velocity (m/s)	ICA/CCA Peak Systolic Ratio
< 50%	$\bar{<}$ 1.5	$\bar{<}$ .50	< 1.8
50–60%	1.5–2.0	.50–.70	$\bar{<}$ 2.2
60–70%	2.0–2.5	.70–.90	2.2–2.8
70–80%	2.5–3.3	.90–1.3	2.8–3.8
80–90%	3.3–4.0	1.3–1.8	3.8–5.0
90–99%	$\bar{>}$ 4.0	> 1.8	$\bar{>}$ 5.0
Occlusion	No ICA flow present Unilateral blunted CCA flow[2]		

[1]These numbers were established using an Acuson XP/128 5.0 MHz multihertz imaging transducer, a 3.5 MHz Doppler frequency, and a consistent 60-degree angle correction.

[2]Blunted CCA flow may also be present with pre-occlusive ICA stenosis (90–99%). Use Doppler at highest sensitivity to rule out slow trickle flow in all vessels suspected of total occlusion. Also, a long segment ICA stenosis may not demonstrate a signficantly high end-diastolic velocity when compared to a short segment stenosis.

CCA = common carotid artery; ICA = internal carotid artery.

aneurysms. Aneurysms that have been identified by ultrasonographic examination but do not warrant surgery are usually examined at 3-, 6-, or 12-month intervals, depending on their size and rate of expansion.

ARTERIAL GRAFT SURVEILLANCE

The function of arterial vein grafts can be determined by direct examination with a duplex scanner. Vein grafts, commonly from the femoral to popliteal or distal arteries, are generally durable. However, even the best centers and surgeons experience early and late failure of grafts; 85% 5-year patency seems to be the upper limit. Vein grafts fail most commonly because intrinsic lesions develop within the graft or at either anastomosis. These lesions represent focal areas of fibrointimal hyperplasia and may occur at old valve sites or previous areas of vein injury. These lesions usually begin within the first few weeks after surgery and are most evident on duplex scanning within 3 months of surgery.

Duplex technology is well suited to identifying these lesions and estimating their severity before flow diminishes to the point that the graft itself is threatened. The entire graft is easily scanned if placed in the in situ position (Figure 39.1–3). Anatomic grafts are usually scanned at fixed intervals. Areas of marked velocity increase (twice that of the immediately proximal region) or reduction, or areas where the flow velocity has dropped below 45 cm/s, may identify grafts that need revision to prevent total occlusion (Figure 39.1–4). Patients should be studied every 3 months following bypass for the first year after surgery, decreasing to biannual and then annual examinations on the second and third years thereafter.

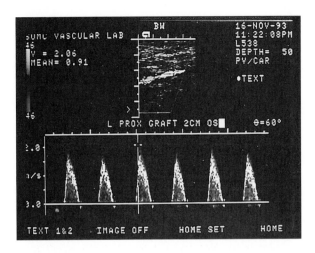

Figure 39.1–4. Graft flow velocity examination of left femoral popliteal bypass graft. Cross-sectional image in the top center identifies the vessel via color flow, and allows Doppler cursor to be placed in the region of interest. Velocity profiles throughout the cardiac cycle are noted below. This image was obtained 2 cm from the proximal anastomosis of a reversed saphenous vein graft. Peak systolic velocity at this point is 2.06 meters/second. The examination is completed by examining representation regions of the remainder of the graft in anatomically tunneled bypass grafts, and imaging the entire vessel for in situ grafts.

VEIN MAPPING

The B-mode image of duplex scanning is well suited to assessing upper or lower extremity peripheral veins as potential bypass graft conduits. When patients have intact in situ greater saphenous veins (GSV) and no history of limb surgery or thrombophlebitis, the vein is assumed to be adequate. However, if some or all of the GSV is missing from either leg, multiple sites may need to be investigated for suitable conduit. This can substantially increase operative time and morbidity if done blindly or on the basis of physical examination alone. Therefore, in patients without an obvious graft source, vein mapping can dramatically improve efficiency and outcome. We generally use veins that are 3 mm or greater with a smooth luminal contour for infrainguinal bypass. Maximum length is critical, as venovenous anastomosis used to connect multiple smaller pieces of vein can severely compromise arterial graft patency.

EVALUATION OF DEEP VEIN THROMBOSIS

Duplex ultrasonography is ideally suited to scanning the deep veins for evidence of deep vein thrombosis (DVT). Color imaging is used to quickly identify the lumen of the vein; then, maneuvers such as distal calf

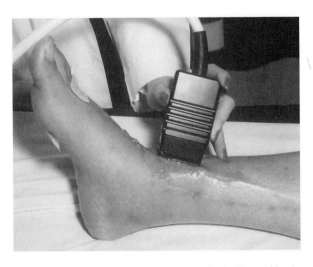

Figure 39.1–3. Duplex scanner placed in the in situ position to determine viability of flow in an arterial graft.

compression, deep breathing, and exhalation against a closed glottis are performed during imaging to confirm the presence and pattern of flow and the presence of luminal filling defects, such as a thrombus. Venous flow in the lower extremities should demonstrate normal respiratory variation with spontaneous respiration and increased flow with calf compression distal to the scan head. The Valsalva maneuver dramatically reduces venous return. If flow is not responsive to these maneuvers, or if the vein itself is not compressible by direct compression with the scan head, the strong probability exists that the lumen is obstructed by clot. Ultrasonographic testing of veins in the lower extremities is rapid, safe, reliable, inexpensive, and generally well tolerated. For these reasons, it is now considered the gold standard examination for DVT.

ADDITIONAL ARTERIAL TESTING

The ability to assess deep visceral arteries via duplex ultrasonographic technology remains a more elusive skill. When performed by experienced technologists, such techniques can recognize and quantitate renal artery stenosis, mesenteric artery stenosis, and distal aortic or iliac stenosis. These techniques have been successfully used to guide interventions, such as catheter-based angioplasty as a stand-alone imaging procedure. Reliable and reproducible criteria now exist to identify SMA stenosis greater than 70%, and hemodynamically significant renal artery stenosis. However, these techniques require patience and considerable technical skill and are not reliable unless performed under the auspices of an accredited vascular laboratory.

Similarly, transcranial Doppler (TCD) ultrasonography can provide accurate information regarding flow in the intracranial carotid and vertebral arteries, the circle of Willis, and its major branches. Scans are performed through the orbit, the base of the skull, and the temporal bone. Although absolute velocities are not obtained using this technique, direction of flow and relative differences between arteries are easily demonstrated and can provide useful information regarding cerebral perfusion. This technology is useful, for example, in studying the frequency and nature of cerebral emboli that may occur during carotid endarterectomy.

ADDITIONAL VENOUS TESTING

Duplex scanning as a direct test has largely replaced indirect tests such as venous photoplethysmography of the lower extremity to assess venous valvular competence. Additionally, duplex scanning is well suited to identifying and marking individual incompetent perforating veins prior to ligation or excision.

NEWER METHODS OF ARTERIAL & VENOUS IMAGING

ROLE OF ARTERIAL IMAGING FOR THERAPEUTIC INTERVENTION

Modern arterial reconstructive surgery is generally safe and effective when performed by experienced surgeons in high-volume centers. More than any other single component of surgery, precision preoperative arterial imaging is paramount to the expectation of success. The sine qua non of arterial reconstructive surgery is "no surprises." Patients and procedures do best when the entire operation can be planned in advance—identification of accessory renal arteries prior to aortic surgery, or clear demonstration of target arteries for bypass at or below the ankle. This essential aspect of vascular surgery stands in marked contradistinction to the approach of the plastic surgeon, where often the ultimate operative strategy is defined during the operation.

CURRENT STATUS & FUTURE PROSPECTS FOR ARTERIOGRAPHIC EXAMINATION

Traditionally, only catheter-based contrast arteriography could provide the necessary preoperative anatomic detail. Thus, every procedure would be preceded by an angiogram. However, the risk and expense of this practice, in addition to rapid and dramatic improvements in alternative, less invasive imaging methods, have led to dramatic changes in "standard" preoperative imaging procedures in the last 5 years. Currently, in our practice, we obtain routine contrast arteriograms for preoperative planning only in infrainguinal arterial reconstructive surgery patients. This is done primarily to identify the optimal bypass target. As such, even for this indication, the term "diagnostic arteriogram" is obsolete. Improvements in magnetic resonance imaging may provide images of sufficient quality for this purpose in the future.

Cerebrovascular arteriography is rapidly becoming obsolete, replaced by the carotid duplex examination and, when patients are symptomatic, CT examination of the head to exclude other causes of symptoms or to confirm cerebral infarction. We now order cerebral arteriograms only when questions regarding the relevant anatomy remain after duplex examination has identified a stenosis. Thus, if the distal end of the internal carotid plaque cannot be identified by ultrasonography, or proximal common carotid lesions are suggested by a low common carotid velocity, arteriography may provide additional, relevant anatomic information. However, for most patients, ultrasonography alone provides sufficient imaging and flow data to ensure safe and successful surgery.

Abdominal aortic imaging, especially for aneurysmal disease, is moving away from catheter-based techniques toward CT or MRI. In patients with aortic occlusive disease, direct injection of contrast into the distal aorta or into significant collateral vessels, such as the internal mammary artery in patients with aortic occlusion, continues to provide the best quality anatomic imaging.

Venous imaging is now primarily performed by ultrasonography. During the last decade, ultrasonic diagnosis of deep venous thrombosis has replaced venography as the "gold standard" diagnostic examination. Today, venography is reserved for patients who are being considered for therapy, such as venous angioplasty or stenting. Further developments in ultrasonography, such as three-dimensional imaging, may further expand the role of noninvasive imaging in the treatment of venous abnormalities.

NEWER IMAGING MODALITIES

Continuous acquisition, or "spiral," CT imaging, is a relatively new method of obtaining computed tomographic images. Acquisition times are remarkably shorter than traditional CT scanning, on the order of 90 seconds. When acquired in this fashion, three-dimensional image sets can be constructed to demonstrate structures as objects in space, where they can be rotated and viewed from any angle. A shaded surface display can be constructed to provide subtle detail regarding aortic luminal contour and shape previously unobtainable from two-dimensional imaging methods, such as biplanar catheter-based aortography. Data can even be displayed in such a fashion that a "fly through" view of structures, such as the thoracic or abdominal aorta, is obtained with remarkable clarity and detail. This technique is especially valuable in sorting out complicated flow channels in aortic dissection patients, for example. While weaknesses remain in luminal versus external diameter imaging, or length of aorta visualized during a single examination, this exciting technology

promises to play an important role in guiding newer interventional techniques, such as aortic stent grafting.

Magnetic resonance imaging also holds immense promise for providing preoperative arterial imaging. In addition to anatomic detail rivaling catheter-based angiographic techniques for lower extremity imaging, MRI can also provide physiologic data on flow volume and oximetric assessment of hemoglobin. Thus, in patients with a possible diagnosis of mesenteric ischemia, the anatomy of the proximal superior mesenteric and celiac arteries can be demonstrated, and flow can be quantified with simultaneous assessment of superior mesenteric venous oxygen saturation to confirm the significance of the anatomic lesions. This exciting technology promises to revolutionize the diagnosis of this frustrating disease, as well as renal vascular hypertension, vasculogenic impotence, and other visceral ischemic syndromes.

SUMMARY

In summary, the evaluation of the patient with vascular disease requires a working knowledge of vascular anatomy, pathology, and pathophysiology. Physical examination is frequently sufficient for diagnosis, especially in the urgent or emergent situation. The noninvasive vascular laboratory complements the physical examination and provides more sensitive methods of assessing progression of vascular disorders or the status of reconstructive procedures than are available by examination alone. Although catheter-based angiographic techniques have guided vascular interventions for more than 60 years, safer and less expensive modalities, such as ultrasonography, CT, and MRI, may represent the future of vascular imaging. Regardless of the method employed, however, the imperative for precise and accurate assessment of arterial and venous anatomy and disorders will remain paramount to the practice of modern vascular surgery.

SUGGESTED READING

Bernstein EF: *Vascular Diagnosis*. Mosby-Yearbook, 1993.
Fann JI, Dalman RL: Genetic and metabolic causes of arterial disease. Ann Vasc Surg 1993;7:594.

Strandness DE: *Duplex Scanning in Vascular Disorders*. Raven Press, 1993.

39.2 Cerebrovascular Occlusive Disease

Christopher K. Zarins, MD, & Ramin E. Beygui, MD

▶ Key Facts

- ▶ Stroke, or CVA (cerebrovascular accident), is the third leading cause of death in the United States.

- ▶ The majority of all strokes, up to two thirds, are caused by atherosclerotic plaques at the carotid bifurcation in the neck.

- ▶ The majority of patients with carotid bifurcation atherosclerosis are asymptomatic.

- ▶ Symptoms of cerebrovascular ischemia may be divided into two categories: carotid territory symptoms and vertebrobasilar symptoms.

- ▶ Stroke is defined as a neurologic deficit lasting more than 24 hours.

- ▶ The surgical treatment of choice for carotid occlusive disease is a procedure known as carotid endarterectomy, which involves the removal of atherosclerotic plaque from the carotid bifurcation.

- ▶ Carotid endarterectomy is the treatment of choice for: (1) patients with carotid stenosis of greater than or equal to 70% and symptoms of TIA (transient ischemic attack) or recent mild stroke in centers where surgical risk of stroke is less than 6%; (2) patients with asymptomatic severe carotid stenosis greater than or equal to 60% in centers where surgical risk of stroke is less than 3%.

- ▶ Complications of carotid endarterectomy include cranial nerve injury, myocardial infarction, bradycardia, hypotension, restenosis, wound problems, and stroke.

GENERAL CONSIDERATIONS

Stroke, or cerebrovascular accident (CVA), is the third leading cause of death in the United States. Approximately 75% of strokes are caused by embolism to the brain. Cerebral emboli can originate from the heart, aortic arch, and great vessels or from the carotid and vertebral arteries. Cardiac sources include intracardiac thrombi in association with atrial fibrillation and ventricular aneurysms. Rarely, emboli can arise from the venous system as paradoxical emboli through a patent foramen ovale or atrial septal defect. The majority of all strokes, up to two thirds, are caused by atherosclerotic plaques at the carotid bifurcation in the neck.

Carotid bifurcation atherosclerosis can cause strokes by one of two mechanisms (1) *embolism* of atherosclerotic plaque, thrombus, or platelet deposits and (2) *stenosis* of the internal carotid artery, causing reduced ipsilateral cerebral blood flow. Emboli or flow disturbances in the posterior cerebral circulation can also cause cerebral ischemia in the distribution of the vertebral or basilar arteries. Stenosis or occlusion of the subclavian artery proximal to the origin of the vertebral artery can result in reversal of flow in the vertebral artery to supply the distal subclavian artery. This flow reversal may cause vertebrobasilar ischemia on exercise of the arm (see Chapter 39.3). Aneurysms of the carotid and vertebral artery may present as a pulsatile neck mass and be a source of emboli or may progress to occlusion. Trauma, fibromuscular disease, vasculitides, and connective tissue disorders can rarely cause stenosis, occlusion, or aneurysmal degeneration of the carotid and vertebral arteries. This chapter primarily addresses the most common causes of cerebrovascular ischemia, which are due to atherosclerotic lesions of the carotid and vertebral arteries. Aneurysms, trauma, and vasculitides are discussed elsewhere in this book.

ETIOLOGY

Carotid bifurcation atherosclerosis is the most common cause of ischemic stroke. Atherosclerotic plaques commonly form in the first portion of the internal carotid artery in the neck (the carotid sinus). Early plaque deposition occurs along the outer wall of the internal carotid sinus. Hemodynamic studies have shown this area to be a region of boundary layer separation and stagnant flow, with relatively low flow velocity and low wall shear stress and oscillation of shear stress direction. These hemodynamic features have been shown to correspond to regions prone to atherosclerotic plaque formation. Plaque enlargement can result in stenosis of the lumen and compromise of flow through the internal carotid artery. Mature atherosclerotic plaques are covered with a fibrous cap that isolates the necrotic core of the atheroma from the lumen. Rupture of fibrous cap covering the plaque may result in embolization of atherosclerotic debris and cause ulceration of the plaque. These lumen irregularities promote the deposition of platelets and thrombi, which may embolize.

Fibromuscular dysplasia is predominantly a disease of Caucasian women of child-bearing age. The cause of fibromuscular dysplasia is unknown, but a number have been hypothesized, including hormonal effects, oral contraceptive use, mechanical injury, and ischemic vessel wall injuries. Fibromuscular dysplasia is associated with abnormal growth and organization of the intima, media, or adventitia, causing stenoses, aneurysms, or dissections of the carotid or vertebral arteries that can cause cerebrovascular symptoms and strokes.

CLINICAL PRESENTATION

The majority of patients with carotid bifurcation atherosclerosis are asymptomatic. Developing stenoses of the carotid artery can produce a cervical bruit. However, only 50% of patients with a cervical bruit have a significant stenosis of the internal carotid artery. Similarly, signifi-

cant stenosis can be present without an audible bruit. The differential diagnosis of cervical bruit includes transmitted cardiac murmurs, venous hums, and external as well as internal carotid stenosis.

Although audible cervical bruit is an important physical finding, it is not a reliable indicator of significant carotid artery stenosis. Cervical bruits should be further investigated with carotid duplex scanning. On funduscopic examination, embolized atheromatous debris in the retinal arteries may be recognized as Hollenhorst plaques.

CLINICAL SYMPTOMS

Symptoms of cerebrovascular ischemia may be divided into two categories: carotid territory symptoms and vertebrobasilar symptoms (Table 39.2–1).

Carotid territory symptoms are produced by embolization or flow reduction in the distribution of the internal carotid artery and its branches. Symptoms include (1) ipsilateral monocular blindness (**amaurosis fugax**) caused by embolization to the retinal artery via the ophthalmic artery, which is the first branch of the internal carotid artery, (2) speech disturbance or aphasia due to flow disturbance to the left middle cerebral artery, which supplies the left parietotemporal lobes containing Broca's and Wernicke's speech areas, and (3) contralateral hemiparesis resulting from ischemia of the parietotemporal lobe supplied by the middle cerebral artery.

Vertebrobasilar symptoms are produced by ischemia of the posterior cerebral or cerebellar arteries that arise from the basilar artery, which is formed by the joining together of the paired vertebral arteries. Symptoms include nonlateralizing neurologic symptoms, such as diplopia, slurring of speech, ataxia, and monoparesis, as well as global symptoms, such as syncope, drop attacks, vertigo, and dizziness.

CLASSIFICATION OF SYMPTOMS

Neurologic symptoms lasting less than 24 hours with complete recovery are classified as **transient ischemic attacks** (TIAs). Reversible symptoms lasting more than 24 and less than 72 hours are known as **reversible ischemic neurologic deficits** (RINDs). The term **crescendo TIAs**

Table 39.2–1. Symptoms of cerebrovascular ischemia.

Carotid Territory Symptoms	Vertebrobasilar Symptoms
Ipsilateral monocular blindness (amaurosis fugax)	Drop attacks/syncope
Expressive aphasia (Broca's aphasia)	Slurred speech
Receptive aphasia (Wernicke's aphasia)	Diplopia/vertigo
Contralateral hemiparesis	Ataxia/monoparesis

Table 39.2–2. Manifestations of cerebrovascular disease.

Asymptomatic
Transient ischemic attack (TIA)
Crescendo TIA
Reversible ischemic neurologic deficit (RIND)
Stroke-in-evolution
Stroke

is used to describe symptoms occurring repeatedly and frequently, with complete resolution between attacks. **Stroke-in-evolution** is a variant of crescendo TIAs when neurologic symptoms do not completely resolve and are progressively more severe with each attack. **Stroke** is defined as a neurologic deficit lasting more than 24 hours. Strokes may be mild, with complete recovery, or severe, with permanent neurologic deficit or death. Ischemic or hemorrhagic stroke can be diagnosed accurately by computed tomography (CT) as well as with magnetic resonance imaging (MRI) (Table 39.2–2).

DIAGNOSIS

The diagnosis of carotid atherosclerosis can be made by auscultation of a bruit in the neck. However, only 50% of patients with neck bruits will have a significant internal carotid stenosis. The degree of internal carotid artery stenosis is a critical factor and must be determined using **carotid duplex ultrasonography**. Carotid duplex scanning is accurate in diagnosing occlusive lesions of the carotid artery and in determining their severity. Blood flow velocity increases across a stenosis, and the degree of velocity elevation reliably predicts the degree of stenosis (Figures 39.2–1 and 39.2–2). Lesions of the vertebral artery can be detected at their origin from the subclavian artery, but lesions higher in the vertebral canal are not easily assessed by duplex scanning. Duplex scanning performed by an experienced operator is becoming the standard diagnostic test for evaluating and following patients with carotid artery disease.

Cerebral arteriography has served as the gold standard for diagnosing lesions of the aortic arch, and carotid, vertebral, and intracranial arteries. The degree of lumen stenosis can be clearly and objectively defined, and specific lesions responsible for producing symptoms can be identified (Figure 39.2–3). Arteriography is an important diagnostic test in assessment and preoperative planning of patients with cerebrovascular disease. Cerebral arteriography, however, carries a 1% risk of stroke and exposes the patient to ionizing radiation and iodinated contrast agents.

Magnetic resonance angiography (MRA) is a noninvasive tool that can reliably image the intracranial and extracranial vasculature and also identify intracranial lesions. It can detect stenotic lesions, and used in conjunction with duplex scanning, has been advocated as a cost-

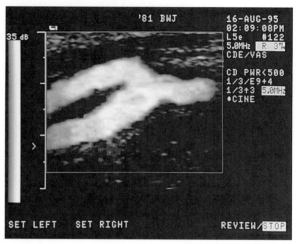

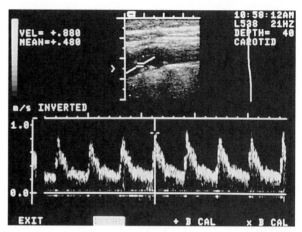

Figure 39.2–1. A: Duplex scan of normal carotid bifurcation; **B:** with normal peak flow velocity. (Reprinted, with permission, from Stanford Vascular Laboratory.)

effective way of obtaining anatomic information without the use of radiation or contrast. Availability of MRA technology and expertise is currently limited to larger medical centers. MRI of the brain can define strokes and is indicated in patients with carotid or vertebrobasilar ischemia to assess presence of infarctions of the cerebral cortex or brain stem.

Transcranial Doppler ultrasonography utilizes natural windows in the cranium to noninvasively study the intracranial circulation. Transcranial Doppler has the potential to evaluate flow in the circle of Willis and assess the integrity of the posterior and anterior communicating arteries. This information is important in surgical management of patients with contralateral carotid stenosis or occlusion.

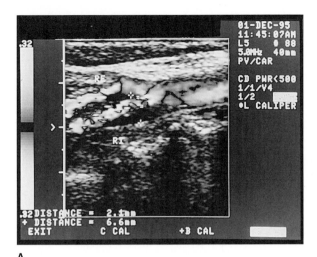

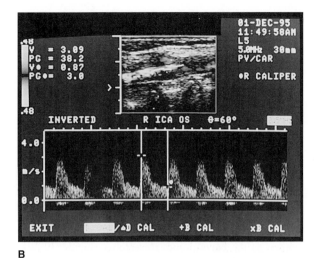

A　　　　　　　　　　　　　　　　　　**B**

Figure 39.2–2. **A:** Duplex scan of carotid bifurcation with high-grade stenosis **B:** elevated peak flow velocity. (Reprinted, with permission, from Stanford Vascular Laboratory.)

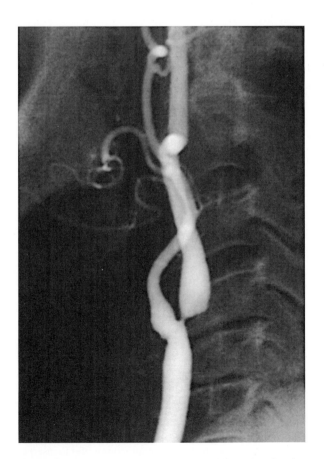

Figure 39.2–3. Arteriogram of the carotid bifurcation showing high-grade stenosis of the origin of internal carotid.

Cerebral CT scanning is useful in evaluating symptomatic patients to determine the presence or absence of acute ischemic or hemorrhagic stroke or space-occupying intracranial lesions. A CT scan is quite accurate in detecting supratentorial infarcts related to carotid circulation. However, the accuracy of CT in detecting infratentorial lesions related to vertebrobasilar ischemia is poor in contrast to MRI.

NATURAL HISTORY

The natural history of patients with carotid atherosclerosis is well defined and is closely related to the degree of stenosis. Patients without significant lumen stenosis of the internal carotid artery (< 50–60%) have a low risk of stroke. The risk increases with increasing stenosis. Patients with severe internal carotid artery stenosis are at significant risk for stroke. Patients with asymptomatic stenosis of greater than or equal to 75% have a risk of stroke of 2–5% per year. Patients with TIA have a risk of stroke of 12% in the first year, with a 5-year risk of stroke of 35%. Patients with a mild stroke and a severe stenosis have a risk of repeat stroke of 25–45% in 5 years. One half of asymptomatic patients who have a stroke have developed a stroke as their first symptom.

The natural history of vertebrobasilar occlusive disease and fibromuscular dysplasia is less defined than that of carotid occlusive disease, and operative procedures are generally performed in symptomatic patients with severe disease.

TREATMENT

CAROTID OCCLUSIVE DISEASE

The treatment strategies are aimed at identifying patients at risk of stroke and reducing the risk. Treatments include both medical and surgical approaches.

Medical treatment consists of antiplatelet therapy, primarily with aspirin, which has been shown to reduce the risk of nonfatal strokes by approximately 2%. Other antiplatelet agents, such as ticlopidine or dipyridamole, have been studied and shown to have little or no added benefit over aspirin therapy.

Surgical treatment involves removal of the atherosclerotic plaque from the carotid bifurcation, a procedure known as the **carotid endarterectomy** (Figure 39.2–4). Several recent prospective, randomized clinical trials involving both symptomatic and asymptomatic patients have clarified the indications for carotid endarterectomy in patients with carotid bifurcation atherosclerosis.

Patient Selection

Carotid endarterectomy is the treatment of choice for several indications. These include patients with: (1) carotid stenosis of greater than or equal to 70% and symptoms of TIA or recent mild stroke in centers where surgical risk of stroke is less than 6% and (2) asymptomatic severe carotid stenosis greater than or equal to 60% in centers where surgical risk of stroke is less than 3% (Table 39.2–3). The effectiveness of carotid endarterectomy in these clinical conditions has been proven to be more effective than medical therapy by prospective, randomized clinical trials. Thus, carotid endarterectomy is generally accepted as the standard of care for these indications.

Carotid endarterectomy is also commonly performed on patients who have had TIAs and have a 50–70% stenosis or on patients with severe carotid ulcerations. These indications have not yet been confirmed with controlled trials; however, clinical results are promising. Currently, trials are underway to determine the efficacy of carotid endarterectomy for patients with lesions of 50–60%. Asymptomatic patients with carotid artery stenosis of less than 50% are not candidates for carotid endarterectomy, as the risk of stroke and complications from the operation surpasses the risk of stroke from a 50% lesion.

Technique of Carotid Endarterectomy

The carotid artery is exposed through an incision anterior to the sternocleidomastoid muscle. Control is obtained of the common, internal, and external carotid arteries, with care being taken to avoid injury to the adjacent cranial nerves. These include the vagus nerve (which contains the recurrent laryngeal nerve), the hypoglossal nerve, the glossopharyngeal nerve, and the marginal mandibular and cervical branches of the facial nerve. Care is taken to avoid

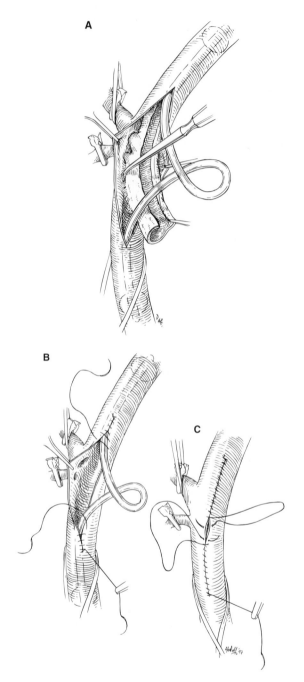

Figure 39.2–4. Carotid endarterectomy: **A:** atherosclerotic plaque is being removed; **B:** plaque removal is completed with shunt in place; **C:** primary arteriotomy closure is in progress.

manipulation of the carotid sinus to avoid dislodging emboli. Intraoperative cerebral function can be monitored directly in awake patients or indirectly with EEG in patients under general anesthesia. Many surgeons prefer to insert an intraluminal shunt to perfuse the distal internal carotid artery during cross-clamping, while others selectively

Table 39.2–3. Proven indications for carotid endarterectomy.

Symptomatic patients with ipsilateral carotid stenosis greater than or equal to 70%
Asymptomatic carotid stenosis of greater than or equal to 60%

shunt based on cerebral function assessment. After cross-clamping the carotid, the carotid artery is opened and the plaque is removed (Figure 39.2–4). The carotid is then either sutured closed primarily or closed with a patch to enlarge the lumen. Meticulous attention to hemostasis and wound closure will help avoid wound complications.

Results

The complications of carotid endarterectomy include cranial nerve injury, myocardial infarction, bradycardia, hypotension, restenosis, wound problems, and stroke. Cranial nerve injury occurs infrequently. Vagus, recurrent laryngeal, hypoglossal, and marginal mandibular branch of the facial are the nerves at risk of being injured. Careful dissection of the carotid sheath and careful placement of retractors may reduce the risk of nerve injury. Postoperative myocardial infarction is correlated with severity of coronary artery disease. Hypertension and bradycardia may occur after carotid endarterectomy but are usually self-limited and treatable.

Early carotid restenosis (< 6 months postoperation) is due to intimal hyperplasia and occurs in 1–2% of patients. Late carotid stenosis is usually due to atherosclerosis. Most early carotid restenoses are mild to moderate (30–70%) and are asymptomatic, thus requiring no further treatment. High-grade or symptomatic restenosis may require repeat operation and patch angioplasty. Wound complications, such as hematoma, occur in 2–5% of patients after carotid endarterectomy.

Stroke within 30 days of carotid endarterectomy occurs in approximately 0.5% of patients. The risk of stroke after carotid endarterectomy is dependent upon the preoperative indication. The risk of stroke during endarterectomy is 1–1.5%. Following successful endarterectomy, the risk of stroke is 1–2% per year for patients with the operative indication of TIAs, and 2–3% for patients with the operative indication of stroke.

VERTEBROBASILAR OCCLUSIVE DISEASE

Symptomatic patients with lesions of the proximal vertebral artery may be treated by reconstruction of the vertebral artery. Three techniques of reconstruction include vertebral to common carotid transposition, subclavian to vertebral bypass using an autogenous interposition graft or vertebral-subclavian endarterectomy. Revascularization of the distal vertebral artery is accomplished by using an interposition graft from the common carotid to the distal vertebral artery. Alternatively, the external carotid artery may be skeletonized and transposed to the distal vertebral artery, or the vertebral artery may be transposed to the distal internal carotid. The success of vertebral revascularization is excellent, with a 5-year patency of up to 85%.

FIBROMUSCULAR DYSPLASIA

Symptomatic patients with fibromuscular disease may be treated with open graduated intraluminal dilatation of the artery. Open balloon angioplasty of the lesions of the carotid artery have been performed with acceptable success. Extensive fibromuscular disease of the proximal internal carotid artery is subject to artery resection and reconstruction with an interposition graft. Percutaneous balloon angioplasty of the fibromuscular disease lesions of the carotid artery has been performed successfully and is a promising therapeutic approach.

SUMMARY

Carotid occlusive disease is the leading cause of stroke. Duplex ultrasonography can reliably determine the presence and severity of carotid occlusive disease. Prospective randomized trials have firmly established carotid endarterectomy as the standard of care for treating significant symptomatic and asymptomatic carotid occlusive disease. Vertebrobasilar revascularization is performed with good clinical success in symptomatic patients. Patients with symptomatic fibromuscular dysplasia may be treated successfully with open dilatation or balloon angioplasty.

SUGGESTED READING

Executive Committee for the Asymptomatic Carotid Atherosclerosis Study: Endarterectomy for asymptomatic carotid artery stenosis. JAMA 1995;273:1421.

Hobson RW et al: Efficacy of carotid endarterectomy for asymptomatic carotid stenosis. N Engl J Med 1993;328:221.

Mayberg MR et al: Carotid endarterectomy and prevention of cerebral ischemia in symptomatic carotid stenosis. JAMA 1991;266:3289.

Moore WS et al: Guidelines for carotid endarterectomy. Stroke 1995;26:188.

North American Symptomatic Carotid Endarterectomy Trial Collaborators: Beneficial effect of carotid endarterectomy in symptomatic patients with high-grade carotid stenosis. N Engl J Med 1991;325:445.

Zarins CK: Carotid endarterectomy: The gold standard. J Endovasc Surg 1996;3:10.

Zarins CK et al: Carotid bifurcation atherosclerosis: Quantitative correlation of plaque localization with flow velocity profiles and wall shear stress. Circ Res 1983;53:502.

39.3 Peripheral Vascular Occlusive Disease

Ramin E. Beygui, MD, & Ronald L. Dalman, MD

▶ Key Facts

- ▶ Arterial diseases affecting the upper extremity include thoracic outlet syndrome, hypothenar hammer syndrome, fibromuscular dysplasia, hypercoagulable states, radiation arteritis, and calcific sclerosis.

- ▶ Connective tissue disorders associated with arterial abnormalities in the upper extremity include systemic lupus erythematosus, progressive systemic sclerosis, and rheumatoid arthritis.

- ▶ Atherosclerosis is an uncommon cause of upper extremity arterial ischemia, but it is the most common cause of ischemia in the lower extremity.

- ▶ Arteriopathies associated with vasculitis that may result in stenosis, thrombosis, aneurysm formation, and distal embolization in the upper

extremity include thromboangiitis obliterans, Takayasu's disease, giant cell arteritis, and polyarteritis nodosa.

- ▶ Claudication is the single most common symptom of mild-to-moderate lower extremity vascular occlusive disease and is defined as reproducible calf pain upon ambulation and cessation of pain at rest.

- ▶ Diagnostic arteriography is essential in the preoperative evaluation of patients who are candidates for revascularization.

- ▶ Treatment of arterial stenosis in the lower extremity includes antiplatelet agents, endovascular procedures, sympathectomy, endarterectomy, bypass operations, and amputations.

UPPER EXTREMITY ARTERIAL DISEASE

PATHOGENESIS & CLINICAL FINDINGS

The pathogenesis of upper extremity ischemia is usually nonatherosclerotic. In general, upper extremity ischemia occurs in younger patients with much more variable etiology, compared to lower extremity ischemia.

Patients with acute upper extremity ischemia may present with pallor, pulselessness, paresthesias, poikilothermia, and pain. Subclavian or brachiocephalic artery aneurysms and ulcerated plaques may cause distal digital embolization, which may progress to digital gangrene. Cold-induced vasospasm (Raynaud's syndrome) may be the early clinical symptoms of connective tissue disorders. Chronic stenosis or occlusion of subclavian or brachiocephalic arteries may be asymptomatic and manifest only as pressure discrepancies, or they may cause forearm fatigue with exercise.

TREATMENT

Selection of treatment for patients suffering from upper extremity ischemia is dependent upon the severity of the symptoms and etiology of the disease. Thrombectomy and thrombolysis (with intra-arterial urokinase or streptokinase) may be the appropriate treatment for arterial thrombosis secondary to hypercoagulable states. Preoperative or intraoperative thrombolysis may also serve as an adjunct to vascular bypass if extensive distal thrombosis is present. For upper extremity bypass procedures, inflow and outflow sites should be selected to minimize the length of conduit while optimizing the quality of inflow and outflow. Reversed autogenous saphenous vein (or nonreversed vein with lysed valves) is the conduit of choice for upper extremity bypass. In the absence of a suitable length of good quality saphenous vein, arm veins or prosthetic grafts may be used. Sympathectomy alone or in conjunction with revascularization may alleviate vasospasm and neuropathic pain associated with upper extremity ischemia. Long-term anticoagulation with warfarin is required in cases of hypercoagulable states or thromboembolic disease. The warfarin dose should be adjusted to achieve a prothrombin time of 2–3 times INR (international normalized ratio).

THORACIC OUTLET SYNDROME

Thoracic outlet syndrome is seen in young athletic adults. The compression of subclavian artery by anatomic structures, such as scalenus anterior muscle, cervical rib subclavius muscle, costoclavicular ligament, pectoralis minor tendon, or the humeral head may cause injury to the artery. This injury may manifest itself as ulceration, aneurysm formation, or occlusion. Distal embolization secondary to aneurysm may occur. causing digital ischemia.

Treatment usually involves repair of the diseased artery and a decompressive procedure at the thoracic outlet. Decompression is accomplished by resection of the first rib alone or in combination with division of the scalenus anterior and resection of the medial head of the clavicle. In case of aneurysm of subclavian artery, exclusion and bypass of the diseased artery should be performed.

HYPOTHENAR HAMMER SYNDROME

Hypothenar hammer syndrome is seen in people, such as mechanics and carpenters, who use their hand forcefully and repeatedly as a hammer. The ulnar artery crossing the wrist passes lateral to the pisiform and hook of the hamate bones and lies close to the skin. Trauma to the ulnar artery causes spasm, aneurysmal degeneration, distal digital embolization, and occlusion. Treatment of a patent aneurysmal ulnar artery is resection and reconstruction, with interposition of an autogenous vein graft. After diagnosis and operation, the patient should be counseled to avoid hand trauma.

CONNECTIVE TISSUE DISORDERS

Systemic lupus erythematosus (SLE) is an autoimmune connective tissue disease with antibodies against double-stranded DNA and Smith antigens. Clinical manifestations are diverse, including malar rash, alopecia, oral ulcers, serositis, and renal failure. Arterial disease may be mediated by immunocomplements. The most common early arterial symptom is cold-induced vasospasm known as **Raynaud's syndrome**. Approximately one third of patients with SLE have antiphospholipid antibodies. Lupus anticoagulant causes prolongation of activated partial thromboplastin time (aPTT). Paradoxically, patients with lupus anticoagulant have thromboembolic disease, as opposed to a hemorrhagic diathesis. Lupus anticoagulant was initially identified in patients with diagnosis of SLE but it is more commonly found in patient without lupus. Anticardiolipin antibody is a related but distinct antibody causing thromboembolic disease with or without association to SLE.

Progressive systemic sclerosis (PSS, scleroderma) is a chronic disorder of fibrosis of the skin and internal organs. A subtype of PSS is characterized by calcinosis cutis, Raynaud's phenomenon, esophageal dismotility, sclerodactyly, and telangiectasia (**CREST syndrome**). Raynaud's phenomenon is seen in 90% of patients with PSS and may represent early symptoms of the disease.

Rheumatoid arthritis (RA) is the most common connective tissue disorder, but it infrequently affects arteries. Arterial abnormalities associated with RA include occlusive disease or hyperemia (hypervascularity). Tapering of subclavian or axillary arteries may be encountered in patients with RA. Arterial occlusions frequently manifest as forearm fatigue.

ATHEROSCLEROSIS

Atherosclerosis is an uncommon cause of upper extremity arterial disease. When atherosclerosis does involve the upper extremity, the subclavian artery is most commonly affected. **Subclavian steal syndrome** occurs with stenosis or occlusion of the subclavian artery proximal to the take off of the vertebral artery. Upper extremity exercise causes retrograde flow in the vertebral artery as the occluded or stenotic proximal subclavian artery cannot accommodate the increased flow. This retrograde flow causes vertebrobasilar ischemia. Ulceration of atherosclerotic plaque may lead to digital embolization. Atherosclerotic aneurysms of the brachiocephalic or subclavian arteries could also present as distal digital embolization.

Stenosis or occlusion of the subclavian artery is a common cause of brachial blood pressure difference in older patients. Asymptomatic patients, in general, do not need treatment. Symptomatic patients may be treated by performing a carotid-subclavian bypass or transposition. Subclavian endarterectomy is less frequently performed. Aneurysms of the subclavian artery causing digital embolization may be ligated and bypassed or resected and reconstructed using prosthetic or autogenous grafts.

FIBROMUSCULAR DYSPLASIA

Fibromuscular dysplasia (FMD) (Figure 39.3–1) is a disease typically seen in young and middle-aged Caucasian women. Various subtypes of this disorder are recognized. The most common subtype is medial fibroplasia, with the arteriographic finding of "string of beads." Carotid and renal arteries are most commonly affected, followed by vertebral, subclavian, axillary, external iliac, and visceral vessels. Symptomatic patients may successfully be treated with balloon angioplasty or surgical bypass and reconstruction of the affected vessel.

VASCULITIDES

This group of diseases is associated with vasculitis that may result in stenosis, thrombosis, aneurysm formation, and distal embolization. Histologic studies of giant cell arteritis, Takayasu's disease, and polyarteritis nodosa demonstrate necrotizing arteritis, whereas thromboangiitis obliterans is characterized by non-necrotizing arteritis.

Thromboangiitis obliterans (Buerger's disease) is an intermittent and segmental disease of the arteries and veins. Arterial thrombosis and migratory thrombophlebitis are characteristics of this disease. Buerger's disease is almost exclusively seen in younger men who use tobacco products. Pathologic findings are thrombus-filled vessels with multinucleated giant cells microabscesses and non-necrotizing arteritis. The vessel wall shows preservation

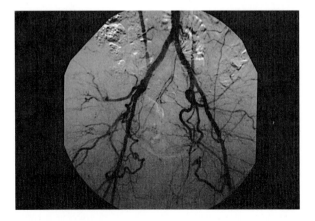

Figure 39.3–1. Bilateral external iliac artery fibromuscular dysplasia.

of internal elastic lamina without necrosis. Arteries of the lower extremity are affected more often than those of the upper extremity.

Cessation of smoking is the most essential aspect of treatment. Sympathectomy for treatment of arterial spasm and rest pain is controversial. Arterial reconstruction may be performed for treatment of gangrene or ischemic rest pain. The results of arterial reconstructions are usually poor and ultimately futile if the patient continues to smoke. Progression of the disease may require amputation. Other treatments, such as aspirin, warfarin, steroids, pentoxifylline, intra-arterial streptokinase, prostaglandin E (PGE), iloprost (PGI_2 analog), and vasodilators have been used with little or no success. Despite extensive limb involvement, the life expectancy of patients with Buerger's disease is the same as for sex- and age-matched controls.

Takayasu's disease is clinically manifested by fever, weight loss, and fatigue. Stenosis and inflammation of the aorta and its major branches may cause arm fatigue, claudication, pulse discrepancies, digital ischemia, congestive heart failure, and impotence. The histology of Takayasu's disease and giant cell arteritis are identical in their acute phase. Takayasu's arteritis predominantly occurs in women under 50 years of age, whereas giant cell arteritis occurs in older patients, with lower female predominance.

Characteristic histologic findings are necrotizing granulomas of the media and adventitia. Segmental narrowing of the major branches of the aorta may present as "pulseless disease." Pharmacologic treatment using nonsteroidal anti-inflammatory drugs (NSAIDs), corticosteroids, and cyclophosphamide are directed at controlling the inflammation. Arterial revascularization may be undertaken when critical end-organ ischemia occurs. Arterial bypass procedures are preferred to balloon angioplasty in the treatment of critical limb ischemia. Noninflamed arterial segments should be selected as inflow and outflow of the bypass graft.

Giant cell arteritis (temporal arteritis) may present as headaches, jaw fatigue, and blindness. This disease is associated with polymyalgia rheumatica in 50% of patients. Ophthalmic arteritis and central retinal artery occlusion may occur, causing blindness. Women are two to four times more commonly affected than men. Involvement of subclavian and axillary arteries may progress to occlusion or rupture and hemorrhage. Erythrocyte sedimentation rate (ESR) is typically elevated. Biopsy of temporal arteries demonstrates necrotizing arteritis, mononuclear infiltrates, and multinucleated giant cells (indistinguishable from Takayasu's disease). The role of surgery is usually limited to bilateral temporal artery biopsy for diagnosis and, rarely, treatment of acute hemorrhage. Corticosteroid administration is the primary mode of treatment.

Polyarteritis nodosa (PAN) is clinically manifested by weight loss, fever, and fatigue. Visceral involvement can cause cholecystitis, arterial hemorrhage, and intestinal infarction and perforation. Renal involvement may be presented as glomerulonephritis and hypertension. Visceral and digital arteries may be affected with aneurysms, fibrosis, hemorrhage, or thrombosis. Occlusion of digital arteries may manifest itself as digital ischemia and gangrene. PAN is associated with seropositivity for hepatitis B or hepatitis C in 30–50% patients. Acute necrotizing inflammation of arterial media with fibrinoid necrosis and inflammation are hallmarks of polyarteritis nodosa. Treatment is immunosuppression for control of inflammation, using corticosteroids, cyclophosphamide, and azathioprine. Only complications of PAN, such as hemorrhage from ruptured visceral aneurysms and intestinal infarction, are treated surgically.

HYPERCOAGULABLE STATES

Hypercoagulable states, acquired or congenital, may cause venous or arterial thromboses. Congenital disorders include antithrombin III and protein C and protein S deficiencies. Homocystinuria (cystathionine synthase deficiency) causes premature atherosclerosis and arterial and venous thromboembolism. Acquired conditions include heparin-induced thrombocytopenia and thrombosis, lupus anticoagulant and anticardiolipin antibodies, oral contraceptive use, malignancy, pregnancy, polycythemia vera, and postoperative states. Most complications of hypercoagulable states are related to venous thrombosis and pulmonary embolism, although arterial occlusion and ischemia may also occur. A single base mutation resulting in substitution of Arg506 with Gln is known as factor V Leiden. This mutation causes activated protein C resistance (APCR). APCR is the most common hypercoagulable state in patients with a diagnosis of deep venous thrombosis.

RADIATION ARTERITIS

Radiation arterial injury usually occurs with doses in excess of 5000 cGy. Acutely, radiation arteritis may cause arterial thrombosis or hemorrhage. Long-term complications are fibrosis, stenosis, and rapidly progressive atherosclerosis. Prompt treatment of exsanguinating hemorrhage or bypass procedures for severe ischemia may be required. Avoidance of the irradiated field and use of autogenous grafts and frequent graft surveillance with duplex ultrasonography decreases the incidence of complications.

CALCIFIC SCLEROSIS

Calcific sclerosis is seen in diabetic patients with renal failure. Rapid calcification is considered to be due to secondary hyperparathyroidism (calciphylaxis). Calcific medial sclerosis (Mönckeberg's) may progress to artery lumen stenosis, arterial obliteration, and digital gangrene.

LOWER EXTREMITY ARTERIAL DISEASE

Acute lower extremity ischemia may be due to embolization from a proximal source or thrombosis of an artery or graft. Unlike upper extremity ischemia, the great majority of cases of chronic lower extremity ischemia are due to atherosclerotic arterial disease. Other uncommon causes of lower extremity ischemia include popliteal artery entrapment syndrome and adventitial cyst.

Classic symptoms of acute lower extremity ischemia are pain, pallor, pulselessness, poikilothermia, and paresthesias. Diseases such as connective tissue disorders, vasculitides, and fibromuscular dysplasia, discussed in conjunction with upper extremity arterial disease, may also involve the arteries of the lower extremities, with similar symptoms (ie, Raynaud's syndrome, claudication, and digital embolization and gangrene).

ACUTE LOWER EXTREMITY ISCHEMIA

Pathogenesis

Acute lower extremity ischemia may occur from thrombosis or embolization to the lower extremity arteries. Arrhythmias, left ventricular aneurysms, cardiovascular instrumentation, proximal ulcerated plaques, and aneurysms predispose to atheroembolism and embolization to lower extremity vessels. Venous thrombosis may cause paradoxical arterial embolization to arteriovenous channels, such as atrial septal defects, patent foramen ovale, or arteriovenous malformations and fistulae. Acute arterial thrombosis may superimpose on a previously present nonocclusive atherosclerotic plaque. Acute bypass graft thrombosis frequently presents as critical lower extremity ischemia.

Clinical Findings

The time between onset of ischemia and treatment is important in determining the etiology and the appropriate treatment. History of claudication or rest pain would be indicative of thrombosis, whereas atrial fibrillation or cardiovascular instrumentation would be more likely to cause embolism. Careful physical examination with attention to level of palpable pulses, pallor, coolness, and neurologic deficit assist in determining the anatomic site of arterial occlusion. Prolonged acute ischemia, in excess of 6–8 hours, may produce acidosis, hyperkalemia, rhabdomyolysis, compartment syndrome, and permanent neuropathy. Myoglobulinuria may cause acute tubular necrosis and renal failure.

Diagnosis

Diagnosis is primarily dependent on physical examination and bedside assessment using a hand-held continuous wave Doppler and determination of the ankle-brachial index (ABI). If necessary, duplex ultrasonography can document presence of arterial embolus or thrombus. It may also identify aneurysms of the aorta, and femoral and popliteal arteries. Arteriography can help to determine the underlying lesion and inflow and outflow targets for the bypass procedure. Arteriography is more important in the diagnosis of acute thrombotic than acute embolic disease. Echocardiography would detect presence of ventricular aneurysm, septal defects, or aortic dissection. Transesophageal echocardiography may be performed in the operating room as a diagnostic adjunct. Magnetic resonance angiography could delineate vascular anatomy and detect presence of thrombus and embolus noninvasively, with versatility in image reconstruction.

Treatment

Embolic Disease. The patient with minimal ischemia may be treated with systemic heparin at a dose of 50–150 units/kg intravenous bolus, followed by 7–17 units/kg/h, maintaining a partial thromboplastin time (PTT) of two-and-a-half to three times normal. Patient with moderate ischemia and viable muscles are candidates for prompt surgical exploration and catheter-based embolectomy. Direct intra-arterial injection of urokinase preoperatively or intraoperatively may accomplish thrombolysis in distal vessels (tibial, peroneal, or pedal arteries) and improve outflow if catheter-based embolectomy is incomplete. Four-compartment fasciotomy (anterior, lateral, deep, and superficial posterior compartments) may be indicated following revascularization of the ischemic limb in order to avoid compartment syndrome.

Compartment syndrome occurs when swelling and muscular edema after reperfusion cause compression of neurovascular bundles, exacerbating ischemia and neuropathy. Severe prolonged limb ischemia should be treated with limb amputation, since if the limb is nonviable, revascularization is futile and delay may cause severe hyperkalemia, acidosis, arrhythmias, myoglobulinuria, renal failure, and death.

Thrombotic Disease. Diagnostic arteriography is essential for recognizing underlying lesions that may have progressed to occlusion, as well as inflow and outflow targets for potential bypass operations. Concurrent thrombolysis with urokinase may improve outflow, providing a target for bypass procedures and improving patency of bypass grafts. This may be particularly helpful in acute thrombosis of popliteal artery aneurysm. Most patients with acute thrombosis of a bypass graft presenting with critical ischemia will require revascularization with a new conduit, as thrombectomy or thrombolysis of a preexisting graft will result in early graft occlusion. Acute thrombosis in the setting of hypercoagulable states should be treated with long-term warfarin therapy after thrombectomy or thrombolysis. A typical dose of intra-arterial urokinase for treatment of acute thrombosis is 2000–5000 units/kg/h for 1–2 hours, followed by a continuous infusion at 1000–2000 units/kg/h. Patients should be observed closely for any evidence of hemorrhage. Serum fibrinogen level, platelet count, and hemoglobin (hematocrit) should be checked prior to initiation of therapy. While the patient is receiving urokinase therapy, venipuncture to obtain blood samples should be severely restricted to avoid hemorrhagic complications. Heparin is frequently infused concurrently with urokinase. Alternatively, recombinant tissue plasminogen activator (rt-PA) or streptokinase may be used as thrombolytic agents instead of urokinase.

CHRONIC LOWER EXTREMITY ISCHEMIA

Pathogenesis & Clinical Findings

Atherosclerosis is the most common cause of symptomatic lower extremity ischemia. Fatty streaking, which represents accumulation of lipid-laden macrophages (foam cells), is seen in children as young as 3 years old. Whether the fatty streak lesion represents early atherosclerosis is controversial. The risk factors for atherosclerosis include smoking, hyperlipidemia, hypertension, obesity, male sex, old age, diabetes, and genetic predisposition. Smoking is the most important controllable risk factor. Certain segments of the arterial system, such as carotid bifurcation, aortic bifurcation, and superficial femoral artery, are prone to deposition of atherosclerotic plaque. Hemodynamic factors, such as low arterial wall shear stress and high tensile stress, may contribute to atherosclerosis.

Progression of atherosclerosis does not necessarily result in arterial stenosis, as compensatory arterial enlargement of up to 140% of the original arterial diameter may occur. Significant pressure gradient and flow reduction occur when arterial diameter reductions of 55% (cross-sectional area reduction of 80%) are reached. This "critical stenosis" is dependent upon flow and varies at different levels of muscle activity. Recently, vascular remodeling in the setting of chronic arterial stenosis has been attributed to matrix metalloproteinases (MMP) released by mononuclear inflammatory cells.

In Latin, the term "claud" means "to limp." **Claudication** is defined as reproducible calf pain upon ambulation and cessation of pain at rest. Claudication is the single most common symptom of mild to moderate lower extremity vascular occlusive disease. Claudication is classified as functional ischemia where blood supply to calf muscles is adequate at rest and inadequate with exercise. The term "rest pain" refers to critical limb ischemia experienced in the distal part of the foot. Typically, patients with ischemic rest pain experience pain at night while recumbent and receive relief and diminution of pain by placing the foot in a dependent position. Physical examination may reveal extremity pallor on elevation and dependent rubor. Patients have thin shiny skin, loss of hair, and hypertrophic nails. Nonhealing ulcers and gangrene represent more advanced ischemia (Figure 39.3–2). Pedal pulses are absent or diminished. Ankle-brachial index (ABI), defined as the ratio of ankle systolic pressure to brachial systolic pressure, is normally greater than one. ABI of 0.5–0.9 is seen in claudicators; below 0.5 is seen in patients with critical ischemia.

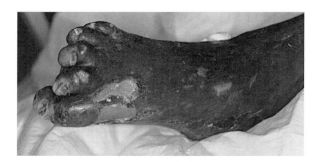

Figure 39.3–2. Advanced chronic lower extremity ischemia with nonhealing ulcerations.

Diagnosis

Diagnostic arteriography is essential in the preoperative evaluation of patients who are candidates for revascularization. Suitable inflow and outflow targets for bypass can be identified by angiography. Short-segment (< 3 cm) stenosis of iliac arteries may be amenable to percutaneous balloon angioplasty, with or without stenting, and could be treated concurrently. Diagnostic arteriography can be performed via percutaneous puncture of femoral or brachial arteries. Digital subtraction angiography can improve the quality of imaging and reduce the amount of contrast used.

Carbon dioxide can be used as contrast medium in patients with renal insufficiency, thus reducing the risk of renal failure due to iodinated contrast. Other complications of angiography include allergic reactions and anaphylaxis, nausea and vomiting, bronchospasm, hypotension, arrhythmias, seizures, and distal atheroembolization. Acute adverse reactions occur in 5–8% of patients, with the majority of complications self-limited and responding well to treatment.

Treatment

Medical Treatment. For patients with functional ischemia (ie, claudication), recommended treatment is cessation of smoking and a regular exercise regimen. Regular exercise appears to improve the efficiency of muscles in extracting oxygen, thus increasing walking distance and reducing calf pain. **Pentoxifylline** is a hemorheologic agent that increases red cell deformity and reduces platelet aggregation. In some studies, 30–40% of claudicators have improved their walking distance while taking pentoxifylline at 400 mg three times a day. Pentoxifylline, however, has not been found to be effective in the treatment of critical ischemia, and its use is limited to treatment of claudication. Aspirin and ticlopidine are antiplatelet agents that have been investigated in prevention of cardiovascular death, but their role in treatment of peripheral vascular disease is, at this point, unclear. Prostaglandin E_1 and iloprost (prostaglandin I_2 analog) have been used to treat ischemic rest pain in some small studies, but their efficacy remains unclear. Newer drugs currently under clinical investigation include Cilastacol (antiplatelet agent) and L-propionyl carnitine (ATP-increasing substance).

Endovascular Procedures. Percutaneous transluminal angioplasty (PTA) with or without stenting is effective in the treatment of focal arterial stenosis. The results are better in shorter stenotic segments (< 3 cm), larger arteries (ie, iliac artery), and in arteries with good runoff. For treatment of more extensive disease and threatened leg, however, bypass operations are superior to PTA (with or without stenting). Endovascular procedures may be appropriate for patients with prohibitive risk for general anesthesia in whom long-term patency may not be critical.

Sympathectomy. Lumbar sympathectomy alone is rarely performed to treat lower extremity ischemia. Sympathectomy may be useful in treatment of vasospastic disorders, digital atheroembolization, Buerger's disease, reflex sympathetic dystrophy (causalgia, post-traumatic sympathetically mediated pain syndrome), and hyperhidrosis.

Endarterectomy. Endarterectomy is currently used infrequently as the treatment of focal aortoiliac occlusive disease in younger patients (< 50 years old). Endarterectomy of profunda femoris artery is performed alone or in combination with patch angioplasty (profundoplasty) as an adjunct to aortobifemoral bypass when the superficial femoral artery is occluded.

Bypass Operations. The treatment of choice for aortoiliac occlusive disease is aortobifemoral bypass. The indication for operation is critical ischemia. A bifurcated prosthetic graft is used to bypass the diseased segment of the aorta or iliac arteries. If preservation of antegrade distal aortic flow is necessary, proximal anastomosis is made in an end-to-side fashion so that the internal iliac arteries remain in continuity with the aorta. Femoropopliteal bypass is used to treat critical lower extremity ischemia with occluded superficial femoral artery and patent popliteal artery. In case tibial and peroneal vessels are stenotic or occluded, the bypass procedure should extend to distal tibial, peroneal, or pedal arteries.

Autogenous saphenous vein is the conduit of choice for femoropopliteal and tibioperoneal occlusive disease. Reversed saphenous vein, harvested nonreversed saphenous vein, or in situ (nonreversed) saphenous vein may be used as conduit. Nonreversed veins may be suitable following valve lysis. Valve lysis may be performed under direct vision in conjunction with angioscopy. Long-term graft patency of bypass procedures using reversed or nonreversed saphenous veins are equivalent. In case no suitable autogenous saphenous vein is available, arm veins may be used as conduits for bypass procedures. Nonautogenous conduits such as expanded polytetrafluoroethylene (ePTFE) or glutaraldehyde-stabilized human umbilical vein may be used if no autogenous conduit is available. In general, prosthetic grafts have unacceptable patency rates if bypass to an infrageniculate artery is necessary.

Extra-anatomic bypass (axillobifemoral, femorofemoral) was initially designed to avoid infected fields (eg, infected vascular grafts, aortoenteric fistulae) or hostile abdomen (eg, multiple previous operations, irradiation). These operations can be performed under local anesthesia and may be the treatment of choice in patients who have severe cardiopulmonary disease and are at prohibitive risk of general anesthesia. The 5-year patency of axillobifemoral bypass is as high as 78%, compared to 85–90% for aortobifemoral bypass. Femorofemoral bypass has a variable reported patency, ranging up to 87% at 5 years.

Amputations. In patients with prolonged extensive acute ischemia or chronic critical ischemia where revascularization is not possible, amputation is indicated. The level of amputation is determined in order to remove all nonviable infected tissue, ensure adequacy of blood supply for healing, and provide appropriate accommodation for a prosthetic limb. Patients with distal digital gangrene may undergo **digital amputation**. If gangrene is extended to the proximal phalanx, the corresponding metatarsal head should also be removed (**ray amputation**). More extensive gangrene may require fore foot amputation (**transmetatarsal amputation**). A **Syme's amputation** involves ankle disarticulation and preservation of distal tibia and fibula. A well-healed Syme's amputation may be less disabling than a **below-knee amputation**. In practice, however, if a transmetatarsal amputation does not provide

adequate healing, it is unlikely that a Syme's amputation will perform substantially better. In these circumstances a below-knee amputation is indicated. Digital, ray, or transmetatarsal amputations may allow the patient to undergo rehabilitation to ambulate without the aid of a prosthesis.

An above-knee amputation is necessary if calf muscles do not provide adequate healing and when knee contractures develop. Preservation of the knee joint is, in general, desirable, as it accommodates a prosthesis well and assists in patient balance and transfer, requiring less energy expenditure. A debilitated, nonambulatory patient with lower extremity gangrene, however, should be considered for above-knee amputation.

AORTOILIAC OCCLUSIVE DISEASE

The triad of gluteal claudication, absent femoral pulses, and impotence (in males) is classically related to aortic occlusion (Leriche's syndrome) and is the hallmark of aortoiliac occlusive disease. Indications for invasive intervention include disabling short-distance claudication and critical ischemia (ischemic rest pain, nonhealing ulceration, and gangrene) (Figure 39.3–3).

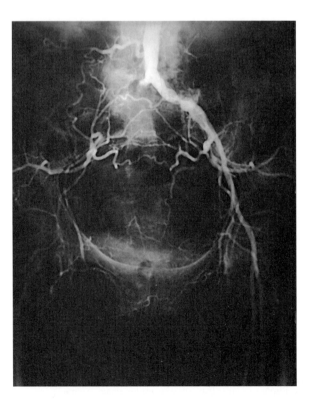

Figure 39.3–3. Aortoiliac occlusive disease. Right common iliac artery occlusion and left common iliac artery stenosis.

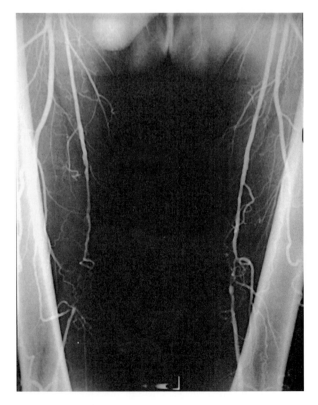

Figure 39.3–4. Femoropopliteal occlusive disease. Right superficial femoral artery (SFA) occlusion and left SFA stenosis at the adductor hiatus.

FEMOROPOPLITEAL OCCLUSIVE DISEASE

Stenosis of the superficial femoral artery is usually at the adductor hiatus (Hunter's canal). Superficial femoral artery stenosis or occlusion usually results in claudication, as the profunda femoris artery (PFA) is an important collateral blood supply to the foot (Figure 39.3–4). Progression of the disease to stenosis and occlusion of PFA or trifurcation of the popliteal artery causes critical ischemia, requiring bypass procedures for limb salvage.

TIBIOPERONEAL OCCLUSIVE DISEASE

This pattern of small artery disease is seen more commonly in diabetic patients. Stenosis or occlusion of tibial or peroneal arteries with critical ischemia generally requires a bypass procedure to the distal tibial, peroneal, or pedal arteries to prevent limb loss.

POPLITEAL ARTERY ENTRAPMENT SYNDROME

Popliteal artery entrapment syndrome is an uncommon cause of lower extremity ischemia and claudication. Anatomic aberrations related to the medial head of the gastrocnemius and course of the popliteal artery cause compression of the artery. Magnetic resonance imaging (MRI) is the diagnostic test of choice, as it provides information about the dynamic anatomic relation between the popliteal artery and muscles and tendons.

The treatment involves division of the medial head of the gastrocnemius and return of the popliteal artery to a normal anatomic position. A damaged artery should be resected or ligated and excluded. Autogenous saphenous vein can be used for popliteal artery reconstruction.

POPLITEAL ARTERY ADVENTITIAL CYST

Popliteal artery adventitial cyst is a rare disorder causing lower extremity ischemia. Gelatinous secretions of the popliteal artery adventitia accumulate, causing popliteal artery compression. Patients are typically young, nonsmoking men. Duplex ultrasonography or conventional arteriography may confirm the diagnosis. CT or MRI may be particularly helpful if duplex scan is equivocal.

Cyst incision, evacuation of gelatinous content, and cyst wall excision is usually an adequate treatment if the popliteal artery is patent. If the popliteal artery is occluded, a simple thrombectomy is not usually adequate. In that case, the artery should be resected and reconstructed with autogenous saphenous vein.

SUGGESTED READING

Brewster DC, Darling RC: Optimal methods of aortoiliac reconstruction. Surgery 1978;84:739.

Dalman RD, Taylor LM Jr.: Basic data related to infrainguinal revascularization procedures. Ann Vasc Surg 1990;4:309.

Dean RH, Yao JST, Brewster DC: *Current Diagnosis & Treatment in Vascular Surgery.* Appleton & Lange, 1995.

Haimovici H: Pattern of arteriosclerotic lesions of the lower extremity. Arch Surg 1967;95:918.

Kempczinski RF: Management of chronic ischemia of the lower extremity. In: Rutherford RB (editor): *Vascular Surgery,* 4th ed. WB Saunders, 1995.

Porter JP et al: Extra-anatomic bypass: A new look (supporting view). Adv Surg 1993;26:133.

Szilagyi DE et al: A thirty-year survey of the reconstructive surgical treatment of aortoiliac occlusive disease. J Vasc Surg 1986;3:421.

Taylor LM, Edwards JM, Porter JM: Present status of reversed vein bypass grafting: Five-year results of a modern series. J Vasc Surg 1990;11:193.

Yao JST: Pathology of upper extremity arterial disease. In: Ernst CB, Stanley JC (editors): *Current Therapy in Vascular Surgery.* Mosby, 1995.

39.4 Aneurysms

Christopher K. Zarins, MD, & Dainis K. Krievins, MD

▶ Key Facts

- ▶ Arterial aneurysms are defined as focal enlargements of arterial diameter 50% greater than normal.

- ▶ A true aneurysm is defined as an enlargement involving all three layers of the aortic wall, whereas a false aneurysm (pseudoaneurysm) is defined as a defect of the aortic wall with absence of the internal elastic lamina, media, and adventitia.

- ▶ Approximately 90% of aneurysms are localized to the infrarenal abdominal aorta.

- ▶ Most patients with abdominal aortic aneurysms (AAA) have evidence of atherosclerosis in the coronary, carotid, and/or peripheral arteries.

- ▶ Patients at the highest risk for developing AAA are those with a family history of aneurysm, cig-

arette smoking, hypertension, chronic obstructive pulmonary disease, and evidence of systemic atherosclerosis.

- ▶ The most precise method of assessing AAA is computed tomography.

- ▶ The principle of operative repair of AAA is exclusion of the aneurysm from the circulation and replacement of the diseased aortic segment with a prosthetic aortic graft.

- ▶ Thoracic aortic aneurysms are less common than AAA and may involve the aortic arch, descending thoracic aorta, and suprarenal aorta.

- ▶ Aneurysms may develop in peripheral areas, such as the femoral, popliteal, carotid, subclavian, renal, celiac, superior, mesenteric, and splenic arteries.

GENERAL CONSIDERATIONS

Arterial aneurysms are defined as focal enlargements of arterial diameter 50% greater than normal. A true aneurysm is defined as an enlargement involving all three layers of the aortic wall. A false aneurysm (pseudoaneurysm) is defined as a defect of the aortic wall with absence of the internal elastic lamina, media, and adventitia. The lumen is contained by external structures or fibrous tissue. Pseudoaneurysms usually are caused by penetrating trauma, such as gunshot or stab wounds, and may develop following arterial catheter insertions or at vascular anastomoses. **Mycotic** or infected aneurysms are pseudoaneurysms that form as a result of aortic wall destruction by an infectious process.

Aneurysms tend to enlarge and are considered clinically significant when they exceed twice the expected normal arterial diameter. Generalized diffuse arterial enlargement is defined as **arterial ectasia** and is not considered an aneurysm with its associated risk for rupture because the enlargement is not focal. Aneurysms may leak and tamponade, allowing time for diagnosis and surgical repair. Aneurysm rupture may result in uncontrolled hemorrhage and death. Death from ruptured abdominal aortic aneurysm is the 13th leading cause of death in the United States. Elective repair of aortic aneurysms eliminates the risk of death from rupture. Therefore, the treatment strategy of arterial aneurysms is to diagnose them when they are asymptomatic, identify those that have a significant risk of rupture, and perform elective aneurysm repair in order to eliminate the risk of rupture. Approximately 90% of aneurysms are localized to the infrarenal abdominal aorta, therefore, the first section of this chapter will focus predominately on the abdominal aortic aneurysm.

ABDOMINAL AORTIC ANEURYSMS

ANATOMY

Abdominal aortic aneurysms are usually localized to the infrarenal aorta and commonly extend to involve the common iliac arteries (Figure 39.4–1). A 1- to 2-cm segment of aorta immediately below the renal arteries is usually spared and is known as the **neck** of the aneurysm. The aortic wall in aneurysms is thin and attenuated, with dis-

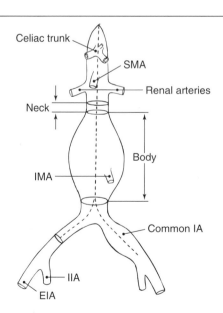

Figure 39.4–1. Schematic anatomy of an infrarenal abdominal aortic aneurysm. The aneurysm usually begins 1–2 cm below the renal arteries and may extend to involve the iliac arteries. The inferior mesenteric artery (IMA) exits from the anterior wall of the aneurysm. SMA, superior mesenteric artery; CIA, common iliac artery; EIA, external iliac artery; IIA, internal iliac artery.

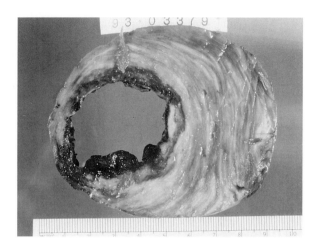

Figure 39.4–2. Laminated mural thrombus removed from abdominal aortic aneurysm.

appearance of elastin from the media and loss of the lamellar architecture of the aorta. The aortic aneurysm sac is usually filled with laminated mural thrombus (Figure 39.4–2), thus making the lumen size smaller than the true size of the aneurysm. The mural thrombus, which may be quite thick, provides no structural support and does not eliminate the risk of rupture.

PATHOGENESIS

A number of factors are thought to be involved in the pathogenesis of abdominal aortic aneurysms, including atherosclerotic aortic wall degeneration, inflammation, proteolytic enzyme activity, and predisposing genetic factors. Most patients with aortic aneurysms have evidence of atherosclerosis in the coronary, carotid, and peripheral arteries, and, thus, abdominal aortic aneurysms (AAA) are commonly called "atherosclerotic aortic aneurysms." Histologic examination of aortic aneurysms demonstrates evidence of atherosclerosis along with disappearance of elastin from the aortic media. Increased matrix metalloproteinases (MMP) and increased mononuclear inflammatory cells have also been demonstrated in aortic aneurysms. Although there is a clear association between the atherosclerotic process and aneurysm formation, a causal relationship has not yet been proved. Genetic factors and cellular and molecular mechanisms are currently under active investigation.

INCIDENCE

Aortic aneurysms are found most commonly in elderly men. Aneurysms begin to appear after the age of 55 in men and appear 10–15 years later in women. Ultrasonographic screening studies defining aneurysm as a 3.0-cm or larger abdominal aorta have shown that the incidence of aneurysm increases continuously after the age of 55 in men and reaches a peak of more than 10% at the age of 75. In women, the highest rate of AAA, approximately 5%, is found in those 85 years of age and older.

The overall prevalence of aortic aneurysm has increased from 2% to 5% per year in the past 30–40 years as the population has aged. Patients at the highest risk of developing AAA are those with a family history of aneurysm, cigarette smoking, hypertension, chronic obstructive pulmonary disease, and evidence of systemic atherosclerosis.

NATURAL HISTORY

Abdominal aortic aneurysms tend to enlarge and rupture. The average rate of aneurysmal enlargement is 0.5 cm per year, but the rate of enlargement is variable and unpredictable. The risk of aneurysm rupture increases exponentially with increasing aneurysm size (Table 39.4–1). The risk of rupture for a 4-cm aneurysm is approximately 4% per year; it is 8% for a 5-cm aneurysm, 10% for a 6-cm aneurysm, and 40% for a 7-cm aneurysm. Approximately 50% of patients with aortic aneurysms who do not undergo operative repair will die of a ruptured aortic aneurysm. Approximately 75% of patients less than 70 years of age with an asymptomatic 4-cm AAA will eventually undergo operative repair due to aneurysmal enlargement or the development of symptoms.

CLINICAL PRESENTATION

Most abdominal aortic aneurysms are asymptomatic and are discovered on routine physical examination or incidentally during ultrasonographic or computed tomographic (CT) examination for other reasons. Enlarging aortic aneurysms may produce symptoms of back or abdominal pain without signs of hypovolemia or hypotension. Such patients are considered to have symptomatic aortic aneurysms and are at risk for aortic rupture. Therefore, patients with symptomatic aneurysms should undergo immediate diagnostic evaluation and urgent aneurysm repair. Patients with ruptured aortic aneurysms usually experience a sudden onset of severe back or abdominal pain, with the development of syncope and hypotension. Approximately 50% of patients with ruptured

aneurysms will die before reaching the hospital. Those that arrive with a pulsatile abdominal mass and hypotension should be taken immediately to the operating room for operative repair.

DIAGNOSIS

Physical examination of patients with asymptomatic AAA may reveal a pulsatile midepigastric abdominal mass. Physical examination tends to overestimate the size of the aneurysm by 1–2 cm, and even large aortic aneurysms may be missed in examining obese patients. Ultrasonography can reliably identify and determine the size of abdominal aortic aneurysms and should be used as the screening procedure of choice to evaluate patients for the presence of aortic aneurysms (Figure 39.4–3). Ultrasonography is also the most useful test for follow-up studies on patients with known abdominal aortic aneurysm and for follow-up determinations of aneurysm size.

The most precise method of assessing aortic aneurysms is computed tomography (Figure 39.4–4). A CT scan with contrast enhancement will allow precise determination of aortic size, extent of mural thrombus, relationship of the aneurysm to the renal arteries, and involvement of the iliac arteries. A CT scan also will reveal the presence or absence of retroperitoneal hemorrhage and will allow identification of other abdominal abnormalities. Newer techniques of spiral CT angiography with a timed contrast bolus injection and three-dimensional reconstruction can provide more precise morphologic information regarding the extent of the aneurysm and its relationship to renal and mesenteric vessels, as well as identify visceral artery stenoses (Figure 39.4–5).

MRI is also a valuable imaging modality for aneurysm

Table 39.4–1. Risk of rupture of abdominal aortic aneurysm.

Size of Aneurysm (cm)	Risk of Rupture (%)
> 4	4
> 5	8
> 6	10
> 7	40

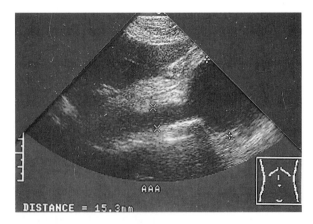

Figure 39.4–3. Duplex ultrasound demonstrating an abdominal aortic aneurysm (AAA) in the longitudinal projection. The AAA is 5.7 cm in size. The neck of the aneurysm is 2 cm in length and has a diameter of 1.5 cm.

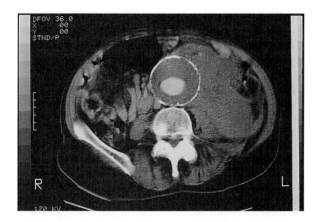

Figure 39.4–4. Spiral CT scan with intraluminal contrast demonstrating the calcified wall of the aneurysm and mural thrombus within the aneurysm. The maximum transverse diameter of the aneurysm is 6.7 cm. The lumen diameter is 2.8 cm.

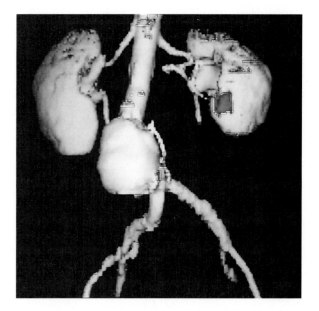

Figure 39.4–5. Three-dimensional reconstruction of spiral CT scan with contrast infusion. The abdominal aortic aneurysm and its relationship to the renal arteries and iliac arteries are clearly demonstrated. The inferior mesenteric artery (IMA) is occluded.

and has the advantage of not utilizing iodinated contrast material. This is particularly useful in patients with renal failure. Contrast arteriography is the most commonly used modality in the evaluation and preoperative planning of patients selected for abdominal aortic aneurysm repair, particularly if there is a question of involvement or stenosis of the renal arteries.

SELECTION OF PATIENTS FOR OPERATION

Patients with ruptured aortic aneurysms should be immediately transferred to the operating room for surgical repair of the ruptured aortic aneurysm. Patients with symptomatic aneurysms should be rapidly evaluated and prepared for urgent surgical repair of the aneurysm. Patients with asymptomatic aortic aneurysms are selected for operation based on an assessment of the risk of aneurysm rupture compared to the risk of elective aneurysm repair.

Since the risk of rupture increases exponentially with aneurysm size, large aneurysms are repaired if there are no prohibitive medical contraindications (Table 39.4–2). Contraindications to repair include recent myocardial infarction, intractable congestive heart failure, severe pulmonary insufficiency, severe renal insufficiency, incapac-

Table 39.4–2. Candidates for abdominal aortic aneurysm operation.

Patients with asymptomatic aneurysms 6 cm or larger
Patients with asymptomatic aneurysms 5–6 cm with increased risk for rupture
Patients with enlarging aneurysms
Patients with symptomatic aneurysms
Patients with ruptured aneurysms

itating stroke, or life expectancy of less than 2 years. Patients with asymptomatic abdominal aortic aneurysms measuring 5 cm or more in diameter without medical contraindications are usually selected for elective aneurysm repair. Occasionally, patients without medical contraindications with aneurysms 4–5 cm that are more than twice the normal diameter of the aorta may be selected for elective aneurysm repair.

OPERATIVE APPROACH

The principle of operative repair of aortic aneurysms is exclusion of the aneurysm from the circulation and replacement of the diseased aortic segment with a prosthetic aortic graft. The aortic aneurysm may be approached through a transperitoneal or left flank retroperitoneal exposure. Proximal control of the aorta is obtained at the neck of the aneurysm just below the renal arteries. Distal control is obtained of the common iliac arteries if the aneurysm is confined to the abdominal aorta. If the aneurysm extends to involve the common iliac arteries, control of the internal and external iliac arteries is obtained below the aneurysm.

Following heparinization, the aorta is clamped proximally, the iliac arteries are clamped distally, and the aneurysm is opened (Figure 39.4–6). The mural thrombus is removed from within the aneurysm, and the lumbar arteries within the aneurysm are oversewn to control retrograde

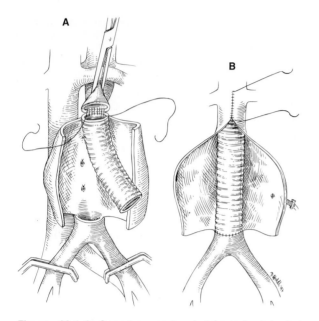

Figure 39.4–6. Operative repair of infrarenal abdominal aneurysm. ***A:*** The proximal infrarenal abdominal aorta and distal common iliac arteries are cross-clamped, and the aneurysm is opened. The proximal anastomosis of the Dacron graft to the infrarenal aorta is performed with nonabsorbable monofilament suture. ***B:*** After complettition of the proximal and distal anastomoses, flow is restored to the iliac arteries. The aneurysm wall is then closed over the Dacron graft.

bleeding. The inferior mesenteric artery is controlled and may be ligated or later reimplanted into the graft. A knitted or woven Dacron graft is selected and sutured end-to-end to the infrarenal aorta using monofilament nonabsorbable suture. If the aneurysm is confined to the abdominal aorta, the distal anastomosis is made to the aorta just above its bifurcation, and this repair is known as a **tube graft repair**. If the aneurysm involves the iliac arteries, a bifurcation graft is used and each limb anastomosed distally to nonaneurysmal iliac arteries below the aneurysm. This repair is known as an **aortoiliac bypass** or **bifurcation graft repair**. Occasionally, the bifurcation graft must be anastomosed to the common femoral arteries as an aortofemoral bypass. The aneurysmal wall is then sewn over the graft as a protective layer to separate the Dacron graft from the abdominal viscera and to prevent the potential late complication of an aortoduodenal fistula. The general techniques of operative repair for elective, urgent, and emergent aneurysm repairs are the same.

RESULTS

Operative mortality for elective aortic aneurysm repair in low-risk patients is 1–2% and increases to 5–10% in high-risk patients. Operative mortality for urgent aneurysm repair in symptomatic patients ranges from 5–10%. Overall mortality rate for patients undergoing repair of ruptured aortic aneurysms is 50% and increases to more than 90% in patients with preoperative shock, acidosis, and renal failure. Complications of aortic aneurysms include myocardial infarction, respiratory failure, and renal insufficiency. Elective aneurysm repair is an effective procedure with an overall operative mortality of 4% (range 1.4–6.5%) in 13 studies from 1956 to 1989 involving 6488 patients.

The long-term outcome of patients undergoing elective aneurysm repair depends on their overall medical condition. Long-term mortality is commonly due to coronary artery disease. Four large studies involving 3226 patients between 1955 and 1989 revealed long-term survival following elective aneurysm repair at 1 year to be 92%, 67% at 5 years, and 40% at 10 years (Tables 39.4–3 and 39.4–4).

THORACIC AORTIC ANEURYSMS

Thoracic aortic aneurysms are less common than abdominal aortic aneurysms and may involve the aortic arch, descending thoracic aorta, and suprarenal aorta. Aneurysms 6 cm in size and greater are considered to be significant. The 1-year survival of nonoperated patients with thoracic aneurysms is 60% and the 5-year survival is 20%. Operative repair of thoracic aortic aneurysms and thoracoabdominal aneurysms is more complex because of the involvement of the visceral branches and the celiac, superior, mesenteric, and renal arteries. In addition, patients undergoing thoracic aortic aneurysm repair are subject to a risk of paraplegia because of ischemia of the anterior spinal artery, which may receive its blood supply from intercostal artery branches arising from the aneurysm at the level of T-10 through L-2. The operative mortality rate for patients undergoing thoracic aortic aneurysm repair is 10–15%.

The thoracic aorta is also prone to **dissection**, which is a separation of the layers of the aortic wall, with creation of a false channel. This may result in obstruction of side branches, producing ischemia, aortic valvular insufficiency, or aortic rupture and death. Aortic dissection is associated with systemic hypertension and degeneration of the aortic media; it is a different disease entity with a different pathogenesis from atherosclerotic aortic aneurysms.

Table 39.4–3. Long-term survival rate after abdominal aortic aneurysm repair.

Follow-up (y)	Survival (%)
1	92
5	67
10	40

Table 39.4–4. Operative mortality of abdominal aortic aneurysms.

Type of Aneurysm	Operative Mortality (%)
Elective: low-risk	1–2
high-risk	5–10
Symptomatic	5–10
Ruptured	50–90

PERIPHERAL ARTERIAL ANEURYSMS

Aneurysms may develop in peripheral arteries such as the femoral, popliteal, carotid, subclavian, renal, celiac, superior, mesenteric and splenic arteries.

The most common peripheral aneurysm is a popliteal aneurysm. Popliteal aneurysms are usually bilateral and are frequently associated with the presence of an abdominal aortic aneurysm. More than 50% of patients with popliteal aneurysms have abdominal aortic aneurysms. Popliteal aneurysms may thrombose, presenting as acute lower extremity ischemia, or they may embolize to the distal tibial arteries, presenting as foot or toe ischemia. They rarely rupture, but may cause compressive symptoms on the adjacent popliteal vein and tibial nerve.

Popliteal aneurysms may be found by palpation as pulsatile masses in the popliteal fossa and confirmed with duplex ultrasonography. Operative repair requires preoperative angiography to identify the extent of the aneurysm and inflow and outflow vessels, and to permit proper planning. Operative treatment includes ligation of the aneurysm to exclude it from the circulation and reversed saphenous vein bypass, usually femoropopliteal, to restore flow. Since untreated popliteal aneurysms carry a significant risk for limb loss, elective repair should be carried out for large popliteal aneurysms.

The most common visceral aneurysm is a splenic artery aneurysm. Splenic artery aneurysms comprise 60% of all visceral aneurysms. Most splenic aneurysms are solitary and usually occur in the distal part of the artery. They are most commonly found in women of child-bearing age and may rupture during pregnancy. Ruptured splenic aneurysms carry up to a 72% maternal and fetal mortality. Splenic artery aneurysms may be identified as a calcified ring on plain x-ray and can be identified on CT scans and angiography. Patients with splenic artery aneurysms greater than 3 cm are candidates for elective operation, which involves ligation of the aneurysm with or without splenectomy.

SUMMARY & FUTURE PERSPECTIVES

Aneurysms of the aorta and peripheral arteries can cause death and disability from rupture, thrombosis, or embolization. By far, the most common aneurysm is the abdominal aortic aneurysm, which is a major cause of significant morbidity and mortality. Death from a ruptured aortic aneurysm can be prevented with early detection and elective aneurysm repair. Aneurysms can be reliably detected with ultrasonographic examination and are present in up to 10% of 75-year-old men. Elective aneurysm repair is a safe and durable treatment that is effective in the prevention of rupture.

New diagnostic and imaging modalities allow precise aneurysm definition, and new treatment modalities are currently being investigated. These treatment modalities include endovascular approaches with endoluminal stent graft repair. These new treatment technologies may enhance the safety and efficacy of elective aneurysm repair in years to come.

SUGGESTED READING

Crawford ES, Denatale RW: Thoracoabdominal aortic aneurysm: Observations regarding the natural course of the disease. J Vasc Surg 1986;3:578.

Cronenwett JL, Sampson LN: Aneurysms of the abdominal aorta and iliac arteries. In: Dean RH, Yao JST, Brewster DC (editors): *Current Diagnosis & Treatment in Vascular Surgery*. Appleton & Lange, 1995.

Graham LM, Mesh CL: Celiac, hepatic, and splenic artery aneurysms. In: Ernst CB, Stanley JC (editors): *Current Therapy in Vascular Surgery*, 3rd ed. Mosby, 1995.

Miller DC, Myers BD: Pathophysiology and prevention of acute renal failure associated with thoracoabdominal and abdominal surgery. J Vasc Surg 1987;5:518.

Panneton JM et al: Ruptured abdominal aortic aneurysms: Impact of comorbidity and postoperative complications on outcome. Ann Vasc Surg 1995;9:535.

Shortell CK et al: Popliteal artery aneurysms: A 25-year experience. J Vasc Surg 1991;14:771.

Zarins CK: Pathogenesis of aortic aneurysms. In: Ernst CB, Stanley JC (editors): *Current Therapy in Vascular Surgery*, 3rd ed. Mosby, 1995.

39.5 Renovascular Hypertension & Mesenteric Ischemia (Visceral Artery Disease)

Cornelius Olcott IV, MD

► Key Facts

- ► Stenosis of one or more renal arteries may produce hypertension that is referred to as renovascular hypertension.

- ► Renovascular hypertension is responsible for 5–10% of all cases of hypertension.

- ► The most common pathological entities responsible for stenotic lesions of the renal arteries are atherosclerosis and fibromuscular dysplasia.

- ► Endovascular procedures for the management of renovascular hypertension include percutaneous transluminal angioplasty (PTA) with or without stenting. Surgical procedures include endarterectomy and bypass grafting.

- ► The hallmark of visceral ischemia is abdominal pain that is characteristically out of proportion to physical findings.

- ► Patients with suspected acute visceral ischemia should have prompt arteriography and emergent laparotomy. An embolectomy or vascular reconstruction with bowel resection may be necessary.

- ► The mortality rate for patients with acute visceral ischemia is 70–90%, depending on the consequences of bowel infarction and the primary disease.

- ► Patients with chronic visceral ischemia should undergo reconstruction of their visceral vessels to prevent progression of their ischemia and development of necrotic bowel.

ANATOMY & PHYSIOLOGY

Arterial lesions producing stenosis may involve the renal arteries or the visceral arteries of the abdominal aorta. Typically, there are single renal arteries to each kidney, however, multiple renal arteries may be present, either unilaterally or bilaterally. There are three visceral arteries—the celiac axis, which branches into the hepatic artery, the splenic artery, and the left gastric artery; the superior mesenteric artery (SMA), which feeds the small intestine and the ascending and transverse colon; and the inferior mesenteric artery (IMA), which supplies the distal colon. The celiac and SMA arise from the anterior surface of the suprarenal aorta and the IMA arises from the left anterior-lateral surface of the infrarenal aorta, approximately one-half way between the renal arteries and the bifurcation of the aorta (Figure 39.5–1).

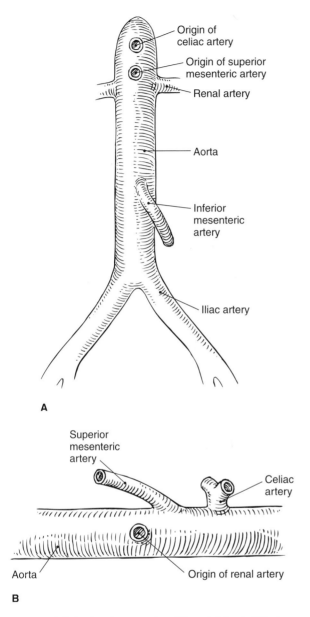

A

B

Figure 39.5–1. Anterior-posterior **(A)** and lateral **(B)** views of the abdominal aorta and visceral and renal arteries. Note that the celiac artery and the superior mesenteric artery arise from the anterior surface of the aorta.

Lesions of the renal arteries that produce stenosis of the lumen of the artery may produce hypertension. This is termed **renovascular hypertension** (RVH). The mechanism of this was first demonstrated by Goldblatt in 1934. The stenotic lesion in the renal artery decreases the perfusion pressure to the kidney, specifically to the juxtaglomerular apparatus. The juxtaglomerular apparatus responds to this decrease in pressure by secreting renin, a proteolytic enzyme. Renin acts on renin substrate (an-

giotensinogen) to form angiotensin I. Converting enzyme then cleaves two amino acids from angiotensin I to form angiotensin II. Angiotensin II produces RVH by two mechanisms—directly through its vasoconstrictor properties and indirectly by stimulating the adrenal to secrete aldosterone. The latter leads to increased plasma volume by sodium and fluid retention.

Occlusive lesions of the visceral arteries may produce visceral ischemia. Typically, this involves the small or large intestine, though the liver, spleen, and stomach may also be involved. The collateral circulation of the visceral vessels is very well developed. Hence, it is believed that at least two of the three vessels need to be involved for chronic visceral ischemia to occur. Acute ischemia may arise from the sudden occlusion of a single vessel, for example, embolic occlusion of the SMA. The primary collateral pathway between the celiac and the SMA is the gastroduodenal artery. The collateral pathway between the SMA and IMA is the marginal artery of Drummond. In cases of visceral artery occlusive disease, these collaterals are prominent and are easily detected on arteriograms.

RENOVASCULAR HYPERTENSION

DIAGNOSIS

It is estimated that RVH is responsible for 5–10% of all cases of hypertension. The diagnosis of RVH should be entertained in any patient with renal artery stenosis and progressive, difficult-to-control hypertension. However, one must keep in mind that the presence of renal artery stenosis does not ensure a renovascular etiology for a patient's hypertension. There are a number of different pathologic entities that may produce stenotic lesions of the renal arteries and result in hypertension (Table 39.5–1). By far the most common are atherosclerosis, which typically occurs in males 50–70 years old, and fibromuscular dysplasia (FMD), which typically occurs in women 35–50 years old. Atherosclerosis typically involves the aorta and proximal renal artery. Its involvement my be either unilateral or bilateral and it occurs more commonly in men than women. There are a number of variants of FMD. The most common is medial fibroplasia, which involves the mid, and occasionally the distal, third of the renal artery and produces a characteristic string-of-beads appearance on arteriography.

Table 39.5–1. Etiology of renal artery stenosis.

Atherosclerosis
Fibromuscular dysplasia
Dissection
Extrinsic compression
Neurofibromatosis
Trauma

The challenge when evaluating a hypertensive patient with renal artery stenosis is to determine whether or not the renal artery stenosis is responsible for the patient's hypertension. A number of tests have been developed over the years to attempt to select those patients who would benefit from renal artery reconstruction or dilatation (angioplasty). Previously employed tests include the intravenous pyelogram (IVP) and split renal function tests. The test most commonly used today is the renal vein renin determination.

In this test, renin levels are determined from each renal vein and the inferior vena cava (IVC). If the renin level in the vein ipsilateral to the arterial lesion is greater than 1.5 times the control level, it is presumed that the stenotic lesion is responsible for the hypertension. Unfortunately, a number of false positive and false negative results do occur, primarily secondary to the patient's antihypertensive medications, to the patient's diet, or to improper handling of the specimen. Other studies that may help predict the presence of RVH include (1) the presence of renal artery stenosis associated with significant ipsilateral collaterals on arteriography, (2) a positive captopril nuclear medicine scan, and (3) evidence of diminished renal artery flow on color flow Doppler examination. The latter is particularly useful in screening patients with hypertension, as it is noninvasive and can be done in the vascular laboratory. The presence of elevated systolic velocities in the renal artery or prolonged acceleration times are compatible with renal artery stenosis of greater than 60%.

A recommended protocol for the evaluation of patients with suspected RVH is outlined in Figure 39.5–2. Patients with hypertension are evaluated in our vascular clinic to see if their history and physical examination are compatible with RVH. Attention is particularly directed to patients in the pediatric age group (< 5 years old), middle-aged women who might have FMD, and patients in the atherosclerotic age group. In our experience, patients with sudden onset of hypertension and/or severe, difficult-to-control hypertension are more likely to have RVH. If a renal vascular etiology seems likely, patients are evaluated by color flow Doppler. If this is positive, or if the history and physical examination strongly suggest a renovascular etiology, the patient is referred for arteriography to document the renal artery anatomy. If an appropriate lesion is identified, then the diagnosis of renovascular hypertension is strongly considered. Renal vein renin studies are reserved for those cases calling for further documentation of a renovascular etiology.

In addition to hypertension, renal artery stenosis may be responsible for renal insufficiency. This has two implications for the surgeon evaluating a patient for renovascular hypertension. First, one must be careful when ordering contrast studies (arteriograms) on these patients, so as not to produce further renal insufficiency/failure as a result of the contrast agent. Second, consideration must also be given to maintaining functioning renal mass. Renal artery reconstruction may be indicated, not only to manage the patient's hypertension, but also to prevent progressive

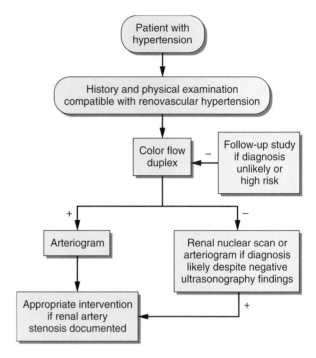

Figure 39.5–2. Algorithm for the work-up of renovascular hypertension.

renal failure. Work by Dean has demonstrated that renal insufficiency may be reversed in appropriately selected patients with renal artery stenosis and renal failure, including patients on dialysis.

MANAGEMENT

The first step in management is to determine if the patient is a candidate for any type of intervention and then to determine the appropriate intervention. Patients are considered for intervention if renal artery stenosis can be established as the most likely cause of their hypertension, or if they have significant renal mass at risk from ischemia; in addition, their age and medical condition must permit the desired intervention to be conducted safely. Failure of medical therapy is not necessary, especially if the patient is a good surgical risk or has experienced complications from medical therapy (eg, progressive azotemia).

Intervention for renovascular hypertension can be broken down into two broad categories: endovascular and surgical. Endovascular procedures include percutaneous transluminal angioplasty (PTA), with or without stenting. Atherectomy has been used but has not been associated with acceptable results. Indications for angioplasty are: FMD or non-ostial atherosclerosis in a patient who is not a candidate for an open, surgical procedure. In fact, angioplasty is the treatment of choice for FMD.

A surgical approach is indicated for: atherosclerosis, recurrent hypertension in patients with FMD not responding to angioplasty, renal artery dissection, extrinsic renal artery compression (eg, by the crux of the diaphragm), or renovascular hypertension in children. Atherosclerotic lesions of the renal artery typically involve the adjacent aorta and, hence, do not usually do well with angioplasty.

Surgical procedures can be grouped into two categories: endarterectomy or bypass grafting. Endarterectomy is typically performed by opening the perirenal aorta from above the SMA to below the renal arteries and endarterectomizing the aorta and involved renal artery or arteries. Endarterectomy is particularly appropriate when multiple renal arteries are affected and when the lesion is limited to the very proximal renal artery. Bypass grafts may be done using autogenous artery (particularly in pediatric or young adult patients or patients requiring an ex vivo repair), saphenous vein, or prosthetic material—either Dacron or PTFE. A prosthetic graft is frequently used when associated aortoiliac graft replacement is required. If branches of the primary renal artery are involved in the stenotic process (eg, in FMD), then an ex vivo approach may be warranted. This technique involves dividing the renal artery and vein and moving the kidney up onto the abdominal wall or to a platform where the kidney may be cooled, perfused with a preservative, and repaired microsurgically, usually using a branched hypogastric artery autograft.

Results for renal artery reconstruction are typically broken down into three categories: (1) cured—off all medications, (2) improved—still mildly hypertensive but on less medications, and (3) failed—no improvement following intervention. Patients with FMD can expect better results than patients with atherosclerosis. Patients with diffuse (multisystem) atherosclerosis do not do as well as patients with focal renal artery disease. Average results for renovascular surgery are outlined in Table 39.5–2.

VISCERAL ISCHEMIA

DIAGNOSIS

The hallmark of visceral ischemia is abdominal pain that is characteristically out of proportion to the physical findings. Visceral ischemia may be either acute or chronic. Acute visceral ischemia usually results from embolic occlusion or from acute thrombosis of a preexisting atherosclerotic lesion. Because of the acute angle that the

SMA takes in arising from the aorta, the SMA is the most frequent artery involved in an embolic occlusion. A diagnostic point in differentiating embolic from thrombotic lesions is that patients with thrombotic lesions will usually have a history of preexisting ischemic symptoms, such as postprandial pain and weight loss. Patients with embolic occlusions typically do not have preexisting symptoms, but do have an embolic source, most frequently a cardiac lesion. The typical presentation of a patient with acute visceral ischemia is outlined in Table 39.5–3.

In over 80% of the cases, chronic visceral ischemia results from atherosclerotic involvement of two or more of the visceral vessels, although extensive disease of the SMA may also produce significant chronic symptoms. Other causes of intestinal ischemia include dissection, fibrodysplastic disease, and compression of the celiac artery by the arcuate ligament of the diaphragm. The typical presentation of a patient with chronic visceral ischemia is postprandial pain with fear of eating and weight loss. These symptoms may also be associated with changes in bowel patterns and with other findings of visceral ischemia, including diffuse, nonhealing gastric erosions, gangrenous acalculous cholecystitis, and unexplained elevation of liver enzymes. Differential diagnosis includes: occult gastrointestinal or pancreatic malignancy, chronic pancreatitis, and peptic ulcer disease.

In addition to fixed-lesion ischemia, nonocclusive mesenteric ischemia may occur. This is simply a low-flow state occasionally associated with vasospasm. This entity presents with a clinical picture similar to acute ischemia of any other origin but in conjunction with entities associated with low-flow states—myocardial infarction, congestive heart failure, arrhythmias, hypovolemia, trauma, and inotropic drugs.

The diagnosis of visceral ischemia depends upon a strong index of suspicion, based on the history and physical examination and angiographic documentation of appropriate visceral artery lesions. The "gold standard" for the diagnosis of visceral ischemia remains biplane angiography. A good lateral view of the aorta is necessary to visualize the origin of the celiac artery, the SMA, and occasionally the IMA (Figure 39.5–1).

Many centers are increasingly using color flow Doppler as a screening examination. This test can easily be performed in the outpatient setting. With experience, the celiac artery and the SMA, and occasionally the IMA, may be visualized. This test is also useful for imaging visceral reconstructions during follow-up. However, this examination is very technician-dependent and is difficult in patients who

Table 39.5–2. Average results of renovascular surgery.

Disease	Cured (%)	Improved (%)	Failed (%)
Atherosclerosis	30–50	40–50	5–20
Fibromuscular dystrophy	55–65	30	2–5

Table 39.5–3. Presentation of acute visceral ischemia.

Sudden onset of severe abdominal pain
May have minimal physical findings early in course, peritonitis later
Associated atherosclerosis or embolic source
Acidosis
WBC > 15,000

are obese or who have excessive bowel gas. Magnetic resonance imaging (MRI) and spiral computed tomography (CT) are also being used for visualizing the visceral circulation. However, results at this time are not as good as with angiography. Experimental use of MRI techniques to physiologically determine the presence or absence of intestinal ischemia looks promising at this time.

MANAGEMENT

Acute Visceral Ischemia

Our present protocol for the management of acute visceral ischemia is outlined in Figure 39.5–3. If the diagnosis of intestinal ischemia is considered, prompt angiography is obtained and emergent laparotomy is indicated. Procrastination and delay will only result in irreversible ischemia of the gut. With the exception of nonocclusive mesenteric ischemia, there is no place for medical management of these patients.

The choice of surgical procedure will be dictated by the etiology of the acute lesion. If an embolic occlusion is responsible, embolectomy of the appropriate vessel is the proper treatment. If the ischemia is a result of acute thrombosis, reconstruction utilizing an autogenous technique, endarterectomy, or vein graft bypass, is the treatment of choice. In either case, the vascular reconstruction should be performed first and the bowel evaluated. All irreversibly ischemic bowel should then be resected. It is generally agreed that a "second look" procedure in approximately 24 hours is necessary to ensure that no further ischemic bowel is present. The risk of incomplete resection justifies this aggressive approach.

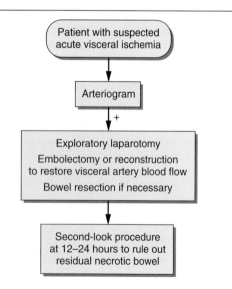

Figure 39.5–3. Algorithm for the management of acute visceral ischemia.

The treatment for nonocclusive mesenteric ischemia is aimed at correcting the primary cause of the low-flow state. Occasionally, intra-arterial vasodilators may also be helpful. Laparotomy may be required to evaluate bowel viability and to resect obviously ischemic or necrotic bowel.

Chronic Visceral Ischemia

Patients with chronic visceral ischemia should undergo reconstruction of their visceral vessels to prevent progression of their ischemia and development of necrotic bowel. Reconstruction may be accomplished either by endarterectomy or bypass grafting. If endarterectomy is used, it is best accomplished by a thoracoabdominal approach or by medial visceral rotation, exposing the left lateral side of the aorta and the proximal visceral vessels. The endarterectomy can then be performed using a transaortic approach, removing the lesion from the aorta and proximal visceral vessels. This approach is particularly useful when only the proximal portion of the celiac or SMA is involved or the adjacent aorta is involved in the atherosclerotic process.

If the stenotic lesion extends distally into the vessel, then a bypass from the supraceliac aorta to the SMA (and to the celiac, if involved) is the usual approach. Prosthetic material (eg, Dacron) has been found to be more durable than vein grafts. For these reconstructions, some surgeons use the distal aorta or iliac artery for inflow. However, most experienced vascular surgeons prefer the supraceliac aorta as the origin for their revascularizations. The aorta at that level is usually free of atherosclerotic disease, and the course of the graft is much more direct. These antegrade grafts have been found to be more durable than grafts arising from the infrarenal aorta or iliac arteries.

Chronic ischemia of the descending colon and rectum can result from occlusion of the IMA, either by atherosclerosis or, more commonly, when this vessel is ligated in conjunction with an aortic reconstruction, such as repair of an abdominal aortic aneurysm or in performing an aortofemoral bypass. At the time of aortic reconstruction, the distal colon should be carefully inspected. If there is any evidence for colon ischemia or if the IMA backbleeding is marginal, then the IMA should be reimplanted into the graft that is used in the aortic reconstruction.

Percutaneous transluminal angioplasty has been utilized in the management of visceral artery occlusive disease. This may be combined with stenting of the lesion. Unfortunately, the rate of recurrent stenosis is high, approximately 40% at 1 year, hence, this technique is usually reserved for those patients not believed to be operative candidates.

Results from the management of visceral ischemia depend upon the etiology of the ischemia. Patients with acute ischemic lesions do not do well. The mortality rate for these patients is 70–90%, due primarily to the consequences of bowel infarction and to the primary disease, for example, cardiac disease. On the other hand, patients with chronic visceral ischemia do reasonably well after reconstruction. The operative mortality rate is 3–4%, early success is approximately 95%, and 5-year patency is 80–90%.

SUGGESTED READING

Dean RH et al: Revascularization of the poorly functioning kidney. Surgery 1979;85:44.

Geelkerken RH, Van Bockel JH: Mesenteric vascular disease: A review of diagnostic methods and therapies. Cardiovasc Surg 1995;3:247.

Hallett JW et al: Recent trends in the diagnosis and management of chronic intestinal ischemia. Ann Vasc Surg 1990;4:126.

Hallett JW et al: Advanced renovascular hypertension and renal insufficiency: Trends in medical comorbidity and surgical approach from 1970 to 1993. J Vasc Surg 1995;21:750.

Hanesn KJ et al: Contemporary management of renovascular disease. J Vasc Surg 1992;16:319.

Kuestner LM, Stoney RJ: The case for renal revascularization. Cardio Surg 1995;3:141.

Standley JC: The evolution of surgery for renovascular disease. Cardio Surg 1994;2:195.

Stanley JC et al: *Renovascular Hypertension*. Saunders, 1984.

Taylor LM: Mesenteric ischemia. In: Rutherford RB (editor): *Seminars in Vascular Surgery*. Saunders, 1990.

Taylor LM, Moneta GL: Intestinal ischemia. Ann Vasc Surg 1991;5:403.

39.6 Venous Disorders

Edmund J. Harris, Sr, MD, & E. John Harris, Jr, MD

▶ Key Facts

- ▶ Varicose veins have traditionally been the most common clinical venous disorder requiring treatment by vascular surgeons.

- ▶ Veins transport the same amount of blood as arteries but have a potential cross-sectional area that is three to four times greater.

- ▶ Normal musculovenous pump function serves to keep venous outflow from the lower limb equal to the arterial inflow.

- ▶ The venous system of the lower limb has three components: superficial veins, perforator veins, and deep veins.

- ▶ Most pathologic changes (75%) found in the venous system develop in the lower extremities.

- ▶ Increased venous pressure causes a corresponding increase in capillary pressure, resulting in skin changes that include swelling, diffuse subcutaneous fibrosis, hyperpigmentation, eczema, and cutaneous ulceration.

- ▶ Primary varicose veins occur only in the superficial veins of the lower limbs, predominantly in the greater saphenous vein and its tributaries.

- ▶ The goal of surgery for varicose veins is interruption of the source of deep-to-superficial vein reflux, and removal of both the main pathway of incompetence and its associated tortuous tributaries.

- ▶ Venous disorders are the predominant cause of skin ulcerations in the lower extremity and occur as a result of increasing interstitial pressure, which interrupts the nutrient flow to the dermis.

- ▶ Deep vein thrombosis is diagnosed in roughly 800,000 new patients per year.

- ▶ Immediately after objective clinical confirmation of deep vein thrombosis, standard heparin therapy should be initiated, followed by warfarin therapy when therapeutic heparin levels have been reached.

GENERAL CONSIDERATIONS

Venous disorders are markers of dysfunction of a complex venous system whose primary function is to return blood from the capillary beds to the right heart. Movement of venous blood in the limbs is dependent on three forces: arterial pressure across the capillary bed, gravity, and pressure created by the musculovenous pumps. Venous blood flow is dependent upon the integrity of the vein wall and venous valves and the maintenance of blood fluidity by the venous endothelial cells that form an intimal monolayer capable of inhibiting blood coagulation and platelet aggregation, and promoting fibrinolysis.

Varicose veins have traditionally been the most common clinical venous disorder requiring treatment by vascular surgeons. Other equally significant venous disorders include: chronic venous insufficiency due to venous valvular dysfunction, venous obstruction, venous compression syndromes, congenital venous malformations, and acute deep venous thrombosis. A deeper understanding of these other venous disorders has led to greater involvement of vascular surgeons in the treatment of such conditions. Excluding thrombosis, the pathophysiology uniting these different venous disorders involves failure of the lower limb muscular venous pumping mechanisms, including the venous valves. To better understand the importance of the musculovenous pump, a brief review of venous hemodynamics and anatomy is provided to preface current therapies for these venous disorders directed at normalizing venous blood flow. A brief review of deep vein thrombosis is also provided.

VENOUS HEMODYNAMICS

Venous pressure is the sum of dynamic pressure produced by the contraction of the left ventricle, hydrostatic pressure produced by the weight of the column of blood within the venous system, and static filling pressure that is related to the elasticity of the venous wall. In most circumstances, static filling pressure is negligible in the venous system. The dynamic pressure within the venous system is low—15–20 mm Hg in postcapillary venules and gradually declining to 0–6 mm Hg in the right atrium. While a subject is supine and quiet, venous blood flow follows this pressure gradient from the postcapillary venules to the right atrium, generally less than 10 mm Hg.

Veins transport the same amount of blood as arteries, but have a potential cross-sectional area that is three to four times greater. Veins are collapsible tubes, a feature providing an important capacitance function for the venous system. As veins fill and distend, their resistance to flow drops markedly, accommodating increased blood flow without significant increases in venous pressure.

Transmural pressure is the difference in pressure between the intramural pressure expanding the vein and the extraluminal tissue pressure acting to collapse the vein. At low transmural pressure, the wall collapses to an elliptical low volume configuration; at higher pressures, it changes to a high volume circular tube. When venous transluminal pressure is increased from 0 mm Hg to 15 mm Hg, the vein volume may increase by more than 250%.

Venous flow from the extremities is not dependent upon properly functioning valves, either in the supine or erect position, since the existing pressure gradient to the heart via the system of communicating conduits is sufficient for normal venous return. The valves in the veins of the lower limb are distributed very unevenly. In the deep veins within leg segments contributing to the musculovenous pump system, valves are much more numerous than in the communicating veins and the superficial veins. No valves are present in the sinusoids. Venous valves function primarily to prevent flow of blood into the superficial venous system during muscle contraction. Venous blood flow should be directed centrally into the deep venous system by the unidirectional valves during exercise.

Venous valves are generally located immediately distal to a point of entry of a major tributary. Each valve has two gossamer-thin but strong cusps that coapt centrally within the vein. This valve apparatus can withstand intraluminal pressures well over 300 mm Hg during experimental attempts to rupture them. The slight expansion of the vein wall at the valve ring, known as the **sinus**, facilitates avoidance of contact of the valve leaflets with the vein wall when the valve apparatus is widely open. This ingenious valve apparatus permits rapid valve closure (0.5 seconds) but requires a short reversal of venous flow with a velocity greater than 30 cm/s for successful closure. Vein walls supporting the cusps are capable of considerable distention or contraction, as a result of the increase of muscle fibers running circumferentially and longitudinally at the base of the cusps.

Venous valves are an essential part of the venous pumping mechanisms to return blood to the heart against gravity and protect the peripheral tissues from hydrostatic and hydrodynamic back pressure when the subject is erect. Muscular exercise is accompanied by increased arterial inflow. Abnormal back pressure on the capillary bed (postcapillary venule congestion) is avoided by ensuring simultaneously an equal venous outflow supporting the Starling equilibrium. Muscle contraction can generate pressures in excess of 200 mm Hg, literally squeezing out the large blood volume from the deep calf veins and venous sinusoids with partial emptying of superficial veins. The proximal valves are forced open; the distal valves and perforator valves close to prevent both caudal flow and retrograde flow into the superficial veins respectively. During muscle relaxation the proximal valves close because of gravitational reflux of blood; the distal deep and perforator valves open. As the hydrostatic pressure column is interrupted, the distal intraluminal pressure falls, and inflow of blood from capillaries and superficial veins occurs.

The musculovenous pump consists of muscles with synchronous effects upon movement in a joint ensheathed by a common fascia, supplied by the same artery and drained by a set of densely valved intramuscular and intermuscular veins that empty into a sparsely valved collecting vein proximal to the unit. Three units are incorporated in the lower leg: (1) the posterior unit, with superficial and deep compartments: the superficial comprising the triceps surae, of which the soleus and gastrocnemius muscles are the major components, and the deep comprising the deep flexor muscles, drained by posterior tibial and gastrocnemius veins; (2) the anterior unit: the anterior tibial muscle and extensors hallucis and digitorum longus component, drained by the anterior tibial vein; and (3) the lateral unit: the peroneal muscles, drained by the peroneal vein. During walking, the contraction of these musculovenous units expels blood into the popliteal vein, alternating rhythmically. Normal musculovenous pump function serves to keep venous outflow from the lower leg equal to the arterial inflow during exercise without significant dilatation of veins of the lower leg, and with low pressure in the input area of the calf pump, the superficial veins, and, particularly, the deep ankle veins.

When the subject changes position from supine to erect, the deep veins continue to fill steadily from arterial inflow, yet additionally from superficial-to-deep vein translocation as the hydrostatic venous pressure rises over the next 30–60 seconds. The orthostatic elevation of venous pressure is the same for the superficial and deep systems and is associated with a shift of 250 mL of blood to each leg. Some dilatation of the dependent veins occurs, since no active venous constriction occurs as a reflex response to orthostasis. In a quiet, standing subject the dynamic pressure across the capillary bed is sufficient to direct venous blood centrally to the heart with a linear flow velocity of a few centimeters per second. In a quiet standing 6-foot subject, the ankle hydrostatic pressure approximates 102 mm Hg, and added to the dynamic venous pressure (15 mm Hg), produces a total resting intravenous ankle pressure of 117 mm Hg. A prolonged rise of capillary and venous pressures to these levels in the foot and ankle region without interruption has undesirable soft tissue consequences.

Calf muscle contraction associated with the slightest movement of the toes or calf initiates a fall in venous pressure in the lower limb. With continuous walking, or ten toe-ups at 1 per second, blood is pumped centrally, emptying the veins in the lower leg very effectively, dropping the total intravenous ankle pressure to a new baseline of 0–30 mm Hg. This is the **ambulatory venous pressure** (AVP). Normal ambulatory venous pressure should be less than 50% of maximal standing intravenous ankle pressure. On ceasing all exercise, the intravenous ankle pressure steadily returns to the resting maximal pressure within 30 seconds during muscle relaxation.

The time required for this return to baseline is known as the venous refilling time. A normal venous refilling time is greater than 20 seconds. A short refilling time, 5–6 seconds, suggests valvular incompetence, as the expelled blood is not supported by normal valves to prevent gravitational reflux and a rapid increase in the hydrostatic component of total intravenous pressure is observed.

In supine patients, the superficial veins drain partly through saphenous vein terminations and partly through communications with the deep veins. Numerous valves in the saphenous veins segment the continuous column of blood into short subsegments, allowing each subdivision to empty inwardly into the deep venous system through its own perforator or communicating vein. Normal deep vein valves also prevent axial reflux. Following vigorous muscular contraction, the resulting fall in deep venous pressure, from 60 mm Hg to 70 mm Hg, attracts flow from the superficial veins to the deep veins. During this muscular contraction each segment of the superficial venous system empties its volume of blood into the deep venous system through its communicating vein.

Respiration has a major influence on venous blood flow in a supine individual. The abdominal cavity performs as a closed container through which the collapsible inferior vena cava passes. Inspiration causes the diaphragm to descend, increasing intra-abdominal pressure and effecting an increase in the transmural pressure gradient across the vena cava, which momentarily prevents venous outflow from the legs. Expiration reverses these effects. This creates the intermittency of venous flow. The venous valves prevent distal reflux during inspiration. In returning venous flow from the head and upper extremities, the "closed container" is the thoracic cavity, and inspiration in this case decreases intrathoracic pressure. Venous blood flow increases during inspiration as the intrathoracic pressure drops and decreases during expiration.

Since slow venous flow, due to the width of the venous bed and long periods of stasis, favors thrombosis, the thromboresistant properties of endothelium play a major role in maintaining venous patency. The endothelial cells synthesize prostaglandin (PGI_2), nitric oxide (NO), thrombomodulin, heparin, and plasminogen activators, all of which are antithrombotic compounds and inhibitors of blood coagulation. The endothelium forms a protective barrier that prevents blood cells and plasma proteins from combining with highly reactive subendothelial components in the deeper vessel wall, unless the vessel is disrupted or severed. Blood coagulation is inhibited on the endothelial cell surface by thrombomodulin and heparan sulfate. Fibrinolysis is initiated by secretion of tissue plasminogen activator (tPA) from the endothelial cell, and then blocked by plasminogen activator inhibitor I (PAI-1). By releasing PGI_2 and NO, endothelial cells produce vasodilatation and inhibit platelet aggregation, further hindering stasis of blood and thrombosis.

ANATOMY

The venous system of the lower limb has three components: superficial veins, perforator veins, and deep veins (Figure 39.6–1). The superficial system is composed of long and short saphenous veins, freely intercommunicating between their tributaries over all limb surfaces. The tributaries of the saphenous system lie epifascial and unsupported by Scarpa's (membranous) fascia, thereby being more prone to gross varicosities. The main saphenous trunk receives some support from Scarpa's fascia and rests on the deep fascia. Smooth muscle layers of the saphenous veins are thicker than those of the deep veins. The distal vein segments have thicker muscle layers than the proximal segments; this is appropriate for the focal differences in venous pressures affected by gravity and deep fascial support.

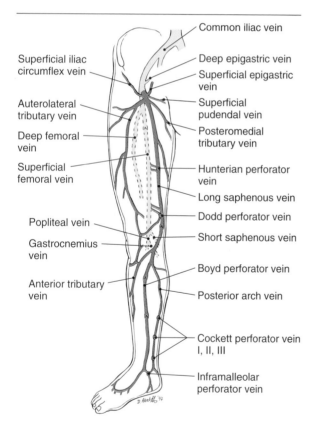

Figure 39.6–1. Anteromedial view of the superficial venous system. The system intercommunicates on all surfaces of the lower limb (see Figure 39.6–2 for posterior view). The three superior branches of the saphenous bulb play a major role in recurrent varicose veins. The anterolateral and posteromedial branches may be independently incompetent. An incompetent Boyd perforator frequently causes the first clinical indication of varicose veins in the long saphenous system.

The labels in the figure read:
- Common iliac vein
- Superficial iliac circumflex vein
- Deep epigastric vein
- Superficial epigastric vein
- Anterolateral tributary vein
- Superficial pudendal vein
- Deep femoral vein
- Posteromedial tributary vein
- Superficial femoral vein
- Hunterian perforator vein
- Long saphenous vein
- Popliteal vein
- Dodd perforator vein
- Gastrocnemius vein
- Short saphenous vein
- Boyd perforator vein
- Anterior tributary vein
- Posterior arch vein
- Cockett perforator vein I, II, III
- Inframalleolar perforator vein

The greater saphenous vein originates in the dorsal venous arch of the foot, ascends anterior to medial malleolus along the medial calf across the posteromedial popliteal space, ascending the medial thigh to terminate in the common femoral vein. From below the medial malleolus, the posterior arch vein ascends the calf and drains into the three Cockett perforator veins. The anterior tributary and posterior tributary calf veins empty into the saphenous vein below the knee. They collect blood from the anterolateral and medial posterior surfaces of the lower leg. The anterolateral and posteromedial thigh veins are the largest long saphenous tributaries. Other tributaries terminating in the saphenofemoral bulb are the superficial external pudendal, the superficial inferior epigastric, and the superficial circumflex iliac veins.

The posterolateral superficial thigh vein and the posterolateral tributary calf vein are inconstant, but very important, posterolateral tributaries (Figure 39.6–2A). Persistence of the lateral veins of the lower limb deserves special mention. Gross anatomic aberrations of superficial veins should suggest the possibility of anomalies or absence of the deep veins. The posterolateral tributary vein of the calf running superficially up the outer side of the leg, joining the anterolateral superficial thigh vein, terminates either in the deep femoral vein or runs with the sciatic nerve into the pelvis to join the internal iliac vein. This massive valveless channel is the main venous outflow of the limb in many patients with Klippel-Trénaunay syndrome.

Posteriorly, the lesser saphenous vein originates in the dorsal venous arch, passes inferiorly posterior to the lateral malleolus, becoming contiguous with the sural nerve. The lesser saphenous vein ascends the mid-posterior calf, penetrating the deep fascia between the middle third of the calf and the popliteal fossa, terminating at variable levels in the popliteal vein (Figure 39.6–2B and C). Two uncommon terminations are the continuation of the lesser saphenous vein as a sciatic vein and multiple connections of the lesser saphenous vein to the gastrocnemial and popliteal veins. The inconstant posterolateral tributary vein is the most important branch of the lesser saphenous system. The lesser saphenous vein through the vein of Giacomini, an upward extension of the lesser saphenous system, may terminate in either the greater saphenous vein or the deep femoral vein. The posteromedial tributary of the greater saphenous vein may communicate directly with the vein of Giacomini.

The deep venous system, beneath the deep investing fascia, has two components: the venous conduits and the venous pumping chambers (sinuses). The deep venous system parallels the major arterial tree of the lower extremity. The venous drainage of the foot is essentially a valveless system with profuse intercommunication between the superficial and deep veins. The venae comitantes of the lateral plantar artery empty into the posterior tibial venae comitantes. The anterior tibial, posterior tibial, and peroneal veins are paired structures, with all three coalescing below the knee joint in 60% of persons to

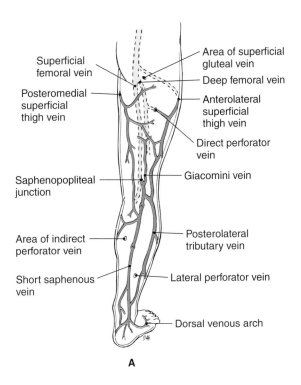

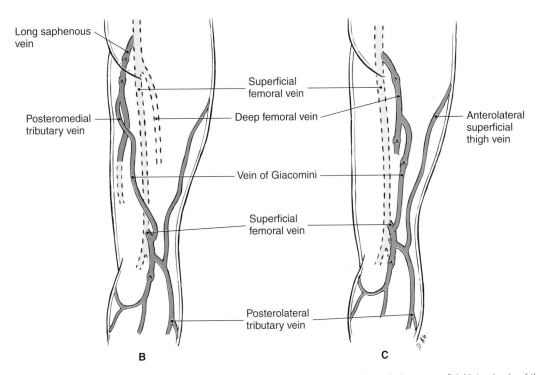

Figure 39.6–2. **A:** Posterolateral view of the superficial venous system. The presence of a valveless superficial lateral vein of the lower limb often indicates the absence of the deep vein system. **B, C:** There are multiple variations of termination of the short saphenous trunk either distal or proximal to the popliteal crease. In association with the vein of Giacomini, it may terminate in different branches, frequently into the long saphenous vein via the posteromedial tributary; it may terminate in the profunda femoral vein or in muscles of the posterior thigh.

form the single popliteal vein. Many variant patterns of coalescence occur. At the adductor canal, the popliteal vein becomes the superficial femoral vein, which continues cephalad to join the deep femoral vein, which drains the thigh muscles, forming the common femoral vein. Above the inguinal ligament it ascends as the iliac vein and inferior vena cava to the heart. These major deep veins and their numerous branches serve as conduits to carry blood from the peripheral tissues to the heart and contribute a limited additional ejection volume with calf muscle contraction. The powerful muscles of the lower limb embody numerous thin-walled capacious sinuses, strongly supported with muscle and investing fascia. The valveless sinuses empty with each muscle contraction into the main conduit veins through connecting veins, which contain a valve in the end of the sinus nearest the heart.

Eponyms, named after authorities first describing them, have been given to the most common perforator veins associated with the greater saphenous vein. Recognizing the anatomy of superficial veins and tributaries, plus the most common perforator vein sources of varicosities, facilitates identification of patterns of varicosities. The site of the perforator in the anteromedial proximal calf has been named after A. M. Boyd. Anatomically, the saphenous nerve and saphenous vein are inseparable distal to the Boyd perforator vein. Along the course of the greater saphenous vein, perforating veins named after John Hunter located in the mid medial thigh, and Harold Dodd in the distal medial third of the thigh, are recognized. The three major perforator veins of the medial gaiter area, named after Frank Cockett, connect the deep veins to the posterior arch vein. The location of the Cockett perforator veins is inconstant. On the medial ankle, the important inframalleolar perforating vein arises.

VENOUS INSUFFICIENCY

Most pathologic changes (75%) found in the venous system develop in the lower extremities. Valvular insufficiency or venous obstruction, both impeding venous return to the heart, lead to the development of increased venous pressure in the distal veins, venules, and capillaries, which is easily recognized and quantified during upright exercising. Failure to lower the ambulatory venous pressure to less than 50% of maximal standing intravenous ankle pressure indicates venous insufficiency.

The fundamental dysfunction of venous insufficiency impairs venous outflow of blood from the affected limb. The increased venous pressure causes a corresponding increase in capillary pressure, resulting in skin changes. Excess capillary transudation of fluid and large protein molecules follow, leading to deposition of fibrin and the formation of a barrier to nutritional exchange between capillaries and interstitial tissues. These skin changes develop over months or years and are found where the venous pressure is highest, unless they are secondary to an arteriovenous fistula. Observable skin changes include (1) swelling of the foot and leg; (2) diffuse subcutaneous fibrosis, varying from slight thickening to chronic hard tissue with venous grooves; (3) hyperpigmentation from hemosiderin, the earliest and most characteristic sign of venous hypertension; (4) eczema, also known as stasis dermatitis; and (5) cutaneous ulceration, where small areas of necrotic tissue coalesce.

Venous insufficiency of the lower extremity related to valvular insufficiency does not represent a well-defined clinical entity, but rather a spectrum of defects with varying clinical signs and symptoms. In the spectrum of valvular insufficiency, the "well-defined" group with primary varicose veins (1 degree VV), involving only the superficial veins, have a normal number of valves, all of which are incompetent. This group responds well to treatment that involves removal of the source of deep-to-superficial venous reflux plus obliteration of the incompetent superficial reflux pathways. At the other end of the valvular insufficiency spectrum is a small group with primary and secondary superficial varicose veins with widespread deficiency of functioning valves in both superficial and deep veins. Patients with these findings are defined as the **primary valve deficiency group**. The primary failure is in the deep vein reflux, overwhelming the calf pump mechanisms and creating a valvular insufficiency too severe to benefit from removal of the incompetent superficial veins. This group responds only to conservative measures to lower venous pressure, such as elevation of the lower limbs and, often, external compression. Ulcerations developing in these patients are often intractable.

Between these two clinically divergent forms of venous insufficiency reside subgroups with definable valve abnormalities and variable clinical symptoms. There is a syndrome of weak vein walls in patients with a history of incompetent superficial veins appearing in their teens. These patients are prone to continuing vein wall dilatation and valvular incompetence. They are also prone to recurrent varicose veins after appropriate surgery and sclerotherapy.

Venous insufficiency symptomatology related to failure or impairment of calf muscle pumping mechanisms is variable and related to the number of residual functioning valves and integrity of the vein walls. Post-thrombotic changes variably interfere with calf muscle pumping, decreasing venous capacitance and diminishing vein wall compliance. Neuromuscular disabilities and loss of ankle mobility can severely decrease muscular contraction. Generally, patients with well-functioning valves in the deep veins have sturdy musculovenous pumping mechanisms that are not easily overwhelmed by significant superficial vein reflux. These patients may have very enlarged superficial veins without venous hypertension. Patients with dysfunctional deep vein valves have a relatively weak calf pumping mechanism that can be overwhelmed by superficial reflux and often develop significant superficial and deep venous hypertension.

Primary varicose veins (1 degree VV) occur only in the superficial veins of the lower limbs, predominantly in the greater saphenous vein and its tributaries (Figure 39.6–3A). Valvular incompetence of the saphenous vein, either at the saphenofemoral junction or along the course of the saphenous veins, allows the generation of venous hypertension in the involved segment when the limb is upright. The column of blood in the saphenous vein is not segmented by competent valves during standing, with gravity-induced reflux encouraged. **Tortuousity**, the hallmark of varicose veins since 1550 BC, identifies veins with intermittent or continuous retrograde flow, indicating a dynamic phenomenon and not merely a static distention. Tortuousity presents in various forms. It may appear as one or more lateral wall bulges located near the termination of the long saphenous vein, in which case it is named **saphena varix (saccule)**. Most commonly, tortuousity appears as small varices zigzagging subdermally down the limbs, or as massive clusters of enlarged twisted subcutaneous veins (Figure 39.6–3B). Tortuousity of secondary varicose veins occurs most commonly in superficial veins conducting reversed collateral flow around obstructed deep veins, such as enlarged tortuous suprapubic veins, acting as collaterals to iliac vein occlusion. This is an acquired response. Enforced reversed flow against the normal direction will cause enlargement and tortuousity in formerly normal veins. In contrast, the long saphenous veins acting as a collateral bypass to an obstructed femoral-popliteal vein enlarge without becoming tortuous, because venous flow follows the normal direction (Figure 39.6–4). Enforced reverse flow seems to be the determining factor. In primary varicose veins, venous tortuousity usually indicates retrograde gravitational downflow in the superficial veins. In secondary varicose veins, tortuousity indicates retrograde collateral flow in superficial veins bypassing deep venous obstruction. Tortuousity is frequently present in lesser branch veins near an arteriovenous fistula (Figure 39.6–4).

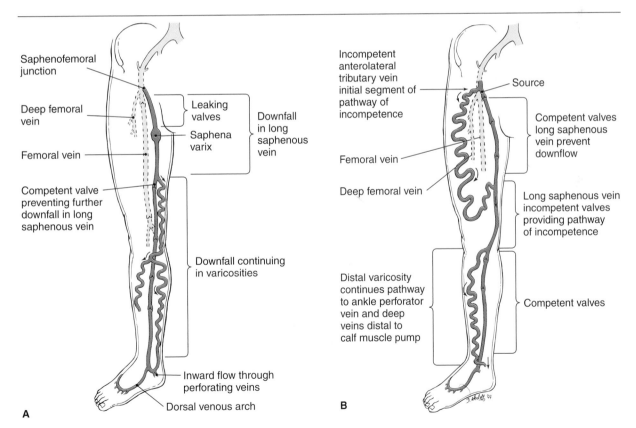

Figure 39.6–3. A: Components of a typical retrograde circuit of flow in superficial vein incompetence: (1) source (saphenofemoral junction), (2) superficial venous pathways of retrograde flow when erect (long saphenous vein and distal tortuous tributaries), (3) reentry point of venous flow to deep veins (perforator veins distal to calf muscle pump), (4) central return pathway in deep veins (activated by musculovenous pump). **B:** Note incompetent valve of the anterolateral tributary vein with competent axial saphenous vein. Reentry into incompetent midsaphenous vein with refluxive downflow in the anterior calf tributary to the ankle perforator. The saphenous trunk may be preserved as a result of competent valve segments.

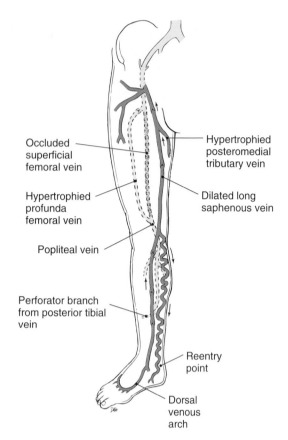

Occluded superficial femoral vein

Hypertrophied profunda femoral vein

Popliteal vein

Perforator branch from posterior tibial vein

Hypertrophied posteromedial tributary vein

Dilated long saphenous vein

Reentry point

Dorsal venous arch

Figure 39.6–4. Deep vein thrombosis (DVT) occludes the superficial femoral vein, increasing venous outflow via the long saphenous vein and the profunda femoral vein. The increased flow in the saphenous vein and tributaries produces hypertrophy of the smooth muscle in the vein wall. The retrograde venous flow in the tortuous posterior calf vein should be prevented by ligation and stripping (stab incisions) to decrease the volume of venous blood in the retrograde circuit of flow in the superficial system.

SCLEROTHERAPY FOR VARICOSE VEINS

The use of sclerotherapy has been expanded by nonsurgical physicians for most forms of varicosities. Its use for axial reflux through the saphenous veins, for large clusters of veins in the thigh, and for varicosities associated with large perforating veins represents a suboptimal indication. Appropriately, it is the only effective treatment for ablation of telangiectasias. It is effective for obliterating postsurgical recurrent and reticular veins and varices less than 4 mm in diameter. Below the knee, sclerosants combined with effective compression can obliterate large varicosities and some clusters of varices not associated with gross saphenous reflux. Since compression is much more efficient against the bony and firm calf than the softer, larger conical-shaped thigh. Proximal superficial vein incompetence and venous hypertension must be controlled first for the best results. In the aged or infirm, sclerotherapy plays a role in palliation of external bleeding from varicose blebs, or in recurrent thrombophlebitis in varicosities to obliterate the diseased vein in the absence of proximal control of venous hypertension.

Indications for sclerotherapy are relief of symptoms and obliteration of pathologic veins. Symptoms include achy leg pain and limb tenderness after prolonged standing or sitting.

In women, these symptoms are exacerbated at both the conclusion of the monthly menstrual cycle and the first day of the menstrual period, when the predominant progesterone level decreases as the estrogen level increases.

The fundamental dysfunction of venous insufficiency is impaired venous blood flow from the affected level, causing pathologic accumulation of interstitial fluid in the affected region. The resulting edema is indicative of an impairment of transcapillary fluid exchange. Recent studies confirm conclusively that the mildest form of 1 degree VV with no clinical edema is associated with increased resting interstitial pressure of deep subfascial tissues of the supramalleolar area, where the earliest and largest trophic changes develop. Therefore, 1 degree VV represents a form of venous insufficiency that should be appreciated by the health care community. Early supportive conservative therapy is indicated.

Knowledge of anatomy and pathophysiology is essential in the treatment telangiectasias. Direct communication of telangiectasias and telangiectatic blemishes with the deep veins occurs in the posterolateral distal third of the thigh, less frequently in the medial thigh. These communicating veins conduct high hydrodynamic pressures from the muscular compartment to the unsupported subdermal reticular veins and the dermal venous network. The abnormal direct venous communications are associated with severe posterior thigh pain with prolonged standing or sitting. The significance of this clinical entity is commonly missed.

The source of these high-pressure communicating veins may be identifiable by careful insonation of the lesion with a continuous wave Doppler ultrasonographic probe. Once identified, the source must be obliterated. Sclerotherapy fails if the sclerosant does not reach the outflow vein from the source in sufficient concentration to effect vein sclerosis. Major contraindications to sclerotherapy include the presence of arterial occlusive disease, venous ulceration, immobile patients, and, finally, unusually large varicosities with large communications to the deep system.

Clinical examination in preparation for sclerotherapy is performed after the patient has been standing for 5–10 minutes. Inspection of the feet through the groin suggests the various patterns of disease. Obesity obscures pathologic veins. The continuous wave Doppler is routinely used to identify sources of venous hypertension, including the saphenofemoral junction, the saphenopopliteal junction, the major perforator veins with eponyms, and areas with nonsaphenous varicosities. Duplex scanning and color flow imaging will be necessary when planning sclerotherapy for complex patterns of disease or inborn venous malformations, such as Klippel-Trénaunay syndrome.

The best results from sclerotherapy follow endothelial destruction, minimal thrombus formation, and fibrosis of the full thickness of the vein wall, avoiding excessive perivenous inflammation. The FDA-approved agents are both detergents and thrombogenic solutions, namely, sodium morrhuate and sodium tetradecyl sulfate. When thrombus results, it must be expressed from the treated veins through a needle stab wound. This procedure is best performed 2–4 weeks after sclerotherapy, at which point the intraluminal thrombus is lysing, to avoid hemosiderin pigmentation in the sclerosed venous segment. Hypertonic saline (11.7%) is preferred as a sclerosant by many dermatologists for spider veins. The FDA has approved it only as an abortifacient. Following injection sclerotherapy, some form of pressure gradient compression over the sclerosed venous segments is recommended.

SURGICAL TREATMENT OF VARICOSE VEINS

The first operation for treatment of varicose veins affords the best opportunity for long-term surgical cure. Responsible surgery for varicose veins is time-consuming. The goal of surgery is removal of the abnormal source of deep to superficial vein reflux, which requires removal of both the main pathway of incompetence and its associated tortuous tributaries. The greater saphenous vein must be ligated flush with the common femoral vein at the saphenofemoral junction. Additionally, careful identification, wide dissection, and ligation of all tributaries of the terminal saphenous vein are essential. Stripping of the main saphenous trunk to just below the knee (**Boyd's perforator area**) is essential if the saphenous valves are functionless. To minimize hemorrhage and hematoma formation in the subcutaneous tunnel created from the groin to below the knee, a strip of vaginal packing soaked with dilute epinephrine solution can be pulled with the stripper through the tunnel.

Incompetent anterolateral tributaries arising from the bulb are treated similarly. The tortuous tributaries are removed through small stab incisions, or occasionally by sclerotherapy. After simple ligation of a valveless saphenous vein, its main-stem remains open as an incompetent conduit extending directly to the low-pressure areas beneath the musculovenous pumps. Commonly, it provides the basis of a new retrograde circuit of incompetence with recurrent varicose veins, if it is not ablated. The presence of the skin changes of venous hypertension indicates an advanced state of venous incompetence. Both gross incompetence of the superficial veins and the post-thrombotic syndrome can be the source for this venous hypertension and cutaneous changes. If these changes are due to superficial vein incompetence they are curable by surgery; if due to the post-thrombotic state, they often can only be palliated. Surgery is preferable to sclerotherapy in the presence of skin changes with large incompetent veins because it confers more lasting benefit.

CHRONIC VENOUS ULCERATION

Chronic venous ulceration (CVI) of the leg causes considerable disability, with major economic consequences for the patients and health care services. Venous disorders are the predominant cause of all skin ulcerations. Considerable variation geographically and within ethnic groups exists. It is essential to identify accurately the source in each patient, since treatment suitable for venous ulceration may jeopardize an ischemic limb. Patients with chronic venous hypertension will develop swelling, induration, fibrosis, eczema, and cutaneous hyperpigmentation in the legs. These "venous stasis" changes will progress to tissue necrosis and skin ulceration without aggressive treatment, usually chronic compression therapy. These characteristic changes are seen in the gaiter areas of legs with chronic venous insufficiency and distal to arteriovenous fistulas, both regions of venous hypertension.

The site of venous ulcers is dependent on the pattern of venous insufficiency and may occur anywhere in the leg. Most commonly, they arise in the medial supramalleolar area where a high level of venous pressure is sustained. Unnaturally high peaks of intravenous pressure from muscular contractions in venous segments without competent valves may be superimposed on the interstitium with exercise. Although no age of adult life is immune, the occurrence of venous ulcers increases with age, possibly due to progressive deterioration of musculovenous pump mechanisms. Venous ulcers develop as interstitial pressures increase to such a level that nutrient flow to the dermis is interrupted and skin slough occurs. Venous ulcers develop healthy granulation tissue, yet are prone to persistent weeping of serous fluid. A fibrinous exudate frequently covers the open wound and provides an ideal media for overgrowth of normal skin flora. Secondary cellulitides are frequent and quite painful when present.

The clinical diagnosis of CVI can be confirmed by continuous wave Doppler in lean patients, but is more reliably diagnosed with duplex scanning or color flow Doppler imaging. Special investigations, such as functional phlebography or varicography, may be needed to define the precise details of complex venous obstruction, heavy reflux in recanalized deep veins, and impaired pumping mechanisms. If ulceration is associated with significant deep venous obstruction or insufficiency, surgical correction of superficial venous incompetence often does not benefit the patient. For deep venous obstruction or severe insufficiency, surgical therapies have been proposed and include: axillary vein valve transposition to the incompetent superficial femoral vein, valvuloplasty of the incompetent superficial femoral vein valves, wrapping incompetent venous valve segments, contralateral saphenous vein crossover bypass for iliofemoral venous obstruction and, most recently, cryopreserved superficial femoral vein by-pass grafts for superficial femoral vein insufficiency or obstruction. To date, none of the surgical therapies directed at deep venous insufficiency or obstruction have experienced durable success.

The mainstay of treatment for CVI is intermittent leg elevation and elastic stocking compression therapy. With insufficiency and no ulcers, 30- to 40-mm Hg below-knee compression stockings are recommended while the patient is up and ambulatory. At night, the stockings are removed and the legs are elevated. Venous ulcerations can be prevented by close compliance with this protocol. The elastic stockings should be replaced every 4–6 months to maintain adequate compression. Once venous ulceration is present, compression therapy should not be abandoned. Vigilant wound care is essential. The ulcer bed is washed with soap and water, after which a dry dressing is applied two to three times per day and the compression stocking is fitted right over the freshly dressed wound. For inframalleolar ulcers, a foam pad can be fashioned to cover the ulcer bed to localize compression from the stocking to the wound. Medicated boots are not superior to this method, but merely represent another form of compression therapy. Once the ulcers have healed, maintenance of compression therapy is critical in preventing recurrence.

RECURRENT VARICOSE VEINS

The recurrence rate of varicose veins after sclerotherapy and surgery is significant. Hurried treatment based on an unconfirmed source, compounded by inadequate dissections, play a major role in postsurgical persistent or truly recurrent varicose veins. Persistent varicose veins are unaltered by surgery and are immediately apparent. They represent branches of a functionally valveless superficial vein still connected to the deep system, without a normally valved vein segment to prevent this high-pressure reflux. Truly recurrent varicose veins reappear in the same distribution within 1–2 years. Usually, these veins result from inadequate ligation of the saphenous termination with the femoral vein, or incomplete removal of incompetent saphenous vein or tributaries. These incompetent superficial veins act as a direct conduit for the reflux from the high-pressure deep venous system down to the low-pressure areas distal to the calf muscle pump. Anatomic reconnections may be formed with the side branches of the saphenous stump. Neovascularization forms a plexus of small veins between the ligated saphenous stump and the unstripped incompetent vein. In the treatment of simple primary varicose veins, it is essential to remove the incompetent saphenous vein (the pathway of incompetence) when the source of incompetence is surgically ligated to avoid development of recurrent varicose veins, via either anatomic reconnection or neovascularization.

The large recurrent varicose veins are the most difficult to treat. Previous surgery has fragmented the anatomy of the superficial veins. The venous patterns are less predictable and often unrecognizable. Usually, there have been several unsuccessful surgical attempts at extirpation or ligation, each event followed by recurrence and worsening symptoms. Many of these patients have also had adjunctive sclerotherapy, providing at best a temporary response.

Careful examination of these patients with continuous wave Doppler, preferably with the patient standing, allows mapping of the overall flow patterns, often with the discovery of several sources of superficial venous reflux on each leg. Areas of reflux can be marked for surgical exploration. Successful surgery for recurrent varicose veins requires careful yet extensive dissections of the saphenofemoral or saphenopopliteal junctions to assure complete ligation of all superficial veins from the deep veins. Additionally, ligation of incompetent perforators and excision of associated varicosities is critical and is facilitated by thorough preoperative duplex evaluation of the recurrent varices.

DEEP VEIN THROMBOSIS

Deep vein thrombosis (DVT) is felt to have a multifactorial etiology, since it is not unusual for it to occur in the absence of a known predisposing event. Acute DVT is a major health problem with two serious outcomes. During the acute course, pulmonary embolism (PE) may be fatal. Over the long term, recurrences of DVT may produce pulmonary hypertension from recurrent embolism, or the post-thrombotic syndrome may develop. Prevention of DVT in high-risk patients is an important priority for the medical profession. DVT is newly diagnosed in roughly 800,000 persons per year. Thirty-five percent of these patients develop the post-thrombotic syndrome, while approximately 5% experience pulmonary embolism.

Studies show a high incidence of congenital or acquired hematologic abnormalities in patients with "idiopathic" DVT, including low levels of antithrombin III (3%), protein C (12%), protein S (1%), heparin cofactor deficiency, and decreased fibrinolytic activity (40%). Testing for the presence of these abnormalities is routine in patients with "idiopathic" DVT. Presently, factor V Leiden mutation is the most commonly identified congenital clotting predisposition, estimated to be present in 6% of the US population. A mutation in the factor V protein occurs that inhibits binding of activated protein C but does not alter binding of this factor V protein to the prothrombinase complex. Leiden factor V can activate prothrombin to thrombin but is not inactivated by activated protein C. Therefore, factor V Leiden defect acts as a protein C deficiency in the setting of normal levels and function of protein C. The spectrum of thrombosis found in patients with factor V Leiden mutation is predominantly venous, with some patients experiencing arterial thrombosis in retinal, intracranial, hepatic, coronary, and renal vessels. Recommendations to evaluate patients suspected to be hypercoagulable by initial screening for Leiden mutation have been proposed because of the frequency of this abnormality. If negative, a subsequent multipanel screen may be done.

The labeled fibrinogen tests of the mid 1960s–70s provided evidence that the incidence of postoperative DVT was much higher than suspected. The natural history of minimal calf vein thrombi of the deep veins suggests that they are usually asymptomatic, common in high-risk hospitalized patients, and clinically unimportant if the thrombi remain confined to the calf. The specific sites within the deep venous system where thrombi originate include the soleal sinuses in the calf, the sinuses of the venous valve cusps, and the iliofemoral venous segment. DVT is most common in hospitalized patients undergoing major general, thoracic, or orthopedic surgeries that require confinement to bed for prolonged periods. Following trauma, particularly when associated with spinal cord injury, or immediately postoperative, activated clotting factors are circulating in the blood as part of a systemic inflammatory response. These activated clotting factors, in combination with areas of venous stasis, produce thrombosis. Stasis in soleal sinuses and valve pockets is considerable in supine patients with immobile legs, where the majority of these thrombi have been identified by labeled fibrinogen.

Most thrombi identified soon after operation disappear through spontaneous lysis or embolize into the pulmonary circulation where they undergo spontaneous lysis. In up to 20% of patients, asymptomatic thrombi may propagate into the popliteal or more proximal veins, with pulmonary embolism detected postoperatively by pulmonary ventilation/perfusion scanning. When calf vein thrombi extend into the proximal veins, they are usually asymptomatic. If they go untreated, these proximal vein thrombi may become symptomatic and the source of large pulmonary emboli that can be fatal. The exact frequency is unknown. Thrombi confined to the soleal or venous valve sinuses incite little inflammation, and, essentially, no trouble results. It is possible for deep vein thrombosis to progress in two different ways. In most instances, the thrombus may totally occlude the involved venous segment, forcing the venous blood to find new collateral pathways to the right heart, as edema develops distally. Less commonly, the progression of thrombus only partially occludes the deep popliteal or femoral veins. This is a treacherous state. Since no limb swelling occurs, the risk of pulmonary embolism can be easily overlooked. This scenario has potential for formation of a friable tail clot that may shower pulmonary emboli at any time.

The diagnosis of DVT cannot reliably be made on symptoms and signs of leg pain, swelling, or calf tenderness, since they are not unique to acute deep vein thrombosis. DVT may be totally asymptomatic. Unilateral leg swelling with pitting edema of the ipsilateral ankle does suggest deep venous thrombi confined to the infrapopliteal vein. Actually, the accuracy for bedside assessment of patients for DVT averages only 50%. Predispos-

ing conditions, such as low antithrombin three levels in women taking oral contraceptives, low levels of urokinase in patients with carcinoma, or low levels of protein C in patients with protein-losing enteropathy or liver disease, should be ruled out. Resistance to activated protein C is ten times more common among patients with DVT than other heritable anticoagulant deficiencies. Its role in recurrent DVT has yet to be defined. A high percentage of these patients with resistance to activated protein C have the Leiden mutation. Generally, the patient's history of any previous venous thrombosis, or family history of thrombosis, plus the clinical evaluation, should alert the physician to the possible presence of DVT. A hypercoagulable panel may be indicated. However, the diagnosis of DVT must be established or excluded by an objective test, before anticoagulation therapy is initiated.

Objective methods for the diagnosis of DVT include both invasive and noninvasive tests. Venography is regarded by many as the gold standard test. Venography produces significant patient discomfort with a low but real risk of potentially serious complications from the contrast injection. Generally accepted incidences are: anaphylactoid reaction 0.1%, contrast reactions 5–8%, fatalities 1/40,000. The incidence of post-phlebographic DVT that is clinically symptomatic and venographically proven is 2–13%. No significant difference has been found between non-ionic and ionic contrast media of comparable concentration with respect to the incidence of this complication. Contrast-induced DVT may be reduced by the infusion of heparin (1000 units in 250 mL of saline) through the venous access site before termination. The expense and discomfort of venography precludes its use for screening and follow-up evaluations of DVT.

Although the indirect noninvasive tests for venous disease provide useful information in the clinical setting, continuous wave Doppler examination, impedance plethysmography, and phleborheography share three general deficiencies. First, they do not differentiate between DVT and other causes of venous obstruction. Second, they cannot reliably detect isolated thrombi in the calf vein. Third, they do not identify thrombi in the more proximal deep veins.

Duplex ultrasonographic imaging, a direct noninvasive test, provides the ability to image the deep venous system with visualization of venous flow characteristics and venous valve cusp movements and to characterize acute deep vein thrombus. Acute thrombus may be differentiated from chronic thrombus, according to the clot echogenicity and vein wall changes, using real time B-mode ultrasonic imaging. Selective evaluation of flow patterns is done by Doppler ultrasonography. Color flow imaging identifies immediately the presence or absence of venous flow and obviates the need for compression maneuvers in the presence of echolucent thrombus. Color flow Doppler helps to distinguish veins from arteries, minimizes use of spectral analysis, and greatly facilitates identification of tibial and peroneal veins. Duplex scanning is especially helpful in precisely documenting the location and severity of reflux often associated with chronic deep vein thrombosis. The use of color flow duplex scanning to detect deep vein thrombosis enjoys an overall sensitivity and specificity greater than 90%, respectively. This safe, reliable, and cost-effective test is best performed by skilled personnel who have established standards of accuracy for their examinations compared against venography.

In addition to ultrasonography, current MRI scanning provides another noninvasive direct examination of the deep venous system that can be used safely in patients with allergies to dye or with impaired renal function, since intravenous contrast agents are not used. MRI can detect thrombi in the pelvic veins when bowel gas or adiposity preclude accurate assessment by color flow duplex imaging.

The acute sequelae resulting from DVT are the obstructed venous segments. The venous resistance increases, causing the most significant increase in peripheral venous pressure. The venous resistance is dependent on the location, length, and number of venous segments obstructed, as well as the adequacy of preexisting collateral channels.

When quietly standing erect, patients with acute phlebitis have foot pressures that are not essentially different from persons without phlebitis. With exercise, however, ambulatory venous pressure drops below 50% of the pre-exercise pressure in normal subjects, while in limbs with phlebitis there is little fall in ambulatory venous pressure. Venous volume and pressure increases in the phlebitic leg, secondary to thrombotic venous obstruction and valvular incompetence. The musculovenous pump mechanism cannot maintain a balanced arterial inflow and venous outflow. The normal and important low pressure period for the calf during exercise is shortened and reduced in magnitude. As a result of this increased venous pressure, there is a concomitant increase in mean capillary pressure, leading to the formation of edema. The degree of swelling is proportional to the rise in venous pressure.

The fate of thrombi after the initial formation is incompletely understood. Studies of acute deep venous thrombosis suggest that venous thrombi undergo a dynamic evolution early after the acute event. Since there is a delicate balance between the coagulation and fibrinolytic systems, this balance might easily be tipped to rethrombosis by continuing stimuli for coagulation, by hypercoagulable states, or by fibrinolytic deficiencies. Recanalization proceeds rapidly in most patients while, simultaneously, this process is balanced by the potential for propagation of thrombus if the thrombotic stimulus remains. Early complete recanalization after acute DVT has been determined to be an important predictor of ultimate valve function in all segments except the posterior tibial vein. For venous segments developing post-thrombotic reflux, the median lysis times were 2.3–7.3 times longer than median lysis times for corresponding venous segments in which valve function was preserved. A small number of patients developed reflux despite early lysis (< 1 month). Conversely, some segments with relatively late lysis (> 9–12 months) will not develop reflux. The possibility of subsequent thrombotic events could explain these observations. Extension of thrombus to contralateral uninvolved segments and rethrombosis of involved segments occur somewhat later, in all but the most proximal venous segments.

Identifying patients at risk for propagation and rethrombosis and preventing their occurrence are important in preventing post-thrombotic syndrome. Unfortunately, to date no clinical or laboratory markers have been identified for thrombus propagation and rethrombosis in patients with DVT. The post-thrombotic syndrome develops in up to 60% of the patients with occluded proximal segments, popliteal to inferior vena cava, with documented valvular incompetence. The remaining 40% of patients with the post-thrombotic syndrome will have normal valve function.

The treatment of DVT has been fairly standard. Immediately after an objective diagnosis, intravenous heparin is started, beginning with a bolus (100 units/kg) followed by continuous intravenous infusion to maintain partial thromboplastin times (PTT) 1.5–2.5 times control values. Prompt and adequate initiation of anticoagulation for acute DVT may also play a role in decreasing the incidence of post-thrombotic syndrome. When inadequate anticoagulation exists for 24 hours or more after the diagnosis is established and treatment is begun, recurrent thromboembolism occurs 15 times more frequently. The patient is started on warfarin as soon as they are therapeutic on heparin. Warfarin therapy is monitored with use of the International Normalized Ratio (INR) system for 3 months in patients with a first episode of proximal venous thrombosis and longer for recurrent thrombosis. Average rates of recurrence are reported to be as high as 20% within 6 months of discontinuation of anticoagulation. There is a need to define the persistent risk factors in patients treated for a first episode of venous thromboembolism so that oral anticoagulation can be continued longer in selected patients at risk for recurrent DVT.

SUGGESTED READING

Bergen JJ, Goldman MP: *Varicose Veins and Telangiectasias: Diagnosis and Treatment.* Quality Medical Publishers, 1993.

Bergen JJ, Yao JS: *Venous Disorders.* Saunders, 1991.

Eklöf B et al: *Controversies in the Management of Venous Disorders.* Butterworth, 1989.

Gardner AM, Fox RH: *Return of Blood to the Heart*, 2nd ed. John Libbey, 1993.

Sumner D: Hemodynamics and pathophysiology of venous disease. In: Rutherford RB (editor): *Vascular Surgery,* 4th ed. Saunders, 1995.

Tibbs DT: Venous disorders, vascular malformations, and chronic ulcerations in the lower limbs. In: Morris PJ, Malt RA (editors): *Oxford Textbook of Surgery.* Oxford University Press, 1994.

39.7 Management of Major Vessel Trauma

E. John Harris, Jr, MD

► Key Facts

- ► Penetrating trauma accounts for 90% of arterial injuries. The remaining 10% are due to blunt trauma.

- ► The incidence of limb morbidity and the amputation rate rises when hard signs of vascular injury (the five "*P*'s") are overlooked.

- ► The most common types of vessel injury are laceration, partial wall injury, complete disruption, stretch injury, pseudoaneurysm, and arterial venous fistula.

- ► The four major types of vessel repair include ligation, primary repair, resection and anastomosis, and interposition graft.

- ► The neck has been divided into three zones for purposes of diagnosis and management of penetrating injuries. These include: zone I, which is considered the base of the neck; zone II extends cephalad from zone I to the angle of the mandible; zone III extends from zone II to the base of the skull.

- ► General management principles for both penetrating and blunt thoracic vascular injuries include establishment of large-bore venous access in the lower extremities for fluid resuscitation, availability of blood products for the operating room, and a wide sterile field to include at least one groin for potential establishment of extracorporeal bypass through the femoral vessels.

- ► Abdominal injuries present clinically as either free intraperitoneal hemorrhage or as a contained retroperitoneal, mesenteric, perinephric, or pelvic hematoma.

- ► Popliteal artery injuries are often associated with blunt trauma to the knee and should be suspected in all patients with knee dislocations, proximal tibial fractures, or supracondylar femoral fractures, and especially in patients with combined femoral shaft and proximal tibial fractures.

GENERAL CONSIDERATIONS

Trauma has become a critical and costly public health problem, and vascular trauma represents a considerable component of the problem. The incidence of vascular trauma is increasing, with the recent rise of violent penetrating trauma among our youth. As a result of improved rapid transport and triage of critically injured patients, many facilities have seen an increase in vascular injuries. Penetrating trauma accounts for 90% of arterial injuries.

The majority of our knowledge regarding the management of penetrating injuries comes from our military experience of the last century, mostly from Vietnam and the Vietnam Vascular Registry. Arterial injuries observed during military conflicts are typically characterized as high-velocity missile injuries and are associated with massive tissue destruction, both along the missile tract and remote from the missile path, as a result of concussive forces and fragmentation of the missile. In contrast, civilian vascular injuries are typically caused by low-velocity weapons, such as handguns, knives, or hand-held instruments. Low-velocity weapons produce injury generally confined to the missile tract, with little destruction of the surrounding tissues. Shotguns can be devastating at close range, but often cause little arterial injury when fired from mid-range. With increasing use of assault weapons in our urban centers, these patterns may change.

Blunt trauma accounts for the remaining 10% of vascular trauma. Blunt vascular injuries result from crushing or stretching forces, most commonly in regions where vascular structures are tethered to bone, tendon, or soft tissues. Fractured bones with displaced fragments and dislocated joints are frequently associated with vascular trauma, often occult on initial evaluation. Deceleration injury is a frequent mechanism for vascular injury.

VESSEL INJURY & REPAIR

SIGNS OF VASCULAR INJURY

The history and physical examination are important tools in the detection of vascular injury. The classic signs of arterial injury rely on the history and physical examination and are characterized by the **five "P's"**: pain, pallor, pulselessness, paralysis, and paresthesias. These signs are typically seen with acute occlusion of poorly collateralized arteries, such as the common femoral or popliteal arteries. In patients with preexistent arterial occlusive disease, these signs may be absent. Therefore, an evaluation of symmetry should be part of the arterial examination. If the noninjured limb has normal pulses, then absence of pulses in the injured limb is significant. If the noninjured limb has absent distal pulses, physical examination of the injured limb

alone is less helpful. A supplemental objective vascular assessment of the two limbs is often indicated and may vary from Doppler-derived ankle-brachial indices to duplex ultrasonographic arterial evaluations to arteriography.

Patients with massive bleeding, an expanding or pulsatile hematoma, obvious signs of ischemia (as outlined by the five "P's"), absent or diminished distal pulses, or a bruit or thrill in the region of injury should be taken directly to the operating room for exploration without additional delay for diagnostic evaluations. In the setting of penetrating extremity trauma, these five "hard signs" are predictive of a vascular injury that requires surgical repair. Active external hemorrhage should be controlled with direct pressure over the site of hemorrhage to preserve collateral flow that would be disrupted with application of a tourniquet. Blind placement of vascular clamps into a bleeding wound is condemned, as this practice often exacerbates the vascular injuries. Embedded or impaling weapons should be left undisturbed until the patient is in the operating room. Removal of these objects often precipitates major hemorrhage. Intraoperative angiography should be available to assist in the management of vascular injuries of the extremities. The incidence of limb morbidity and the amputation rate rise when these hard signs of vascular injury on initial examination are overlooked and diagnosis is further delayed by superfluous evaluations.

For patients with stable vital signs and without active bleeding or acute, limb-threatening ischemia, time is available to more carefully evaluate softer signs of vascular injury as one completes a secondary survey of the patient to prioritize treatment of associated injuries. The physical examination is not as reliable an indicator of vascular injury in the setting of blunt trauma as it is with penetrating trauma. Soft signs of vascular injury include small, stable hematomas in proximity to a vascular structure, injury to an adjacent nerve, unexplained hypotension, a history of hemorrhage at the scene of injury that is not observed in the trauma center, and proximity of a wound to a major vascular structure. Historically, many of these soft signs prompted either surgical exploration or diagnostic angiography, yet a disappointing relationship between these soft signs and extremity vascular injuries was realized. In most instances, these signs were associated with injuries to nearby bone, nerve, muscle, or soft tissues and were only coincidentally present in cases of vascular injury. Currently, the clinical significance of these soft signs remains unclear, and the value of therapies based on these signs alone is debatable.

TYPES OF VESSEL INJURY

Laceration

Simple arterial lacerations do not cause distal ischemia because the vessel remains patent. The typical laceration is full thickness and leads to continued hemorrhage, as the vessel cannot constrict to prevent continued hemorrhage.

Partial Wall Injury

A more substantial laceration can lead to lateral wall disruption; yet, again, the remaining intact vascular wall prevents retraction and thrombosis of the injured ends. Both the simple and severe vessel lacerations commonly present with active hemorrhage or large or pulsatile hematomas.

Complete Disruption

With complete disruption of the arterial wall, the transected ends usually retract, constrict, and thrombose. These patients typically do not show signs of hemorrhage, but rather present with distal ischemia. The arteriographic appearance is one of occlusion and rarely does contrast extravasate from the transected artery.

Stretch Injury

With long bone fractures and joint dislocations, the adjacent artery is often stretched. Different layers of the arterial wall have different compliances, especially as the arteries become atherosclerotic. The adventitia usually remains intact but the intima is frequently torn or completely transected. Intramural hematomas may form, which lead to intimal compression, which can progress to complete occlusion with distal ischemia. Intimal tears can become dissections as the flowing blood elevates the flap and it folds into the lumen to occlude the vessel.

Pseudoaneurysm

The periarterial tissues can often constrict the hemorrhage from a lacerated or punctured artery. This contained hemorrhage is known as a pseudoaneurysm. Pseudoaneurysms may enlarge over time, with risk of rupture associated with continued expansion. Adjacent structures are often compressed, and the compression of these structures can cause symptoms, such as pain or paresthesia. Adjacent venous structures can become obstructed by the mass effect, causing venous outflow obstruction. Typically, there is laminated clot along the wall of the pseudoaneurysm, with to-and-fro blood flow into the pseudoaneurysm from the puncture or laceration site.

Arterial Venous Fistula

Arterial venous (AV) fistulas may develop when there are concomitant arterial and venous injuries in adjacent vessels. The arterial hemorrhage preferentially flows into the venous segment because there is less resistance to flow than in the periarterial space. Pseudoaneurysms can erode into adjacent veins, again leading to AV fistula formation. With both pseudoaneurysm and AV fistula, distal perfusion is intact. The arteriographic appearance of early venous filling is pathognomonic of an AV fistula (Figure 39.7–1).

VESSEL REPAIRS

Ligation

Ligation of the severed ends of arterial segments is the simplest form of repair. Ligation is usually reserved for situations where exsanguination is possible in a patient with multiple critical injuries. In this setting, distal ischemia is acceptable in order to save the patient's life. More commonly, ligation is used for laceration or transection of distal arterial segments when alternative collateral routes are uninjured. A radial artery can be ligated with an intact palmar arch and patent ulnar artery. Similarly, one or two tibial arteries can be ligated below the tibioperoneal trunk if the remaining tibial vessel is patent. If operative exploration is required for other injuries and the patient is otherwise stable, arterial repair rather than ligation is recommended.

Primary Repair

Primary repair is usually reserved for small simple arterial lacerations, where the primary closure does not narrow the vessel lumen more than 25%. Typical injuries repaired primarily include arterial lacerations from catheters and sheaths. The injured wall is debrided prior to closure, usually with interrupted sutures. Proximal and distal arterial control assures adequate debridement and secure closure of the injured arterial segment. For larger lacerations and for partial wall injuries, patch angioplasty is recommended, typically with autogenous vein as the patch material. Patch angioplasty allows repair without reduction in the diameter of the vessel.

Resection & Anastomosis

If the area of vessel injury is limited to a short segment, resection of the area of injury, mobilization of the vessel proximally and distally, and primary anastomosis is appropriate. The debrided vessel ends can be cut perpendicular to the long axis of the vessel or beveled to allow a larger anastomotic circumference. The key to this type of repair is adequate mobilization to assure the anastomosis is tension-free. If branch vessels tether the injured vessel during mobilization, they should not be divided to allow mobilization, as this destroys an important source of collateralization should the repair fail.

Interposition Graft

For vessel injury where debridement of the injured area leaves a large defect, interposition grafting is employed. In most trauma settings, autogenous vein is the preferred conduit. Vein is harvested from a noninjured limb to preserve as much venous outflow in the injured limb as possible. Depending upon the arterial segment to be replaced, saphenous vein is usually reversed and interposed in end-to-end fashion to the debrided ends of the vessel. For larger-caliber proximal arterial segments, the vein can be opened longitudinally and sewn into a panel graft or a spi-

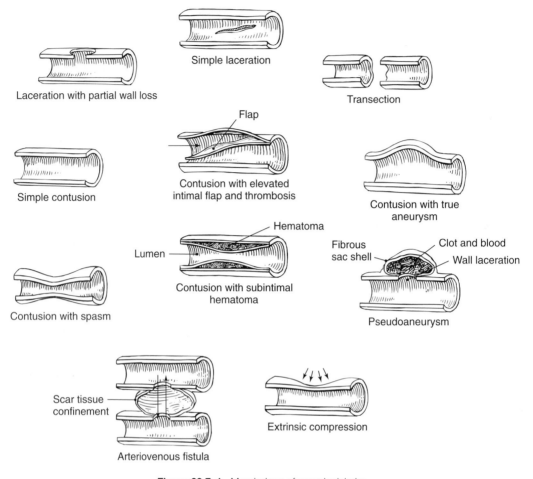

Figure 39.7–1. Morphology of vascular injuries.

ral graft with running monofilament suture to increase the diameter of the vein graft.

Both grafts are created over some form of stent, with the panel graft formed by two running longitudinal suture lines, effectively doubling the diameter of the vein graft. The spiral graft is formed by wrapping the opened vein in a spiral around a stent and running a continuous spiral suture along the edges to create a conduit the diameter of the chosen stent. These grafts are then interposed in the injured vessel. Prosthetic grafts are rarely used in the trauma setting because of their increased risk for graft infection.

VESSEL REPAIR ADJUNCTS

Extra-Anatomic Bypass

Vascular trauma often occurs in association with local tissue loss or adjacent organ injury, leading to potentially contaminated fields for the vascular repair. In this setting, the vessel repair may be exposed to a hostile environment

if carried out in situ. Extra-anatomic bypass is used in these situations. The area of vessel injury is thoroughly debrided and the vessel ligated, usually with monofilament suture in a mattress technique. A bypass is then extended from healthy tissue planes above and below the ligated vessel, to complete the bypass. Thus, the graft and both anastomoses are placed in nontraumatized tissues. Examples include the axillary femoral bypass, the femerofemoral bypass, and an iliac-femoral bypass routed through the obturator foramen. As these bypass grafts typically do not involve violated or infected planes, one can use a prosthetic graft conduit.

Indwelling Shunt

Vessel injuries occurring in association with extremity injuries are difficult to manage because the limb is often unstable as a result of multiple long bone fractures or joint instability. If the limb is critically ischemic from a vascular injury, vascular repair takes precedence before orthopedic stabilization. Orthopedic stabilization facilitates arterial repairs, especially when an interposition graft must be used, and there is a potential for length discrepancy in the graft when the extremity is not stabilized. In this situation, the arterial injury can be explored, the vessel debrided, and an intraluminal shunt placed. The limb is reperfused, the orthopedic stabilization proceeds, and the definitive vascular repair is accomplished once the limb is stable.

Management of Venous Injury

Techniques for venous repair are identical to those for arterial repair. In venous injuries, size mismatch between the saphenous vein and the injured vein is often more severe than in arterial injury. In venous injury without associated arterial injury, ligation is most frequently employed. Ligation is better tolerated in the upper extremity compared to the lower extremity because of a superior collateral network in the upper extremity. Repairs of venous injuries do not increase the risk for deep venous thrombosis or pulmonary embolus.

With combined arterial and venous injuries, repair of the venous injury is indicated. Simultaneous repair of the venous injury improves the results of the arterial repair. Although venous repairs, especially interposition grafts, often fail in the early postoperative period, there are a significant number of repairs that will recanalize in the intermediate postoperative period, with improvement in long-term disability from venous hypertension.

Fasciotomy

Fascial sheaths within the extremities confine muscle groups, their supporting bones, blood vessels, and nerves into osteofascial compartments. A **compartment syndrome** develops when pressure within one of these osteofascial compartments rises, leading to impeded nerve conduction and blood flow through the compartment. If pressures within the compartment exceed arterial inflow pressures, especially in situations of multiple injuries with systemic hypotension, the structures within the compartment can become ischemic. Soft tissue trauma with hemorrhage into the compartment, reperfusion injury following warm limb ischemia, and venous outflow obstruction may all lead to increased compartment pressures. In a traumatized limb, all three situations are often present. Although most commonly seen in the lower leg, compartment syndromes may be seen in the buttock, thigh, foot, upper arm, forearm, or hand. Although individual compartment pressures can be easily measured, the knowledge and equipment necessary to measure compartment pressures is often unavailable. The diagnosis relies significantly on a high index of suspicion and clinical signs, such as pain with passive motion and paresthesias of nerves coursing through the compartment. Loss of arterial pulses is a terminal event, therefore, presence of arterial pulses does not exclude the diagnosis. When measured, compartment pressures above 30–40 mm Hg are diagnostic. Fasciotomy should be performed liberally in extremity vascular injuries, especially when there is extensive soft

tissue trauma, concomitant arterial and venous injuries, or prolonged warm ischemic time prior to revascularization.

PENETRATING NECK TRAUMA

DIAGNOSIS

The overwhelming majority of vascular trauma in the neck is secondary to penetrating injuries, the majority of which are related to gunshot wounds. Injury to the common carotid artery is most frequent, followed by injury to the internal carotid, then the external carotid arteries. Injuries to the vertebral arteries are rare, yet the majority of these are related to penetrating trauma. Associated venous injuries are seen in roughly one third of the cases. Associated injuries most commonly cause mortality in patients with penetrating neck trauma. Injuries to the aerodigestive tract are less frequent than vascular injuries, but all patients with penetrating neck trauma should be evaluated for these potential injuries.

Physical examination remains important in the diagnosis of penetrating vascular injury. The presence of crepitation, hoarseness, or stridor are highly associated with a positive finding at neck exploration. A cervical bruit, especially in a patient less than 50 years of age, and a cervical hematoma are significant physical findings. Neurological deficit contralateral to the side of neck injury, and Horner's syndrome or dysfunction of cranial nerves IX–XII ipsilateral to the side of neck injury, may or may not be present.

For purposes of diagnosis and management of penetrating injuries, the neck has been divided into three anatomic zones (Figure 39.7–2). The definition of zone I has been variably described, but should be considered as the base of the neck. Some choose the cricothyroid membrane as the margin, others the heads of the clavicle, but the zone includes wounds directed toward the chest with the potential for injury to innominate, subclavian, and common carotid arteries. Zone II extends cephalad from zone I to the angle of the mandible. Zone III extends from zone II to the base of the skull.

MANAGEMENT

Arteriography is an important step in the management of penetrating vascular injuries in zones I and III, as vascular injuries in these regions are difficult to expose surgically, and arteriography is essential in formulating an operative plan versus a potential interventional radiologic procedure. If the patient is hemodynamically stable, then arteriography is mandatory for penetrating vascular injuries in zones I and III.

The presence of active external hemorrhage or an expanding cervical hematoma with the potential for airway

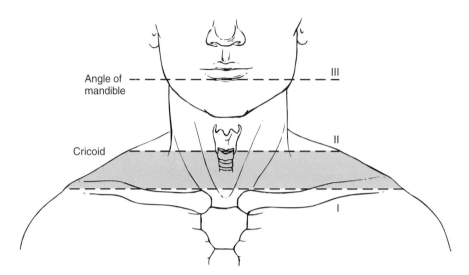

Figure 39.7–2. Anatomic zones of the neck. Zone III is above the angle of the jaw *(dotted line)*. The shaded area depicts the variable border between the sternal notch and the cricothyroid membrane used to define zone I caudally and zone II cephalad.

obstruction mandates immediate surgical exploration, without preoperative arteriography and regardless of zone of injury. For zone I injuries, this requires inclusion of the chest in the surgical field, where potential sternotomy, thoracotomy, or both may be required to gain proximal arterial control.

Penetrating vascular injuries of zone II most frequently involve the common carotid artery, and this vessel is easily exposed surgically. Most advocate immediate surgical exploration for zone II injuries that penetrate the platysma muscle layer. If the patient is stable, without enlarging hematoma or obvious external hemorrhage, others are more selective with operation. Noninvasive carotid duplex ultrasonography has recently been used to define vascular injuries in this setting. Others recommend arteriography, which, of course, will not define all venous injuries. If a selective nonoperative approach is employed with zone II injuries, similar evaluation of the aerodigestive tract with panendoscopy and radiologic esophageal imaging is recommended. Small intimal defects and pseudoaneurysms less than 5 mm in diameter are safely followed with serial carotid duplex examinations. Intimal flaps, larger pseudoaneurysms, and lacerations of the carotid arteries detected by imaging studies should then undergo standard operative repair.

Operative repair is recommended for all penetrating injuries of the carotid artery except in situations where the patient has preoperative evidence of a dense neurologic deficit, or the patient is neurologically intact and the carotid artery is occluded. Penetrating carotid artery injuries are repaired in standard fashion as described earlier. Vein graft interposition grafts are frequently required, therefore, one should prepare a limb for vein harvest in anticipation prior to any exploration for penetrating vas-

cular injuries of the neck. More recently, expanded polytetrafluoroethylene (ePTFE) grafts have been used as interposition grafts for carotid artery injuries. Although synthetic grafts have a theoretically higher risk for graft infection than autologous tissue with penetrating vascular trauma, this risk has not been realized with increasing experience with these grafts.

For patients with preoperative neurological deficit and arterial injury, ligation is recommended. For patients with normal preoperative neurological examination and either a carotid artery occlusion detected by vascular imaging study, or an occlusion diagnosed intraoperatively during exploration, intermediate-term (3–6 months) anticoagulation is recommended. The anticoagulation is used to prevent thrombus propagation up the internal carotid artery into the middle cerebral artery, a potential complication of acute carotid artery occlusions. Attempts at recanalization of the occluded artery are discouraged, as they often increase the risk for development of neurological deficits.

With more frequent use of arteriography and Duplex scanning in penetrating vascular injuries of the neck, vertebral artery injures have been recognized more frequently. Because of their paired contribution to basilar arterial blood flow, unilateral vertebral artery injuries rarely cause symptoms of vertebrobasilar ischemia. Since they are located in the vertebral foramina surrounded by a significant amount of soft tissue, exsanguination from vertebral arterial injuries is rare. Because of the difficult and often hazardous exposure of the majority of the vertebral artery and the paucity of ischemic symptoms following unilateral occlusion of a vertebral artery, ligation rather than repair was historically advised for vertebral artery injuries. More recently, fluoroscopically guided embolization of the injured vertebral artery by interventional radiologists is recommended. Embolization proximal and distal to the site of vertebral artery injury is possible, although not always necessary, since proximal interruption alone may often be sufficient to induce distal thrombosis. Occlusive injuries to the vertebral artery are observed. Primary repair of vertebral artery injuries is employed only when the contralateral vertebral artery is congenitally absent, hypoplastic, or injured. Discussion of repair techniques for vertebral artery injuries is beyond the scope of this chapter.

VASCULAR INJURIES OF THE CHEST

DIAGNOSIS

With the successful development of emergency medical systems for effective prehospital rapid triage of critically injured patients, more patients with critical truncal vascular injuries are surviving long enough to arrive in trauma centers for resuscitation and operative salvage. In urban trauma centers, 90% of thoracic vascular injuries are related to penetrating trauma, and 10% are related to blunt chest trauma.

For penetrating chest trauma, arteriography is essential in hemodynamically stable patients. The roles of contrast enhanced spiral computed tomography (CT) scans and transesophageal echocardiography (TEE) as diagnostic tools for vascular injury in penetrating chest trauma remain incompletely defined, but in experienced centers the results with these techniques are promising. In patients who present with penetrating chest trauma and hypotension, resuscitation with large-bore intravenous lines in the lower extremities is initiated. Those who are resuscitated to a point where systolic blood pressure can be maintained above 70 mm Hg should be transported to the operating room for emergent thoracotomy, sternotomy, or supraclavicular exploration, or a combination of these approaches (Figure 39.7–3). There should be no delay in heading to the operating room for an arteriogram. In patients in whom resuscitation fails to maintain a systolic blood pressure greater than 70 mm Hg, emergency department thoracotomy is indicated. In hemodynamically stable patients, arteriography defines the injured vessels and allows precise planning of the operative intervention.

Diagnosis of blunt chest vascular injuries requires a high index of suspicion. Blunt injuries of the chest cause deceleration tears of the descending thoracic aorta (DTA) at the level just caudal to the origin of the left subclavian artery and of the innominate artery at its origin. Nonrestrained patients in motor vehicle accidents can sustain deceleration injuries of the ascending aorta, yet these tears are almost universally lethal at the scene. Blunt deceleration injuries of the DTA are the most frequent vascular injuries treated in patients with blunt chest trauma, with autopsy series detecting DTA disruption in as many as 15%

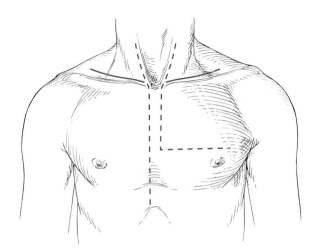

Figure 39.7–3. Cervicothoracic lines of incision for repair of arterial and venous injuries at the base of the neck and in the chest to the innominate artery or veins, common carotid arteries, jugular veins, subclavian arteries and veins, superior vena cava, ascending and transverse arch of the aorta, and the pulmonary arteries.

of victims of fatal motor vehicle accidents. Eighty to ninety percent of patients with DTA transection die at the scene of injury. If these patients arrive at the hospital alive, and the lesion is undetected, one third will die within 24 hours if untreated.

Findings obtained from the patient's history that are suggestive of injury to one of the great vessels include deceleration, usually from speeds in excess of 40–45 miles per hour, and a severe broadside collision. Great vessel injury can occur whether or not a shoulder harness was worn, with innominate, carotid, and subclavian injuries more common with deceleration in restrained passengers, and DTA injury more common with deceleration in unrestrained passengers. Physical examination findings suggestive of blunt aortic transection include pulse asymmetry between the two upper extremities or upper and lower extremities, or unexplained systemic hypotension. Due to the magnitude of the blunt injury, DTA transection is often associated with sternal and rib fractures. Great vessel injuries may present with supraclavicular hematomas.

Chest x-ray provides the most important diagnostic signs of blunt vascular injury, which include a superior mediastinum that is widened to more than 8–9 cm, an obscured or indistinct aortic knob, apical capping, or pleural effusion or hemothorax. With DTA transection, the left main-stem bronchus may be depressed, the trachea may be deviated to the right, or the nasogastric tube (ie, esophagus) may be deviated to the right. Mediastinal widening may be misleading, and films obtained in a supine position should be repeated with the patient upright and leaning slightly forward, if the spine has been cleared for fractures and dislocations. Thoracic spine fractures may mimic DTA transection on plain chest x-ray. Normal chest x-rays may also be seen with DTA transection.

In a stable patient with a possible blunt thoracic vascular injury, further diagnostic evaluation is recommended. The most commonly performed study is transfemoral aortography, to include the aortic arch and DTA. With diminished femoral pulses, a transaxillary approach may be necessary. More recently, contrast-enhanced spiral CT scanning and transesophageal echocardiography (TEE) have been used to detect blunt thoracic vascular injuries with good results. Contrast-enhanced CT scans may potentially miss small aortic tears because of artifact from vessel ectasia. TEE can be performed in the emergency room and can image the thoracic aorta in a continuous fashion; preliminary reports suggest high sensitivity and specificity for TEE in the detection of thoracic aortic tears. Further prospective studies of these new diagnostic modalities are necessary before widespread application can be recommended. To date, a thoracic aortogram remains the gold standard for diagnosis of blunt thoracic vascular injuries.

MANAGEMENT

General management principles for both penetrating and blunt thoracic vascular injuries include establishment of large-bore venous access in the lower extremities for fluid resuscitation, availability of blood products for the operating room, and a wide sterile field to include the entire thorax and neck, the entire abdomen, and at least one groin for potential establishment of extracorporeal bypass through the femoral vessels. Vascular grafts of varying sizes, extravascular heparin-bonded shunts, cardiopulmonary bypass machine, and a centrifugal pump for partial bypass should all be available. Proximal and distal arterial control is obtained prior to entering any hematoma surrounding a great vessel.

Penetrating thoracic vascular injuries are usually treated by debridement and patch angioplasty if partial wall injury is sustained. Great vessel injuries are repaired primarily whenever feasible, yet most injuries will require graft insertion following adequate debridement of the injured wall. Interposition grafts of Dacron or ePTFE are used for innominate, subclavian, or proximal common carotid arterial injuries, both blunt and penetrating, with the proximal graft originating from the ascending aorta in end-to-side fashion and the distal anastomosis end-to-end following transection distal to the area of injury. The origin of the great vessel is oversewn on the aortic arch. Blunt injury to the DTA is repaired primarily if possible, but most tears are treated with a short interposition graft of Dacron. Techniques for repair range from the so-called "clamp and go" method, to hypothermic cardiac arrest with cardiopulmonary bypass. The issue is spinal cord perfusion and protection during repair of the thoracic aorta. Discussion of the various techniques for cord protection are beyond the scope of this chapter. DTA transection should be repaired by a surgeon experienced in thoracic vascular procedures.

ABDOMINAL VASCULAR TRAUMA

DIAGNOSIS

Midline abdominal vascular injuries involve the abdominal aorta and the inferior vena cava, including the retrohepatic vena cava, the mesenteric arteries and veins, and the hepatic artery and portal vein. Lateral abdominal vascular injuries predominantly involve the renal arteries and veins. Pelvic vascular injuries involve the iliac arteries and veins. Abdominal vascular injuries rarely occur as isolated injuries and are frequently associated with hollow and solid visceral injuries.

Abdominal vascular injuries are uncommon with blunt abdominal trauma and in patients with penetrating stab wounds, with roughly 10% of patients with each type of injury having a vascular injury as well. Penetrating abdominal trauma from gunshot wounds is more frequently associated with vascular injury, in up to 30–40% of cases. Abdominal vascular injuries present clinically as either free intraperitoneal hemorrhage or as a contained retroperitoneal, mesenteric, perinephric, or pelvic hematoma. Most often, the diagnosis of abdominal vascular injury is made at laparotomy rather than preoperatively, as the urgency for laparotomy is clear in most patients. Abdominal vascular injury should be suspected in any patient with a penetrating missile wound between the nipples and thighs.

When the abdomen is explored for presumed vascular injury, care should be taken to assure a widely prepped surgical field, from the neck to the knees. Release of the abdominal wall tamponade could lead to sudden decompensation of the patient, therefore, blood should be available in the operating room, and large-bore intravenous access in the arms or shoulders should be obtained for ongoing resuscitation. Autotransfusion equipment and rapid infusion devices with warming capacity are useful adjunctive measures for patients with abdominal vascular injuries.

In patients who have suffered penetrating wounds to the upper abdomen and are not in profound shock, a rapid one-shot intravenous pyelogram (IVP) should be performed on the way to the operating room, especially if hematuria is identified. In patients with blunt abdominal trauma and hematuria, a contrast-enhanced abdominal CT scan provides more information on potential renal trauma than the IVP. Contrast-enhanced abdominal-pelvic CT scans also define pelvic hematomas often associated with blunt pelvic fractures. In unstable patients with suspected abdominal vascular injuries, time must not be wasted on unnecessary diagnostic tests or futile attempts at stabilization in the emergency department.

MANAGEMENT

Injuries to the abdominal vasculature are similar to those previously described and are repaired in a similar manner. The most critical issue is control of active hemorrhage, if present. When the abdomen is entered, the four quadrants are packed to tamponade any hemorrhage from visceral injuries. If massive hemorrhage is encountered, the surgeon should obtain proximal aortic control before searching for a specific injury site. The most common method is aortic control of the supraceliac aorta as it emerges from the diaphragmatic crura. The lesser sac is opened, the esophagus retracted medially, and either direct pressure with a stick sponge or aortic occluder is applied, or the left crus is divided and a vascular clamp is applied across the aorta.

Central hematomas should be explored to rule out potential injuries to the aorta and its branches and to the vena cava and its branches. Medial visceral rotation is the usual maneuver employed to expose the midline vasculature from a transperitoneal midline incision. The left kidney can be rotated or left down, depending upon specific injuries. Most aortic injuries are repaired primarily. If extensive debridement is necessary, interposition grafts are employed unless there is gross contamination in the field. In this setting, the aorta is debrided, then the healthy ends are oversewn in two layers and an extra-anatomic bypass is performed through clean tissue planes. Caval injuries are repaired by lateral venorrhaphy, or ePTFE interposition grafts for large defects. Avulsions of the celiac artery can be safely ligated in young patients. Injuries to the superior mesenteric artery (SMA) injuries can be treated by primary repair with a bypass from uninvolved aorta to uninvolved SMA, or by transposition of the SMA to a more inferior position on the aorta. Inferior mesenteric arterial injuries can usually be treated by ligation.

Perinephric hematomas are not explored if they are not expanding and there is perfusion of the involved kidney on preoperative IVP or CT scan. Expanding perinephric hematomas should be explored with standard repair of identified injuries. In unstable patients with an injured kidney, no ipsilateral perfusion on preoperative imaging and contralateral kidney perfusion, nephrectomy rather than vascular repair is indicated. Renal arterial injuries with less than 4–6 hours of warm ischemia should be repaired in otherwise stable patients.

Pelvic hematomas associated with blunt trauma are usually not explored. Persistent bleeding from pelvic hematomas associated with pelvic fractures is best treated by radiologically guided embolization of the bleeding site, which is identified on arteriography. Pelvic hematomas associated with penetrating trauma should be explored; these injuries are associated with a high mortality rate. Ligation of iliac arterial injuries is associated with a prohibitive rate of limb loss. If ligation is necessary to arrest the hemorrhage, extra-anatomic bypass should be completed once the hemorrhage is controlled. Extra-anatomic bypass, such as a femorofemoral bypass, should also be used when in situ repair would occur in a contaminated field. Care must be maintained to avoid injury to the adjacent ureter and iliac veins when they are not initially injured. Repair of the iliac veins is often problematic, especially on the left side, as the vein lies directly behind the iliac artery. Attempts at proximal and distal control often lead to more tearing of these large veins. The left iliac artery can be divided to gain acces to the left iliac vein, and once the venous injury is controlled, the artery can be reapproximated primarily.

VASCULAR INJURIES ASSOCIATED WITH BLUNT KNEE TRAUMA

DIAGNOSIS

Popliteal arterial injuries are often associated with blunt trauma to the knee and should be suspected in all patients with knee dislocations, proximal tibial fractures, or supracondylar femoral fractures, and especially in patients with combined femoral shaft and proximal tibial fractures (the so-called "floating knee") (Figure 39.7–4). Vascular injuries may or may not be clinically apparent following blunt knee trauma; often, documentation of the vascular status of a patient presenting with severe lower extremity orthopedic trauma is inadequate. The most common cause of delay in treatment is failure to recognize the severity of ischemia. The contralateral limb, if uninjured, should always be used as a reference. Often the patient will have a history of intermittent pulses in the injured limb or return of distal pulses with reduction of the fracture or dislocation. Popliteal arterial injuries associated with blunt knee trauma cannot be ruled out by clinical examination alone, for as many as 50% of patients with documented major arterial damage will present initially with intact distal pulses.

Arteriography is critical in the diagnosis of arterial injuries associated with blunt knee trauma. If the injury to the lower limb is isolated, and the patient is otherwise stable, then biplanar arteriograms in the radiology suite give the most information. With multiple fractures of an extremity, the area of arterial injury is not always adjacent to the fracture site; there may be more than one site of popliteal arterial injury, therefore, complete lower limb runoff is essential. In patients presenting with clear evidence of distal limb ischemia following blunt knee trauma, arteriography is performed in the operating room.

MANAGEMENT

Popliteal arterial injuries following blunt trauma to the knee vary from small intimal defects without flow restriction to complete transection with retraction and thrombosis of the ends of the popliteal artery. The patient should

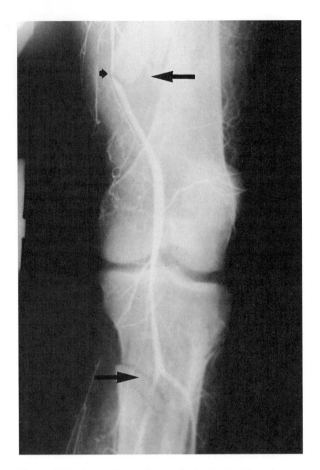

Figure 39.7–4. Arteriogram in a patient with blunt knee trauma following a "floating knee." **Large arrows:** The femur fracture sites. **Small arrow:** Attenuation of the popliteal artery where it is stretched by the displaced femur fragment.

have both lower extremities included in the operative field, from abdomen to toes. The operating room should have fluoroscopy for both operative angiography and to assist orthopedic fixation of the skeletal injuries. When obvious limb ischemia is present, arterial repair takes priority over skeletal fixation. In the rare instance where the lower limb is severely unstable due to multiple fractures, and will require multiple levels of skeletal stabilization,

temporary shunting of the popliteal artery is a useful adjunct, with definitive repair to follow skeletal fixation. If arterial repair precedes skeletal fixation, patency of the repair should be confirmed after the fixation procedure and before the patient leaves the operating room.

Standard repair techniques are used to treat popliteal arterial injuries associated with blunt knee trauma. Mobilization of the popliteal artery with resection of the zone of injury and primary anastomosis is often recommended, yet if geniculate branches must be sacrificed to allow adequate mobilization, we favor an interposition vein graft, which preserves a critical potential for collateralization should the repair fail over time. Saphenous vein is the preferred conduit for interposition grafts and can be harvested from the ipsilateral limb if the ipsilateral popliteal vein is not injured. If the ipsilateral popliteal vein is injured, contralateral harvest of the saphenous vein is recommended. Adjunctive balloon thromboembolectomy of the superficial femoral artery and the distal popliteal and runoff is performed after control and debridement of the area of popliteal arterial injury. If the popliteal vein is disrupted, it should be repaired, either primarily or with interposition vein graft.

Primary amputation is rarely recommended, but should be considered in patients with multiple critical injuries and limb ischemia and in patients with skeletal instability, limb ischemia, and loss of tibial or sciatic nerve function. Most of these trauma victims are young, otherwise healthy, males, and they will do better with a below-knee amputation than an insensate reconstructed limb.

Muscle compartments should be frequently monitored before, during, and after arterial reconstructions associated with blunt knee trauma. One's threshold for performing fasciotomy should be low. Postoperative surveillance of the arterial repair should be frequent and should include both physical examination as well as Doppler evaluation of the repair and its outflow.

The amputation rate associated with blunt trauma to the knee remains high, due mostly to delay in diagnosis and management of arterial injuries. Amputation rates are higher when arterial damage is more extensive and requires interposition vein graft. If ischemia is unrecognized or untreated for more than 12 hours, the amputation rate is higher than 50%. Therefore, the key to successful outcome following blunt trauma to the knee is a high index of suspicion for, and early management of, arterial vascular injuries.

SUGGESTED READING

Burch JM et al: Penetrating iliac vascular injuries: Recent experience with 233 consecutive patients. J Trauma 1990;30:1450.

Dennis JW et al: New perspectives on the management of penetrating trauma in proximity to major limb arteries. J Vasc Surg 1990;11:84.

Fabian TC et al: Carotid artery trauma: Management based on mechanism of injury. J Trauma 1990;30:953.

Flannigan DP: *Civilian Vascular Trauma.* Lea & Febiger, 1992.

Frykberg ER et al: Nonoperative observation of clinically occult arterial injuries: A prospective evaluation. Surgery 1991;109:85.

Johansen K et al: Non-invasive vascular tests reliably exclude occult arterial trauma in injured extremities. J Trauma 1991;31:515.

Mattox KL: Thoracic great vessel injury. Surg Clin North Am 1988;68:693.

Mattox KL et al: Five thousand seven hundred sixty cardiovascular injuries in 4459 patients: Epidemiologic evolution 1958–1987. Ann Surg 1989;209:698.

Mukherjee DM, Inahara T: Another use of the shunt in vascular surgery. Am J Surg 1988;146:385.

Nypaver TJ et al: Long-term results of venous reconstruction after vascular trauma in civilian practice. J Vasc Surg 1992; 16:762.

Perry MO et al: Management of arterial injuries. Ann Surg 1971;173:403.

Rich NM et al: Acute arterial injuries in Vietnam: 1,000 cases. J Trauma 1970;10:359.

Roessler MS et al: The mangled extremity: When to amputate. Arch Surg 1991;126:1243.

40

Transplantation

40.1 Historical Perspectives

Donald C. Dafoe, MD

"Gibson and Medawar demonstrated that a second allograft from the same donor was rejected more rapidly than the first . . . the "second set" phenomenon established that the rejection process was not immutable; instead, it implied an allergic or immunological process which potentially might be manipulated."

——Dr Joseph P. Murray, 1990 Nobel Prize acceptance speech, Stockholm

Historians debate two schools of thought to explain the impetus behind progress. One viewpoint is that enlightened and strong-willed individuals seize circumstances and force progress from inertia. The other perspective maintains that interrelated events (eg, social and political) create the conditions for progress, then certain individuals become facilitators at that propitious time. Both schools of thought are well supported by the history of organ transplantation. For example, heart transplantation could not have occurred without cardiopulmonary bypass. Renal transplantation became more feasible because of dialytic support. Sir Peter Medawar and others are credited with the intellectual conceptus that grew into the field of cellular immunology, which then progressed to clinical transplantation (Figure 40.1–1). Collaboration between basic scientists and transplant surgeons was invaluable, as organ transplantation was first addressed in small and large animal models. The persistence of surgical scientists such as Hume, Shumway, and Starzl provided the combination of energy, intellect, and surgical skill to establish clinical transplantation as a highly effective therapeutic modality (Figures 40.1–2, 40.1–3, 40.1–4).

The landmark event that is often cited as the birth of clinical transplantation occurred in 1954 at Peter Bent Brigham Hospital in Boston (Figure 40.1–5). A successful renal transplant was carried out between identical twins. It was, primarily, a technical feat since rejection would not be an issue, given the genetic identity of the donor and recipient. Nevertheless, this bold endeavor established the feasibility of organ replacement therapy. Dr Joseph Murray headed the team that capitalized on an ideal opportunity in anticipation of future renal allotransplantation. An era of cadaver and living-related donor renal transplants followed, using nonspecific forms of global immunosuppression, such as total body irradiation and antiproliferative drugs. The history of clinical transplantation is the gradual unveiling of interwoven facts, theories, and techniques, but the quantum steps in transplantation, superimposed on steady incline of general medical advances, are due to the discovery of immunosuppressive drugs of increasing specificity (Table 40.1–1).

1960s

In the early 1960s, 6-mercaptopurine (6-MP), an antimetabolite that interfered with cell division, was found by Schwartz and Damashek to have immunosuppressive properties. The use of azathioprine, the imidazole derivative of 6-MP, brought about sporadic success in clinical allotransplantation. By the mid-1960s, when azathioprine was coupled with prednisone as maintenance immunosuppression, 50–60% 1-year renal transplant survival rates were reported for cadaver donor grafts and 70–80% for living-related donor grafts. Acute rejection episodes were found to be responsive to high-dose intravenous steroids.

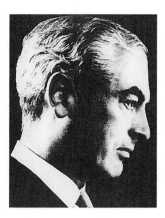

Figure 40.1–1. Sir Peter Medawar (1915–1987). British biologist and 1960 Nobel Laureate. His experimental studies on second-set rejection, cell-mediated immunity, immunosuppressive antibodies, and immunologic tolerance helped to establish the field of transplantation immunology. (Reprinted, with permission, from Terasaki PI: *History of Transplantation: Thirty-Five Recollections.* UCLA Tissue Typing Laboratory, 1991, p. 2.)

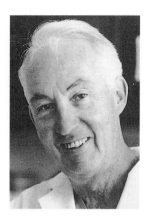

Figure 40.1–3. Norman E. Shumway, MD, PhD (b 1923). Cardiothoracic transplant surgeon. Dr Shumway performed the seminal large animal studies in heart transplantation leading to the first heart transplant in the United States in 1968 at Stanford University Medical Center. Under his guidance, the team at Stanford has done nearly 1000 heart grafts; in the process, many heart transplant surgeons who populate the leadership positions of programs around the globe have received training. (Reprinted, with permission, from Terasaki PI: *History of Transplantation: Thirty-Five Recollections.* UCLA Tissue Typing Laboratory, 1991, p. 436.)

Success in renal transplantation encouraged attempts to transplant other organs (Table 40.1–2). Transplant pioneers were both celebrated and vilified. Their daring actions were justified by the dire condition of their patients and the lack of alternative therapy.

During the 1960s, renal transplant and heart transplant programs proliferated despite high rates of morbidity and mortality. For example, in 1963 the only active renal transplant programs in United States were at the Peter

Bent Brigham Hospital, the Medical College of Virginia, and the University of Colorado; in 1964, there were 25 new programs. Some were not sustained as the glory faded and efforts were stymied by chasms in understanding. About this time, antilymphocyte serum was intro-

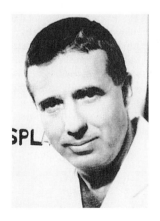

Figure 40.1–2. David M. Hume, MD (1917–1973). Transplant surgeon. As Director of Surgical Research at Harvard from 1951 to 1953, he carried out nine cadaver donor renal transplants in patients with terminal renal failure. Later, when he was Chairman of the Department of Surgery at the Medical College of Virginia, he started one of the early renal transplant programs in the United States. (Reprinted, with permission, from Terasaki PI: *History of Transplantation: Thirty-Five Recollections.* UCLA Tissue Typing Laboratory, 1991, p. 112.)

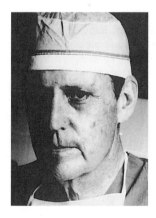

Figure 40.1–4. Thomas E. Starzl, MD, PhD (b 1926). Abdominal organ transplant surgeon. Most notably, Dr Starzl performed the first successful human liver transplant in 1967 and in the 1980s built the largest program in the United States at the University of Pittsburgh. A renowned scientist and prodigious innovator, Dr Starzl has had a major impact on virtually every aspect of transplantation, from inventive techniques to immunobiology. (Reprinted, with permission, from Terasaki PI: *History of Transplantation: Thirty-Five Recollections.* UCLA Tissue Typing Laboratory, 1991, p. 146.)

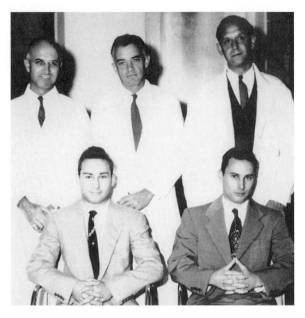

Figure 40.1–5. The main individuals involved in the celebrated first successful renal isograft at the Peter Bent Brigham Hospital in 1954. Richard Herrick, the recipient *(left, seated)* and his brother Ronald Herrick, the donor *(right, seated)*. The physician team was composed of *(left to right)* Dr Joseph Murray, surgeon, Dr John Merrill, nephrologist, and Dr Hartwell Harrison, urologist. Dr Murray won the 1990 Nobel Prize in Medicine for his pioneering work in renal transplantation. (Reprinted, with permission, from Terasaki PI: *History of Transplantation: Thirty-Five Recollections.* UCLA Tissue Typing Laboratory, 1991, p. 128.)

Table 40.1–1. The evolution of clinical immunosuppression.

Agent	Year	Responsible Individual(s)/Site
Total body irradiation	1958	Mannick, Murray[1]/Boston Hamburger/Paris
6-mercaptopurine	1959	Schwartz, Dameshek/Boston Calne[2], Murray/Boston Lee, Zukoski/Richmond
Corticosteroids	1962	Goodwin/Los Angeles Starzl[3]/Denver Kountz/Stanford
Anti-lymphocyte globulin	1966	Waksman, Woodruff/Edinburgh Najarian[4]/San Francisco Monaco, Russell/Boston
Total lymphoid irradiation	1975	Kaplan, Strober/Stanford Levin/San Francisco Myburgh/South Africa
Cyclosporine	1978	Borel/Basel Calne, White/Cambridge Kahan/Houston Starzl/Pittsburgh
OKT3	1980	Goldstein/Raritan Cosimi/Boston
Tacrolimus	1987	Ochiai/Chiba Starzl/Pittsburgh
Mycophenolate mofetil	1990	Nelson/Palo Alto Morris/Stanford Sollinger/Madison

[1]See Figure 40.1–5.
[2]See Figure 40.1–7.
[3]See Figure 40.1–4.
[4]See Figure 40.1–8.

duced. These heterogeneous mixtures of antibodies were produced by injecting human lymphoid cells into horses or rabbits and collecting the animals' serum. One problem was batch-to-batch variation, but the preparations could reverse acute rejection episodes that were unresponsive to high-dose steroids. Scientific and clinical advances challenged societal attitudes and ethics. The concepts of brain death and organ gifting moved from the shadows of mistrust and misunderstanding to legislative codification. Transplant centers with concentrated expertise became Meccas of patient care, clinical training, and research in immunobiology. In the United States, prominent clinical transplant programs, such as the University of Minnesota (Figure 40–6), the University of California at San Francisco, and the University of Pittsburgh, were based on strong laboratory efforts undergirding high-volume clinical efforts.

1970s

Opelz and Terasaki analyzed data from the UCLA Renal Transplant Registry and reported the heretical find-

ing that patients who received multiple random donor blood transfusions had a higher renal allograft acceptance rate. This report generated enthusiasm for a policy of intentional random donor transfusions prior to cadaveric renal transplantation.

A related development was the use of donor-specific transfusions (DSTs) from living-related donors into the prospective recipients as advocated by Dr Oscar Salvatierra of San Francisco. Despite the perceived illogical nature of this approach and the risk of sensitization of the future recipient to donor antigens, better 1-year renal allograft survival was achieved in DST recipients on azathioprine and prednisone immunosuppression. It was reasoned that DSTs either selected out immunologically inharmonious donor-recipient pairs or altered the recipients' immune system by a form of clonal deletion, anti-idiotypic antibody formation, or the induction of suppressor cells.

1980s

In the medical realm, the 1980s has been named the "Decade of Transplantation." Lung transplantation evolved from the first successful en bloc heart/lung transplant by Drs Reitz and Shumway in 1981. Isolated single- or double-lung transplantation was developed, most notably, by the Lung Transplant Group in Toronto. Pancreas transplantation for the treatment of insulin-dependent dia-

Table 40.1–2. The history of first successful vascularized organ allografting.[1]

Transplant	Category	Year	Surgeon(s)	Institution
Kidney	Cadaver D	1945	Hufnagel	PBBH, Boston
	Cadaver D	1946	Hume[2]	PBBH, Boston
	LRD	1951	Kuss	Paris
	Isograft	1954	Murray, Harrison[3]	PBBH, Boston
	LRD	1959	Murray	PBBH, Boston
	Cadaver D	1962	Murray	PBBH, Boston
	Chimpanzee D	1963	Reemtsma	Tulane, New Orleans
	Baboon D	1963	Hitchcock	Minneapolis
	Pediatric R	1963	Najarian[4]	Minneapolis
Liver	Cadaver D	1967	Starzl[5]	Univ Colorado, Denver
	RVG	1984	Bismuth	Villejuif
	LRD RVG	1990	Broelsch	Univ Chicago
	Baboon D	1993	Starzl	Univ Pittsburgh
Pancreas	Segmental	1966	Lillehei, Kelly	Univ Minnesota
	DO	1978	Dubernard	Lyon, France
	ED	1976	Groth	Stockholm
	LRD	1980	Sutherland	Univ Minnesota
	Isograft	1982	Sutherland	Univ Minnesota
	BD	1985	Sollinger	Univ Wisconsin
Intestine	Isolated	1966	Lillehei, Kelly	Univ Minnesota
	Isolated	1989	Deltz	Kiel, FDR
	MV	1989	Starzl	Univ Pittsburgh
	Isograft	1994	Dafoe, Alfrey, Kuo	Stanford
Heart	Chimpanzee D	1963	Hardy	Univ Mississippi
	Orthotopic	1967	Barnard	Capetown, S. Africa
	Orthotopic	1968	Shumway[6]	Stanford
	Heterotopic	1972	Barnard	Capetown, S. Africa
	Baboon D	1985	Bailey	Loma Linda Univ
Lung	Cadaver, single	1963	Hardy	Mississippi
	Cadaver, single	1971	Derom	Louvain
	Cadaver, single	1983	Cooper	Univ Toronto
	Cadaver, double	1988	Cooper	Univ Toronto
	LRD, lobar	1991	Starnes	Stanford
Heart-lung	En bloc	1981	Reitz, Shumway	Stanford
"Domino" heart		1987	Yacoub	Middlesex, UK
			Baumgartner	Johns Hopkins

[1]The definition of success is variable. Success, as applied in the construction of this list, may be the completion of transplant surgery, short-lived or long-term graft, or patient survival. In creating these lists, the author regrets that worthy accomplishments by individuals may have been neglected due to ethnocentrism or simple oversight. Progress in transplantation has been the accretion of knowledge through meticulous experimentation and enlightened practice of many who are deserving of recognition but remain obscure.
[2]See Figure 40.1–2.
[3]See Figure 40.1–5.
[4]See Figure 40.1–6.
[5]See Figure 40.1–4.
[6]See Figure 40.1–3.
BD = bladder drainage; D = donor; DO = duct obstructed; ED = enteric drainage; LRD = living-related donor; MV = multivisceral; PBBH = Peter Bent Brigham Hospital; R = recipient; RVG = reduced-volume graft.

betes attained respectability when the pancreas was transplanted synchronously with a same-donor kidney graft. Technical advances such as drainage of pancreatic secretions into the urinary bladder diminished early complications. The main spokesman for pancreatic transplantation has been Dr David Sutherland of the University of Minnesota, who influenced the field through a combination of experimental studies, clinical trials, and the establishment of the International Pancreas Transplant Registry. The attractive approach of isolated islet transplantation by embolization into the liver did not live up to expectations due to lack of sufficient islet yield from processed pancreata and inadequate engraftment.

The transplant field had slowed to a pace of steady im-

provement until the arrival of cyclosporine. Released in the United States in 1983, cyclosporine provided potent immunosuppression without a dramatic increase in infectious disease. Under cyclosporine-based immunosuppression, the average 1-year graft survival for kidney, pancreas, heart, and liver transplants approached or exceeded 70% (Figure 40.1–7). Usually such an increase in allograft survival would have been accompanied by an increase in patient mortality from infection, but cyclosporine was different. As was later revealed, cyclosporine worked via a more specific mechanism of action. Unlike prior immunosuppressive agents that acted indiscriminately on dividing cells, cyclosporine worked selectively on T lymphocytes by inhibiting interleukin-2 production.

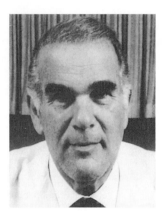

Figure 40.1–6. John S. Najarian, MD (b 1927). Transplant surgeon. Dr Najarian is most highly regarded for his contributions to pediatric renal transplantation and kidney and pancreas transplantation in diabetics. During his reign as Chairman of the Department of Surgery at the University of Minnesota, a large-volume transplant program was developed, characterized by excellent academic transplant surgeons. Large-scale production of Minnesota antilymphoblast globulin made this effective antirejection treatment available to other programs. Clinical activity was complemented by prolific research laboratories. (Reprinted, with permission, from Terasaki PI: *History of Transplantation: Thirty-Five Recollections.* UCLA Tissue Typing Laboratory, 1991, p. 452.)

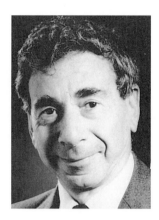

Figure 40.1–7. Sir Roy Calne (b 1930). Abdominal transplant surgeon. Beginning in 1960 with his report of 6-mercaptopurine as an effective immunosuppressant in canine renal allografts, Dr Calne has been influential in all phases of progress in transplantation. Most significantly, his Cambridge team helped realize liver transplantation as a therapeutic modality and brought cyclosporine into the clinical arena. (Reprinted, with permission, from Terasaki PI: *History of Transplantation: Thirty-Five Recollections.* UCLA Tissue Typing Laboratory, 1991, p. 228.)

Next, so-called "triple therapy" emerged. Consisting of cyclosporine, azathioprine, and prednisone, this regimen used lower cyclosporine doses, thereby avoiding troublesome side effects (eg, cyclosporine nephrotoxicity) and incurring less expense. Furthermore, it was reasoned that combination chemotherapy incapacitated the immune system at several levels, resulting in synergistic immunosuppression. With the better results achieved using cyclosporine, the practice of random donor blood transfusions or DSTs prior to renal transplantation fell out of favor—particularly in light of patients' growing fears about human immunodeficiency virus infection.

As success rates increased and mortality decreased, transplantation became the preferred mode of treatment for renal failure. Renal transplantation was found to be more cost-effective and had higher rehabilitation rates than treatment of chronic renal failure with dialysis. One consequence of successful organ transplantation was an exacerbation of the cadaver donor shortage. Recipient waiting times began to stretch from months to years, and many died for lack of organs. Issues of candidate selection, allocation of donor organs, expense of medications, and proliferation of low-volume transplant centers began to draw attention.

During the 1980s, general improvements in medical care and the support of the very ill transplant joined technical advances in the operating room to enhance the outcome for many organ transplant recipients. These efforts were strengthened by improved organ preservation. Cold storage, the exsanguination of organ grafts by purging with preservation solution and immersion in ice, became the standard technique for all organs. In kidney transplantation, this simple and inexpensive technique supplanted the complex hypothermic pulsatile perfusion apparatus that had been employed. A new preservation solution was introduced by Dr Folkert Belzer at the University of Wisconsin (UW) (Figure 40.1–8). Completely synthetic, UW solution replaced Collins or EuroCollins solutions, which had been the standard preservation solutions. UW solution differed from Collins in the substitution of a nonmetabolizable starch for glucose, to provide the high osmolality necessary to inhibit cell swelling from hypothermia-induced paralysis of the sodium-potassium pump. As multiorgan recoveries from heart-beating, brain-dead cadaver donors became commonplace, retrieval techniques matured to in situ perfusion and en bloc procurement. Subsequent dissection or reconstruction of grafts could be completed ex vivo in a basin of iced slush.

In the United States, the National Organ Transplant Act of 1984 established the administrative oversight for organ-sharing, cooperative efforts between regional organ procurement agencies and a national transplant registry. Organ donation from the general public was encouraged through the combined efforts of the government, transplant surgeons/physicians, transplant nurse coordinators, patient advocacy groups, and organ procurement agencies. Another legislative initiative was the mandate of "required request." In most states in this country, this law dictated that whenever there was a potential donor, health

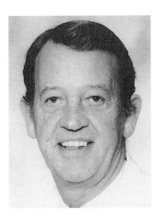

Figure 40.1–8. Folkert O. Belzer, MD (1930–1995). Transplant surgeon. Dr Belzer devoted a lifetime to transplantation and established a balanced program in multiorgan transplantation during his long tenure as Chairman of the Department of Surgery at the University of Wisconsin in Madison. Of his many accomplishments, he will be remembered primarily for his studies in organ preservation culminating in the development of UW solution. (Reprinted, with permission, from Terasaki PI: *History of Transplantation: Thirty-Five Recollections.* UCLA Tissue Typing Laboratory, 1991, p. 596.)

care personnel were legally obliged to offer to the next-of-kin the option of organ donation.

Despite increasing graft and patient survival, uniform success remained elusive. The recipient's immune response against alloantigens regularly penetrated cyclosporine-based maintenance immunosuppression, manifesting as acute rejection. High-dose steroids remained the first line of rejection treatment and antilymphocyte serum was used for steroid-resistant episodes. Chronic rejection continued to be an intractable problem, with a predictable drop in graft survival of approximately 15% in the 5 years following transplantation. Although cyclosporine raised the survival curve to a higher level, the inexorable decrement in graft survival over time ran parallel to the curve of the prior decade.

1990s

Hybridoma technology made possible the production of large quantities of reproducible monoclonal antibody preparations directed at specific cell surface markers on lymphocytes. The promise of monoclonal antibodies in transplantation was fulfilled by OKT3, a molecule designed by Dr Gideon Goldstein of Ortho Biotech and investigated clinically by Dr Ben Cosimi. Rather than intravenous infusions of grams of heterologous antilymphocyte preparations such as ATGAM (Upjohn Co, Kalamazoo, Michigan) and Minnesota antilymphoblast globulin, only 5 mg of OKT3 murine xenoantibody eliminated T

lymphocytes, as detected by fluorescent antibody labelled scanning, within minutes of administration. OKT3 found its niche as a substitute for heterologous antilymphocyte preparations in the treatment of steroid-resistant rejection or as "induction" therapy immediately after transplantation. OKT3 effectively reversed acute rejection the great majority (> 90%) of the time.

As usual, aggressive manipulation of the immune system brought new clinical problems. Chills, fever, and a capillary leak syndrome resulted from the elaboration of cytokines from T cells stimulated by the engagement of OKT3 and its targeted CD3 receptor. A significant proportion of recipients treated with OKT3 formed antibody against the OKT3 xenoprotein. These antibodies neutralized OKT3, rendering it ineffectual against rejection. The injudicious use of OKT3 retaught the lesson of over-immunosuppression manifested as infectious complications and Epstein-Barr virus–related lymphoproliferative disorders.

The 1990s, thus far, have ushered in an era of promising new immunosuppressive agents, such as tacrolimus (FK506) and mycophenolate mofetil. These agents, recently released in the United States by the Food and Drug Administration, are significant additions to the pharmacologic arsenal. As other new immunosuppressants become available, organ-specific immunosuppressive regimens—doses, monitoring, and drug combinations—must be optimized. Other agents on the path to clinical application are mizoribine, deoxyspergualin, brequinar, rapamycin, and leflunomide. The biotechnology industry, through collaboration with university centers, has created monoclonal antibodies with cell targets that are more refined than the pan-T cell CD3 ligand of OKT3.

There has been a renewal of interest in xenotransplantation borne of the union of burgeoning cadaver organ waiting lists and the power of molecular biology. An example is the creation of transgenic pigs as organ donors. Anticomplement factors have been transfected into porcine tissue grafts to interrupt the complement cascade started by naturally occurring IgM xenoantibody in the primate host. A worrisome consequence of xenotransplantation is the risk of zoonoses and the spectre of virulent pathogens spreading from beast to man.

In the United States, the ascension of managed care and governmental cutbacks in health care entitlements has forced consolidation of transplant centers. Economic stringency has brought about a reconsideration of transplant candidate criteria with the balanced goal of equitable access to transplantation for individual patients and cost-effectiveness for the general community.

Transplantation has been a microcosm of the changing world of general medicine and science. It has been a high-profile activity that has raised ethical dilemmas requiring scrutiny by ethicists, clergy, and the general populace. Advances have emanated from all sectors of society, from the basic scientist to the legislator. The once fantastic goal of organ replacement has come to be a daily reality. Two hundred years hence, when end-stage organ failure is prevented or cured with gene therapy, will the era of transplantation be a fascinating aberration? Or, will serial replacement of obsolescent organs with xenogeneic organs be commonplace? With the passing of this millennium, it is likely that immunologic tolerance—donor-specific un-responsivenes—will be routinely induced in recipients. Equally likely is the development of transgenic animals as a source of organ xenografts. In the meantime, transplantation remains a challenging and rapidly evolving discipline.

SUGGESTED READING

Medawar P: *Memoir of a Thinking Radish*. Oxford University Press, 1988.

Phillips MG: *Organ Procurement, Preservation and Distribution in Transplantation*. United Network for Organ Sharing, 1991.

Salvatierra O, Lum CT: *History of the American Society of Transplant Surgeons*. Stanton Publication Services, 1993.

Terasaki PI: *History of Transplantation: Thirty-Five Recollections*. UCLA Tissue Typing Laboratory, 1991.

40.2 Organ Donation

Phyllis G. Weber, RN

▶ Key Facts

▶ A 1993 survey reported that nearly nine of 10 Americans support the concept of organ donation, but fewer than 28% of the respondents had signed a donor card.

▶ Factors suggested as barriers to organ donation include uncertainty about religious beliefs, fear that everything will not be done to save a person's life before the organs are removed, and concern that organ donation may interfere with a regular funeral service.

▶ The organ donation process consists of eight basic components: donor identification and determination of brain death, referral, evaluation, consent, management, organ allocation, organ recovery, and follow-up.

▶ Medical contraindications to organ donation include active sepsis, a history of cancer (with the exception of primary brain tumors and basal cell skin carcinomas), and the presence of transmissible disease, such as the human immunodeficiency virus.

▶ Discussion about organ donation should only be initiated after the family clearly understands that death has occurred despite all attempts to save the patient's life.

▶ Donor management is a labor-intensive process that may take as long as 12–24 hours. The length of time is dependent on the ease or difficulty of placing the organs and the stability of the organ donor.

▶ Information critical to "matching" the donor with waiting recipients includes the donor's height, weight, age, and blood group.

▶ Because of recent advances in organ preservation, the heart and lungs can be preserved for 4–6 hours, the pancreas and liver for 24 hours, and the kidneys for 48 hours.

Organ transplantation for the treatment of patients with end-stage organ disease is severely limited by the availability of cadaveric organ donors. In 1994, with nearly 40,000 patients on a national transplant waiting list, organs were recovered from only 5100 donors. While slightly higher in 1994, the number of organ donors has remained relatively static over the last 5 years. Estimates of organ donor potential throughout the United States vary, but it is widely believed that potential ranges from 10,000 to 15,000 donors per year. This gap between the potential and actual donor supply can be best understood by an evaluation of the complex medical, legal, and social interactions that are involved in the organ donation process.

NATIONAL PERSPECTIVE

The United States organ donor program is a voluntary system that relies on the altruism of our residents. As early as 1968, enabling legislation was enacted by Congress with the Uniform Anatomical Gift Act. This law allows individuals to state their intent to donate by signing an organ donor card. Adopted by all 50 states, the language of the original legislation has been clarified and strengthened, and, recently, some states have begun to develop statewide registries of persons who have expressed a desire to become organ donors at the time of death. The total impact of the donor card is still unknown and may be hindered to some extent by the practice of most organ donation programs to obtain the consent from the next-of-kin, despite the knowledge that a legally executed donor card exists.

Combining the forces of organ donor programs and organ transplant centers was facilitated by the 1984 adoption of the National Organ Transplant Act, P.L. 98-507, an amendment to the Public Health Service Act. This law directed the Secretary of Health and Human Services (HHS) to contract for the establishment of the Organ Procurement and Transplantation Network (OPTN); to establish and direct a Task Force on Organ Transplantation to study and make recommendations to improve the field of transplantation; to direct organ procurement organizations (OPOs) to distribute organs equitably among waiting recipients; and to prohibit the sale of organs. Subsequently, the United Network for Organ Sharing (UNOS) was awarded the federal contract to administer the OPTN and the Task Force recommendations were incorporated into the Omnibus Budget Reconciliation Act of 1986. These recommendations required (1) all hospitals participating in Medicare and Medicaid to establish written protocols for identifying potential donors and assuring that families are aware of the option to donate organs; (2) designation of one OPO per service area; (3) OPOs to meet standards and qualifications in order to receive payment from Medicare and Medicaid; (4) OPOs and transplant centers to allocate organs in accordance with established medical criteria and OPTN requirements.

Since its inception, UNOS has played a critical role in directing national policy. Among its most significant accomplishments are the establishment of minimum training requirements for kidney, liver, and pancreas transplant surgery fellows, membership criteria for transplant centers, the development of a fair and equitable system for organ allocations, and through the Scientific Registry, the collection and publication of the most comprehensive data on the outcome of organs transplanted in the United States from 1987 through 1991.

Members of UNOS comprise all organ procurement organizations and transplant centers as well as histocompatibility laboratories, voluntary health organizations, and the general public. Although still considered voluntary, member compliance with policies developed by its Board of Directors is high. These policies will become binding when final regulations are developed by the Secretary of HHS; such action is anticipated in the fall of 1995.

PUBLIC ATTITUDES TOWARD ORGAN DONATION

The voluntary system of donation practiced in the United States is dependent on decisions of individuals or their families to donate organs to help others. Public attitude surveys consistently confirm support for organ donation. The most recent and largest study of its kind, conducted by the Gallup Organization in 1993, found that nearly nine in ten Americans support the concept of organ donation, but less than half had made a personal decision about donation of their own organs and only 28% of the respondents had signed an organ donor card. Support for organ donation correlated positively with higher levels of education, and was somewhat lower among nonwhite than white respondents. When asked to project their likelihood to donate family members' organs, nearly all respondents would be likely to honor the wishes of the deceased if these wishes were known to them. Since it is the practice of organ procurement organizations to obtain consent from the next-of-kin despite the presence of a donor card, the results of this survey suggest that public education efforts should reinforce the need to obtain information about donation, to make an informed decision, and to share this decision with family members.

Many factors have been suggested as barriers to support for organ donation: uncertainty about religious beliefs; fear that not everything will be done to save a person's life before organs are removed for transplants; and concern that organ donation may interfere with a regular funeral service. These factors were not major impediments when respondents were queried about these issues by Gallup, although nonwhite respondents reflected a slightly higher level of misinformation than white respondents.

Other systems to improve donation have been debated. At least 13 European countries have adopted a presumed consent policy. Practicing under such conditions, physicians are free to recover organs for transplantation without explicit consent, unless the potential donor expressed an objection before death. One of the major problems with this system has been the lack of an adequate method of recording objections (opting out) in a way that is readily available to health care professionals. This failing is similar to the lack of a central donor registry (opting in) in the United States. A slight variation of presumed consent, mandated choice, has been proposed and supported by the Council on Ethical and Judicial Affairs of the American Medical Association. Under mandated choice, individuals would be required to state their preferences regarding organ donation when they renew their driver's license, file income tax forms, or perform some other task mandated by the state. To date, no state has passed such legislation nor implemented such a plan.

Financial incentives for donor families ranging from assistance with funeral expenses to tax credits have been also proposed, but there is no consensus on this issue among transplant professionals, health care workers, donor families, or the general public.

THE ROLE OF ORGAN PROCUREMENT ORGANIZATIONS

Throughout the United Stares and Puerto Rico, 66 OPOs play an essential role in coordinating all aspects of organ donation. Designated by the Health Care Financing Administration (HCFA), they have similar responsibilities (Table 40.2–1), but the size and scope of their operations vary greatly. OPOs differ in geography, population served, the demographics of that population, and the number of transplant centers, transplant patients, and hospitals within their service area. The majority of OPOs are independent not-for-profit organizations; a smaller number of

Table 40.2–1. Responsibilities of the organ procurement organization (OPO).

1. Educate health care professionals about donation criteria so that all potential organ donors are identified.
2. Evaluate the suitability of organ donors referred.
3. Discuss the options of organ donation with family members of potential donors.
4. Manage the care of the potential donor to ensure viability of organs to be recovered.
5. Coordinate the allocation of organs to patients waiting.
6. Assist with the recovery, preservation, and transportation of organs.
7. Provide reimbursement to the hospital for costs incurred during the donor evaluation, management, and organ recovery.
8. Provide outcome information to donor families and health care professionals involved with the donor process.

agencies remain based at a single transplant hospital and generally serve that one transplant center. Funding for OPOs is generated through a fee-for-service system. When a medically suitable organ is recovered, the OPO will bill a standard organ acquisition charge to the transplant center; the transplant center then invoices the primary insurance carrier of the transplant recipient. Additionally, OPOs may receive funding from Medicare as a condition of coverage for patients with end-stage renal disease.

OPO effectiveness is most commonly measured by the number of donors from whom organs are recovered per population. In 1994, the Association of Organ Procurement Organizations (AOPO) reported a range of performance from 10.8 to 33.9 donors per million of population. The variations in OPO performance are not entirely understood but may reflect dissimilar rates of medically suitable potential donors throughout the country and variances in consent rates among different ethnic groups.

The staff of the organ procurement organizations must generate and sustain public and health care professional enthusiasm and support for organ donation. The ability to accomplish these tasks may also contribute to explaining the wide range of performance.

THE DONATION PROCESS

The organ donation process consists of eight basic components: donor identification and determination of brain death, referral, evaluation, consent, management, organ allocation, organ recovery, and follow-up.

IDENTIFICATION

Identification of a potential organ donor may occur in an emergency department or a critical care unit. In the United States, the majority of organs are recovered from patients who have been declared dead by neurologic criteria (commonly referred to as **brain-dead** or **heart-beating cadaver donors** because their hearts are beating at the time of organ recovery). Generally, these persons have had a massive insult to the brain from direct trauma, cerebral hemorrhage, or an anoxic event that has resulted in irreversible cessation of all brain functions, including the brain stem.

The development of mechanical ventilation to sustain respiratory and circulatory function, as well as the advent of transplantation, forced the medical community and the public to reevaluate the standard of determination of death by cardiac cessation. The Harvard Report, published in 1968, followed by the President's Commission for the Study of Ethical Problems in Medicine and Biomedical Research in 1981, were largely successful in defining brain death criteria and proposing clinical tests to assess

Table 40.2–2. Neurologic testing for determination of brain death.

Cessation of cerebral function: deep coma with no clinical response to any physical stimuli
Absence of brain stem functions: absent cranial nerve functions, including pupillary, corneal, oculocephalic, oculovestibular, and oropharyngeal reflexes
No evidence of spontaneous breathing during an apnea test

cerebral and brain stem functions (Table 40.2–2). The diagnosis of brain death requires the clinical assessment of at least one physician; some states require independent assessments by two physicians.

A neurologic examination is the first step in determining brain death. The physician will conduct a thorough examination by testing all cranial and cerebral reflexes. This examination evaluates responses to noxious stimuli, cold water caloric testing, corneal, and cough, and gag reflexes, and doll's eyes, and assesses spontaneous respirations or other deliberate movements. Hypothermic patients should have their temperature normalized before the determination of brain death is made, and the presence of central nervous system depressants or neuromuscular blockers must be carefully assessed prior to the declaration of brain death. Confirmatory testing, such as cerebral blood flow studies, electroencephalograms, and evoked response testing, may be used to support a clinical examination but they are not legal requirements. It is generally recommended that a patient be observed for a minimum of 6 hours prior to the evaluation and determination of brain death. The determination of brain death in children under the age of 2 is usually evaluated under more stringent criteria than adults (Table 40.2–3). The data and time of brain death must be clearly documented in the permanent patient records.

Although limited by "warm ischemia" (injury to organs when the blood supply is interrupted and before the organs can be cooled and reperfused), the recovery of organs from "non–heart-beating cadaver donors" is also practiced by some organ procurement organizations and transplant centers. Such potential donors fall into two primary categories: (1) patients who have suffered a sudden cardiac arrest and whose proximity to a hospital allows for intravascular catheters to be inserted to cool organs, and (2) patients who have requested removal of life support and who are expected to die within a very short time after-

ward. These situations have been referred to respectively as **uncontrolled** versus **controlled circumstances**. Both protocols have advantages and disadvantages, but estimates have been made that this practice could increase the availability of some organs by as much as 20%.

Individuals who do not meet brain death criteria and are not being considered for "non–heart-beating" organ donation may donate tissues, the most common of which are corneas, skin, bone, and heart valves. Tissue donation should also be considered when the potential for organ donation is being evaluated.

Each OPO and transplant center has specific medical criteria for organ donation, but criteria change frequently and donor acceptability is also dependent on the acuity of the waiting transplant recipients. Throughout the country, most OPOs will evaluate referrals of potential donors who range in age from newborns to 70. Organs have been recovered from donors over the age of 70, but these patients are frequently compromised by comorbidity factors that may have contributed to the primary cause of brain death. Medical contraindications to organ donation include active sepsis, a history of cancer with the exception of primary brain tumors and basal cell skin carcinomas, and the presence of transmissible disease, such as the human immunodeficiency virus (HIV). Past medical histories of hypertension, diabetes, and hepatitis B and C are not absolute contraindications; if brain death is suspected, these persons should be referred to the OPO. Potential donors with behavioral or historical risk factors by Centers for Disease Control (CDC) identification (Table 40.2–4) are evaluated carefully, and the risks and benefits of recovering and transplanting their organs are weighed heavily.

REFERRAL

Once a potential donor has been identified, a referral to the regional OPO is made by a physician, nurse, or other health care professional. An organ procurement coordina-

Table 40.2–3. Guidelines for the determination of brain death in children.

Age	Observation Period/Laboratory Tests
7 days–2 months	Two clinical examinations, apnea tests, and electroencephalograms 48 hours apart
2–12 months	Two clinical examinations, apnea tests, and electroencephalograms at least 24 hours apart
> 12 months	Two clinical examinations and apnea tests 12 hours apart

Table 40.2–4. High-risk organ donors by CDC criteria.

1. Men who have had sex with another man in the preceding 5 years.
2. Persons who report nonmedical intravenous, intramuscular, or subcutaneous injections of drugs in the preceding 5 years.
3. Persons with hemophilia or related clotting disorders who have received human-derived clotting factor concentrates.
4. Men and women who have engaged in sex in exchange for money or drugs in the preceding 5 years.
5. Persons who have had sex in the preceding 12 months with any person described in items 1–4 above or with a person known or suspected to have HIV infection.
6. Persons who have been exposed in the preceding 12 months to known or suspected HIV-infected blood through percutaneous inoculation or through contact with an open wound, nonintact skin, or mucous membrane.
7. Inmates of correctional systems.

CDC = Centers for Disease Control.

tor will respond to the call, carefully assess the potential for organ donation, and advise the staff of the next steps in the process. An early referral (before the pronouncement of brain death and before the option of donation is mentioned to the family) gives everyone adequate time to prepare a smooth transition from care of the patient to management of an organ donor.

EVALUATION

An initial evaluation of the potential donor includes a review of the current medical status, the extent of injuries, and any pertinent past medical or social history that is known to the hospital staff. This initial review can take place over the phone or on site at the hospital. Based on these findings, a recommendation will be made to either proceed with a more thorough examination at the hospital or halt the process based on medical unsuitability.

CONSENT

Discussions about organ donation should only be initiated after the family clearly understands that death has occurred despite all attempts to save the patient's life. Premature discussions about donation will not only confuse a family but will also have them question the staff's motivations. Most families who are approached early in the process will refuse to give consent for donation, when what they are denying the most is the death. Given more time to absorb the impact of this tragedy, many families will give consent, particularly if they know the wishes of the deceased. OPO coordinators are well-trained and experienced in conducting such conversations with families, and the ideal approach to a family about donation will always include the coordinator. Family members' questions and concerns must be addressed in a sensitive and compassionate manner. They need to be informed that evaluating the medical suitability of the potential donor, matching organs to appropriate recipients, and recovering the organs may take anywhere from 12 to 24 hours. It should be explained that the organ recovery is similar to any other major surgery—that the body will be treated with respect and that no alterations of the body will be made so that a normal funeral and viewing of the body can take place. Families also need to understand that the costs associated with the evaluation and organ recovery are covered by the OPO. And finally, they need to be reassured that their final decision—to donate or to decline this option—will be honored and respected.

If the family is willing to give consent, a formal consent form is signed by the legal next-of-kin. The order of legal priority is (1) spouse, (2) adult children, (3) parent, (4) sibling, (5) legal guardian, and (6) any person authorized to dispose of the body. While the main goal is to provide organs for transplantation, family members may also agree to donate tissues and organs for research. This infor-

mation should be recorded on the consent form. The OPO coordinator is then responsible for obtaining a thorough medical and social history of the deceased from family and friends. Blood samples for serologic testing of the HIV, hepatitis B and C, human T-cell lymphotropic virus (HTLV-1), cytomegalovirus, and syphilis, mandated for every potential organ donor, will be obtained, as well as blood or peripheral lymph nodes to be used for preliminary histocompatibility testing. If the death of the potential donor falls under the jurisdiction of the medical examiner or coroner, permission from them to proceed with the organ recovery must be obtained.

DONOR MANAGEMENT

Once brain death has been determined and consent for organ donation has been obtained from the family, the management of the donor is coordinated by the OPO staff. Usually the organ procurement coordinator is on site, but in some rural areas, management of the donor may be coordinated by phone with the nursing staff.

The goal of management is to optimize the function of all organs to be recovered, which may be a formidable challenge. Hypotension is the most common problem, and is treated aggressively with colloid and crystalloid replacement and titrated doses of dopamine hydrochloride. Insertion of a central line and frequent monitoring of the central venous pressure (CVP) will help guide fluid replacement. Ideally, the CVP will be maintained between 5 and 10 cm water. Good respiratory care and ventilator management aimed at keeping the PaO_2 greater than 100 on 40% FIO_2 will improve the likelihood of recovering and transplanting the lungs. Adding 5 cm of positive end-expiratory pressure (PEEP) to the ventilator is always recommended. Low urine output in an adequately hydrated donor can be treated with furosemide or mannitol, but more frequently, diabetes insipidus ensues and can be managed with desmopressin (DDAVP). Normothermia should be maintained and frequently requires the use of warming blankets. A broad-spectrum systemic antibiotic should be administered if the donor has been hospitalized more than 72 hours, blood and urine cultures should be obtained before the antibiotic is given (Table 40.2–5).

Frequent monitoring of electrolytes, hematocrit, and arterial blood gases are important components of general donor management. More specific tests, such as liver function studies, chest x-rays, ECGs and echocardiograms, lipases and amylases, BUNs, and creatinines are required to assess the medical suitability of the liver, lungs, heart, pancreas, and kidneys.

Donor management is a labor-intensive process that may take as long as 12–24 hours. The length of time is dependent on the ease or difficulty of placing organs and the stability of the organ donor. The OPO procurement coordinator will be responsible for assisting with this process, and will be in frequent contact with the transplant teams during this time.

Table 40.2–5. Organ donor management.

Hemodynamic Instability
Ascertain sources of instability.
Use blood products to maintain Hgb > 10, Hct > 30.
Use colloid/crystalloid therapy.
Use beta blockade for hypertensive crisis or consider afterload reduction.
Use vasopressors prudently.
Fluid and Electrolyte Management
Replace volume deficits with hypotonic saline/glucose crystalloid solutions.
Replace cc/cc urine > 300 ml/h with solution determined by serum laboratory values.
Consider use of vasopressin where applicable.
Maintain central venous pressure and blood pressure at acceptable levels.
Ventilation and Oxygenation
Institute mechanical ventilation with settings adjusted per donor; add 5 cm of positive end-expiratory pressure (PEEP).
Maintain arterial pH 7.35–7.45.
Initiate aggressive pulmonary care with frequent suctioning and hyperventilation.
Obtain arterial blood gases at least every 4–6 hours and as needed.

ORGAN ALLOCATION

During the management process, measures are taken to allocate organs using a national formula that begins when the OPO coordinator contacts the UNOS organ center to provide information about the donor. Information critical to "matching" the donor with waiting recipients includes the donor's height, weight, age, sex, and blood group. Based on these variables, a national computer matching program is run according to each organ donated. Patients listed with the transplant centers served by the regional organ procurement organization have local priority. If the organs cannot be placed locally, the organs will be offered to programs in a larger region, then nationally. If compatible by blood group and size, the computer matching program will list extra renal recipients sequentially by the acuity of illness and length of time on the waiting list. Kidney allocation requires identification and comparisons of human leukocyte antigens (HLA) between the donor and recipients and serologic tests to determine the absence of preformed cytotoxic antibodies. Blood group compatibility, the degree of HLA matching, a negative cytotoxic antibody crossmatch, and length of time on the list will direct the kidney offer.

ORGAN RECOVERY

In almost all circumstances, the organs will be recovered in the operating room of the donor hospital. While it occurred more frequently in the earlier years of transplantation, it is now rare to transport an organ donor to a transplant facility. The surgical team consists of scrub and circulating nurses and an anesthesiologist from the donor hospital and the visiting transplant surgeons and technicians.

The surgical procedure is similar to a major exploratory laparotomy. The body is prepped and draped in the usual fashion, and a long midline incision is made. Techniques for organ recovery vary slightly, but will be discussed in greater detail in other chapters. When each team is ready to remove the organs, the aorta is cross-clamped and the organs are flushed simultaneously with cold preservation solutions. Because of recent advances in organ preservation, the heart and lungs can be preserved for 4–6 hours, the pancreas and liver for 24 hours, and the kidneys for 48 hours. Extrarenal organs are stored and transported in preservation solutions on ice at temperatures of 4°C. Kidneys may be stored similarly or may be preserved and transported on pulsatile preservation machines. While more cumbersome, expensive, and infrequently used, machine preservation of kidneys can extend the storage time to 72 hours.

FOLLOW-UP

Key hospital personnel involved in the donor assessment, evaluation, management, and organ recovery are apprised of the outcome of the donation. Letters and follow-up visits to the donor hospital by the OPO staff acknowledge the efforts of the staff and encourage their continued participation in the program. Special thanks are sent to the donor family, and they, too, are given general information about the individuals who have benefited from the donation. The confidentiality of organ donors and transplant recipients is maintained by the transplant centers and OPOs, but anonymous correspondence, particularly thank-you notes from the recipients to donor families, are encouraged by many transplant centers and facilitated by the OPOs. Many OPOs have begun grief support and aftercare programs for donor families to provide them with some measure of comfort and to address any unmet needs or problems associated with the donation process. Documentation of the organ donation, organ allocation, and recipient information is provided by the OPO to UNOS.

THE ROLE OF THE PHYSICIAN

Organ donation cannot take place without the active support of physicians. In the critical care setting, the early identification and referral of a potential organ donor will begin a process that may save the lives of as many as seven waiting individuals. If families are treated in a kind and sensitive manner, and if time has been taken to fully explain the facts of the situation in a phased approach, they are more likely to agree to donation. Primary care physicians should routinely provide information about organ donation to patients, encourage their patients to discuss their decision with family members, and document their patients' wishes.

SUGGESTED READING

American Medical Association Council on Ethical and Judicial Affairs: Strategies for cadaveric organ procurement: Mandated choice and presumed consent. JAMA 1994;272:809.

Arnold RM, Younger SJ: Ethical, psychological, and public policy implications of procuring organs from non-heart-beating cadavers. Kennedy Institute of Ethics Journal. 1993;3:103.

Darby JM et al: Approach to management of the heartbeating "brain dead" organ donor. JAMA 1989;261:2222.

Evans RW, Orians CE, Ascher NL: The potential supply of organ donors. An assessment of the efficiency of organ procurement efforts in the United States. JAMA 1992;267:239.

The Gallup Organization: Highlights of public attitudes toward organ donation and transplantation. Princeton, NJ: The Gallup Organization; March 1993:1–8.

Garrison RN et al: There is an answer to the shortage of organ donors. Surg Gynecol Obstet 1991;173:391.

Guidelines for the determination of death. Report of the medical consultants on the diagnosis of death to the President's commission for the study of ethical problems in medicine, biomedical and behavioral research. JAMA 1982;246:2184.

Halevy A, Brody B: Brain death: Reconciling definitions, criteria, and tests. Ann Intern Med 1993;119:519.

Kittur DS et al: Incentives for organ donation? The United Network for Organ Sharing Ad Hoc Donations Committee. Lancet 1991;338:1441.

Mackersie RC, Bronsther OL, Shackford SR: Organ procurement in patients with fatal head injuries: The fate of the potential donor. Ann Surg 1991;213:143.

Mejia RE, Pollack MM: Variability in brain death determination practices in children. JAMA 1995;274:550.

Phillips MG, Mainous PD: Organ procurement coordinator's manual. United Network for Organ Sharing, 1995.

Report of the Ad Hoc Committee of the Harvard Medical School to examine the definition of death. A definition of irreversible coma. JAMA 1968;205:337.

Rogers MF et al: Guidelines for preventing transmission of human immunodeficiency virus through transplantation of human tissues and organs. MMWR 1994;43:1.

Siminoff LA et al: Public policy governing organ and tissue procurement in the United States. Ann Intern Med 1995;123:10.

Spital A: Mandated choice, the preferred solution to the organ shortage? Arch Intern Med 1992;152:2421.

US General Accounting Office: Increased effort needed to boost supply and ensure equitable distribution of organs. GAO/HRD; 93–56. Washington DC, 1993.

40.3 Transplant Immunology

Nancy Krieger, MD, C. Garrison Fathman, MD, & Edward J. Alfrey, MD

► Key Facts

- ► The rejection response against an allograft is elicited when histocompatibility antigens on the transplanted tissue differ from those of the recipient.

- ► The redundancy of the immune response prevents the host from reliance on a single pathway for protection; however, this makes it difficult to paralyze the host's ability to respond to transplant antigens.

- ► Macrophages play an important role in the immune response by ingesting foreign antigen and presenting it to lymphocytes.

- ► T cells are the primary cells that respond to transplantation antigens present on virtually all tissues. Immunosuppressive therapy is, therefore, often targeted at these cells.

- ► The major histocompatibility complex molecules not only serve to present antigens to T cells, but are the major target of activated lymphocytes, which underlie the rejection of allografts.

- ► Antibody production involves interaction between B cells, CD4+ T helper cells, and accessory cells. Unless stimulated by antigen, B cells become senescent.

- ► The ultimate goal in clinical transplantation is to induce a state of donor-specific unresponsiveness or tolerance to the transplanted allograft with full immunocompetence of the recipient to fight infections and to eliminate malignant cells.

Despite recent advances in surgical techniques, organ preservation, and immunosuppressive pharmacologic intervention, transplant rejection remains a formidable obstacle in the field of transplantation. A better understanding of the basic cellular interactions involved in the immune response is critical for understanding the mechanisms that lead to rejection of allograft transplants and will lead to the development of strategies that prevent transplant rejection.

The host's response to a foreign antigen is complex, involving recognition of foreign peptide in the context of major histocompatibility complex (MHC) molecules, cell-to-cell interactions, transmembrane signaling, activation of cellular subsets, and effector functions of the immune system. The cells involved in immune activation are complex and diverse and have many functions that are redundant. The specificity of the immune system provides the host protection against foreign antigens while maintaining unresponsiveness to self-antigen, often referred to as self-tolerance. The redundancy of the immune response prevents the host from reliance on a single pathway for protection. It is, therefore, not surprising that blocking the immune response along one pathway with specific im-

munopharmacologic agents may not paralyze the host's ability to respond to transplantation antigens. This section reviews some of the prominent cellular components and important molecules involved in transplant immunology. The cascade of immune events leading to allorejection is depicted in Figure 40.3–1.

MACROPHAGES & ANTIGEN-PRESENTING CELLS

Macrophages play an important role in the immune response, functioning as accessory cells that ingest foreign antigen and present it to the appropriate lymphocytes. The primary role for macrophages is host defense. These phagocytes ingest and kill intracellular parasites and clear extracellular pathogens from the bloodstream and tissues. Macrophages engulf and process antigen and then present it on their cell surface to lymphocytes in a "reactive" form, thus serving as accessory cells in the activation of lymphocytes. Macrophages exposed to endotoxin on bacterial surface membranes can activate themselves, permitting a rapid immune response to invading microbes.

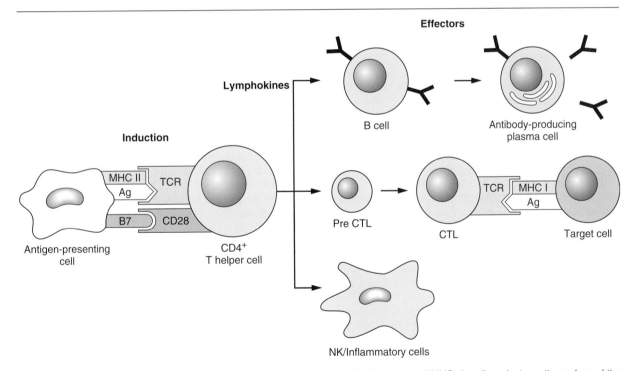

Figure 40.3–1. Interaction of the CD4+ T helper cell with antigen presented in the context of MHC class II products on the surface of the professional antigen-presenting cell in association with co-stimulatory interaction between CD28 and B7 activates the CD4+ T helper cell to produce lymphokines. Such cell free products drive the effector mechanisms of immunity, including the differentiation of B lymphocytes into antibody-producing plasma cells and precursors of cytotoxic T lymphocytes (CTLs) into effector CTLs. In addition, lymphokines drive effector pathways, indicated generally as natural killer (NK)/inflammatory cells. (Reprinted, with permission, from Fathman CG: Editorial overview. Inhibition of immune induction: The target of current transplantation tolerance strategies. Curr Opin Immunol 1992;4:545.)

Activated macrophages are larger, have an increased capacity to adhere to and spread on surfaces, and have increased numbers of vesicles containing cytokines, including tumor necrosis factor, interleukin-1 (IL-1), interferon-β, fibronectin, lysozyme, prostaglandins, elastase, and complement components. IL-1 is an important factor secreted by the macrophage. IL-1 stimulates B cell proliferation and subsequent antibody production, and stimulates production of T cell lymphokines. The increased production of IL-1 by activated macrophages results in an amplification of the immune response.

T LYMPHOCYTES

All T lymphocytes express on their cell membrane surface many copies of an antigen-specific T cell receptor (TCR) that is the antigen-binding site and associated proteins that make up the T cell receptor complex (CD3). The "conventional" T cell receptor contains two polypeptide chains, the alpha (α) and beta (β) chains, which are linked by disulfide bonds. Each chain has a variable region composed of amino acid sequences that makes it antigen-specific, and a constant region. The α chain is encoded on chromosome 14; the β chain on chromosome 7. The TCR is physically associated on the cell membrane with three invariant polypeptides (CD3) and all are collectively referred to as the T cell receptor complex. While the TCR molecule is similar in all T cells, the antigen recognition site is provided by the hypervariable region. The CD3 molecule is an important component of the signal transductive pathways within the cell. The TCR complex is also associated with either the CD4 or CD8 molecule, which are also important in corecognition of the MHC gene products during antigen presentation.

The TCR does not recognize soluble antigen in isolation. Antigen is processed by antigen-presenting cells (APCs) into peptide fragments, either from endogenous protein for MHC class I molecules, or endocytosed exogenous protein for MHC class II molecules. The peptide antigen is bound in the groove of the MHC molecule on the surface of the APC, and this complex activates the T cell via the antigen or peptide-specific TCR (hypervariable region). After ligation of the T cell receptor/CD3 complex with the antigen-charged MHC molecule, signaling occurs through tyrosine phosphorylation. Intracellular calcium is mobilized and protein kinase C (PKC) is translocated, which promotes the expression of several nuclear regulatory proteins. Calcineurin and immunophylins (cyclophylin) also participate in signal transduction to the nucleus.

Ligation of the TCR/CD3 complex and the MHC complex alone does not induce T cell proliferation. Activation of T cells leading to proliferation and cytokine secretion requires two signals: the interaction of the TCR with antigen presented by MHC molecules on the donor APCs or on host APCs (signal one); and co-stimulatory signals provided by molecules such as CD28/B7, LFA-1/ICAM-1, ICAM-2, ICAM-3, and CD2/LFA-3 (signal two). Other intermolecular interactions can also provide down-regulatory co-stimulatory signals, such as B7 molecules on APCs and CTLA4 on T cells. (The ligation of CTLA4 and B7 is a calcium-independent pathway that is not affected by the immunosuppressive drugs cyclosporine and FK506.) Once stimulatory and co-stimulatory signals have been received, IL-2 and other genes are activated along with transcription of multiple T cell-derived cytokines (eg, IL-2 and TNF-β) and enhanced expression of IL-2 receptors on T cells.

Resting T cells express the TCR but do not express high-affinity receptors for IL-2. When TCRs are stimulated by antigen, the MHC/TCR/CD3 complex causes the IL-2R to appear within hours, while CD3 expression on the cell surface is down-regulated. T cell activation results in IL-2 production and secretion by the activated T cells. IL-2 binds to new IL-2Rs on the same and adjacent cells, resulting in the initiation of cell mitosis and proliferation. The magnitude of T cell activation and proliferation is influenced by external antigens through both positive and negative feedback control. T cells are the primary cells that respond to the transplantation antigens present on virtually all tissues, the genes of which are referred to as the MHC locus (see below). As a result, T cells are crucial in the rejection response, and immunosuppressive therapy is often targeted at these cells.

T cells are divided into two distinct T cell subsets: the CD8+ cytotoxic T cells, which lyse target cells and kill cells infected with virus; and the CD4+ immunoregulatory (helper/inducer) T cells, which mediate interactions of T cells, B cells, macrophages, and other cells, primarily through cytokine production. As stated earlier, CD4+ T cells recognize antigen in the context of MHC class II molecules, and CD8+ T cells in the context of MHC class I molecules. CD8+ T cells primarily serve as effectors that mediate cellular cytotoxicity. Almost all CD8+ cells have this potential. If CD8+ T cells recognize antigen bound to the MHC molecule of a cell, they can be activated to kill that cell. This cytotoxicity is paramount to the rejection of allografts and the lysis of cells infected with virus. The CD4+ cells also recognize and bind to specific antigens. CD4+ T helper or immunoregulatory cells mediate their effects through elaboration of cytokine products. These lymphokines stimulate B cells to make antibodies in response to foreign antigens (humoral immunity), activate macrophages to secrete products, and help CD8+ T cells mature from precursors to effector cytotoxic cells. This amplifies the immune response, stimulating cells to proliferate in their immediate vicinity.

CD4+ T cells, and more recently CD8+ T cells, have been shown to possess two different phenotypes, Th1 and Th2, distinguished by the elaboration of distinct cytokine profiles. Th1 cells produce interleukin-2 (IL-2), interferon-gamma (IFN-γ), and tumor necrosis factor-beta (TNF-β), factors that promote cell-mediated immune responses, while Th2 cells produce IL-4, IL-5, IL-6, and IL-10, factors that promote humoral immunity. The two subsets are capable of regulating each other through the elaboration of their respective cytokines: IFN secreted by Th1 cells inhibits Th2 cell proliferation and IL-4 function, and IL-4 and IL-10 secreted by Th2 cells down-regulate Th1 cell responses. The phenotype has been shown to depend upon the microenvironment of the naive T cell where the relative amounts of IL-12 and IL-4 present at the time of antigen priming of naive T cells determines whether a response will be dominated by cells producing IFN-γ or IL-4. In the presence of IFN-γ and IL-12, uncommitted Th0 cells polarize into the Th1 phenotype, while Th0 cells polarize into the Th2 phenotype in the presence of IL-4. In addition, IL-10 has been shown to inhibit proliferation of Th1-type cells by directly inhibiting T cell production of IL-2 and IFN-γ (Figure 40.3–2).

The relationship of Th1 and Th2 phenotypes in rejection and allograft tolerance is not well understood. There is both experimental and clinical evidence that Th1 cytokine profiles are more active in settings of allograft rejection and Th2 profiles in the setting of donor-specific unresponsiveness. Conversely, other experiments have been unable to demonstrate a predominance of Th1 or Th2 profiles in either situation. There is continuing investigation into understanding these important relationships.

THE MAJOR HISTOCOMPATIBILITY COMPLEX

The MHC proteins not only serve to present antigens to T cells, but are the major target of activated lymphocytes, which underlie rejection of allografts. In humans, the MHC genes are found on the short arm of chromosome 6. The MHC genes are divided into three classes: class I, II, and III. The MHC class I genes encode cell surface trans-

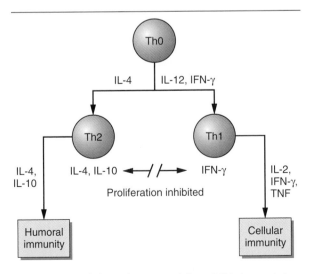

Figure 40.3–2. Schematic representation of T helper polarization.

plant antigens that serve as the primary targets for CD8+ cytotoxic T lymphocytes in graft rejection. They are composed of a polymorphic heavy (α) chain that is responsible for the antigen (peptide) restriction specificity and a nonspecific (constant) monomorphic (β) light chain, β2-microglobulin. The heavy chain contains three extracellular segments and a transmembrane segment in continuity with the cytosol. Class I molecules are ubiquitous, found on almost all nucleated cell types. Red blood cells are enucleated and therefore contain no class I (or class II) molecules. Interferons have been noted to up-regulate class I expression of a variety of cell types, through binding to a specific cell surface receptor. Three major gene loci on chromosome 6 code for the class I molecules designated A, B, and C. However, only HLA-A and -B are used extensively for tissue typing in transplantation (see below). Class I antigens play a major role in eliciting an immune alloresponse and, thus, dominate allograft rejection.

The MHC class II molecules serve as the primary targets for T helper cells. They are made up of an α chain and a β chain. Both of these are transmembrane proteins. The surface segment contains a polymorphic α_1 and β_1 domain responsible for peptide binding specificity and a monomorphic cytosolic segment. The α and β chains of class II molecules comprise the grove for peptide binding, and an invariant chain serves to prevent premature peptide binding during intracellular assembly. After the invariant chain is released, the MHC class II molecules are loaded with peptide in the lysosomal vesicles and transported to the cell surface. Class II molecules are found predominantly on cells of the hematopoietic system, including dendritic cells, thymic epithelial cells, activated T cells, B cells, and macrophages. The class II loci in humans include HLA-DR, -DQ, and -DP. Of the best studied loci for class II, the DR locus is used for tissue typing in transplantation.

Minor transplantation antigens, located on chromosomes outside of the MHC locus, also code for weaker histocompatibility loci. Although they elicit a weaker rejection response, they can have a major impact upon the survival of a transplanted organ. Grafts between HLA-(MHC)-identical siblings will still reject if chronic immunosuppression is not utilized after transplantation because of the presence of these minor transplantation antigens.

MHC class III antigens encode complement components that are beyond the scope of this chapter.

TISSUE TYPING

Tissue typing, also called **HLA typing**, is the determination of the particular MHC alleles expressed by an individual. Matching to minimize differences in histocompatibility is critical, since the more antigenic the graft, the more vigorous the rejection response. The presence of

HLA antigens on a cell surface can be detected both functionally (most specific for class II antigens) and serologically (detects class I antigens). The functional method measures the reactivity of the serum from a potential recipient to the lymphocytes of the donor. The recipient serum is cultured with lymphocytes of the donor and will lyse donor lymphocytes in response to transplantation antigens of the donor, if they recognize them as being foreign. Only HLA (MHC) antigens are detected by this method; the most effective are those of class II MHC. Alloantisera specific for each of the class I loci (A, B, C) are also used for serologic typing of a potential donor and recipient by the use of antigen-specific sera, which reacts only with cells expressing that specific antigen.

B LYMPHOCYTES

B lymphocytes are the set of cells in the immune system generated to produce antibodies. Like T cells, they possess an antigen receptor. In the case of the B cell, the antigen receptor is a surface immunoglobulin molecule. B cells, with help from T cells, produce antibody in response to foreign antigen. Nine different immunoglobulin (Ig) isotypes have been identified: IgM, IgD, IgG_1, IgG_2, IgG_3, IgG_4, IgA_1, IgA_2, and IgE. Each antibody is composed of a heterodimer of two identical heavy chains and two identical light chains. The heavy and light chains have a constant region (Fc) that is identical for antibodies of that class, plus a highly variable binding or recognition site for antigen. The antibody binding site is formed by the association of the variable region of both the heavy and light chains. Each B cell produces only one highly specific antibody, and the variable region of the Ig gives each individual antibody its specific binding characteristics. All the immunoglobulins are glycoproteins. The variable region of the Ig binds antigen, resulting in conformational change of the constant portion which, in turn, stimulates a number of effects, such as complement fixation and histamine release by mast cells.

B cells, with the help of T cells, are stimulated to differentiate and mature into antibody-secreting plasma cells and memory cells only if they encounter antigens that bind to their antigen-specific surface Ig receptor. Unless stimulated by antigen, B cells become senescent. B cells can be activated directly by cross linkage of Ig molecules or indirectly through interactions with T cells. Antibody production involves interaction between B cells, CD4+ T helper cells, and accessory cells (APCs). The antigen-MHC complex on the macrophage cell surface membrane binds to the receptors of a CD4+ T helper cell. This stimulates the APC to produce IL-1 while the CD4+ cell produces IL-4, IL-5, and IL-6, which stimulate the B cell and further T cell proliferation. The first Ig produced by an activated B cell is IgM, which is subsequently switched to either IgA, IgG, or IgE, referred to as an **isotype switch**, without changing its antigen-specificity. Unless stimulated by antigen, the B cells become senescent at this stage of development. B cells are induced by antigen stimulation to mature into both antibody-secreting plasma cells and memory B cells, which are primed cells that remain in reserve. The memory B cells secrete antibody upon restimulation from T cells recognizing the same antigen. In the setting of re-exposure to the same antigen in transplantation, antibody-mediated hyperacute rejection results in the rapid (within 30 minutes) destruction of the allograft. The CD28 molecule present on T cells interacts with the B7 molecules on B cells and provides the second signal necessary for T cell activation. In the absence of this second signal, a state of anergy (antigen-specific unresponsiveness) can exist.

CROSS-MATCHING

In order to optimize transplant outcome and reduce the incidence and severity of acute cellular rejection, all kidney and pancreas transplant patients have their serum tested against the donor's lymphocytes in a cross-match test prior to receiving a transplant. Cross-matching is a test for identification of preformed cytotoxic antibody in the serum of potential allograft recipients, which reacts directly with the lymphocytes of other cells of a potential donor. Donor lymphocytes are cultured with recipient serum in the presence of complement and a vital dye. Lymphocyte destruction by antibody directed against the donor's T cells becomes apparent when the lysed cells take up the vital dye. The presence of these antibodies (a positive cross-match) usually, if not always, contraindicates the performance of transplantation because virtually all such grafts will be subject to a hyperacute rejection, which occurs within minutes after anastomosing the organ graft. Donor-directed antibodies can also be evaluated using flow cytometry but this technique may be too sensitive. It is currently being evaluated in comparison to standard cross-matching tests and clinically important rejection events.

The importance of matching MHC class I and class II antigens is also controversial. While statistically significant improvement in outcome can be demonstrated comparing patients with perfect matches at all six loci (HLA-A, -B, and -DR), this is not a continuum.

THE NATURAL KILLER CELL

The natural killer (NK) cell is a cytotoxic cell capable of killing tumor cells. NK cells are morphologically distinctive due to the presence of large cytoplasmic azurophilic granules that probably mediate tumor lysis. The NK receptor is unknown but is certainly not the T cell receptor. NK cell lysis is nonspecific. NK cells have been characterized as playing a major role in rejection of nonself bone marrow stem cells in bone marrow transplant recipients.

THE CELLULAR BASIS OF ALLOGRAFT REJECTION

The rejection response against an allograft is elicited when histocompatibility antigens on the transplanted tissue differ from those of the recipient. In kidney and pancreas transplantation, ABO blood group antigens will elicit a rapid, fulminant antibody-mediated graft rejection in recipients with preformed cytotoxic natural antibody, representing hyperacute rejection. A similar form of rejection occurs with some xenografts between different species when preformed cytotoxic antibodies are present in the recipient. However, the most common form of rejection encountered in clinical transplantation is acute rejection, which is mediated almost exclusively by T cells in response to MHC or transplantation antigens.

Two separate pathways of allograft recognition have been described. The first pathway of recognition of MHC-incompatible allografts involves a direct pathway in which the host responder T cells are activated by MHC class II-incompatible cells (passenger leukocytes) within the graft. The second, or indirect, pathway involves processing of graft alloantigens in a manner similar to nominal antigen as peptides presented by APC of the host (self–MHC-restricted antigen). Both of these pathways have been demonstrated to be involved in mechanisms of allorejection. Chronic rejection occurs in solid-organ grafts over months to years, and is most likely due to the deposition of anti-MHC antibodies, resulting in a gradual loss of graft function. Host-versus-graft response to the MHC-encoded alloantigens is mediated by both helper and cytotoxic T lymphocytes. Although in vitro work has demonstrated that class I antigens are the primary targets for cytotoxic T lymphocytes and class II antigens are the primary stimulating determinants for helper T lymphocytes, these two T cell subpopulations have been shown to cooperate in the generation of cytotoxic responses in vivo.

When a transplanted organ or tissue has mature T cells, a **graft-versus-host** (GVH) response may occur. Lymphocytes of donor origin recognize the transplanted antigens of the host as foreign, and allorejection of the host ensues. This occurs only in transplantation of tissue and organs that contain mature T lymphocytes, and is most common in bone marrow or small bowel transplants. This GVH response is primarily mediated by T cells and is controlled by the same nonspecific immunosuppressive regimens that treat graft-versus-host rejection.

Monoclonal antibodies directed at T cell subpopulations have been helpful in dissecting the sequence of events involved in rejection. Experimental transplantation utilizing monoclonal antibodies directed against either cell surface CD4+ or CD8+ molecules has suggested that depletion or blocking of CD4 prevents allorejection. This is confirmed with studies in mice that lack either the CD4 or CD8 gene, where even skin allograft rejection is prevented in the complete absence of CD4+ T cells. This supports the hypothesis that CD4+ cells are central to the induction of immune rejection, while CD8+ T cells play perhaps a specialized, but not essential, role in host defense.

By understanding the basis of immune recognition of allografted tissue, it has been possible to develop novel strategies to attempt to supplement current pharmacologic intervention for long-term maintenance of allografted tissue. The current nonspecific immunosuppressive agents have made transplantation possible, though their nonspecific function is antecedent with infections and the possibility of developing fatal tumors. Investigative efforts are now being directed to identify more specific therapies to manipulate the immune response to prevent allograft rejection. The ultimate goal in clinical transplantation is to induce a state of donor-specific unresponsiveness or tolerance to the transplanted allograft with full immunocompetence of the recipient to fight infections and to eliminate malignant cells.

SUGGESTED READING

Alberts B et al: *The Cell*, 2nd ed. Garland Publishing, 1989.

Fathman CG: Editorial overview. Inhibition of immune induction: The target of current transplantation tolerance strategies. Curr Opin Immunol 1992;4:545.

Paul WE: *Fundamental Immunology,* 3rd ed. Raven Press, 1993.

Schwartz JA, Schwartz RS: Structure and function of the immune system. In: Hoffman R et al (editors): *Hematology,* 2nd ed. Churchill Livingstone, 1995.

Sell S: *Immunology, Immunopathology, and Immunity.* Elsevier, 1987.

40.4 Transplant Immunopharmacology

Edward J. Alfrey, MD, & Randall E. Morris, MD

▶ Key Facts

- ▶ Most transplant centers use "triple therapy" for maintenance immunosuppression, which consists of prednisone, azathioprine, and cyclosporine.

- ▶ Quadruple therapy is the addition of either a polyclonal or monoclonal antibody preparation at the time of engraftment, which is continued for 10–14 days.

- ▶ Cyclosporine A is very effective at preventing the onset of acute cellular rejection in combination with prednisone and azathioprine when compared to dual therapy without cyclosporine A.

- ▶ Tacrolimus has been shown to reverse acute cellular rejection episodes that are refractory to treatment with steroids and anti–T cell antibodies.

- ▶ Steroids have been used as immunosuppressants for over 30 years. In addition to combination immunosuppressive therapy with cyclosporine and azathioprine, they are also the first line of therapy to treat acute rejection in most patients.

- ▶ Muromonab-CD3 (OKT3) and antithymocite globulin are primarily used as a second-line treatment for rejection in organ transplantation patients, but they are also used for induction immunotherapy in some centers.

- ▶ Immunosuppressants currently being developed include cyclosporine analogues, rapamycin, leflunomide, brequinar sodium, deoxyspergualin, and CD4 monoclonal antibodies.

Immunosuppressive strategies for solid organ transplantation have improved over the last 15 years such that 1-year patient and graft survival for most organ transplant recipients is now greater than 80%. Most transplant centers use "triple therapy" for maintenance immunosuppression, which consists of prednisone, azathioprine, and cyclosporine (Figure 40.4–1). Quadruple therapy is the addition of either a polyclonal or monoclonal antibody preparation at the time of engraftment, which is continued for 10–14 days. Since 1994, two new small molecules have been approved by the FDA for use in organ transplantation, tacrolimus and mycophenolate mofetil. Several other small molecules are in different phases of experimental trials and may be approved soon. There are also several new antibody preparations currently in evaluation. In the next decade we expect to see several new drugs available for prevention and treatment of rejection in organ transplantation.

CYCLOSPORINE A

Cyclosporine A (CsA) is a lipophilic cyclic polypeptide that acts on T lymphocytes to suppress cell-mediated immunity. CsA blocks early events in T cell activation by interfering with the transcription of the interleukin-2 (IL-2) gene and other cytokines in T helper cells. CsA does not ef-

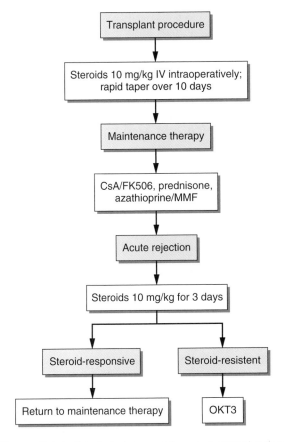

Figure 40.4–1. A typical strategy of immunosuppressive therapy for solid organ transplant recipients. CsA = cyclosporine; MMF = mycophenolate mofetil.

cellular rejection in combination with prednisone and azathioprine when compared to dual therapy without CsA. In the early 1980s when CsA was first introduced in liver transplantation, survival improved from approximately 30% at 1 year to 70%. CsA has become the primary immunosuppressant over the last 10 years, but has always been used in combination with prednisone (Figure 40.4–2).

Cyclosporine is poorly absorbed after oral administration. Absorption occurs in the small intestine. The bioavailability varies between 5% and 70%, which makes dosing between individual patients more difficult. Bile increases CsA absorption. Cyclosporine is metabolized in the liver by the cytochrome P450 system and then excreted in the bile. Clearance is increased in children. A new form of cyclosporine, Neoral, has more reliable bioavailability.

The side effects of CsA include nephrotoxicity, gingival hyperplasia, hypertrichosis, hypertension, hyperlipidemia, diabetes mellitus, and gastrointestinal and neurological events. Nephrotoxicity is secondary to CsA vasoconstrictor effects on the afferent arteriole and the proximal tubule. CsA whole blood levels are monitored to optimize the therapeutic effects and minimize the adverse effects. There are several accepted assays to measure CsA.

TACROLIMUS (FK 506)

Tacrolimus is a macrolide immunosuppressant that is 10–100 times more potent than cyclosporine in vitro and inhibits both cell-mediated and T cell–dependent humoral immunity. Like cyclosporine, tacrolimus binds to a cytosolic binding protein, FK506 binding protein (FKBP). This interaction inhibits calcineurin and blocks calcium-dependent molecules in signal transduction pathways, which then prevents the transcription of interleukin 2 and other cytokine genes. Cytokines produced after T cell activation, however, are not blocked by tacrolimus. In the thymus tacrolimus appears to inhibit thymocyte differentiation. Tacrolimus also inhibits IgM and IgG production by poke weed mitogen–stimulated B cells.

fect membrane signaling. Events that occur after activation of the IL-2 gene are not altered. CsA binds cyclophylin in the cytoplasm and targets calcineurin, a calcium-dependent phosphatase. Calcineurin is an intermediate in the cellular influx of calcium during nuclear gene expression.

CsA is very effective at preventing the onset of acute

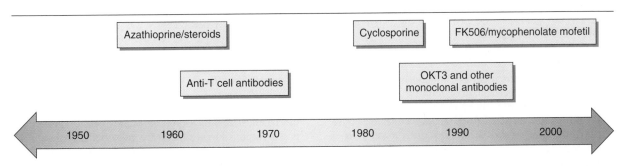

Figure 40.4–2. Approximate time periods when different immunosuppressive drugs were used in transplant patients.

Both in vitro and in vivo tacrolimus is far more potent than cyclosporine. This may be due to the fact that tacrolimus binds with much greater affinity to FKBP than cyclosporine binds to cyclophyllin. It is also possible that tacrolimus partitions more efficiently into the cytoplasm than cyclosporine. Tacrolimus has been shown to reverse acute cellular rejection episodes that are refractory to treatment with steroids and anti-T cell antibodies. The ability of tacrolimus to suppress ongoing rejection distinguishes it from cyclosporine. Currently, tacrolimus is the drug of choice for liver transplantation and is gaining more widespread use for pancreas transplantation as primary maintenance therapy.

Tacrolimus is lipophilic and metabolized extensively in the liver. It has a maximum peak absorption when given fasting or 1 hour prior to a meal. Pediatric patients have a higher clearance of tacrolimus but similar absorption to adults. Serum levels are measured and the dose adjusted to decrease toxicity. The side effects of tacrolimus include neurotoxicity, nephrotoxicity, gastrointestinal distress, and new-onset diabetes.

AZATHIOPRINE

Azathioprine was one of the first drugs used in transplantation for maintenance therapy. After its conversion to 6-mercaptopurine, it acts as an antimetabolite and suppresses lymphocyte proliferation by inhibition of DNA and RNA synthesis. Because it is a purine analog, 6-mercaptopurine is utilized as a precursor of RNA and DNA synthesis. Azathioprine is well absorbed from the gastrointestinal tract. Azathioprine was used in combination with prednisone as primary therapy until the early 1980s, when cyclosporine became available. It has since been used as triple therapy in combination with cyclosporine and prednisone.

The major side effects of azathioprine are leukopenia, thrombocytopenia, nausea, vomiting, pancreatitis, and hepatitis. Liver function studies and white blood cell counts are monitored and the dose of azathioprine is reduced or discontinued if either bone marrow suppression or hepatotoxicity occurs.

CORTICOSTEROIDS

Steroids have been used as immunosuppressants for over 30 years. One mechanism of action is the prevention of IL-1 and IL-6 production by macrophages. Glucocorticoids are rapidly absorbed from the gastrointestinal tract. At the time of engraftment, a high dose of steroids is given, followed by a rapid taper over the next 7–10 days. Maintenance doses are much lower. Steroids are currently used for maintenance immunosuppressive therapy in combination with cyclosporine and azathioprine. Steroids are also the first-line therapy to treat acute rejection in most transplant recipients.

Side effects of steroids include peptic ulcer disease, cataracts, metabolic bone disease, Cushing's syndrome, hyperlipidemia, mood swings, and poor wound healing.

MYCOPHENOLATE MOFETIL

Mycophenolate mofetil (MMF) is converted to mycophenolic acid, which is the active metabolite. Mycophenolic acid (MPA) uncompetitively inhibits inosine monophosphate dehydrogenase, which blocks the de novo synthesis of the purine guanosine, a requirement for DNA synthesis. The proliferation of T and B cell synthesis is extremely sensitive to MMF. However, the synthesis of IL-2 is not inhibited. Although lymphocytes require guanine nucleotides for DNA synthesis, other nonimmune cells compensate for the antiproliferative effects of MMF by producing purines via the salvage pathway. Therefore, MMF has been shown to be less myelotoxic than other immunosuppressive drugs in patients with psoriasis. MMF, marketed as CellCept, was recently approved for use by the FDA in organ transplantation. It is highly bioavailable, but large doses are required to suppress the alloimmune response. The low potency may result from its effective conversion into an inactive metabolite, its low binding to inosine monophosphate dehydrogenase, or perhaps because plasma proteins compete with inosine monophosphate dehydrogenase for binding to MPA. MMF is now being substituted for azathioprine for use in triple therapy in some transplant centers.

ANTIBODY TO T CELLS

MUROMONAB-CD3 (OKT3)

Muromonab-CD3 (OKT3) is a murine antihuman monoclonal antibody to the CD3 molecule found on human T cells. The CD3 molecule is a complex of invariant polypeptide chains that represents the signal transduction segment of the T cell receptor. OKT3 is produced by the hybridoma technique and is, therefore, derived from a single clone, which prevents the lot-to-lot variation seen with polyclonal antibody preparations. Because it is highly specific for mature T cells there is no nonspecific binding. By forming a complex with the CD3 antigen, OKT3 blocks the function of mature T cells. However, it also activates the T cell, which then promotes mitogenesis. This activation is responsible in part for the side effects seen after the first dose of OKT3. Inhibition of T cell antigen recognition occurs as a result of the receptor blockade. OKT3 coats the circulating T cells, which are then removed from circulation. It may also modulate the CD3 molecule, which results in the removal of the molecule from the cell surface. Because the CD3 molecule is modulated, several days after initiation of OKT3 therapy T cells that express CD4 and CD8 but not CD3 molecules may appear.

OKT3 is eliminated by binding to mature T cells. It is only administered by intravenous infusion. The effect of OKT3 is monitored by evaluating the absolute number of CD3$^+$ T cells by flow cytometry. An absolute number of greater than 10 CD3$^+$ T cells/mm^3 necessitates a doubling of the dose. Because OKT3 is a monoclonal antibody, a smaller dose of immunoglobulin can be given. In general, adults are initially treated with 2.5–5.0 mg/d. Pediatric patients receive 2.5 mg/d. Within 10 minutes of the initial dose, T cells are removed from the circulation. However, the effect on central lymphoid compartments is unclear at the present. Additionally, patients who develop antimouse antibodies will require increased doses.

OKT3 was initially approved by the FDA for treatment of steroid-resistant rejection in renal transplant recipients. It is now primarily used as second-line treatment for rejection in all organ transplant patients. However, OKT3 is also used in some centers for "induction" immunotherapy, given at the time of transplantation and continued for up to 10–14 days posttransplant, although it has not been approved by the FDA for such use. Approximately 50% of all transplant patients will develop a rejection episode within the first 90 days posttransplant, and 50–80% of these will respond to steroids ("**steroid sensitive**"). Of the patients who are steroid resistant, 80–90% will respond to OKT3. When used as induction therapy, OKT3 delays the time to first rejection from 2 weeks to 4 weeks. It is probably most useful for induction therapy in pancreas transplant patients, and kidney transplant patients who are highly sensitized.

Because OKT3 specifically binds to the CD3 molecule, myelosuppression is not seen in patients receiving this antibody. However, after the first two doses, patients usually have a constellation of flu-like symptoms. The symptoms are related cytokines released after the lysis of the T cells, particularly tumor necrosis factor (TNF), interleukin-2 (IL-2) and IL-6, and interferon-gamma (IFN-γ). The increase in IL-2 can be abated with corticosteriods administered concomitantly with OKT3. Symptoms in patients receiving OKT3 include fever, headache, nausea, vomiting, diarrhea, hypertension, and fatigue. Aseptic meningitis can occasionally be seen. Steroids, antihistamines, and antipyretics are administered concurrently with OKT3 to reduce the symptoms associated with the initial doses. Steroids not only decrease the severity of the patients' response to TNF, IL-2, and IFN-γ but also decrease the production of these cytokines. Mild to severe pulmonary edema can occur after the first dose of OKT3. It is recommended that patients who are more than 3% above their dry weight (postdialysis weight) be diuresed or dialyzed prior to administration of OKT3. A humanized chimeric anti-CD3 monoclonal antibody is being evaluated that does not have associated cytokine release or the anti-idiotypic re-

sponse seen with OKT3. In addition, mouse IgM monoclonal antibody directed to the T cell receptor is in clinical trials; it does not produce the cytokine release syndrome.

ANTITHYMOCYTE GLOBULIN

Antithymocyte globulin (ATGAM) is an equine antihuman gamma globulin made from hyperimmune serum extracted from horses immunized with human thymus lymphocytes. It is used for the treatment of steroid-resistant rejection in most centers but is also used for induction immunotherapy. After systemic administration, a reduction in the number of circulating thymus-dependent T cells is observed. It also depletes lymphocytes in the spleen and lymph nodes. It must be administered into a central venous line or a dialysis fistula or shunt. The white blood cell count is monitored daily and the dose adjusted for leukopenia.

Side effects of ATGAM include fever, chills, leukopenia, thrombocytopenia, rash, and pruritus. Rarely, dyspnea, headache, diarrhea, or hypotension is seen. An intradermal test dose should be given prior to the first dose. Patients usually receive 10–30 mg/kg for 10–14 days as therapy for steroid-resistent rejection.

IMMUNOSUPPRESSANTS IN DEVELOPMENT

CYCLOSPORINE ANALOGUES

Two analogues have been recently evaluated in clinical trials: cyclosporine G (CsG) and IMM125. Both analogues effectively suppress immune responses in preclinical models in vitro and in vivo, but have been discontinued from further development.

RAPAMYCIN

Part of this molecule has the same structure as the segment of tacrolimus that binds to FKBP, so it is not surprising that rapamycin (RPM) also binds to FKBP. The structural similarity between FK506 and RPM prompted the first studies of RPM in transplantation. In fact, RPM, like CsA and FK506, is a prodrug that must first complex with its immunophilin before it can block immune cell activation. RPM blocks cell proliferation caused by growth factors by preventing cells from progressing from the G$_1$ to the S phase of the cell cycle by affecting the proteins that are required for cell cycle progression. The precise molecular targets for the RPM-FKBP complex are unknown, but may involve kineses: RPM affects T and B cells directly by preventing cytokines from activating these cells.

Since RPM appears to be capable of blocking only cell proliferation stimulated by growth factors, the actions of

RPM are more restricted than many antiproliferative drugs that halt the division of all cells. Phase II studies in cadaveric renal transplant patients have shown RPM to reduce the incidence of biopsy-proven rejection substantially.

LEFLUNOMIDE

Leflunomide (LFM) has been used in hundreds of patients in Europe for the treatment of rheumatoid arthritis and only recently has been considered for use in transplantation. After oral absorption, LFM is converted in the blood into its active form, A77 1726 (a malononitrilamide). LFM was developed as a prodrug to reduce the gastrointestinal irritation caused by ingesting A77 1726. Very little is known about how LFM suppresses the actions of immune cells other than recent data which suggest that tyrosine kinases associated with growth factor receptors and the de novo pathway for pyrimidine biosynthesis are inhibited by this drug. At the cellular level, LFM has been shown to inhibit immune cell proliferation. Like RPM, LFM blocks the action of IL-2 and other immune cytokines as well as the mitogenic effects of growth factors on nonimmune cells.

Although much more preclinical work needs to be done to understand the potential roles of LFM as a suppressant of graft rejection, there are several reasons to continue to evaluate its potential: (1) it has been well tolerated in patients at blood levels required to treat rheumatoid arthritis; (2) its ability to inhibit cytokine and growth factor action defines an unusual mechanism of action similar to RPM; (3) its actions are not limited to T cells, since it very effectively blocks antibody synthesis; (4) it effectively prolongs allograft survival in small and large animal models; and (5) since it produces neither myelotoxicity nor nephrotoxicity, it should be able to be used in combination with other drugs to minimize their toxicities without sacrificing overall immunosuppressive efficacy. While LFM will be restricted to use in autoimmune diseases, malononitrilamide analogs are being evaluated for transplantation.

BREQUINAR SODIUM

Brequinar sodium (BQR) inhibits T and B cell proliferation by interfering with nucleotide biosynthesis. BQR inhibits the action of dihydroorotate dehydrogenase in the de novo biosynthetic pathway leading to the synthesis of pyrimidines needed for DNA and RNA synthesis. Evidently, the salvage pathway in T and B cells cannot compensate for the reduction in pyrimidine synthesis caused by the inhibition of the de novo pathway by BQR. Inhibition of the de novo synthesis of uridine by BQR could reduce plasma levels of uridine, which is a substrate for the salvage pathway in lymphocytes. Like MMF, BQR decreases the function of adhesion molecules on lymphocytes in vitro, because glycosylation of adhesion molecules requires pyrimidine—as well as purine—sugar intermediates.

The efficacy of BQR as an immunosuppressant has been primarily determined from work in rodents. These experiments have shown that BQR effectively prolongs the survival of organ allografts when the dose and schedule are modified to minimize toxicity and maximize efficacy. BQR has also been shown to reverse ongoing rejection. BQR very effectively controls antibody synthesis by its direct action on B cells, and it is one of the most effective drugs available for the treatment of two forms of antibody-mediated rejection.

There is no question that BQR very effectively inhibits the actions of T and B cells that cause different forms of graft rejection. Since its mechanism of action does not allow it to be completely lymphocyte-specific, its utility in clinical transplantation will depend on how much more sensitive lymphocytes are to its antiproliferative effects than cells in the marrow and gastrointestinal tract. Based on current knowledge, it is unlikely that BQR can replace CsA as a primary immunosuppressant. Used with CsA, however, BQR could play an important role as an inhibitor of antigraft antibody and as a means of reversing intractable rejection. Its clinical development is currently on hold.

DEOXYSPERGUALIN

Deoxyspergualin (DSG) has little in common with the other new immunosuppressive drugs. It can be administered only parenterally, and typical treatment schedules last 5–10 days. It does not inhibit the synthesis of IL-2 but does reduce IL-1 synthesis. By blocking the maturation of T and B cells, DSG halts the development of cytotoxic T cells and the development of B cells into antibody-secreting cells. DSG can be added several days after stimulation of immune cells in vitro without loss of efficacy. How DSG causes these effects is unknown, but the recent finding that DSG binds to a cytoplasmic heat shock protein may ultimately give a clue about this drug's mechanism of action.

Despite numerous clinical studies of DSG in transplant patients in Japan, the ultimate role of DSG in transplantation remains to be seen. For now, its predicted uses might include treatment of ongoing rejection and prevention or suppression of unwanted primary or secondary antibody responses.

CD4 MONOCLONAL ANTIBODIES

The CD4 molecule is expressed on immature T cells in the thymus and on mature T helper cells in humans. However, the CD4 molecule is also found on monocytes, macrophages, Langerhans cells, eosinophils, endothelial cells in the hepatic sinusoids, and sperm cells. Therefore, monoclonal antibodies (MAbs) directed at the CD4 molecule can have a wide spectrum of activity. The CD4 molecule recognizes the MHC class II antigen on T cells. CD4+ T cells assist in B cell activation, differentiation, and proliferation. CD4 MAbs may act by preventing the interaction between T cells and antigen-presenting cells.

Initial experience with CD4 MAbs in organ transplantation suggests that they must be administered prior to antigen stimulation for effect. This may result from the fact that after B cells are stimulated they no longer require T helper cells for activity. Whether or not the CD4$^+$ T cells need to be eliminated or just modulated is not clear from the current experience. In a human clinical trial conducted by the National Institutes of Health, 19 patients received 0.5 mg/kg of murine OKT4 for 12 days in addition to routine triple therapy (CsA, prednisone, azathioprine). Seven (37%) of the patients were treated for rejection within the first 90 days posttransplant, a rate somewhat lower than routine. There were no adverse side effects, which supports the need for further clinical investigation of these MAbs.

INFECTIOUS & MALIGNANT COMPLICATIONS OF IMMUNOSUPPRESSIVE THERAPY

Infectious and malignant complications are increased in patients after transplantation as a result of the use of immunosuppressive therapy. The risk for these complications is directly related to the dose and length of time patients are taking these medications. In the early posttransplant period, the type of infectious complication is similar to nonimmunosuppressed patients, but by the first month, opportunistic infections begin to appear. Prophylactic regimens are used to reduce the morbidity and mortality from infections after transplantation. While all types of malignant complications increase after transplantation, viral-associated malignancies such as lymphomas show the greatest increase. Posttransplant lymphoproliferative disorder (PTLD) is directly related to the amount of immunosuppression and the recipient pretransplant and donor serological status. Children who are negative for the Epstein-Barr virus (EBV) and receive an EBV-positive donor graft have a very high incidence of PTLD (11% in liver transplant patients receiving FK506 maintenance therapy). The time to development of PTLD and its virulence and incidence have increased in some centers since the introduction of OKT3 in the late 1980s. Other centers have reported no change in the pattern of PTLD since OKT3 has been added to the therapeutic strategies at their centers.

SUGGESTED READING

Chatenoud L, Bach JF: Monoclonal antibodies to CD3 as immunosuppressants. Immunology 1990;2:437.

Morris RE: New immunosuppressive drugs. In: Busuttil RW, Klintmalm GB (editors): *Transplantaion of the Liver*. Saunders, 1996.

Morris RE: New small molecule immunosuppressants for transplantation: Review of essential concepts. J Heart Lung Transplant 1993;12:S275.

Sablinski T et al: CD4 monoclonal antibodies in organ transplantation—a review of progress. Transplantation 1991;52:579.

Schreiber SL, Crabtree GR: The mechanism of action of cyclosporin A and FK506. Immunol Today 1992;13:136.

Thomson AW, Starzl TE: New immunosuppressive drugs: Mechanistic insights and potential advances. Immunol Rev 1993;136:71.

40.5 HLA & Histocompatibility Testing

Alan Ting, PhD

► Key Facts

- ► Human leukocyte antigens (HLAs) are involved in the initiation of the immune response and act as targets of the host's rejection response.

- ► The three main histocompatibility tests used in transplantation are HLA type and match, HLA antibody screen, and HLA crossmatch.

- ► HLA antibodies are not "naturally occurring" and only develop after a sensitizing event. These antibodies bind to the appropriate antigens on endothelial cells lining the blood vessels, causing immediate (hyperacute) rejection.

- ► Acute rejection (occurring in the first week after transplantation) may be caused by "weak" HLA antibodies not detected by standard crossmatch methods.

- ► Crossmatch techniques with greater sensitivity to detect weak HLA antibodies include antihuman globulin (AHG) augmentation of cytotoxicity, B lymphocyte cytotoxicity, and flow cytometry.

- ► The importance of the three histocompatibility tests varies among kidney, heart, and liver transplants.

HLA & ITS CLINICAL IMPORTANCE

HLA stands for "human leukocyte antigen." It was given this designation because the antigens were first detected on the surface of leukocytes, in the mid-1950s.

HLA antigens are clinically important because they are the major cell surface antigens that are recognized as foreign on a transplanted allograft. These antigens are involved in the initiation of the immune response and act as targets of the host's rejection response. Therefore, HLA antigens are major histocompatibility antigens, and the HLA system is the human major histocompatibility complex (MHC). The ABO blood group system is also a major histocompatibility system. Transplants carried out across the ABO barrier are mostly rejected immediately, because of the presence of preexisting antibody in the recipient that binds to the ABO blood group antigens on the endothelial cells lining the blood vessels of the transplanted organ.

GENETIC STRUCTURE OF THE HLA SYSTEM

The HLA system is located on the short arm of chromosome 6. It is divided into three regions (designated class I, II, and III), based primarily on differences in molecular structure, function, and tissue distribution. Well over 100 genes have been mapped to the HLA region, so far. The eight genes that are the most important in histocompatibility are shown in Figure 40.5–1.

CLASS I REGION

Over 50 genes have been mapped to this region, including the A, B, and Cw genes. Class I antigens were the first HLA antigens detected. Each antigen is made up of two polypeptide chains, one with a molecular weight (MW) of 45,000 and the other 11,000. The heavy chain is polymor-

REGION: CLASS II CLASS III CLASS I

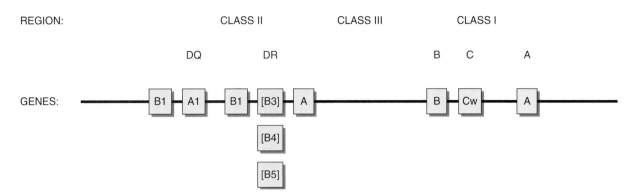

Figure 40.5–1. Genetic structure of the HLA region on chromosome 6. The eight genes that are most important in transplantation are shown. In the DR region, the B3, B4, and B5 genes occupy the same position on the chromosome, and each chromosome has only one of these genes.

phic, confers the "specificity," and is encoded by the HLA gene. The 11,000 MW chain is B_2 microglobulin, which is nonpolymorphic, and is encoded by a gene on chromosome 15. Class I antigens have a widespread distribution, and are found on virtually all nucleated cells, including endothelial cells lining the blood vessels. These antigens are primary targets of immune attack, both by cellular and antibody mechanisms.

CLASS II REGION

Over 30 genes have been mapped to this region, including the DR and DQ genes. Class II antigens also are made up of two polypeptide chains (alpha [A] and beta [B]). The alpha chain has a MW of 33,000 and the beta chain 28,000. Both molecules are encoded by HLA genes. The DR beta genes are highly polymorphic, encoding multiple alleles, whereas the DR alpha gene codes only two alleles. The DQ alpha and beta genes are both polymorphic, but it is the product of the DQB gene that confers "specificity." Class II antigens have a more restricted tissue distribution than class I. For example, they are not found on T lymphocytes, and are less dense on endothelial cells than class I antigens. Class II antigens are primarily involved in the initiation of the immune response.

CLASS III REGION

About 30 genes have been mapped, including many complement genes, such as Bf, C_2, and C_4 (not shown in the figure). The 21-hydroxylase enzyme gene is also found in this region. Class III genes will not be discussed in this chapter.

DETECTION OF HLA ANTIGENS & ALLELES

The HLA type of an individual can be determined at two levels: antigen and allele. An **HLA antigen** is a molecule made up of two polypeptide chains and found on the cell surface (previously described). HLA antigens are detected by antibody-dependent serologic tests. An **HLA allele** is a polypeptide chain that is encoded by an HLA gene. Alleles are detected by molecular DNA techniques, which identify the unique nucleotide sequence of DNA corresponding to the region of the polypeptide that confers the "allele specificity."

SEROLOGIC HLA TYPING

HLA class I and II antigens are detected by the lymphocyte cytotoxicity test. Class I typing uses T lymphocytes as targets and class II typing uses B lymphocytes (this is because T lymphocytes do not have class II antigens). In brief, lymphocytes are isolated from whole blood by attachment to immunomagnetic beads coated with monoclonal antibodies to T cells (CD2 or CD8) or B cells (CD19), and then labeled with carboxyfluoroscein diacetate (CFDA), which stains the live cells green. These cells are incubated with reagent antisera in microtest trays. Complement (rabbit serum) is added, and then ethidium bromide (EB). EB is taken up by dead cells (which have been killed by antibody-antigen reaction and complement). The tests are examined with fluorescent microscopy for positive reactions (dead cells that stain red), and negative reactions (live cells that stain green).

Most reagent antisera are obtained from multiparous women. Other sources include monoclonal antibodies from mouse and human hybridomas, and from Epstein

Barr virus–transformed antibody-secreting human B cell lines.

MOLECULAR DNA TYPING

Routine clinical DNA typing for HLA class II alleles (DR and DQ) is relatively new, and a number of techniques are being used or evaluated by different laboratories. Not all laboratories use DNA techniques, some still rely on serologic techniques. Class I DNA typing techniques are currently being developed and will probably be in routine clinical use within the next few years.

All DNA techniques require extraction of DNA (usually from whole blood) and a DNA amplification step to obtain sufficient material for analysis. Amplification is carried out in a thermal cycler with Taq polymerase enzyme and two oligonucleotide primers flanking the DNA segment to be amplified. This is the **polymerase chain reaction (PCR)**. The principles of the three most commonly used techniques are briefly described.

Sequence-Specific Primers

PCR amplification of DNA is carried out with sequence-specific primers (SSPs) against each HLA allele, separately. Only DNA that hybridizes with a primer set is amplified, and the amplified DNA is detected as a band by agarose gel electrophoresis. The "specificity" determination is part of the DNA amplification step.

Sequence-Specific Oligonucleotide Probes

PCR amplification of genomic DNA is carried out with biotin-labeled primers specific for the DR (or DQ) gene. The amplified DNA is then hybridized with sequence-specific oligonucleotide probes (SSOPs), which have been immobilized on nitrocellulose strips, for each allele separately. Detection of hybridization consists of streptavidin/alkaline phosphatase conjugate, which binds to biotin-labeled hybrids, and BCIP/NBT chromogen substrate, which forms a purple precipitate. The test is examined visually, and the pattern of positive stripes is interpreted. The "specificity" determination is carried out as a post-DNA amplification step.

Oligonucleotide Sequencing

The nucleotides of the DR (or DQ) gene are directly sequenced. This method gives the highest resolution of class II typing but it is very labor intensive (and costly). High-resolution HLA typing is used in bone marrow transplants from unrelated donors and is not normally used in solid organ transplantation.

DNA techniques have a number of advantages over serological analysis. These include greater reproducibility, no need for live cells, and possibility of automation; in addition, the primers and probes are synthetically made and can be easily standardized and used repeatedly. On the other hand, serological typing reagents for many specificities are difficult to obtain in large quantities and their stan-

dardization can be difficult. There is no doubt that DNA techniques will replace serological analysis in the routine laboratory within the next few years.

RELATIONSHIP BETWEEN GENE, ALLELE, & ANTIGEN

One antigen can have many alleles, and most of these differences between alleles cannot be detected serologically. For example, 20 different alleles of the antigen DR4 can be detected by molecular DNA techniques but none can be detected by serological analysis. All alleles of an antigen have a common amino acid sequence, which confers the "antigen specificity." In addition, each allele has its unique amino acid sequence, which confers the "allele specificity." The relationship between the gene, allele, and antigen is represented in Figure 40.5–2. Nomenclature of HLA antigens and alleles are specified in Table 40.5–1.

INHERITANCE OF HLA ANTIGENS & ALLELES

HLA antigens are codominantly inherited. The A, B, Cw, DR, and DQ genes are closely linked, and the encoded antigens and alleles are normally inherited together. Recombination occurs at a rate of about 1% between A and B, and 0.8% between B and DR. Each individual has two A, two B, two Cw, two DR, and two DQ antigens. The degree of HLA match among immediate family members can be precisely determined, and these are defined as: **HLA identical** (siblings who have inherited the same HLA haplotype from both parents). A **haplotype** is the HLA antigens/alleles encoded by the HLA genes of one parental chromosome; **HLA haploidentical** (siblings who share one haplotype). Parents and offsprings are haploidentical; and **HLA mismatched** (siblings who share no haplotypes).

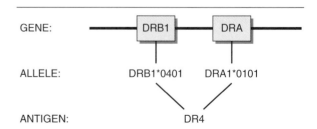

Figure 40.5–2. The relation between gene, allele, and antigen. The product of the DRB1 gene is the polypeptide chain (allele) DRB1*0401, and the product of the DRA gene is DRA*0101. These two polypeptide chains combine to form the antigen DR4.

Table 40.5–1. Nomenclature of HLA antigens and alleles.

Antigen
[Gene] + [number for the specificity] Examples are: A2, B27, DR4, DQ1

Allele
[Gene] + [*] + [2-digit number for the specificity] + [2-digit number for the allele] Examples are A*0201, B*2701, DRB1*0401, DQB1*0602

HISTOCOMPATIBILITY TESTING

The three main histocompatibility tests used in transplantation are HLA type and match, HLA antibody screen, and HLA crossmatch.

HLA TYPE & MATCH—RATIONALE FOR CLINICAL USE

Graft outcome is improved if the donor and recipient are matched for their HLA antigens. However, finding completely HLA-matched pairs within an unrelated population (most solid organ transplants are from unrelated cadaver donors) is extremely rare because of the enormous polymorphism of HLA antigens and alleles. Fortunately, not all HLA antigens are important in transplantation—only A, B, and DR. Furthermore, the relative strengths of these antigens is different; DR is "stronger" than B, which is "stronger" than A. That is, matching the donor and recipient for DR antigens has the greatest impact on graft survival, followed by matching for B, and then matching for A. To illustrate this point, data from the United Network for Organ Sharing (UNOS) are shown in Table 40.5–2.

UNOS is responsible for administering organ procurement and allocation, and the collection of scientific data in the United States. The data show a clear correlation between the quality of donor-recipient HLA match and graft

Table 40.5–2. 1- and 2-year graft survival rates for recipients of first cadaver grafts, according to degree of HLA match or mismatch.[1]

Group	No. Patients	Graft Survival (%)	
		1-year	2-year
6-antigen match	1239	89	83
0 A,B,DR mm	195	89	83
0 B,DR mm	618	84	73
1 B,DR mm	3988	83	72
2 B,DR mm	10,206	81	69
3 B,DR mm	9369	79	67
TOTAL	32,003	81	69

[1]Data from the United Network for Organ Sharing (UNOS) for transplants performed 10/1/87–12/31/92.
mm = mismatch.

survival at 1 and 2 years. The 6-antigen matched (matched for two A, two B, and two DR antigens) and zero A, B, and DR mismatched grafts have the same (and highest) survival rates. Then follows a correlation between the number of B, DR mismatches and graft survival rates. The importance of HLA matching in kidney transplantation, however, is only relative, and not an absolute prerequisite for a successful transplant. In fact, the vast majority of transplants are HLA-mismatched to some extent, and most are successful (about 85% at 1 year after transplantation). This is because all patients receive posttransplant maintenance immunosuppression (eg, cyclosporine, FK506, steroids, azathioprine, etc), without which all grafts would fail (except those from monozygotic twins). A short cold ischemia time after organ procurement and the use of potent immunosuppressive drugs (eg, antithymocyte globulin [ATG] and anti-T-cell monoclonal antibodies [OKT3]) for the treatment of rejection episodes are additional factors that contribute to the high success rate of cadaveric donor kidney transplants.

HLA ANTIBODY SCREEN & CROSSMATCH—RATIONALE FOR CLINICAL USE

HLA antibodies are not "naturally occurring" and develop only after a sensitizing event. These antibodies can bind to the appropriate antigens on the endothelial cells lining blood vessels of the transplanted organ, causing immediate (hyperacute) rejection. This association between preexisting HLA antibodies and immediate graft rejection was first demonstrated in the mid-1960s by Patel and Terasaki, and proved to be the most important finding made in histocompatibility. Based on this finding it became necessary to screen patients for HLA antibodies on a regular basis prior to transplantation, and particularly after a sensitizing event. Furthermore, a pretransplant crossmatch (react the patient's serum against the donor's lymphocytes to detect donor-specific HLA antibodies) is always carried out, and a positive crossmatch result is a strict contraindication to transplantation.

Causes of Sensitization to HLA
Patients can develop HLA antibodies after sensitization by pregnancies, blood transfusions, and a previous failed graft. About 50% of women with multiple pregnancies develop HLA antibodies; their presence in the serum may be brief (days to months) or, frequently, prolonged (many years). About 30–40% of multiply-transfused patients develop antibodies. Up to 90% of patients develop HLA antibodies after a failed graft, particularly if the graft is removed. The HLA antibodies that develop after these modes of sensitization are mostly IgG. Occasionally, IgM HLA antibodies are found in nontransfused, nontransplanted male patients, and it is thought that their occurrence is due to viral infections. Additionally, patients may develop IgM HLA (and non-HLA) antibodies after transplantation while receiving immunosuppressive therapy.

HLA Antibodies & Hyperacute Rejection

Hyperacute rejection (rejection occurring within hours after revascularization) is generally considered to be caused by IgG HLA class I antibodies. These antibodies bind to the appropriate HLA antigens on the endothelium lining the small blood vessels of the transplanted organ. This binding causes complement fixation, platelet aggregation, and fibrin deposition. This cascade leads to occlusion of the vessels and death of the tissues and organ. IgM HLA class I antibodies probably do not cause hyperacute rejection, and there is even some evidence that they do not damage kidney allografts at all.

HLA Antibodies & Acute Rejection

Acute rejection (rejection occurring in the first week after transplantation) may be caused by "weak" HLA antibodies not detected by the "standard" crossmatch method. In the standard cytotoxic test the patient's serum and donor's cells are incubated for 30 minutes, complement is added and incubated for a further 60 minutes, and an indicator system is added to the test to distinguish positive reactions (dead cells) and negative reactions (live cells). More sensitive crossmatch techniques have been developed to detect weak HLA antibodies, and the most commonly used are:

1. *Anti Human Globulin (AHG) Augmentation of Cytotoxicity.* An anti-kappa antibody is added to the cells-serum mixture, and allows the detection of antibodies that normally do not fix complement, in addition to complement-fixing antibodies.
2. *B Lymphocyte Cytotoxicity.* B lymphocytes have a higher density of class I antigens than do T cells. Weak HLA class I antibodies can react with B cells but not T cells. One major drawback of using B lymphocytes, however, is that class II antibodies also react with B lymphocytes, and their impact on graft outcome is still not fully understood. It is impossible to tell whether a positive B lymphocyte crossmatch is due to weak class I antibodies or to class II antibodies.
3. *Flow Cytometry.* This technique is a binding assay that can detect binding antibodies that are not cytotoxic. Furthermore, the flow cytometer can detect very low numbers of antibody molecules bound onto cells. It is the most sensitive crossmatch method and is in routine use by most laboratories.

HLA Class II Antibodies

HLA class II antigens are less dense on endothelial cells than class I antigens. Anti-DR and anti-DQ antibodies, whether IgG or IgM, probably do not cause hyperacute rejections, although they may cause acute rejections or be associated with a lower long-term graft survival rate. These conclusions are controversial, and most histocompatibility laboratories neither screen nor crossmatch for class II antibodies, based on the assumption that they are benign to an allograft.

APPLICATIONS OF HISTOCOMPATIBILITY TESTING IN SOLID ORGAN TRANSPLANTATION

The relative importance and use of the three histocompatibility tests varies among kidney, heart, and liver transplants, and each will be discussed in turn.

KIDNEY & KIDNEY-PANCREAS TRANSPLANTATION

In the majority of cases in which a pancreas is transplanted, a kidney is simultaneously transplanted from the same cadaver donor; therefore, the "rules" that apply to kidney transplants also apply to the pancreas.

The kidney can be procured from a cadaver or a living donor. In the United States about 25% of all kidney transplants are from living donors, although in some centers it can be as high as 50%.

Cadaver Donor Kidneys

The procurement and allocation of all cadaveric donor kidneys in the United States is carried out on a regional basis by the local Organ Procurement Organization (OPO), which is accredited by UNOS (currently there are 60–70 OPOs in the United States). The policy of organ allocation is based on an equal balance between medical utility and justice. Medical utility means that the outcome of all transplants as a whole should be maximized (that is, factors known to increase the likelihood of graft success should be implemented). Justice means that all patients should have equal access to all organs.

In practice, a donor kidney procured by an OPO is HLA typed and crossmatched by the local laboratory, with all patients of the identical ABO blood group. Zero A, B, and DR antigen–mismatched kidneys must be mandatorily shared nationwide. A list of all patients with their HLA types is held at UNOS. Kidneys that are not shared are allocated locally. The crossmatch-negative patients in the OPO's jurisdiction are ranked according to the UNOS allocation algorithm, which assigns points to each patient based on: (1) quality of HLA match between donor and recipient; (2) length of waiting time for a donor organ; (3) HLA sensitization status (highly sensitized patients receive extra points); (4) age of the recipient (pediatric patients receive extra points).

The patient with the highest number of points is offered the kidney, provided that the crossmatch is negative. If the offer is turned down (for acute medical or other reasons), the kidney is offered to the patient with the next highest number of points, and so on until both kidneys have been placed. Because of the extreme shortage of donors, most patients will wait at least 2 years before receiving a transplant.

Not all transplant professionals support the use of HLA

matching in the allocation algorithm, because they have not found that HLA-matched grafts have a better survival rate than HLA-mismatched grafts in their own centers. As a consequence, OPOs can apply to UNOS for a local variance to the UNOS allocation algorithm. These may be granted, provided that the policy takes into account medical utility and justice. One such variance is to allocate kidneys based essentially on waiting time alone.

Living Donor Kidneys

During the medical work-up, patients are HLA-typed for A, B, and DR, and screened for HLA antibodies. Family members who wish to be considered as donors are HLA-typed and crossmatched. If all other factors are equal (eg, medical and psychological fitness, willingness to donate, etc), an HLA-identical sibling is usually selected (if such a donor is available), since grafts from these family members have the best chance of long-term success (survival rate is ~95% at 1 year) compared with lesser matched grafts. A sensitive crossmatch technique (eg, flow cytometry) may be used in transplants that have a potential for high immunological risk, such as offspring to mother, because of possible presensitization, and in highly sensitized patients (patients with broadly reactive HLA antibodies).

Because of the extreme shortage of cadaver donors, many transplant centers advocate the use of distant relatives (eg, cousins, aunts, and uncles), and genetically unrelated individuals, such as spouses, as donors. The success rates of these transplants are extremely high (~90–95% at 1 year), although most will be a poor HLA match (Terasaki, 1995). The histocompatibility tests performed for these transplants are the same as for living related donors, and a sensitive crossmatch is often used, particularly if the transplant is from a husband to his wife.

HEART, HEART-LUNG, & LUNG TRANSPLANTATION

Retrospective analyses have shown that HLA-matched heart and lung grafts, particularly those matched for DR antigens, have a better survival rate than mismatched grafts. However, HLA matching is not used in the selection of donor-recipient pairs because of logistic difficulties, such as patient medical urgency status, short allowable cold ischemia time of the organ once procured, and size match between donor and recipient.

Preexisting HLA antibodies can cause hyperacute rejection and acute rejection of cardiac grafts; therefore, all patients are screened for HLA antibodies at medical evaluation. A pretransplant crossmatch is performed in patients who have HLA antibodies. If the crossmatch is positive, the transplant is not performed in that patient.

The major factors considered in heart, heart-lung, and lung allocation are (1) ABO blood group compatibility; (2) negative HLA crossmatch (in patients with HLA antibodies); (3) patient medical urgency status; and (4) size match between donor and recipient.

LIVER TRANSPLANTATION

Prospective HLA matching is not used for the same logistic difficulties listed for heart transplantation, and because there is not clear evidence that HLA matching significantly improves graft survival. On the contrary, some published data show that HLA-matched transplants have a poorer graft survival rate than HLA-mismatched transplants! One proposed explanation is that matched grafts are more susceptible to viral infections, so that the graft is lost not because of rejection, but patient death.

The role of HLA antibodies on liver transplants is not clear. Some studies have shown that they can cause acute rejection, while other studies have shown that they are completely benign. Many centers do not screen their patients for HLA antibodies or perform a prospective crossmatch. There is no doubt that the liver is more resistant to antibody-mediated rejection than other solid organs. It has been well-documented that circulating HLA antibodies are cleared from the patient's blood after successful liver transplantation, although the precise mechanism is unknown. There have even been reports of highly sensitized patients who received both a liver and kidney transplant in spite of a positive crossmatch. In these cases, the liver is transplanted first, then the kidney from the same donor is transplanted once the HLA antibodies are removed from the circulation (presumably by the liver). These kidneys have not suffered hyperacute or acute rejection.

The major factors considered in liver allocation are (1) ABO blood group compatibility; (2) patient medical urgency status; and (3) size match between donor and recipient.

SUGGESTED READING

Bodmer J et al: Nomenclature for factors of the HLA system, 1995. Hum Immunol 1995;43:149.
Campbell RD, Trowsdale J: Map of the human MHC. Immunol Today 1993;14:349.
Iwaki Y, Yoshida Y, Griffith B: The HLA matching effect in lung transplantation. Transplantation 1993;56:1528.

Manez R et al: The influence of HLA donor-recipient compatibility on the recurrence of HBV and HCV hepatitis after liver transplantation. Transplantation 1995;59:640.
Nikaein A et al: HLA compatibility and liver transplant outcome. Improved patient survival by HLA and cross-matching. Transplantation 1994;58:786.

Opelz G, Wujciak T: The influence of HLA compatibility on graft survival after heart transplantation. N Engl J Med 1994;330:816.

Patel R, Terasaki PI: Significance of the positive crossmatch test in kidney transplantation. N Engl J Med 1969;280:735.

Terasaki PI et al: High survival rates of kidney transplants from spousal and living unrelated donors. N Engl J Med 1995; 333:333.

Ting A, Welsh K: HLA matching and crossmatching in renal transplantation. In: Morris PJ (editor): *Kidney Transplantation. Principles and Practice*, 4th ed. WB Saunders, 1994.

40.6 Kidney Transplantation

Oscar Salvatierra, Jr, MD

▶ Key Facts

▶ Kidney transplantation is the most common transplant performed.

▶ Candidates for renal transplant are patients with end-stage renal failure who require dialysis for maintenance of life or are near the dialysis requirement phase.

▶ Diabetes, hypertension, and chronic glomerulonephritis are the principal etiologies of renal failure in the adult, but in children congenital abnormalities of the urinary tract or the kidney itself are more common etiologies.

▶ Graft survival in kidney transplantation is primarily dependent upon the histocompatibility match between donor and recipient.

▶ The presence of acute tubular necrosis, secondary to prolonged cold storage or warm ischemia, appears to enhance the occurrence rate of rejection, leading to poorer graft survival.

▶ Next to meticulous detail to technique in the vascular anastomosis, the most important considerations for good early renal function after transplantation are efforts to limit cold and warm ischemia and good renal perfusion.

▶ The two most commonly used immunosuppressive protocols for renal transplantation are (1) cyclosporine, prednisone, and mycophenolate mofetil; and (2) FK506 and prednisone.

▶ Rejection is initially treated with high-dose steroids. If this is not satisfactory, then a monoclonal antibody is most often employed.

▶ Nationally, patient survival with living donor transplantation is approximately 97% at 2 years, while patient survival with cadaveric transplantation is 94%.

Kidney transplantation is the most common organ transplant. More than 11,000 per year are currently being performed in the United States.

The first successful renal transplant with implantation of the organ graft in the abdomen was performed between identical twins on December 23, 1954, at the Peter Bent Brigham Hospital. Prior to this, there were 13 attempts at kidney transplantation with anastomosis of the kidney vessels to the femoral vessels, but these all failed because of infection and lack of immunosuppression. However, these early efforts underscored the fact that the immune response to the grafted organ would need to be controlled pharmacologically, except in the identical twin donor-recipient situation.

From 1958 through 1962, various attempts were made to provide the necessary immunosuppression to avoid graft rejection. Initially, total body irradiation was used, but this uniformly resulted in over-immunosuppression and death of the graft recipient from infection. However, the introduction of azathioprine in 1962 and its combined use with prednisone heralded a new era of transplantation. Cadaver transplantation could now be successfully performed, albeit with only 50% graft survival at 2 years. With living-related transplantation from a sibling or parent, 2-year graft survival of 75% could be obtained. Nevertheless, infectious complications from what we now consider to be crude conventional immunosuppression prevented renal transplantation from becoming the therapy that it is today for end-stage renal failure. It was not until the advent of cyclosporine and some additional, more specific immunosuppressants that the current era of greatly enhanced graft survival was achieved.

ETIOLOGY OF RENAL FAILURE

Candidates for renal transplantation are patients with end-stage renal failure who require dialysis for maintenance of life or are near the dialysis requirement phase. The acceptable age range for transplantation generally varies from approximately 6 months to just over 70 years. Transplantation in the older age group is certainly not as common as that in patients in the 15–65 age range. Transplantation in infants and small children is performed in specialized centers.

The principal contraindications to transplantation are the presence of active infection, substance abuse, and a history of cancer. A patient must be free of cancer for 2–5 years, dependent on the cancer type and extent. A relative contraindication is the cardiovascular status of the potential transplant recipient where symptomatic coronary artery disease would require definitive treatment prior to the patient receiving a kidney transplant.

The etiology of end-stage renal failure is very different in adults as compared to children (Figure 40.6–1). Diabetes, hypertension, and chronic glomerulonephritis are the principal etiologies of renal failure in the adult, but these three causes make up only a small fraction of the renal failure population in children. In children, congenital abnormalities of either the urinary tract or the kidney itself are responsible for the greater majority of patients receiving kidney transplants. Focal segmental glomerular sclerosis (FSGS) is also much more common in children than in adults, which has significance because of a 20–30% rate of recurrence in the transplanted kidney, especially in younger patients.

DONOR SOURCE & HISTOCOMPATIBILITY

The kidney graft may come from either a cadaveric or living donor source. In 1995, there were 11,767 kidney transplants performed in the United States, of which 8593 utilized cadaver kidneys and 3174 living donor sources. Most living donor sources are from the immediate family, with parents, siblings, or children (aged 18 or greater) most often serving as donors. Distant family members can also be living donors. Recently, because of the organ donor shortage and the initial higher graft survival rates of kidney transplants from spousal and living unrelated donors, this source of organ donors is being increasingly

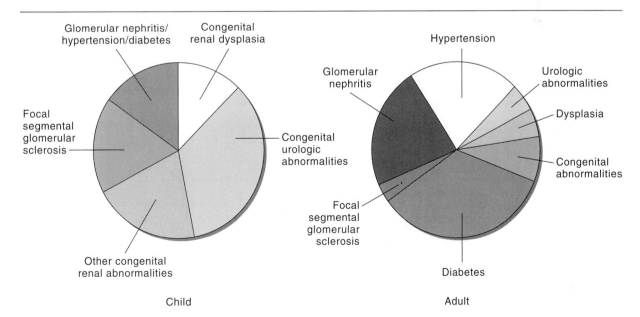

Figure 40.6–1. Etiology of renal failure in adults and children.

utilized. Currently, at least 5% of living donor transplants are from spouses and 2.5% are from other unrelated donors. In both these cases, a meaningful relationship between donor and recipient or recipient family has to be established.

In addition, with the use of any living donor, a thorough medical evaluation must precede the donation to assure that the donor will not suffer undue risk and that his or her life after the donation will remain essentially unchanged. All donors, whether living or cadaver, are comprehensively screened for any communicable disease or virus, with particular attention paid to the human immunodeficiency virus (HIV) and hepatitis B and C viruses.

Graft survival in kidney transplantation is largely dependent upon the histocompatibility match between the donor and recipient. In general, a 2-haplotype match will produce a better result than a 1-haplotype match, which in turn will produce a better result than a 0-haplotype match. An individual's HLA antigen combination on the major histocompatibility complex (MHC) on chromosome 6 is known as an **HLA haplotype** and is inherited from parent to child as a unit, carrying the three principal antigens from the A, B, and DR loci. Figure 40.6–2 demonstrates the possible haplotype combinations within a family and from an unrelated donor source, whether living donor or cadaver donor. As can be seen from the figure, there is a 25% chance that a potential kidney recipient will have a 2-haplotype match (HLA-identical sibling). There is, likewise, a 25% chance that he will have a 0-haplotype sibling. By definition, a potential recipient would be a 1-haplotype match with a parent, and, in addition, would also have a 50% chance of being a 1-haplotype match with a sibling.

A potential kidney recipient, in general, will be a 0-haplotype match with an unrelated living donor or cadaver donor. However, a number of antigens can be shared with a cadaver donor, but these antigens will be organized in different fashion than the recipient's antigens on the MHC and respective HLA haplotypes.

Even though debated over the years, HLA matching now does seem to make a difference in cadaver graft survival, particularly if a 6-antigen match can be achieved. Graft survival at 1 year in recipients with a 6-antigen match to their cadaver donors is approximately 10% better when compared to the nonmatched group, and this difference in graft survival becomes progressively greater with

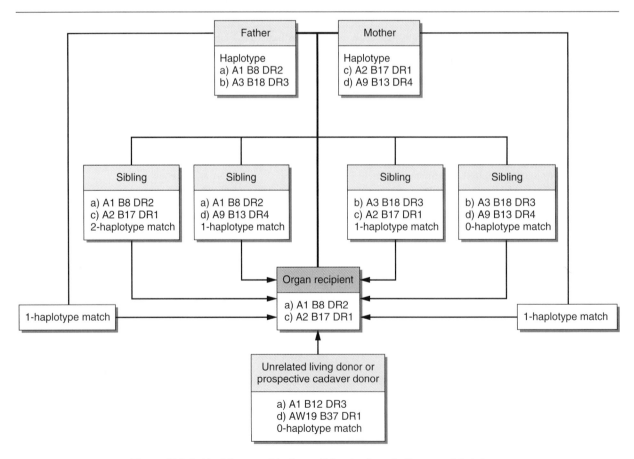

Figure 40.6–2. Haplotype combinations within a family and with an unrelated donor.

ensuing years. In regards to spousal and living unrelated donors of similar match grade to cadaveric grafts, graft survival in the former is significantly better than the latter, primarily because of the absence of prolonged cold storage and varying degrees of secondary acute tubular necrosis (ATN) in the cadaver group. The presence of ATN appears to enhance the occurrence rate of rejection, leading to poorer graft survival.

RECIPIENT OPERATION

The adult recipient procedure for implantation of the kidney graft is essentially unchanged from the technique employed with the first successful renal transplant in 1954. A curved oblique incision is employed in either the right or left lower abdominal quadrant, through which the iliac vessels and the urinary bladder can be exposed through an extraperitoneal approach. The medial extent of the incision is at the lower lateral border of the rectus abdominis muscle, while the upper lateral extent of the incision lies approximately 1 inch above the anterior superior iliac spine. The implantation of the kidney generally involves an end-to-side anastomosis of the renal vein to the iliac vein and an end-to-side anastomosis of the renal artery to external iliac artery after an appropriate oval arteriotomy has been created in the recipient artery.

Alternatively, the internal iliac artery is sometimes used in an end-to-end anastomosis with the renal artery. Either 5-0 or 6-0 vascular sutures are used for these anastomoses. Figure 40.6–3 depicts the vascular anastomoses in an adult recipient.

In an infant or small child, the recipient iliac vessels are too small for anastomoses to the larger donor renal vessels. In addition, better results are obtained in children with larger or adult-sized kidneys. In this situation, the most appropriate method for graft implantation employs a midline incision from xiphoid to symphysis pubis with reflection of the right colon, followed by mobilization of the vena cava and distal aorta. In these small patients, vascular anastomosis involves an end-to-side anastomosis of the renal vein to the vena cava and an end-to-side anastomosis of the renal artery to the aorta. Figure 40.6–4 demonstrates the vascular anatomy of a large kidney in a small child, while Figure 40.6–5 shows an intravenous pyelogram of an adult kidney transplanted in an infant.

Next to meticulous detail to technique in the vascular anastomoses, the most important consideration for good early renal function is the effort to limit both cold and warm ischemia as well as to provide good early renal perfusion. For the latter, it is imperative that adequate crystalloid and colloid infusion be achieved prior to revascularization of the kidney, so that optimum blood pressures are maintained following reestablishment of circulation to the kidney graft. In small children receiving adult kidneys, it is important to obtain a central venous pressure of 18–20 cm of water prior to release of the vascular clamps and reestablishment of kidney circulation. The early initiation of urine production by the kidney graft is also encouraged by the administration of intravenous Lasix or mannitol at the time of revascularization of the graft.

After the vascular anastomoses, the next step involves mobilization of anterior and lateral aspects of the urinary bladder for anastomosis of the ureter (**ureteroneocystostomy**). This can be done either by an extravesical or intravesical approach. If the anastomosis is to be performed extravesically, a longitudinal incision is made on the anterolateral aspect of the bladder. Here the muscular layer of the bladder is opened for an approximate distance of 2.5–3.0 cm, exposing the bladder mucosa. An additional

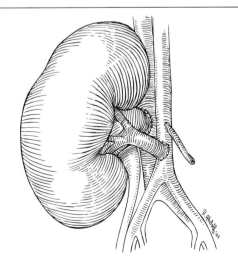

Figure 40.6–4. Vascular anastomoses of adult-size kidney in a small child.

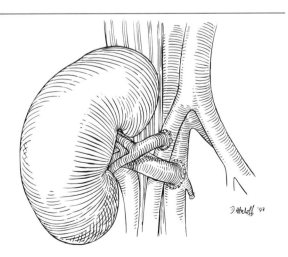

Figure 40.6–3. Vascular anastomoses in an adult recipient.

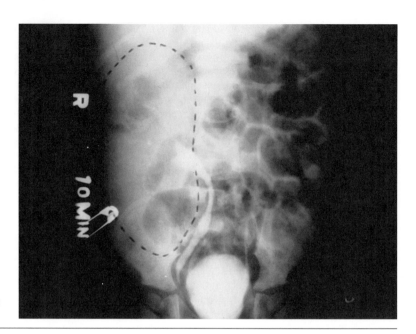

Figure 40.6–5. Intravenous pyelogram of an adult transplant kidney in an infant.

1-cm incision is made in the distal portion of the bladder mucosa, to which the distal end of the spatulated ureter will be anastomosed with a running 6-0 monofilament absorbable suture. Next, the bladder musculature is closed over the distal aspect of the ureter with interrupted absorbable sutures.

The alternative procedure for the ureteroneocystostomy is the intravesical modified Leadbetter-Politano anastomosis. This is accomplished through an anterior cystotomy incision, opening the bladder for approximately 2 inches. The transplant ureter is then brought through the bladder wall into an intravesically fashioned submucosal tunnel on the posterior lateral aspect of the bladder. Anastomosis of the spatulated end of the ureter is accomplished intravesically, just lateral to the ipsilateral native ureteral orifice, with interrupted 5-0 or 6-0 absorbable suture. The anterior cystotomy is then closed in two layers, each utilizing 3-0 absorbable suture. The modified Leadbetter-Politano procedure requires a little more time than the extravesical approach, but it appears to provide a uniformly better submucosal tunnel and, therefore, appears to be a better antireflux procedure.

IMMUNOSUPPRESSION & REJECTION

Transplant immunopharmacology has been covered in a previous section (see Chapter 40.4). This has been a very dynamic area in organ transplantation and, as indicated in the introduction to this chapter, the status and improvements in immunosuppression management have portended the progressive improvement in graft survival success since the first successful kidney transplant in 1954.

Current strategies for renal transplantation generally involve one of the following two immunosuppressive protocols: (1) cyclosporine (Neoral), prednisone, and mycophenolate mofetil (Cell Cept); or (2) FK506 (Prograf) and prednisone. Most renal transplant centers are using the former combination, which appears to be associated with a very low incidence of acute rejection episodes requiring additional immunosuppression for treatment. Both protocols seem possible of rendering the transplant recipient, in a certain percentage of cases, free of steroids. In instances of cadaveric renal transplantation where the recipient is experiencing ATN, cyclosporine and FK506 may be initially withheld because of their nephrotoxicity potential until there is evidence of resolving ATN. To afford the recipient maximum protection at the time of antigen presentation in these cases, a murine antihuman T-cell monoclonal antibody (OKT3) has been very effective as an early bridge until cyclosporine or FK506 can be used.

In regards to an acute rejection episode, this is generally manifest by a rising serum creatinine, which must be differentiated from cyclosporine or FK506 nephrotoxicity. This is most appropriately done by a renal biopsy to confirm the diagnosis before cycling higher-dose immunosuppressive medication to control the rejection episode. A rejection episode is usually treated initially with high-dose steroids, but, if refractory to this therapy, a monoclonal antibody preparation is most often employed. In turn, if the rejection episode does not respond to the antibody, then a rescue strategy with other immunosuppressive medication can be tried.

Immunosuppression is the area of transplantation that

has seen the greatest advancement during the past decade and a half. A number of clinical trials are currently in progress evaluating other new immunosuppressants. The difference between the current and early prednisone-azathioprine immunosuppression eras is that the newly developed agents are more specifically targeted to the major components of the allograft immune response. They are, therefore, more effective in the control of rejection, while at the same time sparing the transplant recipient the previous high incidence of infectious complication seen with early, totally nonspecific immunosuppression. Thus, large numbers of successful kidney transplant recipients are today being fully rehabilitated to normal lives.

COMPLICATIONS

Complications from renal transplantation generally fall into two categories: technical and nontechnical. Both categories have early and late components. Fortunately, technical complications related to graft implantation are minimal at the present time. Early technical complications of kidney transplantation can include hemorrhage, vascular thrombosis, urinary leak from the site of ureteral anastomosis or from ureteral necrosis, ureteral obstruction, perigraft lymphocele, and spontaneous graft rupture. The most common late technical complications include ureteral stenosis with secondary obstruction and graft hydronephrosis as well as renal artery stenosis with secondary hypertension.

Nontechnical complications are currently minimized through judicious use of immunosuppressive therapy but can include any of the following infectious complications associated with the immunocompromised host: cytomegalovirus, common bacteria, fungi, and protozoa such as *Pneumocystis carinii*. In addition, diabetes mellitus, hypertension, aseptic joint necrosis, and an increased risk of neoplasia can be attributed to the immunosuppression. Chronic liver disease may be an additive consequence of immunosuppression upon prior exposure to hepatitis viruses. Currently, almost all chronic renal patients are immunized against hepatitis B virus, but hepatitis C virus continues to be a problem in a small percentage of patients.

RESULTS

The results of both cadaver and living donor transplantation have steadily improved throughout the years. The advent of newer immunosuppressive agents and a better understanding of the immunologic, technical, and medical aspects of renal transplantation have led to the current outstanding results. This has allowed most kidney recipients to essentially return to normal life with a quality of life that could not be achieved by any other treatment modality.

Nationally, patient survival with living donor transplantation is approximately 97% at 2 years, while patient survival with cadaveric transplantation is 94%. The primary difference in patient survival is related to an overall lesser requirement of immunosuppressive medication in the liv-

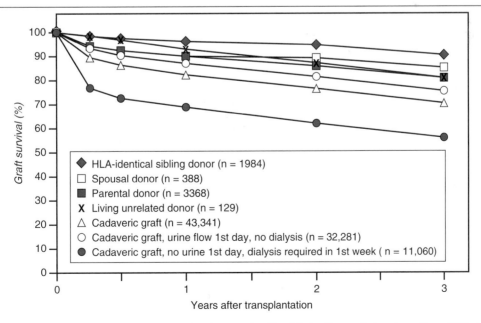

Figure 4.6–6. Survival of first kidney living donor and cadaver grafts. (Reprinted, with permission, from: Terasaki PI et al: High survival rates of kidney transplants from spousal and living unrelated donors. N Engl J Med 1995;333:334.)

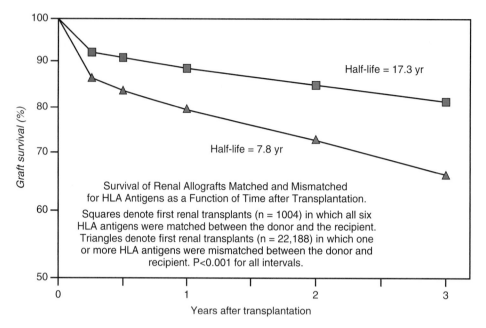

Years after transplantation

Figure 40.6–7. Survival of cadaver grafts matched and mismatched for six HLA antigens as a function of time after transplantation. *Squares* denote first renal transplants in which all six HLA antigens were matched between the donor and the recipient. *Triangles* denote first renal transplants in which one or more HLA antigens were mismatched between the donor and recipient. (Reprinted, with permission, from: Takemoto S et al: Survival of nationally shared, HLA-matched kidney transplants from cadaveric donors. N Engl J Med 1992;327:834.)

ing donor group because of generally better histocompatibility matching and absence of ATN.

Graft survival is also greatly influenced by histocompatibility match and absence or presence of ATN. The best graft survival is obtained in the rare identical twin transplant where no immunosuppression is required because of complete similarity between donor and recipient.

Survival of first kidney grafts is depicted in Figure 40.6–6. HLA identical sibling transplants (2-haplotype match) enjoy the best survival rates. Even though the donor and recipient share the same haplotypes, they are different from identical twin transplants because of minor histocompatibility differences that require immunosuppression. Parental donors (1-haplotype match) and 1-haplotype-match siblings are the next most desirable transplants. Spousal and other unrelated donors (0-haplotype match) have comparable early graft survival rates with other 1-haplotype match transplants, but they are fewer in number and are currently generally performed at larger centers. Long-term graft survival is yet to be determined in this group, but it is expected that it will be only slightly less than that achieved with 1-haplotype-matched living related transplants.

Cadaveric graft survival is especially influenced by the presence or absence of ATN. In addition, as shown in Figure 40.6–7, the presence or absence of a 6-antigen match also significantly influences graft survival. Because of national transplantation policy to award any pro-cured cadaver kidney to a 6-antigen match recipient, approximately 5% of patients on the national waiting list can receive such a kidney by national sharing.

Retransplantation is also possible in patients who have lost their first transplant. Graft survival is worse in those patients who had early kidney loss from rejection, whereas second graft survival approaches first kidney graft survival in those patients who attained long-term kidney function with their previous transplant.

SUMMARY

Renal transplantation is currently very successful and provides the best potential for return to normal life for patients with end-stage organ failure. Dialysis may serve as a bridge to maintain patient life until transplantation is possible, but the primary therapy for suitable patients should be a kidney transplant, preferably from a living donor but otherwise a cadaver graft.

In addition, it would be important that patients themselves be aware of the graft survival possibilities with both living and cadaver donor organs as described in this chapter, so that an appropriate informed choice of therapy can be made; if a cadaver graft is to be used, every effort should be made to avoid ATN.

SUGGESTED READING

Flye MW: *Atlas of Organ Transplantation*. WB Saunders, 1995.

Takemoto S et al: Survival of nationally shared, HLA-matched kidney transplants from cadaveric donors. N Engl J Med 1992;327:834.

Terasaki PI et al: High survival rates of kidney transplants from spousal and living unrelated donors. N Engl J Med 1995; 333:333.

40.7 Pancreas Transplantation

Donald C. Dafoe, MD

▶ Key Facts

- ▶ More than 6000 pancreas transplantations have been carried out worldwide between 1965 and 1995.

- ▶ Type I diabetes mellitus is characterized by insulinopenia, lean body habitus, and a tendency toward ketosis, with an age of onset typically in the teenage years. Type II diabetes is characterized by a strong family history, obesity, and a history of initial treatment with diet or oral hypoglycemic agents. Pancreatic transplantation is not indicated in those with type II diabetes.

- ▶ Pancreatic transplantation is designed to restore a functional beta cell mass, thereby establishing near-normoglycemia with resultant metabolic benefits, improved sense of well-being, and stabilization or retardation of diabetic neurovascular complications.

- ▶ Heartbeating, brain-dead cadaver donors must be free of overt diabetes, and there must be ABO compatibility and a negative crossmatch with the recipient.

- ▶ Because of the strong likelihood of vigorous rejection, potent immunosuppressive regimens have been devised for pancreas transplantation patients. These include anti-lymphocyte serum or anti-T cell monoclonal antibody on top of combined agents: cyclosporine or tacrolimus, azathioprine or mycophenolate mofetil, and prednisone.

- ▶ Currently, the average 1-year graft survival, defined as independence from exogenous insulin, is 74%. The survival rate is 91% at 1 year after transplantation, with myocardial infarction being a major cause of death.

Pancreas transplantation may be indicated in highly selected patients with type I diabetes mellitus. The goal is the establishment of near-normoglycemia, thereby improving the recipient's sense of well-being and, possibly, altering the inexorable progression of neurovascular damage.

The incidence of type I diabetes mellitus (insulin-dependent diabetes mellitus, juvenile-onset diabetes) is 13–16 per 100,000 population for ages 0–29 years. The prevalence in the United States has been estimated to be 600,000–1,000,000. Type I diabetes is characterized by insulinopenia, lean body habitus, and a tendency toward ketosis, with an age of onset typically in the teenage years. The disease has sporadic incidence within families, but there is a definite genetic predisposition, as shown by linkage with certain human leukocyte histocompatibility antigens (HLAs). Usually, it is not difficult to distinguish type I diabetes mellitus from type II diabetes (adult-onset diabetes). Type II is typified by a strong family history, obesity, and a history of initial treatment with diet or oral hypoglycemic agents. Occasionally, the lines between type I diabetes and type II are blurred; in those cases, the native beta cells' ability to make insulin can be determined by an assay of serum C-peptide. Type II diabetes is characterized by a major component of peripheral insulin resistance, therefore, C-peptide levels are not markedly depressed or absent (as in type I diabetes), and pancreatic transplantation is not currently applied to this group.

The etiology of type I diabetes mellitus is an autoimmune attack on native islets of Langerhans and destruction of the beta cells. Pancreatic transplantation is designed to restore a functional beta cell mass, thereby establishing near-normoglycemia with resultant metabolic benefits, improved sense of well-being, and stabilization or retardation of diabetic neurovascular complications.

CANDIDATE SELECTION

Currently, most pancreas transplant candidates have end-stage diabetic nephropathy (ESDN) and are referred for a renal or simultaneous renal-pancreas transplant (SPK). The prototypic candidate is 30–40 years of age and developed diabetes in the mid-teens. Proteinuria was detected several years prior, followed by progressive renal insufficiency, despite a protein-restricted diet and treatment with angiotensin-converting enzyme inhibitors, leading to ESDN. Candidates usually have retinopathy, gastroparesis, and peripheral neuropathy. They often have orthostatic hypotension as a result of autonomic neuropathy. There may be a history of coronary artery disease. Since neuropathy may dampen the herald sign of chest pain and dialysis dependence may render the patient sedentary, coronary artery disease may be occult, despite critical lesions.

The goal of pancreas transplantation is prevention of diabetic neurovascular complications, such as retinopathy and macrovascular disease. Most candidates receive an SPK (from the same cadaver donor) as treatment of both renal failure and diabetes. It has been reasoned that ideal candidates are patients with harbingers of organ dysfunction (eg, microalbuminuria) who do not have irreversible damage. However, preemptive pancreatic transplantation (**pancreas transplant alone**, or PTA) is not widely practiced because of a high technical failure rate (eg, graft thrombosis) of 18% overall and vigorous rejection episodes. In addition, there is an overall success rate of only about 50% at 1 year after transplantation, according to the International Pancreas Transplant Registry (IPTR). With optimization of HLA matching, the success rate for PTA at the University of Minnesota, the most experienced pancreas transplant center in the world, has approached 70% at 1 year after transplantation.

Another candidate group are those individuals with type I diabetes who already have a successful kidney transplant from a living-related or cadaver donor. Pancreatic trans-

plantation sequential to kidney transplantation (**pancreas after kidney**, or PAK) accounts for only 6% of the pancreas transplantations carried out from 1987 to 1994, as reported to the IPTR. There is a favorable selection bias for PAK candidates, since they have demonstrated the ability to accept an allograft, and tolerate surgery and immunosuppression. Nevertheless, success rates are lower than with simultaneous pancreas-kidney (SPK) transplant.

This discrepancy, higher success rates for SPK, has been attributed to the immunosuppressive and anticoagulation effects of uremia. Furthermore, with SPK transplants, incipient acute rejection of the pancreas allograft can be diagnosed early using the familiar signs and symptoms of acute renal transplant rejection. A simultaneous, same-donor renal allograft usually undergoes rejection in synchrony with the pancreas allograft and a rise in serum creatinine is premonitory of the late signs of pancreas transplant rejection, such as flagrant hyperglycemia. In other words, in the SPK recipient, the renal allograft acts as the "miner's canary" to the pancreas graft, with confirmation of suspected rejection by percutaneous renal transplant biopsy. When the pancreas transplant is PAK or PTA, acute pancreas rejection is suggested by fever, hyperamylasemia, elevated white blood cell count, and graft tenderness. If the pancreas graft was drained into the urinary bladder, a common technique, pancreas transplant rejection is associated with a fall in urinary amylase production and, sometimes, gross hematuria. The pancreas graft may either be biopsied transcystoscopically or percutaneously under ultrasonic guidance. The histological features of acute rejection are endovasculitis and a mononuclear cellular infiltrate of the pancreas graft.

In the 1980s, when pancreatic transplantation made the transition from experimental to accepted therapy, myocardial infarction claimed lives after successful transplantation. It is important to investigate possible occult coronary artery disease in candidates, most reliably with cardiac catheterization, and correct significant coronary artery lesions in preparation for surgery.

DONOR ISSUES & PROCUREMENT

Heartbeating, brain-dead cadaver donors must be free of overt diabetes. Mild hyperglycemia in a cadaver donor is not uncommon as a result of a hormonal environment rich in counter-regulatory hormones, such as epinephrine, and the treatment of cerebral edema with steroids. In addition to generic contraindications (eg, active infection, malignancy), pancreatitis and overt glucose intolerance are contraindications to pancreas donation. The preferred technique of procurement is in situ perfusion and en bloc procurement with minimal manipulation of the pancreas graft (Figure 40.7–1). Cold-storage in University of Wisconsin (UW) solution provides satisfactory pancreas graft preservation for up to 24 hours.

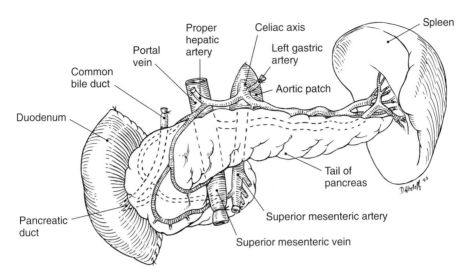

Figure 40.7–1. The whole organ pancreas graft as procured from a cadaver donor. The arterial blood supply originates from the celiac axis and superior mesenteric artery based on a Carrel patch. The venous drainage is via the portal vein. Pancreatic secretions exit into the graft duodenum that is anastomosed to the recipient urinary bladder or bowel.

There must be ABO compatibility and a negative cross-match (no significant microcytotoxicity of donor cells when incubated with recipient serum and complement) between the donor and recipient if hyperacute rejection is to be avoided. An analysis of IPTR data demonstrated that HLA matching is associated with better graft survival in PTA recipients.

SURGICAL TECHNIQUES

The technical aspects of the transplantation of a vascularized pancreas graft have been through several variations. During the 1970s, segmental pancreas grafts were used. These grafts were composed of the tail of the pancreas only, with blood supply based on the splenic artery and vein. The pancreatic duct was occluded with polymers or drained into a Roux-en-Y limb. Segmental grafts gave way to the whole organ grafts to maximize islet mass. In whole pancreas transplantation, the arterial blood supply originates from the celiac axis and superior mesenteric artery (SMA) (Figure 40.7–2). In the frequent circumstance of a cadaveric multiorgan donation, the celiac axis goes with the liver graft. The pancreas receives arterial blood from the splenic artery and SMA following reconstruction with a donor iliac artery Y graft (Figure 40.7–3). After reconstruction of the pancreas graft in an iced basin, the donor common iliac artery is anastomosed to the recipient external iliac artery in an end-to-side fashion similar to a kidney transplant. Venous drainage is via graft portal vein end-to-side anastomosis into the recipient external iliac vein.

Difficulties with the handling of exocrine secretions led to the technique of drainage into the urinary bladder via a segment of donor duodenum. The urinary bladder provides a sterile repository for exocrine secretions and the thickened bladder wall of the diabetic recipient makes for a secure anastomosis. Leak rates are low and monitoring of urinary amylase has been touted as an index of graft function—a fall in urinary amylase has been correlated with acute rejection. When the patient receives an SPK from the same cadaver donor, the value of urinary amylase in the diagnosis of rejection is superseded by the predictive role of the kidney allograft. Since urinary bladder drainage has resulted in problems (eg, urinary tract infections, urethritis, volume depletion, and acidosis resulting from bicarbonate loss), enteric drainage has recently gained acceptance.

COMPLICATIONS

Complications of pancreatic transplantation include bleeding, graft thrombosis, graft pancreatitis, pancreaticocutaneous fistulae, wound infection, and perigraft collections. Intraperitoneal placement of the pancreas transplant has improved morbidity. Subfascial wound infections, for example, were relatively frequent after extraperitoneal placement in the iliac fossa. This complication has been greatly reduced by intraperitoneal placement because of the absorptive capacity of the peritoneum and the protective effects of the omentum.

Graft thrombosis is a poorly understood entity that causes the demise of the pancreas graft in about 10% of cases. The use of UW preservation solution and cumulative

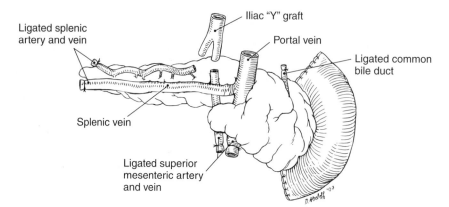

Figure 40.7–2. Reconstruction of the pancreas transplant with a Y graft using the donor iliac artery. This technique facilitates the procurement of liver and pancreas from the same cadaver donor.

experience of pancreas transplant teams have decreased the rate of thrombosis from that of 25% a decade ago. This complication is seldom due to surgical error, but apparently originates within the graft parenchyma as a result of local hypercoagulability, often with propogation of clot into the

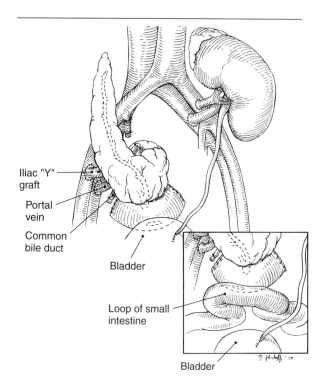

Figure 40.7–3. A simultaneous kidney-pancreas transplant. The pancreas graft is placed intraperitoneally. The vessels of both grafts are sewn end-to-side into the corresponding iliac vessels of the recipient. In this depiction, the graft duodenum is drained into the urinary bladder. **_Inset:_** Alternatively, the pancreas graft is drained into the small bowel.

portal vein. Various anticoagulation regimens have been unsuccessful in preventing this potentially life-threatening complication. Thrombosis requires urgent graft pancreatectomy to minimize the physiologic insult from hemorrhagic pancreatitis and consumptive coagulopathy. Also, pulmonary embolus threatens when the graft portal vein clot propagates into the recipient iliac vein.

Urinary bladder drainage of pancreas transplant secretions results in bicarbonate wasting. The tendancy toward metabolic acidosis is exacerbated by a poorly functioning renal transplant. Salt loss and dehydration in a patient with orthostatic hypotension and noncompliant vessels must be aggressively countered. Mineralocorticoid administration, bicarbonate replacement, and generous oral fluid intake are necessary. These measures may be insufficient, especially since the oral intake of fluid may be limited by diabetic gastroparesis. In the early period after pancreas transplantation, prophylactic adminstration of intravenous normal saline may be warranted on a routine basis in the outpatient clinic. Pancreatic trypsinogen can be activated to trypsin by the enterokinase produced by the graft duodenum. Trypsin may alter the protective mucous layer of the bladder, resulting in an increased susceptibility to urinary tract infections. Enzymatic digestion of the urethral epithelium may also cause urethritis. A leak at the pancreaticoduodenocystic anastomosis requires intervention. The leak site must be drained to create a controlled fistula. Closure of the fistula will be aided by the pharmacologic shutdown of exocrine secretions with somatostatin treatment.

CLINICAL IMMUNOLOGY

A great deal of knowledge has been gained from the clinical immunology of pancreatic transplantation. Recurrent diabetes was demonstrated in segmental pancreas graft recipients from nondiabetic identical twin donors by the University of Minnesota team. The histologic finding of insulitis, a lymphocytic infiltrate of islets, provided irrefutable evidence for the autoimmune pathogenesis of type I diabetes mellitus. Transplantation of SPK grafts has been found to stimulate more acute rejection episodes than renal transplant alone. It has been hypothesized that immune cells within the composite grafts (eg, lymph nodes, duodenal lymphoid patches) present a large passenger leukocyte load, evoking a vigorous host response. The immunocompetence of passenger leukocytes in the pancreas graft has been shown by the natural experiment of transplantation of an ABO blood group O graft into a blood group A recipient, leading to hemolytic anemia—a form of graft-versus-host disease.

Because of the strong likelihood of vigorous rejection, potent immunosuppressive regimens have been devised for pancreas transplantation. The use of adjuvant anti-lymphocyte serum or anti-T cell monoclonal antibody has been associated with an improved success. This so-called "induction" therapy is given on top of combined agents, such as cyclosporine or tacrolimus, azathioprine or mycophenolate mofetil, and prednisone. Ironically, many of these immunosuppressants are diabetogenic. Tacrolimus, for example, may induce hyperglycemia, raising the concern of possible pancreas allograft rejection.

FUNCTION OF THE GRAFT

The main rationale for pancreatic transplantation is glycemic control. The desired outcome is the prevention or retardation of diabetic neurovascular complications. After a successful pancreas transplant, the recipient will have fasting blood glucose that is typically 80–90 mg/dL, and 120–130 mg/dL 2 hours postprandially. Hour-to-hour blood glucose determinations in a successful pancreas transplant recipient reveal a metabolic profile that is comparable to a nondiabetic renal transplant recipient; that is, glucose clearance is not completely normal. There may be mild hyperglycemia after meals. The other suboptimal metabolic milieu in pancreas transplant recipients is peripheral hyperinsulinemia, because it is thought to promote atherosclerosis and insulin resistance. Hyperinsulinemia has been largely attributed to systemic venous drainage of insulin rather than physiologic portal vein drainage that lowers insulin levels by hepatic extraction. Nevertheless, the glycemic control experienced by pancreas transplant recipients is unsurpassed, and superior to a regimen of multiple daily insulin injections and repeated glucose monitoring throughout the day.

The long awaited results of the Diabetes Control and Complications Trial showed that a sustained regimen of glucose control improved neurovascular diabetic complications, such as nephropathy. This trial supported the widely held belief that "tight control" will help to stave off the devastating complications that type I diabetics experience following a 10- to 15-year grace period. Not surprisingly, the beneficial effects of metabolic control in pancreas transplant recipients have also been documented. Several reports have shown an improved sense of well-being in pancreas transplant recipients. This is probably due to easing of the psychological burden of daily concern about glycemic control, insulin injections, and dietary constraints. Another benefit of a successful pancreas transplant has been documented by serial renal transplant biopsies in SPK recipients. The contemporaneous renal grafts do not develop the light and electron microscopic changes that presage recurrent nephropathy; these findings are in contrast to serial biopsies in diabetic recipients of a renal transplant only. Comparison studies are hindered by the absence of an ideal control group and the logistical impossibility of a randomized study. However, clinical investigators have generated support for other salutary effects of pancreas transplantation.

Autonomic neuropathy (eg, improved gastric emptying), peripheral neuropathy, myocardial dysfunction, and retinopathy are ameliorated. Also, pancreas transplant recipients develop a less atherogenic lipid profile, particularly when a variation in technique is used that directs the venous effluent of the graft into the recipient portal vein. Despite encouraging data, many of the current candidates have advanced diabetic complications. It is important for the pancreas transplant candidate to have realistic expectations. It would be unrealistic to expect that established neurovascular complications, years in the making, would reverse or stop abruptly after a successful pancreas transplant. Ideally, this intervention would be applied earlier in the disease course.

RESULTS

According to the IPTR, more than 6000 pancreas transplantation procedures were carried out between 1965 and 1995, worldwide. Currently, the average 1-year graft survival, defined as independence from exogenous insulin, for SPK recipients is 74%, with an associated renal graft survival of 84% (Figure 40.7–4). The patient survival rate was 91% at 1 year after transplantation. The major causes of mortality are cardiovascular and infectious.

THE FUTURE

The transplantation of isolated pancreatic islets by inoculation into the portal vein and embolization into the liver is an attractive alternative to transplantation of the entire organ. Since 1972, when transplanted islets were shown to reduce glycosuria in diabetic rats, many groups have pursued islet transplantation. The main difficulty has been the

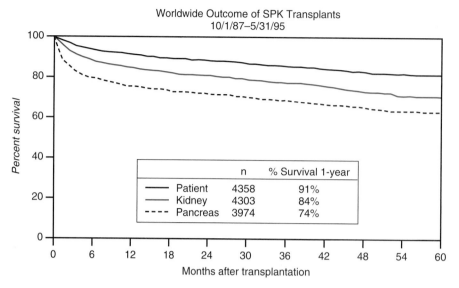

Worldwide Outcome of SPK Transplants
10/1/87–5/31/95

	n	% Survival 1-year
Patient	4358	91%
Kidney	4303	84%
Pancreas	3974	74%

Figure 40.7–4. Patient and graft survival data in recipients of SPK transplants (simultaneous pancreas and kidney transplant from the same cadaver donor) as reported to the International Pancreas Transplant Registry and the United Network for Organ Sharing.

recovery of adequate numbers of islets from pancreata with sufficient purity for transplantation. Despite a clinical experience of more than 200 attempts worldwide, long-term insulin independence has been rare. In the 1990s, fewer than 10% of islet recipients were rendered independent of exogenous insulin at 1 year after transplantation. Other strategies of islet transplantation are encapsulation, isolation in immunologically privileged chambers, and islet xenografts. It is conceivable that genetic engineering will create islet surrogates that sense glucose and secrete insulin appropriately. If donor-specific tolerance could be induced through immunological manipulation (avoiding chronic immunosuppression),

pancreas transplantation, as currently practiced, could be employed at an appropriate time in the progression of diabetes-induced neurovascular complications. As success rates progressively increase, candidate criteria for pancreas transplantation must be redefined. Timely intervention—not too early in the deteriorative course of diabetes, yet not too late to have an impact on established complications—is the aim. Ultimately, preventative treatment, such as vaccination of genetically predisposed individuals to the offending autoantigen or treatment of autoimmunity, will end the need for transplantation of a functional islet cell mass.

SUGGESTED READING

Douzdjian V et al: Renal allograft and patient outcome after transplantation: Pancreas-kidney versus kidney-alone transplants in type I diabetic patients versus kidney-alone transplants in nondiabetic patients. Am J Kidney Dis 1996;27:106.

London NJ et al: Human pancreatic islet isolation and transplantation. Clin Transplantation 1994;8:421.

Ricordi C: Vth Congress of the International Pancreas and 1st Transplant Association; "Cure of Diabetes by Transplantation." Transplant Proc 1995;27:2971.

Sollinger HW et al: Two hundred consecutive simultaneous pan-

creas-kidney transplants with bladder drainage. Surgery 1993;114:736.

Stratta RJ et al: Surgical treatment of diabetes mellitus with pancreas transplantation. Ann Surg 1994;220:809.

Sutherland DE, Gruessner A: Pancreas transplant results in the United Network for Organ Sharing (UNOS) United States of America (USA) registry compared with the non-USA data in the international registry. In: Terasaki PI, Cecka JR (editors): *Clinical Transplants*, 1994. UCLA Tissue Typing Laboratory, 1994.

40.8 Liver Transplantation

Carlos O. Esquivel, MD, PhD, Waldo Concepcion, MD, & Samuel K.S. So, MD

▶ Key Facts

- ▶ Important factors implicated in the evolution of hepatic transplantation include improved immunosuppression, development of the University of Wisconsin (UW) solution for cold preservation of the liver, improvements in surgical technique, proper selection of patients, and advances in critical care.

- ▶ Indications for liver transplantation include acute liver failure, chronic liver failure, liver malignancies, metabolic diseases, and graft failure.

- ▶ Key components to candidacy for liver transplantation include: acute or chronic end-stage liver disease, absence of alternative therapy, full understanding of the process of liver transplantation, and an understanding of the long-term financial implications.

- ▶ Scarcity of donors is the limiting factor in liver transplantation; 14–17% of candidates die while waiting for a liver allograft.

- ▶ Effective and safe immunosuppression is a delicate balance between infection and rejection. Except for technical complications, the onset of infection in a liver transplantation recipient implies over-immunosuppression.

- ▶ The most common surgical complications after liver transplantation include biliary tract strictures or leaks, vascular complications, and primary graft nonfunction.

- ▶ The overall patient survival after hepatic transplantation in adults and children at Stanford is 93%.

- ▶ Indications for retransplantation fall into five broad categories: chronic rejection, vascular complications, primary graft nonfunction, recurrence of underlying liver disease, and miscellaneous.

DIAGNOSTIC INDICATIONS

There are more than 30 different diagnostic indications for liver transplantation (Table 40.8–1). Almost all these diagnostic indications are associated with irreversible liver injury. However, in a few cases, a metabolic defect based in the liver may lead to fatal extrahepatic complications, such as in primary amyloidosis, primary hypercholesterolemia, and primary oxalosis, although the function and histologic architecture of the liver may be normal. Primary hypercholesterolemia and primary amyloidosis may be associated with coronary artery disease and amy-

loid cardiomyopathy, respectively. Primary oxalosis leads to renal failure, bone fractures, and early death unless treated with simultaneous liver and kidney transplantation. Liver transplantation will correct the metabolic defect.

The incidence of hepatocellular carcinoma is particularly high in patients with tyrosinemia and hemochromatosis, but any chronic liver injury may be associated with the development of this complication. Therefore, patients with chronic liver disease must be screened with alpha-fetoprotein and radiologic studies for early detection of liver cancer.

Certain liver disorders demand special considerations.

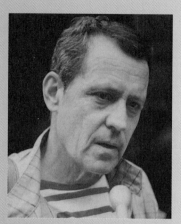

Thomas E. Starzl, MD, PhD (b 1926). (Courtesy of the University of Pittsburgh.)

Hepatic transplantation had its beginnings in the mid-1950s in the research laboratories of Dr Jack Cannon at the Department of Surgery, University of California, Los Angeles (UCLA). Soon after, Dr Thomas E. Starzl began to pursue his dream of making liver transplantation a clinical reality. After several years of animal experimentation, Dr Starzl performed the first liver transplantation in a 3-year-old child on March 1, 1963. This first transplant, as well as the next six, failed. Such disappointing results forced him to impose a moratorium on the clinical program to redefine the transplantation procedure. In 1967, Dr Starzl reinitiated the clinical program, but in contrast to the previous experience, the new results were encouraging, since some of the patients survived long periods of time. Still, the morbidity and mortality were significant, mainly due to complications brought about by rejection from the lack of effective immunosuppressive drugs. The immunosuppression consisted of a combination of azathioprine and prednisone, a regimen copied from the kidney transplantation experience.

In 1980, a new immunosuppressive agent, cyclosporine, was introduced to clinical transplantation; over a short time span, the combination of cyclosporine and corticosteroid became the conventional immunosuppressive regimen for more than a decade. The much improved results prompted a National Consensus Meeting sponsored by the National Institutes of Health in 1983 to evaluate the progress of liver transplantation and create guidelines for the use of this therapy in patients with acute and chronic end-stage liver disease. An important conclusion of this meeting was that liver transplantation should no longer be considered an experimental procedure but rather the accepted mode of therapy for those patients with liver failure.

In 1984, human clinical trials were begun to assess the efficacy and safety of the monoclonal antibody OKT3 in reversing refractory rejection. OKT3 was found to be effective in reversing refractory rejection in two thirds of patients with steroid-resistant rejection. Moreover, OKT3 was found to be useful in providing adequate immunosuppression in patients with postoperative acute renal failure, allowing the renal function to recover before treatment was instituted with the nephrotoxic drug, cyclosporine. In subsequent trials, OKT3 was noted to be an effective drug in preventing rejection when used as induction therapy (see Chapter 40.4).

In 1985, another milestone marked the progress of hepatic transplantation. A new preservation solution was developed by Belzer and coworkers at the University of Wisconsin. This solution, which contains lactobionate and other components, has become the standard in experimental and clinical organ preservation.

Table 40.8–1. Indications for liver transplant.

Acute Liver Failure

Viral hepatitis
Toxic injury (paracetamol, halothane, mushroom, others)
Ischemic injury (shock, heart failure)
Massive steatosis

Chronic Liver Failure

Cholestatic disease (primary biliary cirrhosis, primary sclerosing
   cholangitis, biliary atresia, familial cholestatic syndromes)
Hepatocellular disease (viral hepatitis, alcoholic cirrhosis, toxic
   injury, autoimmune cirrhosis)
Vascular disease (Budd-Chiari, veno-occlusive disease)

Liver Malignancies

Hepatocellular carcinoma
Hepatoblastoma
Hemangioendothelioma
Metastatic neuroendocrine tumor
Sarcoma

Metabolic Diseases

Alpha$_1$ antitrypsin deficiency
Wilson's disease
Tyrosinemia
Hemochromatosis
Glycogen storage disease types I and IV
Cystic fibrosis
Erythropoietic protoporphyria
Crigler-Najjar syndrome
Oxalosis
Urea cycle enzyme deficiency
Protein C deficiency
Hemophilia A

Graft Failure

Rejection (acute, chronic)
Primary graft failure
Technical failure

Arteriohepatic dysplasia (Alagille's syndrome) is frequently complicated by peripheral pulmonic stenosis. The severity of the pulmonary hypertension must be carefully assessed for candidacy. Hemochromatosis is often accompanied by cardiomyopathy from iron deposition. During the postoperative period, patients with hemochromatosis may experience cardiac arrhythmias that may be life-threatening. Alcoholic patients may also be at risk of developing arrhythmias during the postoperative period, caused by alcohol-induced cardiomyopathy.

Alcoholic cirrhosis, chronic hepatitis B, primary hepatic malignancies, old age of recipient, and multiple organ system failure at the time of transplantation are controversial indications. The grounds for the controversy are the potential risk of alcohol recidivism, recurrence of primary disease, and potential waste of organs in patients with poor chances of survival. Lacking a universal criteria for inclusion or exclusion of patients with controversial indications, most transplant centers have created their own guidelines for the proper selection of these patients and the prevention of negative media information that may damage the effort for organ donation.

EVALUATION OF RECIPIENT

Candidacy for liver transplantation is determined by a careful evaluation of the potential candidates. Parameters that must be present to proceed with an evaluation are: acute or chronic end-stage liver disease, absence of alternative therapy, full understanding of the process of liver transplantation, and an understanding of the financial implications. Upon referral, the diagnosis of the liver disease must be confirmed. This will require careful review of medical records, radiologic studies, and laboratory tests, including biopsies. On occasion, patients may require additional studies. The timing for transplantation is determined to create a plan for the evaluation of candidacy. Patients in acute liver failure require an expeditious evaluation, whereas patients with well-compensated cirrhosis may require a more leisurely evaluation. Patients are seen in consultation by transplant hepatologists and surgeons, social workers, and financial counselors. Consultants from other specialties, including psychiatry, may be necessary. On completion of the work-up, cases are discussed in a multidisciplinary meeting, and a consensus is reached in regards to patients' candidacy.

Patients accepted for transplantation are placed on a waiting list and a status is assigned based on medical condition following the revised UNOS (United Network of Organ Sharing) recommendations effective January 20, 1997, as follows: (1) status 1—life expectancy under 7 days due to sudden or complete liver failure as a result of acute viral hepatitis or reactions to prescription or over-the-counter drugs; this category also includes patients who have received a transplant that has immediately failed and pediatric patients with liver disease that would result in irreversible neurologic damage without transplantation; (2) status 2—patients with continuous hospitalization necessary; (3) status 3—patients with continuous medical care necessary, hospital or home; and (4) status 7—temporarily inactive.

CONTRAINDICATIONS

Table 40.8–2 shows a list of absolute contraindications that pose little trouble in the patient selection for liver transplantation. Nevertheless, there is a longer list of relative contraindications that create significant problems, such as the alcoholic patient with marginal family support, or the alcoholic patient with a sobriety period of less than 6 months, or patients with recent drug abuse. Another relative contraindication is the presence of a primary liver malignancy. Thus, in a patient with a hepatocellular carcinoma the selection for transplantation should be individualized and other factors taken into consideration, including size of the tumor, age of the patient, and other co-morbid factors, such as renal dysfunction and cardio-

Table 40.8–2. Contraindications for liver transplantation.

Absolute
Patient unable to understand and comply with immunosuppression
Active extrabiliary sepsis
Unresectable hepatobiliary carcinoma
Advanced cardiopulmonary disease
Active alcoholism and drug addiction
Acquired immunodeficiency syndrome
Documented anatomical anomalies precluding transplantation

Relative
Age above 70 years
Active sepsis of hepatobiliary origin
Active infection of extrahepatic organs
Retransplantation for recurrence of hepatitis C
Cholangiocarcinoma
Peptic ulcer disease
Renal insufficiency
Severe malnutrition
Diabetes mellitus with coronary artery disease
Thrombosis of the splanchnic venous system
Hepatocellular carcinoma in the setting of chronic hepatitis B
Multiple organ failure requiring cardiopulmonary support
Patients in coma stage IV
Mental retardation
Epilepsy
Marginal support system

Table 40.8–3. Exclusion criteria for donors.

Absolute
Infection
Untreated sepsis
Acquired immunodeficiency syndrome
Viral hepatitis
Viral encephalitis
Tuberculosis
Intravenous drug abuse
Hepatobiliary disease
Cancer

Relative
Diabetes mellitus
Previous abdominal surgeries
Chronic alcoholism
Abdominal trauma
Prolonged cardiopulmonary arrest
Age over 75 years
High-risk sexual activities

vascular problems. Other relative contraindications are: elderly patients with several medical problems rendering them as a high-risk population, patients with multiple organ system failure requiring cardiopulmonary support, patients in coma stage IV, retransplantation for recurrence of hepatitis C, patients with metastatic neuroendocrine tumors, patients with mental retardation, epilepsy, recent Epstein-Barr virus infection, and polycystic liver disease with normal hepatic function. Other relative contraindications are listed in Table 40.8–2.

DONOR OPERATION

The success of a donor operation depends on the technique as well as the proper selection of the donor. Unfortunately, it is difficult to predict organ function based on criteria commonly used in clinical transplantation. Nevertheless, with the introduction of the Wisconsin solution and modifications in the donor operation, the rate of primary graft nonfunction has dropped from 15–20% to 2–10%. The evaluation of the donor must be done carefully, but expeditiously, since some of the donors may be hemodynamically unstable. A careful history must be obtained from the next of kin, relatives, and medical records. A list of exclusion criteria in the selection process is given in Table 40.8–3. The clinician should also perform an individual assessment of the recipient's medical status and the donor's relative contraindications. The scarcity of donors is the limiting factor in liver transplantation, and

14–17% of candidates die while waiting for a liver allograft; thus, the benefits must be weighed against the risks.

The extraction of the liver may be accomplished by performing a careful dissection of the hilar structures before the infusion of preservation solution, or by performing an en bloc procurement at the same time that the liver and the other abdominal organs are being perfused. This method of procurement is also known as a **rapid infusion technique** and has been subjected to several modifications. We prefer the en bloc technique since it can be carried out expeditiously and safely, minimizing the injury to the vascular structures in the hilum. The following steps summarize the technique:

1. Dissection and cannulation of the superior mesenteric vein and infrarenal aorta.
2. Circulatory arrest by clamping supraceliac aorta.
3. Drainage of venous effluent through the intrapericardial inferior vena cava or through the infrarenal inferior vena cava through a cannula.
4. Transection of esophagus and proximal jejunum with removal en bloc of the stomach, duodenum, liver, pancreas, kidneys, and spleen.
5. Separation of different organs in the back table.

The hilar structures are dissected out at the "back table" in a controlled environment. Our incidence of primary graft nonfunction with this method of procurement is 2%. Furthermore, there are no repercussions to the kidneys, pancreas, or small bowel when procured with this technique. Figure 40.8–1 depicts the most important steps of the en bloc extraction.

Liver reductions are often needed in pediatric transplantation because of scarcity of pediatric donors. A liver reduction consists of "cutting down" the liver allograft from a much larger donor to be accommodated in the small abdomen of a pediatric recipient. A drawback of this particular technique is the potential risk of bleeding or

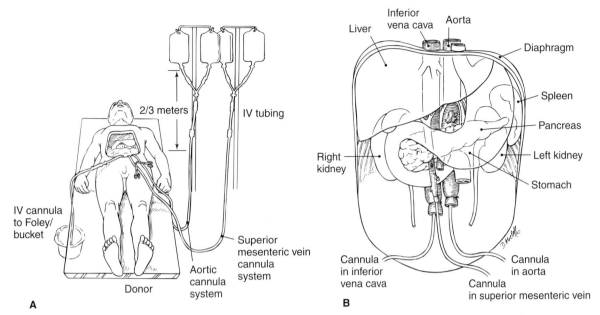

Figure 40.8–1. A: Gravity perfusion system for the delivery of preservation fluid. **B:** Contents of the en bloc resection. Superiorly, the diaphragm, inferior vena cava, aorta, and esophagus. Laterally, the liver and right kidney, and the spleen and left kidney. Inferiorly, the distal aorta, distal inferior vena cava, small intestine, and ureters. Posteriorly, the retroperitoneum, posterior abdominal aorta, and inferior vena cava.

biliary leaks from the raw surface of the liver. These complications have been minimized by the use of a staple device applied to the resection margin. Smaller vessels not included in the staple line are oversewn with 5-0 Prolene sutures. Teflon strips have been also used for hemostasis by "sandwiching" the cut edges with 3-0 Prolene. This technique has evolved into split liver transplantation whereby the liver is divided, resulting in two grafts: the right lobe is then transplanted in an adult patient and the left lateral segment of the left lobe is transplanted into a child. In living-related liver transplantation, the parenchyma of the liver is divided with the ultrasonic dissector (CUSA) and electrocoagulation. This technique results in excellent hemostasis and very little risk of biliary leaks.

RECIPIENT OPERATION

The recipient operation begins with the proper preparation of the recipient before the surgical procedure. Table 40.8–4 demonstrates the standard preoperative orders at Stanford University Medical Center. In the operating room the patient is positioned in a well-padded bed lying on a heating blanket. The lower extremities are also wrapped in Webril with the feet resting softly on a footrest board. In children, the extremities and the head are also wrapped in plastic to maintain the body temperature. The left arm is left out to allow access to the axillary vein, should venous bypass be needed. Careful positioning of the arm, avoiding hyperextension, is of utmost importance to prevent brachial plexus injury. It is recommended to sew the drapes to the patient to prevent them from sliding in lengthy operations. A cesarean drape, which holds the fluids in a pocket around the operating field, is particularly useful in keeping the patient dry and warm during the operation.

HEPATECTOMY

Figure 40.8–2 depicts the incisions commonly used in hepatic transplantation. The skin is barely incised with a scalpel and then the incision is continued with the electrocautery to maximize hemostasis. An upper hand retractor applied to the table is utilized for exposure. The hepatectomy could be a formidable task, particularly in patients with severe portal hypertension, coagulopathy, and previous abdominal surgery. The hepatectomy, including removal of the retrohepatic inferior vena cava, may be performed without a venous bypass if interruption of the venous return by transiently cross-clamping the portal vein and infrahepatic cava is not associated with significant hemodynamic changes. If this maneuver is not well tolerated, the use of venous bypass is strongly recommended.

Table 40.8–4. Preoperative orders for adult liver transplant recipients.[1]

Nursing Orders
Admit to transplant unit
Diagnosis: end-stage liver disease
Diet: nothing by mouth
Activity: ad lib
Weight: weigh patient and record on vital sign sheet
IV: per anesthesia
Pre-op Hibiclens shower

Studies
Stat: complete blood count (manual differential), platelets, renal panel, electrolytes, prothrombin time, partial prothrombin time
Routine: hepatic panel
Type and cross for: 10 units packed red blood cells
10 units fresh frozen plasma
10 units platelets
12-lead ECG
Chest x-ray, posterior-anterior and lateral
Urinalysis and microscopic (urgent)

Medications
Ampicillin 1 g intravenously on call to operating room
Ceftriaxone 1 g intravenously on call to operating room

[1]From Stanford University Hospital Multi-Organ Transplant Center.

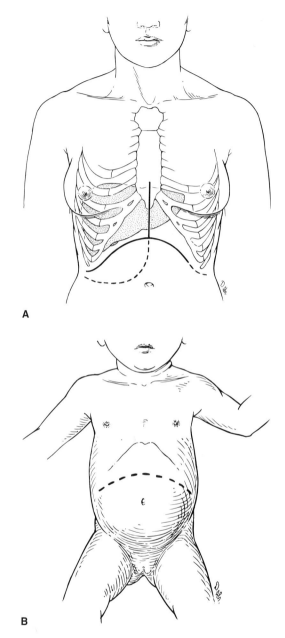

Figure 40.8–2. Most common incision used for the recipient of an orthotopic liver graft. **A:** The most frequently used incision, a right subcostal incision with a midline extension (solid line), or a Reynold's flap ("hockey stick") sometimes used for patients with a small liver. **B:** A bilateral subcostal incision without a midline extension, used for pediatric patients.

VASCULAR RECONSTRUCTION

Three venous and one arterial anastomoses are required for revascularization of the liver (Figure 40.8–3). The venous anastomoses consist of the suprahepatic vena cava, infrahepatic vena cava, and portal vein. In children, these anastomoses are performed with absorbable sutures to permit growth of the anastomotic lumen as the child grows. In adults, the venous anastomoses may be carried out with either nonabsorbable or absorbable sutures. The arterial anastomoses are always performed with nonabsorbable sutures, using a running or an interrupted technique in adults and children, respectively.

Unusual vascular reconstructions may be necessary in cases with abnormal congenital anomalies (eg, numerous hepatic arteries) or thrombosis or atresia of the portal vein. Iliac vessels from the donor function well as vascular conduits. The immunosuppression prevents these conduits from being rejected; thus, degeneration and aneurysm formation are rarely observed. For reconstruction of the hepatic artery, iliac arteries from the donor are then used as interposition vascular grafts between the aorta and the allograft hepatic artery. For the reconstruction of the portal vein, the donor iliac veins are placed between the junction of the superior mesenteric and the splenic veins and the allograft portal vein, or between the superior mesenteric vein and the allograft portal vein.

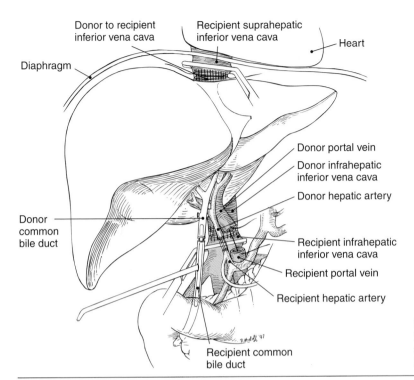

Figure 40.8–3. Recipient organ transplantation. Three venous and one arterial anastomoses are required for revascularization of the liver.

PIGGYBACK LIVER TRANSPLANTATION

A technique that we have adopted is piggyback transplantation. With this method, the vena cava of the recipient is left intact; therefore, the venous return is maintained throughout the operation. The surgeon separates the liver from the vena cava, using a meticulous technique to ligate the tributaries to the vena cava. The right hepatic vein is divided and oversewn with a nonabsorbable suture. A clamp is placed across the confluence of the middle and left hepatic vein, and the hepatectomy is completed. A cuff of the middle and left hepatic veins is created.

There are only two venous anastomoses in the piggyback technique. The first anastomosis between the cuff of the recipient hepatic veins and the cuff of the suprahepatic vena cava is carried end-to-end. This is followed by the portal vein reconstruction, which is also performed end-to-end. The liver is flushed by allowing splanchnic blood from the portal vein to go through the liver and out the infrahepatic vena cava of the allograft, getting rid of the intrahepatic preservation solution and air bubbles. The allograft infrahepatic vena cava is immediately ligated. The vascular clamps are then removed. Lastly, the hepatic artery reconstruction is made end-to-end, which completes the vascularization of the liver (Figure 40.8–4).

The piggyback technique, in our experience, has been associated with better intraoperative hemodynamics, shorter stays in the intensive care unit and hospital, and reduced intraoperative blood requirements. In fact, 20% of our liver transplantation operations are carried out with no blood transfusions.

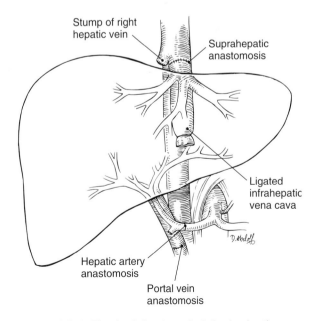

Figure 40.8–4. Piggyback liver transplantation leaving the vena cava intact.

COMMON BILE DUCT RECONSTRUCTION

Two methods of reconstruction of the common bile duct are used: an end-to-end choledochocholedochostomy for those recipients with a normal extrahepatic biliary system and an end-to-side choledochojejunostomy for those patients with absence of the common bile duct (eg, biliary atresia), diseased bile duct (primary sclerosing cholangitis), or size mismatch. The anastomoses are stented with either a T-tube or a silastic tube, respectively. Absorbable sutures are placed in an interrupted fashion. The choledochocholedochostomy may also be performed with no stenting (Figure 40.8–5).

IMMUNOSUPPRESSION

PROTOCOLS

Table 40.8–5 provides a summary of the most common immunosuppressive protocols used in hepatic transplantation. This is a very dynamic aspect of transplantation as new drugs are discovered and added to the antirejection armamentarium. There is also a great deal of physician preference, which makes it difficult to compare different protocols for efficacy and safety. As previously mentioned, the combination of cyclosporine and prednisone has been known as the conventional protocol. Some centers strongly favor adding azathioprine to this regimen (**triple drug therapy**) to enhance the immunosuppressive effect of cyclosporine. Other centers have recommended induction therapy with a polyclonal agent for 7–10 days, to which cyclosporine, prednisone, and sometimes azathioprine are added. This regimen is known as **quadruple therapy**, or sequential induction therapy. Proponents of this protocol believe that the utilization of a polyclonal antilymphocyte preparation spares the use of cyclosporine during the immediate perioperative period, benefiting patients with renal dysfunction by allowing them time to recover their renal function. The incidence of rejection seems to be the same compared to other protocols, but the onset is delayed 4–6 weeks, as opposed to 1–2 weeks with the conventional protocol.

A combination of a potent immunosuppressive agent, tacrolimus (FK506), and low-dose prednisone is gaining acceptance by many transplant centers around the world. The incidence of side effects with tacrolimus is similar to that of cyclosporine; however, tacrolimus has been more effective in reducing the rate of acute rejection.

REJECTION

Effective and safe immunosuppression is a delicate balance between infection and rejection. Rejection of the liver may be acute or chronic. Acute rejection or acute

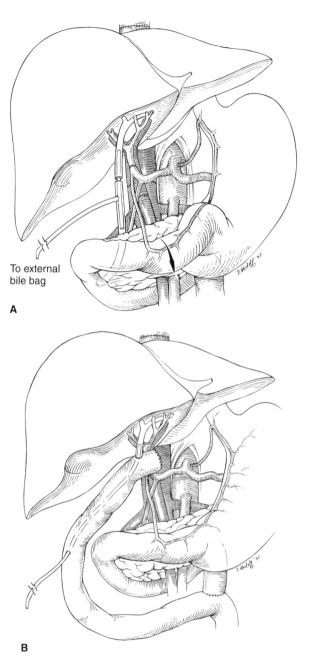

Figure 40.8–5. Biliary reconstruction. **A:** Most common biliary reconstruction, choledochocholedochostomy. **B:** Biliary reconstruction used in pediatric patients and patients with an abnormal or diseased native biliary system, choledochojejunostomy utilizing a Roux-en-Y limb.

cellular rejection is characterized by a mixed lymphocytic infiltrate involving the portal triads, with destruction of biliary canaliculi and arterioles. The incidence of acute cellular rejection in the liver transplant recipient has been reported to be between 50% and 100% and depends on the

Table 40.8–5. Immunosuppressive protocols
in liver transplantation.

Induction Therapy
Cyclosporine and prednisone
Cyclosporine, prednisone, and azathioprine
Antilymphocyte globulin (ALG) or OKT3 and prednisone, then cyclosporine
Tacrolimus and prednisone

Maintenance Therapy
Cyclosporine alone
Cyclosporine and prednisone
Cyclosporine and prednisone and azathioprine
Cyclosporine and azathioprine
Tacrolimus alone
Tacrolimus and prednisone

intensity of immunosuppression. Rejection must be diagnosed early and treated immediately. The differential diagnosis of acute cellular rejection is listed in Table 40.8–6. Acute cellular rejection is usually observed between the first and the second week post-transplantation, with a mean of 10 days, although it may be observed any time after transplantation. Its treatment is shown in an algorithm in Figure 40.8–6. The incidence of chronic rejection is much lower, with a rate of 8–15% reported in the literature. Chronic rejection may also occur any time after transplantation, although it is usually observed much later. The **vanishing bile duct syndrome**, or **ductopenic rejection**, are terms being used for chronic rejection and have the connotation of irreversible injury; however, clinicians know now that this concept is no longer true. Hyperacute rejection of the liver has rarely been observed in liver transplantation and, thus, is of little clinical significance. In fact, successful liver transplantation across ABO groups has been performed, particularly in children. There is, however, a slight drop in patient and graft survival in recipients with positive cytotoxic crossmatches. But the shortage of organs is so serious that the benefit of subjecting a patient to transplantation with a positive crossmatch outweighs the risk.

Table 40.8–6. Differential diagnosis in rejection of the liver.

Acute Rejection
Acute viral hepatitis
Acute cholangitis
Drug-induced hepatotoxicity
Hemolysis
Systemic sepsis
Neoplastic liver diseases

Chronic Rejection
Recurrence of viral hepatitis
Acute chronic cholangitis
Drug-induced hepatotoxicity

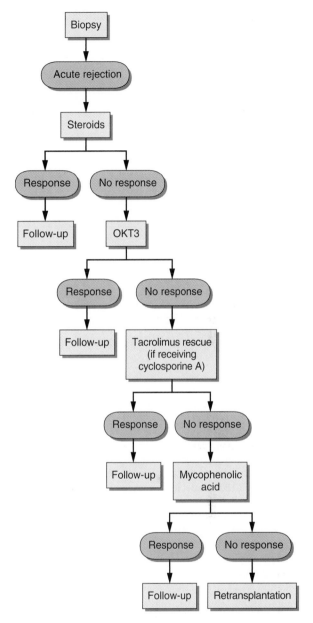

Figure 40.8–6. Algorithm for the treatment of acute cellular rejection of a liver transplant.

INFECTION

Infections that may occur during the post-transplant course are described in Table 40.8–7. The rate of infections has changed considerably as more selective immunosuppressive agents and better antibiotics have been discovered. Still, the incidence of infection is high, particularly viral infections. Epstein-Barr virus (EBV) infections in small children may be complicated by develop-

Table 40.8–7. Infections in liver transplant recipients at different times in the post-transplant course.

First Month Post-Transplant
Infections present in recipient prior to transplant (eg, hepatitis, bacterial infections, tuberculosis, influenza).
Infections transmitted with the allograft (eg, hepatitis, human immunodeficiency virus, acute bacterial infection, fungal infection).
Infections related to technical complications of the transplant procedure (eg, pneumonia, wound infection, liver abscess, biliary sepsis).

1–6 Months Post-Transplant
Lingering effect of infections acquired earlier.
Viral infections (eg, cytomegalovirus, Epstein-Barr virus, hepatitis).
Opportunistic infections (eg, *Pneumocystis, Listeria*).

More than 6 Months Post-Transplant
Chronic (reactivation of) cytomegalovirus, Epstein-Barr virus, and herpetic infections.
Patients with good graft function and minimal immunosuppression have a risk for community acquired infections (eg, influenza, pneumococcal pneumonia).
Patients with chronic rejection and excess immunosuppression are at risk for opportunistic infections (eg, *Cryptococcus, Listeria, Pneumocystis, Aspergillus*).

ment of post-transplant lymphoproliferative disorders. Except for technical complications, the onset of infection in a liver transplant recipient implies over-immunosuppression. In addition to the institution of antibiotic therapy, the immunosuppression must be reduced and may require readjustment as the infection is brought under control.

SURGICAL COMPLICATIONS

Table 40.8–8 lists the most common surgical complications observed in the liver transplant recipient. Surgical complications must be diagnosed early and treated promptly, since they will lead to increased morbidity and mortality. In decreasing order of frequency, the most common complications observed in the liver transplant recipient are: biliary tract strictures or leaks, vascular complications, and primary graft nonfunction.

BILIARY TRACT COMPLICATIONS

The incidence of biliary tract complications ranges from 6% to 27%. The clinical presentation depends on the type of complication. Biliary strictures may involve the anastomosis or the intrahepatic biliary branches. In the former, the cause is usually an ischemic phenomenon from leaving the donor bile duct unnecessarily long, ren-

dering it ischemic. This complication is prevented by trimming the bile duct until bleeding from the transected edge occurs, indicating adequate blood supply. The mechanism of injury for intrahepatic biliary strictures is different, although probably ischemic as well. This is usually associated with severe preservation damage of the liver allograft.

Other factors implicated in the etiology of this complication are: rejection, cytomegalovirus hepatitis, thrombosis of the hepatic artery, and recurrence of primary sclerosing cholangitis. Patients with strictures usually experience multiple episodes of cholangitis, particularly if the bile duct reconstruction consists of a choledochojejunostomy. At times, this problem may be erroneously labeled as rejection. The laboratory chemistries may show elevation of the alkaline phosphatase and gamma glutamyl transferase (GGT). The total bilirubin may also be elevated in the presence of tight strictures.

The treatment for anastomotic strictures consists of balloon dilatation first and surgical revision if the dilatation fails. The prognosis is generally good. In contrast, intrahepatic strictures pose a significant management problem, since they are not amenable to dilatation or surgical revision. In the case of a dominant intrahepatic stricture, percutaneous stenting may be considered. In addition, the administration of prophylactic antibiotics such ciprofloxacin, trimethoprim-sulfa, or ampicillin may prevent further episodes of cholangitis. The administration of ursodeoxy-

Table 40.8–8. Surgical complications in liver transplantation.

Biliary	
Early:	Late:
Anastomotic leak	T-tube site fistula
Bile duct necrosis	Anastomotic stricture
	Intrahepatic stricture
	Extrahepatic obstruction
	Lithiasis

Vascular	
Early:	Late:
Acute hepatic artery thrombosis	Hepatic artery stenosis
Acute portal vein thrombosis	Portal vein thrombosis
	Portal vein stenosis
	Suprahepatic inferior vena cava stenosis/Budd-Chiari syndrome

Primary graft nonfunction	

Others	
Wound-related:	Abnormal fluid collection:
Infection	Abscess
Dehiscence	Biloma
Herniation	Infected ascites
Intestinal:	Chylous
Perforation	
Obstruction	

cholic acid has been recommended, although its efficacy has not been clearly defined. The poor quality of life or the development of secondary biliary cirrhosis in some of these patients is a strong indication for retransplantation.

Biliary leaks are unusual and are usually caused by necrosis of the bile duct from thrombosis of the hepatic artery or occur following removal of the t-tube. The former is a formidable problem since the complication is associated with the development of infected bilomas; these may be temporarily managed with percutaneous drainage and antibiotics, but retransplantation is inevitable in the majority of these patients. On the other hand, a leak following removal of the t-tube occurs from a torn sinus tract; although these patients may require a laparotomy to treat the bile peritonitis, the prognosis is excellent. At laparotomy, placement of a single stitch to close the sinus tract is all that is needed. Some transplant surgeons recommend nonsurgical treatment consisting of nasobiliary tube suctioning and antibiotics, but this approach may prolong the hospital stay unnecessarily. There is also the risk of developing an intra-abdominal abscess with its associated morbidity, particularly in an immunosuppressed patient.

VASCULAR COMPLICATIONS

The most common vascular complication is thrombosis of the hepatic artery, with an incidence of 6% but ranging from 2% in adult patients to up to 20% in children. Several factors have been implicated in the etiology of this complication, such as technical problems, arterial anomalies, the utilization of vascular conduits, high postoperative hematocrit, and acute rejection. The presentation is usually within the first 10 postoperative days. There may be an abrupt elevation of the liver enzymes, although this is not a reliable sign. Thrombosis of the artery results in necrosis of the bile duct and hepatic infarcts with subsequent abscess formation. A rare complication is gangrene of the liver caused by *Clostridium* infection, due to thrombosis of the hepatic artery and portal vein. These patients are toxic and develop multiple organ system failure quickly. Urgent retransplantation is the only chance for survival; however, in the absence of a donor, a total hepatectomy and creation of a portocaval shunt may be a lifesaving temporary procedure as a bridge to transplantation. The longest time for an anhepatic patient was 76 hours, with full recovery following retransplantation. The overall patient survival after retransplantation for thrombosis of the hepatic artery is approximately 50%.

Portal vein thrombosis is the second most common vascular complication, with a reported incidence of 1–4%. The incidence is slightly higher in patients receiving reduced-size livers. The clinical presentation depends on the time of onset. Thrombosis occurring during the early postoperative period is associated with acute portal hypertension, coagulopathy, and frequently gastrointestinal (GI) bleeding. The liver enzymes may or may not change. The

onset of GI bleeding should raise the suspicion of portal vein thrombosis and be evaluated by emergency Doppler ultrasonography. When the diagnosis is made early, thrombectomy and revision of the vascular reconstruction may salvage the liver allograft. Late thrombosis or stenosis of the portal vein may also present with GI bleeding, but, unlike the early presentation, the synthetic function of the liver is not compromised. Stenosis of the portal vein may be treated with percutaneous dilatation or excision of the stenotic area. Late thrombosis is managed by the creation of a portosystemic shunt. Retransplantation is rarely needed.

Stenosis of the suprahepatic vena cava anastomosis is seldom seen and often occurs late, with the clinical manifestation being that of Budd-Chiari syndrome. The treatment of choice is balloon dilatation with placement of a Wall stent. The clinical response is immediate and the long-term prognosis is good.

PRIMARY GRAFT NONFUNCTION

Primary graft nonfunction is defined as acute liver allograft failure following transplantation. Patients develop severe coagulopathy followed by other symptoms and signs of liver insufficiency, such as hypoglycemia, metabolic acidosis, progressive encephalopathy, multiple organ system failure, and death unless emergency retransplantation is performed. The overall patient survival following retransplantation is approximately 35%.

Other surgical complications that may require invasive procedures observed during the immediate postoperative period are listed in Table 40.8–8.

RESULTS

Patient and graft survival after hepatic transplantation may be influenced by the underlying liver disease, age of the patient, primary versus retransplantation, the indication for retransplantation, the medical status of the patient, and the experience of the liver transplant team. At our institution, the overall patient and graft survival for adult patients at 1 year is 93% and 85%, respectively. In children, the overall patient and graft survival at 1 year is 93% and 83%, respectively. The long-term administration of hepatitis B immunoglobulin has been associated with improvement in the prognosis, with the survival approaching that of cholestatic liver disease. The patient and graft survival is significantly compromised in high-risk elderly patients and patients of any age with multiple organ system failure. In children, the age or the weight of the recipient at the time of transplantation bears no influence on patient survival. Nonetheless, graft survival is decreased in infants weighing less than 10 kg receiving full-size livers. On the other hand, a comparison between reduced-size and full-size liver transplants in the entire patient population showed no significant difference between the two groups. In our experience the patient and graft survival in living-related liver transplantation has been 100%, and good results have also been published by other transplant centers.

RETRANSPLANTATION

For didactic purposes, the indications for retransplantation may be divided into five broad categories: chronic rejection, vascular complications, primary graft nonfunction, recurrence of underlying liver disease, and miscellaneous reasons. The overall patient and graft survival depends on the indication. The patient survival for retransplantation for chronic rejection is 60–70%; for thrombosis of the hepatic artery, 50%; and for primary graft nonfunction, 35%. The prognosis is rather poor when retransplantation is performed for recurrence of hepatitis C.

QUALITY OF LIFE

Quality of life in liver transplant recipients warrants as much concern as does patient survival. Close to 90% of liver transplant recipients will return to a much improved quality of life compared to the preoperative status. Many of these patients do require extensive rehabilitation, particularly patients with cholestatic liver disease, such as primary biliary cirrhosis in adults and biliary atresia in children. Patients afflicted with this type of liver disease often suffer from osteoporosis and rickets, not infrequently complicated by multiple fractures. Children with biliary atresia also show signs of motor and mental delay, which improves after transplantation although the improvement does not become noticeable until the first year after transplantation.

With proper selection of alcoholic patients, the incidence of recidivism is approximately 15% and usually amounts to very transient drinking. More importantly, 80% of our alcoholic liver transplant recipients returned to part-time or full-time work.

The type of immunosuppression has also had an impact on quality of life. Patients receiving tacrolimus usually do not experience the hirsutism observed with cyclosporine.

Furthermore, over half of the patients on tacrolimus do not require prednisone, resulting in a much improved appearance by eliminating the moon facies, hirsutism, and truncal obesity commonly caused by chronic administration of steroids.

SUMMARY

The consequences of end-stage liver disease are devastating. Patients suffer from problems associated with portal hypertension, osteoporosis, and rickets. Children experience mental and motor retardation and adult patients become incapacitated, unable to work and take care of themselves. Liver transplantation offers a chance for survival. Furthermore, it is cost-effective, since the majority of the patients are reinstated back into society and become active participants in the work force.

Better immunosuppression was not the only factor contributing to the progress of hepatic transplantation. Other important factors were the development of the Wisconsin solution for cold preservation of the liver, improvements in surgical techniques for the donor and recipient operations, proper selection of patients, and advances in critical care. Still, there are many problems to be overcome in hepatic transplantation. The main problem is the shortage of organs, which is the limiting factor in liver transplantation. Approximately 17% of patients on the waiting list die while waiting for a suitable organ. The use of reduced-size or living-related transplants has not solved the problem. The future calls for the use of split livers, in which a single liver is "split" for transplantation in two recipients. Unfortunately, this procedure has not evolved into a common practice because of its increased morbidity, especially in an era of cost containment.

Efforts are being made to find ways to abrogate rejection from organs across species, but this continues to be within the realm of experimental surgery, not clinical reality. Although tolerance has not been addressed in this chapter, it is a topic of great interest, since several liver transplant recipients have acquired enough tolerance to discontinue immunosuppression for several years without experiencing rejection. The main problem is identifying those patients who have become immunotolerant. This has been actively investigated, since it will permit safe withdrawal of immunosuppression without jeopardizing the patient's life.

SUGGESTED READING

Blumgart LH: *Surgery of the Liver and Biliary Tract*, 2nd ed. Churchill Livingstone, 1994.

Bussutil RW, Klintmalm G: *Transplantation of the Liver.* Saunders, 1996.

Maddrey WC, Sorrell MF: *Transplantation of the Liver.* Appleton & Lange, 1995.

Neuberger J, Adams D: *The Immunology of Liver Transplantation.* Little, Brown, 1993.

Starzl TE, Demetris AJ: *Liver Transplantation: A 31-Year Perspective.* Year Book Medical Publisher, 1990.

40.9 Intestinal Transplantation

Donald C. Dafoe, MD

► Key Facts

- ► Candidates for small intestinal transplantation suffer from short-gut syndrome with insufficient intestinal absorptive capacity to maintain nutrition or electrolyte balance.

- ► The primary disease leading to intestinal failure is loss of intestine due to surgical resection, vascular catastrophe, or functional disturbances, such as generalized Hirschsprung's disease.

- ► Contraindications to intestinal transplantation include unresectable cancer, active infection, insufficient cardiorespiratory reserve or renal failure, long-standing diabetes with severe neurovascular complications, inadequate social support, major psychiatric disease, ongoing substance abuse, or an inability to appreciate the magnitude of the operation and its sequelae.

- ► Sepsis with multiorgan system failure is the primary cause of death in patients with an intestinal

transplantation, followed by lymphoproliferative disorders, thrombosis of the blood supply, or a leak in the gastrointestinal anastomosis.

- ► Sepsis is a frequent complication in patients with intestinal transplantations given the debilitated, malnourished state of the patient, the combination of immunosuppression, and a large bacterial burden.

- ► As of June 1995, there have been approximately 180 intestinal transplants (with liver grafts or multivisceral) performed worldwide. Overall, the patient survival rate is 50–60% after 1 year.

- ► Despite an estimated 600 candidates for intestinal transplantation generated each year, it is unlikely that intestinal transplantations will be widely applied in the near future.

Small bowel transplantation is carried out as treatment for the patient with short-gut syndrome. Intestinal transplantation is a clinical endeavor that is slowly recapitulating the history of other organ allografts. Lillehei began transplanting bowel grafts in dogs in 1959 at the University of Minnesota. In 1966, Lillehei and Kelly did the first human small bowel transplant. Between 1964 and 1970 seven cases of clinical intestinal transplant were reported; each ended in the death of the recipient. Approximately 1 decade later, the introduction of cyclosporine brought a resurgence in clinical small intestinal transplantation but the outcome was still dismal. In 1989 the transplant team at the University of Kiel reported the first successful case of small bowel transplantation; success was defined as discontinuation of total parenteral nutrition (TPN) and sustenance by oral alimentation. The immunosuppressive regimen consisted of anti-lymphocyte globulin induction and maintenance on cyclosporine and steroids. Sporadic reports of success have given way to steady gains in graft and patient survival with the new immunosuppressive agent tacrolimus.

Notably, during the 1980s, a technique of pancreatic transplantation was devised that included the whole donor pancreas and 6 cm of donor duodenum, which drained into the urinary bladder. The majority of duodenopancreatic grafts survived for at least at 1 year after transplantation, with excellent healing at the interface of donor duodenum and recipient bladder. Thus, successful small intestinal transplantation in the form of a 5- to 6-cm segment was commonplace; yet intestinal grafts of greater length were usually lost from rejection, despite stronger immunosuppressive protocols. These disparate results suggested a "dose" effect. The length of intestine transplanted has immunologic relevance insofar as more length includes more immunocompetent donor cells, a greater microbial load, and increased immunogenicity due to enterocytes that express abundant major histocompatibility complex (MHC) class II antigen. The burden of passenger leukocytes also raises the possibility of graft-versus-host disease (GVHD). Clinically, GVHD has been found to be primarily a theoretical concern. Host-versus-graft, better known as rejection, is the main barrier to success.

CANDIDATE SELECTION

Candidates for small intestinal transplantation suffer from short-gut syndrome, with insufficient intestinal absorptive capacity to maintain nutrition or electrolyte balance. The incidence of appropriate candidates has been estimated at two per million population annually, with an equal distribution between adults and children. These patients can be maintained on TPN but recurrent sepsis, progressive liver bone disease, intractable chronic diarrhea, electrolyte imbalance, and loss of access make intestinal transplantation the only remaining therapeutic option. The primary disease leading to intestinal failure is loss of intestine due to surgical resection (eg, inflammatory bowel disease, necrotizing enterocolitis in children, radiation enteritis), vascular catastrophe (eg, midgut volvulus, trauma), or functional disturbances, such as generalized Hirschsprung's disease. In children, congenital abnormalities, such as gastroschisis and intestinal atresia, may be responsible. Before intestinal transplantation is attempted, medical measures such as TPN support, glutamine (a gut-specific fuel), growth hormone, and a high-carbohydrate/low-fat diet are advisable. The passage of time will allow for intestinal adaptation. The patient is likely to escape a lifetime of TPN if more

than 100 cm of small intestine remains, particularly if the portion remaining is ileum and the ileocecal valve is intact.

If the patient also has advanced liver disease, often due to hepatitis or cholestatic injury from TPN, combined liver and intestinal transplantation may be warranted. Based on the known protective effect of a liver graft on a synchronously transplanted same-donor kidney graft, it has been reasoned that the liver allograft might wield a similar influence on the intestinal component. In practice, it appears that bowel graft survival is better when done in isolation. A consensus is developing that candidates should be referred for isolated small bowel transplantation prior to the development of end-stage liver disease. The transplant team at the University of Pittsburgh under the guidance of Dr Thomas E. Starzl expanded intestinal transplantation to multivisceral "cluster" transplants. Encouraging results in the research laboratory using large animal models and tacrolimus immunosuppression provided the impetus for clinical trials. These complex grafts have consisted of upper abdominal organs, such as the liver, stomach, pancreas, small bowel, and colon. Problems with hemorrhagic pancreatitis caused the cluster graft to be altered by removal of the pancreas from the composite graft. In some cases, the pancreas was processed, then returned, as isolated islets, via the portal vein into the transplanted liver. The colon has also been identified as a significant risk factor. The length of intestine distal to the ileocecal valve should be minimized. Multivisceral transplants were done following abdominal exenteration as an en bloc resection for cancer. Early outcomes have been comparable to single organ grafts. However, vigorous immunosuppression has resulted in a high incidence of lymphoproliferative disorders (LPD) and recurrent metastatic disease.

Generic contraindications to intestinal transplantation include unresectable cancer, active infection, insufficient cardiorespiratory reserve or renal failure, long-standing diabetes with severe neurovascular complications, inadequate social support, major psychiatric disease, ongoing substance abuse (many of these patients have narcotic addiction), and inability to appreciate the magnitude of the operation and its sequelae, including long-term immunosuppression. Relative contraindications that are specific to intestinal transplant candidates relate to technical difficulty, such as thrombosis of the inferior vena cava, portal vein, multiple prior surgeries, and fistulae.

DONOR ISSUES & PROCUREMENT

There are a few case reports of living-related donor (LRD) intestinal transplantation. The author and colleagues reported the unique case of intestinal transplant between identical twins—a rare opportunity—with an excellent outcome. There are advantages of LRD grafts over cadaveric, such as histocompatibility leukocyte antigen (HLA) compatibility and elective surgery. There is minimal risk to the donor. Nevertheless, heart-beating, brain-dead cadaver donors are the usual source of bowel grafts.

The technique of intestinal retrieval is in situ perfusion of the distal aorta with University of Wisconsin (UW) preservation solution and en bloc resection as part of multiple organ donor recovery. Prior to procurement, oral antibiotics (eg, nystatin, neomycin, trimethoprim-sulfamethoxazole), and intravenous antibiotics have been used to bring about "gut decontamination." In addition, some clinical investigators have pretreated the donor with lymphocyte-depleting agents, such as anti-T cell monoclonal antibody, in an effort to decimate passenger leukocyte load. There is no evidence that this practice reduces GVHD, LPD, or rejection. Cold-storage in ice after flushing with UW preservation solution will provide adequate preservation for up to 12 hours.

Contraindications to donation, in addition to generic reasons (eg, malignancy, infection, prolonged hypotension, extensive vascular disease), include a history of malabsorption, inflammatory bowel disease, and prior surgery with multiple adhesions.

The donor-recipient must be compatible with regard to ABO blood type and **crossmatch** (non-killing of donor cells by recipient serum and complement). HLA matching, of undeniable value in renal transplantation, is not of proven worth in bowel transplantation.

SURGICAL TECHNIQUES

The isolated small bowel graft may be transplanted in the orthotopic position. Arterial blood is supplied via an anastomosis between the recipient's superior mesenteric artery (SMA), often on a Carrel patch of donor aorta, and infrarenal aorta. The venous drainage from the superior mesenteric vein (SMV) or donor portal vein empties into the recipient portal vein (Figure 40.9–1). Alternatively, the graft may be drained into the infrahepatic vena cava. Physiologic portal venous drainage is preferred because the venous effluent from the bowel graft provides hepatotrophic substances to the liver. Also, hepatic filtration is important in the clearance of translocated bacteria from the lumen. Each small bowel graft end may be either exteriorized as an ostomy or connected to the native gastrointestinal (GI) tract. The flow of succus entericus stimulates the absorptive surface and thereby maintains the barrier to

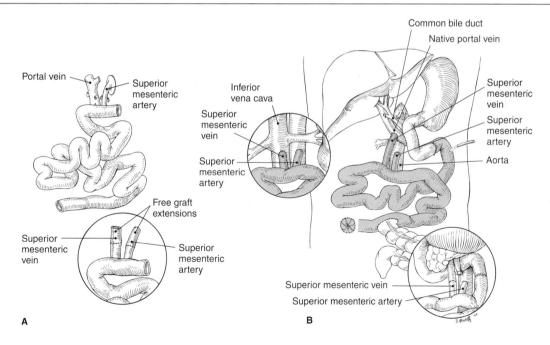

Figure 40.9–1. **A:** The isolated small bowel graft as prepared from the donor. **(Inset)** Vascular extension grafts using donor vessels can be added to provide length, thereby facilitating transplantation. **B:** Implantation techniques include: **(main panel)** donor superior mesenteric artery anastomosed to the infrarenal aorta of the recipient, venous drainage via the donor superior mesenteric vein into the native portal vein, proximal gastrointestinal recipient-to-donor continuity, enterostomy tube and "chimney" ileostomy; **(left inset)** venous drainage into the recipient inferior vena cava; or, **(right inset)** venous drainage into the Superior mesenteric vein below the pancreas.

bacteria. Exteriorization of transplanted gut allows access for monitoring rejection and other changes by serial mucosal biopsies. Some surgeons have created a "chimney," a limb of defunctionalized bowel graft that exits through the abdominal wall to the skin, and GI continuity is reestablished by way of an intraperitoneal anastomosis between donor and recipient. An ostomy is helpful for biopsy and endoscopy access. Inclusion of the ileocecal valve in the graft is recommended to slow intestinal transit and promote adaptation. Early feeding is facilitated by the placement of an enterostomy tube.

The surgical technique is different in combined liver/intestinal or multiple visceral transplantation (Figure 40.9–2). The arterial blood supply of a liver/intestinal transplant arises from an anastomosis between a Carrel patch of donor aorta that incorporates visceral arteries (celiac axis and SMA) and the recipient infrarenal aorta. Rather than a Carrel patch, a cylinder of donor aorta can be used. The retrohepatic vena cava segment of the graft is interposed between the recipient caval ends following hepatectomy and bowel resection. Another technique for routing of the venous blood is the so-called **piggyback technique** used by some transplant centers in liver transplantation. During hepatectomy, the recipient vena cava is left intact, thereby leaving retroperitoneal varices undisturbed and venous return to the heart uninterrupted. The diseased liver is peeled off the recipient's retrohepatic vena cava by suture-ligating small hepatic veins and caudate lobe branches. Then the suprahepatic vena cava of the graft is sewn into a venous confluens constructed from recipient hepatic veins. The infrahepatic vena cava of the liver graft is simply tied off. Venous drainage from the intestinal graft flows into the portal vein through the en bloc liver graft and out the suprahepatic vena cava. The donor bile duct is anastomosed either to the graft duodenum or a Roux-en-Y limb of bowel. The native portal vein that drains the remnant GI tract is decompressed into the graft portal vein.

COMPLICATIONS

Sepsis with multisystem organ failure is the primary cause of death. LPD is another major source of mortality. Thrombosis of the blood supply secondary to kinking or technical imperfection results in graft loss. A leak at a GI anastomosis is a disastrous occurrence that is predisposed by poor nutrition, rejection, and steroids. Hemorrhage, obstruction, and perforation are other adverse outcomes. High graft enterostomy output can rapidly lead to dehydration.

CLINICAL IMMUNOLOGY

In the immunologic tug-of-war between GVHD and host-versus-graft in intestinal transplant recipients, rejec-

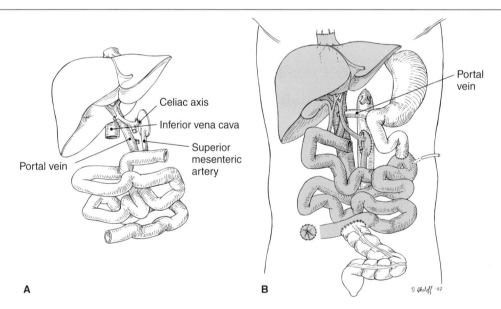

A **B**

Figure 40.9–2. Combined liver-intestine transplant. The prepared composite graft from the donor **(A)** and after transplantation **(B)**. Note several features: the arterial supply is from a Carrel patch of donor aorta encompassing the celiac artery and superior mesenteric artery; the retrohepatic donor cava is interposed between the caval ends, the suprahepatic cava, and the inferior vena cava of the recipient; the bile duct remains in situ, emptying into the graft duodenum; the native portal vein from the remnant gut is decompressed into the graft portal vein beyond the proximal anastomosis of donor and recipient gut an enterostomy tube is placed for early feeding; and the distal bowel is exteriorized as a "chimney" for endoscopy and biopsy access and connected to the native sigmoid colon.

tion regularly emerges as the victor. GVHD, manifested by skin rash and fever, has been reported but acute rejection has an extremely high incidence in the weeks after transplantation. Clinical evidence of small bowel rejection includes fever, high stoma output, and gut atony. During rejection, gross examination of the stoma of exteriorized bowel graft reveals an ulcerated, friable mucosa with a pseudomembranous appearance. Endoscopically, the mucosa is edematous and hyperemic, with flattened villi. Since no reliable screening test for acute rejection exists, a biopsy (endoscopic biopsies are preferred to misleading stomal biopsies) is necessary to make the definitive diagnosis. The histologic features of acute rejection include cryptitis, vasculitis, and a mononuclear cellular infiltrate. Probes for Epstein-Barr virus (EBV) are important to distinguish acute rejection from LPD.

Chronic rejection is characterized by fibrosis of lamina propria, loss of goblet and Paneth cells, villus atrophy, and vascular thickening. Microchimerism has been demonstrated in the months after successful engraftment by fluorescent-activated cell sorting of lymphocytes from the recipient's peripheral blood and antibodies directed against donor HLA. This finding correlates microchimerism with long-term graft survival and suggests that donor lymphocytes may be active mediators of donor-specific hyporesponsiveness.

The intestinal graft is denervated, lacking in lymphatic connections and damaged as a result of nonspecific injuries, such as preservation and reperfusion. Therefore, immunosuppression of the intestinal transplant recipient is complicated by the variable absorption of medications by the altered graft. Parenteral delivery of immunosuppressive agents is mandatory in the early post-transplant days. Tacrolimus-based immunosuppression (which appears to be superior to cyclosporine for intestinal transplantation) has been coupled with prednisone. Induction therapy with OKT3 or heterologous anti-lymphocyte serum is usually given. Acute rejection is treated with high-dose steroids or anti-T cell preparations, often followed by a step-up in maintenance immunosuppression. Recipients also receive intravenous antibiotics, anticytomegalovirus (CMV) agents (eg, ganciclovir), and the antifungal fluconazole or low-dose amphotericin.

Immunologic injury to the transplanted gut results in loss of barrier function and bacterial translocation. Given the debilitated, malnourished state of the patient, combination immunosuppression, and large bacterial burden, it is not surprising that sepsis is a frequent complication of small intestinal transplantation. In the early post-transplant period, bacterial infections are most common. Early feeding via a enterostomy tube placed at the time of transplantation preserves barrier function. Nonabsorbable oral antibiotics are used to "decontaminate" the gut—lower intraluminal bacterial counts—with alterations of antibiotics depending on quantitative stool cultures. Viral infections with DNA viruses, such as CMV, have been problematic. Prophylactic ganciclovir followed by high-dose acyclovir maintenance or a regimen of passive immunization with hyperimmune anti-CMV globulin is efficacious in the prevention of CMV disease. Long-term trimethoprim-sulfamethoxazole protects against *Pneumocystis carinii*. EBV-related LPD has a reported incidence of as high as 20% in some series. Treatment consists of an antiviral agent, decrease or discontinuation of immunosuppression, resection of the tumor, if possible, and chemotherapy if the LPD undergoes malignant transformation to lymphoma.

FUNCTION OF THE GRAFT

Success in intestinal transplantation is operationally defined as independence from parenteral nutrition and maintenance of body weight on enteral feeds. Within 3–6 weeks after the transplant, enteral feeds are often tolerated and TPN can be stopped. Blood levels of tacrolimus or cyclosporine, serum albumin levels, and measurement of fat-soluble vitamins can be used as surrogates of graft function. Carbohydrate absorption has been studied using D-xylose. Steatorrhea and quantitative stool fat determinations reflect fat absorption. Within weeks after transplantation, peristalsis and transit time are normalized.

RESULTS

According to the Intestinal Transplant Registry, as of June 1995, approximately 180 intestinal transplants (with liver grafts or multivisceral) have been performed worldwide in 170 patients (Figure 40.9–3). Overall, the patient survival rate is 50–60% at 1 year after transplantation. At some centers, a 1-year graft survival of 70% has been achieved for isolated small bowel transplants. The University of Pittsburgh has the largest experience in the world. A report of their experience with 63 intestinal transplants using tacrolimus-based immunosuppression from 1990–1995 included recipients of isolated small intestine (22), hepatic-intestinal composites (30), and multivisceral transplants (11). Patient survival at 1 year was 75% and graft survival was 67%. Common causes of death included CMV infection, fungal and bacterial infections, rejection, and lymphoma.

In summary, success rates at experienced centers are beginning to equal that of other organ grafts. Intestinal transplantation has repeated the history of other transplants with gradually increasing success, albeit, after a 15-year lag due to unique immunologic complexities. Intestinal transplantation can now be considered a viable therapeutic treatment for patients who have gut failure.

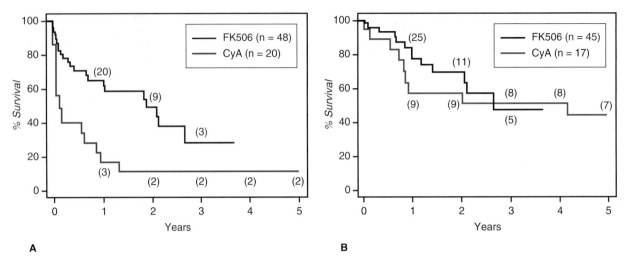

Figure 40.9–3. Graft **(A)** and patient **(B)** survival data from the Intestinal Transplant Registry (1985–1995). FK506 = tacrolimus; CyA = cyclosporine.

THE FUTURE

An estimated 600 candidates for intestinal transplantation are generated each year in the United States. In the near future, it is unlikely that intestinal transplants will be widely applied. However, since short-gut syndrome is a debilitating disease for the individual and extremely expensive to society, intestinal transplants will find a niche in the therapeutic armamentarium. Success rates will continue to improve with refinements in immunosuppression and, ultimately, tolerance induction. Most advances will occur in the prevention of short gut by improved treatment of inflammatory bowel disease and a better understanding of the mechanisms underlying native bowel adaptation.

SUGGESTED READING

Asfar S et al: Small bowel transplantation. Surg Clin North Am 1994;74:1197.

Byrne TA et al: A new treatment for patients with short-bowel syndrome: Growth hormone, glutamine, and a modified diet. Ann Surg 1995;222:243.

Todo S et al: Outcome analysis of 71 clinical intestinal transplantations. Ann Surg 1995;222:270.

Tzakis AG et al: Intestinal transplantation. Ann Rev Med 1994;45:79.

40.10 Cardiac Transplantation

David D. Yuh, MD, & Bruce Reitz, MD

▶ Key Facts

▶ Between 2500 and 3500 cardiac transplantations per year were performed at over 200 centers worldwide between 1990 and 1994.

▶ Most cardiac transplant patients suffer from end-stage coronary artery disease or idiopathic cardiomyopathy.

▶ The contraindications to cardiac transplantation include irreversible hepatic, renal, or pulmonary dysfunction, active infection, recently diagnosed cancer of uncertain stage, psychiatric illness, and severe systemic disease.

▶ Cardiac donor evaluation consists of a directed history and physical examination, arterial blood gas measurements, echocardiogram, serologic screening, and viral screening for hepatitis, herpes simplex virus, and cytomegalovirus.

▶ In the postoperative period, cardiac function generally normalizes within 3–4 days, during which time parenteral inotropes and vasodilators can be weaned.

▶ Currently, conventional immunosuppression in cardiac transplant recipients consists of a "triple-drug" combination of cyclosporine, azathioprine, and prednisone.

▶ Accelerated graft coronary artery disease is a major limiting factor for long-term survival in cardiac transplant patients, while infection is the leading cause of morbidity and mortality.

▶ A review of 496 heart transplant patients at Stanford between 1980 and 1993 placed 1-, 5-, and 10-year actuarial survival estimates at 82%, 61%, and 41%, respectively.

PREOPERATIVE CONSIDERATIONS

RECIPIENT SELECTION

Adherence to strict recipient selection criteria has played an important role in achieving the excellent results observed in cardiac transplantation today. However, recent advances in the management of these patients, both before and after transplantation, have been accompanied by a relaxation of certain criteria, including upper age limits, concomitant disease, and level of disability. Although a wider range of patients has benefited from this expansion of eligibility, the perennial problem of donor organ shortage has been exacerbated. Most transplant centers observe mortality rates between 20% and 30% among patients on their waiting lists. Consequently, current efforts are directed toward refining recipient evaluation methods and selection criteria to channel heart grafts to those patients who are in most immediate need while maintaining good short-term and long-term outcomes.

As a general rule, those patients suffering from severe cardiac disability despite aggressive medical management, but who are otherwise healthy, are considered for cardiac transplantation. Most cardiac transplant recipients suffer from end-stage coronary artery disease or idiopathic cardiomyopathy (Figure 40.10–1). Other diagnoses include defined cardiomyopathy (eg, viral, postpartum, fa-

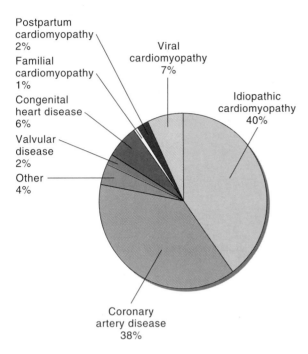

Figure 40.10–1. Indications for adult cardiac transplantation at Stanford (1980–1993).

Table 40.10–1. Contraindications to adult cardiac transplantation.

Significant systemic or multisystem disease (eg, peripheral or cerebrovascular disease, diabetes mellitus)
Active or extrapulmonary infection
Significant irreversible pulmonary, hepatic, or renal dysfunction
Severe pulmonary hypertension
Incurable malignancy
Cachexia or obesity
Current cigarette smoking
Psychiatric illness or history of medical noncompliance
Drug or alcohol abuse

milial), congenital disease, and valvular disease. Disabling symptoms typically include those found in congestive heart failure (eg, dyspnea, fatigue, peripheral edema), although recurrent malignant arrhythmias and severe ischemic symptoms are frequently observed.

The upper recipient age limit of 50 years originally established at Stanford has been raised to 60 at most centers, as a result of accumulating evidence that older recipients experience survival rates and an improved quality of life comparable to younger recipients. In fact, few transplant centers would disqualify an otherwise favorable candidate based solely upon advanced age. The assessment of a potential recipient's emotional stability, compliance, and socioeconomic environment is important as substantial emotional, medical, and financial demands are placed upon the recipient and family.

There are several well-established contraindications to cardiac transplantation (Table 40.10–1). These include irreversible hepatic, renal, or pulmonary dysfunction, active infection, recently diagnosed cancer of uncertain stage, psychiatric illness or history of medical noncompliance, and severe systemic disease that would significantly limit survival or rehabilitation. Severe or fixed pulmonary hypertension has recently been identified as a significant independent risk factor for early mortality after orthotopic cardiac transplantation, presumably a consequence of acute right ventricular failure. Retrospective studies at Stanford and the University of Pittsburgh clearly showed that early post-transplantation mortality was threefold

higher in cardiac transplant recipients with a preoperative pulmonary vascular resistance greater than or equal to 5 Wood units or a transpulmonary pressure gradient (mean pulmonary artery pressure minus mean pulmonary capillary wedge pressure) greater than or equal to 15 mm Hg. Patients with severe pulmonary hypertension are considered for combined heart-lung transplantation.

Significant attention has been directed toward developing a more discriminative method of stratifying patients awaiting transplantation in order to channel hearts to those patients in most immediate need. In the past, a left ventricular ejection fraction of less than 20% was relied upon as an indicator of severe cardiac dysfunction amenable to transplantation; however, refinements in medical management, particularly aggressive vasodilator therapy, has rendered this parameter less representative of severe patient disability or predictive of imminent death. In fact, a review of 152 patients at the UCLA Medical Center with ejection fractions less than or equal to 20% who did not receive transplants showed that survival was not predicted by the severity of hemodynamic compromise at referral, but rather by the success of tailored medical therapy designed to lower the pulmonary artery wedge pressure. Despite the poor status of this group at the time of referral, the 1-year survival rates without transplantation were 63% overall and 83% in patients who achieved low pulmonary wedge pressures. These patients frequently achieved functional capacities typically attained after transplantation. These results suggest that there may exist a substantial subset of potential transplant recipients with severe cardiac dysfunction who, with close medical management, could be placed at a lower priority without significantly affecting survival or functionality. Furthermore, it has been suggested that cardiac transplantation can be safely deferred in ambulatory patients with severe left ventricular dysfunction and peak exercise oxygen consumption of more than 14 mL/min/kg. Until there is sufficient clinical follow-up of these newly defined patient subsets, however, the well-established selection criteria for cardiac transplantation will prevail.

Patients deemed suitable for cardiac transplantation are categorized on the basis of clinical status, time on the waiting list, body size, and ABO blood group. Clinical status is comprised of two broad classes and separate waiting lists: the status I designation is applied to patients who require an intensive care unit (ICU) setting receiving parenteral inotropic drugs or mechanical assist devices to maintain adequate circulatory function. Status II comprises all other patients.

DONOR SELECTION & MANAGEMENT

Donors must have sustained irreversible brain death, usually as a result of blunt and penetrating head trauma or intracranial hemorrhage. Donor evaluation consists of a directed history and physical examination, chest roentgenogram, 12-lead electrocardiogram, arterial blood gases, echocardiogram, serological screening (ie, human immunodeficiency virus [HIV], hepatitis B surface antigen [HB$_s$Ag], hepatitis C antibodies, herpes simplex virus, cytomegalovirus [CMV], and *Toxoplasma*) and direct inspection and palpation of the heart at explantation. Normal cardiac function and the absence of a significant cardiac history and significant coronary atherosclerosis must be established. A donor age of less than 50 years is preferred, although potential donors aged 55 years and older are considered at most centers with a more detailed evaluation, sometimes to include coronary angiography, to rule out significant cardiac disease. At Stanford, a retrospective review showed that older donor age (greater than 25 years) was associated with an increased risk of graft atherosclerosis after cardiac transplantation.

Absolute contraindications for donation include severe coronary or structural heart disease, prolonged cardiac arrest, prior myocardial infarction, a carbon monoxide-hemoglobin level greater than 20%, arterial oxygen saturation less than 80%, metastatic malignancy (sometimes excluding primary brain and skin cancers), and positive HIV status. Relative contraindications include thoracic trauma, sepsis, prolonged severe hypotension (ie, mean arterial pressure less than 60 mm Hg for more than 6 hours), noncritical coronary artery stenosis, HB$_s$Ag or hepatitis C antibodies, multiple resuscitations, severe left ventricular hypertrophy, and a prolonged high inotropic requirement (eg, dopamine in excess of 20 µg/kg/min for 24 hours). It is important to rule out correctable metabolic or physiologic causes of cardiac rhythm disturbances and electrocardiographic anomalies (eg, brain herniation, hypothermia, hypokalemia).

The overriding goal of managing the cardiac donor is the maintenance of hemodynamic stability. Patients suffering from acute brain injury are often hemodynamically unstable due to neurogenic shock, excessive fluid losses, and bradycardia. Continuous arterial and central venous pressure monitoring, aggressive fluid resuscitation, vasopressors, and inotropes are usually required.

Judicious fluid management serves to both prevent intraoperative blood pressure instability and minimize the need for inotropes and vasopressors, which are myocardial stressors. Intravascular volume should be given to maintain the central venous pressure between 5 and 12 mm Hg. Diabetes insipidus is common in organ donors,

requiring the use of intravenous vasopressin (0.8–1.0 U/h) to reduce excessive urine losses.

To maintain adequate perfusion pressures, dopamine is the standard inotropic agent used although alpha agonists (ie, phenylephrine) are often appropriate. Blood transfusions should be used sparingly to maintain the hemoglobin concentration at around 10 g/dL to ensure adequate myocardial oxygen delivery. Hypothermia should be avoided, as it predisposes to ventricular arrhythmias and metabolic acidosis.

DONOR-RECIPIENT MATCHING

Currently, donor-recipient matching parameters include ABO compatibility and body size. ABO compatibilities are strictly adhered to, because isolated episodes of hyperacute rejection have been observed after cardiac transplantation procedures performed across this barrier. Although fairly wide limits are acceptable, size matching and graft ischemic time are particularly important for recipients with an elevated pulmonary vascular resistance (greater than 6–8 Wood units). Generally, grafts from donors whose weight is less than 80% of that of the recipient or those with ischemic times greater than 2 hours are avoided for both adult and pediatric recipients with pulmonary hypertension. There is no upper size limit in adults due to the typically enlarged recipient pericardial space resulting from congestive cardiac enlargement.

Once an appropriate donor-recipient pairing is made, the recipient is screened for preformed antibodies against a panel of random donors. A percent reactive antibody (PRA) level greater than 5% prompts a prospective specific crossmatch between the donor and recipient. Although several retrospective studies have shown that the degree of human leukocyte antigen (HLA) mismatching between donor and recipient influences survival after cardiac transplantation, HLA matching is currently not feasible on a prospective basis in heart or lung transplantation.

ORGAN PRESERVATION

The use of cold crystalloid cardioplegic infusions coupled with topical cooling has permitted safe distant procurement of heart grafts. A commonly used cardioplegic solution is the Stanford formulation comprised of potassium chloride 30 meq/L, sodium bicarbonate 44.6 meq/L, and mannitol 12.5 g/L in 5% dextrose in water. Graft cold ischemic times typically range between 3 and 4 hours, although ischemic times up to 6 hours have not significantly affected graft function or patient survival. These preservation techniques coupled with streamlined donor and recipient protocols have permitted heart procurements as far as 1000 miles from the transplant center. Extensive communication and coordination must be maintained between the organ procurement agency, donor and recipient operative teams, medical centers, and abdominal organ procurement teams. The major procurement agencies in existence are the United Network for Organ Sharing (UNOS) in the United States, Multiple Organ Retrieval (MORE) in Canada, and The EURO Transplant Organization in Europe.

OPERATIVE TECHNIQUES

The current technique for orthotopic cardiac transplantation has remained essentially unchanged from its initial description by Shumway and Lower in 1960. This technique is summarized below and illustrated in Figure 40.10–2.

DONOR OPERATION

After the chest is entered through a median sternotomy, a retractor is placed and the pericardium is opened. The heart is inspected and palpated for contusions, perforations, thrills, and coronary atherosclerosis. If the heart is deemed satisfactory, its final acceptance is immediately communicated to the recipient team. The aorta and pulmonary artery are dissected superiorly to the level of the arch and bifurcation, respectively, to ensure adequate length for implantation. The superior vena cava is then mobilized superiorly to the origin of the azygous vein and encircled with two ligatures. An adequate length of the inferior vena cava is dissected free from its pericardial reflection and is surrounded with an umbilical tape. The aorta is then encircled with an umbilical tape and a 14-gauge cardioplegia perfusion cannula is inserted into its ascending segment. Intravenous heparin is administered at a dose of 300 U/kg and allowed to circulate for 3–5 minutes.

Excision of the heart commences with ligation of the superior and inferior venae cavae. The ascending aorta is then clamped distal to the perfusion cannula at the level of the innominate artery and a hyperkalemic cardioplegic solution at 2–4 °C is rapidly infused into the aortic root at a pressure of 150 mm Hg with the concurrent application of topical cold saline into the pericardial well. The inferior vena cava is divided, decompressing the right heart now filling with cardioplegia. When the heart is fully arrested, cooled, and perfused with cardioplegia, it is elevated from the pericardial well and each of the pulmonary veins are divided at their pericardial reflections. The pulmonary artery and aorta are divided at the level of the bifurcation and innominate artery, respectively. The explanted heart is placed in two sterile plastic bags with a cold saline interface. This, in turn, is placed within an airtight container filled with ice-cold saline and transported in a standard ice-filled cooler.

RECIPIENT OPERATION

After anesthesia is induced and arterial and venous lines are placed, the supine patient's chest and groin areas are prepped and draped. Central venous access via the left internal jugular vein is usually obtained, sparing the right side for future endomyocardial biopsies. After a median sternotomy is performed and the pericardium is opened, the patient undergoes routine cannulation of the aorta and both venae cavae. The arterial cannula is inserted in the most distal aspect of the ascending aorta. The venous cannulae are both placed laterally in the high right atrium near the superior vena caval junction. After institution of cardiopulmonary bypass with moderate hypothermia (28–30°C) and snugging of caval snares, the ascending aorta is cross-clamped and 50–100 mL of cardioplegic solution is rapidly infused into the aortic root, causing diastolic arrest. The aorta and pulmonary arteries are separated and divided at the level of the semilunar valve commissures. The atria are then transected at the level of their atrioventricular grooves, excluding the atrial appendages, leaving two recipient atrial cuffs.

Placing the donor heart in a bowl of cold saline, the left atrium is opened by connecting the pulmonary veins, fashioning the donor atrial cuff. The aorta and pulmonary arteries are completely separated from each other. Under continuous application of topical cold saline into the pericardial well, implantation begins with the direct anastomosis of the donor and recipient left atrial cuffs. The donor right atrium is then opened with an incision extending from the inferior vena caval orifice superiorly in a curvilinear fashion into the base of the right atrial appendage. Through this incision, an intact tricuspid valve and fossa ovalis are inspected and assured. The right atrial cuff anastomosis is then performed followed by an end-to-end anastomosis of the donor and recipient pulmonary arteries. Systemic rewarming is initiated at this time and caval snares are released, permitting blood into the heart and lungs, displacing any air trapped in the left-sided chambers. The end-to-end aortic anastomosis follows this maneuver. Just before completing the aortic anastomosis, additional attempts are made to vent any residual air by agitating the heart. Topical cold saline is then discontinued, 200 mg lidocaine is infused into the bypass circuit, the aortic cross-clamp is removed, and a needle vent is placed in the ascending aorta. Although spontaneous defibrillation usually occurs at this time, electrical defibrillation is effected as necessary. Still under cardiopulmonary bypass, all suture lines are inspected for hemostasis before bypass is weaned. The superior vena caval cannula is drawn back into the right atrium and the inferior vena caval cannula is removed just prior to discontinuation of bypass. An isoproterenol infusion (0.005–0.01 µg/kg/min) is titrated to achieve a heart rate of 90–110 beats/min to chronotropically and inotropically maximize cardiac output and to lower pulmonary vascular resistance. Temporary atrial pacing wires are placed on the donor right atrium. The pericardium is left open. The right pleural

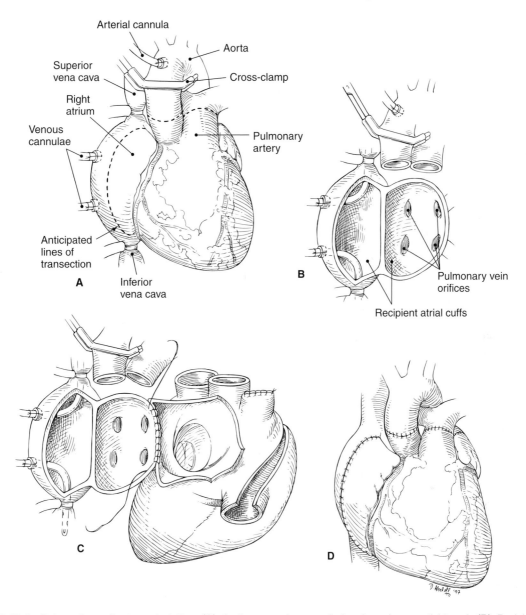

Figure 40.10–2. Orthotopic cardiac transplantation. **(A):** Aortic cross-clamp applied and caval snares tightened. **(B):** Recipient atrial cuffs and great arteries. **(C):** Left atrial anastomosis begun at the left superior pulmonary vein. **(D):** Completed operation with suture lines shown.

space is opened and chest tubes are placed in the right chest and the mediastinum. The sternum and overlying fascia and skin are closed in the usual fashion.

TOTAL ORTHOTOPIC CARDIAC TRANSPLANTATION

Transesophageal echocardiographic analyses of hearts grafted using the standard technique described above have revealed some physiologic abnormalities arising from the donor to recipient atrial cuff anastomoses. Asynchronous contraction of the two atrial cuffs with distortion and asynchronous opening of the tricuspid and mitral valves, resulting in atrioventricular regurgitation and turbulent flow, has been reported. Subclinical atrial mural thrombi have also been observed. These findings have led to a modification of the standard operation developed by Shumway and Lower. The technique of total orthotopic cardiac transplantation employs direct end-to-end anastomoses of the vena cavae and pulmonary veins. By eliminating the heterogeneous atrial cuff anastomoses, this total

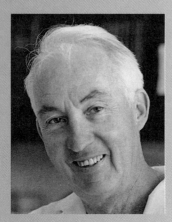

Norman E. Shumway, MD, PhD (b 1923).

The origins of heart transplantation date back to the early 1900s when Alexis Carrel, engaged in experimental vascular surgery at the University of Chicago (see Chapter 39), described the transplantation of a puppy's heart into the neck of an adult dog. In the Soviet Union, V.P. Demikhov developed numerous anatomic variants of intrathoracic heterotopic cardiac transplantation in the mid 1940s, establishing the technical feasibility of these operations. Encouraged by this early experimentation, several laboratories pursued orthotopic cardiac transplantation in the late 1950s. In a landmark *Surgical Forum* presentation in 1960, Norman Shumway and Richard Lower at Stanford University described an elegantly simple method of orthotopic heart transplantation through anastomosis of the atrial cuffs, pulmonary artery, and aorta. The Stanford group reported extended recipient survival from 6–21 days in five of eight dogs, with a return to normal activity until death by homograft rejection. Interestingly, the technique of orthotopic cardiac transplantation has remained essentially unaltered since its initial description. Subsequent investigation by Shumway and others laid the groundwork for methods of graft monitoring, preservation, and physiology.

heart transplantation method was designed to permit a more physiologic atrial contribution to ventricular filling, less distortion of the mitral and tricuspid annuli, and synchronous valve action. The long-term benefits of this modification have yet to be seen.

HETEROTOPIC CARDIAC TRANSPLANTATION

Originally described by Demikhov, heterotopic transplants account for about 2.5% of the cardiac transplantation procedures currently performed. The operative technique bypasses the left heart and involves anastomoses between the left atria, aorta, pulmonary arteries, and donor superior vena cava to recipient right atrium. The major indication for this operation is the presence of irreversible, severe pulmonary hypertension whereby the native right heart continues to work against the elevated pulmonary vascular resistance while the graft bypasses the left heart. Other indications include cases where diminished donor heart function is anticipated due to size mismatch or pro-

longed ischemic time and where the graft is a temporary support in the setting of reversible cardiac failure.

POSTOPERATIVE MANAGEMENT

EARLY POSTOPERATIVE PERIOD

The acute postoperative management of the cardiac transplant patient resembles that of other cardiac patients. Upon completion of the cardiac transplantation procedure, the intubated transplant patient is transported immediately to the ICU, where cardiac rhythm and arterial and central venous pressures are monitored. Swan-Ganz pulmonary artery balloon catheters are usually reserved for those recipients with significant pulmonary hypertension. Strict isolation precautions, previously enforced to reduce the incidence of infection in these immunocompromised patients, are no longer required; simple handwashing and face masks are now considered sufficient.

The world's attention was captivated on December 3, 1967, upon news of the first human heart transplantation procedure performed at the University of Capetown in South Africa. Christiaan Barnard and his colleagues transplanted the heart of a 24-year-old automobile accident victim into a 54-year-old man plagued with severe coronary artery disease and repeated myocardial infarctions. The recipient survived for 18 days before expiring from pneumonia. Subsequent heart transplantations by Kantrowitz at Maimonides Hospital in Brooklyn and Shumway at Stanford University generated enthusiasm for the procedure in the United States and around the world, as the number of centers performing the procedure grew exponentially between December 1967 and March 1971.

Cardiac transplantation experienced its darkest days in the early 1970s. Numerous postoperative complications stemming from acute rejection and infection led to a mere 15% 1-year survival rate, driving the morbidity and mortality of this most unnatural of procedures to near unacceptable levels. Under the guidance of Shumway, the Stanford group continued to pursue cardiac transplantation through the 1970s, as the majority of other transplant centers stepped back during these difficult early years. Between 1974 and 1981, Stanford's clinical cardiac transplant program, involving 140 patients, achieved postoperative survival rates of 63% and 39% at 1 and 5 years, respectively. This clinical experience coupled with painstaking laboratory experimentation produced many of the current techniques and management philosophies used in cardiac transplantation today.

The discovery of the immunosuppressant cyclosporine A by Jean Borel in 1972 and its first use in heart transplant patients at Stanford in 1980 launched the rebirth of cardiac transplantation as the 1- and 5-year survival rates surged to over 80% and 60%, respectively. The number of cardiac transplantations grew from fewer than 360 before 1980 to more than 3200 in 1995.

Simply put, a primary objective in the immediate postoperative period is to maintain adequate perfusion in the recipient while minimizing cardiac work. Approximately 10–20% of transplant recipients experience some degree of transient sinus node dysfunction in the immediate perioperative period, often manifested as sinus bradycardia, which usually resolves within a week. Because cardiac output is primarily rate-dependent after transplantation, the heart rate should be maintained between 90 and 110 beats/min during the first few postoperative days, using temporary pacing or isoproterenol (0.005–0.01 µg/kg/min) as needed. Although rarely seen, persistent sinus node dysfunction and bradycardia may require a permanent transvenous pacemaker. The systolic blood pressure should be maintained between 90 and 110 mm Hg, with afterload reduction in the form of nitroglycerin or nitro-

prusside used if necessary. Renal dose dopamine (3–5 µg/kg/min) is frequently used to augment renal blood flow and urine output. The adequacy of cardiac output is indicated by a urine output greater than 0.5 mL/kg/h without diuretics and warm extremities. Cardiac function generally normalizes within 3–4 days, during which time parenteral inotropes and vasodilators can be weaned. Hypovolemia, cardiac tamponade, sepsis, and bradycardia should be considered and treated expeditiously in the event of reduced cardiac output and hypotension.

Several factors may contribute to some form of depressed global myocardial performance in the acute postoperative setting. The myocardium is potentially subject to prolonged ischemia, inadequate preservation, or catecholamine depletion prior to implantation. Furthermore, the newly grafted heart may be called upon to work against a significantly elevated pulmonary vascular resistance in the recipient.

The maintenance of adequate pulmonary function is another critical objective in the acute postoperative period. Upon arrival in the ICU, an anteroposterior chest x-ray is obtained and the ventilator is typically set to a 100% fractional inspired oxygen content (FiO_2) of 100%, tidal volume of 10–15 mL/kg, an assist-control rate of 10–14 breaths/min, and positive end-expiratory pressure (PEEP) of 3–5 cm H_2O. These settings are adjusted every 30 minutes to achieve an arterial oxygen pressure (PaO_2) greater than 75 mm Hg with an FiO_2 of 40%, arterial carbon dioxide pressure ($PaCO_2$) between 30 and 40 mm Hg, and pH between 7.35 and 7.45. Ventilatory weaning is initiated after the patient is deemed stable, awake, and alert. Usually, weaning is accomplished through successive decrements in intermittent mandatory ventilation rate followed by a trial of continuous positive airway pressure. Once ventilatory mechanics and arterial blood gases are deemed acceptable, the patient is extubated, usually within the first 24 hours after operation. After extubation, pulmonary care consists of supplemental oxygen for several days, aggressive pulmonary toilet, and serial chest x-rays.

Expedient removal of vascular lines has been shown to reduce the incidence of line sepsis. Pleural and mediastinal chest tubes are removed when drainage has fallen off to less than 25 mL/h and atrial pacing wires are removed 7–10 days after operation provided pacing is not required. After several days, barring significant complications, the patient is transferred from the ICU to a standard cardiac surgery ward for the remainder of the hospital stay.

GRAFT PHYSIOLOGY

During procurement, the heart graft is separated from the sympathetic and parasympathetic cardiac plexus of nerves located between the tracheal bifurcation and aortic arch. Normally, this plexus autonomically regulates the heart rate, contractility, and coronary arterial tone. The denervated heart graft is, therefore, isolated from normal autonomic regulatory mechanisms. The resting heart rate is generally higher due to the absence of vagal tone, and sinus arrhythmia and carotid reflex bradycardia are absent. Interestingly, the denervated heart graft develops an increased sensitivity to catecholamines, apparently due to an increase in beta-adrenergic receptor density and a loss of norepinephrine uptake in postganglionic sympathetic neurons. This augmented sensitivity plays an important role in maintaining an adequate cardiac response to exercise and stress.

Cardiac output and index of cardiac allografts are at the low end of the normal range and the measured cardiac response to exercise or stress is subnormal. Nevertheless, the response of the cardiac allograft is adequate for almost all activities. During exercise, the cardiac transplant recipient experiences a steady but delayed increase in heart rate due primarily to a rise in circulating catecholamines. This

initial rise in heart rate is subsequently accompanied by an immediate increase in filling pressures resulting from augmented venous return. These changes result in an augmentation of stroke volume and cardiac output sufficient to sustain the increase in activity.

The ability of the coronary circulation to dilate and increase blood flow in response to increased myocardial oxygen demand is normal in the cardiac transplant recipient. Conversely, graft coronary vasodilator reserve is abnormal in the presence of rejection, hypertrophy, or regional wall motion abnormalities.

Finally, the atrial cuff anastomoses also result in abnormal cardiac physiology. The normal atrial contribution to ventricular end-diastolic filling is impaired by the dissociation between recipient and donor atrial contractions. Moreover, the atrial anastomoses may partially deform the atrioventricular annuli, leading to mitral and tricuspid regurgitation (Table 40.10–2).

IMMUNOSUPPRESSION

Currently, conventional immunosuppression in cardiac transplant recipients consists of the "triple-drug" combination of cyclosporine, azathioprine, and prednisone. Initially, high doses of these drugs are given, with eventual tapering for chronic administration. A typical dosing protocol employed at the Stanford University Hospital is outlined in Table 40.10–3. Cyclosporine is titrated to maintain a trough serum concentration between 150 and 250 ng/mL in the first few weeks after transplantation and from 100–150 ng/mL thereafter. Azathioprine dosages are adjusted to maintain the white blood cell count greater than 4000/mm^3.

In 1987, the Stanford cardiac transplant program added prophylactic induction therapy with **OKT3 monoclonal antibodies** to its standard triple-drug regimen. Directed against the T-cell (CD3) receptor, OKT3 antibodies rapidly remove circulating T lymphocytes without affecting erythrocytes, granulocytes, or platelets. OKT3 induc-

Table 40.10–2. Structural and functional aspects of the transplanted heart.

Denervation from sympathetic and parasympathetic cardiac plexus
Higher resting heart rate
Absence of sinus arrhythmia and carotid reflex bradycardia
Increased chronotropic and inotropic sensitivity to circulating catecholamines
Cardiac output normal at rest and subnormal during exercise
Slower initial rise in heart rate in response to exercise or stress
Normal coronary flow reserve in the absence of rejection
Dissociated contractions between donor and recipient atrial cuffs
Impaired atrial contribution or "kick" to ventricular end-diastolic filling
Possible distortion of atrioventricular annuli, leading to mitral or tricuspid insufficiency

Table 40.10–3. Typical immunosuppression protocol for heart and lung transplant recipients.

Immunosuppressant	Early Postoperative Period	Late Postoperative Period
Cyclosporine A	6–10 mg/kg/d orally[1,2] or 0.5–2 mg/kg/d intravenously	3–6 mg/kg/d orally[3]
Methylprednisolone	500 mg intravenously after cardiopulmonary bypass followed by 125 mg intravenously for three doses	None
Prednisone	1 mg/kg/d orally tapered to 0.4 mg/kg orally	0.1–0.2 mg/kg/d orally
Azathioprine	2 mg/kg/d orally[4]	1–2 mg/kg/d orally[4]
OKT3	5 mg/d intravenously for 14 days	None

[1]Intravenous dose only if preoperative serum creatinine > 1.5 mg/dL.
[2]Maintain trough serum concentration between 150 ng/mL and 250 ng/mL.
[3]Maintain trough serum concentration between 100 ng/mL and ng/mL.
[4]Maintain white blood cell count greater than 4000/mm^3.

tion therapy has delayed the time to first rejection and has reduced early rejection rates but has not resulted in significant differences in the total number of rejection episodes, rates of infection, graft coronary artery disease, renal function, or overall recipient survival.

Judicious doses of these drugs are usually well tolerated by patients, however, each is associated with side effects. Cyclosporine is commonly associated with nephrotoxicity, hypertension, hepatotoxicity, hirsutism, and an increased incidence of lymphoma. The primary toxicity of azathioprine is generalized bone marrow depression manifested as leukopenia, anemia, and thrombocytopenia. Steroids are associated with myriad side effects, including the appearance of cushingoid features, hypertension, diabetes, osteoporosis, and peptic ulcer disease. Initial doses of OKT3 may cause significant hypotension, bronchospasm, or fever, presumably due to T-cell–mediated release of lymphokines. Patients receiving OKT3 are, hence, closely monitored and premedicated with acetaminophen, antihistamines, and corticosteroids. Most of these adverse effects are readily manageable or reversible with dosage reduction, however, their prevalence emphasizes the inadequacies of pharmacologic immunosuppression. Active experimental and clinical research is directed toward developing more potent, less toxic immunosuppressive agents. FK506 (tacrolimus) and mycophenolate mofetil are two promising drugs recently approved for use in organ transplantation by the Food and Drug Administration.

POSTOPERATIVE COMPLICATIONS

Infection and graft rejection are the predominant postoperative complications seen after cardiac transplantation. Causes of operative and overall deaths among cardiac transplant recipients at Stanford from 1980–1993 are shown in Figure 40.10–3.

ACUTE REJECTION

Acute graft rejection is a major cause of death following cardiac transplantation. The incidence of acute graft rejection is highest during the first 3 months after transplantation. At Stanford Hospital, 84% of cardiac transplant recipients receiving triple-drug therapy without OKT3 induction experience acute rejection during this period. The addition of OKT3 therapy reduces this figure to about 75%. After this initial 3-month period, the incidence of acute rejection averages about one episode per patient-year.

Despite good attempts at developing noninvasive means for the timely detection of acute rejection, the endomyocardial biopsy developed by Philip Caves and associates in 1973 remains the diagnostic gold standard. The technique, performed under local anesthesia, involves the percutaneous introduction of a Caves-Schultz bioptome into the right ventricle, usually via the right internal jugular vein, under fluoroscopic guidance. Alternative access sites include the right subclavian and both femoral veins. Multiple biopsy specimens are taken from the interventricular septum per session. Safe, simple, and relatively well tolerated by the patient, endomyocardial biopsies of the transplanted heart commence 7–10 days after transplantation and are repeated periodically.

Acute rejection is histologically characterized by lymphocytic infiltration and myocytic necrosis (Figure 40.10–4). The classic Stanford classification developed by Margaret Billingham in 1979 was the first grading system widely used to characterize rejection severity. Since then, many grading systems have evolved from different transplant groups, culminating in a uniform criteria developed by the International Society for Heart and Lung Transplantation in 1990. Both the Stanford classification and International Grading Systems are outlined in Table 40.10–4.

At Stanford, the timing and severity of rejection episodes dictate therapy according to an algorithm illustrated in Figure 40.10–5. Rejection episodes occurring within the first 3 months or that are graded moderate or severe are treated by pulse steroid dosing. Methylprednisolone is given intravenously at a dose of 1000 mg/d for

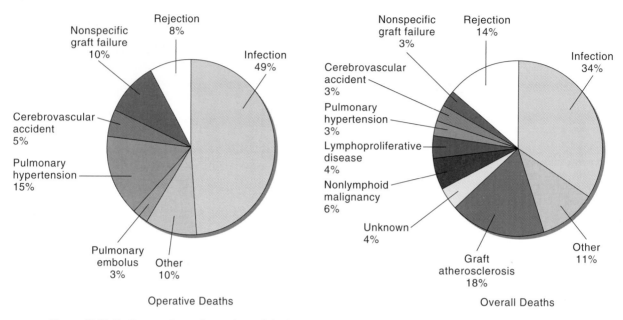

Operative Deaths

Overall Deaths

Figure 40.10–3. Causes of operative and overall deaths among cardiac transplant recipients at Stanford (1980–1993).

3 consecutive days. Episodes occurring after the first 3 months or those that are mild are initially treated by merely increasing the oral prednisone dosage to 100 mg/d for 3 consecutive days followed by a taper back to baseline dosages over 2 weeks. Acute rejection refractory to steroid therapy is treated with antilymphocyte preparations in the form of antithymocyte globulin (ATG) or OKT3 monoclonal antibody. Potent second-line therapies

that are used in especially difficult, persistent cases of rejection include methotrexate and total lymphoid irradiation. Endomyocardial biopsies are repeated 10–14 days following antirejection therapy to assess efficacy.

CHRONIC REJECTION

Accelerated graft coronary artery disease (CAD), or atherosclerosis, is a major limiting factor for long-term survival in cardiac transplant recipients. Significant graft CAD resulting in diminished coronary blood flow may lead to arrhythmias, myocardial infarction, sudden death, or impaired left ventricular function with congestive graft failure. Classic angina due to myocardial ischemia is not usually noted in transplant patients because the cardiac graft is essentially denervated. At Stanford, the prevalence of graft CAD at 1 and 5 years after transplantation is 25% and 80%, respectively. Clinically observed risk factors for developing this condition include donor age greater than 35 years, incompatibility at the HLA-A1, A2, and DR loci, hypertriglyceridemia (serum concentration greater than 280 mg/dL), frequent acute rejection episodes, and documented recipient CMV infection.

Multiple causes for graft CAD have been proposed, but they all focus upon chronic, immunologically mediated damage to the coronary vascular endothelium. In fact, elevated levels of anti-endothelial antibodies have been correlated with graft CAD. Unlike coronary occlusive disease in the native heart, which tends to be focal in nature, transplant atherosclerosis represents a more diffuse vascu-

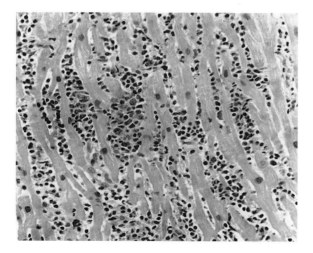

Figure 40.10–4. Moderate acute cardiac allograft rejection. There are extensive perivascular and interstitial mononuclear cell infiltrates (H & E × 300).

Table 40.10–4. Histologic grading systems for acute cardiac rejection.

The Stanford Classification	
Grade	**Histologic Characteristics**
Mild rejection	Interstitial and endocardial edema Scanty perivascular and endocardial lymphocytic infiltrate Pyroninophilia of endocardial and endothelial cells
Moderate rejection	Interstitial, perivascular, and endocardial lymphocytic infiltrate Early focal myocytolysis
Severe rejection	Interstitial hemorrhage Infiltrate of lymphocytes and polymorphonuclear leukocytes Vascular and myocyte necrosis
Resolving rejection	Active fibrosis Residual small lymphocytes, plasma cells, and hemosiderin deposits
The International Grading System	
Grade	**Histologic Characteristics**
Grade 0	No rejection
Grade 1A	Focal (perivascular or interstitial) infiltrate without necrosis
Grade 1B	Diffuse but sparse infiltrate without necrosis
Grade 2	One focus with aggressive infiltration or focal myocyte damage
Grade 3A	Multifocal aggressive infiltrates or myocyte damage
Grade 3B	Diffuse inflammatory process with necrosis
Grade 4	Diffuse aggressive polymorphous with or without infiltrate, edema, hemorrhage, or vasculitis Necrosis

lar narrowing extending symmetrically into distal branches. Histologically, transplant arteriopathy is characterized by concentric intimal proliferation with smooth muscle hyperplasia (Figure 40.10–6).

Coronary angiograms are performed on a yearly basis to identify recipients with accelerated CAD. Because graft CAD manifests as diffuse coronary intimal thickening, in-tracoronary ultrasonography has been advanced as a more sensitive means to detect graft atherosclerosis because of its ability to assess vascular wall morphology in addition to luminal diameter.

Percutaneous transluminal coronary angioplasty and coronary artery bypass grafting have been used to treat discrete proximal lesions in some cases of graft CAD,

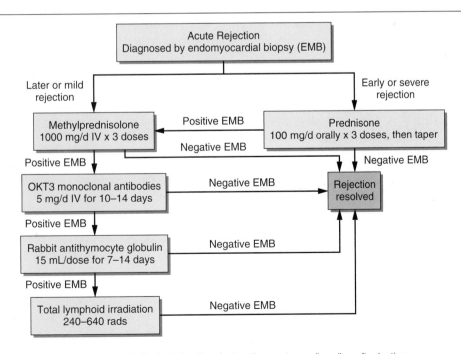

Figure 40.10–5. Typical algorithm for treating acute cardiac allograft rejection.

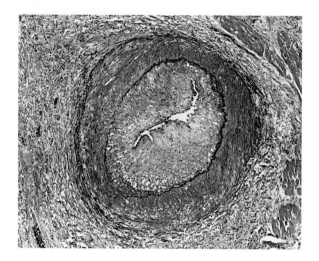

Figure 40.10–6. Cardiac graft atherosclerosis. Note the concentric intimal proliferation with smooth muscle hyperplasia (EVG × 100).

however, the only definitive therapy for diffuse disease is retransplantation. Effective prevention of graft CAD will rely upon developments in improved immunosuppression, recipient tolerance induction, improved CMV prophylaxis, and inhibition of vascular intimal proliferation.

INFECTION

Infection is the leading cause of morbidity and mortality after cardiac transplantation. The risk of infection and infection-related death peaks early during the first few months after transplantation and rapidly declines to a low persistent rate thereafter. At Stanford, the actuarial freedom from any infection at 3 months, 1 year, and 5 years was 40%, 27%, and 15%, respectively. (By 5 years, 85% of patients will have experienced some form of infection.) The actuarial freedom from infection-related death at 3 months, 1 year, and 5 years was 95%, 93%, and 85%, respectively.

Postoperative infections can be broadly classified into those that occur early and late after transplantation. Early infections occurring during the first month after transplantation are commonly bacterial (especially gram-negative bacilli) and manifest as pneumonia, mediastinitis, catheter sepsis, and urinary tract and skin infections. Typical nosocomial organisms are listed in Table 40.10–5. Treatment of these infections generally involves characterization of the infective agent (eg, cultures, antibiotic sensitivities), source control (eg, catheter removal, debridement), and appropriate antibiotic regimens. In the late post-transplantation period, opportunistic viral, fungal, and protozoan pathogens become more prevalent (Table 40.10–5). The lungs, central nervous system, gastrointestinal tract, and skin are the usual sites of invasion.

CMV infection is widely recognized as the most common and important viral infection in transplant patients, with an incidence of 73–100% in cardiac transplant recipients. It presents either as a primary infection or reactivation of a latent infection, most commonly 1–4 months after transplantation. By definition, primary infection results when a previously seronegative recipient is infected via contact with tissue or blood from a seropositive individual. The donor organ itself is thought to be the most common vector of primary CMV infections. Reactivation

Table 40.10–5. Infections in cardiac transplant recipients.

Early Post-Transplant Infections	Late Post-Transplant Infections

Pneumonia
    Gram-negative bacilli
	Viral
	    Cytomegalovirus
	    Herpes simplex
	    Varicella-zoster
	    Hepatitis C

Mediastinitis
    Staphylococcus epidermidis
    Staphylococcus aureus
    Gram-negative bacilli	

	Bacterial
	    Listeria
	    Nocardia
	    Legionella
	    Mycobacterium

Catheter sepsis
    Staphylococcus epidermidis
    Staphylococcus aureus
    Gram-negative bacilli
    Candida albicans	

	Fungal
	    Aspergillus
	    Cryptococcus
	    Candida
	    Mucor (Phycomycetes)

Urinary tract infections
    Gram-negative bacilli
    Enterococcus
    Candida albicans	

Skin infections
    Herpes simplex
	Protozoan
	    Pneumocystis carinii
	    Toxoplasma gondii

infection occurs when a recipient who is seropositive prior to transplantation develops clinical CMV infection during immunosuppressive therapy. Seropositive recipients are also subject to infection by new strains of CMV. Clinically, CMV infection has protean manifestations including leukopenia with fever, pneumonia, gastroenteritis, hepatitis, and retinitis. CMV pneumonitis is the most lethal of these, with a 13% mortality, while retinitis is the most refractory to treatment, requiring indefinite treatment. The significance of CMV as an infective agent becomes clear when one realizes that it is implicated as a trigger for accelerated graft CAD and as an inhibitor of cell-mediated immunity.

Diagnosis of CMV infection is made by direct culture of the virus from blood, urine, or tissue specimens, by a fourfold increase in antibody titers from baseline, or by characteristic histologic changes (ie, markedly enlarged cells and nuclei containing basophilic inclusion bodies). Most cases respond to ganciclovir (DHPG) and hyperimmune globulin. Both of these agents have been used prophylactically, especially in seronegative patients receiving a graft from a seropositive donor. Prophylaxis has been shown to decrease the incidence of clinical CMV infections in recipients who were seropositive prior to transplantation, but not in the seronegative patients.

Fungal infections are less common than bacterial or viral infections, however, the importance in recognition stems from the fact that these infections are generally more refractory to current therapy and are, therefore, more lethal. Therapy consists of antifungal agents, including amphotericin B, fluconazole, and flucytosine.

Infection prophylaxis in cardiac transplant patients is comprised of vaccinations, perioperative broad-spectrum antibiotics, and long-term prophylactic antibiotics. Pretransplant inoculation with pneumococcal and hepatitis B vaccines as well as DPT (diphtheria–pertussis–tetanus) boosters are recommended. Immunization with live MMR (measles–mumps–rubella) and polio vaccines should be performed prior to transplantation in the pediatric population. All cardiac transplant recipients should also receive annual influenza vaccinations. Perioperative antibiotic regimens vary widely between transplant centers, however, first-generation cephalosporins (eg, cefazolin) or vancomycin are commonly used. Long-term prophylaxis typically includes nystatin mouthwash for thrush, sulfamethoxazole-trimethoprim for opportunistic bacterial and *Pneumocystis carinii* infections, and antivirals, such as acyclovir or ganciclovir.

NEOPLASM

Organ transplant recipients possess a significantly greater risk for developing cancer, undoubtedly due to chronic immunosuppression. Tumors to which recipients are predisposed include skin cancer, B cell lymphoproliferative disorders, carcinoma in situ of the cervix, carcinoma of the vulva and anus, and Kaposi's sarcoma. On the other hand, neoplasms of the breast, lung, prostate, and colon do not appear to be increased in these patients. On average, tumors appear approximately 5 years after transplantation.

The incidence of B cell lymphoproliferative disorders in transplant patients is a staggering 350 times greater than seen in the normal age-matched population. Diagnosis is established by lymph node biopsy. Lymphomas are frequently observed in younger recipients (younger than 20 years) within a year after transplantation, carrying an 80% mortality over the 3 months following diagnosis. Older recipients (older than 45 years) diagnosed with lymphoma tend to present several years after transplantation, with an average survival of 9 months following diagnosis. Thought to be caused by unchecked Epstein-Barr virus infection in the setting of T cell suppression, B cell lymphoproliferative disorders are generally treated with a reduction in immunosuppression and administration of an antiviral agent, such as acyclovir or ganciclovir. A response rate of 30–40% can be expected, with recurrence being uncommon. Chemotherapy and radiotherapy have been used successfully in some cases. Of course, close monitoring of the graft with echocardiography along with clinical assessment of tumor status is important during therapy.

RETRANSPLANTATION

The primary indications for cardiac retransplantation are graft failure due to accelerated graft atherosclerosis or recurrent acute rejection. Patients in need of retransplantation are generally held to the same standard criteria as initial candidates. Survival rates after retransplantation are significantly diminished compared to those achieved in primary transplant patients. At the Stanford University Medical Center, 1-year survival was 55% after cardiac retransplantation.

RESULTS

According to the Registry of the International Society for Heart Transplantation, between 2500 and 3500 heart transplantations per year were performed at over 200 transplant centers worldwide between 1990 and 1994. A review of 496 heart transplantations performed at Stanford between 1980 and 1993 placed 1-, 5-, and 10-year actuarial survival estimates at 82%, 61%, and 41%, respectively (Figure 40.10–7). Most cardiac transplant patients are fully rehabilitated to New York Heart Association functional class I status. When one considers the prognosis of these patients without transplantation, the benefits of this procedure are clear.

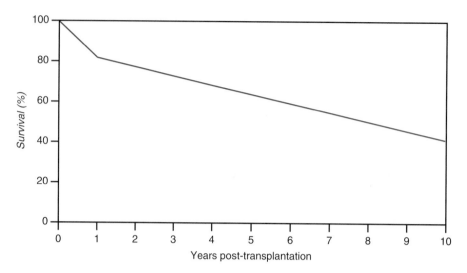

Figure 40.10–7. Actuarial survival of adult cardiac transplant recipients at Stanford (1980–1993).

PEDIATRIC CARDIAC TRANSPLANTATION

Cardiac transplantation is now an accepted therapeutic option for infants and children with end-stage heart disease. The number of children undergoing heart transplantation has increased rapidly, from about 200 pediatric transplantations performed between 1978 and 1986 to ap-

proximately 320 performed in 1993, with over 100 recipients being less than 1 year old. The leading indications for cardiac transplantation in children are acquired dilated cardiomyopathy and congenital heart disease (Figure 40.10–8). Contraindications for transplantation in this group closely resemble those seen in adults, with the addition of some complex venous drainage anomalies (Table 40.10–6).

Blood type and donor size are the most important considerations in donor-recipient matching. The paucity of pediatric heart donors, wider ranges of patient size, and severe disability of many waiting pediatric patients have resulted in an expanded range of accepted donor-to-recipient weight ratios. At Stanford, the average ratio is 1.4 ± 0.45, ranging from 0.75 to 3.54. Moderately oversized heart grafts are preferred for recipients with an elevated pulmonary vascular resistance.

The operative technique of orthotopic heart transplantation in the pediatric population is similar to that used in adults, with some exceptions in certain cases of congenital heart disease (eg, aortic arch or venous drainage reconstruction). Likewise, immunosuppressive regimens are similar to those employed in adults, namely, triple-drug therapy with or without antilymphocytic induction. Steroids are tapered more quickly in pediatric recipients to

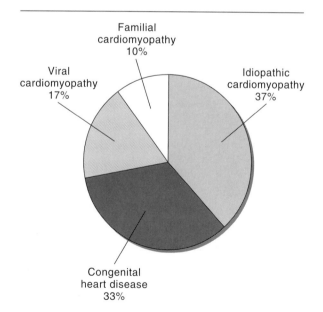

Figure 40.10–8. Indications for pediatric cardiac transplantation at Stanford (1977–1993).

Table 40.10–6. Contraindications to pediatric cardiac transplantation.

Elevated pulmonary vascular resistance (> 8 Wood units)
Active systemic infection
Malignancy (active or in remission)
Recent pulmonary embolism or infarction
Remote organ failure
Inadequate psychosocial resources
Some complex venous drainage anomalies

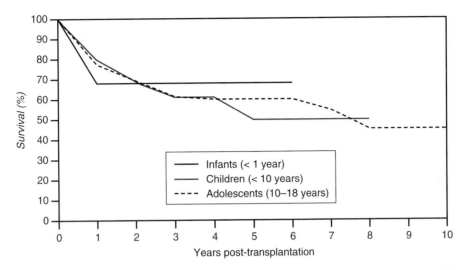

Figure 40.10–9. Actuarial survival of pediatric cardiac transplant recipients at Stanford (1977–1993).

minimize growth retardation and infectious complications.

Acute rejection rates in children and adolescents do not appear to differ significantly from those encountered in adults, although rejection may be less frequent in the neonatal population as a result of immune system immaturity. Acute rejection in children is often suspected from a spectrum of clinical signs, including fever, tachycardia, anorexia, and restlessness coupled with echocardiographic abnormalities (eg, left ventricular free wall thickening, decreased function). Although routine endomyocardial biopsies for rejection surveillance are performed less frequently in neonates and small children, they are still used to confirm the diagnosis of rejection. As in adults, acute rejection in children is initially treated with pulsed steroids, with antilymphocyte preparations, total lymphoid irradiation, and methotrexate reserved for refractory cases. Graft CAD in children occurs at a frequency comparable to that found in the adult population and constitutes a significant cause of death.

The cumulative experience at Stanford between 1977 and 1993 has yielded satisfactory medium-term results of pediatric cardiac transplantation. Actuarial 1-, 5-, and 10-year survival estimates are 75%, 60%, and 50%, respectively, with most survivors achieving New York Heart Association functional class I (Figure 40.10–9). Accumulating experience in pediatric cardiac transplantation suggests that a normal somatic growth rate can be maintained in these recipients and, likewise, that normal cardiac chamber dimensional growth also occurs. Nevertheless, the perennial difficulties in adult cardiac transplantation still hold in the pediatric population. Causes of death in these recipients resemble those seen in the adult population, with infection and rejection leading the list, followed by graft atherosclerosis and pulmonary hypertension. Improved results will undoubtedly parallel advances in the postoperative management of these special patients.

SUGGESTED READING

Barnard CN: A human cardiac transplant: An interim report of a successful operation performed at Groote Schuur Hospital, Capetown. S Afr Med J 1967;41:1271.

Billingham ME: Some recent advances in cardiac pathology. Hum Path 1979;10:367.

Carrel A, Guthrie CC: The transplantation of veins and organs. Am J Med 1905;10:1101.

Caves PK et al: Percutaneous endomyocardial biopsy in human heart recipients. Ann Thorac Surg 1973;16:325.

Demikhov VP: *Experimental Transplantation of Vital Organs.* New York Consultants Bureau, 1962.

Lower RR, Shumway NE: Studies on the orthotopic homotransplantation of the canine heart. Surg Forum 1960;11:18.

Sarris GE et al: Cardiac transplantation: The Stanford experience in the cyclosporine era. J Thorac Cardiovasc Surg 1994; 108:240.

Sarris GE et al: Pediatric cardiac transplantation: The Stanford experience. Circulation 1994;90(part 2):II-51.

40.11 Lung & Combined Heart-Lung Transplantation

David D. Yuh, MD, & Bruce Reitz, MD

▶ Key Facts

▶ Most lung transplant candidates suffering from end-stage lung disease, with or without concomitant cardiac dysfunction, are considered for three broad categories of transplant operations: single-lung, bilateral single-lung, and heart-lung transplantation.

▶ Single-lung transplantation is ideally suited for patients with fibrotic lung disease, bilateral single-lung transplantation is intended for patients suffering from septic lung disease, while heart-lung transplantation was developed for patients suffering from pulmonary vascular disease but has since broadened to include patients with end-stage lung disease and intercurrent cardiac dysfunction.

▶ Because the lungs are susceptible to infection and edema, particularly in the setting of brain death and trauma, suitable lungs are more difficult to obtain than other organs.

▶ Donor-to-recipient lung volume matching is based upon the vertical (apex to diaphragm along the midclavicular line) and transverse (level of the diaphragmatic dome) radiologic dimensions on chest x-ray, as well as body weight, height, and chest circumference.

▶ Chronic lung rejection most commonly presents as obliterative bronchiolitis, a pulmonary corollary to cardiac graft atherosclerosis.

▶ The 1- and 2-year actuarial survival rates for adult single and bilateral single-lung transplants performed worldwide between 1988 and 1993 were 70% and 60%, respectively.

▶ In adult and pediatric lung and heart-lung recipients, long-term survival is limited by infection, obliterative bronchiolitis, and accelerated graft coronary artery disease.

PREOPERATIVE CONSIDERATIONS

RECIPIENT SELECTION

The overriding objective in recipient evaluation is to select individuals with progressively disabling cardiopulmonary or pulmonary disease possessing the capacity for full rehabilitation after transplantation. Most recipients suffering from end-stage lung disease with or without concomitant cardiac dysfunction are considered for three broad categories of transplant operations: single-lung, bilateral single-lung, and heart-lung transplantation. The lists of indications for each operation are evolving with accumulating clinical experience (Table 40.11–1).

Single-lung transplantation is most ideally suited for patients with fibrotic lung disease because the low compliance and increased vascular resistance of the native lung ensure that both ventilation and perfusion are preferentially diverted to the transplanted lung. Emphysematous lung disease is also a major indication for this procedure.

Bilateral single-lung transplantation is intended for pa-

Table 40.11–1. Indications for adult single-lung, bilateral single-lung, and heart-lung transplantation.

Single-Lung Transplantation
Pulmonary fibrosis
Emphysema
Bronchopulmonary dysplasia
Primary pulmonary hypertension without significant right heart dysfunction
Post-transplant obliterative bronchiolitis

Bilateral Single-Lung
Cystic fibrosis/bronchiectasis without cardiac decompensation)
Emphysema/chronic obstructive pulmonary disease without cardiac decompensation

Heart-Lung Transplantation
Severe primary pulmonary hypertension with right ventricular decompensation and/or cardiomyopathy
Severe Eisenmenger's syndrome with right ventricular decompensation or uncorrectable congenital heart disease (eg, truncus arteriosus, large ventricular septal defect)
Intercurrent cardiac and pulmonary disease

Table 40.11–2. Contraindications to adult lung and heart-lung transplantation.

Age > 60 years (lung) or > 50 years (heart-lung)
Significant systemic or multisystem disease (eg, peripheral or cerebrovascular disease, diabetes mellitus)
Active or extrapulmonary infection
Significant irreversible hepatic or renal dysfunction
Incurable malignancy
Corticosteroid therapy > 10 mg/d
Cachexia or obesity
Current cigarette smoking
Psychiatric illness or history of medical noncompliance
Previous cardiothoracic surgery (considered on a case-by-case basis)
Drug or alcohol abuse
Severe osteoporosis

tients suffering from septic lung disease, including cystic fibrosis and bronchiectasis, or from chronic obstructive pulmonary disease. Single-lung transplantation is avoided in patients with septic lung disease because the associated chronic bilateral pulmonary infections would place such recipients at high risk for infection from the retained native lung. It is also important to note that the extra pulmonary reserve and potential survival advantage afforded by bilateral single-lung compared to single-lung transplantation must be weighed against the benefits of providing lungs to two patients versus one.

Heart-lung transplantation was initially developed for patients suffering from severe pulmonary vascular disease, specifically, pulmonary hypertension and Eisenmenger's syndrome secondary to congenital heart disease. Subsequently, the indications for this procedure have broadened to include patients with end-stage lung disease and intercurrent cardiac dysfunction as well as patients with cystic fibrosis and bronchiectasis.

Other permutations of cardiopulmonary replacement have recently been developed. In the so-called "domino" transplant operation, the explanted heart of a heart-lung recipient is transplanted into another patient in need of a cardiac transplant. In patients who have had prior thoracic surgery, heart–single-lung transplantation has been successfully employed to avoid extensive adhesions in a previously treated pleural cavity. Finally, lobar lung transplantation (from living-related and cadaveric donors) has been developed to expand the effective donor pool, readily provide healthy lung tissue to patients with severely limited life-expectancy, and accommodate the small chest dimensions of pediatric patients.

Contraindications to lung and heart-lung transplantation are similar to those in cardiac transplantation (Table 40.11–2). Among most lung and heart-lung transplant programs, upper age limits typically range between 50 and 60 years, with projected life expectancies limited to less than 12–18 months despite the use of appropriate medical or alternative surgical strategies. With some pulmonary diseases, survival without transplantation has been estimated using certain parameters. For example, in patients with primary pulmonary hypertension, elevated right atrial pressure, diminished cardiac output, and elevated pulmonary artery pressure correlate with diminished survival. Despite these estimations, however, clinical judgment is often required to determine when transplantation is appropriate. Mortality while on the waiting list remains considerable, ranging from 10–30%.

Patients suffering from systemic disease with significant renal or hepatic dysfunction, acute illness, unresolved malignancy, or psychiatric illness are not offered transplantation. Relative contraindications include cachexia or obesity and a recent history of active peptic ulcer disease. Patients requiring systemic corticosteroids are tapered to the lowest tolerable level before transplantation. Cigarette smokers must quit smoking and be off cigarettes completely for at least several months before transplantation. During the early years of heart-lung transplantation, previous cardiothoracic surgery or pleurodesis were considered absolute contraindications to heart-lung transplantation because of bleeding from chest wall adhesions and difficulty preserving the vagus, recurrent laryngeal, and phrenic nerves. With improved surgical technique, however, these cases are now being considered for transplantation. Of course, a stable, supportive socioeconomic environment is an important consideration.

Since adequate cardiac function is the most important determinant of whether single-lung or bilateral single-lung transplantation will be tolerated, preoperative evaluation includes echocardiography with Doppler and saline-contrast flow studies, radionuclide angiography and, when indicated, Holter monitoring and cardiac catheterization.

DONOR SELECTION & MANAGEMENT

Because the lungs are susceptible to infection and edema, particularly in the settings of brain death and trauma, suitable lungs are more difficult to obtain than other organs. Fewer than 25% of nonthoracic organ donors possess lungs suitable for donation. Potential lung donors must be ABO-compatible, be free of infection, demonstrate good pulmonary gas exchange, and lack a significant smoking history. Lung volumes similar to or less than that of the intended recipient are generally preferred, however, larger single lungs can be placed on the left side where greater hemidiaphragmatic excursion is permitted.

As in cardiac transplantation, donor evaluation consists of a history and physical examination, ABO compatibility testing, a percent reactive antibody (PRA) panel, and infectious serologic screening. A donor chest roentgenogram must be entirely clear, and the PaO_2 should exceed 300 mm Hg on an FiO_2 of 100% and positive end-expiratory pressure (PEEP) of 5 cm H_2O. Bronchoscopy should assure the absence of purulent secretions or signs of aspiration. For infection prophylaxis, donors receive broad-spectrum antibiotics. Donor-to-recipient lung volume matching is based upon the vertical (apex to diaphragm along the midclavicular line) and transverse (level of the diaphragmatic dome) radiologic dimensions on chest x-ray, as well as body weight, height, and chest circumference. The recipient's nominal predicted thoracic volume is used. Medical management of the donor is as described in cardiac transplantation.

ORGAN PRESERVATION

On-site lung procurement was considered essential between 1981 and 1984 because of inadequate lung preservation techniques. Since then, active research and clinical experience have produced several different preservation protocols that have permitted distant procurement. Nevertheless, current techniques are far from ideal, as inadequate lung preservation still remains a significant cause of early graft dysfunction after lung and heart-lung transplantation. Commonly, lung grafts are flushed via the pulmonary artery with a modified Euro-Collins cold crystalloid solution and a vasodilator, such as prostaglandin E_1 (PGE_1). Euro-Collins solution is of essentially intracellular composition and is the most commonly used of several different lung perfusates. The vasodilator is intended to counteract reflex pulmonary vasoconstriction resulting from the cold flush and to permit uniform distribution of the perfusate throughout the lung. Heart-lung blocs are typically preserved with a modified Euro-Collins pulmonary artery flush in conjunction with standard crystalloid cardioplegic arrest, topical hypothermia, intravenous PGE_1 infusion, and subsequent cold storage. Generally, with proper preservation technique, cold ischemia times of up to 6 hours appear to be consistently well tolerated.

Longer ischemic times increase the risk of significant post-transplant pulmonary edema, alveolar damage, and early graft dysfunction.

Experimental studies suggest improved graft function when the lung is inflated, when 100% oxygen is used, when the lung is transported at 10°C, and when PGE_1 is administered before perfusion of the modified Euro-Collins solution. The development of improved lung preservation has recently focused upon the reduction of injurious oxygen free radicals via scavengers and leukocyte depletion techniques and the use of colloid-based perfusates. Based upon experimental evidence that donor lymphocytes play a role in ischemic lung graft injury, methylprednisolone is given intravenously to the donor in an effort to inactivate them.

OPERATIVE TECHNIQUE

Single-lung, bilateral single-lung, and heart-lung operations are summarized below and illustrated in Figures 40.11–1 and 40.11–2.

LUNG & HEART-LUNG DONOR OPERATIONS

In single-lung and bilateral single-lung procurement operations, the chest is entered via a median sternotomy. Donor lungs are usually procured in conjunction with the heart. First, the aorta and venae cavae are encircled with umbilical tapes in preparation for inflow occlusion and cardioplegic arrest. Then, for each lung to be procured, the pleura is opened longitudinally and the entire pericardium is excised from the diaphragm to the pleural apex, extending posteriorly through the phrenic nerve to the hilum. The inferior pulmonary ligament is incised to the inferior pulmonary vein. The right or left pulmonary artery is then dissected free from the pulmonary artery bifurcation to the pulmonary hilum. Pulmonoplegia, most commonly Euro-Collins solution at 2–4°C, is rapidly flushed into the main pulmonary artery simultaneously with cardioplegic infusion into the ascending aorta. Iced saline is then poured over the heart and lungs. The superior and inferior vena cavae, ascending aorta, and common pulmonary artery are divided, leaving the heart attached only to the pulmonary veins. In single-lung procurement, the contralateral pulmonary veins are divided and a left atrial cuff surrounding the two remaining pulmonary veins is created (Figure 40.11–1A). In bilateral single-lung procurement, all four pulmonary veins are left intact with the atrial cuff. After the heart is removed, the trachea is clamped or stapled at its midpoint and divided.

In combined heart-lung transplantation, the heart and lungs are excised en bloc through a median sternotomy that is extended into the abdomen. Both pleural spaces are entered anteriorly and the pericardium is trimmed, leaving

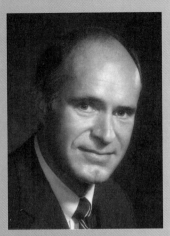

Bruce Reitz, MD (b 1944).

Early attempts at lung transplantation met with little clinical success. James Hardy at the University of Mississippi performed the first human lung transplant in 1963. The patient, suffering from both squamous cell carcinoma of the left lung and emphysema, received a single left lung transplant and survived for 18 days, dying of renal failure. Over the next 18 years, 37 more single-lung transplants were attempted, with the longest survivor dying after just 10 months. Although many of these recipients were poor transplant candidates by today's standards, the majority of these patients expired from early graft dysfunction caused by inadequate preservation, rejection, or bronchial anastomotic complications (eg, breakdown and leakage). These early results helped set priorities for subsequent improvements in lung preservation, immunosuppressive management, and surgical technique.

In 1981, after extensive experimentation with nonhuman primates and cyclosporine A in the laboratory, Bruce Reitz and colleagues at Stanford University performed the first successful human heart-lung transplantation in a 45-year-old woman suffering from primary pulmonary hypertension. This success rejuvenated worldwide efforts in lung and heart-lung transplantation. Successful efforts in human single-lung transplantation soon followed in 1983, when Joel Cooper and the Toronto Lung Transplant Group performed a successful right lung transplant in a patient suffering from pulmonary fibrosis. The Toronto group used an omental wrapping technique to improve collateral blood flow to the bronchial anastomosis.

En bloc double-lung transplantation was successfully applied clinically in the middle to late 1980s. This technique, originally intended for patients with chronic obstructive lung disease, arose from concern about preferential hyperinflation and herniation of the emphysematous native lung and mediastinum that might occur with single-lung transplantation. Nevertheless, since 1989, chronic obstructive lung disease has been effectively treated with single-lung transplantation and currently constitutes a major indication for this procedure. When en bloc double-lung transplantation was extended to patients with septic lung disease, particularly cystic fibrosis, significant mortality resulted from bleeding complications in the poorly visualized posterior mediastinum. As a result, bilateral sequential lung transplantation was developed, with marked reductions in bleeding and airway complications, and has become the preferred technique for double-lung transplantation today.

Since the initial clinical success by the Toronto Lung Transplant Group in 1983, over 2700 lung transplants have been registered by the International Lung Transplant Registry. The number of centers performing lung and heart-lung transplantation is steadily growing.

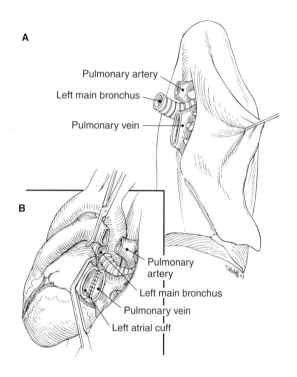

A

Pulmonary artery

Left main bronchus

Pulmonary vein

B

Pulmonary artery

Left main bronchus

Pulmonary vein

Left atrial cuff

Figure 40.11–1. Single-lung transplantation. **A:** Left lung procurement. The pulmonary veins are detached from the heart along with a cuff of left atrium. The left pulmonary artery is then transected from the main PA. Finally, the left main bronchus is transected between two staple lines. **B:** Lung graft implantation begins with anastomosis of the donor pulmonary vein to a left atrial cuff fashioned in the recipient. The transplant is completed with bronchial and pulmonary artery anastomoses.

both phrenic nerves on pedicles. After the heart is cannulated, cardiopulmonary bypass is instituted and ventilation is stopped to facilitate the remainder of the operation. After inflow occlusion and cardioplegic arrest, the ascending aorta, pulmonary artery, and venae cavae are dissected free. The innominate artery and vein are ligated and divided, thereby facilitating exposure of the underlying trachea. The trachea is divided about 6–8 cm above the carina. The heart-lung bloc is dissected free from the esophagus, both pulmonary ligaments are divided inferiorly, and the posterior hilar attachments are divided.

The respective organ(s) are removed from the chest after clamping of the trachea and immersed in a bag containing ice-cold saline solution at 2–4°C which is, in turn, transported in an ice-filled cooler.

SINGLE-LUNG & DOUBLE-LUNG RECIPIENT OPERATIONS

The single-lung transplant procedure is performed under single-lung anesthesia with the aid of a bronchial blocking device or double-lumen endotracheal tube. The side receiving the lung graft is not ventilated during implantation. Cardiopulmonary bypass is usually not required, but is often indicated in cases of significant pulmonary hypertension. A posterolateral thoracotomy is used for single-lung grafting. Bilateral single-lung transplants are performed through a bilateral anterothoracosternotomy or "clamshell" incision.

Excision of the recipient's diseased lung commences with the temporary occlusion of the ipsilateral pulmonary artery. If the patient's blood pressure, contralateral pulmonary artery pressure, and arterial blood gases are satisfactorily stable during this maneuver, the case can proceed. If significant peturbation of one or more of these parameters occurs, cardiopulmonary bypass will be required. The pulmonary veins are isolated lateral to the pericardium and the mainstem bronchus is mobilized just proximal to the upper lobe bronchus. After complete hilar mobilization, cardiopulmonary bypass is instituted, if needed; otherwise, the pulmonary artery is clamped as proximally as possible and divided just distal to the first upper lobe branch. The two pulmonary veins are ligated extrapericardially. The mainstem bronchus is then divided just proximal to the upper lobe bronchus and the recipient's diseased lung is removed from the chest.

Lung graft implantation begins by clamping the recipient's left atrium in such a way as to isolate the ligated pulmonary vein stumps. The recipient left atrial cuff is then fashioned and, after the graft is placed in the chest, anastomosed to the donor cuff (Figure 40.11–1B). The bronchial anastomosis is then completed end-to-end with a running polypropylene suture. At Stanford, omental wrapping of the bronchial anastomosis is not performed. The pulmonary artery anastomosis is constructed end-to-end, leaving the running suture untied to permit flushing and backbleeding. The left atrial clamp is gradually released, permitting backbleeding through the untied pulmonary artery suture line. After the pulmonary artery clamp is momentarily opened to flush the pulmonary artery, the suture line is tied and the clamp is removed, restoring circulation to the lung graft. The graft is then ventilated. A second sequential lung transplant is performed in the same manner. After all anastomoses are completed and hemostasis is assured, the patient is weaned from bypass, if it was required. Thoracostomy tubes are placed and the chest is closed. All bronchial anastomoses are checked endoscopically before the patient leaves the operating suite.

HEART-LUNG RECIPIENT OPERATION

Heart-lung transplantation is performed using cardiopulmonary bypass. After the chest is entered through a median sternotomy, both pleural spaces are opened anteriorly. The anterior surface of the pericardial surface is excised, preserving the lateral segments to support the heart and to protect the phrenic nerves (Figure 40.11–2). The ascending aorta and both venae cavae are cannulated and

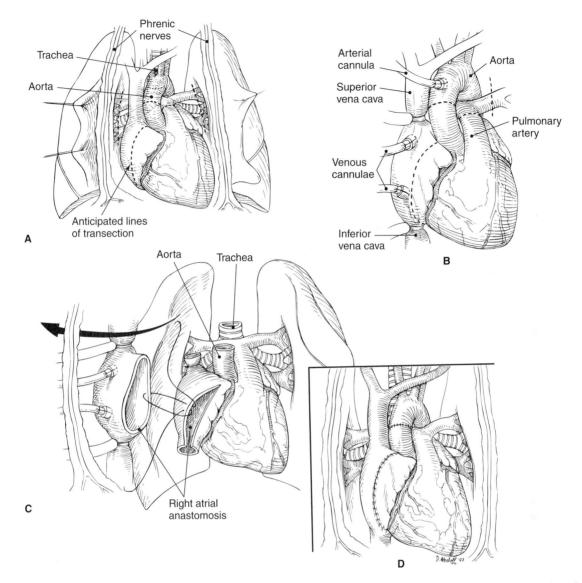

Figure 40.11–2. Heart-lung transplantation. **A:** Preparation of the recipient for heart-lung transplantation with preservation of the phrenic nerves on pedicles. Anticipated lines of transection are illustrated. **B:** Recipient cannulation for cardiopulmonary bypass. Separate vena caval cannulae are placed in the lower right atrium, and the arterial cannula into the ascending aorta. **C:** The recipient right atrium is retained, including a portion of the intra-arterial septum, and anastomosed to a right atrial cuff fashioned on the graft. Note that the right lung is passed behind the vena cava and right phrenic nerve pedicle. **D:** Final appearance of the transplant procedure with completed atrial, aortic, and tracheal anastomoses.

hypothermic cardiopulmonary bypass is instituted, cooling the patient to about 30°C.

The native heart and lungs are excised from the thorax. The native heart is arrested and excised by dividing the ascending aorta just above the aortic valve, the main pulmonary artery, and both atria. After the left and right phrenic nerves are dissected free, the pulmonary ligaments are divided inferiorly and the pulmonary artery and vein are divided in each hilum. The left and right bronchi are stapled and divided, permitting removal of the native lungs. Of note, a portion of the pulmonary artery is left in-

tact adjacent to the underside of the aorta near the ligamentum arteriosus to preserve the recurrent laryngeal nerve.

The donor heart-lung graft is then prepared by irrigating, aspirating, and culturing the tracheobronchial tree and by trimming the trachea to leave one cartilaginous ring above the carina. The heart-lung graft is then lowered into the chest, positioning the right lung below the right atrial cuff and right phrenic nerve. After opening the recipient trachea just above the carina, the tracheal anastomosis is performed with a running polypropylene suture. Next, a donor right atrial cuff is constructed and anastomosed to the retained recipient right atrial cuff. At this point, the patient is rewarmed toward 37°C and the aortic anastomosis is performed, completing the implantation. After the ascending aorta and pulmonary artery are cleared of air, the aortic cross-clamp and caval tapes are removed. As in cardiac transplantation, isoproterenol is usually initiated on graft reperfusion to increase the heart rate and lower pulmonary vascular resistance. Ventilation is resumed, starting with an FiO_2 of 50%. Cardiopulmonary bypass is discontinued and decannulation performed after normothermia and satisfactory cardiopulmonary function have been achieved. Temporary right atrial and ventricular pacing wires are placed. Right and left pleural chest tubes are placed, followed by chest closure. The tracheal anastomosis is checked endoscopically before transporting the patient to the intensive care unit (ICU).

POSTOPERATIVE MANAGEMENT

EARLY POSTOPERATIVE PERIOD

Ischemia and reperfusion injury in the transplanted lung result in increased vascular permeability as well as impaired mucociliary clearance mechanisms, prompting specific considerations in postoperative management. After the operation, the patient remains intubated and is transported immediately to the ICU. Monitoring of the recipient includes a pulmonary artery catheter, a peripheral arterial catheter, pulse oximeter, and end-tidal CO_2 monitor.

Proper ventilator management is of paramount importance during this period, as barotrauma and high airway pressures that might compromise bronchial mucosal flow must be avoided. Lower tidal volumes and flow rates may be necessary to limit peak airway pressures to less than 40 cm H_2O. Pulmonary toilet with endotracheal suctioning is an effective means of reducing mucus plugging and atelectasis.

A diffuse interstitial infiltrate is often found on early postoperative chest x-rays. Previously referred to as a "reimplantation response," this finding is better defined as graft edema due to inadequate preservation, reperfusion injury, or early rejection. It appears that the degree of edema is inversely related to the quality of preservation. Judicious administration of fluids and loop diuretics are required to maintain fluid balance and minimize this edema.

After the patient is fully awake, the patient is weaned from the ventilator and extubated when blood gases and ventilatory mechanics are satisfactory. Most patients are extubated within 3 days and weaned from supplemental oxygen by 10 days after transplantation. Early ambulation is encouraged.

Early lung graft dysfunction manifested by persistent marginal gas exchange without evidence of infection or

rejection occurs in less than 10% of transplants. Histologic analysis revealing diffuse alveolar damage suggests this phenomenon is a result of ischemia or reperfusion injury. Of course, technical causes of graft failure must always be considered.

IMMUNOSUPPRESSION

Immunosuppression protocols for lung and heart-lung transplant recipients are similar to those used in cardiac transplantation. Commonly, 500–1000 mg of intravenous methylprednisolone is administered to the recipient just before graft reperfusion. Triple-drug therapy immediately commences postoperatively and is tapered according to standard protocols. Depending on the transplant center, induction therapy with antilymphocytic antibody preparations may be used.

POSTOPERATIVE COMPLICATIONS

Early morbidity and mortality after lung and heart-lung transplantation is most commonly caused by infection, graft failure, and heart failure. Late mortality after 1 year is most commonly caused by obliterative bronchiolitis, infection, and malignancy.

ACUTE REJECTION

As in cardiac transplantation, the majority of acute rejection episodes in lung transplant recipients occur in the first 3 months after transplant. Biopsy-proven rejection occurs in 60–70% of patients in the first month. In the early post-transplant period, the diagnosis of acute rejection is usually based on clinical parameters. Signs of rejection include fever, dyspnea, impaired gas exchange manifested by a decrease in PaO_2, a diminished forced expiratory volume during 1 second (FEV_1, a measure of airway flow), and the development of an interstitial infiltrate on chest x-ray. Fiberoptic bronchoscopy with transbronchial parenchymal lung biopsy and bronchoalveolar lavage is used routinely and when clinically indicated to diagnose acute rejection or rule out infection. A standardized nomenclature has been reported for the grading of lung biopsies (Table 40.11–3).

In the case of heart-lung transplantation, the results of simultaneous surveillance endomyocardial and transbronchial biopsies were recently compared at Stanford. Pulmonary and cardiac rejection presented asynchronously in most cases. Transbronchial biopsies produced a sensitivity of 89% in predicting cardiac rejection, while endomyocardial biopsy yielded a sensitivity of only 34% in predicting lung rejection. Based on these findings, surveillance endomyocardial biopsies have been abandoned

Table 40.11–3. Histologic grading system for acute lung rejection.

Grade	Histologic Appearance (Transbronchial Biopsy)
0	No significant inflammation; normal specimen
1	Small, infrequent perivascular infiltrates with or without bronchiolar lymphocytic infiltrates
2	Larger, more frequent perivascular lymphocytic infiltrates with or without moderate bronchiolar lymphocytic inflammation; occasional neutrophils and eosinophils
3	Extension of infiltrates into alveolar septa and alveolar spaces with or without bronchiolar mucosal ulceration

in heart-lung transplant recipients at Stanford in whom transbronchial biopsies can be reliably performed.

Episodes of acute rejection are treated with a short course of intravenous steroid boluses, specifically, methylprednisolone 500–1000 mg daily for 3 consecutive days. Clinical improvement following steroid therapy is often rapid and dramatic and is considered confirmatory of rejection. Persistent rejection is treated with ATG or OKT3 monoclonal antibodies.

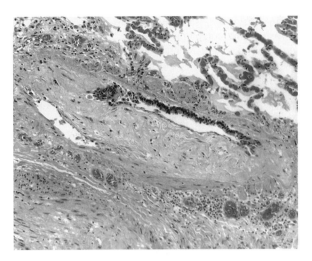

Figure 40.11–3. Bronchiolitis obliterans. Note the dense eosinophilic submucosal scar tissue resulting in partial obliteration of the airway lumen (H & E × 200).

CHRONIC REJECTION

Chronic lung allograft rejection is the greatest limitation to the long-term benefits of lung and heart-lung transplantation. Chronic lung rejection most commonly presents as obliterative bronchiolitis (OB), a pulmonary corollary to cardiac graft atherosclerosis.

Diagnosed in 20–50% of long-term lung transplant survivors, OB is histologically characterized by dense eosinophilic submucosal scar tissue that partially or totally obliterates the lumen of small airways (Figure 40.11–3). Physiologically, OB manifests as decreases in PaO_2 and FEV_1. A working formulation for the clinical staging of chronic lung graft dysfunction based on the ratio of the current FEV_1 to the best post-transplant FEV_1 has been proposed by Cooper and associates at Toronto (Table 40.11–4). Interestingly, there is often no correlation between the histologic and physiologic manifestations of OB.

As to the etiologies of OB, experimental and clinical evidence points to injury of the bronchial epithelium by one or more mechanisms. These include infection, particularly by cytomegalovirus (CMV), toxic fume inhalation, chronic foreign body exposure stemming from impaired mucociliary clearance, and immunologic mechanisms.

Currently, there is no effective treatment for OB. Augmentation of immunosuppression constitutes current therapy. Pulmonary function can be stabilized in most patients, however, significant improvement is infrequent. Unfortunately, relapse rates are greater than 50% and progressive pulmonary failure or infection resultant from increased immunosuppression are the most common causes of death in lung transplant patients after the second year. Efforts at preventing the development of OB focus upon

improved immunosuppression, the aggressive treatment of acute rejection episodes, and infection prophylaxis.

INFECTION

Bacterial, viral, and fungal infections are the leading causes of morbidity and mortality in lung and heart-lung recipients. Bacterial infections, particularly caused by gram-negative bacteria, predominate during the early postoperative period, although the risk of bacterial pneumonia persists throughout the recipient's course. Most common are pulmonary bacterial infections involving the allograft. The absence of the cough reflex in the denervated lung, abnormal mucociliary clearance mechanisms, and deficiencies in lymphatic drainage predispose grafted lungs to infection. From 75% to 97% of bronchial washings obtained from donor lungs before organ retrieval will culture at least one organism. Post-transplant invasive infections frequently will be caused by organisms cultured from the donor. Conversely, bacterial infections develop-

Table 40.11–4. Working formulation for obliterative bronchiolitis syndrome.

0a or b	No significant abnormality: $FEV_1 \geq 80\%$ of baseline
1a or b	Mild obliterative bronchiolitis syndrome: FEV_1 66–80% of baseline
2a or b	Moderate obliterative bronchiolitis syndrome: FEV_1 51–65% of baseline
3a or b	Severe obliterative bronchiolitis syndrome: $FEV_1 \leq 50\%$ of baseline

a = without pathologic evidence of obliterative bronchiolitis; b = with pathologic evidence of obliterative bronchiolitis.

ing in patients with septic lung disease, particularly cystic fibrosis, most commonly originate from the recipient's airways and sinuses. Therapy is comprised of identifying the offending organism and instituting antibiotic therapy based upon sensitivity studies.

As in heart transplant recipients, CMV is the most common and clinically significant viral pathogen. Infections occur most frequently between 2 weeks and 100 days after transplantation. Primary and reactivation CMV infections in lung transplant recipients encompass a wide range of severities and variegated clinical presentations. Primary infection in previously seronegative recipients are generally more serious than reactivation or reinfection in seropositive patients. The diagnosis of CMV pneumonitis, usually the most severe manifestation of CMV infection, is made from a positive viral culture or cytologic evidence obtained from bronchoalveolar lavage or transbronchial biopsy, respectively. Ganciclovir is the treatment of choice. Herpes simplex pneumonia, which presents similarly to CMV pneumonitis, is treated with acyclovir.

In one series, CMV infections developed in approximately 90% of seronegative recipients who received lungs from seropositive donors, compared to about 10% who received lungs from seronegative donors. CMV infections occur in the majority of patients who are seropositive before lung transplantation. Because of organ scarcity, most transplant centers perform transplants across CMV serologic barriers. CMV prophylaxis includes ganciclovir, acyclovir, and polyvalent immune globulin.

Lung and heart-lung transplant patients are also at an increased risk for developing lymphoproliferative disease, particularly in association with Epstein-Barr virus infection. Treatment consists of lowering immunosuppression and the administration of acyclovir. Certain lymphomas

have been successfully treated with chemotherapy and radiotherapy.

Fungal infections, the most infrequent but most deadly of infectious complications in transplant patients, peaks in frequency between 10 days and 2 months after transplant. Fungal species encountered in these patients include *Candida albicans* and *Aspergillus*. Treatment is with fluconazole, itraconazole, or amphotericin B.

Pneumocystis carinii pneumonia has been effectively prevented in lung transplant patients since the institution of prophylaxis, specifically oral trimethoprim-sulfa or inhalational pentamidine for sulfa-allergic patients. The highest risk of infection with *Pneumocystis* occurs during the first transplant year, however, infections do occur late after transplant, prompting most transplant programs to continue prophylaxis indefinitely.

AIRWAY COMPLICATIONS

Improvements in surgical technique and post-transplant management have resulted in a relatively low incidence of airway complications after lung and heart-lung transplantation. The rates of lethal airway complications and late stricture have recently been reported at 3% and 10%, respectively. The most common airway complications are partial anastomotic dehiscence and stricture. Such complications are usually diagnosed during bronchoscopic examination. Airway dehiscence is treated by reoperation or close observation and supportive care. Strictures are treated with laser ablation or dilatation with rigid bronchoscopy or balloon and bougie dilators. Most strictures are stented after dilatation. Cystic fibrosis patients appear

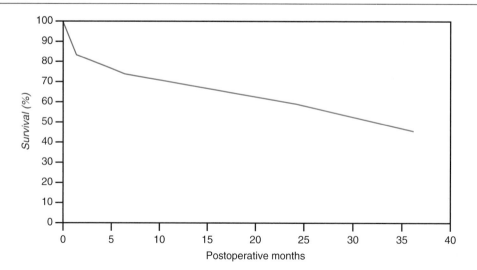

Figure 40.11–4. Actuarial survival of adult lung transplant recipients worldwide (1988–1993).

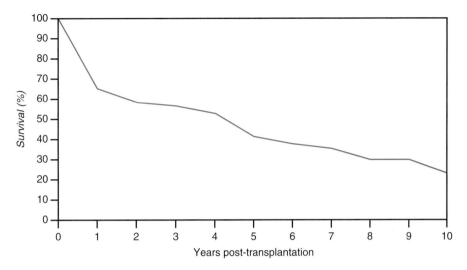

Figure 40.11–5. Actuarial survival of adult heart-lung transplant recipients at Stanford (1981–1994).

to be at a higher risk for developing airway complications after transplantation.

RETRANSPLANTATION

Retransplantation in patients who have developed end-stage OB has generally yielded poor results. In a collected series of pulmonary retransplantation performed at centers in North America and Europe, actuarial 1- and 2-year survival rates were 41% and 33%, respectively. The most common causes of death after retransplantation were infection and OB.

RESULTS

According to the International Heart-Lung Registry, the 1- and 2-year actuarial survival rates for adult single-lung and bilateral single-lung transplants performed worldwide between 1988 and 1993 are 70% and 60%, respectively (Figure 40.11–4). At Stanford, the 1-, 5-, and 10-year actuarial survival rates after adult heart-lung transplantation performed between 1981 and 1994 were 68%, 43%, and 23%, respectively (Figure 40.11–5). Most recipients are able to resume active lifestyles without supplemental oxygen. Pulmonary function measured by spirometry and arterial blood gases is markedly improved in patients after transplantation, with a normalization of ventilation and gas exchange after 1–2 years. The improvements in these parameters are generally greater in bilateral versus single-lung transplant recipients, however, significant differences in exercise testing parameters have not been observed.

PEDIATRIC LUNG & HEART-LUNG TRANSPLANTATION

More than 200 children have undergone single-lung, bilateral single-lung, or heart-lung transplantation worldwide since 1985. At Stanford, pediatric heart-lung and lung transplantation began in 1986 and 1989, respectively. Heart-lung transplantation is indicated for children suffering from end-stage pulmonary vascular or parenchymal diseases, particularly pulmonary hypertension (primary and associated with congenital heart defects) and cystic fibrosis (Table 40.11–5). Single-lung or bilateral single-lung transplantation has become an established option in such cases with preserved right ventricular function.

Table 40.11–5. Indications for pediatric heart-lung or lung transplantation by age.

Infants (0–1 year)
Complex congenital heart disease with pulmonary hypertension
Pulmonary atresia
Bronchopulmonary dysplasia

Children (1–10 years)
Congenital heart disease with pulmonary hypertension (Eisenmenger's syndrome)
Primary pulmonary hypertension
Postviral end-stage parenchymal lung disease
Cystic fibrosis

Adolescents (10–18 years)
Cystic fibrosis
Eisenmenger's syndrome
Primary pulmonary hypertension
End-stage cardiopulmonary disease

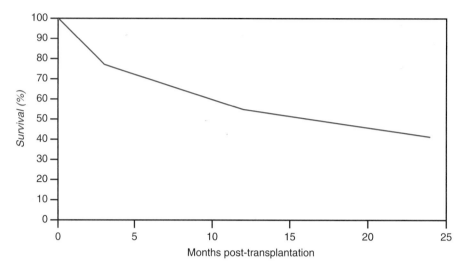

Figure 40.11–6. Actuarial survival of pediatric lung and heart-lung transplant recipients at Stanford (1986–1993).

The general selection criteria for pediatric recipients are similar to those used in adult lung and heart-lung transplantation. Potential recipients generally have a life expectancy of less than 12 months, have normal hepatic and renal function, are free from active systemic infection, and are in a stable psychosocial environment. Blood group and size are the primary criteria used for donor-recipient matching. Size matching is particularly difficult in the pediatric population because of wider size disparities. The recent development of lobar transplantation has permitted the grafting of lung lobes from living-related or cadaveric adult donors into children. Early experience with lobar transplantation, particularly at the University of Southern California, has been encouraging.

The operative techniques for lung and heart-lung transplantation in children are essentially the same as those used in adult thoracic transplantation. Likewise, triple-drug therapy is the mainstay of postoperative immunosuppression. Some centers, including Stanford, also use OKT3 induction therapy.

The incidence of acute rejection in pediatric lung and heart-lung patients does not differ significantly from that seen in adults. Surveillance for rejection in children and adolescents consists of serial transbronchial biopsies with lavage and pulmonary function studies. Routine invasive bronchoscopy is not performed in neonates for technical reasons, shifting emphasis on clinical and radiographic signs in diagnosing pulmonary rejection. The diagnosis of acute pulmonary rejection in the pediatric population, as in adults, is based upon a combination of clinical signs, laboratory tests, and histologic analysis. Pyrexia, fatigue, dyspnea or oxygen desaturation, an interstitial or perihilar infiltrate on chest radiography, and a decreasing FEV_1 are suggestive of rejection.

As in adult recipients, long-term survival in pediatric lung and heart-lung recipients is limited by infection, OB, and accelerated graft CAD. For pediatric lung and heart-lung transplants performed at Stanford between 1986 and 1993, actuarial 3-, 12-, and 24-month survival rates of 78%, 55%, and 41%, respectively, have been observed (Figure 40.11–6). Somatic growth in the pediatric transplant population is generally improved after transplantation, despite the harmful effects of steroids and cyclosporine on bone metabolism. This is most likely due to the marked improvement in cardiopulmonary status after transplantation. Corresponding growth of the transplanted organs also appears to occur.

CONCLUSIONS

The ascent of heart and lung transplantation from rudimentary laboratory experimentation to its current prominence as an accepted therapy for end-stage cardiopulmonary disease is a product of ingenuity, perseverance, skill, and courage. Many debilitated patients, both adult and pediatric, now have an opportunity to resume full and active lifestyles after transplantation. Nevertheless, significant hurdles have yet to be overcome, particularly graft rejection, infection, and a limited donor pool. Important advances on the horizon include cross-species transplantation, improved immunosuppression, the induction of immunologic "tolerance" to foreign tissue, and improved organ preservation techniques.

SUGGESTED READING

Armitage JM et al: Pediatric lung transplantation: The years 1985 to 1992 and the clinical trial of FK506. J Thorac Cardiovasc Surg 1993;105:337.

Hardy JD et al: Lung homotransplantation in man: Report of the initial case. JAMA 1963;186:1065.

Marshall SE et al: Selection and evaluation of recipients for heart-lung and lung transplantation. Chest 1990;98:1488.

Reitz BA et al: Simplified operative method for heart and lung transplantation. J Surg Res 1981;31:1.

Reitz BA et al: Heart and lung transplantation: Autotransplantation and allotransplantation in primates with extended survival. J Thorac Cardiovasc Surg 1980;80:360.

Reitz BA et al: Heart-lung transplantation: Successful therapy for patients with pulmonary vascular disease. N Engl J Med 1982;306:557.

Sarris GE et al: Long-term results of combined heart-lung transplantation: The Stanford experience. J Heart Lung Transplant 1994;13:940.

Starnes VA et al: Heart-lung transplantation in infants, children, and adolescents. J Pediatr Surg 1991;26:434.

Toronto Lung Transplant Group: Unilateral lung transplant for pulmonary fibrosis. N Engl J Med 1986;314:1140.

41

Plastic Surgery

Paul N. Manson, MD

► Key Facts

- ► Plastic surgeons are commonly called upon to evaluate wounds that do not heal.

- ► The stages of wound healing include the "substrate phase," the "proliferative phase," and continuous wound repair and tissue remodeling over a period of 1 year.

- ► Factors that adversely affect wound healing include ischemia, reduced blood supply, formation of fibrous scar tissue, hematoma, infection, chronic illness, steroid treatment, cancer, and the presence of nonviable material.

- ► Survival of skin grafts, which are partial or full thickness pieces of skin used to close large wounds, depends on diffusion of nutrients into the graft ("plasmatic inhibition") and a revascularization process, which should occur within 5 days ("inosculation").

- ► A flap (most commonly, musculocutaneous) is a thickness of tissue that may be transferred from one site to another for wound closure.

- ► Plastic surgeons are often called upon to assess and excise skin lesions. Basal cell carcinoma is the most common form of skin cancer, but malignant melanoma causes the majority of skin cancer morbidity.

- ► The treatment of keloid scars includes intralesional steroid injections, pressure, excision, and, occasionally, radiotherapy.

- ► Anomalies and injuries of the head and neck that may require reconstructive surgery include cleft lip and palate, ear and craniofacial anomalies, mandible deformities, and facial trauma.

- ► Reconstruction of the breast following mastectomy is accomplished with the use of local flaps, tissue expansion, silicone implants, or soft tissue from another location.

- ► Reconstruction is important in reestablishing body image.

- ► The management of hand injuries and infections should always include a careful history and examination of the sensory, motor, and vascular supply to the hand.

- ► The treatment of leg ulcerations includes dressing changes, hygiene, correction of venous pressure, arterial evaluation, or a skin graft for larger lesions.

- ► The most common aesthetic surgical procedures are treatment of the skin to reduce wrinkling and procedures to remove excess skin, such as those performed on the eyelids and face.

Plastic and reconstructive surgery deals with the repair, replacement, and rejuvenation of the skin and subcutaneous tissues, which may include the correction of congenital defects, acquired defects (such as surgical wounds or skin tumors), or cosmetic defects. Plastic surgeons are commonly called to evaluate wounds that do not heal. The nature of plastic surgery requires meticulous attention to detail, delicate tissue handling, gentle dissection, and precise and timely hemostasis.

WOUNDS

Wounds can be regarded as a disruption in the normal structure of tissue as a result of disease or injury. The injury may result from trauma or pressure or may be the result of surgical wounds that fail to heal. There are certain stages or phases of wound healing. The first stage begins with the "substrate phase," where cells and blood products are brought to the site of the injury. These cells remove clot, debris, bacteria, and other impediments to wound healing. A "proliferative phase" then begins, which results in collagen synthesis from fibroblasts. Wound repair results in a rapid gain of tensile strength for the next 60 days. The wound repair tissue then remodels over a period of 1 year.

Traumatic wounds may be closed primarily with placement of suture material to avoid dead space by closure in layers. Small superficial wounds may heal by spontaneous or **secondary healing**, the result of the dual processes of wound contraction and epithelialization (Figure 41–1). Epithelialization generally occurs at the rate of 1 mm a day; contraction occurs from forces generated in the wound margin by myofibroblasts. Many surgeons let some wounds heal secondarily, such as pilonidal sinus excisions in the perineum. **Tertiary wound healing** is delayed wound closure after the wound has been intentionally left

open to allow for contamination and infection to subside. A number of factors adversely influence wound healing, including ischemia, diseases that reduce blood supply, the formation of mature fibrous scar tissue, hematoma, infection, chronic illnesses, steroid treatment, the presence of cancer, and the presence of nonviable material.

For initial closure of traumatic wounds, one considers cleansing them with irrigation or light scrubbing to remove dirt and foreign material. Hematoma or blood clots should be removed. The edges of the wound or laceration are then trimmed so that a precise repair can be performed in anatomical layers. Closure of the deep and superficial tissues is obtained with the smallest appropriate suture material. Careful attention to wound alignment will minimize scar formation, as will removal of devitalized tissue at the edge of the wound and elimination of dead space. Overaggressive debridement may result in deformity or inability to close the wound. Anatomical landmarks provide keys to laceration alignment, such as the vermilion border, the nostril sill, and ear cartilage framework.

For amputated parts, replacement may be attempted within 6 hours by microvascular anastomosis. The amputated part should be placed in a plastic bag and the bag should be placed on ice.

The management of contaminated wounds includes mechanical or sharp debridement, irrigation, antibiotics, dressing changes, and consideration for delayed closure. For chronic wounds, topical and systemic antibiotics, dressing changes, debridement, and, eventually, a flap or a graft as mechanism of closure. Wound dressings may provide light pressure, debridement, and splinting of the wound, or deliver antibacterial medication. Dressings should be changed frequently. The "wet to dry" saline dressing is a debriding dressing, while the "wet to wet" dressing is gentler to the wound surface and is not as debriding. Many "designer" compounds now exist to provide specific environments for the wound surface area that

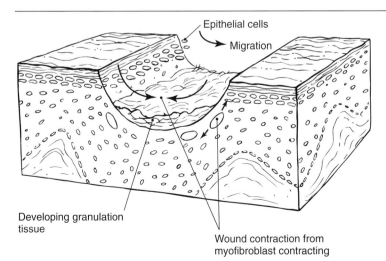

Epithelial cells

Migration

Developing granulation tissue

Wound contraction from myofibroblast contracting

Figure 41–1. Wounds may be closed secondarily by the spontaneous mechanisms of wound contracture from myofibroblasts and epithelial proliferation from the wound edges. Epithelialization requires a level granulating tissue base.

encourage specific properties, such as epithelialization. Wounds resulting in significant loss of tissue have to be closed with grafts or flaps.

The skin is an important structure protecting the body from invasive organisms, such as bacteria. It also prevents the loss of important body fluids. The skin includes the epidermis, the dermis, and the subcutaneous tissue (Figure 41–2). Small wounds heal by spontaneous epithelialization. Large wounds may have to be closed by a graft or a flap. Skin grafts are pieces of skin of various thicknesses (partial to full thickness), depending on the need.

Partial-thickness skin grafts are harvested with a dermatome; they include epidermis and part of the dermis. After a partial-thickness graft is harvested, some dermal appendages remain at the donor site from which spontaneous epithelialization and healing occur. Partial-thickness skin grafts are used on open wounds, as the survival is more predictable with a thinner graft. Thinner grafts contract more than thicker grafts. Partial-thickness grafts are used in large areas of skin loss, such as burns and on open granulating tissue beds, such as a leg ulcer.

Full-thickness skin grafts provide the full layer of the dermis and the epidermis. They are generally placed only into immediately created surgical wounds, as they do not survive in contaminated wounds. Full-thickness grafts provide better coverage, but are less likely to survive than partial-thickness skin grafts. They are used on the face for the purpose of achieving better color match and thickness. Their use is limited by the need to close the donor site primarily. The selection of donor site is made by determining the amount and thickness of skin needed, color match, and the presence of hair.

Skin graft survival initially depends on diffusion of nutrients into the skin graft ("plasmatic imbibition"), then on a revascularization process that occurs within 5 days where vessels from the host invade the vascular system of the graft ("inosculation"). Grafts do not take when bacterial counts in the wound exceed 10^5/g. Generally, a graft is temporarily immobilized by sutures or dressings so that no interference with vascular invasion occurs. Care is taken to prevent hematoma from occurring between the graft and the bed, which prevents revascularization. Graft losses occur from hematoma, sheering, poor recipient sites, and infection.

A **flap** is a thickness of tissue that can be transferred from one site to another. It generally consists of skin and subcutaneous tissue and may include fascia, muscle, bone and other tissues, such as the omentum. Flaps can be clas-

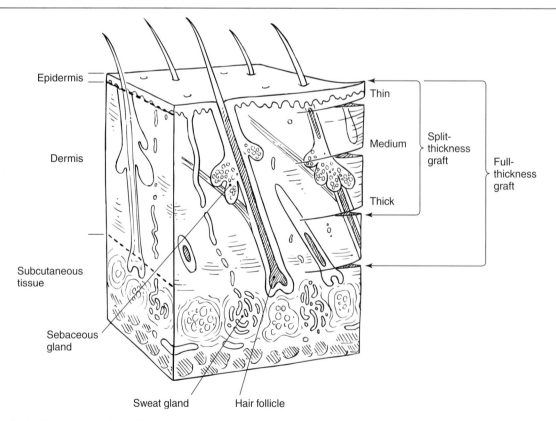

Figure 41–2. The structure of the skin includes the epidermis, the dermis, and skin appendages. The dermis consists of several layers of cells. Capillary and lymphatic circulation begin in the dermis.

sified by the tissue contained and by the pattern of their circulation. **Random pattern** skin flaps (Figure 41–3A) are those where skin blood supply is provided by the dermal and subdermal plexus. They are rotated or advanced into position, have a pedicle or base that remains attached to adjacent tissue, and therefore have a limited size. The base section remains attached to provide blood supply. Flaps that contain a direct artery and vein are called **axial pattern** or **arterial flaps** (Figure 41–3B). The artery can be left intact or divided, whereby the flap may be moved to another location and the vessels reanastomosed with microsurgical techniques. An "island" (axial pattern) flap implies the division of the skin in the pedicle but not the vessels.

Musculocutaneous flaps are the most commonly used flaps for reconstruction. They are flaps that are "compound" and consist of skin, subcutaneous tissue, and muscle. The blood supply comes from the muscle, which often has a single dominant vascular pedicle. The entire compound flap can be moved around the axis of the muscular vascular pedicle or it may be disconnected and reanastomosed at another location. Such flaps are often used to bring in better blood supply to an ischemic area, such as a chronic radiation wound. They can even be designed to provide specialized tissue such as bone or provide padding for pressure sore reconstruction.

Other tissues are often used as grafts. For instance, tendon grafts replace damaged segments of tendons; bone

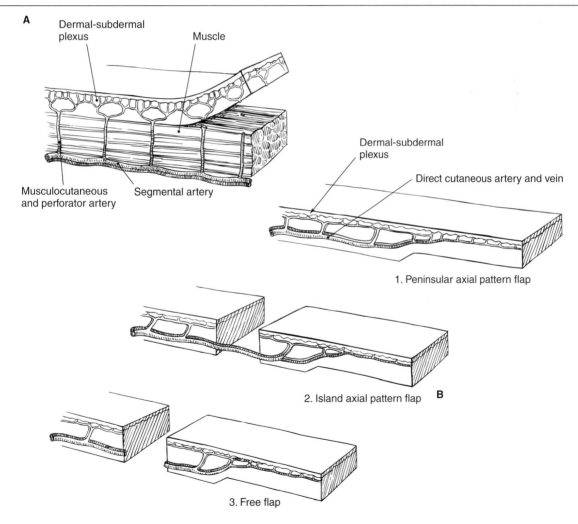

Figure 41–3. Skin flaps may include **A:** random pattern skin flaps where the circulation is provided by a subdermal and dermal circulation through the pedicle or base of the flap is seen on the right; a musculocutaneous circulation is seen at left; **B:** axial/arterial pattern skin flaps. **1.** In a peninsular axial pattern, the flap contains a dominant artery, vein, skin, and subcutaneous tissue. **2.** The island axial pattern flap is most often connected to the body only by an artery and vein. **3.** A free flap can have its dominant artery and vein transected, permitting anastomosis in a remote location. This is a "free tissue transfer."

grafts (either vascularized or nonvascularized) are used to repair bone defects. Cartilage may be taken from ribs, nose, or ears to repair cartilage defects, such as congenital absence of the ear. Fascia may be used for reconstruction of abdominal wall strength. Dermis is sometimes used to increase bulk for contour restorations and in scar repair. Nerves are commonly used to span nerve defects. Vessels such as veins can be used to bridge arterial defects. Fat may be obtained to restore contour defects or to augment areas where fat is deficient. The "take" of tissues depends on a number of factors, including vascularity and the absence of infection.

SKIN TUMORS

Skin tumors are removed to alleviate symptoms from benign tumors and to distinguish and treat skin malignancy. Excision of small lesions is planned in the relaxed lines of skin tension so that scar formation is optimal. Layered closures are performed, including dermal and skin sutures.

Common benign tumors include warts of viral origin, benign nevi, and lipomas. **Nevi** (or moles) are cellular rests classified on the basis of their location within the dermis and their activity. Junctional nevi, large surface nevi, and dysplastic nevi (> 5 mm with irregular borders, variegation in color, and variations in surface height) are more likely to develop into malignant melanoma.

Malignant melanoma is a serious malignancy requiring early diagnosis. The clinical appearance usually involves a history of recent change and enlargement, elevation of a portion of the lesion, bleeding, or itching. Melanoma colors represent combinations of reds, browns, and blacks (Figure 41–4). The surface characteristics of these lesions are irregular in outline. Excisional biopsy is recommended.

Keratoses are brown, "greasy" feeling, thickened areas of the skin that respond to superficial electrodesiccation or liquid nitrogen treatment. Actinic keratoses result from sun damage. They are crusting, reddish areas that have superficial inflammation. Biopsy is indicated to exclude basal cell or squamous cell carcinoma. The skin is often affected by epidermal inclusion cysts. These should be excised with the overlying skin attachment containing the duct of the blocked gland. If inflamed, they should be drained and the cyst excised when the inflammation has subsided.

Lipomas are subcutaneous, fatty tumors that are not adherent to the overlying skin. **Fibromas** are brownish-red lesions within the dermis. **Vascular lesions** affecting the skin include hemangiomas, which are common in infancy, capillary angiomas, and lymphatic and vascular malformations. Many hemangiomas grow rapidly for 6–7 months, then begin to regress over several years. The treatment of most of these vascular lesions is observation. Pulsed steroid administration may be indicated for rapidly enlarging hemangiomas.

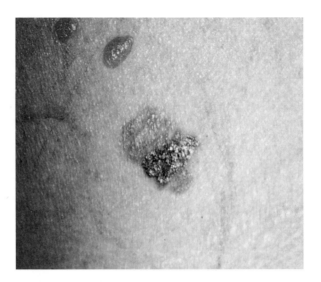

Figure 41–4. The typical appearance of a melanoma consists of shades of brown, black, red, or blue pigmentation (not readily seen in black and white photo), irregular borders, and irregular surface height. Such lesions indicate the need for biopsy.

Port-wine stains are "birthmarks" that consist of reddish pink or purple areas of skin. Laser treatment is recommended for port-wine stains to improve appearance. **Arteriovenous malformations** show progressive increase in size and extent. Their treatment is embolization and surgical excision. **Lymphatic abnormalities** include cystic hygroma, which results from lymphatic obstruction and may be localized, massive, and disfiguring. Lymphatic malformations may be mixed with arteriovenous malformations. Treatment involves subtotal surgical excision.

Basal cell carcinoma is the most common form of skin cancer (Figure 41–5). It can be either nodular or flat and may show a variety of pigmentation. It is usually seen on the face or other sun-exposed areas. It grows slowly, destroys by local invasion and rarely metastasizes. Surgical excision with frozen section control of the margins is indicated, followed by appropriate reconstruction. **Squamous cell carcinoma** (Figure 41–6) grows more rapidly and has the potential for metastasizing to regional lymph nodes or through the blood stream when it is over 2 cm. It generally occurs on sun-exposed areas of the body and can also occur either in areas treated by x-ray or in chronic nonhealing wounds. The treatment is surgical excision with margin control and reconstruction.

Malignant melanoma causes the majority of skin cancer morbidity. Its classification and potential for spread relate to its Clark's level and Breslow depth of invasion (Table 41–1). Histologic staging is performed on the basis of the biopsy. Melanoma is at first superficial, growing radially, and at this stage is "superficial spreading melanoma."

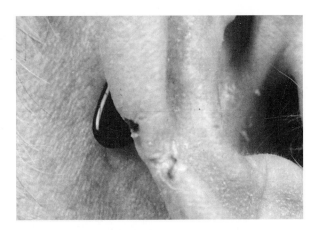

Figure 41–5. Basal cell skin cancers are reddish lesions with opaque borders, umbilicated centers, ulceration, and flaking. Here, the helix of the ear has been eroded by an infiltrative lesion.

This variety accounts for about 70% of melanoma types, and metastasis is not common until the vertical growth phase occurs. Nodular melanomas are characteristically blue back in color, grow rapidly and vertically, and have significant potential for metastatic involvement. Acral lentiginous melanoma is a type of melanoma that is con-

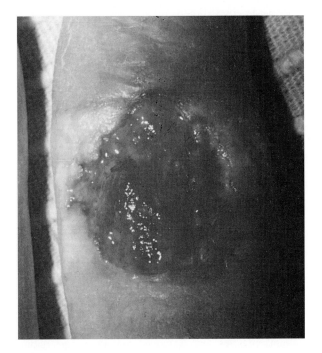

Figure 41–6. Squamous cell carcinoma presents as ulcerated areas with raised peripheral borders. Here a lesion is present on the dorsum of a finger.

Table 41–1. Clark's levels of cutaneous invasion.

Level I	(In situ) above the basement membrane—node metastases extremely rare
Level II	In the papillary dermis—metastases in 2.5%
Level III	To the junction of papillary and reticular dermis—metastases in up to 20%
Level IV	Into the reticular dermis—metastases in 40%
Level V	Into the subcutaneous tissue—metastases in 70%

fined to the skin surface of the distal extremities. Lentigo maligna is a less common early melanoma lesion and consists of a patch of thickened, pigmented skin.

Melanomas usually do not metastasize until a Breslow thickness of 0.76 mm is exceeded. Over 1.5 mm Breslow thickness, metastases are seen in 50% of cases. Melanomas are staged according to thickness, involvement of regional nodes, or systemic dissemination. Melanomas require wide surgical excision with at least 2-cm margins. Thicker lesions may have regional lymph nodes removed "prophylactically." Node dissection is performed for any palpable nodes. Immunotherapy is commonly employed, but its benefit has not been established.

SCARS

Hypertrophic scars are those that display increased thickness and growth, but still remain proportionate to and within the boundaries of the original scar. Their treatment is by elastic pressure and intralesional steroids. **Keloids** grow irregularly beyond the boundaries of the original scar, a characteristic that results in their differentiation from hypertrophic scars. Keloid treatment requires intralesional steroid injections, pressure, excision, and, occasionally, radiotherapy.

CLEFT LIP & PALATE

The structures of the lip and palate are affected by congenital abnormalities that create unilateral incomplete or complete clefting and bilateral incomplete or complete clefting. Cleft lip occurs in approximately 1 in 700 births, and cleft palate in 1 in 1000. Children of involved parents have a risk for the disorder ranging from 4% to 14%, depending on extent of involvement and family history. The etiology is multifactorial.

The primary palate forms at 4–6 weeks of age due to mesenchymal fusion. The secondary palate forms by fusion at 7–12 weeks of age. Clefts of the lip create problems in appearance, lip seal, and eating. A lack of continuity of the skin, muscle, and mucous membrane is repaired by a layered closure involving z-plasties and rotation of tissues. Generally, closure is performed about 3 months of age.

Defects of the palate create inadequate oronasal seal.

Air escapes through the nose in speech, and some sounds cannot be articulated. The palate is generally repaired between 6 months to 1 year of age. Closure of nasal mucosa and mucoperiosteum is performed by flaps created from existing structures. Velopharyngeal insufficiency is hypernasal speech. The syndrome creates the need to add length to the palate so that air does not leak into the nose.

EAR DEFORMITIES & CONGENITAL CRANIOFACIAL ANOMALIES

The ear may be absent, unusually prominent, or have vestigial parts. Some conditions, such as hemifacial microsomia, include absent or hypoplastic ears and mandibular ramus deformities. The treatment for absence of the ear is by ear reconstruction with cartilage grafts at 4–5 years of age. The most common congenital ear deformity is protrusion, resulting both from the lack of an antihelical fold and a tall concha.

Less common craniofacial deformities include craniosynostosis, which may affect a single suture or multiple sutures. Synostosis creates, for the skull, the inability to grow so that brain growth is restricted and intracranial pressure may be elevated. The more severe craniosynostosis deformities include Crouzon's and Apert's syndromes, which have multiple suture synostosis, and skull base and midface growth restrictions resulting in shallow orbits, exophthalmos, and midface retrusion. Children with Apert's syndrome have hypertelorism, multiple suture craniosynostosis, and congenital anomalies of the hands.

FACIAL INJURIES

The soft tissues and the bones of the face are frequently injured. Soft tissue injuries include bruises, hematomas, lacerations, and contusions. Repair of nerves and skin lacerations, and drainage of hematoma, are important in preserving facial appearance. The bones of the face consist of the nose, the maxilla, the zygoma, the frontal bone, and the mandible (see Chapter 33). These bones may be fractured as isolated entities or in combination.

The diagnosis of facial fractures is suspected when bruising, epistasis, asymmetry, and bone mobility are present as well as symptoms such as double vision, sensory loss, malocclusion of the teeth, and local pain. The diagnosis is established by physical examination and computed tomography (CT). The principles of treatment include reestablishing normal occlusion by the use of intermaxillary fixation, plating reduced fractures with small plates and screws, bone grafting of bone defects, and fabrication of dentures or splints. The reduction and immobilization of fractures in anatomical position is accomplished through incisions designed for frontal, orbital, midface, or mandibular exposure.

CONGENITAL DEFORMITIES

Deformities of the face include those of the mandible: **retrognathia**—retrusion of the lower jaw; **prognathia**—protrusion of the lower jaw: **micrognathia**—underdevelopment of the lower jaw; and open bite or cross bite. In **open bite**, the anterior or lateral teeth cannot be brought into apposition; in **cross bite**, the lower teeth are lateral to the upper teeth (the reverse of the normal relationship). The maxilla may also show deficient growth. The diagnosis is established by physical examination and an evaluation of the occlusion with appropriate x-rays called **cephalometrograms**, which access relative proportions of the facial bones. Corrective osteotomies can be performed, with repositioning of bone segments in conjunction with orthodontic corrective measures.

Facial paralysis results in loss of facial nerve function. Significant asymmetry of the face occurs, with drooling, drying of the cornea, and deformity. The etiology may be idiopathic, congenital, traumatic, or result from tumor removal. The treatment includes protective measures, muscle transfers, static suspension procedures, reestablishment of facial nerve function by nerve repair, or transfer of contralateral nerves (**cross-facial nerve graft transfers**) or combined nerve and muscle grafts.

CHEST WALL & ABDOMINAL RECONSTRUCTION

Reconstructive surgery of the chest and abdomen is performed to restore cutaneous cover and structural integrity, or to re-create form, such as in breast reconstruction. Chest wall reconstruction is often indicated for loss of areas of chest wall structures, such as ribs. Sternal infection and dehiscence is a common sequel to 1% of open heart operations; it is managed with sternal debridement, followed by pectoralis muscle flap closure to provide vascularized tissue to combat infection, and cutaneous advancement closure.

BREAST RECONSTRUCTION

Reconstruction of the breast after mastectomy for cancer is important in reestablishing body image. The mastectomy defect includes absence of the breast mound and nipple areolar complex. The treatment includes local flaps, tissue expansion, silicone implants, or soft tissue reconstruction. Commonly, the lower abdomen provides both skin coverage and breast volume by transfer of living tissue (**transverse rectus abdominis muscle**, or TRAM flap). The flap is based on one or both of the rectus abdominis muscles and is moved into the breast region (Figure 41–7). This tissue is then sculptured to approximate the existing breast shape on the contralateral side. Nipple areolar reconstruction is generally performed with

HISTORICAL FACTS

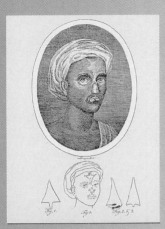

Figure from an article that appeared in 1794 in *The Gentleman's Magazine* published in London, describing Hindu methods of nose reconstruction using a patch from the forehead. The article came to the attention of the English surgeon Joseph Constantine Carpue (1764–1846), who promoted the Hindu method and reestablished rhinoplasty in the West. (Reprinted, with permission, from *The Gentleman's Magazine* 1749;64:891, Jeremy Norman & Co, Inc.)

*I*t [surgery] is eternal and a source of infinite piety, imparts fame and opens the gates of Heaven to its votaries, prolongs the durations of human existence on earth, and helps men in successfully fulfilling their missions, and earning a decent competence, in life.

—Sushruta

Sushruta (uncertain, from 800 BC to 600 BC) is not only the author of the first textbook on surgery, entitled *Sushruta Samhita* (or *The Collection of Sushruta*), but he is also considered the father of plastic and reconstructive surgery. Although he practiced all types of surgery, including laparotomy, tonsillectomy, hernia repairs, vesicolithotomy, and anal fistulotomies, he pioneered the art of rhinoplasty. Physical mutilation was a common punishment for a number of different offenses in India and cutting off the nose was the usual penalty for adultery. For this reason, Indian surgeons had wide experience in developing techniques for nasal reconstruction.

Sushruta describes his methods for rhinoplasty in detail:

"Now I shall deal with the process of affixing an artificial nose. First, the leaf of a creeper, long and broad enough to fully cover the whole of the severed or clipped part should be gathered; and a patch of living flesh, equal in dimension to the preceding leaf should be sliced off from the region of the cheek and, after scarifying it with a knife, swiftly adhered to the severed nose. Then the cool-headed physician should steadily tie it up with a bandage decent to look at and perfectly suited to the end for which it has been employed. The physician should make sure that the adhesion of the severed parts has been fully effected and then insert two small pipes into the nostrils to facilitate respiration, and to prevent adhesioned flesh from hanging down . . ."

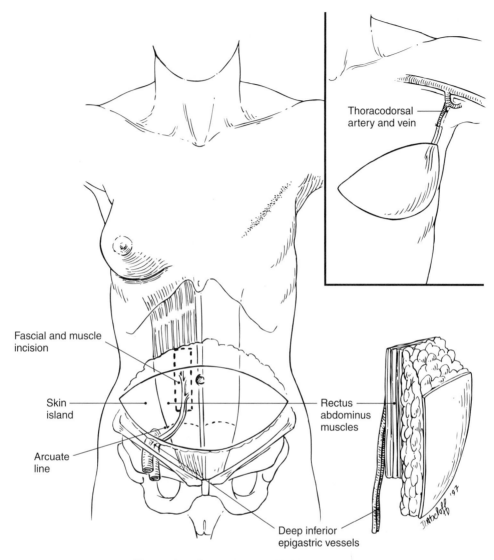

Thoracodorsal artery and vein

Fascial and muscle incision

Skin island

Arcuate line

Rectus abdominus muscles

Deep inferior epigastric vessels

Figure 41–7. Detail of the free TRAM flap dissection.

local flaps, followed by tattoo pigment some months after the primary reconstruction.

BREAST REDUCTION

Marked enlargement of the breasts creates functional problems, such as shoulder and back pain and submammary intertrigo. Patients also complain of personal embarrassment and psychological problems. A variety of procedures can reduce breast size significantly. The procedures all involve moving the nipple areolar complex to a superior position, and removing the lower portions of the breast. Scarring consists of vertical and horizontal scars that surround the areola and cross the inframammary fold.

PRESSURE SORES

Pressure sores are wounds that are created by abnormal pressure persistently in a single area. The tissue dies and becomes infected, and a deep hole is created, which extends to the underlying bone surface. Common sites include the greater trochanter, the ischial tuberosity, the sacrum, and the heel. Paraplegics and those that have absent sensation are most susceptible to pressure sore development.

Pressure sores may be prevented by keeping the skin clean and dry and frequently relieving pressure from an area by turning the patient every half hour. Foam cushions and mattresses may additionally protect the skin. Once a wound is established, the dead tissue is debrided until the wound begins to granulate. It then usually requires flap reconstruction with partial resection of the underlying bony prominence.

UPPER EXTREMITY & HAND

The treatment of hand problems requires specialized knowledge. The hand is supplied by radial, median, and ulnar nerves. Motor power for flexion is derived by flexor tendons to the fingers and thumb. Extensor tendons provide finger extension. Hand injuries should always be splinted in the "safe position," which is the position from which maximal motion and function can be performed. The wrist is extended 45 degrees, the metacarpal phalangeal joints are flexed 60 degrees, and the interphalangeal joints are extended. The thumb is abducted and rotated.

The management of hand injuries includes taking a history and examination of the sensory, motor, and vascular supply to the hand. Both sharp and dull sensitivity and two-point discrimination (utilizing a paper clip) are assessed. One must test the sensory areas of the median, ulnar, and radial nerves and test both sides of the fingers. Transection of the median nerve will result in absent sensation in the thumb, index, and middle finger flexor surfaces. The patient will be unable to abduct the thumb against resistance. Transection of the ulnar nerve produces absent sensation in the flexor surface of the little and ring fingers and inability to abduct the index or little fingers against resistance. Injury to the radial nerve affects the dorsal surface of the thumb and index finger and the extensor tendons. Vascular injury to the hand produces absence of capillary refill or absent pulses. Bleeding is controlled by direct pressure. The hand should be placed in the safe position, splinted and elevated for transfer.

Definitive treatment of hand injuries includes cleansing of the wound and repair under "tourniquet hemostasis" with anesthesia. Tendons and nerves are repaired; fractures and dislocations are reduced, pinned, and splinted. Bone repair may be provided with pins and wires or plates and screws. Postoperatively, the hand is immobilized with a dressing in a safe position. Edema is controlled by elevation.

Fingertip amputations are common injuries. After cleansing the area, avulsed segments of the nail should be replaced as a splint after the nail bed has been repaired. If the amputation involves a significant portion of the fingertip, reconstruction is accomplished with local or regional flaps.

Hand infections are serious, as tissue may be destroyed within a few hours. Any localized pus should be drained, and appropriate elevation, warmth, antibiotics, and rest should be provided. Surgical drainage should be undertaken with tourniquet control in the operating room. Smears and cultures determine offending organisms and selection of appropriate antibiotics.

The **paronychia** is an infection at the side of the nail, which should be drained and local antibiotics and soaks provided for treatment. The felon is pus in the pulp space of the pad of the finger. This is a serious infection that can impair blood supply and result in gangrene. Lateral incisions for drainage avoid nerve injury must be appropriately designed to prevent skin necrosis. Subcutaneous abscesses usually come to the surface on the palm or fingers and require drainage; one should avoid incisions that might injure the health of the digital arteries or nerves.

Tenosynovitis is a serious infection of tendon sheaths, which is diagnosed by the "signs of Kanavel." The finger is held in slight flexion, and there is fusiform swelling of the finger, pain with passive extension, and tenderness over the flexor sheath. This infection requires hospitalization, intravenous antibiotics, and drainage with irrigation.

Human bites are serious because of the vigor of inoculated organisms. Their treatment includes debridement, irrigation, cultures, and broad-spectrum antibiotics, and often initially involves leaving the wounds open.

Fractures should be assessed by physical examination and x-rays performed in two directions to access displacement. Fractures should be accurately reduced, with fixation utilized where appropriate, and splinted while healing occurs. If early motion is possible, joint stiffness is minimized. Often, k-wires or plates and screws are utilized for fracture immobilization.

The most common tumor of the hand is a **ganglion**, a cyst frequently located on the radial-dorsal aspect of the wrist. These are synovial-lined cystic lesions that commonly originate from the scapholunate ligament. They also occur at the interphalangeal joints, and in this area are called **mucus cysts** where they might create a nail deformity. Sometimes they occur in the palmar surface of the hand, arising from the tendon sheath near the distal palmer skin crease. Their management is excision. **Glomus tumors** are uncommon but painful tumors of vascular origin presenting under the nail region with pain, localized tenderness, and temperature sensitivity.

Dupuytren's contracture is a fibrous thickening of the palmar fascia, creating nodules or bands in the palm that contract and limit the ability of the fingers to extend. The treatment is surgical excision when joint restriction exceeds 30 degrees from full motion.

LOWER EXTREMITY RECONSTRUCTION

Plastic surgeons are often called upon to reconstruct open wounds of the lower extremity with defects of skin and bone. These wounds may occur from leg ulcerations, trauma, tumors, and ischemia.

Leg ulcers are an erosion in the epithelial and subcutaneous tissues. The most common cause is venous stasis or venous hypertension related to venous valvular incompetence. These ulcers are usually formed on the medial aspect of the ankle; the patient has dark discoloration in the surrounding skin, edema, and itching. Ischemic ulcers are secondary to proximal artery occlusion; the lesions are usually painful, in contrast to the lack of pain with venous stasis ulcers. Edema is usually absent. Ischemic ulcers are more common on the lateral aspects of the foot and ankle. Surrounding pigmentation is absent. Ankle-brachial indices of less than 0.3 are pathognomonic of an ischemic etiology. Neurotrophic ulcers are seen in the feet of diabetics with decreased sensation. They usually occur on the plantar surface of the foot and relate to changes in the posture of the foot resulting from lack of sensory nerve and motor nerve function that lead to collapse of the arch of the foot, excess pressure, and ulcerations.

Each type of ulcer requires an accurate diagnosis and specific treatment related precisely to the etiology, with a skin closure designed to protect tissue under the wound defect. The care of the wound differs according to the etiology and location. Some ulcers of the lower extremity will heal with dressing changes, hygiene, and correction of venous pressure by elastic wrapping. Surgical intervention is sometimes appropriate for certain lesions. Venous stasis ulcers are usually treated with "pressure boot" bandages and topical antimicrobials. A skin graft can be performed for larger lesions. Ischemic ulcers require revascularization based on angiographic findings. Diabetic ulcers require resection of the underlying bony prominence, special shoes, or casting.

Trauma to the lower extremity often results in compound fractures. Those fractures that are open over a fractured tibia and fibula with soft tissue loss require reconstruction by vascularized tissue transfer. This can be accomplished with local myocutaneous flaps in proximal and middle third leg defects by transferring the gastrocnemius or soleus muscle or by micro surgical tissue transfer for larger lesions or in lower third leg defects.

Lymph edema is a congenital or acquired swelling in an extremity secondary to accumulation of protein and fluid in subcutaneous tissue. It is not only disfiguring but debilitating. Primary or idiopathic lymph edema results from congenital maldevelopment of lymphatics. Usually, the disease is seen in females and occurs at puberty or in early childhood. It is managed by pressure garments and, rarely, subcutaneous surgical excision. Secondary or acquired lymph edemas are due to infections or surgical removal of regional lymph nodes. Elevation, elastic support, and skin hygiene are the main components of treatment.

BURNS

Thermal destruction of the skin can be either partial or full thickness. The amount of tissue destruction is based on the temperature and time of exposure. The burn size should be evaluated by the percent body surface area, which differs in children versus adults. Burns at the ex-

tremes of age carry a greater risk of morbidity and mortality. The depth of the burn is established by physical examination. First-degree burns are epidermal and second-degree burns are either superficial or deep partial-thickness skin injuries. Third-degree burns include the full-thickness injuries of the skin, and so-called "fourth-degree" burns extend to the level of muscle and bone.

The treatment of first-degree burns (which have an initial white and then red appearance) with intact sensation and capillary refill includes cleansing and topical antimicrobials. Second-degree burns have superficial blisters with clear fluid, intact skin sensation, and capillary circulation. Blister debridement and antibacterial creams are utilized topically; these burns heal spontaneously from regeneration of epithelium from remaining living sweat glands and hair follicles. Third-degree burns have absent skin sensation and circulation and black, yellow, white, or severely discolored skin that has a "parchment" quality. They require excision of burn eschar (dead skin) and split-thickness skin grafting if the area of injury is more than a few centimeters. Patients with large burns develop circulatory shock and require precise replacement of fluids, electrolytes, and protein, and management of respiratory distress (see Chapter 18).

Burn shock can be prevented by administration of fluid, electrolytes, and protein. Precise replacement formulas relate the hourly amount of electrolyte solution to be administered over the first few days to the percent body surface area and depth of burn. The patient's pressure, pulse, urine output, and sensorium provide indices of proper fluid replacement. Less common types of burns include chemical burns, which may be produced by agents such as acids, phosphorous, or phenol, and electrical injuries. Electrical injuries create severe deep fourth-degree burns, with markedly damaged deep tissues. The tissue is literally heated by the current, and coagulation necrosis occurs.

Smoke inhalation injury must be suspected in burns and can be identified by history of closed quarters burn, burned nasal hairs, carbon particles in the mouth, nose, or pharynx, hoarseness, and conjunctivitis. Frequently, patients with burns have associated fractures from injuries sustained while trying to escape the burn.

FROSTBITE & IMMERSION FOOT

Thermal injury may also be produced by cold or freezing. **Frostbite** is produced by formation of ice crystals in tissue. The circulation to the area ceases with decreasing temperature. Upon rewarming, reperfusion of tissue occurs but then ceases over several days because of progressive thrombosis of the microcirculation, and tissue death follows. Frostbite is treated with rapid rewarming in a 40°C water bath. Physical therapy, hygiene, vasodilators, and prevention of infection minimize tissue loss. Generally, nonviable tissue is allowed to dry and slough spontaneously over a period of weeks.

Immersion foot is a cold injury that occurs from exposure to nonfreezing temperatures. Treatment is similar to frostbite.

PRIMARY TUMORS OF THE OROPHARYNX, TONGUE, & FLOOR OF MOUTH

Mucosal tumors of the oropharynx, tongue, and floor of mouth commonly are squamous cell carcinomas. These typically present as ulcerated lesions with indurated edges that are exophytic and infiltrative. The incidence of these intraoral tumors increases with tobacco and alcohol use. Tumors are classified by the size of the primary tumor (T) involvement of regional nodes (N) and presence of metastatic disease (M).

Intraoral tumors are sometimes preceded by **leukoplakia**, literally a white patch that is considered to be a premalignant lesion. As more dysplasia occurs, the lesion evolves toward redness (**erythroplakia**) and frank malignancy. Erythema surrounding the white patch is particularly significant of advancing disease. Squamous cell carcinomas are often located in the floor of the mouth and tonsillar area. They metastasize to regional nodes and elsewhere via the blood stream. The site and size of the lesion determines the treatment choice. Small lesions are excised or irradiated. More advanced lesions receive surgical excision. Lesions that are large (T3 or T4), with extensive nodal metastasis, or lesions where excision is incomplete, should have supplemental radiation treatment. Small lesions may be managed with radiation alone. The tonsillar area, tongue, and floor of the mouth are common sites for squamous cell cancer.

PRIMARY TUMORS OF THE SALIVARY GLANDS

Salivary tumors may be benign or malignant. They constitute approximately 6% of all head and neck cancers.

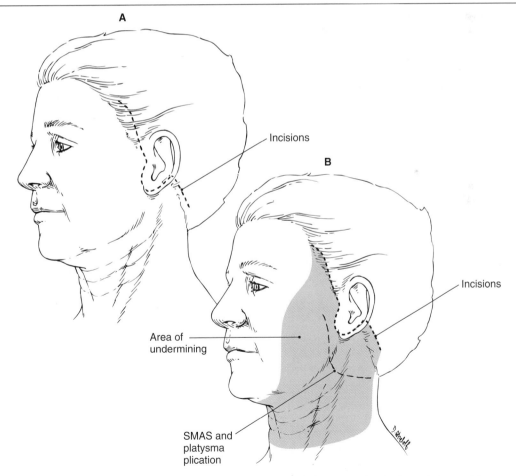

Figure 41–8. **A** and **B:** In the rhytidectomy procedure, an incision beginning in the temporal region is carried around the ear and into the posterior hair. The skin is undermined and the underlying platysma muscle and its surrounding fascia is tightened. Excess skin is excised.

The parotid gland is the primary site of tumor occurrence in 80% of patients. The minor salivary glands, such as the submaxillary gland, are involved in 5–10% of patients. About three fourths of parotid tumors are benign, whereas 60–80% of minor salivary gland tumors are malignant. Salivary gland tumors are identified by the presence of a mass and are identified by palpation. CT and magnetic resonance imaging are utilized to diagnose extent of disease and lymph node involvement, as with tumors of the oropharynx and neck. Ninety percent of benign parotid tumors are pleomorphic adenomas. They are composed of various proportions of epithelial and mesenchymal elements and have their peak incidence at age 50. Other benign tumors include Warthin's tumors, adenolymphoma, and eosinophilic adenoma.

Malignant tumors are commonly mucoepidermoid carcinomas and are classified by histologic grade. Adenoid-cystic carcinomas are the most common submaxillary salivary gland malignancy. Adenocarcinomas are the next most frequently encountered malignancy in the minor salivary glands. Acinic cell carcinoma is a low-grade tumor that occurs primarily in the parotid. Tumors of the salivary gland should be evaluated for tumor size, local extension or nerve invasion, spread to regional nodes, and distant metastases. Treatment involves resection of the primary tumor by total **parotidectomy**, or gland removal, usually with facial nerve preservation. Regional lymph nodes are removed for high-grade lesions, and supplemental radiotherapy may be considered.

AESTHETIC SURGERY

Aesthetic surgery is performed to address changes associated with aging, especially involving the face or eyelids, or to change the shape and appearance of a facial or other bodily feature, such as an overly enlarged nose or breast.

The most common aesthetic surgical procedures are treatments of the skin to reduce wrinkling, such as dermabrasion, chemical peel, or laser treatment, and procedures to remove excess skin, such as those performed on the eyelids and face (**blepharoplasty** and **rhytidectomy**).

Procedures to reduce facial skin wrinkling act to smooth wrinkles and surface irregularities by producing minor damage to the skin surface. The best candidates for **chemical peel** are patients with fair complexions, as the complications involve hypertrophic scarring, hyperpigmentation, or irregular pigmentation.

The most commonly performed procedure in aesthetic surgery is **liposuction**. In this procedure, fat is aspirated from areas of excess through the use of small suction cannulas.

The elimination of excess facial skin involves excision, which is called **rhytidectomy**. Fat can be contoured simultaneously by excision or suction (Figure 41–8). In the eyelid area, skin excision is combined with fat excision, which improves the "puffy" appearance. In the face, an incision surrounding the lower ear, extending into the hairline anteriorly and posteriorly, is used to dissect a skin flap (Figure 41–8). After extensive undermining of the face and neck area, the underlying superficial musculoaponeurotic system (consisting of superficial fascia and platysma muscle) is tightened. Excess skin is excised to remove redundant skin and tighten underlying muscle, smoothing the neck. This greatly improves the appearance of aging in the neck, jowl, and nasal labial fold region.

Excess skin and fat can also be excised from the thighs (**thigh and buttock lift**) and the abdomen (**abdominoplasty**). Scars from these procedures can be prominent. In the abdominoplasty procedure, the rectus abdominis muscle is plicated and any diastasis between the muscles is repaired by muscle plication, which improves abdominal contour. Skin redundancy is resected.

SUGGESTED READING

Ariyan S: *Cancer of the Head and Neck.* Mosby, 1987.

Bostwick J: *Plastic & Reconstructive Breast Surgery.* Quality Medical Publishing, 1994.

David D, Simpson D: *Craniofacial Trauma.* Churchill Livingstone, 1995.

Farmer E, Hood A: *Pathology of the Skin.* Appleton & Lange, 1990.

Georgiade N, Georgiade G, Reifkohl R: *Plastic Reconstructive and Maxillofacial Surgery.* Williams & Wilkins, 1991.

Green T: *Operative Hand Surgery,* 3rd ed. Churchill Livingstone, 1994.

Lister G: *The Hand: Diagnosis and Indications.* Churchill Livingstone, 1994.

McCarthy JG: *Plastic Surgery.* Saunders, 1990.

Millard DR: *Cleft Craft.* Little, Brown, 1976.

Rees R, LaTrenta GS: *Aesthetic Surgery.* Saunders, 1994.

Ruberg R, Smith D: *Plastic Surgery: A Core Curriculum.* Mosby, 1994.

Smith J, Aston S: *Grabb and Smith's Plastic Surgery.* Little, Brown, 1991.

Strickers R et al: *Craniofacial Malformations.* Churchill Livingstone, 1990.

Williams J, Rowe NL: *Rowe and Williams' Maxillofacial Injuries,* 2nd ed. Churchill Livingstone, 1995.

42

Orthopedic Surgery

Glen S. O'Sullivan, MD

▶ Key Facts

- ▶ Axis is a term used to describe the orientation of the bones and joints, particularly in the lower extremity. It is an important concept when planning for an osteotomy or total joint replacement.

- ▶ The five main maneuvers of examination of any joint are (1) inspection; (2) palpation; (3) joint movement; (4) strain and stress maneuvers of the joint; and (5) radiographs.

- ▶ Two views of a joint are routinely taken with plain radiographs: an anterior-posterior view and a lateral view. Radiographs of a bone should include the joints above and below.

- ▶ In recent years, magnetic resonance imaging has proven invaluable in the early diagnosis of muscular skeletal abnormalities, as it reveals the bony cortex and describes the fluid content, both in the bone and in the soft tissues.

- ▶ There is a trend toward early active range-of-motion exercises for musculoskeletal injuries to maintain strength and motion with the use of isometric and closed chain eccentric exercise programs.

- ▶ The most common orthopedic procedures include osteotomy, arthrodesis, arthroplasty, epiphysiodesis, and arthroscopy.

- ▶ Comminution is the presence of more than two fragments in a fracture. The greater the comminution and violence involved in creating the fracture, the greater the chance for complications.

- ▶ The classification of open injuries is based on the size of the wound and the amount of soft tissue injury and ranges from Grade I to Grade III.

- ▶ The most common bone and joint infections include acute hematogenous osteomyelitis, subacute osteomyelitis, chronic osteomyelitis, and septic arthritis.

- ▶ Tumors of the musculoskeletal system are uncommon. Benign tumors are more common than malignant ones.

- ▶ The classification of a surgical procedure for an orthopedic neoplasm is based on the surgical plane of dissection in relation to the tumor (intracapsular, marginal, wide, or radical).

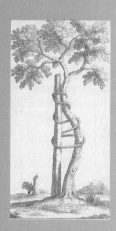
ORTHOPEDIC TERMINOLOGY

Nicholas Andry in 1741 coined the term "orthopedics" in a book on the art of preventing and correcting deformities in children, combining the terms *orthos* (straighten) and *pais* (child). Several deformities are frequently encountered in the clinical setting. **Angulation** or **bowing deformities** refer to the direction in which the apex of the angle points (rather than the direction in which the distal fragment points). The deformity may be described as anterior, posterior, medial, or lateral. **Varus** and **valgus** are terms used mainly to describe deformities of a bone or joint causing angulation of the limb distal to the point of deformity. Angulation away from the midline is a valgus deformity, whereas angulation toward the midline is referred to as a varus deformity (Figure 42–1).

Axis is a term used to describe the orientation of the bones and joints, particularly in the lower extremity. It is an important concept when planning for an osteotomy or total joint replacement. The various types can be defined as follows: (1) **mechanical axis** is a line passing from the femoral head to the center of the ankle; (2) **vertical axis** is a line passing from the center of gravity of the body to the ground; (3) **anatomic axis** is a line joining the shaft of the femur and tibia (Figure 42–2).

The mechanical axis is 3 degrees valgus from the vertical axis. The anatomic axis of the femur is 6 degrees of valgus from the mechanical axis. The anatomic axis of the tibia is 3 degrees of varus from the mechanical axis. When considering arthrodesis of the knee, the surgeon should probably place the fusion in 0–7 degrees of valgus and 10–15 degrees of flexion.

Anteversion and **retroversion** are deformities referring to the relationship between the neck of the femur and the femoral shaft. Normally, this relationship is approximately 20 degrees of anteversion. If a fractured neck of femur is pinned in a retroverted position, the fixation is bound to fail. If a hip prosthesis is placed in a retroverted

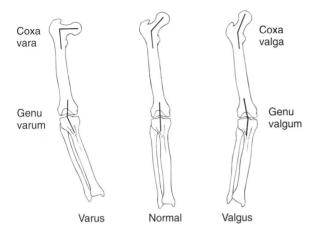

Figure 42–1. Varus and valgus deformities of a bone or joint, which cause angulation of the limb distal to the point of the deformity.

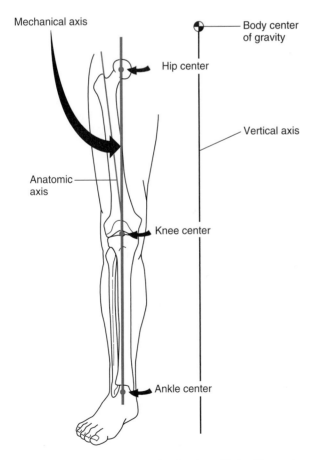

Figure 42–2. Knee axes. (Reprinted and modified, with permission, from Rohr WL: Primary total knee arthroplasty. In: *Chapman's Operative Orthopedics.* Lippincott, 1988, p. 718.)

position, there is an increased incidence of dislocation of the artificial joint.

Supination and **pronation** describe movements of rotation in the forearm or forefoot. The motion of supination describes moving the palmar surface upwards for the hand or placing the forefoot in inversion. Pronation describes the opposite direction of movement, downwards for the hand or eversion for the foot.

Calcaneus describes a deformity in which the foot is maintained in a dorsiflexed position on weightbearing so that only the heel touches the floor. **Equinus** is a deformity in which the foot is maintained in a plantar flexed position on weightbearing, resulting in pressure on the undersurface of the forefoot. **Pes cavus** describes an exaggeration of the instep of the foot (a high arch). The combined deformity of calcaneus of the hindfoot and equinus or plantar flexion of the forefoot is called **calcaneocavus**. **Pes planus** describes a flattening of the arch in a flat foot deformity.

BONE GROWTH & DEVELOPMENT

The human skeleton begins life as a cartilaginous template laid down in utero. Primary areas of ossification begin in the center of the cartilage anlage and progress towards either end by intramembranous bone formation. Secondary centers of ossification appear in the cartilaginous ends of the bone during the first few years of life. The **physis** is a thin area of cartilage remaining unossified between the primary and secondary areas of ossification. This growing cartilage layer produces length of the bone by enchondral ossification (Figure 42–3).

Diaphysis is the area between the physis. This is the site of primary ossification in vitro. The **epiphysis** is the area beyond the physis. This is the secondary center of os-

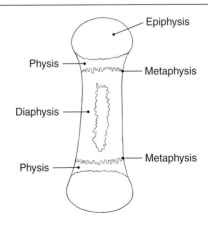

Figure 42–3. Diagram of developing long bone.

sification and eventually supports the joint cartilage. The **metaphysis** is an expansion of the diaphysis close to the physis made up of spongy cancellous bone.

Many orthopedic conditions during childhood affect specifically one part of the developing bone. For example, the metaphysis with its diminished blood flow is prone to osteomyelitis. A fracture involving the growth plate can lead to late deformities, with altered growth in the limb around the joint. The Saltar-Harris classification is used to describe physeal fractures (Figure 42–4) (Table 42–1). A fracture line passing across the growth plate is more prone to late complications.

Various conditions affecting skeletal growth and development may occur, including abnormalities of cartilage anlage formation and conversion to primary ossification, such as proximal focal femoral deficiency (sporadic occurrences), cleidocranial dysostosis presenting as hypoplastic clavicles and pubic rami, and Apert's syndrome (sporadic) syndactyly and premature cranial synostosis (Figure 42–5). Failure of formation of the secondary centers of ossification (**epiphysis**) may present as multiple epiphyseal dysplasia (MED) early joint deformity and arthritis mimicking Perthes disease, spondyloepiphyseal

Table 42–1. Salter-Harris classification of physeal fractures.

Type	Description	Characteristics
I	Transverse fractures through physis	Younger children
II	Fractures through physis with metaphyseal fragment	Children > 10 years
III	Fractures through physis and epiphysis	Intra-articular
IV	Fractures through epiphysis, physis, and metaphysis	Migration/growth arrest
V	Crush injury of physis	Growth arrest late
VI	Injury to perichondrial ring	Bridging/angular deformity

Reprinted, with permission, from Miller MD: *Review of Orthopedics,* Saunders, 1992, p. 275.

dysplasia similar to MED with platyspondylia (vertebral flattening), and diastrophic ("to bend") dwarfism, which is a short-limbed dwarfism with joint contractures and spinal kyphosis.

The **groove of Ranvier** is a thickening in the perichondrium occurring at the physis. Abnormalities at this location can cause dysplasia epiphysealis hemimelica, which often presents as an asymptomatic epiphyseal osteochondroma. Osteochondroma can be solitary or multiple, and can act like a growth plate during childhood, but ceases growth after skeletal maturation. This presents as a palpable mass and may occasionally compress a nerve or artery.

Abnormalities of chondroid calcification in the physis result in the **Ricket's defect**. This defect causes a buildup of hypertrophic chondroblasts with minimal amounts of calcified chondroid. There are wide unmineralized osteoid seams. The bones are soft and brittle and bend and bow. The patient usually has short stature. Radiographs reveal physeal cupping and widening with an absent provisional zone of calcification. The treatment is usually vitamin D and calcium for all types of rickets, which include (1) vitamin D-dependent; (2) vitamin D-resistant; (3) renal osteodystrophy; (4) gastrointestinal rickets (malabsorption syndrome); and (5) anticonvulsant-induced rickets.

Abnormalities affecting normal osteoid production in the physis and affecting normal intramembranous osteoid production of the periosteal cambium layer include osteogenesis imperfecta. With this abnormality, the cortical bone is not organized and lacks strength. There is generalized osteoporosis with pathological fractures. Scurvy is caused by inadequate dietary intake of vitamin C required for conversion of proline into hydroxyproline in the collagen fibrils, resulting in inadequate amounts of osteoid and collagen. Granulation tissue fills in the juxtaphyseal areas of the metaphysis, producing the lucent x-ray scorbutic zone, clinically presenting with swollen, tender joints, bleeding of blood vessels, and subperiosteal bleeding.

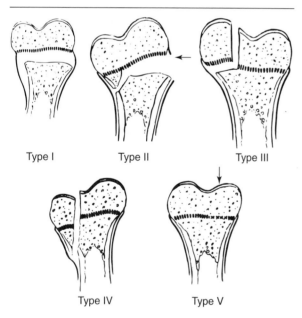

Type I   Type II   Type III

Type IV   Type V

Figure 42–4. Salter classification of epiphyseal plate fractures. Type I: separation of epiphysis. Type II: fracture–separation of epiphysis. Type III: fracture of part of epiphysis. Type IV: fracture of epiphysis and epiphyseal plate; bony union causing premature closure of plate. Type V: crushing of epiphyseal plate; premature closure of plate on one side with resultant angular deformity. (Reprinted, with permission, from Garland J: *Fundamentals of Orthopaedics,* 3rd ed. Saunders, 1987, p. 90.)

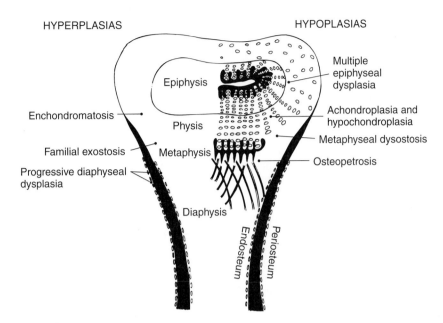

HYPERPLASIAS   HYPOPLASIAS

Figure 42–5. A diagram of the location of failure of appropriate growth with regard to the particular dysplasia seen. The dysplasia may be due to overactivity of the area or underactivity. (Reprinted, with permission, from Rodrigo JJ: *Orthopaedic Surgery: Basic Science and Clinical Science.* Little, Brown, 1986, p. 441.)

HISTORY & PHYSICAL EXAMINATION

Most patients who seek advice from an orthopedic surgeon complain of pain or deformity with swelling or wasting, or altered range of motion of a joint or joints. It is important for the physician to determine causation, location and radiation, duration, degree of pain with aggravating and relieving factors, and the extent of a patient's reaction to the pain. The patient should be examined standing, walking, and lying down. For comparison, the contralateral limb should be examined along with the affected limb. Particular attention should be paid to the spine or other structures innervated from the same segment of the spine. The five main maneuvers of examination of any joint are (1) inspection (look); (2) palpation (feel); (3) movement of the joint (active and passive); (4) strain, stress maneuvers of the joint; and (5) radiographs.

During inspection one should be cognizant of the position of the joint (eg, a painful hip is usually held in a flexed position), degree of swelling or joint effusion, the presence of scars or sinuses, associated deformities around the joint, and degree of muscle wasting. In palpation of the joint, attention should be directed toward increased temperature, local tenderness, the degree of swelling, and the presence of crepitus in the joint. The patient should first be asked to move the joint actively, and the joint should be compared to the contralateral joint. Occasionally, a painful arc of motion will be discovered; loss

of a few degrees of motion may suggest intra-articular pathology. Forces can be applied across the joint to determine any evidence of instability or provocation of pain. The joint itself may be injected with local anesthetic and reexamined.

Diagnostic studies are very important. Two views of a joint with plain radiographs, an anterior-posterior (AP) and lateral view, are routinely taken. It is important to have radiographs that include the joint above and below the suspected level of pathology. Weight-bearing or stress x-rays are also very valuable, and, occasionally, oblique x-rays are necessary. Computed axial tomography may be extremely useful in complex situations in determining three-dimensional anatomy, such as pelvic and spinal pathology.

In recent years, magnetic resonance imaging has proven invaluable in the early diagnosis of muscular skeletal pathology. Although the CT scan may give better definition of bony cortex, the MRI describes the fluid content, both in the bone and in the soft tissues. It is invaluable in the diagnosis of intra-articular and periarticular pathology, such as rotator cuff tears in the shoulder, and anterior cruciate ligament and meniscal tears in the knee, and in determining the presence of avascular necrosis in the femoral head. Occasionally, bone scan studies are helpful if one is suspicious of malignancy or stress fractures or wishing to determine the activity of heterotopic ossification.

No examination is complete without a thorough neurovascular examination to rule out the presence of neurologic involvement and to guarantee the adequacy of the peripheral circulation. Measurements that should be taken include limb girths to rule out muscle atrophy, grip strengths bilaterally, range-of-motion of the joints in question, and leg lengths, the clinician being aware of apparent and true shortening by squaring the pelvis. Finally, it is important to observe gait, noting any use of a cane or ambulation device, such as a walker. Particular gaits are (1) hemiplegic gait, occurring in cerebral palsy and following cerebral vascular accidents; (2) scissoring gait, caused by overactivity of thigh adductors occurring in cerebral palsy; (3) athetoid gait, or uncontrolled, purposeless movements with loss of coordination, usually occurring in cerebral palsy; (4) drop foot gait, particularly seen in polio patients, resulting in a high-stepping gait with the foot in an equinus position when off the ground; (5) Trendelenburg gait, a lurch toward the weight-bearing side, due to either pain or weakness of the abductors of the hip; and (6) antalgic gait, an antipain gait, typically caused by osteoarthritis of the hip or knee and characterized by the patient hurrying off one lower limb and spending a greater part of the walking cycle on the other. At the conclusion of a history and physical examination and review of the diagnostic studies, one can develop a differential diagnosis based on the classic VITAMIN format (Table 42–2).

TREATMENT OPTIONS IN ORTHOPEDICS

NONOPERATIVE TREATMENT

Many musculoskeletal afflictions may be treated by conservative management. Often, inflamed tissues respond to a period of rest or immobilization. The use of a temporary splint, for example, is helpful in repetitive stress syndromes like tennis elbow (lateral epicondylitis), which responds well to an elbow splint, or carpal tunnel syndrome (median nerve compression at the wrist), which responds well to the use of night splints. An extremity may require support for a ligamentous injury, such as an injury to the ankle, which would require the use of a splint or air cast. Physiotherapy is very helpful, utilizing passive range-of-motion exercises to avoid joint stiffness or continuous passive motion machines. There is a trend toward early active range-of-motion exercises to maintain strength and motion with the use of isometric and closed

Table 42–2. Development of a differential diagnosis with the classic VITAMIN format.

V — Vascular diseases
I — Infection
T — Tumor
A — Arthritis
M — Metabolic
I — Injury
N — Neurodevelopmental disorders

chain eccentric exercise programs. Other modalities include the use of local heat or electrical stimulation, application of ultrasonography together with steroids (**iontophoresis**), and local massage.

Injections of steroids and anesthetics to tender points or trigger points can be helpful in alleviating local inflammation or pain. Joint aspiration allows analysis of synovial fluid (Figure 42–6), and the introduction of anesthetic allows an examination of the joint free from pain to determine the degree of stability of the joint. The most common medications used in orthopedic surgery for muscular skeletal inflammation are nonsteroidal anti-inflammatory agents.

OVERVIEW OF OPERATIVE TREATMENTS

Osteotomy

Osteotomy is a division of a bone to correct angular or rotatory deformity. This may be done to shorten or lengthen a bone. The different procedures include wedge osteotomy, rotation osteotomy, and displacement osteotomy. Following completion of an osteotomy, fixation is usually achieved with metal plates or screws, or occasionally with the use of an external fixator (especially in limb-lengthening procedures).

Arthrodesis

Arthrodesis is the procedure for fusion of a joint. It is usually used to relieve pain in arthritic conditions, such as post-traumatic arthritis in young patients. It is important to have good functioning joints above and below the arthrodesis joint, as increased stress across those joints is anticipated. Most common sites are hip, knee, wrist, and ankle. The position of the fusion is critical.

Arthrodesis, or fusion, is also used to prevent progression of a deformity or to hold a deformity in alignment following correction of that deformity, such as scoliosis surgery, where a release of the spine and insertion of instrumentation is carried out to realign the spinal curvature. Arthrodesis of the spine is then accomplished to prevent it from deforming further.

One of the largest complications of arthrodesis is inability to achieve a solid fusion. This depends on multiple factors, such as the length of the fusion, the patient's smoking status, the use of instrumentation, and the selection of autologous or allograft bone. The best bone graft is autologous bone, which is usually harvested from the iliac crest. Complications from this can include persistent donor site pain and, occasionally, fractures of the pelvis itself.

Arthroplasty

Arthroplasty is the creation of a new joint, which may be accomplished with several different techniques: (1) excisional arthroplasty is the removal of the joint, resulting in a gap at the location of the joint, usually with a reduction in pain but an abnormally functioning joint; (2) inter-

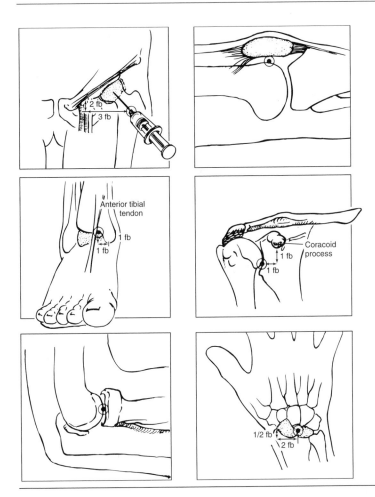

Figure 42–6. Sites for introduction of a needle for arthrocentesis of various joints. Fingerbreadth, approximately 1.5 cm. (Reprinted, with permission, from Rodrigo JJ: *Orthopaedic Surgery: Basic Science and Clinical Science.* Little, Brown, 1986, p. 226.)

positional arthroplasty is the placement of soft tissue material in the site of the joint; (3) hemiarthroplasty, removal of one half of the joint, is the replacement of the humeral or femoral head following a traumatic situation, with preservation of the articular glenoid or acetabular surface, respectively; and (4) total joint arthroplasty is the most common procedure performed for arthritic changes of the hip and knee.

In most cases, the prosthesis is cemented into position. Many improvements in cement technique have reduced the rate of loosening of the prosthesis. There has been a trend towards use of uncemented prostheses with specially made implants that allow bony ingrowth. There is also a trend in total hip replacement to perform a hybrid procedure, that is, an uncemented replacement of the acetabular component and placement of a cemented femoral component.

The most common complication with lower extremity arthroplasty is deep vein thrombosis, with an incidence of up to 60%; prophylaxis, therefore, is important. Other risks include infection (prophylactic antibiotics are given), dislocation, and loosening of the prosthesis.

Epiphysiodesis

Epiphysiodesis is the ablation of the growth plate, which is carried out in an attempt to prevent further growth. This may be done to equalize a leg length discrepancy or, in an area such as the spine, to prevent further angulation of a deformity.

Arthroscopy

Arthroscopy is a surgical technique that has dramatically changed the management of many joint conditions. Techniques employing an arthroscope result in reduced morbidity from surgery. Previously impossible or technically demanding procedures can now be undertaken, such as repair of a posterior meniscal tear. Advances in this technology include the use of a rigid arthroscope. The most commonly used scope is a 30 scope, with 4-mm scopes for large joints and 1.7-mm and 2-mm scopes for smaller joints. The use of a fiberoptic light source and miniature cameras with corresponding television monitors have improved visualization. A variety of hand-operated and powered instruments are used, including electrocautery and lasers.

The general indications for arthroscopy include joint diagnosis and assessment, synovial biopsy, removal of loose bodies, incision of osteophytes, irrigation of septic arthritis, drilling or shaving within the joint, and synovectomy. In the knee, not only can the meniscus be repaired or shaved, but the cruciate ligament can be reconstructed. The most common portals are a medial and lateral parapatellar portal. In the shoulder, labral tears can be repaired or excised and subacromial decompressions carried out. The most common portal in the shoulder lies posteriorly in the soft spot between the infraspinatus and teres minor, located 2 cm inferior and 2 cm medial to the posterolateral corner of the acromion. The trocar is directed towards the coracoid. An anterior portal can be made with the use of a guiding rod.

A NOTE ON TOURNIQUETS

The width of a tourniquet cuff is important. In the upper extremity the cuff should be 20% wider then the diameter of the upper arm. The pressure should not be elevated more than 50 mm Hg higher than the systolic blood pressure. In the lower extremity, the cuff width should be 40% wider than the diameter of the thigh and the pressure elevated to twice the level of the systolic blood pressure. The tourniquet should not be elevated for longer than 2 hours.

Contraindications to the use of an automatic pneumatic tourniquet include peripheral arterial disease with large vessel atheromatosis plaques, severe crushing injuries with compromised vasculature, and sickle cell disease. The extremity may be exsanguinated by elevation prior to inflation of the tourniquet or by expression with the use of an Esmarch's bandage. Expression of the extremity is contraindicated in cases with venous thrombosis, malignancy, or infection for fear of embolization.

ORTHOPEDIC EMERGENCIES & TRAUMA

A **fracture** can be described as a break in the continuity of a bone. **Comminution** indicates more than two fragments. The greater the comminution and violence involved to create the fracture, the greater chance of complications, such as difficulties fixing the fracture or delay in bone healing. A transverse fracture is usually caused by a direct force, while a spiral or oblique fracture is usually caused by an indirect force transmitted from a distance. A greenstick fracture occurs in children, whose bones are more compliant. A crush fracture occurs in cancellous bone from direct compression, while burst fracture occurs from a greater impaction axial loading force. Avulsion fractures are caused by traction, usually by a tendon or ligament tearing off a bony fragment attachment. Fracture dislocations or subluxations involve joints, resulting in malalignment of joint surfaces and resulting in higher

risks of post-traumatic arthritis. A compound fracture is the description for an open injury with a much higher potential for infection or delay in healing.

The classification of open injuries is based on the size of the wound and amount of soft tissue injury. Grade I is a low-energy injury with less than 1 cm of open skin defect. Grade II is a defect less then 10 cm with moderate involvement of energy. A grade-III injury has a wound of greater then 10 cm, involves high energy (such as a shotgun wound), a very contaminated wound (such as a barnyard injury or segmental fracture), a neurovascular injury, or a wound that has been open for longer than 8 hours. A grade-III open fracture can be further classified as type A with adequate soft tissue coverage, type B with massive soft tissue destruction and bony exposure, and type C with repairable vascular injury. The infection rate for grade-III open injuries is approximately 25% versus 1–2% for a grade-I open injury (Figure 42–7).

When a patient presents with orthopedic traumatic injuries, it is important to assess the overall status of the patient. Assuring that the patient's breathing, pulmonary function, and circulation are stable are priorities. It should be emphasized that improvements in trauma and resuscitation have stemmed from early diagnosis and treatment of shock with fluid replacement, monitoring of blood gases, and the use of ventilator support. The establishment of emergency medical services and regional trauma centers have led to a 40% improvement in preventing deaths.

Once the trauma victim has been stabilized, four major questions must be addressed to adequately evaluate and treat the orthopedic injury:

1. *Is the injury an isolated fracture or are multiple systems involved?* There is a trend to rapidly stabilize patients with multiple injuries. This allows early mobilization and avoids the risks of adult respiratory distress syndrome and pulmonary failure. Rapid fixation of extremity shaft fractures, such as the femur, within 12 hours has reduced the incidence of pulmonary complications.

2. *What is the state of the skin?* Is this an open or closed fracture? As described earlier, an open or compound fracture may involve more soft tissue loss, a higher degree of kinetic energy, and a greater degree of fracture comminution. Wound care *must* be addressed rapidly, with swift irrigation and debridement within 8 hours. Intravenous antibiotics should be given for at least 48 hours; these include cephalosporin, aminoglycosides, and possibly penicillin. Depending on the state of the injury, immobilization or fixation should be considered, and early flap coverage may be necessary within 48 hours. Tetanus prophylaxis should not be forgotten.

3. *What is the stability of the fractured part?* Stability of a fractured extremity depends on the degree of kinetic energy absorbed, and the degree of soft tissue damage and bony comminution, as well as the orientation of the fracture line (whether there is a propensity for the fracture to slip or be grossly unstable). The greater the

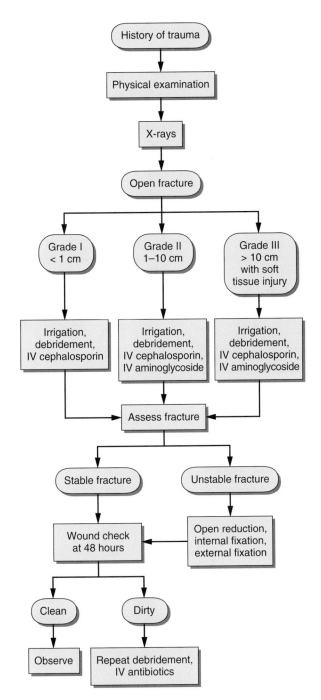

Figure 42–7. Algorithm for management of open fractures. (Reprinted and modified, with permission, from Wiesel SW et al: *Essentials of Orthopedic Surgery.* Saunders, 1993, p. 91.)

comminution, the more likely fixation is necessary to preserve the bony alignment and protect the neurovascular structures. It is imperative to know the neurovascular status. The presence of a neurologic injury is important, especially when one is considering the spinal column. A potentially unstable vertebral column requires rapid restoration of alignment and fixation to prevent further neurologic deterioration and injury. A good quality cervical spine x-ray should include visualization of C7/T1. If there is an associated vascular injury, a work-up for this, including arteriogram, is necessary.

A hemodynamically unstable patient with a disrupted pelvic ring will require rapid stabilization of the pelvis to control venous bleeding. This is successful, in most cases, with the use of an external fixation frame in the immediate situation. If the patient continues to be hemodynamically unstable, an arteriogram may be necessary to isolate an arterial bleeder that may require embolization or open ligation. Associated visceral injuries with a pelvic fracture have a high rate of complications and mortality and also require early stabilization to mobilize the patient (Figure 42–8).

An arterial injury with an associated fracture or dislocation can be devastating. Often, blood flow is restored by just realigning the fracture fragments or reducing the dislocated joint. A high index of suspicion is necessary in the presence of a possible arterial injury, and arteriograms should be performed. This is particularly true in the case of a suspected knee dislocation or elbow fracture dislocation. Early diagnosis and repair of an arterial injury with concomitant compartment fasciotomies is necessary to avoid soft tissue ischemia.

Compartment syndrome is increased pressure within an enclosed soft tissue compartment and can lead to serious sequelae. This is particularly true following high-energy injuries to the forearm and leg. The presence of pain (especially with passive flexion of the digits, the earliest and most reliable indicator), pallor, paralysis, paresthesia, and lack of pulse are indicators of elevated pressure. A compartment pressure of greater then 40 mm Hg or within 10–30 mm Hg of the diastolic pressure confirms the diagnosis of compartment syndrome. The pressures are measured with a White side or indwelling catheter device.

4. *What is the location of the fracture?* Is the fracture midshaft at the diaphysis? Does it involve the metaphysis and articular surface of a joint? Periarticular injuries require anatomic restoration and bone grafting to support the joint. Rapid fixation is essential to allow early mobilization of the joint to prevent the long-term risks of post-traumatic arthritis. Radiographs should include the joint above and below the injury; a floating joint with a fracture above and below requires immediate fixation.

Reducing a fractured bone can be accomplished by closed technique, either manually with local or general

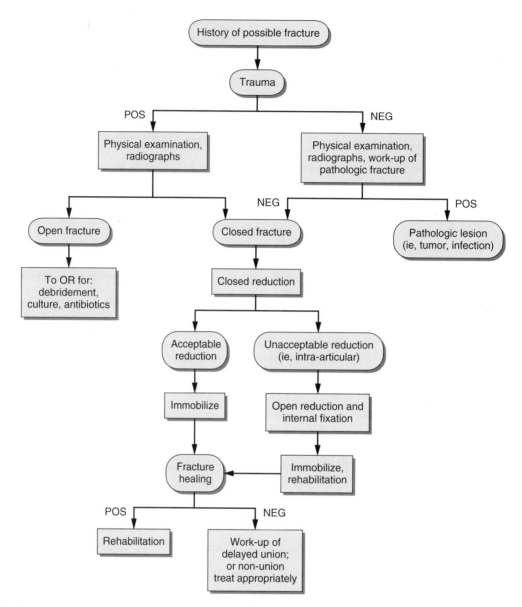

Figure 42–8. Fracture management algorithm. (Reprinted and modified, with permission, from Wiesel SW et al: *Essentials of Orthopedic Surgery*. Saunders, 1993, p. 45.)

anesthetic or indirectly with the use of skeletal traction. The reduction can be maintained with the use of skeletal traction or the application of a splint or cast. In the acute setting, the cast should be univalve to accommodate swelling and avoid the risks of compartment syndrome. External fixation can also be used to maintain alignment of the bones. The other technique is a surgical open reduction, and internal or external fixation may or may not be used. **External fixation** involves the placement of wires or pins through the skin, transfixing the bone and holding the fracture alignment in place with an external frame. This allows minimal soft tissue dissection. There has been a trend towards minimal open techniques in conjunction with **hybrid fixation** (small wires close to the joint and larger pins in the shaft). Wires are also used in a tension band technique to restore alignment of avulsed fragments. Screw fixation is very helpful and can be used in an interfragmentary fashion. Newer cannulated systems are available.

Screws alone may not be enough to maintain fixation

and may require a backup of a fixator, metal plate, or external splint. Several **plate fixation devices** are available. They can be used in a buttress fashion to prevent gliding of fracture fragments or used as a neutralization device to protect the interfragmentary fixation of a screw. There are semitubular plates for fixation of small bones, such as the fibula. There are reconstruction plates, which are long and can be more easily contoured for pelvic fractures. Condylar, clover leaf, and spoon plates are helpful for metaphyseal/diaphyseal injuries that involve a joint. Dynamic compression plates come in either small or large sizes and allow a degree of compression across the fracture site. Also available are rigid blade plates and dynamic screw and side plate devices. The dynamic screw and side plate allows settling at the fracture site in hip fractures.

Finally, intramedullary fixation can be achieved by multiple means. Solid or cannulated interlocking nails have become invaluable in the treatment of long bone injuries, especially in the lower extremities. Reconstruction nail devices allow fixation of both hip and shaft fractures. The interlocking capabilities provide rigid fixation for early mobilization in these complex injuries. The weight-sharing properties of the intermedullary nails allow early weight-bearing and produce few complications, as opposed to the older plate techniques. The main concern is whether the intramedullary canal should be reamed to place a nail in the presence of an open injury (periosteal blood supply has been compromised) because the reaming technique will further compromise the blood supply to the bone by disturbing the intramedullary blood source. There is a trend toward fixing the open shaft fractures with intramedullary devices, but in severely contaminated situations external fixation may be more prudent.

Fat emboli syndrome occurs in 0.5–2% of trauma victims within 24–72 hours following multiple fractures. It is believed to be caused by the systemic release of bone marrow fat, possibly a change in the chylomicrons' stability of the free fatty acids. The patient presents with an increase in heart rate and temperature, breathing rapidly with hypoxia, mental state changes, oliguria, and preticia rash. Treatment includes early fracture stabilization within 24 hours and pulmonary support.

BONE & JOINT INFECTIONS

ACUTE HEMATOGENOUS OSTEOMYELITIS

Acute hematogenous osteomyelitis is most commonly caused by blood-borne organisms, particularly involving children and more common in boys than girls. *Staphylococcus aureus* is the most common organism. Anaerobe infections also occur. The most frequent site is the metaphysis of long bones. Radiographs may not be impressive, and it takes more than 2 weeks for demineralization to be noticed on x-ray. Soft tissue swelling may be apparent.

The patient presents with loss of function and pain, soft tissue swelling, or abscess. Laboratory findings include elevated white cell counts and sedimentation rates, as well as positive blood cultures. A bone scan is usually positive. Gallium studies are helpful in the spine, and indium is helpful in difficult extremity cases. MRI is extremely sensitive. Finally, aspiration may be the key to the diagnosis (Figure 42–9).

Treatment usually involves immobilization of the affected part. Intravenous antibiotics should be followed by oral antibiotics for at least 6 weeks or until sedimentation rate falls to normal. Surgical drainage may be necessary in persistent cases or if destructive lesions are present.

SUBACUTE OSTEOMYELITIS

Subacute osteomyelitis may present as a painful limp in a patient with no other local or systemic signs. Radiographs may demonstrate a Brodie's abscess, which is a localized lucency. The blood work may be totally normal. The differential diagnosis may be difficult and includes tumors, such as Ewing's sarcoma. Surgical drainage and antibiotics are often necessary.

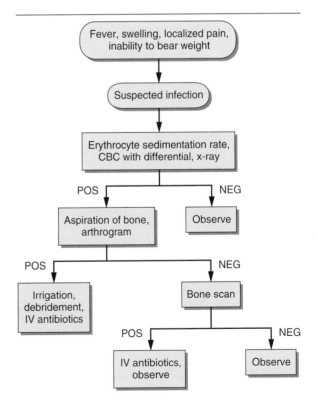

Figure 42–9. Acute osteomyelitis. (Reprinted and modified, with permission, from Wiesel SW et al: *Essentials of Orthopedic Surgery*. Saunders, 1993, p. 88.) POS = Positive; NEG = negative.

Table 42–3. Staging system for bone tumors.

	Stage	Grade	Site	Metastasis
Benign				
1	Inactive	G_0	T_0	M_0
2	Active	G_0	T_0	M_0
3	Aggressive	G_0	T_{1-2}	M_{0-1}
Malignant				
IA	Low-grade, intracompartmental	G_1	T_1	M_0
IB	Low-grade, extracompartmental	G_1	T_2	M_0
IIA	High-grade, intracompartmental	G_2	T_1	M_0
IIB	High-grade, extracompartmental	G_2	T_2	M_0
IIIA	Low- or high-grade, intracompartmental, with metastases	G_{1-2}	T_1	M_1
IIIB	Low- or high-grade, extracompartmental with metastases	G_{1-2}	T_2	M_1

Reprinted and modified, with permission, from Enneking WF: *Musculoskeletal Tumor Surgery.* Churchill Livingstone, 1983, p. 80.

CHRONIC OSTEOMYELITIS

Chronic osteomyelitis may follow an acute episode of osteomyelitis. It is especially likely in the elderly or immunosuppressed, patients with diabetes, or intravenous drug abusers. Aggressive treatment may be necessary, including surgical excision, bone grafting, and use of vascular flaps for coverage. On occasion, amputation may be necessary.

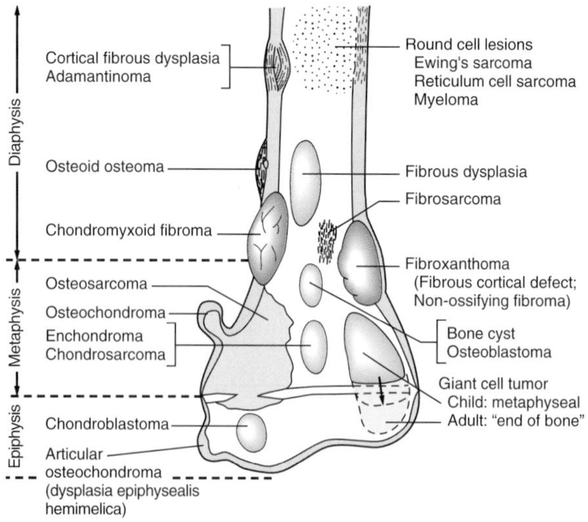

SEPTIC ARTHRITIS

Septic arthritis may either be caused by hematogenous spread or extension of an osteomyelitis focus at the metaphyseal location. It is very common in the infant, especially involving the hip, and in the knees of young children. *Haemophilus influenzae* is often the offending

Figure 42–10. Location of common bone tumors. (Reprinted and modified, with permission, from Madewell JE et al: Radiologic and pathologic analysis of solitary bone lesions. Part I: Internal margins. Radiol Clin North Am 1981;19:715.)

Table 42–4. Musculoskeletal disease: Relationship to site.

Location/Site	Typical Pathologic Findings
Epiphyseal	Chondroblastoma, chondrosarcoma, giant cell tumor, infection
Metaphyseal	Any lesion
Diaphyseal	Osteoblastoma, Ewing's, eosinophilic granuloma, lymphoma, adamantinoma, fibrous dysplasia
Pelvis	Metastasis, myeloma, Ewing's, chondrosarcoma, Paget's
Proximal humerus	Chondroid lesions
Knee	Osteosarcoma, adamantinoma, chondromyxoid fibroma
Ribs	Metastasis, myeloma, Ewing's, chondrosarcoma, fibrous dysplasia
Spine (vertebral body)	Metastasis, myeloma, eosinophilic granuloma, chordoma, Paget's, hemangioma
Spine (posterior elements)	Aneurysmal bone cyst, osteoid osteoma, osteoblastoma
Parosteal	Myositis, osteosarcoma, chondrosarcoma, chondroma
Multiple lesions	Metastasis, myeloma, hemangioma, fibrous dysplasia, osteochondromas, enchondromas, histiocytosis X

Reprinted and modified, with permission, from Miller MD: *Review of Orthopedics,* Saunders, 1992, p. 168.

organism in a child under 5 years old, while *S aureus* occurs in a child over 5 years. In adults, gonococcus is the most likely offending organism. Arthroscopic or open surgical drainage is the treatment of choice, including placement of drains and the use of intravenous antibiotics.

TUMORS OF THE MUSCULOSKELETAL SYSTEM

Tumors of the musculoskeletal system are uncommon. Benign tumors are more common than malignant ones. Benign tumors are subclassified as latent, active, or aggressive. Malignant tumors are subclassified as lowgrade

or highgrade, based on their behavior. Tumor spread is by the hematogenous route. Satellite lesions are caused by local spread of tumor within the pseudocapsule (reactive zone). **Skipped metastases** are nodules located within normal tissue outside the reactive zone. Both these entities may be responsible for local recurrence following tumor resection.

The **GTM system** (grade, tumor site, metastasis) is the Enneking system for staging tumors. G0 describes benign tumors, malignant tumors are either low-grade G1 or high-grade G2. G0 lesions have distinct margins on x-ray but can be divided into latent, active, and aggressive forms. G1 lesions have frequent mitoses and moderate differentiation and can be invasive but do not have satellite lesions. G2 lesions have more frequent mitoses, anaplastic, pleomorphic and hyperchromatic cells.

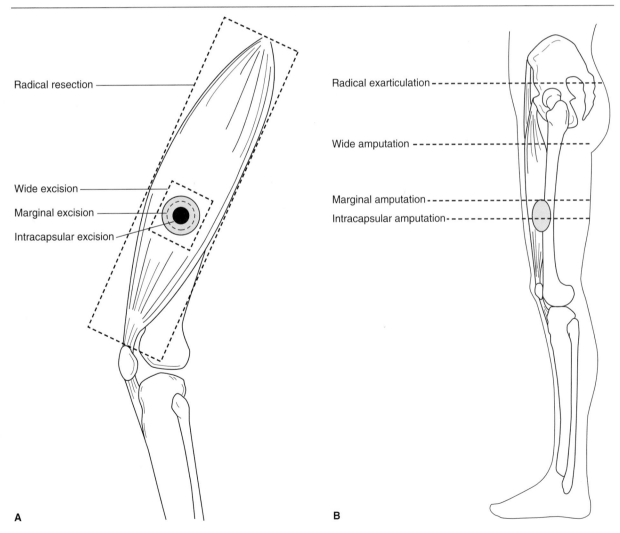

A

B

Figure 42–11. *A* and ***B:*** Tumor margins. (Reprinted, with permission, from Enneking WF: A system of staging musculoskeletal neoplasms. Instr Course Lect 1988;37:8.)

Table 42–5. Characteristics of soft tissue tumors.

Tumor	Common Sites	Clinical Presentation	Histology	Treatment	Prognosis
Fibrous Tumors					
Juvenile aponeurotic fibroma	Hands & wrists	Painful masses	Disorganized fibrous tissue, cartilage islands	En bloc excision	Moderate recurrence
Aggressive fibromatosis	Trunk	Infiltrative, aggressive spread	Spindle cells, dense collagen	Wide excision	High recurrence
Nodular fasciitis	Volar forearm	Tender, rapidly growing nodules	Fibroblasts, myxoid; inflammatory cells	Excision	Moderate recurrence
Malignant fibrous histiocytosis	Thigh	Mass	Spindle cells/histiocytes, storiform pattern	Wide/radical excision ± XRT, ± chemo	Poor
Fibrosarcoma	Thigh/arm	Lobulated deep mass	Spindle cells, herringbone pattern	Wide/radical excision ± XRT, ± chemo	Poor
Fatty Tumors					
Lipoma	Shoulder, proximal thigh	Well-defined, painless, mobile mass	Mature lipocytes, myxoid	Marginal excision	Low recurrence (except angiolipoma)
Liposarcoma	Shoulder, proximal thigh	Large, painful mass	Lipoblasts, myxoid or pleomorphic	Wide/radical excision ± XRT, ± chemo	Poor
Neural Tumors					
Neurilemmoma	Peripheral nerve (upper extremity > lower)	Enlarged nerve	Antoni A & B areas	Marginal excision (shell out)	Good
Neurofibroma	Multiple	Multiple nodules	Nodules (Verocay bodies)	Excision if painful	Malignant degeneration
Neurofibrosarcoma	Multiple	Multiple painful nodules	Palisading pleomorphic spindle cells	Wide/radical excision ± XRT, ± chemo	Poor
Muscle Tumors					
Leiomyoma	Multiple	Subcutaneous mass	Normal smooth muscle cells	Excision	OK
Leiomyosarcoma	Deep	Painful mass	Wavy mitotic cells	Wide/radical excision	Moderate–poor
Rhabdomyosarcoma	Extremities	Painful mass	Pleomorphic spindle cells, parallel bundles, giant cells	Wide excision, chemo, ± XRT	Poor
Vascular Tumors					
Hemangioma	Thigh, intramuscular	Purple mass, thrill	Epithelium-lined vessels	Observation	Good
Glomus tumor	Hands & feet	Blue-red skin discoloration, nail changes	Abundant vessels	Marginal excision	Good
Angiosarcoma	Extremities	Painful, purple mass	Vessels, pleomorphic cells	Wide/radical excision ± XRT, ± chemo	Poor
Kaposi's sarcoma	Hands & feet	Like pyogenic granuloma, AIDS	Spindle cells, vascular spaces, phagocytic cells	Chemotherapy/ excision	High recurrence
Synovial Tumors					
Ganglia	Wrist	Painless, cystic nodule	Collagenous tissue with few cells, myxoid fluid	Aspiration/excision	Good
PVNS	Knee	Painful boggy joint	Vascular villi, hemosiderin-stained giant cells	Synovectomy	High recurrence
Synovial chondromatosis	Large joints	Pain, swelling, stiffness	Nests of cartilage, stalks, free bodies	Synovectomy	Moderate recurrence
GCTTS	Hands & feet	Firm nodules, flexor surface	Round cells, spindle cells, giant cells, xanthoma cells	Marginal excision	Good
Synovial sarcoma	Long bone joints	Multinodular, radiographic calcification	Biphasic: spindle & epithelioid	Wide/radical excision ± XRT, ± chemo	Poor–moderate

Table 42–5. Characteristics of soft tissue tumors. (continued)

Tumor	Common Sites	Clinical Presentation	Histology	Treatment	Prognosis
Lymphatic Tumors					
Lymphangioma	Skin, subcutaneous	Subcutaneous masses	Lymph, vessels, smooth muscles	Avoid excision	Moderate
Lymphangiosarcoma	Skin, subcutaneous	Painful subcutaneous masses	Like angiosarcoma	Wide/radical excision ± XRT, ± chemo	Poor
Other					
Epithelioid sarcoma	Hand	Firm multinodular mass	Granulomatous, focal necrosis, inflammatory	Wide excision	High recurrence
Clear cell sarcoma	Foot & ankle	Multinodular mass near tendons	Nests of round cells with clear cytoplasm ± pigment	Wide/radical excision, chemo, ± XRT	Poor–moderate
Alveolar cell sarcoma	Skeletal muscle	Multiple nodules	Glandular nest of PAS + cells	Wide/radical excision	Moderate–poor

GCTTS = giant cell tumor of the tendonous sheath; PVNS = pigmented villonodular synovitis.
Reprinted and modified, with permission, from Miller MD: *Review of Orthopedics,* Saunders, 1992, p. 171.

The site of the tumor is determined by radiography, nuclear studies, CT scan, and MRI studies. T0 lesions are confined within the capsule and within their compartments of origin. T1 tumors have extracapsular extension into the reactive zone around them. Both the tumor and the reactive zone are confined within the compartment of origin. T2 lesions extend beyond the anatomic compartment of origin by direct extension. A tumor that involves major neurovascular bundles is classified always as a T2 lesion. Regional and distal metastases have worse prognoses. No metastases is designated M0 and the presence of metastases or skipped metastases as M1. Staging of sarcomas are based on these parameters (Table 42–3).

Four factors should be considered when radiographics are reviewed:

(1) Anatomic location and site (Figure 42–10) (Table 42–4).
(2) Effect of the lesion on the bone. Malignancies have large destructive lesions, associated soft tissue masses, and irregular margins. MRI is helpful in determining the size of these features.
(3) Response of bone to the lesion. Internal margins can be well circumscribed (geographic) and either sclerotic or nonsclerotic, or poorly defined. Multiple staggered holes is given the description "moth eaten." Multiple oval or cortical lucencies are described as "permeative." The reaction of periosteum is also a measure of the degree of the malignancy. The periosteum can be continuous and destructive with a thin shell, or exaggerated with onion skin appearance. The periosteum can be interrupted, creating a Codman's triangle, or it can have a complex sunburst ("hair on end") appearance, as is typical with osteosarcoma. Finally, the extracellular substance that is produced by the tumor causes certain appearances on a radiograph. Osteoid is cloud-like; chondroid calcification may have a ring-like appearance; and fibroid may look like ground glass.

Other radiographic correlations with tumors include a flattened vertebra plana with eosinophilic granuloma, vertebral striations or jail house vertebra hemangioma, a picture frame vertebra caused by Paget's disease, or an ivory vertebra caused by lymphoma, Paget's, or osteoblastic metastases. The shepherd's crook deformity of the proximal femur is caused by fibrous dysplasia. A nidus in an oval lesion is osteoid osteoma. A fallen leaf sign (a fracture through a bone cyst) with fluid-filled level on CT is consistent with an aneurysmal bone cyst, and an eccentric soap bubble appearance is characteristic of non-ossifying fibroma.

Five conditions can mimic almost anything and should always be considered in the differential diagnosis: (1) metastases; (2) infection; (3) cartilage tumors; (4) fibrous dysplasia; and (5) eosinophilic granuloma.

Laboratory studies may not be helpful, but a complete blood count to determine elevated white cell count or sedimentation rate may be useful in making a diagnosis. Calcium, phosphate, alkaline phosphate levels, liver function tests, blood urea nitrogen, creatinine, and urinalysis may also be helpful. Serum/urine protein electrophoresis or immunoelectrophoresis can help determine the presence of myeloma. Bone scans may be helpful to determine the presence of metastatic disease. Some tumors may present with a cold scan with little reaction, including multiple myeloma, eosinophilic granuloma, lymphoma, and sarcomas. CT scans and MRI are very useful in evaluating bone lesions. Chest CT studies are helpful to determine any evidence of lung metastases. Malignant neoplasms have high intensity on T2 weighted images with MRI studies. An-

Table 42–6. Characteristics of bone tumors.

Tumor	Decade	Common Site	Location[1]	Radiographs	Histology	Treatment	Prognosis
Osteogenic							
Osteoid osteoma	2	Proximal femur	M/D	Nidus with sclerotic rim	Trabeculae, giant cells, fibrovascular stroma	Observation, marginal excision	Rare recurrence
Osteoblastoma	2	Vertebrae (posterior elements)	(P)V	Lucent, thin reactive rim > 2 cm in size	Trabeculae, giant cells, fibrovascular stroma	Marg. excision ± cryo-surgery	Rare recurrence
Osteoma	2–5	Mandible, maxilla tibia	Flat	Ossified protrusion	Lamellar bone	Observation	Rare recurrence
Ossifying fibroma	2	Tibia, fibula	D(Ec)	Bowing	Fibrous tissue, bone, giant cells	Observation	Good
Paget's	3–5	Sacrum, spine, femur	Flat	Ivory vertebrae, cotton wool, bowing	Incr. blasts & clasts mosaic appearance	Calcitonin, diphosphonates	6% malignant degeneration
Osteosarcoma:							
Central	2	Knee, prox. humerus	M	Lytic and/or blastic, soft tissue mass	Hypercellular, anaplastic spindle cells making osteoid	Radical/wide excision/ adjuvant chemotherapy	Poor
Parosteal	3	Distal posterior femur	M	Lobulated ossified mass	Low-grade, fibroblastic stroma	Wide excision	Good
Periosteal	2	Femur, tibia	D	"Scooped out," partial calcification	Chondroid with osteoid spicules	Wide local excision, reconstruction	Moderate
High-grade surface	2	Femur	M/D	Cortical destruction	Chondroid, spindle osteoid, pleomorphic, freq. mitosis	Radical/wide excision, adjuvant chemotherapy	Poor
Chondrogenic							
Enchondroma	2–5	Hands, feet	IM	Medullary, punctate, calcification	Hypocellular cartilage	Observation, curettage, bone graft	Rare recurrence
Periosteal chondroma	2–4	Prox. humerus	M/D	Shallow cortical defect < 3 cm in size	Cartilage lobules	En bloc excision	Rare recurrence
Osteochondroma	2	Distal femur, tibia, humerus	M	Contiguous projections, calcification cartilage cap	Marrow connects to bone, disorg. epiphyseal cartilage	Observation, excision at maturity	Rare recur., 1% malignant degeneration
Chondromyxoid fibroma	2–3	Prox. tibia	M(Ec)	Eccentric, elongated, radiolucent	Chondroid (stellate cells), myxoid & fibrous areas	Curettage, graft, or marg. excision	Rare recurrence
Chondroblastoma	2	Prox. humerus, knee	E	Lucent, small, sharp margins	Fibrochondroid islands, giant cells, chicken wire calcification	Curettage, bone graft	10% recurrence
Chondrosarcoma							
Central	4–6	Pelvic/shoulder girdle	M/D	Partial calcification, cortical erosion	Chondroid, cellular, pleomorphic binucleation	Wide excision	Histology dependent
Peripheral	3–4	Ilium, humerus, femur	M	Osteochondroma with change, lytic	Cytologic atypia, stringing of matrix	Wide excision	Histology dependent
Mesenchymal	3	Pelvis, ribs, jaw	D	Poor margins, cortical destruction, calcification	Bimorphic: hyaline cartilage, round/spindle cells	Wide excision	Poor
Dedifferentiated	5–7	Femur, pelvis	M/D	Like central with aggressive area	Bimorphic: hyaline cartilage, high-grade spindle cells	Radical/wide excision ± chemo, ± XRT	Poor
Clear cell	3–4	Prox. femur	E	Epiphyseal, ± marginated	Lobulated, mononuclear clear cell, giant cells	En bloc resection	Good

	Age (yr)	Location	Site[1]	Radiographic	Histology	Treatment	Prognosis
Fibrogenic							
Simple cyst	1–2	Prox. humerus/femur/tibia	M	Sharply marginated, "fallen leaf"	Thin fibrous lining, macrophages, giant cells	MPA injections, curettage & bone graft	40–50% recurrence
Aneurysmal bone cyst	2	Vertebrae, femur, tibia	M	Cystic expansion, sclerotic rim	Cavernous space, fibrous walls giant cells	Curettage & bone graft	15% recurrence
Fibrous dysplasia	2–3	Skull, ribs, femur	M/D	Ground glass, expansile, bowing	Fibrous tissue, irregular woven bone	ASX: observation; SX: curettage & bone graft	Variable recurrence
Fibrous cortical defect	2	Distal femur, tibia	M(Ec)	Oval, sharp margins, multilocular	Fibrous tissue, clusters of giant cells, lipophages & macrophages	Observation	Rare recurrence
Malignant fibrous histiocytosis	2–7	Distal femur, tibia	M/D	Lytic, cortical destruction, soft tissue mass	Spindle cell, storiform pattern, giant cells	Radical/wide excision ± chemo, ± XRT	Poor
Fibrosarcoma	2–7	Knee, humerus	M/D(Ec)	Lytic, cortical destruction, soft tissue mass	Spindle cell, herringbone pattern, giant cells	Radical/wide excision ± chemo, ± XRT	Poor
Hematopoietic							
Eosinophilic granuloma	1–2	Pelvis, femur, spine	D	Lytic, vertebra plana	Histiocytes + eosinophils, giant cells	Observation, chemotherapy	Rare recurrence
Myeloma	5–7	Spine, pelvis, ribs	(B)V	Multiple lytic lesions	Plasma cells, amyloid	Chemo ± XRT, prophylactic stabilization	Solitary: Moderate
Malignant lymphoma	3–7	Femur	D	Permeative, lytic, poor margins	Lymphocytes, cleaved nucleus strands	XRT ± chemo	Poor
Vascular							
Hemangioma	3–7	Skull, spine	(B)V	"Jailhouse" vertebrae	Cavernous, vascular spaces	ASX: observation; SX: curettage & bone graft	Rare recurrence
Angiosarcoma	2–7	Long bones, vertebrae	(B)V	Lytic, multifocal	Atypical endothelial cells	Wide/radical resection ± chemo, ± XRT	Unknown
Hemangiopericytoma	3–6	Pelvis	Flat	Lytic ± honeycomb	Increased oval cells, thin "staghorn" vessels	Wide resection	Unknown
Neurogenic							
Chordoma	5–7	Sacrum/skull	(B)V	Asymmetrical destruction, soft tissue mass	Lobulated cords of physaliforous cells, chondroid	Wide excision	High recurrence
Neurilemmoma	2–7	Mandible	Flat	Discrete, erosive	Hypocellular spindle cells, Verocay bodies	Marginal excision	Protracted
Other/Unknown:							
Giant cell	3–4	Knee, distal radius	E	Expansive lytic lesion	Giant cells w/nuclei in mononuclear cells	Excision ± cryosurgery/phenol bone graft vs. polymethyl methacrylate (bone cement)	30% recurrence, 5% malignant degeneration
Adamantinoma	2–3	Tibia	D	Multicentric lucency, expansion	Epithelial nests w/nuclear palisading (spindle)	Wide local excision	Good
Ewing's	1–2	Pelvis, fibula, femur	D	Permeative, lytic, onion skin	Small blue cell, fibrous strands, pseudorosettes	Chemo, wide excision vs. XRT	Poor
Metastases	4–7	Proximal	D/M	Multiple lucencies	Glandular (breast, prostate, lung, kidney, thyroid) or squamous	Tailored to patient	Poor

[1]M = metaphyseal; D = diaphyseal; (P)V = posterior vertebral; IM = intramedullary; E = epiphyseal; M(Ec) = metaphyseal (eccentric); M/D(Ec) = metaphyseal/diaphyseal (eccentric); (B)V = vertebral body. POS = positive; NEG = negative.
Reprinted and modified, with permission, from Miller MD: *Review of Orthopedics*, Saunders, 1992, p. 177.

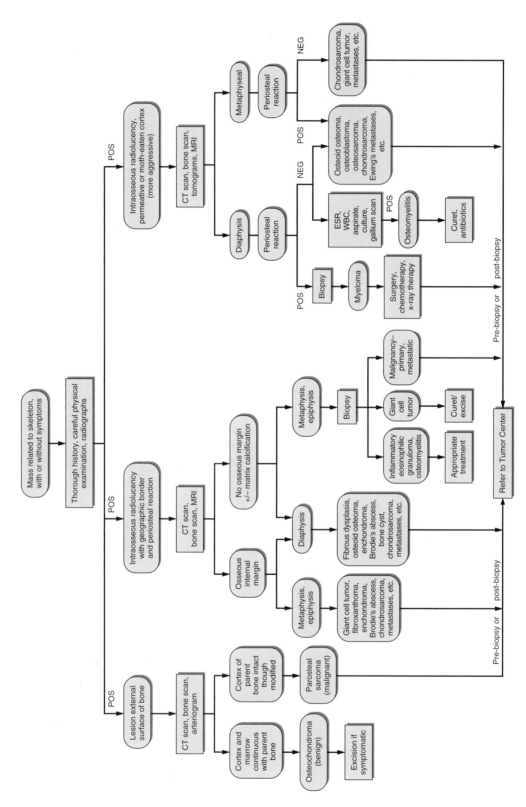

Figure 42–12. Algorithm for management of skeletal tumors. POS = positive; NEG = negative. (Reprinted and modified, with permission, from Wiesel SW et al: *Essentials of Orthopedic Surgery*. Saunders, 1993, p. 111.)

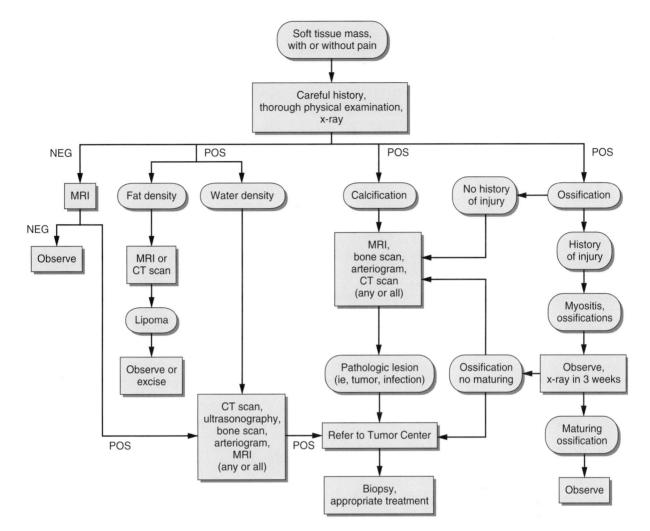

Figure 42–13. Algorithm for management of soft tissue tumors. POS = positive; NEG = negative. (Reprinted and modified, with permission, from Wiesel SW et al: *Essentials of Orthopedic Surgery.* Saunders, 1993, p. 114.)

giography may be helpful in planning tumor surgery and response of the tumor to chemotherapy.

Surgical procedures include biopsy, which should be done after staging procedures. Longitudinal incisions are necessary and the biopsy should be intramuscular. Care must be taken not to contaminate potential soft tissue planes. Needle biopsies may not be accurate. Most biopsies are incisional. Excisional biopsies are reserved for benign-appearing lesions. The classification of surgical pro-

cedure is based on the surgical plane of dissection in relation to the tumor (intracapsular, marginal, wide, or radical) (Figure 42–11). A comprehensive list of soft tissue tumor sites, presentation, histology, treatment, and prognosis can be found in Table 42–5. Table 42–6 contains similarly comprehensive information concerning bone tumors. Finally, chemotherapy and radiation therapy are very important in delaying the onset of metastases and in reducing local recurrence (Figures 42–12 and 42–13).

SUGGESTED READING

Adams JC: *Outline of Orthopedics,* 12th ed. Churchill Livingstone, 1995.

Miller MD: *Review of Orthopedics.* Saunders, 1992.

Salter RB: *Textbook of Disorders and Injuries of the Musculoskeletal System,* 2nd ed. Williams & Wilkins, 1983.

Wiesel SW et al: *Essentials of Orthopedic Surgery.* Saunders, 1993.

43

Neurosurgery

Mark C. Watts, MD, & Henry Brem, MD

► Key Facts

- ► The brain is divided into cortex, brainstem, and cerebellum. The cortex is divided into dominant and non-dominant hemispheres, which are further divided into four lobes. The brainstem is composed of three sections known as the midbrain, pons, and medulla.

- ► The volume within the skull is fixed so that any change requires immediate compensatory action to maintain constant pressure within the skull.

- ► The four types of herniation syndromes that may occur when intracranial pressure continues to rise are cingulate, uncal, central, and tonsillar.

- ► Increasingly, neurosurgery has come to rely on newly available radiologic modalities such as CT, MRI, angiography, sonography, myelography, and nuclear medicine studies to aid in the diagnosis of neurologic disease.

- ► Brain abscess has a variety of etiologies, including systemic illness, direct contiguous spread, sepsis, immune deficiency, hereditary hemorrhagic telangiectasia, cardiac arteriovenous shunting, and bacterial endocarditis.

- ► Linear, nondisplaced skull fractures require no surgical intervention, while compound fractures often require surgical exploration and debridement.

- ► Closed head trauma generally results in three types of primary brain injury: contusion, laceration, and axonal shear injury.

- ► The three most common types of cerebral hematoma include intracerebral hematomas, epidural hematoma, and subdural hematoma.

- ► Each year about 180,000 patients are diagnosed with brain tumors in the United States. This estimated figure includes both primary and metastatic tumors.

- ► In general, brain tumors produce three types of symptoms: seizure, headache, and focal neurologic deficits.

- ► Intracranial vascular malformations can be divided into four groups based on their intrinsic anatomy: capillary telangiectasias, venous malformations, cavernous malformations, and arteriovenous malformations.

- ► Rupture of a cerebral aneurysm results in approximately 28,000 subarachnoid hemorrhages (SAH) in North America each year.

- ► The current trend in treating SAH is toward early surgical intervention with clip placement to prevent rebleeding.

- ► Back pain is one of the most common reasons patients seek medical care.

- ► The three major types of pain are nociceptive, deafferentation, and sympathetically maintained pain.

- ► Neurologic developmental anomalies include arachnoid cysts, craniosynostosis, Chiari malformations, spinal dysraphism, and hydrocephalus.

ANATOMY

The anatomy of the nervous system is exquisitely complex. A comprehensive understanding of the brain and its coverings is best obtained by starting superficially and working toward the brain.

SCALP

The scalp is composed of five layers: the skin, connective tissue, galea aponeurotica, loose connective tissue, and periosteum of the skull (Figure 43–1). The rich anastomotic layer of blood vessels, branches of the external carotid artery, course through the loose connective tissue adjacent to the galea. At the anterior and posterior aspects of the cranium the galea is effectively stretched between the frontalis and occipitalis muscles. Consequently, a tear in the galea results in copious bleeding, not only because of the anastomotic network, but also because the vessels are pulled apart, preventing clot formation.

SKULL

The skull is composed of an inner table and an outer table of dense cortical bone. These layers sandwich a thin layer of cancellous bone known as the **dipole** (Figure 43–1).

MENINGES

Inside the skull are the layers of the meninges: the dura, the arachnoid, and the pia. The dura defines two important potential spaces: the epidural space and the subdural space. Beneath the arachnoid and above the closely adherent pia is a real space known as the **subarachnoid space** (Figure 43–1).

BRAIN

The surface of the brain is a series of undulating convolutions in which the hills are gyri and the valleys are sulci. The brain is divided into cortex, brainstem, and cerebellum.

Cortex

The cortex is subdivided into dominant and non-dominant hemispheres by a leaf of dura known as the **falx cerebrum**. Each hemisphere is further subdivided into four lobes: frontal, occipital, parietal, and temporal, the functions of which are listed in Table 43–1 (Figure 43–2). Lesions of a particular lobe result in deficits in the function ascribed to that lobe.

Brainstem

The brainstem is divided into three sections: the midbrain, the pons, and the medulla. Throughout the brainstem are the longitudinal collections of cells, the **reticular formation**, which govern wakefulness. The brainstem contains cell bodies for 11 of the 12 cranial nerves and is also the conduit for the long fiber tracks carrying information to and from the brain and the rest of the body (cell bodies of the optic nerves are in the retina).

Cerebellum

The cerebellum is attached to the posterior aspect of the brainstem. Its hemispheres are separated from those of the cortex by a leaf of dura, the **tentorium cerebelli**. The cerebellum's main function is to coordinate and modulate muscle movement and to maintain the body's equilibrium.

SPINAL CORD

At the distal end of the medulla lies the spinal cord, which begins at the foramen magnum and ends at L1 or L2. There are eight cervical, 12 thoracic, five lumbar, and five sacral pairs, and one coccygeal pair of nerve roots exiting the spinal cord. At the end of the spinal cord the nerve roots travel distally along the cauda equina to exit at

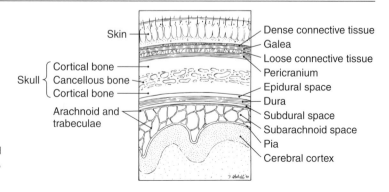

Figure 43–1. Layers of the scalp, skull, and meninges. Important spaces include the subgaleal, epidural, and subdural.

Table 43–1. Major functions of the lobes of the brain.

Lobe	Function
Frontal	Emotional affect, planning and sequencing of movement, and voluntary eye movement. The dominant frontal lobe subserves the motor component of speech (Broca's area).
Temporal	Olfaction, auditory and visual perception, memory and learning, and olfaction. The dominant temporal lobe subserves comprehension of speech (Wernicke's area).
Parietal	Motor control and cortical sensation. The dominant parietal lobe subserves motor programs and the non-dominant lobe subserves spatial orientation.
Occipital	Visual perception and involuntary eye movements.

the appropriate spinal interspace. The spinal cord contains the long fiber tracks that carry information to and from the body, as well as cell bodies of the nerves that activate individual muscle groups.

ARTERIAL ANATOMY

The brain derives its blood supply from the paired carotid arteries and the paired vertebral arteries that form the **circle of Willis**, an anastomotic loop at the base of the brain. The diameter of the circle of Willis is equivalent to the diameter of a nickel. The circle of Willis enables continued supply of blood to the brain, even if one of the major feeding vessels is occluded. The branch points around the circle of Willis are the common location of cerebral aneurysms (Figure 43–3).

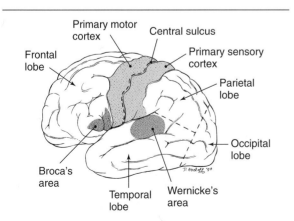

Figure 43–2. Lobes of the brain. Broca's area, Wernicke's area, and primary motor cortex. The primary sensory areas are shaded.

VENOUS ANATOMY

The brain contains both superficial and deep drainage systems. The deep drainage system consists of the internal cerebral veins that drain into the vein of Galen, where it is joined by the inferior sagittal sinus; these vessels, in turn, drain into the straight sinus. The superficial drainage system consists of cortical veins that traverse the subarachnoid space to drain into the superior sagittal and transverse sinuses. The confluence of the sagittal, straight, and transverse sinuses is the torcula. Blood ultimately exits the skull via the paired internal jugular veins that receive blood from the paired transverse sinuses via the paired sigmoid sinuses.

VENTRICULAR ANATOMY

The ventricular system comprises two paired lateral ventricles that connect with a midline third ventricle via the paired foramina of Monro. The third ventricle connects with the midline fourth ventricle via the narrow aqueduct of Sylvius. **Cerebrospinal fluid** (CSF) is a transudate of the blood made principally by the choroid plexus located in the lateral ventricles and the fourth ventricle. CSF made in the lateral ventricles traverses the ventricular system, foramina, and aqueduct to the fourth ventricle, where it exits the brain via the foramina of Luschka and Magendie. The CSF bathes the spinal cord and subsequently the convexity of the brain, where it is reabsorbed into the sagittal sinus via the arachnoid granulations. Approximately 500 mL/d of CSF are made in the adult (Figure 43–4).

PHYSIOLOGY

The anatomic constraints imposed by the skull, its dural attachments, and the brain itself have important physiologic implications. The skull is, by nature, a rigid structure. The major intracranial compartments include the brain (parenchyma and interstitial fluid), CSF, and blood. Since the volume within the skull is fixed, a change in one of the components or the addition of a fourth component (eg, tumor, blood clot) requires a compensatory decrease in the other compartments to maintain constant pressure within the skull. This principle is known as the **Monro-Kellie doctrine**. In the physiologically normal system, the introduction of a mass lesion causes compensatory extrusion of blood and CSF from the cranial vault. Naturally, these compensatory changes have limits. Initially, small changes in volume have little effect on intracranial pressure (ICP). As volumes increase, the compensatory mechanisms are exhausted and even minute changes in volume result in considerable increases in pressure (Figure 43–5).

The importance of ICP relates to its effects on cerebral

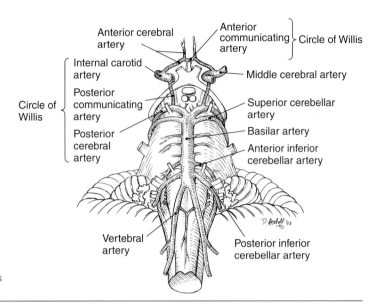

Figure 43–3. The circle of Willis and the major arteries of the brain.

blood flow (CBF): CBF = MAP (mean arterial blood pressure) – ICP. Normal CBF ranges from 55 to 60 mL/100 g brain tissue/min. Deviations from this have physiologically important implications for brain function, as highlighted in Table 43–2.

The **blood-brain barrier**, another physiologically important anatomic feature, is formed by tight junctions between the cerebral endothelial capillary cells and restricts the flow of molecules to the delicate neural tissue. Water-soluble substances cross the barrier via carrier-mediated transport, whereas fat-soluble substances are transported via pinocytic vesicles. Disruption of the tight junctions of the endothelial cells of the capillaries, as seen with brain tumors, causes leakage of plasma components, resulting in vasogenic edema.

CONTROL OF INTRACRANIAL PRESSURE

Various treatments are utilized to control ICP and, therefore, maintain an adequate CBF. Their mechanisms of action are based on the concepts described by the

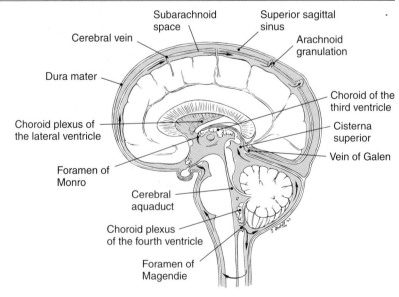

Figure 43–4. Circulation of cerebrospinal fluid and major venous structures.

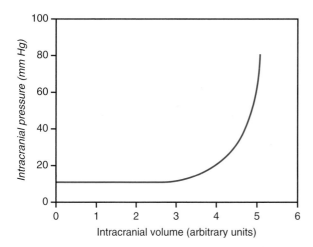

Figure 43–5. Plot of intracranial volume versus pressure. Small changes in volume at low total volumes do not result in significant changes in pressure. At a critical volume, minute changes in volume result in significant changes in pressure. (Reprinted, with permission, from Way LW: *Current Surgical Diagnosis & Treatment,* 10th ed. Appleton & Lange, 1994, p. 813.)

Monro-Kellie doctrine and the unique anatomic features of the brain vasculature.

Raising the head of the bed with the patient's head in a neutral position provides a reasonable compromise between cerebral blood flow and venous drainage. Increased elevation impedes blood flow by reducing blood pressure at the brain, while lowering the elevation impedes venous drainage. Without the head in a neutral position, venous drainage is potentially impaired by the impedance of blood flow through the jugular veins.

Mannitol has been used primarily as an osmotic agent. Intravenous introduction of mannitol causes a transient increase in serum osmolarity that results in a shift of fluid from the brain parenchyma to the serum, thereby decreasing the size of the brain compartment. Mannitol requires an intact blood-brain barrier to function effectively; without the barrier, mannitol leaks into the interstitium and fails to establish an osmotic gradient.

Loop diuretics (eg, Lasix) have a similar effect to mannitol. Induction of the loss of free water through diuretic effect on the kidney raises the serum osmolarity and decreases total body water. Loop diuretics are also thought to potentiate the effects of mannitol as well as decrease the rate of CSF production.

Table 43–2. Cerebral blood flow and cerebral physiology.

CBF (mL/100 g brain tissue/min)	Physiologic State
50–65	Normal
25	EEG flatten
15	Physiologic paralysis
10	Cell death

Hyperventilation works primarily on the blood compartment by causing cerebral vasoconstriction, thereby reducing the volume of blood within the cerebral vasculature. This, however, has the potentially deleterious effect of reducing CBF. At high intracerebral pressures, blood flow to the brain is already reduced. Further reductions in CBF could induce cerebral ischemia. In addition, the vasoconstrictive effects of hyperventilation are short-lived because of the body's intrinsic metabolic compensatory mechanisms. Thus, hyperventilation is useful only in response to acute changes in ICP and for short periods of time. A modest reduction of PCO_2 to 28–32 mm Hg provides a reasonable balance between cerebral blood flow and ICP.

Corticosteroids (dexamethasone) reduce vasogenic edema associated with brain tumors, but do not reduce cytotoxic edema associated with trauma. Corticosteroids are thought to stabilize cell membranes of endothelial cells, thereby restoring their normal permeability, which in turn reduces plasma leakage and consequent vasogenic edema.

Ventricular drainage is the most direct way to reduce one of the intracranial components. A ventricular catheter placed into the ventricle enables the clinician both to monitor ICP and actively reduce the volume of the CSF component. Placement of a ventricular catheter poses modest risk of further parenchymal injury and subsequent infection.

Barbiturates can be used to reduce ICP. One of their mechanisms of action is to slow the metabolism of the brain, thereby reducing the nutritive needs of the parenchyma. They are also thought to have a protective effect on the neural substrate. Because of their profound deleterious effects on hemodynamic stability, barbiturate therapy is generally used when ICP is refractory to other therapies.

HERNIATION SYNDROMES

The Monro-Kellie doctrine is useful in an idealized space. The brain, however, is not sitting within an idealized space. The rigid dura of the falx and the tentorium cerebelli compartmentalize it and lend it support. Clinically, these structures give rise to herniation syndromes when ICP continues to rise (Figure 43–6).

Cingulate herniation is the displacement of the medial aspect of the hemisphere, the cingulate gyrus, across the midline under the inferior edge of the falx, caused by mass lesion in the cerebral hemispheres. No specific clinical signs or symptoms are associated with this type of herniation. Its radiographic appearance indicates significant increased intracranial pressure.

Uncal herniation is the displacement of the medial aspect of the temporal lobe, the uncus, over the edge of the tentorium cerebelli, caused by a mass in the region of the temporal lobe. The classic syndrome of impaired con-

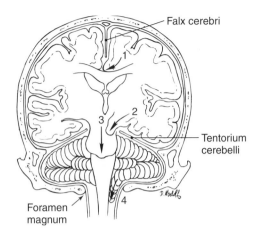

Figure 43–6. Herniation syndromes. Cingulate hernation (1), uncal herniation (2), central herniation (3), and tonsillar herniation (4).

sciousness secondary to compression of brainstem reticular cells, contralateral hemiparesis secondary to compression of the corticospinal tract in the brainstem, and ipsilateral pupillary dilation secondary to compression of parasympathetic fibers carried with the third cranial nerve, represents this form of herniation.

Central herniation is the downward displacement of the midbrain through the tentorium cerebelli acete caused by central or bilateral mass lesions. The clinical syndrome is highly variable. Small pupils, Cheyne-Stokes respirations, loss of vertical gaze, and obtundation are common findings.

Tonsillar herniation is the downward displacement of medial cerebellar structures, the cerebellar tonsils, through the foramen magnum, typically caused by mass lesions in the region of the cerebellum below the tentorii cerebelli. The clinical syndrome is associated with compression of the medulla, resulting in bradycardia, hypertension, and respiratory irregularity. Collectively, these symptoms are known as **Cushing's triad**.

NEURORADIOLOGY

Increasingly, neurosurgery has come to rely on newly available radiologic modalities to aid in the diagnosis of neurosurgical disease. Each modality has intrinsic advantages and limitations. The neurosurgeon must choose the appropriate imaging study based on the patient's history, signs and symptoms, and physical examination. The choice of the appropriate imaging study results in the most efficient and cost-conscious care of the patient.

PLAIN RADIOGRAPHS

Plain radiographs of the skull have played a diminishing role in the diagnosis of neurosurgical disease. Their utility in cranial trauma has decreased with the advent of computed tomography (CT), largely because the findings on skull radiographs do not correlate with the extent of intracranial damage. In the subacute setting, they are often unreliable in the diagnosis of sinus infection. Plain films are, however, invaluable in the diagnosis of bony trauma to the cervical, lumbar, and thoracic spine, and are also useful in the evaluation of degenerative conditions of the spine, and for intraoperative localization during spinal surgery.

COMPUTED TOMOGRAPHY

Since 1972, successive generations of CT scanners have provided higher resolution images and in shorter amounts of time. At present, CT remains the most efficient means of screening patients with head trauma and is the most sensitive imaging study for the detection of subarachnoid hemorrhage. It is invaluable for evaluation of the paranasal sinuses, the bony orbit, and the temporal bone.

MAGNETIC RESONANCE IMAGING

Since the late 1980s, magnetic resonance imaging (MRI) has become the preferred initial imaging study for suspected lesions of the brain and spinal cord and their coverings. Its ability to detect and delineate intracranial lesions is enhanced by utilizing contrast agents. The superb images obtained with magnetic resonance, however, have their limitations. MRI is insensitive to subarachnoid blood and is less sensitive than CT for calcifications. It provides little information in purely bony disease, except for detection of replacement of bone marrow that often accompanies metastasis. In addition, patients with pacemakers, suspected metallic foreign bodies, and non–MRI-compatible implants or clips cannot undergo MRI. Magnetic resonance angiography (MRA) provides noninvasive information on the vasculature of the brain and spinal cord.

CEREBRAL ANGIOGRAPHY

Cerebral angiography remains the gold standard for evaluation of the cerebral vasculature and vessels of the neck. Angiography is essential for the diagnosis and evaluation of carotid vessel disease, aneurysms, arteriovenous malformations, and a variety of intracranial vasculitides. It also has an adjunctive role in assessing vascularization and vessel patency in brain tumors. This procedure may be used therapeutically to decrease the vascularity of tumors and vascular malformations by injection of agents that obstruct feeding vessels (embolization) and by endovascularly treating select aneurysms.

MYELOGRAPHY

Myelography with subsequent CT is useful in patients who cannot undergo MRI, critically ill patients, and patients whose MRI studies are equivocal in terms of delineating a primarily bony disorder.

SONOGRAPHY

Ultrasonography is a superb screening test for plaques and stenosis of carotid arteries; the addition of color flow Doppler provides excellent information about flow direction, velocity, and turbidity. In the neonate and infant, ultrasonography is sensitive for both intraventricular and parenchymal hemorrhage as well as in the assessment of ventricular size. Ultrasonography is useful in the detection of congenital malformations manifested as changes in the size and shape of parenchymal and fluid spaces in both the pre- and postnatal periods. It is also useful for intraoperative localization of brain and spinal cord lesions.

NUCLEAR MEDICINE

Nuclear medicine studies are commonly used in the diagnosis of specific neurosurgical disease states. Technetium pertechnetate is useful to confirm the absence or presence of blood flow to the brain in brain death studies. Indium injected into the CSF space is useful in the detection of sinonasal CSF leaks.

Positron emission tomography (PET) with fluorine-labeled deoxyglucose may distinguish recurrent tumor from radiation necrosis in recurrent brain tumors. Finally, single photon emission computed tomography (SPECT) utilizes specific tracers to evaluate blood flow and metabolism. These agents have been used experimentally in the study of stroke and dementia.

CRANIAL INFECTION

Infection of the brain and its coverings can be localized in any of the layers covering the brain. Infections of the scalp are rare because of its ample vascularization. Similarly, osteomyelitis of the skull is rare. Most infections of the skull are the result of contiguous spread or penetrating trauma. The most common offending organisms are *Staphylococcus aureus* and *S epidermidis*. Treatment with antibiotics alone is rarely curative. Definitive therapy includes open surgical debridement and excision of infected bone. Surgery is generally followed with antibiotics for 6–12 weeks.

Subdural and epidural empyema (purulent infection) are generally due to contiguous spread from a nidus of local infection. The clinical presentation for subdural empyema includes fever, focal neurologic deficit, nuchal rigidity, headache, and seizures. Nuchal rigidity in tandem with unilateral hemisphere dysfunction should raise suspicion of subdural empyema. CT or MRI with contrast are the most useful radiographic studies, but subdural empyema is at times difficult to visualize. Lumbar puncture can be hazardous and is of limited value. Once the diagnosis is made, urgent craniotomy is indicated to debride the infected region. Aerobic streptococci and staphylococci are the usual offending agents. Antibiotics are continued for several weeks. The mortality from this entity approaches 20%.

Brain abscess has a variety of etiologies, including systemic illness, direct contiguous spread, sepsis, immune deficiency, hereditary hemorrhagic telangiectasia, cardiac arteriovenous shunting, and bacterial endocarditis. Typically, patients present with signs of increased ICP, seizure, lethargy, or focal neurologic deficits. CT and MRI remain the diagnostic studies of choice, which can discern whether abscesses are single or multiple, mature or immature. This has therapeutic implications: multiple and immature abscesses are treated primarily with systemic antibiotics, whereas mature solitary abscesses are usually treated with excision, if accessible, or aspiration, if inaccessible. In either case, antibiotics are continued and the lesion is followed with serial MRI or CT until it fully regresses. The use of corticosteroids to control edema remains controversial: although they help control edema associated with abscess, they may also retard maturation of the abscess. Overall mortality from brain abscess approaches 20%, while the rate of significant neurologic disability is nearly 45%.

CRANIOCEREBRAL TRAUMA

Head trauma is among the leading causes of death among young people in United States. Twenty-five percent of all closed head trauma results in a surgical lesion. Brain injuries seen in conjunction with closed head trauma are a result of the anatomic relationships between the brain and the skull and the force of the impact. Injuries to the scalp and skull may belie the full extent of intracranial damage.

SCALP LACERATIONS

Lacerations to the scalp, because of its rich vascular supply, can result in extensive loss of blood. Simple linear lacerations require only minimal debridement, copious irrigation, and closure with nonabsorbable monofilament sutures. Deep sutures that encompass the galea serve to staunch bleeding and reduce the incidence of subgaleal hematoma. More complex stellate or degloving injuries may require skin grafting or the use of vascularized pedicle flaps. Fortunately, the vascularity of the scalp enables rapid healing and serves as a competent barrier to infection.

SKULL FRACTURES

The greatest importance of the presence of a skull fracture is as a gauge of the forces involved during the injury. CT has supplanted plain films in diagnosis and management. Palpation of skull fractures can be fraught with difficulty, since a subperiosteal hematoma of the skull can mimic skull fractures.

Simple linear, nondisplaced skull fractures require no surgical intervention, but patients should be observed for 24 hours for delayed neurologic compromise. Children should receive additional follow-up to ensure that the arachnoid has not insinuated itself within the fracture, resulting in a leptomeningeal cyst or a "growing" fracture. Compound fractures in which the skull is fractured and the overlying scalp is lacerated often require surgical exploration and debridement, although some can be managed in the same fashion as linear skull fractures.

Depressed skull fractures in which the outer table of the skull of one side is depressed below the inner table of the skull of the adjacent side should be elevated, particularly if a neurologic deficit is present. If, however, the fracture is over eloquent cortex and no neurologic deficit is present, it is prudent not to elevate the fracture. Elevation of a fracture does not reduce the incidence of post-traumatic seizures.

Basilar skull fractures are common and are often diagnosed clinically by the presence of raccoon's eyes or Battle's sign (postauricular ecchymosis). On CT, fluid in the mastoid air cells is seen more commonly than an actual fracture. Usually these fractures do not require treatment. If, however, a CSF leak develops, antibiotic therapy to prevent meningitis is recommended. Rarely, cranial nerve injury results from basilar skull fracture. An immediate seventh nerve palsy, which often requires immediate surgical attention, suggests compression of the nerve from a bony fragment, whereas delayed seventh nerve palsy often represents swelling of the nerve. In all cases a CT of the temporal bone and possible surgical exploration are warranted.

CLOSED HEAD INJURY

Closed head trauma results in essentially three types of primary brain injury: contusion, laceration, and axonal shear injury. A significant blow to the head results in deformation of the skull with subsequent contusion of the underlying brain. This is a **coup injury**. If the brain is set into motion as a result of the blow, the brain's impact on the dural attachments or skull opposite the initial impact can also result in contusion. This is a **contrecoup injury**. Areas of contusion are often found at the frontal and temporal poles where the brain is relatively fixed by the skull. In more severe head injury, such as those resulting from automobile accidents, acceleration, deceleration, and rotational forces come into play. Acceleration and deceleration forces, when rapid, not only can result in contusion, but can also result in laceration of the brain. Disruption of the delicate bridging vessels traveling through the pia and arachnoid can result in hemorrhage outside the brain. Rotational injuries result in the shearing of axons within the white matter.

In the comatose patient, once the ABCs (airway, breathing, and circulation) are established, immediate evaluation of the neurologic status must be undertaken. The best initial assessment of the neurologic status of any patient is the 15-point Glasgow Coma Scale (GCS) (Table 43–3), which easily conveys information among examiners with a high rate of reproducibility. A more detailed neurologic examination with emphasis on pupillary symmetry and reactivity, extraocular motility, and symmetry of muscular strength in the extremities is appropriate for the noncomatose patient. In trauma, the depressed level of consciousness is likely to be secondary from the trauma itself, but the possibility remains that an underlying medical disorder precipitated the trauma. Routine examinations are helpful in elucidating factors that may have precipitated the trauma.

Once initial stabilization and evaluation are complete, the patient should obtain a CT of the brain. Contusions of the brain have a range of appearances from punctate to well-circumscribed areas of high signal. On the initial CT, axonal injury is not apparent, but punctate regions of high signal in the white matter tracts of the superior brainstem and the corpus collosum suggest axonal shear. Patients should undergo repeat CT if there are acute changes in neurologic examination or if the initial CT shows intracranial damage.

Table 43–3. Glasgow Coma Scale.

Points	Motor
6	Obeys commands
5	Localizes pain
4	Withdraws to pain
3	Flexor posturing to pain
2	Extensor posturing to pain
1	No response
Points	**Verbal**
5	Oriented
4	Confused
3	Inappropriate speech
2	Incomprehensible speech
1	No response
Points	**Eye Opening**
4	Spontaneous
3	To speech
2	To pain
1	No response

Patients with head injury should be closely monitored. Those with severe head injury (GCS < 9), should be monitored in an ICU setting. In addition to the general care required by the trauma patient, routine tests and specific care for the head-injured are provided in Tables 43–4 and 43–5.

The decision to monitor intracranial pressure is based in theory on whether meaningful serial neurologic examinations can be obtained. A GCS of less than 9 usually precludes a reliable neurologic examination. The initial attempt to monitor ICP should begin with placement of a ventricular drain, because if the ICP is indeed elevated, CSF can be drained from the ventricles in an attempt to lower the ICP (see previous section on Physiology). In some cases, ventricular drainage is not possible and one of several forms of electronic ICP monitors can be placed in the epidural space, the subdural space, or the brain parenchyma. Electronic monitors have proven more reliable than fiber optic systems. The Richmond screw (subarachnoid bolt) is still used in some centers, but is mostly of historical importance.

Management of the intracranial pressure is crucial to the prevention of secondary damage to the brain after initial injury. Swelling from intracranial damage can be virtually immediate in its onset and can last several days. Therapeutic maneuvers used to lower ICP have been previously discussed. In addition, sedation and paralysis can reduce muscular tone and cough. There is no role for corticosteroid therapy in trauma.

CEREBRAL HEMATOMAS

Intracerebral Hematomas

Intracerebral hematomas (Figure 43–7) are collections of blood within the substance of the brain and are often a result of the coalescence of contusions. They are relatively uncommon to present alone, but are generally seen in conjunction with epidural and subdural hematomas. Diagnosis is based on CT and the clinical course resembles that of closed head injury. Surgical treatment of intracerebral hematomas is controversial, because potentially normal brain must be traversed to evacuate the clot. Surgical intervention is considered when the clot presents in ineloquent cortex or in a location that may precipitate a clinically significant herniation syndrome.

Epidural Hematomas

Epidural hematomas (Figure 43–7), collections of

Table 43–4. Routine tests for the head-injured patient.

Serum electrolytes
BUN glucose
Complete blood count
Toxicology screen
Electrocardiogram
Chest x-ray

BUN = blood urea nitrogen.

Table 43–5. Specific care of the head-injured patient.

1. Raise head of bed 30 degrees.
2. Position head in neutral position.
3. Monitor serum electrolytes, serum glucose, and arterial blood gases.
4. Monitor blood pressure.
5. Provide aggressive respiratory care.
6. Feed via alimentary tract as soon as possible.
7. Monitor intracranial pressure if indicated.

blood between the dura and skull, usually result from laceration of a meningeal vessel; typically, laceration of the middle meningeal artery by a fracture of the squamous portion of the temporal bone. Classically, epidural hematomas are associated with a brief loss of consciousness, followed by a lucid interval, and a subsequent decline in level of consciousness, although this occurs in only 30% of cases. Diagnosis is based on CT, where the classic biconvex lens-shaped area of high signal is seen adjacent to the skull. The mainstay of treatment is rapid surgical decompression. Some small epidurals can be managed conservatively with serial CT scans, provided the patient is not neurologically compromised by the insult. Epidurals are also caused by rupture of the transverse or sagittal sinuses. Generally, the clinical course assumes a slower pattern, and surgical decompression remains the mainstay of therapy.

Subdural Hematomas

Subdural hematomas (Figure 43–7) are blood collections that occur in the potential space between the dura and the arachnoid. Generally, they are the result of the tearing of bridging veins that pass between the cerebral cortex and the cerebral sinuses. In elderly or alcoholic patients with cerebral atrophy, the precipitating trauma may be as minor as stepping off a curb. The clinical presentation can range from agitation to modest headache to coma. The management of subdural hematomas depends on the size, age, and the neurologic consequences of the clot. Large clots exhibiting mass effect and producing neurologic deficits require surgical removal. Smaller asymptomatic clots can be managed conservatively with serial CT. Chronic subdurals can form when the subdural blood is insufficiently reabsorbed. A friable membrane forms on the chronic subdural, which is prone to rebleeding. Layers of subdural hematomas and their associated membranes can be seen at the time of presentation, suggesting multiple episodes of bleeding.

There are no absolute predictors of outcome in closed head injury. Generally, more severe injuries have a poorer prognosis. The overall incidence of post-traumatic seizure is roughly 5% of closed head-injured patients. At present, seizure prophylaxis in patients with hemorrhagic injury is indicated within the first week after the injury with therapeutic levels of phenytoin (Dilantin). After the first week, the drug may be discontinued. If a seizure disorder subsequently develops, antiseizure therapy can be resumed.

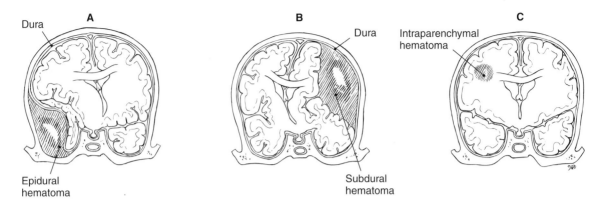

Figure 43–7. *A, B, C:* Intraparenchymal, epidural, and subdural hematomas.

Once acute management is complete, head-injured patients require the full spectrum of rehabilitation services.

BRAIN TUMORS

Each year an estimated 180,000 patients are diagnosed with brain tumors in the United States, including primary tumors that arise from the brain and its coverings, and metastatic tumors that originate elsewhere in the body (Figure 43–8). Primary tumors can be benign and malignant. Overall metastases are the most common lesions, representing nearly 50% of all brain tumors, with glioma, meningioma, and pituitary tumors following in descending order of frequency. The common metastases include tumors that originate in lung, breast, skin (melanoma), colon, and kidney. Melanoma is unique in that it has a relatively low incidence but an extremely high predilection for metastasizing to the brain.

In general, brain tumors produce three types of symp-

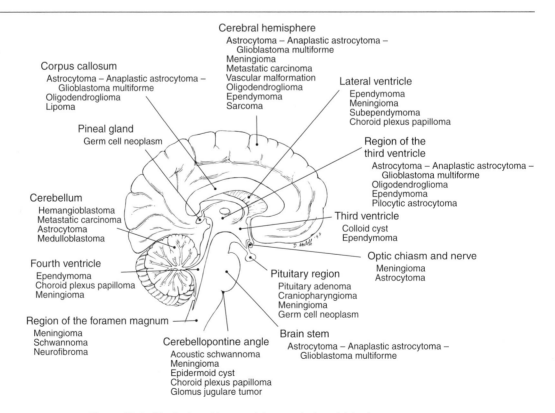

Figure 43–8. Distribution of intracranial tumors in the adult brain.

toms: seizure due to cortical irritation; headache due to increased ICP secondary to mass, edema, hemorrhage, or hydrocephalus; or focal neurologic deficits due to mass effect, edema, or destruction of neural tissue. Recognizing the group of patients with increased ICP is essential, because these patients require urgent evaluation and treatment.

The evaluation of a patient with a suspected brain tumor begins with a detailed history and physical examination. In older patients, where the incidence of metastatic disease is high, screening tests, including chest x-ray, urinalysis, stool guaiac tests, liver function tests, prostate-specific antigen, and breast examination and mammography, should be undertaken in the initial evaluation. In patients with known disease elsewhere at the time of presentation, chest-abdominal-pelvis CT and a bone scan should be obtained to evaluate the extent of disease. Many patients with metastasis have no known primary tumor.

The mainstay of radiography in brain tumors is MRI, with and without contrast, in sagittal, coronal, and axial planes. Triplanar imaging is useful to localize the tumor. A comprehensive history and physical examination and an adequate MRI enable the surgeon to provide a presumptive preoperative diagnosis. CT is helpful in delineating the extent of bony involvement of a tumor and in patients who cannot undergo MRI. Angiography is helpful in evaluating the vascularity of a tumor or a tumor's involvement with major vascular structures. MRA, however, is increasingly supplanting traditional angiography, except in cases in which embolization of a vessel is being considered.

The mainstay of brain tumor therapy remains surgery. The goal of surgery is to obtain a diagnosis and to remove as much tumor as possible without creating a new deficit. An alternative to conventional surgery is stereotactic biopsy, which is indicated in deep-seated lesions, lesions in eloquent cortex, multiple lesions, and in patients who cannot otherwise tolerate craniotomy.

Stereotactic radiosurgery, where precisely guided irradiation is directed at a tumor, is being evaluated in the treatment of brain tumors, including meningiomas, acoustic neuromas, primary gliomas, and metastases. Diagnosis is based on the imaging characteristics, history, and physical examination.

The perioperative management of brain tumor patients includes prophylactic administration of antiseizure medications (Dilantin 300 mg/d), corticosteroids (dexamethasone, 4 mg every 6 hours), and a histamine-2 (H_2) receptor blocker (ranitidine 150 mg twice each day). Postoperatively, patients are closely observed in an ICU setting overnight. Brain tumor patients are at extreme risk of developing deep venous thrombosis (DVT). If a DVT develops it is generally safe to start anticoagulation hours after surgery. A CT scan to rule out postoperative bleeding at the tumor site is helpful. Patients who are not candidates for anticoagulation therapy should undergo placement of Greenfield filters.

Radiation is the principal adjuvant therapy for brain tumors; it is reserved for malignant tumors or some benign tumors that cannot be totally resected. The addition of systemic chemotherapy with 1,3-bis-(2-chloroethyl)-1-nitrosourea (BCNU) or methyl-1-(2-chloroethyl)-3-cyclohexyl-1-nitrosourea (CCNU) has made a minimal improvement in survival. Novel therapies, including BCNU-impregnated biodegradable polymer wafers (Gliadel), have significantly improved survival in glioma patients. Other novel therapies, including biologic response modifiers, anti-angiogenesis agents, and immunotherapeutic agents, all hold some promise in the treatment of brain tumors. The incidence and survival rates of brain tumors are summarized in Figure 43–9.

VASCULAR DISEASE

VASCULAR MALFORMATIONS

Intracranial vascular malformations can be divided into several groups based their intrinsic anatomy: capillary telangiectasias, venous malformations, cavernous malformations, and arteriovenous malformations.

Capillary telangiectasias are small tangles of histologically normal capillaries typically found in the pons, which often measure less than 1 cm in diameter. They are angiographically occult, asymptomatic, and are occasionally discovered as an incidental finding on MRI. No therapy is required for these lesions.

Venous malformations are essentially anomalous veins coursing through normal neurologic structures. They are considered benign lesions that are not likely to hemorrhage. There are, however, case reports of hemorrhage associated with venous malformations, but in these cases the venous malformation is thought to be in association with other malformations.

Cavernous malformations are cystic vascular lesions lined by a single layer of epithelial cells. There is no neural tissue within the mass. These lesions have a characteristic appearance on MRI, but are often angiographically occult. They occasionally clinically present as spontaneous intracerebral hemorrhage.

Arteriovenous malformations are lesions in which the most prominent feature is the direct shunting of blood from the arterial system to the venous system. Histologically, the arteries and veins are abnormal, and there is generally no normal intervening parenchyma. More than 50% of AVMs present with spontaneous intracerebral hemorrhage; seizure and headache are also common presentations. The risk of hemorrhage in an unruptured AVM approaches 4% per year. The diagnosis of AVM is initially made with CT or MRI at the time of presentation, but definitive evaluation requires angiography.

There are several therapeutic options in the treatment of AVMs. The decision to intervene is based on the risk of hemorrhage versus the risks associated with the treatment and the likelihood that the treatment will be successful.

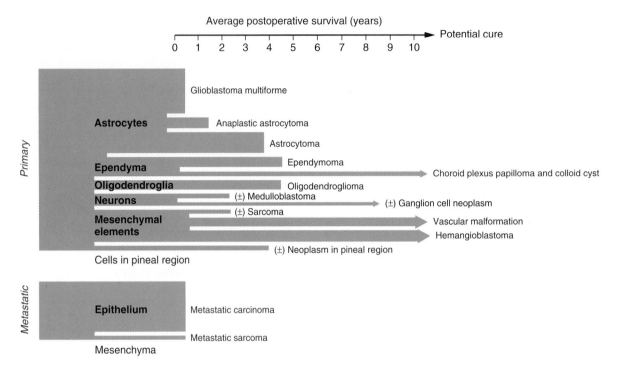

Figure 43–9. Incidence and survival rates of tumors of the brain and its coverings. The relative incidences and average postoperative survivals are indicated, respectively, by the width and length of individual arms. Primary and secondary neoplasms are shown on separate scales. (Reprinted, with permission, from Way LW: *Current Surgical Diagnosis & Treatment,* 10th ed. Appleton & Lange, 1994, p. 835.)

Surgery, endovascular embolization, and stereotactic radiosurgery alone or in various combinations form the mainstay of approaches to vascular malformations. The perioperative management includes phenytoin for seizure prophylaxis and corticosteroids for brain edema.

A variety of etiologies and conditions underlie spontaneous intracerebral hemorrhage (Table 43–6).

ANEURYSMS

Congenital defects (connective tissue disorders, arterial wall defects) and a variety of environmental effects (cigarette smoking, hypertension) play a role in the formation

Table 43–6. Conditions and disease states associated with intracerebral hemorrhage.

Trauma
Hypertension
Aneurysms (berry, mycotic, neoplastic)
Vascular malformations
Coagulopathies
Tumors
Cerebral amyloid angiopathy
Cerebral infarction
Illicit drugs (cocaine, methamphetamine)

and rupture of cerebral aneurysms. Rupture of a cerebral aneurysm results in approximately 28,000 subarachnoid hemorrhages (SAH) in North America each year. The classic clinical presentation in SAH is the sudden onset of "the worst headache in life," often accompanied by nausea, vomiting, focal neurologic deficits, seizures, or apoplexy. Nuchal rigidity, photophobia, and back pain are also common. Among several clinical grading systems for SAH, the Hunt-Hess grading system is most commonly used (Table 43–7). CT confirms the presence of SAH in 95% of aneurysmal ruptures. Patients with a strong history suggesting aneurysmal rupture and a negative CT require lumbar puncture (LP) (Table 43–8). MRI is insensitive to SAH. Once the SAH is confirmed, conventional angiography remains the gold standard for defining the location and position of the aneurysm.

The current trend in neurosurgery is toward early surgical intervention with clip placement for aneurysmal rupture because of the considerable risk of rebleeding in the first 24 hours. Several centers have begun the use of endovascular occlusion of aneurysms with detachable coils. This treatment strategy is in its nascent stages of development. The perioperative management for patients with SAH includes monitoring in an ICU setting, arterial line, antiseizure prophylaxis (phenytoin), corticosteroids (dexamethasone), analgesics (codeine), calcium channel block-

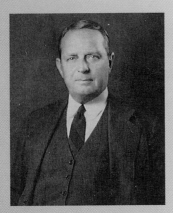

Walter Dandy (1886–1946). (Courtesy of the Congress of Neurological Surgeons.)

Walter Dandy's (1886–1946) numerous contributions to the field provided the basis for the development of modern neurosurgery. As a resident at Johns Hopkins, in 1918 Dandy discovered ventriculography and one year later pioneered pneumoencephalography. Not only were these procedures the first practical approach to directly imaging the brain, they remained a mainstay of preoperative radiographic localization of intracranial lesions until the widespread use of computed tomography in the early 1970s.

Dandy's work in anatomy and physiology was also equally important. He was the first to describe the pathway of egress of the cerebral spinal fluid as well as the organs that subserved its production. This work was the basis for classifying hydrocephalus into communicating and noncommunicating types. Dandy also described in detail the neural and vascular anatomy of the pituitary gland and the pituitary hypophysis as well as the pineal gland.

As a surgeon, Dandy pioneered many of the modern approaches to the treatment of neurosurgical diseases. Dandy can be credited with the first complete removal of an acoustic neuroma, the posterior fossa approach, sectioning of the trigeminal nerve for tic douloureux, and the first clipping of the neck of a carotid cerebral aneurysm. Dandy's genius rested in his ability to bring experimental studies from the laboratory to the clinic, resulting in a variety of new and safe operative approaches.

The breadth and depth of the work done by Dandy during his lifetime has been unparalleled and rightfully stands out as one of the great pioneers of neurosurgery.

Table 43–7. The Hunt-Hess grading system for subarachnoid hemorrhage.

Grade	Description
0	Unruptured aneurysm
1	Asymptomatic, or mild headache and slight nuchal rigidity
1a	No acute meningeal/brain reaction, but with fixed neurologic deficit
2	Cranial nerve palsy, moderate to severe headache, nuchal rigidity
3	Mild focal deficit, lethargy, confusion
4	Stupor, moderate to severe hemiparesis, early decerebrate rigidity
5	Deep coma, decerebrate rigidity, moribund appearance

Reprinted and modified, with permission, from Greenberg MS: *Handbook of Neurosurgery,* 3rd ed. Greenberg Graphics, 1994, p. 714.

ers (nimodipine), H_2 blockers (ranitidine), and a stool softener (Colace). The ultimate goal is to minimize any stresses that might induce an acute rise in blood pressure and subsequent aneurysmal rebleed.

After successful clip placement, the patient must be observed closely for signs of vasospasm, hydrocephalus, or hyponatremia, the three most common complications of subarachnoid hemorrhage. Approximately 30% of all SAH patients develop symptomatic cerebral vasospasm, which is manifested with lethargy, confusion, or focal neurologic deficits. The mainstay of treatment for vasospasm is hypervolemic-hypertensive therapy in order to maximize blood flow through the spastic vessels. Hydrocephalus leading to increased intracranial pressure occurs in 15% of patients with SAH. It is caused by failure to

Table 43–8. Features of cerebrospinal fluid in lumbar puncture in subarachnoid hemorrhage.

1. Grossly bloody, with little change in red blood cell count in successive tubes.
2. Supernatant xanthochromic.

rarely	< 2 hours
70%	< 6 hours
90%	12 hours

3. Fluid usually does not clot.
4. Opening pressure usually elevated.

reabsorb CSF at the arachnoid granulations. Treatment is with serial LPs or, in refractory cases, ventriculoperitoneal shunting. Hyponatremia following SAH is often transient and at times requires oral salt supplementation. Only one third of patients with SAH return to a virtually normal life and the 30-day mortality approaches 46%.

STROKE

The neurosurgeon's role in the treatment of stroke in addition to intracerebral hemorrhage is primarily limited to that caused by atherosclerotic carotid artery disease. Carotid artery disease can be symptomatic or asymptomatic. Symptoms include: amaurosis fugax, transient ischemic attacks (TIA) and reversible ischemic neurologic deficit (RIND), and cerebrovascular accident (CVA) (Table 43–9). The evaluation of symptomatic patients begins with Doppler ultrasonography to rule in carotid involvement and is followed by conventional angiography in Doppler-positive cases.

Medical therapy (anticoagulation and antiplatelet) and carotid endarterectomy are the two principal treatments for occlusive carotid artery disease. Carotid endarterectomy significantly lowers the incidence of stroke when compared to maximal medical therapy in patients with more than 70% carotid artery stenosis and previous symptoms referable to the ipsilateral side. Asymptomatic patients with more than 60% carotid artery stenosis also show decreased incidence of stroke with carotid endarterectomy. In patients who fall outside these criteria, an-

Table 43–9. Definitions of symptoms in stroke.

Amaurosis fugax	Ipsilateral monocular blindness that is temporary or permanent
TIA	Transient ischemic attack: a focal neurologic deficit that lasts < 24 hours
RIND	Reversible ischemic neurologic/deficit lasting > 24 hours but < 1 week
CVA	Cerebrovascular accident: a permanent neurologic deficit caused by inadequate profusion of the brain or brainstem

Modified, with permission, from Greenberg MS: *Handbook of Neurosurgery,* 3rd ed. Greenberg Graphics, 1994, p. 776.

tiplatelet therapy and anticoagulation are the treatments of choice.

SPINE

LUMBAR SPINE

The most common condition to affect the lumbar spine is back pain. Overall, back pain is one of the most common reasons patients seek medical care. Low back pain can be divided into two types: radiculopathic and mechanical. **Radiculopathy** is a constellation of findings, including pain, weakness, numbness, and hypoactive reflexes in the leg that can be ascribed to one particular nerve root. Mechanical back pain is the axial back pain that often has a musculoskeletal etiology.

Evaluation of the patient with low back pain involves a careful history and neurologic examination, with attempts to ascribe symptoms to a particular nerve root. Plain radiographs of the spine are not helpful unless trauma, infection, or malignancy are likely in the differential diagnosis. MRI is the imaging study of choice because it provides superior views of the anatomy. Myelography with CT is a useful adjunct in patients who require better delineation of the bony anatomy or who cannot tolerate MRI. Electromyelography (EMG) and nerve conduction studies (NCS) are useful diagnostic adjuncts.

Lumbar Disc Herniation

Lumbar disc herniation is most common at the lower vertebral levels. The constellation of clinical findings for each nerve root is given in Table 43–10. In general, patients with herniated lumbar discs have considerably more leg pain than axial back pain. If back pain is the primary complaint, other etiologies should be investigated. The management of herniated lumbar discs is primarily conservative, including bed rest, NSAIDs, and low levels of narcotics. Surgery is reserved for those patients who fail at least a 6-week period of conservative therapy. Indications for urgent surgery include a progressive motor deficit, intolerable pain, or cauda equina syndrome, which is caused by a central disc herniation compressing the cauda equina. The constellation of clinical findings includes saddle anesthesia, bowel or bladder incontinence or retention, or decreased anal tone; this syndrome is a neurosurgical emergency.

Lumbar Stenosis

Lumbar stenosis usually presents as the clinical syndrome of neurogenic claudication: bilateral or unilateral buttock, hip, or thigh pain exacerbated by standing and ambulation and relieved by sitting or recumbency. This syndrome generally affects older adults and consequently it must be differentiated from pseudoclaudication, which results from vascular insufficiency; patients with vascular

Table 43-10. Lumbar radicular syndromes.

Disc space	L3–4	L4–5	L5–S1
Root compressed	L5	L5	S1
Reflex diminished	Knee jerk	–	Ankle jerk
Motor weakness	Knee extension	Great toe dorsiflexion	Ankle plantiflexion
Sensory deficit	Medial ankle	Medial foot	Lateral foot
Pain	Anterior thigh	Posterior leg	Posterior leg

claudication usually have trophic changes and poor pulses in the feet and their symptoms are in the distribution of muscle groups. Management of lumbar stenosis is largely conservative with the use of NSAIDs and physical therapy. For patients with symptoms refractory to conservative management, lumbar laminectomy is appropriate.

CERVICAL SPINE

Degenerative cervical spine disease can be divided into categories based on the constellation of clinical symptoms: myelopathy, radiculopathy, and myeloradiculopathy. Evaluation of the patient with neck and arm symptomatology includes a detailed history and neurologic examination. Unlike back pain, plain radiographs of the cervical spine are helpful in determining canal width, foraminal size, and alignment of the spine. MRI provides excellent images of the neural structures within the canal. CT with myelography is useful in patients who are unable to undergo MRI imaging. In cases where the physical exam is equivocal, electrical studies, including EMG and NCS, may provide additional information.

Cervical Disc Herniation

Cervical disc herniation can produce all three categories of symptoms. The radiculopathic syndromes are summarized in Table 43–11. In general, patients with herniated cervical discs have painful limitation of neck movement in addition to their extremity symptoms: 95% of patients with predominantly radiculopathic symptoms respond to conservative therapy in the form of analgesics, NSAIDs, and cervical traction. Surgery is reserved for those who fail conservative therapy or who manifest a progressive neurologic deficit. Surgical approaches can be anterior or posterior.

Table 43-11. Cervical radicular symptoms.

Disc space	C4–5	C5–6	C6–7	C7–T1
Root compressed	C5	C6	C7	C8
Motor weakness	Deltoid	Bicep	Tricep	Hand intrisics
Sensory deficit	Shoulder	Arm and thumb	Fingers 2 and 3	Fingers 4 and 5

Cervical Stenosis

Cervical stenosis is usually a result of spinal degeneration and subsequent canal narrowing. The resulting clinical syndrome is usually myelopathy: **myelopathy** is the insidious progression of weakness and wasting of the hands, hyperreflexia progressing toward spasticity, and occasionally mild sensory loss in the hands. The pathophysiology of myelopathy is multifactorial and can be related to the spinal canal impinging on the cord, compression of vasculature feeding the cord, or multiple minor traumas to the cord associated with movement. The management of cervical stenosis is controversial, as is the decision to make an anterior or posterior approach. In general, the indication for surgery is a progressive myelopathy, since surgery is thought to halt such progression. Surgical outcome studies, however, demonstrate that about 20% of patients have progressive symptoms despite surgery.

SPINE TRAUMA

Trauma to the spine encompasses a variety of different injuries that are a result of the mechanisms of injury, the forces applied during the injury, and the unique anatomy of the spinal vertebrae.

The management of spine injuries begins at the site of the injury. In general, any patient who has significant trauma is at risk for spinal cord injury (SCI) until proven otherwise. In the field, rigid collars, spine boards, straps, sandbags, maintenance of blood pressure, and adequate oxygenation are required for the care of patients at risk for SCI. A brief neurologic examination in addition to standard trauma care is useful. In the hospital, management then focuses on diagnosing the SCI. Continued immobilization is required while the examiner takes a focused history and a focused neurologic examination, including GCS, motor strength in the major muscle groups, sensory examination that includes level and perianal sensation, reflex examination, rectal tone evaluation, and palpation over the spine. Close monitoring of blood pressure is required, because interruption of the spinal sympathetics can result in labile blood pressure.

Plain radiographs of the entire spine are the first step in rapid radiographic assessment. Any region of abnormality should have CT with two-dimensional reconstructions. MRI or CT myelogram is utilized in patients with neurologic deficits, whose neurologic examination and radiographic abnormalities are inconsistent, or who have deficits without bony abnormalities.

Spinal cord injuries can be loosely divided into two groups, complete and incomplete. Complete injury is defined as the absence of motor or sensory activity below the level of the lesion. Only 3% of patients with an initially complete examination will show improvement at 24 hours. All patients with a neurologic deficit should be given the methylprednisolone protocol for spinal cord injury in the following regimen: 30 mg/kg intravenously over 15 minutes, wait 45 minutes, then begin 5.4 mg/kg/h for the next 23 hours, then discontinue. This regimen is beneficial if started within 8 hours of the injury.

Cervical Trauma

The cervical spine is the segment most vulnerable to injury, and 42% of spine injuries occur in this region. In children, nearly two thirds of cervical spine injuries occur between the occiput and C3. Injury to the cervical spine can be particularly devastating, given the presence of the spinal cord. The complex anatomy of C1, C2, and their anatomic relationship to the occiput, coupled with the momentum generated by the head during trauma, can result in a variety of complex fractures and fracture dislocations. Management of these injuries is based on the type of injury sustained. Complete lesions require stabilization. The primary goal of surgery is to stabilize the spine in preparation for mobilization and rehabilitation of the patient. In incomplete injuries, rapid assessment and emergent decompression of the cord and other neural structures in conjunction with stabilization are required. A variety of anterior and posterior approaches are utilized, as are a number of plate, screw, and wiring systems.

Lumbar Trauma

The great majority of lower spine fractures occur at the thoracolumbar junction, T12–L1. Fractures can be classi-

fied into four groups; burst, compression, seat-belt type flexion, and fracture dislocation. Although the mechanical forces that result in each fracture differ widely, ultimately the same questions must be answered: (1) Is the fracture stable? and (2) Is there any neurologic compromise? Stability is often determined by using the three-column model of the spine (Figure 43–10). If two or more columns are disrupted based on plain films, CT, or MRI, the spinal injury is likely to be unstable. A careful neurologic examination, including detailed sensory testing, sphincter testing, and post-void residuals, must be undertaken to exclude neurologic injury. A patient with stable injuries and no neurologic deficits can be managed conservatively with bracing, rest, and analgesics. Patients with neurologic deficits or spinal instability require surgery with decompression or fusion, utilizing plates and screws.

Peripheral Nerve Trauma

The most widely used schema to grade injury to peripheral nerves is the Sunderland grading system (Table 43–12), which is based on the anatomy of the peripheral nerve. The key to management of peripheral nerve injury is an accurate clinical history and physical examination. Most injuries to peripheral nerves show maximal deficit at the time of the injury. The mechanism of injury plays a significant role in the decision for immediate surgical exploration. Sharp lacerations should be explored immediately and repaired primarily. Crush, stretch, and gunshot wounds can be explored at a later time. Two weeks from the time of injury, EMG can be performed. If it is normal, the injury sustained was, in fact, a stretch injury, and full recovery can be expected. If the EMG is abnormal, surgical repair may be required. The goal of surgery is to restore continuity between the proximal and distal axons. After transection, the distal portion of the axon dies off in what is known as **Wallerian degeneration**. Regrowth of the proximal portion of the axon proceeds at a rate of 1 mm/d or 1 in/mo. Six weeks after the nerve repair, aggres-

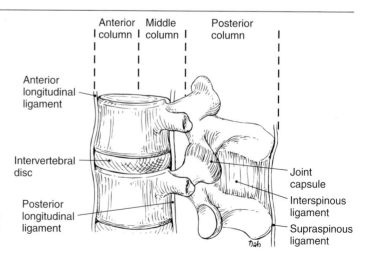

Figure 43–10. Three-column model of the spine. Damage to two or more columns is suggestive of spinal instability.

Table 43–12. Sunderland classification of nerve injury.

Grade	Description
I	Loss of axonal conduction
II	Loss of axonal continuity
III	Loss of axonal and endoneurial continuity
IV	Loss of perineurial continuity with fascicular disruption
V	Loss of continuity of entire nerve trunk

sive physical therapy is started to prevent contractures and the freezing of joints. As the nerves regenerate, progress can be monitored by following the extent of sensation along the cutaneous path of the nerve. Adjuvant surgery, including joint fusions and tendon transfers, can maximize limb function.

Entrapment Neuropathies. Because of their superficial pathways, peripheral nerves can also be subjected to entrapment neuropathies (Table 43–13). The most common of these are **carpal tunnel syndrome**, in which the median nerve is compressed by the transverse carpal ligament and **ulnar nerve entrapment** by tendons at the level of the elbow. The clinician must take time to distinguish entrapment neuropathies from other systemic causes of neuropathy, such as rheumatoid arthritis and diabetes mellitus.

The clinical signs and symptoms of carpal tunnel syndrome include: pain or numbness in the thumb, index, and middle fingers and radial side of the ring finger, weakness of the hand, and pain at site of the transverse carpal ligament. EMG and NCS can confirm the neuropathy. Mild cases can be managed conservatively with splinting, rest, and NSAIDs. Refractory cases may require surgical decompression.

Ulnar nerve compression is manifest as pain, numbness, or hypoesthesia in the little finger and the ulnar half of the ring finger, hand weakness, and pain at the medial aspect of the elbow. Conservative therapy is attempted in mild cases, while surgical decompression and ulnar nerve transposition are reserved for more refractory cases.

PAIN

The surgical relief of chronic pain can be a vexing problem for the neurosurgeon in that pain is a subjective phenomenon. Attempts to develop scales to objectify pain

Table 43–13. Important entrapment neuropathies.

Nerve	Syndrome
Median nerve entrapment	Carpal tunnel syndrome
Ulnar nerve entrapment	
Entrapment of the lateral femoral cutaneous nerve	Meralgia paresthetica
Posterior tibial nerve entrapment	Tarsal tunnel syndrome

have met with some success (see Chapter 5). There are three major types of pain: nociceptive, deafferentation, and sympathetically maintained pain.

Nociceptive pain can be further subdivided into somatic and visceral. **Somatic pain** is well localized and is often described as sharp, stabbing, aching, or cramping. It generally results from tissue injury or nerve compression. **Visceral pain** is poorly localized regional pain with various qualities. **Deafferentation pain** is the perception of disabling pain in an area that is totally or partially devoid of sensation and occurs with amputation, paraplegia, and quadriplegia. **Sympathetically maintained pain** is the triad of burning pain, autonomic dysfunction, and trophic changes.

The diagnosis and treatment of each of the pain syndromes are complex. The surgical procedures for pain are listed in Table 43–14. A variety of pain procedures can be utilized in patients with nociceptive pain who fail to respond to oral analgesics. Deafferentation pain rarely responds to oral analgesics, but often responds to the dorsal root entry zone lesion (DREZ) procedure. Sympathetically maintained pain rarely responds to medical therapy, including oral analgesics and tricyclic antidepressants. Surgical sympathectomy provides relief in 90% of cases.

PEDIATRICS

DEVELOPMENTAL ABNORMALITIES

The development of the nervous system is a complex interplay of embryonic dermal layers. Occasionally, embryogenesis and subsequent development goes awry and developmental anomalies occur.

Arachnoid Cysts

Arachnoid cysts, pockets of CSF, arise from an abnormal splitting of the arachnoid membrane during develop-

Table 43–14. Surgical relief of pain.

Electrical stimulation
  Deep brain stimulation
  Spinal cord stimulation

Intraspinal drug administration
  Epidural
  Intrathecal

Intracranial ablative procedures
  Cingulotomy

Spinal ablative procedures
  Cordotomy
  Commisural myelotomy
  Dorsal root entry zone lesion (DREZ)

Sympathectomy

Reprinted and modified, with permission, from Greenberg MS: *Handbook of Neurosurgery*, 3rd ed. Greenberg Graphics, 1994, p. 380.

ment. Most symptomatic arachnoid cysts present in early childhood. The symptoms commonly include headache, seizure, craniomegaly, and focal neurologic deficits. Diagnosis is based on routine MRI or CT. Occasionally, CSF dye studies are useful in elucidating the connection of the cysts to normal CSF pathways. The treatment of arachnoid cysts remains controversial: options include one-time needle aspiration of the cyst, fenestration of the cyst into normal CSF pathways, shunting of the cyst to the peritoneum, or a combination of these options.

Craniosynostosis

Craniosynostosis is the premature closure of skull sutures that prohibits the normal development of the skull. Diagnosis is usually made by inspection of a misshapen skull. True craniosynostosis can generally be distinguished from flattening of the skull secondary to infant positioning by instructing the parents to keep the infant off the flattened side for a period of weeks. Other diagnostic clues include: palpation of a ridge over the synostotic suture, failure of motion to gentle palpation between bony plates, and absence of lucency at the suture on plain skull radiographs. CT studies are helpful in confirming the deformity and ruling out hydrocephalus which occasionally accompanies craniosynostosis. The treatment for craniosynostosis is cranial expansion and reconstruction, with the main goal of preventing the psychological sequelae associated with deformities. In some cases of multiple suture involvement, surgery can permit the resumption of normal brain growth in an otherwise noncompliant skull.

Chiari Malformations

There are four types of hindbrain disorders known as Chiari malformations:

1. **Chiari 1**: Displacement of the cerebellar tonsils below the level of the foramen magnum. The age of presentation is midadulthood and the most common symptoms are headache, pain, and weakness or numbness of one or more of the extremities.
2. **Chiari 2**: Displacement of the cerebellar tonsils, the medulla, pons, and fourth ventricle. Absence of the septum pellucidum, hydrocephalus, and myelomeningocele often accompany this malformation. Presentation in infancy is a rapidly progressive neurologic decline with apneic spells, swallowing difficulties, and weakness. Presentation as a young child has a more insidious course.
3. **Chiari 3**: Displacement of the entire contents of the posterior fossa into the cervical canal. This deformity is incompatible with life.
4. **Chiari 4**: Hypoplasia of the cerebellum without displacement of the hindbrain structures. This is a rare anomaly.

MRI is the diagnostic modality of choice for Chiari malformations. Treatment is surgical decompression at the level of the foramen magnum with ventriculoperi-toneal shunting of the hydrocephalus and repair of the myelomeningocele as indicated.

Spinal Dysraphism

Spinal dysraphism falls into three entities, based on progressive exposure or agenesis of the posterior spinal elements. **Spina bifida occulta** is the congenital absence of spinous processes and various portions of the spinal lamina. It affects up to 30% of the population and is often considered an incidental finding. Very rarely it is associated with developmental anomalies of the spinal cord.

Meningocele is the congenital absence of the posterior elements, with cystic distention of the meninges. Although neural structures are not displaced, 30% of patients have a neurologic deficit.

Myelomeningocele (MM) is the congenital absence of the posterior elements with cystic distention of the meninges and displacement of the neural elements. Most patients have Chiari 2 malformations, and 80% of these patients develop hydrocephalus.

The diagnosis of MM can be made in utero based on increased serum alpha-fetoprotein, prenatal ultrasonography, and amniotic fluid AFP levels. These patients require extensive work-up for a host of associated abnormalities, and their management requires a multidisciplinary approach, including neonatologists, pediatric cardiologists, pediatric urologists, social workers, geneticists, and pediatric neurosurgeons. The defect should be closed by the neurosurgeon within the first 24 hours of birth. After this time, colonization of the skin by bacteria raises the incidence of postoperative infection. Patients with hydrocephalus at birth should undergo simultaneous shunting. The remaining patients should be watched closely for signs of hydrocephalus.

Hydrocephalus

Hydrocephalus is the abnormal accumulation of CSF within the ventricular system. It is generally caused by a failure in the reabsorption of the CSF produced, rather than overproduction of CSF. The reabsorption failure can occur at any point along the production pathway: foramen of Monro, third ventricle, aqueduct of Sylvius, fourth ventricle, or arachnoid granulations. The etiology can be acquired (a tumor causing mass effect on aqueduct of Sylvius) or congenital (Dandy-Walker cyst, failure of development of the foramina of Luschka and Magendie). CSF overproduction is most commonly associated with choroid plexus papilloma, and removal of the papilloma treats the hydrocephalus in two thirds of cases. MRI and CT are the main imaging tools used to diagnose hydrocephalus. Clinical presentations, which vary depending upon the age at presentation, include lethargy, nausea, vomiting, headache, irritability, and diplopia.

The treatment for hydrocephalus is shunting. Ventricular shunts most commonly have their distal ends placed in the peritoneum, but the pleural space, atrium of the heart, and ureter can all be used. Communicating hydrocephalus can sometimes be treated with a lumbar-peritoneal shunt.

The patient with a shunt for hydrocephalus and suspected shunt failure should be treated as an emergency. Rapid evaluation requires history, physical examination, CT, and plain radiographs of the shunt system. If the radiographic studies are equivocal, some shunting systems permit the introduction of a needle to assess the fluid dynamics. Surgical revision should rapidly follow the diagnosis of a malfunctioning shunt.

SUGGESTED READING

Apuzzo M: *Brain Surgery Complication Avoidance and Management*. Churchill Livingstone, 1993.

Burger P et al: *Surgical Pathology of the Human Nervous System*, 3rd ed. Churchill Livingstone, 1991.

Boldrey E et al: Intracranial aneurysms. In: Way L (editor): *Current Surgical Diagnosis & Treatment*, 10th ed. Appleton & Lange, 1994.

Bonica J: *The Management of Pain*, 2nd ed. Lea & Febiger, 1990.

Carpenter M: *Neuroanatomy*, 4th ed. Williams & Wilkins, 1991.

Cheek W: *Pediatric Neurosurgery: Surgery of the Developing Nervous System*, 3rd ed. Saunders, 1994.

Duus P: *Topical Diagnosis in Neurology*, 2nd ed. Thieme, 1989.

Edwards M: Brain tumors. In: Way L (editor): *Current Surgical Diagnosis & Treatment*, 10th ed. Appleton & Lange, 1994.

Frymoyer J: *The Adult Spine: Principles and Practice*. Raven Press, 1991.

Greenberg M: *Handbook of Neurosurgery*, 3rd ed. Greenberg Graphics, 1994.

Hoff J: Diagnosis and management of depressed states of conciousness. In: Way L (editor): *Current Surgical Diagnosis & Treatment*, 10th ed. Appleton & Lange, 1994.

Mackinnon S, Dellon A: *Surgery of the Peripheral Nerve*. Thieme, 1988.

Pitts L, Perkins R: Craniocerebral trauma. In: Way L (editor): *Current Surgical Diagnosis & Treatment*, 10th ed. Appleton & Lange, 1994.

Rengechary S, Wilkins R: *Principles of Neurosurgery*. Wolfe, 1994.

Rolak R: *Neurology Secrets*. Hanley and Belfus, 1993.

Rothman R, Simeone F: *The Spine*, 3rd ed. Saunders, 1992.

Way L: *Current Surgical Diagnosis & Treatment*, 10th ed. Appleton & Lange, 1994.

Weingart J, Brem H: Brain tumors: Diagnosis and surgical management. In: Niederhuber J (editor): *Current Therapy in Oncology*. Decker, 1992.

Youmans J: *Neurological Surgery*, 4th ed. Saunders, 1996.

44

Urologic Surgery

Gregory P. Zagaja, MD, & Gary D. Steinberg, MD

▶ Key Facts

- ▶ Flank pain associated with renal disorders may be continuous or intermittent. Intermittent pain (renal colic) is most commonly associated with an obstructing stone in the ureter, while continuous flank pain may be related to distention of the renal capsule or acute renal ischemia.

- ▶ Urinary incontinence is the involuntary loss of urine due to an increase in bladder pressure that exceeds urethral pressure.

- ▶ Microscopic examination of the urinary sediment is essential in the evaluation of hematuria. The examination should be performed on a freshly voided specimen; greater than 3–5 RBC/HPF requires further investigation.

- ▶ Impotence is divided into two categories: psychogenic (caused by emotional stress or psychiatric disease) and organic (vascular, neurologic, or endocrine disease).

- ▶ The most common causes of male infertility include varicocele, obstruction of the vasa differentia, testicular abnormalities, endocrine dysfunction, genetic factors, cryptorchidism, toxins, and chronic disease.

- ▶ Urinary tract infections are categorized as specific (associated with a specific bacteria, ie,

syphilis and tuberculosis) and nonspecific (infections that manifest themselves similarly, regardless of causative bacteria, ie, coliform bacteria).

- ▶ Acute pyelonephritis is most commonly caused by gram-negative bacteria that gain access to the kidney by ascent from the lower urinary tract.

- ▶ Approximately 10% of all trauma cases involve the genitourinary tract. Hematuria is the single best indicator of renal injury, occurring in approximately 90% of cases.

- ▶ Benign tumors of the kidney are relatively uncommon but may include oncocytoma, angiomyolipoma, hemangioma, lipoma, and leiomyoma.

- ▶ By age 80, 100% of men will have histologic benign prostatic hypertrophy, 50% will have prostatic enlargement, and 25% will have symptomatic bladder outlet obstruction.

- ▶ Carcinoma of the prostate is the most common cancer in American men, with approximately 300,000 new cases and 40,000 deaths per year.

ANATOMY & PHYSIOLOGY

KIDNEY

The kidneys are paired bean-shaped organs located in the retroperitoneum lateral to the psoas muscle. The approximate adult size measures 11.5 cm in length by 6 cm in width and 2.5–3 cm in thickness. On the medial aspect of the kidney there is a central convexity, the **renal hilum**, through which pass the renal vein, artery, and renal pelvis. The interior of the kidney is referred to as the **renal sinus**, comprising the major renal collecting structures, minor calyces, major calyces, and the renal pelvis. The substance of the kidney is divided into the **cortex** (where the glomeruli are located) and the **medulla** (where the renal concentrating mechanism is located). The kidneys and adrenal glands, which are located superior and medial to the upper pole of the kidneys, are encased in a relatively thick layer of retroperitoneal connective tissue and fat known as **Gerota's fascia**. Other organs do not directly encroach on the kidney because of this fibrous fatty tissue. However, there are many visceral organs in close proximity to this paired organ, including the spleen, tail of the pancreas and descending colon on the left, and liver, duodenum, and ascending colon on the right.

Vasculature

There is usually one renal artery, though there may be two or more, arising from the lateral aspect of the aorta just caudal to the superior mesenteric artery and the main renal artery and most commonly supplying the lower pole of the kidney. The renal artery divides into anterior and posterior branches, which may occur before they enter the renal parenchyma. The right renal artery lies behind the inferior vena cava and the right renal vein, and the left renal artery is located posterior to and slightly superior to the left renal vein.

The renal arteries are all end arteries, typically one posterior and three to four anterior branches. The anterior branches provide superior, anterior, inferior, and usually apical segmental arteries. Within the substance of the kidney the arteries divide into interlobar, arcuate, and interlobular arteries. It should be noted that all renal arteries are end arteries and the more proximal they are occluded the greater the extent of devascularized tissue. The veins usually accompany the arteries. They differ from the arteries in that they intercommunicate. If an intrarenal vein is ligated, the segment drained by that vein will drain through another venous channel. The right renal vein has few or no extra renal connections. The left renal vein, however, has two major branches entering it, the left adrenal vein cranially and the left gonadal vein caudally. Additionally, a lumbar vein may enter the renal vein posteriorly.

Innervation

The innervation is derived from the renal autonomic plexus and accompanies the renal vessels throughout the renal parenchyma. The kidney receives preganglionic sympathetic input from the eighth thoracic through the upper lumbar segments. Postganglionic fibers arise primarily from the celiac and aorticorenal ganglia. Parasympathetic innervation is from the vagus plexus of nerves. Efferent nerve endings within the kidney are mainly vasomotor and end in close proximity to renal vessels, glomeruli, and tubules. Sympathetic activity produces vasoconstriction, whereas parasympathetic activity results in vasodilation. Sensory fibers from the kidney are primarily from the renal pelvis and accompany the sympathetic nerves. They are stimulated by nociceptors sensitive to increased tension or pressure in the renal capsule, renal collecting system, or ureter.

RENAL PELVIS & URETER

The renal pelvis may be entirely intrarenal or vary in the extent to which a portion of it is extrarenal. Medially and inferiorly, the renal pelvis tapers to form the **ureter**, which courses anterior to the psoas muscle and crosses over the bifurcation of the iliac arteries as they descend into the pelvis. Rarely, the right ureter crosses behind the vena cava (the "circumcaval ureter"), and this may result in ureteral compression and obstruction. Anteriorly, the right ureter is related to the terminal ileum, cecum, appendix, and ascending colon and their mesenteries; the left ureter is related to the descending and sigmoid colon and their mesentery. Either ureter is at risk of injury during surgery involving any of these structures. Midline retroperitoneal lesions, including aortic aneurysm or massive lymphadenopathy, may deviate the ureters laterally.

In the female, the pelvic ureter courses behind the ovary and lies in the uterosacral ligament. It then continues inferiorly in a portion of the broad ligament that is closely related to the uterine cervix. Injury may occur during ligation of the ovarian vessels, or during a vaginal hysterectomy the most inferior portion of the ureter may be occluded with a clamp or suture.

Vasculature

The ureteric blood supply is mainly longitudinal but it also derives arterial input from adjacent structures. The pelvis and upper ureter receive contributions from the renal arteries. The central portion of the ureter derives a blood supply from the gonadal vessels and the aorta. The more distal portions of the ureter are supplied by branches from the aorta, the common iliacs, the internal iliacs, and ureteric branches from the superior and inferior vesical arteries. Venous drainage is via paired vessels following the course of their respective arteries. As is seen with renal tumors, the lymphatics from the left kidney and pelvis drain to the renal hilar lymph nodes and then to the para-aortic lymph nodes. On the right side the lymphatic drainage is to the hilar lymph nodes and then to the interaortocaval and lateral paracaval lymph nodes. Crossover, though infrequent, is more common from right to left. The central portion of the left ureter drains to the lateral aortic nodes whereas the central portion of the right ureter drains primarily to the right paracaval and interaortocaval lymph nodes. In the pelvis, the distal ureters drain to the internal, external, and common iliac nodes.

BLADDER

The bladder is a hollow muscular organ assuming a spherical shape in the pelvis when full. It is comprised of three layers—an outer longitudinal, a middle circular, and an inner longitudinal layer—which create an intricate network of muscular tissue. The **trigone** is a triangular-shaped muscle comprised of the ureteric musculature as it blends with the inner longitudinal layer and spreads towards the vesical neck. The bladder is supported inferiorly by the pelvic diaphragm, composed of the obturator muscle, levator ani (pubococcygeus, iliococcygeus, and ischiococcygeus), and coccygeus muscles. Superiorly, the medial umbilical ligament (urachus) attaches to the umbilicus and contributes to the support mechanism.

Vasculature

The blood supply is derived predominantly from the internal iliac artery, which further branches into the superior and inferior vesical arteries. Variably a middle vesical artery is present. As in the surgical dissection for a cystectomy, starting from the superior aspect of the bladder, the obliterated umbilical artery and then the superior and inferior vesical branches are transected. Care should be given to avoid transection of the entire anterior branch of the internal iliac artery during this dissection in order to prevent vasculogenic impotence by compromising blood flow through the internal pudendal artery. The superior gluteal artery, the first branch of the internal iliac artery, supplies the gluteus muscle. Injury to the superior gluteal artery will result in claudication of the buttocks. The venous drainage is via a complex plexus primarily on the posterior surface and base of the bladder that terminates in the internal iliac veins. The lymphatics of the bladder drain into the obturator, external, internal, and common iliac nodes; in addition, some lymph may go directly to the sacral nodes. Clinically, metastases from bladder cancer predominantly spread to the obturator and the external iliac nodes, although the sacral nodes have been noted in some studies to be involved in more than 20% of cases. The limits of the pelvic lymph node dissection, therefore, include the node of Cloquet distally, the genitofemoral nerve laterally, the bifurcation of the common iliac artery superiorly, and the lateral fascia of the rectum medially.

Innervation

The bladder is richly innervated from both divisions of the autonomic nervous system. The sympathetic innerva-

tion originates from the lower thoracic and the upper lumbar segments, mainly T11–L2. Preganglionic fibers arising from sacral segments S2–S4, the nervi verified, form the rich pelvic parasympathetic plexus. These fibers then pass through the hypogastric plexus, derived from the 1st to 3rd sacral splanchnic nerves before terminating in ganglia within the detrusor muscle. The sensation of fullness in the bladder is via the pelvic parasympathetics, and the sensations of pain, touch, and temperature are carried along the sympathetic pathways. The sympathetic adrenergic nerve endings are both alpha- and beta-adrenergic, with alpha-adrenergic predominance in the bladder base and proximal urethra and beta-adrenergic preponderance in the bladder dome and lateral walls. Alpha-adrenergic blockers are used clinically to decrease the smooth muscle tone in the bladder neck to improve micturition in men with bladder outlet obstruction due to benign prostatic hyperplasia.

PROSTATE

The prostate is a chestnut-shaped fibromuscular and glandular organ just below the urinary bladder. The normal prostate, though age-dependent, weighs about 20 g. It is supported anteriorly to the pubis by the puboprostatic ligaments and inferiorly by the urogenital diaphragm. Posteriorly the prostate is separated from the rectum by **Denonvilliers' fascia**, the obliterated remnant of the peritoneal cul de sac. The prostate is made up of five segments or zones: the peripheral zone, a central zone, a transition zone, an anterior segment, and a preprostatic sphincter zone. Benign prostatic hyperplasia (BPH) develops in the transition zone, which is periurethral, while the peripheral zone is where the majority of adenocarcinomas of the prostate develop.

Vasculature

The main arterial supply to the prostate is from the inferior vesical artery, a branch of the anterior division of the hypogastric artery. The artery terminates in two branches, the urethral and capsular arteries to the prostate. The capsular branches, within the lateral pelvic fascia, travel posterolateral to the prostate, supplying branches that course dorsally and ventrally to supply the outer portion of the prostate. Histologically, the neurovascular bundle from the pelvic plexus, which supplies the corpora cavernosum of the penis and is responsible for erectile function, is in close proximity to the capsular vessels. Consequently, the capsular artery acts as a landmark during the dissection for radical prostatectomy. Accessory vessels may arise from the middle hemorrhoidal and internal pudendal arteries. The venous drainage of the prostate is via a periprostatic plexus of veins (plexus of Santorini) that has connections with the deep and superficial dorsal veins of the penis, and the internal iliac veins. Lymphatics from the prostate drain into the obturator, internal iliac, external iliac, hypogastric, vesical, sacral, and periaortic lymph nodes.

Innervation

The innervation of the prostate is via the **pelvic plexus**, composed of sympathetic fibers from T11–L2, as well as parasympathetic fibers from the sacral center (S2–S4), and is mostly responsible for the secretory element of the prostate. The pelvic plexus provides visceral branches to the bladder, ureter, seminal vesicles, prostate, rectum, membranous urethra, and corpora cavernosa. The nerves innervating the prostate travel outside the capsule of the prostate and Denonvilliers' fascia until they perforate the capsule and enter the prostate. Branches to the membranous urethra and corpora cavernosa similarly travel outside the prostatic capsule within the lateral pelvic fascia, coursing dorsolaterally between the prostate and the rectum. The capsular vessels to the prostate are used as a landmark, during radical prostatectomy, to preserve the neurovascular bundle to the penis, when possible. The recognition of this anatomy by Walsh at Johns Hopkins has helped to decrease the incidence of impotence associated with radical surgery of the prostate and bladder.

PENIS & URETHRA

The penis is comprised of paired, dorsally located corpora cavernosa that intercommunicate. On the ventral aspect is the corpus spongiosum, through which traverses the urethra. The corpora are capped distally by the glans penis. Each corpus is enclosed in a fascial sheath, the **tunica albuginea**, and all are surrounded by a thick fibrous envelope known as **Buck's fascia**, within which the neurovascular bundle is located on the dorsal aspect of the penis. Buck's fascia, except when disrupted by infection or trauma, forms an impenetrable membrane limiting extravasation and hematoma from either the bulbous or pendulous urethra. Beneath the skin of the penis is the superficial penile fascia, which is continuous with the dartos muscle of the scrotum and Scarpa's fascia of the lower abdomen. Posteriorly it continues into the perineum and becomes recognizable as **Colles' fascia**. Colles' fascia limits urinary extravasation, hematoma, or abscess formation following trauma to the bulbo membranous urethra. This layer creates a barrier to the dissection of blood and urine that may occur after trauma to the penis.

The male urethra has three anatomical segments: (1) the prostatic urethra, which traverses the substance of the prostate, (2) the membranous urethra, that portion which passes through the urogenital diaphragm, and (3) the penile or anterior urethra, which extends from the level of the suspensory ligament to the meatus. The prostatic and membranous portions make up the posterior urethra, and the same embryological precursors account for the entire female urethra. The **urethral bulb** is an area in the proximal penile urethra that is slightly wider and serves to collect semen prior to expulsion via contraction of the surrounding bulbospongiosus muscle. The fixation and curvature of the bulbous portion of the urethra, as well as its proximity to the underside of the symphysis pubis, make it more vulnerable to injury than the distal segment. Numerous glands of Littre open into the urethra along its dorsal aspect, and the ducts from Cowper's glands drain into the bulbous urethra.

Vasculature

The penis and urethra are supplied by the internal pudendal arteries, branches of the internal iliac artery. The internal pudendal artery becomes the penile artery as it courses through the urogenital diaphragm. This further divides into three branches—the bulbourethral artery and the cavernous artery before ending as the dorsal artery of the penis. Considerable variation can be found: for example, an accessory internal pudendal artery may arise from the obturator artery, the inferior vesical artery, or the contralateral superior vesical artery. This alternate but essential blood flow may be inadvertently divided during prostatectomy or cystectomy and result in vasculogenic impotence.

The venous drainage is by the superficial dorsal vein of the penis within dartos fascia, and the deep dorsal vein of the penis, which lies between the dorsal arteries deep to Buck's fascia. These veins connect with the prostatic plexus, which drain into the internal pudendal vein and then to the internal iliac vein.

The lymphatic drainage of the penis involves three sequential groups of lymph nodes: (1) the superficial inguinal lymph nodes, (2) the deep inguinal lymph nodes, and (3) the pelvic or iliac nodes. The lymphatics of the penile skin drain via a superficial lymphatic system to the superficial inguinal nodes. However, lymphatic drainage from the glans and penile urethra drain into the deep inguinal nodes and occasionally into the external iliac nodes. The lymphatic drainage from both sides of the penis coalesce into a major collecting duct dorsally and then enter the presymphyseal plexus. With this degree of lymphatic intercommunication, it would not be atypical for a tumor on the left side of the penis to metastasize to the right groin.

Innervation

The somatic nerve supply to the penis is via the pudendal nerve (S2–S4), which branches to form the perineal and dorsal nerve of the penis after passing through Alcock's canal. The dorsal nerve of the penis then passes through the deep transverse perineal muscle to course on the dorsolateral aspect of the penis before terminating in multiple branches in the glans. The main cutaneous nerve supply to the penis and scrotum comes from the dorsal and posterior branches of the pudendal nerve and the ilioinguinal nerve. The autonomic innervation of the penis consists of sympathetic input from the lumbar nerves (L1 and L2) and parasympathetic nerves from sacral nerves (S2–S4). The cavernous nerve arises as many fibers from the pelvic plexus. These are mixed nerves, with sympathetic fibers producing vasodilation and parasympathetic

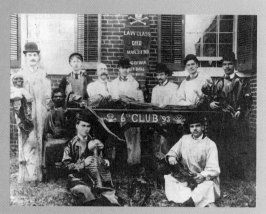

Hugh Young (c 1893) (extreme left) as a medical student at the University of Virginia. This photograph appears to have been taken to celebrate victories over the law students in a tug of war and in football and baseball. (Reprinted, with permission, from Landes RR, Bush RB, Zorgniotti AW (editors): *Perspectives in Urology: The Official American Urological Association History of Urology.* **American Urological Association, 1976.)**

Hugh Hampton Young (1870–1945) has long been considered the "father of American urology." Young was born in San Antonio, Texas, but, like his father, he attended the University of Virginia. In a period of just four years he completed his BA and MA degrees and was also awarded an MD. This was the first time (and probably the last) that such an amazing feat was accomplished. He began to practice in San Antonio, but quickly learned that he needed additional training in order to be a successful surgeon. He went to Baltimore at the age of 21.

Dr Young's long and illustrious career as a professor of urology at Johns Hopkins, under the leadership of William Steward Halsted, began in 1897 when he turned a corner and

" . . . ran into Dr Halsted with great force and almost knocked him down. I caught him before he hit the floor and began to apologize profusely. Dr Halsted, still out of breath, said, 'Don't apologize, Young. I was looking for you, to tell you we want you to take charge of the Department of Genito-Urinary Surgery.' I thanked him and said, 'This is a great surprise. I know nothing about genitourinary surgery.' Whereupon Dr Halsted replied, 'Welch [William Henry Welch] and I said you didn't know anything about it, but we believe you could learn.'" (From Young, HH: *Hugh Young: A Surgeon's Autobiography.* Harcourt, Brace and Co, 1940.)

fibers producing vasoconstriction. The cavernous nerve runs with branches of the prostatovesicular artery and veins as the so-called **neurovascular bundle**. Here, the neurovascular bundle passes anterior to Denonvilliers' fascia, between the posterolateral surface of the prostate and the rectum, before entering the perineum and eventually entering the base of the corresponding corpus.

EPIDIDYMIS

The epididymis is a markedly coiled ductal structure that is contiguous with numerous efferent ducts from the testis at its upper pole and the vasa deferentia at the lower pole. The epididymis lies posterolateral to the testis. The blood supply is from the internal spermatic artery and the artery of the vas deferens. Venous drainage is via the pampiniform plexus to the spermatic vein. Lymphatic drainage is to the pelvic lymph nodes.

TESTIS & SCROTUM

The scrotum is composed of two layers, and the testicular coat has three layers. The five layers surrounding the testis are (1) rugous skin, (2) dartos muscle, (3) external

Subsequently, Young was to prove Halsted and Welch wise judges of aptitude by pioneering the specialty of urology. Having developed the perineal prostatectomy for the relief of bladder-outlet obstruction in 1903, his logical progression was to the radical perineal prostatectomy for cancer of the prostate. This operation was first performed by Young (with Halsted assisting) in 1904. Young then reported on the punch prostatectomy in 1913 and the first demonstrated vesiculography in 1920.

The Brady Urologic Institute at Johns Hopkins opened in 1915, giving Young an excellent opportunity to develop a complete clinical and research staff in the discipline of urology. In addition to organizing an exemplary urologic residency program, he initiated and edited the *Journal of Urology* for many years, and in 1926 published his book entitled *Young's Practice of Urology* (WB Saunders).

He served in World War I with the American Expeditionary Forces, achieving the rank of Colonel and winning the Distinguished Service Medal. He was president of many medical societies, including the American Urological Association, American Association of Genito-Urinary Surgeons, Medical Chiurgical Faculty of the State of Maryland, and the Clinical Society. In 1937, the American Association of Genito-Urinary Surgeons awarded him their Keyes Medal. A friend of Young, Edward L. Keyes is reported to have stated, "The prostate makes most men old, but it made Hugh Young."

spermatic fascia (a continuation of the external oblique fascia), (4) cremasteric fascia and muscle (an extension of the internal oblique and transversus abdominis), and (5) internal spermatic fascia (an extension of the transversalis fascia). The adult testes are paired ovoid gonadal organs, in the male measuring 4.5 cm × 3 cm × 2 cm. They have a dense fibrous covering, the tunica albuginea, which invaginates the testis posteriorly to form the mediastinum testis. The testis is covered anteriorly and laterally by the visceral layer of the tunica vaginalis, which is continuous with the parietal layer that separates the testis from the scrotal wall.

Vasculature

The testicular artery arises from the aorta just below the renal artery. After coursing through the inguinal canal with the spermatic cord, the testicular artery divides into three branches: the vasal artery to the head of the epididymis and the internal and inferior testicular arteries. Venous drainage is via the pampiniform plexus to the corresponding spermatic vein. The right testicular vein enters the anterolateral surface of the vena cava just below the right renal vein, whereas the left testicular vein enters the

left renal vein at a right angle, usually lateral to the junction with the adrenal vein. Embryologically, the testes have a retroperitoneal origin shared with that of the kidney, the urogenital ridge, and they migrate during development to the scrotum. Hence, the primary lymphatic drainage is to the retroperitoneum. The right testis drains to the interaortocaval lymph nodes and subsequently to precaval, preaortic, and paracaval lymph nodes. The common drainage of the left testis is to the left para-aortic nodes just below the level of the renal vein and then to the preaortic nodes.

GENITOURINARY SIGNS & SYMPTOMS

A thorough understanding of urologic signs and symptoms is critical to the proper evaluation and treatment of the patient. A description of common signs and symptoms follows, with an emphasis on mechanism and differential diagnosis.

PAIN

The mechanism by which pain is elicited in the urinary tract is based on distention with an increase in the intraluminal pressure. The severity of the pain is related to the time course involved. Sudden distention of the ureter or renal pelvis causes severe pain, whereas a more gradual onset would produce little to no pain.

Flank pain may be continuous or intermittent. Intermittent pain is often referred to as **renal colic** and is most commonly associated with an obstructing stone in the ureter. The patient with severe renal colic commonly presents with associated nausea and vomiting. Alternative diagnoses include a congenital ureteropelvic junction obstruction, passage of a blood clot, or a ureteral tumor. Continuous flank pain is typically associated with distention of the renal capsule (pyelonephritis, chronic obstruction, or tumor) and acute renal ischemia. However, it also occurs in up to 50% of patients with distention of the ureter, renal pelvis, or calyces.

Pain impulses from the kidney and ureter are carried via visceral afferent fibers that are in close proximity to the somatic neurons, therefore, the pain may be diverted to somatic neurons, with the brain interpreting the impulse as cutaneous in origin (**referred pain**). Spinal cord segments T11 and T12 receive sensory fibers from both the upper ureter and the testis, so distention in the upper ureter may be referred to the ipsilateral testis. Referred pain may occur in the presence or the absence of true visceral pain.

SYMPTOMS RELATED TO URINATION

Symptoms associated with urination are divided initially into those related to obstruction and those related to an irritative etiology.

Obstructive symptoms are hesitancy, intermittency, nocturia, weak stream, dribbling, incomplete voiding, straining to void, and acute urinary retention. BPH is the most common cause of bladder outlet obstruction. Other causes include bladder neck contracture secondary to trauma or surgery, urethral stricture, carcinoma of the prostate, posterior urethral valves in boys, meatal stenosis, and atonic bladder. Pharmacologic agents, such as phenothiazines and anxiolytics with anticholinergic properties, may precipitate urinary retention or exacerbate obstructive symptoms. Similarly alpha-adrenergic agonists, such as pseudoephedrine, ephedrine, and phenylpropanolamine contained in many cold remedies, may cause acute urinary retention.

Irritative symptoms include frequency, urgency, urge incontinence, dysuria, nocturia, and, occasionally, enuresis. Irritative symptoms are precipitated by an irritable focus within the bladder. Occasionally, the focus may be extravesical or due to a central neurologic defect. Acute bacterial infection is by far the most common cause of bladder inflammation. Other causes include bladder cancer, calculi, BPH, urethral stricture, drugs (eg, cyclophosphamide) or radiation, nonbacterial cystitis (viral, fungal, parasitic, or interstitial), neurogenic bladder, and extravesical inflammatory lesions, such as diverticulosis, inflammatory bowel disease, or tumor.

URINARY INCONTINENCE

Incontinence is the involuntary loss of urine. The mechanism by which continence is achieved is based on the intraurethral pressure (70–80 cm of water) being greater than the intravesical pressure (10–20 cm of water). When this pressure gradient is lost and bladder pressure exceeds urethral pressure, urinary incontinence occurs.

Stress incontinence is defined as the loss of urine associated with physical strain, coughing, sneezing, laughing, or other activities that cause a sudden increase in intra-abdominal pressure. These patients are usually women who have lost some of their urethral support, with deficient transmission of intra-abdominal pressure to the urethra. This is also often the type of incontinence associated with prostate cancer surgery.

Urge incontinence is associated with a sudden uncontrollable urge to urinate, followed by the involuntary loss of urine. The cause of urge incontinence is an involuntary detrusor contraction that is usually intermittent, but with significant pressure causing leakage. This not infrequently occurs with inflammation in or near the bladder, or longstanding bladder outlet obstruction (eg, BPH) and is a common symptom of upper motor neuron lesions.

Overflow incontinence is caused by chronic failure of bladder emptying secondary to obstruction, or, less commonly, inadequate detrusor contractions of the flaccid bladder. This form of incontinence is most commonly seen in men with obstruction due to BPH, chronic obstruction, or diabetes mellitus.

True incontinence is the loss of urine without warning. These patients have little to no pressure gradient between the bladder and the urethra, and urine leakage occurs independent of stress or the desire to void. Clinically, true incontinence occurs iatrogenically with disruption of the urethral sphincter (post-radical prostatectomy), after anti-incontinence surgery in women or secondary to radiation to the pelvis, in a bypassed sphincter (urinary fistula or ectopic ureter in the female), in cases of an absent sphincter (epispadias or exstrophy), or in congenital and acquired neurogenic disease.

HEMATURIA

The causes of hematuria are vast, ranging from completely benign to malignant. However, since the degree of hematuria does not always correlate with the seriousness of the underlying cause, all hematuria warrants some degree of investigation.

Evaluation & Management of Hematuria

Hematuria is usually categorized as gross (visible to the unaided eye) or microscopic (greater than 5 cells/HPF). Gross hematuria is more commonly urologic in origin, whereas microscopic hematuria is more often associated with a nephrologic cause. The presence of dysmorphic red blood cells (RBC) on phase microscopy in addition to RBC casts is indicative of a glomerular source. Epithelial RBC usually have an even distribution of hemoglobin, with either a round or crenated shape. The presence of epithelial RBCs in the urine suggests a nonglomerular source, and they are frequently shed by tumors.

Hematuria may also be described as initial, terminal, or total. **Initial hematuria** is indicative of a source distal to the external sphincter. Prostatitis may present with initial hematuria as well as irritative voiding symptoms.

Terminal hematuria refers to blood noted chiefly at the end of urination. Terminal hematuria is often secondary to bleeding from the prostatic urethra, bladder neck, or trigone, which occurs when the bladder finally compresses these areas at the end of micturition. Causes include cystitis, prostatitis, and, less commonly, bladder calculi.

Total hematuria, a uniformly bloody urine, suggests a source in the bladder, ureters, or kidneys. The presence of epithelioid RBCs on microscopic analysis suggests tumor as the potential source, particularly in the absence of pain. Other common causes of total hematuria include infection and renal calculous disease whose diagnosis is often made with the aid of a good history, physical examination, and intravenous pyelogram (IVP). Less common causes are trauma, sickle cell disease, glomerulonephritis, tuberculosis, renal infarction, renal vein thrombosis, coagulation deficiencies, and vascular malformations.

Gross painless hematuria is often the first manifestation of a urinary tract tumor, particularly a bladder tumor. The bleeding is often episodic and may be associated with blood clots. The configuration and size of the blood clots may help to localize the source of bleeding. For example, thin "worm-like" blood clots indicate blood clotting in the ureter, and, therefore, represent bleeding from the upper urinary tract (kidney or ureter).

Microscopic hematuria is more commonly associated with a nephrologic cause, however, a significant percentage of patients with microscopic hematuria (12.5%) are diagnosed with tumor. Microscopic hematuria, therefore, may be reflective of significant underlying disease, commonly infection, stones, and tumor, and less commonly trauma, sickle cell disease, nephropathy, tuberculosis, renal infarction, and vasculitis.

Pain, urinary frequency, and dysuria are frequently associated symptoms; depending on their pattern of presentation, they may assist with localization of the hematuria. The patient presenting with flank pain and hematuria likely has renal colic secondary to an obstructing stone, whereas the patient with irritative voiding symptoms and many bacteria on urinalysis has the working diagnosis of a urinary tract infection.

Discerning a Diagnosis

When a patient presents with the complaint of hematuria, the initial step is to confirm the presence of red blood cells in the urine. Urine should be collected using the clean-catch midstream method. If a satisfactory specimen cannot be obtained, catheterization should be performed. The commonly available reagent strips may be employed to determine urinary pH, protein, glucose, and hemoglobin levels. The reagent strips are not specific for red cells and will also react positively in the presence of hemoglobin or myoglobin. Microscopic examination of the urinary sediment is absolutely essential in the evaluation of hematuria. The exam should be performed on a freshly voided specimen and the presence of greater than 3–5 RBC/HPF is significant hematuria, requiring further investigation. Dysmorphic erythrocytes suggest an origin from a glomerular or tubulointerstitial source, while cells from a nonglomerular source are round or ghost cells having lost their hemoglobin. Red blood cell casts are cylindrical clumps of RBC in the shape of the renal tubules and are pathognomonic of a renal source.

Further investigation for those patients with gross hematuria includes a plain film of the abdomen along with an intravenous urogram to identify a calculus or a filling defect within the collecting system, cystoscopy to examine the bladder, and urinary cytology to identify the presence of cancer cells in the urine. To rule out a renal parenchymal mass, ultrasonography or computed tomography (CT) is recommended. Following these noninvasive studies, further diagnostic studies may be warranted (Figure 44–1).

Intravenous pyelography is an important part of the work-up in patients presenting with gross hematuria. In the event that the upper tracts are not adequately visualized, a retrograde pyelogram should be performed at the time of cystoscopy. Cystourethroscopy is indicated in many patients with hematuria. When possible, cystoscopy should be performed in all patients with gross hematuria to increase the likelihood of identifying the source. All suspicious lesions are biopsied for histopathologic exam. Urinary cytology may be obtained as part of the evaluation of hematuria and may be helpful in diagnosing urothelial malignancies. Cytology is more sensitive in patients with high-grade tumors, however, it may be falsely negative in 20%. False-positive cytologic findings occur in 1–12% of patients. The bladder is the source of bleeding in 40% of patients presenting with gross hematuria. Overall, approximately 20% of patients will be found to have a neoplasm, most commonly bladder carcinoma; 25% will have infections as the cause; and 25% will have calculi.

Dividing hematuria into glomerular, renal, urologic, and hematologic causes we can further associate the cause with certain disease states (Table 44–1). The evaluation of microscopic hematuria in almost all instances is initiated with the appearance of 3–5 RBC/HPF or greater. The evaluation initially involves a plain film of the abdomen with IVP; if no apparent cause is evident, ultrasonography or CT is recommended to rule out a renal parenchymal le-

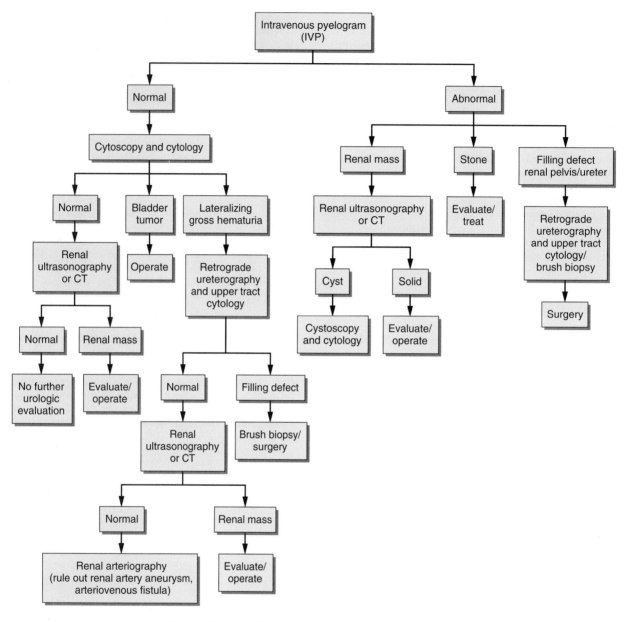

Figure 44–1. Algorithm for the evaluation of essential hematuria.

sion. Cystourethroscopy and bladder washings are indicated in the evaluation of many patients presenting with microscopic hematuria. As many as 5–10% of patients with hematuria will have no identifiable cause, even after an extensive urologic evaluation. Although the vast majority of these patients probably have insignificant disease, they should be monitored regularly. If an episode of gross hematuria occurs, cystoscopy should be performed to localize the source. As long as microscopic hematuria persists, the patient should be followed every 6–12 months with at least a urinalysis, possibly urinary cytology, assessment of renal function, and blood pressure. Repeat intravenous pyelography and cystoscopy are also recommended every other year.

PROTEINURIA

Proteinuria indicates a urinary excretion of greater than 150 mg of protein per 24 hours. The urinary excretion of

Table 44–1. Causes of hematuria.

Glomerular
Acute glomerulonephritis
Lupus nephritis
Benign familial hematuria
Berger's disease
Exercise-induced hematuria

Renal
Polycystic kidney disease
Medullary sponge kidney
Papillary necrosis
Renal infarction or embolus
Inflammation and infection
Arteriovenous fistula

Urologic
Neoplasms
Calculi
Infection
Benign prostatic hyperplasia
Urethral stricture
Endometriosis
Diverticulitis
Appendicitis

Hematologic
Coagulopathies
Sickle cell trait/disease

Factitious
Vaginal bleeding

False Hematuria
Food pigments
Drug-related

protein is about 80 mg/24 h. The major protein constituent is Tamm-Horsfall mucoprotein secreted by the thick ascending loop of Henle. Greater than 95% of the filtered protein is reabsorbed by the proximal tubules. There are four types of proteinuria: glomerular, tubular, overflow, and physiologic.

Glomerular proteinuria is the most common form of proteinuria, found in all patients with significant glomerular damage. It is predominantly an albuminuria, and urinary excretion exceeds 2 g/d.

Tubular proteinuria is usually secondary to tubular or interstitial disorders of the kidney, with the tubules unable to resorb the normal filtered load of protein. Total protein excretion is usually 1–2 g/d.

Overflow proteinuria is the consequence of abnormally elevated quantities of low molecular weight proteins that are filtered across the glomerular membrane and saturate the proximal tubular reabsorptive mechanism. Bence Jones proteins from multiple myeloma, myoglobinuria, and hemoglobinuria may overburden the resorptive mechanism in this way.

Physiologic proteinuria occurs in the absence of any detectable renal or systemic disease. This form of proteinuria is characteristically intermittent and mild, with urinary excretion rarely exceeding 1 g/d. Clinical states that may give rise to functional proteinuria include fever, exercise, stress, and congestive heart failure.

PNEUMATURIA

The passing of gas in the urinary stream strongly suggests a fistula between the urinary tract and the bowel. These occurrences are typically associated with diverticulosis, colorectal cancer, Crohn's disease, or trauma. Because air is lighter than water, it rises to the top of the bladder and is passed at the end of micturition. Recent instrumentation of the urinary tract may also give a similar picture. Enterovesical fistulas may be diagnosed by CT, barium enema, cystogram, or cystoscopy.

IMPOTENCE

Impotence is defined as the inability to obtain and maintain an erection sufficient for sexual intercourse. Impotence is usually divided into **psychogenic impotence**, that caused by emotional stress or psychiatric disease, and **organic impotence**, that caused by vascular, neurologic, or endocrine disease. In order to quickly ascertain the type of impotence, it is important to determine if the patient ever has normal erections (eg, early in the morning or during sleep). If a patient does have normal erections in the morning or during sleep, the impotence is more likely associated with a psychogenic cause. Typically, patients with organic impotence complain of loss of morning erections in addition to the gradual development of erectile dysfunction.

Vasculogenic impotence is either arterial or venous in origin. Atherosclerosis accounts for most impotence in men older than 60 years. The risk factors are similar to those associated with coronary artery disease, diabetes mellitus, hypercholesterolemia, and smoking. **Venogenic impotence**, failure of corporal occlusion, may be either primary or secondary to atherosclerosis, trauma (fractured penis), or Peyronie's disease.

Neurologic impotence is frequently associated with spinal cord injuries to varying degrees, depending on the level of the injury. Other neurologic diseases associated with impotence include multiple sclerosis, tabes dorsalis, myelodysplasia, and peripheral neuropathy of any cause.

Endocrine disorders are responsible for fewer than 5% of instances of impotence. Causes include testicular failure, pituitary failure, and hyperprolactinemia.

Other causes of organic impotence are related to trauma, postoperative/iatrogenic factors (vascular surgery with impaired flow through the internal iliac arteries, radical prostatectomy, abdominoperineal resection, and sacral rhizotomy). A number of medications cause impotence; the most frequently implicated are the antihypertensives, especially beta-blockers, alpha-blockers, clonidine, and thiazide diuretics.

INFERTILITY

Infertility is the inability to achieve a pregnancy resulting in live birth after 1 year of unprotected intercourse. Pertinent information obtained on history and physical include any history of undescended testicles, previous surgery (eg, herniorrhaphy, retroperitoneal surgery), mumps, diabetes, and gynecomastia. Post-pubertal mumps results in mumps orchitis in approximately 30% of patients. Testicular atrophy may develop within months to years after the infection.

The surgically correctable forms of male infertility include varicocele of the spermatic vein and obstruction of the vasa differentia. A **varicocele** is a dilated tortuous internal spermatic vein found in approximately 30% of male patients presenting with infertility. It is the most common surgically correctable cause of male infertility. Varicocele is more common on the left side (90%). The mechanism by which varicoceles lead to infertility is not completely understood, however, an elevation in testicular temperature secondary to refluxing blood in the internal spermatic vein has been implicated.

Clinically, a varicocele may be palpated as a soft mass above the testicle when the patient stands or strains. Typically, the varicocele disappears in the supine position. Patients with sudden onset of a varicocele, a right-sided varicocele, or one that does not reduce when the patient is supine, should be investigated with ultrasonography or CT prior to varicocele repair to rule out a renal or retroperitoneal tumor obstructing the internal spermatic vein.

Bilateral absence of the vasa differentia is rare but may occur in up to 2% of presenting patients. There is a higher association of absence of the vas in patients with cystic fibrosis. Congenital absence of the vas may be associated with renal anomalies, such as ipsilateral renal agenesis. Inflammation is the most important cause of acquired obstruction of the vasa, most commonly from gonorrhea or nonspecific urethritis. A careful evaluation of the azoospermic male includes, initially, a serum LH, FSH, and testosterone level to rule out gonadal dysfunction. Follow-up studies would include a testicular biopsy to differentiate ductal obstruction from abnormal spermatogenesis. Vasography would be performed on those men with normal spermatogenesis and presumptive obstruction. Vasography localizes the level of obstruction prior to surgical repair. If ejaculatory volume is decreased, transrectal ultrasonography may document ejaculatory duct obstruction that may be amenable to transurethral resection.

Other etiologic causes of male infertility include (1) testicular abnormalities (maturation arrest, germinal aplasia, and hypogonadotropic hypogonadism), (2) endocrine abnormalities (excess androgen, estrogen, thyroglobulin, prolactin, and glucocorticoid), (3) genetic (Klinefelter's syndrome (XXY)), (4) cryptorchidism, (5) toxins (chemotherapy, radiation, alcohol, marijuana, cigarettes, and caffeine), and (6) chronic disease (spinal cord injury, uremia, liver disease, myotonic dystrophy).

EVALUATION OF A FLANK MASS

The differential diagnoses for a flank mass are shown in Table 44–2. With the greater use of ultrasonography and CT, approximately two thirds of all locally confined renal masses are found serendipitously. Traditionally, IVP with nephrotomography was the initial step in evaluation of a flank mass. With current advances in ultrasonography and CT, these radiologic methods are used more frequently as the initial study. Ultrasonography has the advantage of being able to distinguish among solid, cystic, and complex masses. Any lesion not meeting the ultrasonographic criteria of a simple cyst, smooth and round with no internal echoes, must be studied further with CT. It is very rare that a simple renal cyst will contain carcinoma, but rather, it is the more complex cyst that may harbor carcinoma. Highly echogenic masses are rare, and most are angiomyolipomas or hemangiomas. CT has the advantage of accurately distinguishing cystic and solid lesions, detecting extracapsular extension of tumor, detecting renal vein or vena caval involvement, and assessing lymph nodes.

EVALUATION OF A SCROTAL MASS

In the evaluation of the scrotum and its contents, it is important to be able to differentiate the testis from the epididymis and cord structures. Most testicular masses are malignant, whereas most masses arising from the cord are benign. A combination of history, particularly with regard to onset, progression, and associated pain, along with physical findings, will help in the diagnosis (Table 44–3).

Testicular torsion results in twisting of the spermatic cord and occlusion of the spermatic vein and artery. The onset is acute, with unrelenting testicular pain. If not treated emergently, within 4–6 hours, complete infarction of the testis results, followed by atrophy of the testis. Prepubertal and pubertal males are most affected, but it may occur in adults and newborns. Clinically, the patient presents with sudden onset of severe testicular pain and tenderness, sometimes associated with nausea and vomiting. The patient is usually unable to find a comfortable position. The main condition in the differential diagnosis is epididymo-orchitis, which usually has a more gradual onset and is accompanied by a urinary tract infection or

Table 44–2. Differential diagnosis of a flank mass.

Benign renal tumors (oncocytoma, angiomyolipoma, lipoma, and fibroma)
Malignant renal tumors (renal cell carcinoma, transitional cell carcinoma of the pelvis, nephroblastoma [Wilms' tumor], sarcoma, lymphoma, and secondary malignant tumors)
Cyst (solitary, unilateral multiple, pyogenic [xanthogranulomatous pyelonephritis])
Vascular (hemangioma, hemartoma, lymphangioma)
Adrenal (adenoma, adrenocorticocarcinoma)

Table 44–3. Differential diagnosis of a scrotal mass.

Trauma
Testicular torsion
Epididymo-orchitis
Incarcerated hernia
Torsion of testicular or epididymal appendix
Tumor
Varicocele
Hydrocele
Spermatocele

prostatitis. On physical examination, the testicle may be distinguished from the epididymis and cord, especially if the patient seeks prompt medical attention. In this scenario one can localize the pain to the testicle on palpation. The testis will likely have a horizontal rather than a vertical orientation. Other differentiating signs may be: (1) the cremasteric reflex is absent on the affected side and (2) elevation of the testis increases pain (Prehn's sign). When medical attention has been delayed, the scrotum and testis will have significant swelling, making it difficult to distinguish from epididymo-orchitis. Diagnosis may be aided by duplex ultrasonography or by radionuclide scan. However, if diagnosis by these procedures causes significant delay in the evaluation, the patient may best be served by scrotal exploration.

A **hydrocele** is a collection of fluid between the tunica vaginalis and the tunica albuginea of the testis. Hydroceles may occur as a congenital abnormality when the processus vaginalis fails to obliterate. Congenital hydroceles are more common in infants and young children. In adults, hydroceles are more frequently associated with infection, tumor, or trauma, or are idiopathic. Transillumination of the scrotal mass is helpful in distinguishing it from a solid mass. Since tumors may be a cause of hydroceles, it is important to evaluate the testicle when a patient presents with a hydrocele. Ultrasonography will help differentiate the normal from the abnormal testicle, within the hydrocele.

INFECTIONS OF THE GENITOURINARY TRACT

Urinary tract infections are separated into specific and nonspecific. **Specific infections** are those that are associated with a specific bacteria that elicits a specific pathologic response (ie, syphilis and tuberculosis). **Nonspecific infections** manifest themselves similarly regardless of the causative bacteria (ie, coliform bacteria). The bacteriostatic properties of the urothelium as well as the relative irrigation of the urinary tract contribute significantly to the urinary tract's natural defenses.

Furthermore, urinary tract infections can be subgrouped into uncomplicated and complicated infections. Uncomplicated infections typically occur in the afebrile patient with a structurally and functionally normal urinary tract. The majority of these patients are women with isolated or recurrent cystitis occurring sporadically or potentially linked to sexual activity. A complicated urinary tract infection describes a patient with pyelonephritis or a structural or functional abnormality that would decrease the efficacy of antimicrobial agents.

TUBERCULOSIS

Tuberculous infection reaches the genitourinary tract by hematogenous dissemination. Currently, pulmonary tuberculosis and genitourinary tuberculosis are increasing in prevalence, especially in HIV-infected and other immunosuppressed patients. The kidney is affected most often, with caseating tubercles forming within the parenchyma and eventually communicating with the collecting system. The possibility of tuberculous urinary tract infection should be suspected in the patient with sterile pyuria. Up to 20% of cases are associated with a concomitant *Escherichia coli* infection of the lower urinary tract.

The diagnosis may be suspected in the individual with a history of pulmonary tuberculosis, though evidence of pulmonary infection is not always present. Occasionally, the presenting symptom of tuberculous infection is a painful swollen testis, which is to be distinguished from an acute epididymo-orchitis. When the epididymis is infected bilaterally, infertility may result and the testis may become involved by direct extension. On examination, a thickened, nontender epididymis or nodular prostate may be palpable. Sterile pyuria is indicative of tuberculosis until proved otherwise, and a high index of suspicion is necessary in order to make an accurate diagnosis. Diagnosis is made by performing a tuberculin test in conjunction with three urine cultures to identify the infecting organism.

Medical treatment includes the use of multidrug therapy (eg, pyrazinamide, isoniazid, and rifampin) daily for 2 months, followed by isoniazid and rifampin 3 times per week for 2 additional months. A fourth drug, streptomycin, may be added initially in the patient with severe infection or bothersome bladder symptoms. The fibrosis and scarring typical of tuberculosis often leads to obstruction of the ureter or urethra and contracture of the bladder. The only place for the use of corticosteroids in the treatment of tuberculosis is in the patient with acute ureteral obstruction, who may respond to a short course of steroid treatment (20 mg three times a week for 3 weeks). Unresolving stricture will require a stent or percutaneous nephrostomy tube, with eventual surgical repair. The indications for nephrectomy are a nonfunctioning kidney and extensive disease of the kidney, together with hypertension or pelviureteric obstruction.

ACUTE PYELONEPHRITIS

Pathogenesis & Etiology

Acute pyelonephritis is caused most commonly by aerobic gram-negative bacteria that gain access to the kidney by ascent from the lower urinary tract. Common etiologic factors include vesicoureteral reflux; obstruction, either congenital (ureteropelvic junction) or acquired (ureteral calculus); or hematogenous dissemination. Hematogenous infection of the kidney occurs with organisms such as staphylococci from the skin and is more likely to occur in the obstructed kidney. During pregnancy, ureteral obstruction is more common on the right side than on the left, due to the protective effects provided by the sigmoid colon.

Diagnosis

The signs and symptoms of acute pyelonephritis include abrupt onset of fever and chills, flank and lower abdominal pain, dysuria, nausea, and vomiting. Physical examination reveals moderate to severe costovertebral angle tenderness, abdominal tenderness, and, occasionally, rebound tenderness. Ultrasonography should be done or an intravenous pyelogram obtained at the time of diagnosis to rule out obstruction. If obstruction is present, percutaneous nephrostomy or ureteral stenting will be required. The causative organism can usually be identified from the urine or blood cultures. The differential diagnosis includes acute cholecystitis, acute appendicitis, and acute pancreatitis. In women the symptoms may mimic pelvic inflammatory disease.

Management

The most important aspect of treatment is to recognize and treat complicating factors, such as obstruction. Intravenous antimicrobial therapy should consist of ampicillin 2 g every 4 hours and an aminoglycoside (tobramycin 1.5 mg/kg every 8 hours). If this regimen is favorable, it should be continued for 5 days and then the patient switched over to an appropriate oral antibiotic for 2 weeks.

CHRONIC PYELONEPHRITIS

Pathogenesis & Etiology

Characteristic findings are those of renal parenchymal scarring overlying dilated calyces, generalized chronic inflammation of the kidneys, and glomerular fibrosis. Progressive parenchymal scarring leads to atrophy, with decreased concentrating ability and excretion as seen on IVP. The condition appears to be the result of infection in childhood, especially when associated with vesicoureteral reflux. Rarely has nonobstructive uncomplicated urinary tract infection alone been found to be the cause of renal insufficiency.

Diagnosis & Management

The patient is usually asymptomatic until renal insufficiency occurs, and then the symptoms are the same as with any other form of chronic renal failure. Similarly, physical findings are nonexistent. Radiologic findings as demonstrated by pyelography consist of asymmetry and irregularity to the kidney outline, blunting and dilation of one or more calyces, and cortical scars over the deformed calyx.

Treatment involves intense antibiotic therapy when infection is present, prevention of future infections, and monitoring and preservation of renal function.

Xanthogranulomatous pyelonephritis is a form of unilateral chronic pyelonephritis seen commonly in patients with diabetes mellitus and characterized by multiple parenchymal abscesses, pyonephrosis, renal calculi, and poor or absent renal function. The inflammatory response typically includes xanthogranulomas that contain lipid-laden macrophages. Bacteriuria and pyuria are almost always present, with *E coli* and *Proteus mirabilis* being the most common organisms. Radiographically, these lesions may be difficult to distinguish from a renal cell carcinoma. With a loss of renal function and difficulty in excluding renal cell carcinoma, nephrectomy is considered the treatment of choice.

RENAL & PERIRENAL ABSCESS

Pathogenesis & Etiology

A renal abscess may arise by hematogenous spread from a distant site, with *Staphylococcus aureus* being the most common infective organism, or it may result directly from pyelonephritis. During the past two decades, gram-negative organisms have been implicated in the majority of adults with renal abscesses. Ascending urinary tract infection associated with tubular obstruction from infection or calculi appears to be the primary pathway for establishing gram-negative abscesses. Complicated urinary tract infections associated with stasis, calculi, pregnancy, neurogenic bladder, and diabetes mellitus may also predispose the patient to abscess formation. The renal abscess is typically located in the cortex of the kidney.

Diagnosis & Management

The patient will often present with fever, chills, flank pain, and occasionally weight loss and malaise. Treatment should be initiated promptly with appropriate intravenous antibiotics (initially ampicillin 2 g every 4 hours and an aminoglycoside). Any obstruction of the urinary tract must be relieved. If the abscess is localized, percutaneous drainage should be performed. Perinephric abscess, with an associated 44% mortality rate, should always be drained, either percutaneously or surgically.

CYSTITIS

Pathogenesis & Etiology

Bacteriuria and urinary tract infections are common in females. Acute cystitis, in the majority of cases, occurs by urethral ascent of bacterial organisms that are colonizing the vaginal and urethral mucosa. Women resistant to urinary tract infections carry specific vaginal antibody against their own fecal *E coli*, whereas those who are susceptible have substantially less vaginal antibody directed against their colonizing strains of fecal bacteria. Additionally, such factors as hormonal status, sexual activity, antibiotic usage, and genetic traits all appear to play a role. Infection in females typically occurs during three stages of development: childhood (toilet training years), onset of sexual activity, and menopause.

Diagnosis & Management

Symptoms include frequency, urgency, dysuria, and suprapubic pain. Urinalysis reveals pyuria in nearly all cases of bacterial infection. Microscopic hematuria is present in 50% of women with acute cystitis. In the absence of complete obstruction and stasis, cystitis is self-limiting and resolves in 24–48 hours with appropriate antibiotic therapy. The probability is very high that infection is caused by *E coli*, therefore, empiric therapy with (1) trimethoprim 160 mg with sulfamethoxazole 800 mg orally twice a day, or (2) nitrofurantoin 50 mg orally four times daily, is usually satisfactory. In cases of recurrent infection, 99% are caused by a new infection with a different organism; these cases can be prevented with prophylactic antibiotics, such as oral nitrofurantoin 50 mg 4 times daily.

URETHRITIS

Urethritis is classified into two groups, gonococcal urethritis and nongonococcal urethritis (Table 44–4). The most common presentation is acute purulent urethritis. Symptoms typically occur 3–10 days after sexual contact, but may be as long as 3 months. The patient presents with urethral discharge and dysuria.

With gonococcal urethritis, there is a 35–40% incidence of concurrent chlamydial infection. It is, therefore, recommended that these cases be treated for both infections. The sexual partner of the patient should also be treated at the initiation of therapy.

ACUTE PROSTATITIS

Pathogenesis & Etiology

Acute prostatitis is common in sexually active men 20–40 years old. Infection of the prostate is usually acquired secondary to a lower genitourinary tract infection by direct reflux of infected urine into the prostatic ducts. Microabscesses occur early in the disease; rarely, they may coalesce into a large abscess as a late complication.

Diagnosis & Management

Acute bacterial prostatitis is associated with the onset of fever, chills, severe irritative voiding symptoms, dysuria, generalized malaise, and varying degrees of bladder outlet obstruction. On rectal examination the prostate is exquisitely tender, swollen, boggy, and warm to the touch. A localized fluctuant, tender region may indicate a prostatic abcess. The prostate should never be massaged for secretions in acute prostatitis. Massage is extremely uncomfortable for the patient and may disseminate bacteria through the vas deferens, causing secondary epididymitis, or, more significantly, produce a gram-negative septicemia. A prostatic abscess usually requires drainage performed transurethrally.

Initially, broad-spectrum IV antibiotics (ampicillin 2 g every 6 hours and an aminoglycoside), an oral agent can be started 24 hours after the patient is afebrile and continued for 2–4 weeks. Prostatic abscesses, when present, may be drained transurethrally.

CHRONIC PROSTATITIS

Pathogenesis & Etiology

Although chronic prostatitis may arise secondary to an episode of acute prostatitis, many men have no history of acute bacterial prostatitis. Typically, chronic prostatitis is heralded by recurrent urinary tract infections by the same pathogen. Infected prostatic calculi may be the source of bacterial persistence and relapsing infection. The organism persists in prostatic fluid during therapy because most antibiotics accumulate poorly in the prostate. During

Table 44–4. Classification of urethritis.

	Gonococcal	Nongonococcal
Pathogen	*Neisseria gonorrhea*	*Chlamydia trachomatis* *Ureaplasma urealyticum* *Trichomonas*
Incubation period	Usually 3–10 days	1–5 weeks
Symptoms	Purulent discharge	Thin, mucoid
Gram's stain	Gram-negative intracellular diplococci	Negative
Therapy twice daily x 7 days	Quinolone	Doxycycline, 100 mg

therapy the urine is sterilized, however, reinfection often occurs after discontinuation of therapy.

Diagnosis & Management

Clinical features include variable irritative voiding symptoms, dysuria, and pain perceived in various sites within the distribution of the pelvis and genitalia. Physical examination of the prostate is normal or slightly tender. Massage for prostatic secretions usually demonstrates clumps of white cells without bacteria. Treatment is often empiric with either doxycycline or a quinolone for 1 month; perineal pain can be treated with oral ibuprofen 400–600 mg three times a day.

NONBACTERIAL PROSTATITIS

Pathogenesis & Etiology

Nonbacterial prostatitis is the most common cause of the prostatitis syndrome. It is an inflammatory condition involving the prostate with no specific etiologic agent.

Diagnosis & Management

Symptoms include urinary frequency, nocturia, dysuria, and pain and discomfort perceived in the pelvic and genital areas. Physical findings are nonspecific. Repeated attempts to isolate a causative organism from the prostatic expressate are negative. Empiric therapy is often tried, very often with no effect. If an infection with ureaplasma or chlamydia is suspected, a trial of doxycycline might be reasonable. The main goal of therapy is to educate the patient, give reassurance, and relieve anxieties and concerns while treating symptoms. Symptoms of pain and discomfort are often treated with oral ibuprofen 600 mg three times daily and sitz baths.

URINARY STONES

Pathogenesis & Etiology

Urinary calculi often are idiopathic but may be related to geography, climate, diet, genetics (cystinuria), or other medical conditions (Crohn's disease and renal tubular acidosis). Eighty percent of urinary stones are composed of calcium, with 35% being calcium oxalate, 10% calcium phosphate, and 35% mixed calcium oxalate and phosphate. Other urinary stones are composed of struvite (due to infection) (10%), uric acid (8%), or cystine (1%). Renal calculi occur more frequently in men and are rare in children and African-Americans. Renal and ureteral stones are usually only symptomatic when they are obstructing the ureter, with subsequent increased pressure and distention of the kidney.

The formation of renal calculi is based on two theories: (1) supersaturation of the solute leads to crystal formation,

and (2) inhibitors of stone formation (peptides, nephrocalcin, uromucoids, citrate, and pyrophosphates) are lacking.

Diagnosis

Symptoms begin when the calculi becomes trapped, with a resultant back pressure leading to distention proximal to the obstruction. Stones typically become lodged in four areas: in the calyx, at the ureteropelvic junction, where the ureter crosses the iliac artery, and at the ureterovesical junction. Symptoms include colicky flank pain, which radiates along the course of the ureter to the scrotum and medial thigh or labia in women, hematuria, nausea, and vomiting. Urinalysis often demonstrates blood in the absence of pyuria. A urinary pH greater than 7.5 implicates urea-splitting organisms as the potential etiologic cause. A pH less than 6.5 is associated with uric acid calculi or, possibly, renal tubular acidosis. Potential complications include infection, obstruction with loss in renal function, and, occasionally, ureteral stricture formation.

With the aid of radiologic imaging, the level of the stone can be identified as well as the degree of obstruction, as evidenced by hydronephrosis. On plain film of the abdomen radiopaque stones (calcium phosphate, calcium oxalate, struvite, and cystine) may be easily seen. Radiolucent stones (uric acid) may only be appreciated as filling defects in a collecting system filled with contrast. On IVP there is delayed visualization of the nephrogram on the affected side, and delayed films may be necessary to determine the level of the obstruction. CT scan or ultrasonography of the abdomen may be helpful in localizing uric acid stones.

Renal stones may be observed if they are small and asymptomatic. If, however, they are associated with recurrent urinary tract infections, decreased renal function, pain, or sepsis, then surgical removal will be necessary. Extracorporeal shock wave lithotripsy (ESWL) is ideal for stones up to 2 cm in size. Multiple stones, stones greater than 2 cm, or stones composed of cystine or hydroxyapatite/brushite generally require percutaneous or ureteroscopic nephrolithotomy.

Management

Factors that affect treatment options for ureteral stones include size of the stone, location of the stone, duration and degree of obstruction, fever, infection, and pain not controlled with oral analgesics. Ureteral stones that are small (< 5 mm) accompanied by infrequent attacks of colic but not by infection or progressive hydronephrosis can generally be observed, with approximately 95% of the stones passing spontaneously with hydration. Any patient presenting with an obstructing stone and signs of infection should be treated promptly by placement of a ureteral stent or percutaneous nephrostomy tube. Surgical treatment varies by size and location of the stone. A stone 1–2 cm lodged at the ureteropelvic junction might best be managed by manipulating the stone back into the renal pelvis, then fragmenting it with ESWL. The lower the stone is in the ureter, the less successful are the results with ESWL. Initially, only small distal ureteral stones were considered for treatment by ureteroscopy. Now, with the aid of smaller diameter ureteroscopes and intraureteral lithotripsy, more bulky stones anywhere in the ureter are being considered for treatment ureteroscopically.

Once the stone has passed or has been removed, a metabolic evaluation may be necessary to discover the etiology of stone formation in the patient. Which patient deserves a full metabolic work is controversial, however, the patient with recurrent urolithiasis or a child with his first stone episode should be evaluated (eg, 24-hour urine for calcium, phosphate, oxalates, uric acid, creatinine, citrate, Na^+, pH, and volume; and serum levels of calcium, phosphate, uric acid, creatinine, Na^+, K^+, and protein). Parathyroid hormone levels are indicated if hyperparathyroidism is suspected in patients with elevated urinary and serum calcium. The majority of stones are secondary to dietary factors and decreased fluid intake.

TRAUMA

Approximately 10% of all trauma cases involve the genitourinary tract, however, the urinary tract is rarely injured without concomitant intra-abdominal, thoracic, or skeletal injuries. Hematuria is the single best indicator of renal injury, occurring in 90% of cases. The degree of hematuria does not entirely correlate with the severity of injury, that is, renal pedicle avulsion (artery and vein) may be associated with the absence of hematuria.

RENAL

Renal trauma is divided into two categories based on the mechanism of injury—blunt trauma or penetrating trauma. Renal trauma ranges in severity from contusion to parenchymal tear to avulsion of the renal artery or vein (Table 44–5).

Blunt renal injuries usually result from automobile

accidents (rapid deceleration), falls, contact sports, and assaults, and are responsible for 80–90% of renal trauma.

High-speed motor vehicle accidents may result in major renal trauma from rapid acceleration/deceleration and cause major vascular injury. Blunt renal injury may be further classified based on the hemodynamic stability of the patient in the field and on presentation to the emergency room.

Clinical findings that suggest a renal injury from blunt trauma are flank tenderness, flank ecchymosis (Grey Turner sign), lower rib fracture, or a flank mass. Hematuria, defined as more than 5 RBCs/HPF, is almost always present in the patient presenting with renal trauma. A palpable abdominal mass may be suggestive of a rapidly evolving retroperitoneal hematoma from a significant renal parenchymal or renal vascular lesion. Rapid deceleration injuries usually are not limited to the kidney. However, the renal injury in such cases may be a renal pedicle avulsion or acute thrombosis of the renal artery. Hematuria may not be present and the diagnosis must be made from a high index of suspicion, given the mechanism of injury. IVP or abdominal and pelvic CT scan are, therefore, recommended in all patients involved in a rapid deceleration accident. If the patient is hemodynamically stable, CT scan is preferable to IVP because of the ability to identify associated intra-abdominal injuries. If a renal vascular injury is identified, arteriography or immediate surgical exploration may be warranted.

Penetrating renal injury accounts for 10% of all cases of renal trauma. Seven percent of penetrating wounds to the abdomen involve the kidney. Conversely, 80% of all penetrating renal injuries will involve injury to other intra-abdominal structures. Most gunshot wounds are associated with intra-abdominal injury, usually involving the stomach, small intestine, colon, and liver. Stab wounds have less frequent involvement of other organ systems. Stab wounds posterior to the anterior axillary line only involve other intra-abdominal organs 12% of the time. Peritoneal lavage may be helpful in evaluating intra-abdominal stab wound injuries. Renal imaging should be done in all patients with stab injury posterior to the anterior axillary line, regardless of the presence of hematuria. Patients with gunshot wounds to the chest and abdomen often present in hemorrhagic shock. Rapid resuscitation is essential, and urgent exploratory surgery may preclude diagnostic imaging studies.

Radiographic staging, either IVP or CT scan with intravenous contrast, should be contemplated in all trauma patients with hematuria or a significant mechanism of injury. Intravenous pyelography should establish the presence or absence of one or both kidneys, define the renal parenchyma, and outline the collecting systems and ureters. Nephrotomograms will aid in the detection of renal lacerations, hematomas, and poorly vascularized renal segments. All children in whom renal injury is suspected should undergo renal imaging studies.

Table 44–5. Classification of renal trauma.

Grade	Description
I	Contusion or subscapular hematoma without parenchymal laceration
II	Nonexpanding perirenal hematoma with cortical laceration < 1 cm
III	Cortical laceration > 1 cm deep without urinary extravasation
IV	Laceration extending through the corticomedullary junction into the collecting system or thrombosis of a segmental renal artery
V	Shattered kidney with multiple lacerations or avulsions/thrombosis of the main renal artery or vein

1. BLUNT RENAL INJURY

History, physical examination, and urinalysis for hematuria are the initial studies in evaluating renal trauma. Three parameters guide the need for radiographic imaging: (1) clinical indicators of flank trauma, including a direct blow, deceleration injury, or associated intra-abdominal injuries, and signs of flank trauma (contusions, seat belt marks, lower rib fractures, or fractures of the lumbar transverse processes), (2) the initial blood pressure, and (3) the presence or absence of hematuria.

The hemodynamically stable patient. Studies have shown that patients presenting with stable blood pressure (systolic > 90 mm Hg) and microscopic hematuria have only a 0.5% chance of sustaining a major renal injury. Therefore, the adult patient with blunt renal trauma, microscopic hematuria, and in stable condition may not require radiographic imaging. However, all pediatric patients with positive clinical findings of renal trauma and a significant mechanism of action, irrespective of their hemodynamic status, require radiographic evaluation. Renal imaging is required in all patients with greater than 5 RBC/HPF, penetrating injury with hematuria, or in any pediatric patient with a suspected renal injury. Clinical evaluation and mechanism of injury are important factors in deciding if the stable adult patient with microscopic hematuria may forego radiologic imaging.

X-ray examination of the kidneys, ureter, and bladder (KUB) may reveal a large radiodense area in the region of the injured organ, along with absence of the psoas shadow. IVP may demonstrate impaired function with delay or absence in visualization of all or a portion of the kidney, or evidence of extravasation. CT accurately stages renal trauma, with valuable information about renal perfusion, urinary extravasation, and potential intraperitoneal involvement. The evaluation and management of renal trauma is shown in (Figure 44–2). The extent of renal injury typically seen in the stable patient with blunt renal injury may range from a renal contusion to major renal laceration.

Contusions represent approximately 85% of blunt renal injuries. Adult patients with no clinical indication of flank trauma, stable blood pressure, and microscopic hematuria are considered to have minor renal injuries (contusions and minor lacerations) and are best managed expectantly. The management of minor lacerations, and even major lacerations in the stable patient, can be managed expectantly with serial hematocrits and blood pressure monitoring. An exception to this would be a patient with a major laceration and a large devascularized segment of kidney. In this case, either a partial or simple nephrectomy may be necessary. The absolute indications for surgical exploration of the kidney include an expanding or pulsatile hematoma. Relative indications include urinary extravasation, vascular injury, nonviable parenchyma, and incomplete staging.

The hemodynamically unstable patient. The he-

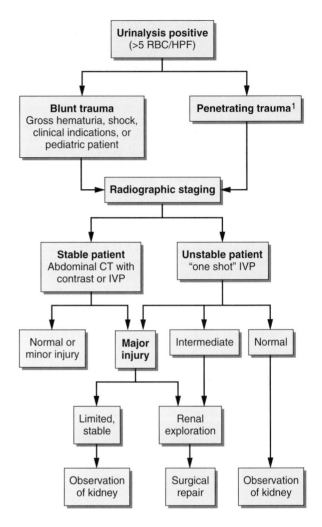

¹The vast majority of patients with penetrating trauma to the kidney should be explored.
CT, computed tomography; IVP, intravenous pyelogram.

Figure 44–2. Algorithm for the evaluation of renal trauma.

modynamically unstable patient is defined as a patient with a systolic blood pressure less than 90 mm Hg recorded at any time in the field. This patient often will respond to fluid resuscitation. Many of these cases are the result of rapid deceleration injuries and involve multiple organ trauma. On physical examination, evidence of flank trauma with an expanding hematoma or abdominal distention may be present. The condition of the patient may preclude a thorough radiologic evaluation, however, a one-shot IVP should be obtained prior to surgical exploration to confirm the presence of a normally functioning contralateral kidney.

2. PENETRATING RENAL INJURY

On physical examination, stab wounds to the kidney usually have their entrance in the lower thorax, upper abdomen, or flank area. Careful abdominal examination may reveal marked tenderness and possible peritoneal signs, suggesting an associated bowel injury. Hemorrhagic shock is a common presenting sign, and fluid resuscitation is of prime importance in the initial treatment. Peritoneal lavage is useful in evaluating intra-abdominal injury after stab wounds to the torso. Hematuria, frequently gross, is usually present with major parenchymal injuries.

The incidence of associated intra-abdominal injuries varies greatly and may be related to the entrance site. A major laceration or vascular injury is a common occurrence in patients who have sustained penetrating renal injury. The majority of these injuries require operative exploration. Only when preoperative staging clearly demonstrates that the extent of injury is minor can the patient be managed expectantly.

URETER

Most ureteral injuries are iatrogenic and are the result of pelvic or abdominal surgery, or endoscopic surgery of the ureter. Other causes of ureteral injury include external trauma (penetrating or blunt) and radiation. In the setting of postoperative anuria, bilateral injury to the ureters must be ruled out. A differential diagnosis for anuria in the postoperative patient will include post-renal obstruction, acute tubular necrosis, and injury to the renal artery. Symptoms of ureteral injury may include persistent flank pain, fever, symptoms of ileus, or drainage of urine from the surgical drain site or vagina. Hematuria is present in only a minority of cases. In the setting of anuria, ureteral obstruction must be ruled out. The combination of IVP and retrograde urography will demonstrate partial or complete obstruction of the ureter and the level of the injury. Ureterovaginal leakage can be distinguished from a vesicovaginal fistula by intravesical injection of methylene blue. A tampon is then inserted in the vagina. If on removal of the tampon there is staining with methylene blue, a vesicovaginal fistula is indicated. In iatrogenic injuries, the ureter is most commonly injured at the level of the pelvic brim where the lower ureter courses closely to the uterine artery, iliac vessels, and the broad ligament of the uterus. Identifying the ureter at this point in its course helps to avoid injury. Extensive pelvic surgery might best be planned, with preoperative placement of ureteral stents to better identify the ureters during the surgical dissection.

There are four major criteria to consider when managing ureteral trauma:

1. *Site* (upper, middle, lower). Ureteroureterostomy may be performed for upper and middle third ureteral injuries. Injury to the lower third of the ureter should be treated by ureteral reimplantation when possible or by transureteroureterostomy. In each case, the ureter is stented and the anastomotic site is drained.

2. *Nature of injury*. A high-velocity projectile may be associated with a significant degree of blast injury. Involvement of more than 7 cm of ureter may require mobilization of the bladder and the kidney to decrease the amount of tension placed on the anastomotic site. For massive destruction of the lower ureter, a transureteroureterostomy or, alternatively, an ileal interposition graft may be necessary.

3. *Time of recognition*. If the injury is recognized early, repair is immediate, while late recognition is managed with proximal diversion of the urinary stream, drainage of the urinoma, and delayed repair of the ureteral injury.

4. *Associated injuries*. For example, if prosthetic vascular grafts are needed, the risk of urinary extravasation, infection, and disruption of the vascular anastomosis may make nephrectomy a more appropriate treatment option.

BLADDER

Blunt trauma to the distended bladder is the most common cause of injury and is frequently associated with pelvic fractures. Bladder rupture can be either **intraperitoneal** (rupture of the dome or anterior bladder wall) or **extraperitoneal** (rupture of the posterior wall, trigone, or bladder neck). The dome of the bladder is most susceptible to rupture because it is mobile and lacks a fixed structural attachment.

A patient with an intraperitoneal bladder rupture may have a pelvic fracture, suprapubic tenderness, or abdominal distention with possible peritoneal signs. The patient may also be unable to void. Extraperitoneal injuries will often cause lower abdominal pain. Hematuria is a hallmark finding with bladder injuries. Gross hematuria occurs in 95% of cases, with microscopic hematuria present in the remaining cases.

If blood is present at the urethral meatus in males, an associated urethral injury must be ruled out before placing a Foley catheter. This can be evaluated with a retrograde urethrogram. If there is no apparent urethral injury, the Foley catheter may be advanced into the bladder and a cystogram obtained by instilling approximately 300 mL of contrast material and obtaining radiographs at volumes of 100 mL and 300 mL of filling. Anterior/posterior (A/P), lateral, and oblique views should be obtained. The bladder should then be drained completely and a postdrainage radiograph obtained. It should be noted that the cystogram phase of an IVP or CT scan is not satisfactory to evaluate the bladder for rupture.

An intraperitoneal leak must be differentiated from an extraperitoneal leak. An intraperitoneal leak is confirmed on cystogram by the demonstration of contrast outlining loops of bowel or contrast filling the colic gutter (especially on the right with the patient in Trendelenburg). In most cases, the peritoneal cavity is explored, the injury is repaired, and the bladder is drained. A small extraperitoneal leak can be managed by Foley catheter drainage of the bladder for 5–7 days, followed by repeat cystogram.

URETHRA

The least mobile portions of the male urethra are the bulbous urethra and the membranous urethra. Consequently, these are the areas most susceptible to injury. The membranous urethra is fixed to the symphysis pubis and is most commonly injured in association with pelvic fractures. Bulbar urethral injuries are usually the result of a straddle type injury where the urethra is compressed between a hard object and the pubic arch, resulting in partial or complete tear. Additionally, there may be blood present at the urethral meatus. Instrumentation or catheterization is contraindicated prior to the performance of a retrograde urethrogram.

Most patients with a ruptured urethra will have blood at the meatus, and many of them will have swelling and ecchymosis of the penis, scrotum and perineum. In addition, the patient may be unable to void. On rectal examination there may be a high-riding prostate due to its elevation by pelvic hematoma and disruption from the symphysis pubis or membranous urethra.

A retrograde urethrogram is essential to the diagnosis and management of urethral injuries. Retrograde urethrography can be performed by placing a Foley catheter approximately 2 cm into the urethral meatus to the fossa navicularis and filling the balloon with 1–2 mL of saline. Then, 25 mL of contrast material is gently instilled and radiographs are obtained in the oblique position, preferably under fluoroscopic control.

A partial tear of the urethra may be converted to a complete tear by Foley catheterization. Thus, the conservative management of these injuries is with the placement of a suprapubic tube. Posterior urethral injuries have been traditionally managed in a staged fashion. Initially the urinary stream is diverted and once the swelling and hematoma subsides (3–6 months) repeat urethrography and cystography are performed to assess the injury. Treatment may be endoscopic realignment or open surgical reconstruction. The complication most frequently associated with these injuries is recurrent urethral stricture.

PENIS

Trauma to the penis may occur from gunshot wounds, stab wounds, and machinery accidents. Spontaneous penile fracture during intercourse may result in rupture of the tunica albuginea of the corpora cavernosum.

Penetrating injury to the penis is managed with debridement, hemostasis, and repair of the injury. Avulsion of the penile skin, as in machinery-type accidents, requires careful debridement and grafting with split thickness skin grafts. Corporal disruption as with penile fracture should be repaired promptly to minimize penile curvature during erection from scar formation in the corpora cavernosum.

SCROTUM

Scrotal and testicular injuries may occur as degloving-type accidents from machinery or may be the direct result of blunt or penetrating trauma. Severe blunt trauma to the testis may result in testicular rupture. Rarely, a spontaneous rupture of the testis may occur with little or no trauma, especially in association with underlying pathology (eg, testicular carcinoma). Following rupture of the tunica albuginea, there is bleeding into the tunica vaginalis around the testis, with hematocele formation.

The patient usually presents with a history of trauma to the testis, with the finding of a tender swollen scrotal mass that does not transilluminate. If a degloving injury occurs, the testis or the penis will appear with little to no dermal covering. In cases of blunt injury to the testis, ultrasonography should be performed to determine the extent of injury.

Degloving injuries will require debridement, intravenous antibiotics, and coverage with residual scrotal tissue or split-thickness skin flaps from the perineum or thigh. Orchiectomy is usually not required in such cases. In patients complaining of little or no trauma, an underlying carcinoma may be suspected. Ultrasonography may confirm the presence of an intratesticular lesion. Exploration of the testis, with a suspected malignant lesion, should be performed using the inguinal approach. Patients with severe bleeding should undergo scrotal exploration, evacuation of clot, and repair of the testis, if possible. Those patients in whom there is a clear history of trauma, but with minimal hematoma formation, may be treated conservatively with elevation, analgesics, and ice packs. When disruption of the tunica albuginea of the testis occurs, as with a close-range gun shot wound, meticulous debridement and copious irrigation is necessary prior to primary closure if the testicle is deemed salvageable.

TUMORS

KIDNEY

Benign tumors of the kidney are relatively uncommon but may include oncocytoma, angiomyolipoma, hemangioma, lipoma, and leiomyoma. Most malignant renal tumors are adenocarcinomas, either clear cell, granular cell, chromophobe, papillary, or sarcomatous variants of renal cell carcinoma. Renal cell carcinoma usually affects those over the age of 50, with the incidence increasing through the eighth decade of life. There are approximately 25,000–30,000 new diagnoses of renal cell carcinoma in the United States annually and 9000 deaths. Men are affected twice as often as women. Possible risk factors include tobacco, cadmium exposure, and genetic predisposition, such as patients with vonHippel-Lindau disease. Chromosome *3p* abnormalities occur commonly in patients with renal cell carcinoma. Renal cell carcinomas originate from the proximal renal tubular epithelium. These tumors are vascular and tend to spread either by direct invasion through the renal capsule into Gerota's fascia or by direct extension into the renal vein. Renal cell carcinoma usually does not invade adjacent organs except for the sarcomatous variants. The most common site of distant metastasis is the lung, however, liver, bone, adrenal, and ipsilateral lymph nodes are frequently involved.

Diagnosis

On presentation, flank or abdominal pain and hematuria are common signs of renal tumors. Symptoms may result from local tumor growth, paraneoplastic syndromes, or metastatic disease. The classic triad of pain, hematuria, and flank mass is rarely seen. An increased number of tumors are being diagnosed while clinically localized to the kidney since the widespread utilization of ultrasonography and CT; however, approximately 30% of patients present with metastatic disease. Recent onset of a varicocele, especially one that does not reduce when the patient is supine, may be indicative of a tumor in the kidney that has invaded the renal vein or caused obstruction of the vena cava. Paraneoplastic syndromes associated with renal carcinoma include erythrocytosis, hypercalcemia, hypertension, and nonmetastatic hepatic dysfunction (Stauffer syndrome).

Staging evaluation may include a chest x-ray or chest CT, and abdominal CT. On CT, the cancer is characteristically a solid mass that is less dense than the surrounding parenchyma, and enhances with the administration of intravenous contrast. Further evaluation with either duplex ultrasonography, magnetic resonance imaging (MRI), or venacavography may be indicated when involvement of the renal vein and vena cava is suspected. Complex cystic masses in the kidney may be best evaluated with a combination of CT and ultrasonography. Approximately 4–10% of patients present with tumor thrombus in the renal vein or inferior vena cava. Bone scans are indicated in patients with either an elevated serum calcium or alkaline phosphatase. The most widely used staging system is the TNM classification (Table 44–6).

Management

Treatment involves radical nephrectomy (removal of kidney, adrenal gland, and surrounding perinephric fat and Gerota's fascia) with regional lymphadenectomy for tumors stage T1 and T2 (confined to Gerota's fascia) without evidence of distant metastatic spread. The 5-year survival rate is 70–90% for stage I and 50–70% for stage II disease. Overall, patients who have tumor extension into the vena cava, especially those with tumor thrombus

Table 44–6. TNM classification of renal tumor.[1]

T	**Primary Tumor**
TX	Primary tumor cannot be assessed
T0	No evidence of primary tumor
T1	Tumor 2.5 cm or less in greatest dimension, limited to kidney
T2	Tumor > 2.5 cm, limited to kidney
T3	Tumor extends into major veins, or invades adrenal gland or perinephric tissues but not beyond Gerota's fascia
T3a	Tumor invades adrenal gland or perinephric tissue but not beyond Gerota's fascia
T3b	Tumor grossly extends into renal vein(s) or vena cava
T4	Tumor invades beyond Gerota's fascia
N	**Regional Lymph Nodes**
N0	No identifiable nodes on clinical assessment
N1	Metastasis in single lymph node, 2 cm or less in greatest dimension
N2	No metastatic lymph node to exceed 5 cm in greatest dimension
N3	Metastasis in a lymph node > 5 cm in greatest dimension
M	**Distant Metastasis**
M0	Tumors without distant metastasis
M1	Tumors with distant metastasis

[1]1987 UICC (International Union Against Cancer) stage.

above the diaphragm, have approximately a 15–20% 5-year survival, however, some patients with pathologic T1 or T2 renal cell carcinoma and involvement of the renal vein or inferior vena cava may have prolonged survival. Patients presenting with or developing metastatic disease have a poor prognosis, with only 5–10% surviving 2 years. Performance status, weight loss, serum calcium, and the presence of anemia are prognostic factors. Radical nephrectomy is generally recommended for those patients in whom all tumor can likely be excised; surgery rarely prolongs survival in patients with advanced local disease, adrenal or adjacent organ involvement, or nodal metastases.

The treatment of metastatic disease with chemotherapy has been unsuccessful, however, the use of immunotherapy with agents such as interferon and interleukin-2, alone and in combination with cis-retinoic acid or 5-fluorouracil, have shown some promise. In addition, clinical trials are underway utilizing gene therapy and cytokine-treated tumor infiltrating lymphocytes (TIL) that have been grown in culture, harvested, and reinfused. In general, the role of radical nephrectomy in lymph node-positive or metastatic disease is limited to participation in gene therapy or TIL cell protocols, palliation of pain, or refractory hypercalcemia.

RENAL PELVIS & URETER

Tumors of the renal pelvis and ureter are rare, accounting for only 4% of urothelial cancers. The mean age at diagnosis is 65, with a male-to-female ratio of 3:1. Urothelial cancer often presents as a multifocal urothelial abnormality, with the risk of subsequent bladder cancer as high as 30–50%. The risk of contralateral involvement is approximately 5%. Etiologic factors associated with urothelial cancers are tobacco, aniline dyes, aromatic amines, nitrates, and analgesics. The majority of upper tract tumors are transitional cell carcinomas, with squamous carcinomas accounting for approximately 10%. Squamous cell cancers tend to invade and metastasize early, however, stage-for-stage prognosis is similar to transitional cell carcinoma. Staging of renal pelvic and ureteral tumors is based on the depth and extent of invasion (Table 44–7). However, the histologic grade of the tumor is of equal importance in determining prognosis and recurrence rates.

Diagnosis

At presentation, symptoms usually include total gross painless hematuria and, occasionally, symptoms of renal colic if the tumor or blood is obstructing the collecting system. An IVP will often demonstrate a filling defect in the renal pelvis or the "goblet sign" when the tumor is in the ureter. Cystoscopy and retrograde pyelography are useful in evaluating the tumor and also aid in evaluating any synchronous lesions. Confirmatory diagnosis may be obtained with cytologic analysis of ureteral washings, brushings, or ureteroscopic biopsy. Staging of the tumor may be assessed with CT of the abdomen and pelvis, chest x-ray or CT scan, and possibly bone scan.

Management

In most cases, a nephroureterectomy is performed with the removal of a cuff of bladder at the ipsilateral ureteral orifice. A regional lymphadenectomy is also usually performed. Less extensive surgical procedures have been reserved for patients with solitary kidneys, bilateral tumors, or compromised renal function. Some low-grade papillary tumors may be treated endoscopically. Ureteral lesions in the distal ureter may be managed with partial ureterectomy and ureteral reimplantation. In general, higher-grade tumors are managed aggressively with surgical extirpation, however, lower-grade tumors may be treated conservatively with local excision and reanastomosis, endoscopic resection, fulguration, or topical immunotherapy.

Conservatively treated lesions require careful surveillance with the frequent performance of an IVP, cystoscopy, retrograde pyelogram, and urinary cytology.

BLADDER

Bladder cancer comprises 90% of the urothelial tumors. There are approximately 50,000 new cases and 10,000 deaths due to bladder cancer per year in the United States. Approximately 70% of all bladder tumors are superficial, confined to the mucosa and submucosa; 25% are invasive, into the muscular wall of the bladder; and 5% are metastatic at the time of diagnosis. In the United States, approximately 90% of bladder tumors are transitional cell carcinoma. Other tumor types include adenocarcinoma (2%), squamous (5–10%), and undifferentiated cancers (2%).

The age and sex distribution is similar to that of the renal pelvic tumors. Etiologic factors identified for bladder cancer are similar to that of the renal pelvic tumors and include cigarette smoking, aniline dyes, sodium cyclamate, and cyclophosphamide. States with the highest per capita cigarette consumption have the highest incidences of bladder cancer in the United States. Squamous cell carcinoma of the bladder may be due to chronic inflammation or infection, especially secondary to schistosomiasis, or neurogenic bladders with chronic indwelling catheters. Adenocarcinomas may be urachal in origin or arise elsewhere in the bladder. Transitional cell carcinoma of the bladder may be associated with chromosome 9, 11, 13, 17, and 18 abnormalities. Advanced tumors may have *p53* tumor suppressor gene mutations. The TNM staging of bladder cancer is based on the depth and extent of tumor invasion (Table 44–8).

The frequency of tumor invasion, recurrence, and progression is strongly correlated with tumor grade and stage; progression is noted in 10–20% of grade 1, 19–37% of grade 2, and 33–67% of grade 3 tumors. Survival rates are similarly affected, with a 10-year survival of 98% in patients with low-grade tumors and only 35% in those with high-grade lesions. The vast majority of patients with low-grade tumors have low-stage disease.

Bladder cancer spreads via pelvic lymphatics and hema-

Table 44–7. TNM classification of renal pelvic and ureteral carcinomas.[1]

Ta, Tis	Confined to mucosa
T1	Invasion of lamina propria
T2	Invasion of muscularis
T3	Extension through muscularis into fat or renal parenchyma
T4	Spread to adjacent organs
N1–3	Lymph node metastases
M1	Distant metastases

[1]1987 UICC (International Union Against Cancer) stage.

Table 44–8. TNM classification of bladder carcinoma.[1]

Tis	Carcinoma in situ
Ta	Tumor confined to the epithelium
T1	Invasion of lamina propria (submucosa)
T2	Invasion of superficial muscle
T3a	Deep muscle invasion
T3b	Tumor invades perivesical fat
T4	Spread to contiguous organs (prostate, uterus, colon)
N1–3	Lymph node metastases
M1	Metastases

[1]1987 UICC (International Union Against Cancer) stage.

togenously with metastases to lung, liver, and, less commonly, bone.

Diagnosis

Intermittent painless hematuria, either gross or microscopic, is present in 85% of patients at presentation. Patients may complain of irritative voiding symptoms, such as urgency, frequency, and dysuria. In patients with total gross painless hematuria, a bladder tumor must be ruled out. On IVP or ultrasonography, a filling defect may be noted in the bladder or there may be hydronephrosis and ureteral obstruction. Advanced tumors involving the posterior wall of the bladder may be palpable by bimanual examination.

The diagnosis is typically established with an IVP, urinary cytology, cystourethroscopy, and resection of the bladder tumor. It is important for staging purposes to determine the level of invasion with deep biopsies at the tumor base. In patients with suspected invasive disease, CT or MRI of the pelvis should be performed prior to biopsy to optimize staging information. Urinary cytology is commonly used as a screening test when there is a history of bladder cancer and in the evaluation of new cases. Cytologic examination is highly sensitive and specific in diagnosing high-grade carcinoma, but is less sensitive in the diagnosis of low-grade bladder tumors. Clinical staging of bladder cancer is performed by bimanual examination under anesthesia, transurethral resection of the bladder tumor, IVP, CT scan of the abdomen and pelvis, and chest x-ray or CT of the chest. In some patients bone scans are also obtained.

Prognostic Factors

For superficial disease (Ta, T1, and Tis), tumor grade has been shown to be the single most important determinant of tumor progression, with high-grade, poorly differentiated tumors having a worse prognosis. Tumor grade is also an important determinant of tumor recurrence and patient survival. Pathologic tumor stage is of prognostic significance, with tumor recurrence in 70% of stage pT1 lesions compared with 48% of pTa tumors. Progression to muscle invasive cancer occurs in 3% of pTa tumors and 24% of pT1 tumors. Patients with recurrent T1 tumors or patients failing intravesical therapy have a high risk of tumor progression. Larger T1 tumor size, associated carcinoma in situ, aneuploid tumors, and superficial tumors with mutation of the *p53* tumor suppressor gene are associated with a poor prognosis. Patients who exhibit symptoms of a paraneoplastic syndrome, either from metastatic or localized disease, usually have a poor outcome.

Management

Superficial disease (stages Ta, T1, and Tis). Treatment of superficial disease Ta and T1 is initially with transurethral resection and accurate staging of the tumor. The initial resection provides important information about the depth of invasion and grade of the tumor and directs further therapy. Surveillance cystoscopy and bladder wash cytology should be performed every 3 months for 2 years, then every 6 months for 2 years, and yearly thereafter if there is no recurrence. IVP to assess the upper tracts may be obtained periodically. Carcinoma in situ (CIS), recurrent superficial tumors (Ta and T1), multiple tumors, and high-grade tumors are at risk of recurrence and, therefore, may be treated with intravesical therapy.

Intravesical chemotherapeutic agents presently include Adriamycin, mitomycin C, and thiotepa. Intravesical immunotherapeutic agents include bacillus Calmette-Guérin (BCG), the "gold standard," and, experimentally, interferon and tumor necrosis factor. The goal of intravesical therapy is (1) to treat residual tumor in the bladder after an incomplete transurethral resection of the tumor (TURBT), (2) to provide prophylaxis to prevent recurrences, and (3) to treat carcinoma in situ. BCG currently is the most effective intravesical agent for patients with CIS. Patients who fail treatment with one intravesical agent may respond to an alternative agent. The dosing regimen is dependent on the agent used, but typically involves weekly bladder instillation for 6–9 weeks. Patients with tumor progression, recurrent CIS, or high-grade T1 lesions require more aggressive therapy, such as radical cystectomy. Patients with recurrent low-grade and low-stage disease may require frequent resections or fulgurations of tumors.

Invasive disease (stage T2 and T3). Diagnosis and staging is performed by TURBT, making sure to adequately sample the bladder muscle. CT scan and MRI are useful in the evaluation of the local extent of the tumor as well as for metastatic disease. Pelvic lymphadenectomy plays an important role in the staging of bladder cancer. In general, CT or MRI should be performed prior to TURBT to minimize postsurgical changes seen by imaging studies that may decrease staging information. The surgical boundaries of lymphadenectomy for bladder cancer include the genitofemoral nerve laterally, the obturator foramen inferiorly, the obturator fossa posteriorly, and the bifurcation of the iliac vessels superiorly.

Treatment options for invasive bladder cancer are either (1) surgical extirpation and urinary tract reconstruction, or (2) bladder-sparing techniques with either aggressive TURBT, partial cystectomy, external beam radiotherapy with or without radiosensitizing chemotherapy, or primary chemotherapy alone.

In general, **radical cystectomy** (removal of the bladder and prostate in men, anterior pelvic exenteration in women) is the gold standard among urologic surgeons. Nerve-sparing modifications and continent urinary diversion, especially **orthotopic continent diversions** (attachment of the intestinal neobladder to the membranous urethra), have made cystectomy more acceptable to patients and physicians. The majority of patients, however, continue to have ileal conduit urinary diversions that require an external ostomy appliance. It may be necessary to remove the remaining urethra in men with cancer in the prostatic urethra or recurrent transitional cell carcinoma in the urethra.

However, despite advances in surgical therapy, 50% of patients that undergo cystectomy are dead of disease in 5 years. Patients with pathologic T0–T3a disease may have 10-year survival rates in the 70–80% range. External beam radiation therapy used as a single treatment modality has only a 20–40% 5-year survival rate. Bladder-sparing techniques using combinations of surgery, radiation therapy, and chemotherapy continue to be updated and require careful follow-up. Approximately one third to one half of patients eventually require cystectomy after attempting to initially spare the bladder. In one series, only 25% of patients are disease-free and have retained their bladders at follow-up of 5 or more years.

The role of adjuvant or neoadjuvant chemotherapy in the treatment of invasive bladder cancer is still being investigated. Presently, there is no clear evidence that chemotherapy is of any benefit except in small subsets of patients.

Metastatic bladder cancer is associated with a poor prognosis, with a 5–10% survival rate at 2 years. Combination chemotherapy is the mainstay of treatment with MVAC (methotrexate, vinblastine, Adriamycin, and cisplatin) as the standard. Initial studies reported 70% response rates, however, subsequent studies demonstrate durable responses in only 10–15% of patients. A number of newer agents and combinations are currently being investigated for the treatment of advanced bladder cancer.

PROSTATE

1. BENIGN PROSTATIC HYPERPLASIA

Histologic BPH begins in men over the age of 35 and the incidence increases with age. By age 80, 100% of men will have histologic BPH, 50% will have prostatic enlargement, and 25% will have symptomatic bladder outlet obstruction. When the hyperplastic tissue encroaches on the urethral lumen, it produces symptoms of urethral obstruction that may progress to urinary retention in 1–2% of men per year. Urethral obstruction may result in incomplete emptying of the bladder, giving rise to urinary stasis, urinary tract infection, and bladder calculi.

Diagnosis. Symptoms due to BPH are either obstructive or irritative in nature. Obstructive symptoms include hesitancy, straining to void, decreased force and caliber of the urinary stream, postvoid dribbling, the sensation of incomplete bladder emptying, and urinary retention. Irritative symptoms include urinary frequency, nocturia, dysuria, urgency, and urge incontinence. The majority of patients with symptomatic BPH have obstructive and irritative voiding symptoms. On physical examination, you may be able to palpate the distended bladder of the patient in urinary retention. On rectal examination, the prostate will be variably enlarged and rubbery in texture. The entire surface of the gland should be examined for evidence of induration, which may be suggestive of prostatic cancer.

Evaluation of the patient with BPH includes a careful history, physical examination that includes digital rectal examination, urinalysis, and possibly a serum prostate specific antigen (PSA) blood test to help diagnose prostate cancer. Additional tests are a voiding questionnaire, urinary flow rate, assessment of postvoid residual, and, possibly, cystoscopy, urodynamics, and ultrasonography or IVP. The goals of treatment for BPH are symptomatic improvement, preservation of renal function, and avoidance of infection and incontinence.

Management. The most common treatment for BPH is partial prostatectomy, however, the rate of surgical therapy has been decreasing since the advent of medical therapy. The relative indications for prostatectomy are (1) urinary retention, (2) bothersome symptoms to the patient, (3) recurrent urinary tract infections, (4) compromised renal function due to hydronephrosis from prostatic obstruction, (5) recurrent gross hematuria with no other explanation, and (6) urge incontinence. Urge incontinence, however, may be worsened with a partial prostatectomy or transurethral resection of the prostate (TURP), and urodynamics may help to ascertain the potential benefits of prostatectomy. A partial prostatectomy attempts to reestablish the channel from the bladder neck to the urethra by selectively removing the adenomatous tissue. This can be accomplished transurethrally (TURP) or by open enucleation of the adenoma, depending on the size of the gland. Adenomas less than 80 g are usually resected transurethrally. Possible complications of surgery include bleeding (10%), urethral strictures (10%), infections (10%), retrograde ejaculation (up to 100%), incontinence (1%), and impotence (1%).

Alternatively, patients can be managed with medical therapy, including sympathetic α-adrenergic inhibitors doxazosin and terazosin or antiandrogen therapy. Sympathetic blockade relieves obstruction by inhibiting α-adrenoreceptor-mediated contractions of the prostatic capsule, adenoma, and bladder neck. Antiandrogen therapy relieves prostatic obstruction by causing atrophy of the prostatic epithelium and stroma. The prostate can be expected to shrink up to 30% in size within 6 months of therapy, however, regrowth occurs quickly with cessation of therapy.

2. PROSTATIC CARCINOMA

Carcinoma of the prostate is the most common cancer in American men, with approximately 300,000 new cases and 40,000 deaths per year. It rarely occurs in men under the age of 40, and its incidence increases with advancing age. Etiologic factors cited in the pathogenesis of prostate cancer include race, aging, familial aggregation or genetic inheritance, hormonal factors, high-fat diet, and environmental factors (decreased exposure to ultraviolet radiation).

Prostate cancers are predominantly adenocarcinomas

(95%) that arise from prostatic acinar cells predominantly in the peripheral zone of the prostate. Thus, early prostatic carcinoma is asymptomatic, whereas BPH commonly produces symptoms of urethral obstruction. Prostate cancer may produce ureteral obstruction by direct spread into the bladder trigone or urethral obstruction in cases of advanced disease; thus, patients with locally advanced prostate cancer have symptoms of BPH. Distant spread occurs through lymphatic and hematogenous routes. Prostatic cancer commonly metastasizes to the pelvic lymph nodes and the axial skeleton. Visceral metastases occur rarely and typically late in the course of the disease, most commonly involving the lungs, liver, and adrenal glands. Prostatic carcinoma has an unpredictable natural history, progressing slowly in some men, while others suffer early metastatic disease and death. Prostatic cancer doubling time may vary from 1 to 6 years. Approximately 10% of men with metastatic prostate cancer survive 10 years, however, the median survival for men with metastatic prostate cancer is 2.5 years.

Diagnosis. Localized carcinoma of the prostate is typically asymptomatic. As the disease progresses, the patient may experience symptoms of urinary obstruction (which are indistinguishable from those produced by BPH); symptoms of uremia from ureteral obstruction; and skeletal pain or pathologic fracture from metastatic disease. Most prostatic cancers are detected by digital rectal examination, where the prostate feels harder than normal and the normal boundaries of the gland may be obscured, or by an elevated level of serum PSA. About 33% of firm areas within the prostate prove to be malignant; others are caused by prostatic calculi, inflammation, infarction, or changes secondary to partial prostatectomy for BPH. The serum PSA normal range for men aged 50–65 is 1–4 ng/mL. Slightly higher normal values may be seen in the older age group. PSA is made by prostatic epithelium and is, thus, prostate-specific, not cancer-specific.

Because of the lack of effective therapies for men with advanced prostate cancer, many urologists believe that the early diagnosis of prostate cancer is critical. The American Urological Association (AUA) recommends that all men over the age of 50 should have a yearly digital rectal examination and serum PSA measurement. Patients with a family history of prostate cancer or African Americans may begin screening at age 40. PSA levels, in combination with digital rectal examinations (Table 44–9), as well as the rate of change of PSA with time and PSA density (serum PSA divided by the volume of the prostate gland), have increased clinicians' ability to detect prostate cancer

when it is still confined to the prostate. Confirmatory diagnosis is obtained with transrectal ultrasonography and biopsy, which is more than 90% accurate. A staging evaluation includes the digital rectal examination and transrectal ultrasonography, histologic Gleason sum, serum PSA prior to biopsy, bone scan, and, in some cases, CT or MRI scan.

Prostate cancers are graded according to the **Gleason system**, which is based on the degree of glandular differentiation and growth pattern in relation to the stroma. Histologically, five Gleason patterns have been described and range from 1 to 5. Gleason pattern 1 is the most well differentiated and 5 is the most undifferentiated pattern. The Gleason "score" is the sum of the two most prominent histologic patterns. The Gleason score aids in the prediction of the presence of lymph node metastasis and prognosis. Staging of prostatic carcinomas is based on the TNM system (Table 44–10).

Management. Treatment options for clinically localized prostate cancer include (1) watchful waiting, delaying hormonal deprivation until symptomatic disease progression, (2) radical prostatectomy, or (3) external beam radiation or brachytherapy. Treatment decisions depend on life expectancy, histologic Gleason grade, tumor stage, and serum PSA level. Additional factors include the morbidity and mortality of treatment, including the risks of impotence and incontinence. Improved surgical techniques have decreased the risks associated with surgery. Presently, up to 90% of men may recover urinary continence after prostatectomy, with only 3–5% suffering severe urinary incontinence. The recovery of sexual function depends on the age of the patient and stage of the tumor. Approximately 50–70% of patients may recover sexual function after radical prostatectomy. In general, men who are otherwise healthy with a life expectancy of 10–15 years and localized T1 and T2 prostate cancer are excellent candidates for radical prostatectomy. No randomized trial has been performed to date comparing radiation therapy to surgery for survival or disease-free survival from prostate cancer. Presently, a large-scale 15-year study is being performed comparing radical prostatectomy versus watchful waiting for men with localized prostate cancer.

Radiation therapy is an alternative for early prostate cancer. Similar overall 10-year survival rates have been quoted with radiation and surgery, however, the percentage of men who die from prostate cancer within 10 years after radiation therapy is approximately 35%, compared with 15% for those with radical prostatectomy. Addition-

Table 44–9. Cancer detection rate related to levels of serum PSA.

DRE	PSA < 4 ng/mL (%)	PSA 4–10 ng/mL (%)	PSA > 10 ng/mL (%)
Normal	0–2	10–20	31
Abnormal	10	38	65

DRE = digital rectal examination; PSA = prostate specific antigen.

Table 44–10. TNM staging system of prostate cancer.[1]

To	No evidence of primary tumor
T1a	TURP < 5% of resected tissue
T1b	TURP > 5% of resected tissue
T1c	Nonpalpable tumor identified on biopsy because of an elevated PSA or abnormal ultrasonographic finding
T2	Tumor involves only one lobe
T3a	Unilateral extracapsular extension
T3b	Bilateral extracapsular extension
T3c	Tumor invades seminal vesicles
T4	Tumor invades adjacent organs
N	Lymph node metastases
M	Metastases

[1]1987 UICC (International Union Against Cancer) stage.
PSA = prostate-specific antigen; TURP = transurethral prostatic resection.

ally, up to one third of those patients treated with radiation therapy have residual cancer detectable on biopsy. Given these findings, current enthusiasm for radiation therapy has lessened. Radiation therapy for early prostate cancer may be recommended for patients refusing radical prostatectomy or those at high risk for perioperative complications.

In patients with comorbid health problems, advanced age, well-differentiated tumors, or small-volume disease, "watchful waiting" or no treatment may also be a reasonable alternative. Patients with pelvic lymph node metastases have a systemic disease and, in general, do not benefit from radical prostatectomy or radiation therapy.

The mainstay of treatment for metastatic prostate cancer is castration achieved either by orchiectomy or medically with LHRH agonists (leuteinizing hormone-releasing hormone) and/or antiandrogens, which block the androgen receptor site within the prostate. The aim is to shrink both primary and metastatic lesions by depriving prostate cells of circulating androgens. Pain from bony metastases that does not resolve with hormonal deprivation (castration) may be palliated with local radiation. Nearly all men eventually relapse with hormone-insensitive prostate cancer, and the mean survival after relapse is approximately 1 year. Unfortunately, to date there is no effective chemotherapy available for the treatment of hormone refractory prostate cancer. Multiple novel therapeutic agents are currently being tested.

TESTIS

Testis cancer is the most common solid tumor in males aged 15–35 years, with about 5000 new cases per year. Men with testis cancer have approximately a 2–4% chance of developing cancer in the contralateral testis. Patients with a history of cryptorchidism have a 40- to 70-fold increased risk of developing testis cancer, especially patients with an intra-abdominal cryptorchid testis. Testicular cancer is relatively rare in African Americans. Tumors arising from the right testis metastasize primarily to

the interaortal caval and pericaval lymph nodes below the level of the renal hilum. Left-sided tumors metastasize primarily to the para-aortic lymph nodes below the renal hilum. Hematogenous spread to the lungs, liver, mediastinum, or other organs may also occur. Testis tumors are initially classified as germinal in origin, which are further differentiated into seminomatous and nonseminomatous tumors, and testis tumors of nongerminal origin (Table 44–11).

Diagnosis

Testicular tumors usually present as an asymptomatic swelling or mass in the scrotum. Some patients present with infertility or presumed epididymal orchitis. All masses arising from the testis should be considered carcinoma until proven otherwise. Systemic symptoms from metastatic disease or hormone production (ie, human chorionic gonadotropin β-subunit (β-HCG) and gynecomastia are rare. On physical examination there is usually a palpable testicular mass, but in 10% of cases this may be obscured by an associated hydrocele.

Scrotal ultrasonography is a sensitive and specific diagnostic tool in the evaluation of a scrotal mass. Diagnosis is confirmed by surgical exploration through an inguinal incision and radical orchiectomy. Trans-scrotal exploration or needle biopsy is contraindicated because of the possibility of altering the lymphatic drainage of the scrotal skin. Tumor markers for testis cancer are alpha-fetoprotein (AFP), which is elevated in yolk sac tumors, embryonal cell carcinomas, and teratocarcinomas. AFP is not elevated in pure seminoma or choriocarcinoma. β-HCG may be produced by all tumor types, however, markedly elevated levels are associated with teratocarcinoma and choriocarcinoma. Staging evaluation consists of serum for AFP, β-HCG, and CT of the abdomen, pelvis, and chest. The differential diagnosis includes a hydrocele, varicocele, or spermatocele. Benign scrotal masses may be differentiated from malignant masses by physical examination with the aid of a flashlight and ultrasonography. Most benign scrotal masses are cystic or fluid-filled and are easily transilluminated.

Management

Treatment after orchiectomy is based on type and stage

Table 44–11. Testis tumors, age of onset, and incidence

Histologic Characteristics	Age	Incidence
Seminoma		
Classic	35–39	35%
Anaplastic	35–39	5–10%
Spermatocytic	> 50	2–12%
Embryonal	25–35	20–25%
Teratocarcinoma	25–35	5–10%
Choriocarcinoma	20–30	1–2%
Yolk sac	0–15	1–2%

of tumor (Table 44–12). Approximately 80–85% of patients with seminoma present with clinical stage I disease.

Seminoma is exquisitely radiosensitive, and external beam radiotherapy is the mainstay of treatment for low-volume disease (stage I–IIA), with a greater than 95% cure rate. Stages IIB, IIC, and III are best treated with cisplatin-based combination chemotherapy, bleomycin, etoposide, and cisplatin (BEP), with greater than 85% overall cure rate.

Nonseminoma clinical stage I tumor is treated by radical orchiectomy and either nerve-sparing or modified template retroperitoneal lymph node dissection (RPLND) or a surveillance regimen. There is approximately a 30–40% relapse rate with surveillance alone. Patients who are pathologic stage II/clinical stage I may be treated with adjuvant chemotherapy or surveillance. The treatment of clinical stage II tumors depends on the cell type and the volume of retroperitoneal disease and may include either RPLND or chemotherapy.

Clinical stage III and IV tumors are treated with four cycles of BEP chemotherapy and salvage chemotherapy, if necessary. Patients with residual masses after chemotherapy require a RPLND to resect residual disease. Complications of RPLND include bowel obstruction and loss of antegrade ejaculation. Modified templates of dissection and nerve-sparing techniques have been developed that spare the sympathetic ganglia from T10 to L2 and, thus, preserve antegrade ejaculation.

Patients treated for testis cancer require serial AFP and β-HCG measurements, chest x-rays, and CT scans to monitor recurrence of the cancer. In patients that have undergone a RPLND, disease recurrence is usually in the chest. Overall survival rate for all patients with testis cancer is approximately 95–98%. Patients who have no evidence of disease 5 years after treatment are most likely cured, however, there are increasing reports of patients suffering relapses after being disease-free for more than 5 years.

PENIS

Carcinoma of the penis is extremely rare in the United States, accounting for only 1% of genitourinary cancers.

The incidence is much higher in Central and South America, Puerto Rico, and Asia. Invasive carcinoma is almost never seen in men who are circumcised in the neonatal period, suggesting that chronic irritation and inflammation from smegma may play a causative role. A viral factor, notably the human papilloma virus, has also been implicated since there is a higher incidence of penile cancer in men whose sexual partners have cancer of the uterine cervix. The primary lesion usually occurs on the glans penis or inner surface of the foreskin. Metastatic spread is primarily to the inguinal lymphatics (superficial and deep inguinal nodes) and then to the pelvic or iliac nodes and hematogenously to the lungs and liver.

Diagnosis

The presenting sign is typically a visible, painless penile lesion or nonhealing ulcer on the glans, coronal sulcus, or the prepuce. Alternatively, patients may present with a penile mass and phimosis. The mass may be exophytic or ulcerated and is often associated with infection. Approximately 50% of patients have palpable inguinal lymph nodes at the time of presentation, but these may be due to inflammation or infection rather than neoplasia. Delayed presentation is not uncommon, with the mean delay to diagnosis being 8 months.

The diagnosis is established by excisional biopsy of the primary tumor. The vast majority of tumors of the penis are squamous cell carcinomas, with invasive lesions penetrating the basement membrane. The differential diagnosis includes syphilitic chancre, chancroid, condyloma acuminata, and the Buschke-Löwenstein tumor, which is not malignant but causes local destruction and requires excision. Further staging studies include physical examination, CT scan of the abdomen and pelvis, and x-ray or CT of the chest. The strongest prognostic indicators for survival are the presence or absence of metastasis and stage and grade of tumor. The staging system most currently used is the TNM classification (Table 44–13). The only abnormal laboratory finding is that of hypercalcemia, which occurs in the absence of bony metastases and is felt to be secondary to the bulk of the disease.

Management

The treatment of carcinoma of the penis is dependent on the stage and grade of the tumor. The local lesion is excised with a 2-cm margin, and this may involve partial penectomy up to total penectomy and perineal urethrostomy.

Superficial disease (Tis, T1), especially lowgrade, is associated with lymph node metastasis in less than 10% of patients. After control of the local tumor with either partial penectomy, laser ablation, or radiation therapy, if inguinal adenopathy occurs it should be treated with bilateral inguinal lymph node dissection.

Patients with T1 Nx M0 moderately or poorly differentiated tumors, or T2–T3 Nx M0 tumors and nonpalpable inguinal lymph nodes, are treated with bilateral inguinal lymph node dissections after treatment of the primary le-

Table 44–12. Pathologic staging of testis cancer.

Stage	Description
I	Disease limited to the testis
IIA	Microscopic retroperitoneal nodes (< 5 nodes and all < 2 cm)
IIB	Moderate retroperitoneal disease (> 5 nodes or any node > 2 cm but < 5 cm)
IIC	Bulky retroperitoneal disease
III	Nodal disease above the diaphragm or extranodal metastases
IV	Visceral metastases

Table 44–13. TNM classification of penile carcinoma.[1]

Primary Tumor (T)	
T0	No evidence of primary tumor
Tis	Carcinoma in situ
T1	Tumor invades subepithelial connective tissue
T2	Tumor invades corpus spongiosum or cavernosum
T3	Tumor invades urethra or prostate
T4	Tumor invades other adjacent structures
Regional Lymph Nodes (N)	
N0	No regional lymph node metastasis
N1	Metastasis in a single superficial inguinal lymph node
N2	Metastasis in multiple or bilateral superficial inguinal lymph nodes
N3	Metastasis in deep inguinal or pelvic lymph node(s)
Distant Metastases (M)	
M0	No distant metastases
M1	Distant metastases

[1]1987 UICC (International Union Against Cancer) stage.

sion. If positive lymph nodes are found, the dissection is extended to include the pelvic lymph nodes.

Tumors with palpable lymph nodes (Tis, T1–T3, N1–N3, M0) are initially managed with control of local tumor and treatment with antibiotics for 4 weeks. If adenopathy resolves, lymph node dissection is based on stage of tumor. If adenopathy persists, then bilateral inguinal lymph node dissection is recommended, and a pelvic lymphadenectomy is performed if the inguinal lymph nodes have metastatic disease.

Complications of inguinal lymph node dissection include wound infection, flap necrosis, and lymphedema of the lower extremities.

Metastatic tumors (any T, any N, M1) are treated with palliative external beam radiation or chemotherapy. The most effective systemic chemotherapeutic agents available to date are cisplatin and methotrexate.

SUGGESTED READING

Fowler JE Jr: *Mastery of Surgery: Urologic Surgery*. Little, Brown, 1992.

Gillenwater JY et al: *Adult and Pediatric Urology*, 3rd ed. Mosby, 1996.

Marshall FF: *Operative Urology*, 2nd ed. Saunders, 1996.

TNM Atlas: *Illustrated Guide to the TNM/p TNM-Classification of Malignant Tumors*, 3rd ed. Springer-Verlag, 1989.

Walsh PC et al: *Campbell's Urology*, 6th ed. Saunders, 1992.

45

Gynecologic Surgery

Jeffrey Warshaw, MD, & John A. Rock, MD

► Key Facts

- ► Organs of the pelvic cavity include the uterus, fallopian tubes, ovaries, bladder, lower half of ureters, urethra, vagina, and rectum.

- ► Pelvic inflammatory disease (PID) is a nonspecific term denoting upper female genital tract infection. Diagnostic precision is often difficult to achieve at the time of clinical presentation.

- ► Long-term sequelae of PID include infertility, subsequent ectopic pregnancies, chronic pelvic pain secondary to adhesions, and postinflammatory masses requiring future surgical exploration.

- ► Effective and aggressive antibiotic therapy for PID has made surgical intervention less common.

- ► The most useful laboratory test for determination of ectopic pregnancy is the β-hCG assay, while transvaginal ultrasonography has become the preferred imaging method for diagnosis.

- ► Laparoscopy is the standard method for confirming the diagnosis of ectopic pregnancy and for the surgical treatment of tubal gestations.

- ► The most common tumors found in the pelvis are leiomyomas, which occur in roughly 25% of women of reproductive age and are present in up to 50% of women at autopsy.

- ► Diagnosis of myomas is usually first suggested by a history of irregular and heavy periods and by pelvic examination in which an enlarged or irregularly shaped uterus is palpated or a large central pelvic mass is found.

- ► Surgical therapy for myomas can either be conservative, with preservation of the uterus (myomectomy), or definitive, in the form of hysterectomy.

- ► The most common ovarian enlargements occurring during the reproductive years are cysts that respond physiologically to sex steroid and gonadotropin stimulation.

- ► Surgery is indicated if ovarian cysts persist over two cycles, if excessive peritoneal fluid is present, if the cyst has significant solid elements or measures greater than 8 cm on ultrasonography, or if the signs and symptoms progress such that expectant management can no longer be entertained.

ANATOMY OF THE PELVIS

The bony pelvis is formed by the articulation of the two large innominate bones with the sacrum posteriorly and with one another anteriorly at the pubic symphysis. Each innominate bone has three subparts: the ilium, the ischium, and the pubis.

The organs of the pelvic cavity include the uterus, fallopian tubes, ovaries, bladder, lower half of the ureters, urethra, vagina, and rectum. The uterus is composed of a muscular fundus and a fibrous cervix. The portion of the uterus where the fundus narrows into the cervix is termed the **uterine isthmus**. The cervix implants into the anterior wall of the vagina. The peritoneum of the pelvis drapes over the pelvic viscerae to form a vesico-uterine fold anterior to the uterus and the cul-de-sac (pouch of Douglas) posterior to the uterus. The cul-de-sac is the most dependent portion of the pelvic cavity in the upright position.

From the superior lateral surface of the uterine fundus, in an area termed the **uterine cornu**, there arise—from anterior to posterior—the round ligament, fallopian tube, and utero-ovarian ligament. The peritoneum draping over these structures forms the broad ligaments (Figure 45–1). The round ligaments sweep anteriorly to the pelvic side wall, where they exit through the internal inguinal ring lateral to the inferior epigastric vessels. The fallopian tubes exit the uterus just posterior and rostral to the origination of the round ligaments and sweep posteriorly to hang into the cul-de-sac. The portion of the broad ligament that folds around the tube to form its mesentery is termed the **mesosalpinx**. The ovary is similarly enshrouded by the pelvic peritoneum, attached by its own mesovarium to the posterior surface of the broad ligament. Vessels emanating from the medial and lateral poles of the ovary are similarly enshrouded by the pelvic peritoneum, which medially forms the ovarian ligament and laterally forms the infundibulopelvic ligament (suspensory ligament of the ovary).

The main support structures of the uterus lie at the base of the broad ligaments. The cardinal ligaments, though they often are not discretely observable, provide considerable support to the uterus, cervix, and upper vagina. These ligaments, formed by a condensation of the endopelvic fascia and perivascular connective tissue at the base of the broad ligaments, span from a lateral origination on the pelvic side walls near the greater sciatic foramen to the cervix and upper vaginal vault medially. The **uterosacral ligaments** are two fibromuscular bands that emanate from the posterior cervix and pass posteriorly, beneath the pelvic peritoneum; they are seen again on either side of the pouch of Douglas, and ultimately fan out over a broad insertion into the lower part of the anterior sacrum. On the pelvic side wall, in the retroperitoneum of the pouch of Douglas, running just superior to the uterosacral ligaments, lies the lower course of the ureters.

Coursing within the superior portion of the cardinal ligament at the base of the broad ligament lies the uterine artery (Figure 45–2), which arises from the internal iliac artery and joins the uterus at the level of the internal cervical os or uterine isthmus. There it diverges into a marginal artery that ascends along the side of the uterus to anastamose with the ovarian blood supply, and another branch that descends along the side of the cervix and vagina. Other pelvic branches of the internal iliac artery include the obturator, internal pudendal, inferior gluteal, superior vesical, and middle rectal arteries.

The ureter crosses over the pelvic brim at the level of the bifurcation of the internal and external iliac arteries,

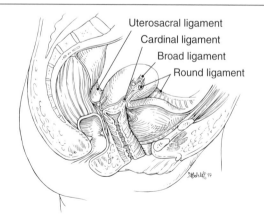

Figure 45–1. Ligamentous supports of the uterus.

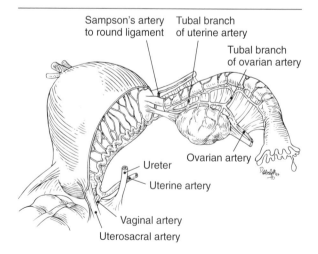

Figure 45–2. The uterine artery arises from the internal iliac artery and courses within the superior portion of the cardinal ligament. It has branches to the cervix and vagina, then ascends into the serosal surface of the uterus before anastomosing with the medial end of the ovarian artery.

just medial to the ovarian vessel. It then descends into the pelvis, attached to the pelvic peritoneum and posterior leaf of the broad ligament, and courses just below the ovarian vessels. Nearing the uterus, it can be seen running just above the uterosacral ligament to finally disappear into a tunnel through the cardinal ligament. If the posterior leaf of the broad ligament and peritoneum of the cul-de-sac are peeled away from the side wall, the ureter will remain attached to the peritoneum and will not be found lying attached to the major vessels of the pelvic retroperitoneum. The ureter enters the cardinal ligament tunnel, crossing just beneath the uterine artery, then passes within 1 cm of the superior lateral border of the cervix to lie on the anterior vaginal wall of the lateral vaginal fornix, and finally terminates in the bladder. Common sites of injury to the ureter include the area near the pelvic brim on the pelvic side wall during clamping of the ovarian vessels with oophorectomy and the area between the uterine artery and the bladder base during the removal of the cervix at the time of hysterectomy.

Table 45–1. Common pathogens isolated in pelvic inflammatory disease.

Neisseria gonorrhoeae
Chlamydia trachomatis
Aerobic bacteria
Garderella vaginalis
Gram-negative enterobacteriaceae
Escherichia coli
Klebsiella species
Proteus mirabilis
Group B streptococci
Anaerobic bacteria
Peptostreptococcus species
Peptococcus species
Bacteroides species
B fragilis
B bivius
B disiens
B melaninogenicus
Mycoplasma hominis
Ureaplasma urealyticum

Reprinted, with permission, from Droegemueller W: Benign gynecologic lesions. In: Droegemueller W et al (editors): *Comprehensive Gynecology.* Mosby, 1987.

PELVIC INFLAMMATORY DISEASE

Pelvic inflammatory disease (PID) is a nonspecific term denoting upper female genital tract infection. More precise diagnoses, such as endometritis, parametritis, salpingitis, and oophoritis, are preferred; however, this degree of diagnostic precision is often difficult to achieve at the time of clinical presentation. The severity of infection can be variable, ranging from mild inflammation of the endometrium (endometritis) and endosalpinx (salpingitis), to a pelvic abscess encompassing the posterior cul-de-sac, ovaries, and fallopian tubes.

The vast majority of cases of PID represent an ascending infection originating from the vagina and cervix (lower genital tract) and spreading up into the endometrial cavity and out into the fallopian tubes and peritoneal cavity. In very rare cases, PID can result from the contiguous intraperitoneal spread of infection from an inflamed nongenital-tract structure, such as the appendix or the colon (diverticulitis).

Sexually transmitted pathogens, such as *Neisseria gonorrhoeae* and *Chlamydia trachomatis*, are the most common initiators of upper genital tract infection, although clinically evident upper genital tract infections are, in the great majority of cases, polymicrobial in nature. A variety of anaerobic and aerobic organisms indigenous to the flora of the vagina are often found in these mixed infections (Table 45–1).

An episode of PID can have a grave impact on a patient's future reproductive health. Long-term sequelae of PID include infertility, subsequent ectopic pregnancies, chronic pelvic pain secondary to adhesions, and postinflammatory masses requiring future surgical exploration.

Patients at risk for PID include those already at risk for

contracting sexually transmitted infections. These risks include early age of first coitus, multiple sexual partners, age less than 25 years, residence in an area with a high prevalence of sexually transmitted diseases, and lack of contraceptive use.

Barrier methods of contraception, by decreasing the spread of sexually transmitted diseases, reduce the incidence of PID. Oral contraceptives, by thickening the cervical mucus, appear to reduce the ascendance of lower genital tract organisms into the upper genital tract, thereby reducing the incidence of PID. Colonization of the cervix (lower genital tract) by sexually transmitted organisms, however, appears to be increased in users of oral contraceptives.

Users of the Dalkon Shield intrauterine device (IUD) experienced an increased risk of PID. With the currently available IUDs, the increased risk of IUD-associated PID appears to be limited to the first 2 to 3 months after insertion, apparently the result of iatrogenic introduction of organisms into the upper genital tract during the insertion process. Any procedure that accesses the upper genital tract via the vagina and cervical canal carries a risk of PID.

Washout of the endocervical mucus barrier during menstruation appears to provide an opportunity for ascent of vaginal organisms into the upper genital tract. A majority of PID cases present during or soon after a menstrual period. Amenorrheic women seldom develop PID; in postmenopausal women who are amenorrheic, the diagnosis of PID should only reluctantly be entertained after other potential diagnoses are first ruled out. Pelvic inflammatory disease, when truly present in postmenopausal women, is often associated with genital tract malignancy. In the case of an intrauterine pregnancy, the combination of amenorrhea, thickened cervical mucus, and growing obstruction of the endometrial cavity by the enlarging conceptus makes ascending colonization of the upper genital tract after the first trimester fairly unlikely, and this combination usually would be associated with signs of a septic abortion.

DIAGNOSIS

Diagnosis begins with a complete medical history, involving a thorough assessment of the risk factors previously mentioned. The date of last menstrual period, contraceptive history, sexual history, and past sexually transmitted disease history all are important elements of this evaluation.

The symptoms associated with PID are fairly nonspecific (Table 45–2). Lower abdominal pain is the most common symptom, usually beginning as mild dull discomfort that slowly progresses in intensity. Acute pain is less common, and the differential diagnosis in a patient with this presentation must consider ectopic pregnancy, appendicitis, ovarian torsion, and rupture of an ovarian cyst as possibilities. Endometriosis, pelvic adhesions, and irritable bowel syndrome can give similar chronic pelvic pain symptoms. Vaginal discharge is a common complaint, occurring in roughly 65–75% of patients with PID. The discharge is often yellow, homogeneous in consistency, and without any characteristic malodor. Complaint of a fever is present in less than half of patients. Nausea and vomiting are relatively uncommon (< 15%), unless diffuse peritonitis is present. Right upper quadrant pain from perihepatitis (Fitz-Hugh-Curtis syndrome) is an inconsistent finding (< 10%) and must be differentiated from pneumonia, cholecystitis, and pyelonephritis. Endometritis can result in irregular vaginal bleeding in 40% of patients with PID.

PHYSICAL EXAMINATION

As is the case with symptomatology, the objecive findings in PID can also be fairly nonspecific (Table 45–3).

The abdominal examination in patients with PID can run the spectrum from relatively benign findings, with mild tenderness on deep palpation in the lower quadrants, to that of a surgical abdomen with diffuse peritonitis, involuntary guarding, and rebound.

On speculum examination of the cervix, there invariably will be some evidence of cervicitis or abnormal vaginal discharge. Cervical erythema, friability of the cervical mucosa, or mucopurulent discharge from the cervical os are frequently seen. Wet mount examination of the vaginal discharge will reveal numerous white blood cells. Indeed, the presence of PID is extremely unlikely in a patient with absence of white cells on wet mount and with clear mucous per os. Conversely, in many populations, the incidence of mucopurulent cervicitis is so high that the finding has low positive predictive value for the presence of upper genital tract infection.

Cervical motion tenderness and adnexal tenderness are the hallmark findings on pelvic examination in a patient with PID. However, the specificity of these findings is diminished by the fact that almost any intraperitoneal irritation, whatever its etiology, can yield similar findings. Bilateral adnexal tenderness alone has a high specificity for PID (92%), but is less sensitive (58%) because not all cases of salpingitis are bilateral. Indeed, any determination of PID on clinical grounds is confirmed only 65–70% of the time when laparoscopy is used to confirm the diagnosis. Of patients with a clinical diagnosis of PID whose diagnosis is not confirmed at laparoscopy (30%), roughly one third will demonstrate some other pathology, and the other two thirds actually will have a normal pelvis. Pelvic disorders causing a false-positive diagnosis of PID are listed in Table 45–4.

Table 45–2. Frequency of various symptoms as reported by patients in acute PID and visually normal groups (first-time PID patients).

Symptom	Acute PID (No. = 414)		Normal (No. = 138)		P Value
	No.	%	No.	%	
Lower abdominal pain	411	99.3	135	98.6	NS
Vaginal discharge	287	69.3	85	61.6	NS
Temperature ≥ 38°C	142	34.4	34	24.6	0.05
Irregular bleeding	165	40.0	54	39.1	NS
Urinary symptoms	82	19.8	29	21.8	NS
Vomiting	43	10.4	13	9.4	NS
Proctitis symptoms	30	7.3	4	2.9	NS
Other	33	8.0	8	5.8	NS

Reprinted, with permission, from Hadgu A, Weström L, Brooks CA, et al: Predicting acute pelvic inflammatory disease: A multivariate analysis. Am J Obstet Gynecol 1986;155:956.
PID = pelvic inflammatory disease.

Table 45–3. Frequency of various objective findings at admission in acute PID and visually normal groups.

Clinical Findings at Admission	Laparoscopic Diagnosis					
	Acute PID (No. = 414)		Normal (No. = 138)		P Value
	No.	%	No.	%	
Bimanual examination					
Marked tenderness	395	95.4	128	92.8	NS
Palpable mass or swelling	198	47.8	36	26.1	0.001
Erythrocyte sedimentation rate > 15 mm/h	336	81.2	78	56.5	0.001
Abnormal vaginal discharge	337	81.4	80	58.0	0.001
Fever (38°C)	146	35.3	21	15.2	0.001

Reprinted, with permission, from Hadgu A, Weström L, Brooks CA, et al: Predicting acute pelvic inflammatory disease: A multivariate analysis. Am J Obstet Gynecol 1986;155:956.
PID = pelvic inflammatory disease.

Not only are the clinical signs and symptoms nonspecific; laboratory measures also are nonspecific for the diagnosis of PID. Specimens for the diagnosis of *N gonorrhoeae* and *C trachomatis* should be obtained from the cervix. Wet mount evaluation of the vaginal discharge should reveal numerous white blood cells, as noted above. White blood cell count and sedimentation rate are too nonspecific to be of value. Of patients with PID, fewer than one half will have white counts above 10,000/mm.

C-reactive protein levels, although not helpful in diagnosis, can be followed during the course of therapy; falling levels indicate therapeutic success. A sensitive test for the beta subunit of human chorionic gonadotropin (hCG) should be obtained to rule out intrauterine or ectopic pregnancy.

Ultrasonographic evaluation is often useful in patients suspected of having PID. The exquisite adnexal pain often associated with moderate to severe infection will, in many cases, render accurate bimanual assessment of the adnexae impossible. Up to 30% of patients with PID who are thought to have a pelvic abscess on bimanual examination are found not to have an abcess at surgery. Conversely, many tubo-ovarian abscesses go undetected on physical examination, secondary to pain and guarding. Ultrasonographic imaging and pelvic CT scans have excel-

lent sensitivity for the presence of pelvic abscess or pyosalpinx, and, in cases in which either of these conditions is suspected or in which an adequate examination is not possible, either imaging modalities can aid in the diagnosis. Ultrasonography of the pelvis in cases of mild to moderate infection without abscess is often unremarkable.

Diagnostic criteria for the treatment of PID have been established by the Centers for Disease Control (CDC) (Table 45–5). In the realization that many cases present with subacute signs and symptoms leading to no treatment or delayed treatment, and with the desire to minimize the impact on reproductive health by early intervention in the course of disease, the CDC has established fairly broad minimum diagnostic criteria for antibiotic therapy, even though many patients without PID consequently will be overtreated. For patients in whom the severity of the clinical presentation mandates greater diagnostic precision in order to avoid morbidity associated with mistreatment, additional criteria have been established. Confidence in the diagnosis of PID will increase with the number of these additional criteria that can be met.

MANAGEMENT

The goals of treatment in PID are, first, to resolve the upper genital tract inflammation and colonization and to eradicate the genital tract of sexually transmitted pathogens, and, second, to minimize the permanent reproductive health sequelae from the infection. To these ends, early institution of treatment to reduce tubal damage will be warranted, even in equivocal cases. Diagnostic imprecision in the clinical diagnosis of PID necessitates overtreatment in roughly 30% of cases.

Ideally, treatment would involve hospitalization of all patients for intravenous antibiotic therapy; however, bed availability and costs often preclude this. Patients with evidence of severe infection should be hospitalized, as should those who are unlikely or unable to adhere to the follow-up requirements of outpatient treatment. CDC-recommended guidelines for hospitalization are shown in Table 45–6. Laparoscopy should be used liberally for

Table 45–4. Laparoscopic findings in patients with false-positive clinical diagnosis of acute PID but with pelvic disorders other than PID.

Laparoscopic Findings	No. Patients
Acute appendicitis	24
Endometriosis	16
Corpus luteum bleeding	12
Ectopic pregnancy	11
Pelvic adhesions only	7
Benign ovarian tumor	7
Chronic salpingitis	6
Miscellaneous	15
Total	98

Reprinted, with permission, from Jacobson LJ: Differential diagnosis of acute pelvic inflammatory disease. Am J Obstet Gynecol 1980;138:1007.
PID = pelvic inflammatory disease.

Table 45–5. CDC clinical criteria for diagnosis of PID.

Minimum Criteria (all three should be met)

Lower abdominal tenderness
Adnexal tenderness
Cervical motion tenderness

Additional Criteria
(the more met, the greater the accuracy of the diagnosis)

Routine
Oral temperature > 38.3°C
Abnormal cervical or vaginal discharge
Elevated erythrocyte sedimentation rate
Elevated C-reactive protein
Laboratory documentation of the cervical infection with
N gonorrhoeae or C trachomatis
Elaborate
Histopathologic evidence of endometritis on endometrial
biopsy
Tubo-ovarian abscess on sonography or other radiologic
tests
Laparoscopic abnormalities consistent with PID

Reprinted, with permission, from the Centers for Disease Control
and Prevention: 1993 Sexually Transmitted Diseases Treatment
Guidelines. MMWR 1993;42 (No. RR-14):75.
PID = pelvic inflammatory disease.

Table 45–7. CDC inpatient treatment regimens for PID.

Regimen A

Cefoxitin 2 g intravenously every 6 hours or cefotetan 2 g
intravenously every 12 hours,
PLUS
Doxycycline 100 mg intravenously or orally every 12 hours

Followed by oral doxycycline 100 mg twice daily to complete
14 days of therapy

Regimen B

Clindamycin 900 mg intravenously every 8 hours,
PLUS
Gentamycin loading dose intravenously or intramuscularly
(2 mg/kg of body weight) followed by a maintenance dose
(1.5 mg/kg) every 8 hours

Followed by oral doxycycline 100 mg twice daily or oral
clindamycin 450 mg twice daily to complete 14 days of
therapy

Reprinted, with permission, from the Centers for Disease Control
and Prevention: 1993 Sexually Transmitted Diseases Treatment
Guidelines. MMWR 1993;42 (No. RR-14):75.
PID = pelvic inflammatory disease.

equivocal cases to improve the accuracy of the diagnosis.
Some centers use laparoscopy to confirm all suspected
cases of PID.

Antibiotic therapy for PID takes into account the
polymicrobial nature of this infection and the anaerobic
species involved. The CDC-recommended treatment
guidelines for inpatient and for outpatient therapy are
shown in Tables 45–7 and 45–8. Inpatient intravenous
therapy should continue until the patient is afebrile and
clinically improved for at least 48 hours, at which time
oral doxycycline treatment (100 mg twice daily for 14
days) should be instituted.

Effective and aggressive antibiotic therapy has made
surgical intervention for PID less common than it once
was. Patients discovered by diagnostic laparoscopy to
have salpingitis certainly should be allowed to respond
first to a standard course of antibiotic therapy before pro-

ceeding with extirpative surgery. Antibiotic therapy cures
well over 90% of uncomplicated salpingitis cases.

Patients diagnosed as having PID but who do not improve within 48–72 hours of appropriate antibiotic therapy most often have a tubo-ovarian abscess or have been
misdiagnosed. Roughly 5–15% of patients hospitalized
for treatment of PID will have a tubo-ovarian abscess. In
one study, 42% of patients presenting with a tubo-ovarian
abscess had recently undergone outpatient treatment of

Table 45–6. CDC criteria for hospitalization of patients with PID.

Diagnosis uncertain
Pelvic abscess
Pregnancy
Adolescent (poor outpatient compliance)
HIV infected
Severe illness or nausea and vomiting
Unable to follow or tolerate an outpatient regimen or return in 72
hours for follow-up
Failure to respond clinically to outpatient therapy

Reprinted, with permission, from the Centers for Disease Control
and Prevention: 1993 Sexually Transmitted Diseases Treatment
Guidelines. MMWR 1993;42 (No. RR-14):75.
PID = pelvic inflammatory disease.

Table 45–8. Outpatient treatment regimens for PID.[1]

Regimen A

Cefoxitin 2 g intramuscularly plus probenecid 1 g orally in a single dose concurrently, or ceftriaxone 250 mg intramuscularly
or other parenteral third-generation cephalosporin
PLUS
Doxycycline 100 mg orally 2 times a day for 14 days

Regimen B

Ofloxacin 400 mg orally 2 times a day for 14 days
PLUS
Either clindamycin 450 mg orally 4 times a day, or metronida-
zole 500 mg orally 2 times a day for 14 days

[1]Patients receiving outpatient therapy should be evaluated again
in 72 hours. Those not showing substantial clinical improvement
should be hospitalized for intravenous therapy and possibly further diagnostic work-up. Patients receiving intravenous therapy
should show improvement within 72 hours. Signs of improvement
include an element of defervescence (not necessarily complete),
decreasing peritoneal signs, decreasing C-reactive protein or
white blood cell count, and decreasing uterine or adnexal tenderness.
Reprinted, with permission, from the Centers for Disease Control
and Prevention: 1993 Sexually Transmitted Diseases Treatment
Guidelines. MMWR 1993;42 (no. RR-14):75.
PID = pelvic inflammatory disease.

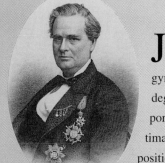

J. Marion Sims (1813–1883) wearing decorations he received from European royalty.

J. Marion Sims (1813–1883) is considered the first great American gynecologist. He was born in South Carolina and received his medical degree from Jefferson Medical College in 1835. His influential article reporting the cure of several vesicovaginal fistulas appeared in 1852. He ultimately succeeded at the procedure by using silver sutures, the knee-chest position for improved exposure, and a vaginal speculum of his own design. He relocated from the South to New York City in 1853 and within a few years established the Women's Hospital in the state of New York. Many advances in gynecologic surgery were made in this facility and were presented in Sims' treatise, *Silver Sutures in Surgery*, which appeared in 1858. Soon after that publication appeared, another important article of his was published, describing a method of cervical amputation (1861).

Within his lifetime, Sims was able to establish a truly international reputation. He was well received in Europe and completed a number of key publications abroad, including an important paper on vaginismus (1862), and his most important clinical text, *Clinical Notes on Uterine Surgery* (1866). Sims served as president of the American Medical Association in 1876 and the American Gynecological Society in 1880. His name is closely linked with a position used to facilitate vaginal examination and with a double "duckbill" vaginal speculum.

PID. Tubo-ovarian abscesses are unilateral in up to 70% of cases.

Medical treatment of tubo-ovarian abscesses fails to avert surgical intervention in anywhere from 30–60% of cases. The need for surgical intervention during the initial hospitalization for intravenous antibiotic therapy, referred to as an early failure of medical therapy, occurs in 10–30% of patients with tubo-ovarian abscesses. Another 20–30% of patients will have late failure of medical therapy, requiring surgical intervention secondary to postinfectious sequelae sometime after the initial hospitalization. Fertility rates following successful treatment of a tubo-ovarian abscess are in the range of 10–15%.

Computed tomography (CT) or ultrasonography of the pelvis can help determine whether an abscess is present and can be used to guide percutaneous drainage of an abscess cavity. Antibiotic therapy plus drainage of a pelvic abscess appears to be superior to antibiotic therapy alone. Laparoscopically guided drainage of tubo-ovarian ab-

scesses has also been described. If drainage of an abscess is not possible, or if no abscess is present, then lack of response after 72 hours of appropriate antibiotic coverage will mandate surgical exploration. Any worsening of a patient's condition during the course of antibiotic therapy will also require exploration, as will increasing abscess size despite antibiotics. Sudden clinical decompensation in patients receiving intravenous antibiotics for a tubo-ovarian abscess is suggestive of spontaneous rupture of the abscess; this mandates immediate stabilization and then laparotomy in order to decrease the high mortality rate associated with this complication.

Although cul-de-sac abscesses are less common in this present era of modern antibiotics, they do still occasionally dissect the rectovaginal septum and present as soft fluctuant masses in the midline of the posterior vaginal wall. Occasionally, such an abscess will rupture and drain spontaneously into the rectum, with subsequent improvement in symptoms. Iatrogenic drainage of such an abscess via incision of the vaginal mucosa overlying the area of midline fluctuance (**colpotomy**) will also speed recovery. Colpotomy should be used only to drain an abscess that is dissecting the rectovaginal space, thus allowing extraperitoneal drainage to occur. Colpotomy to reach and drain an abscess higher in the pelvis will result in intraperitoneal spillage of the abscess contents, which is associated with increased morbidity and mortality.

When intravenous antibiotic therapy for PID fails, and surgical intervention is required, the classic procedure has been to perform a total abdominal hysterectomy with bilateral salpingo-oophorectomy ("pelvic clean out"). This practice has been based partly on the finding that one third of apparently normal-appearing adnexae in patients with a contralateral tubo-ovarian abscess demonstrated microabscesses on pathological evaluation. Subsequent data concerning tubo-ovarian abscess have shown that unilateral adnexectomy, together with continued antibiotic therapy, is curative in roughly 85% of patients, with a subsequent 15–20% fertility rate. About 15% of patients fail this conservative surgical intervention and require subsequent definitive surgery. Conservative surgical treatment is, therefore, appropriate only for patients desirous of future fertility and willing to accept a 15% reoperation rate.

There has also been some success with conservative surgery for ruptured tubo-ovarian abscesses. Irrigation of the pelvis and abdomen with drainage of the ruptured abscess cavity has been shown to successfully deter more extensive surgery in 80% of such cases. Even when bilateral salpingo-oophorectomy for bilateral tubo-ovarian abscesses is required, retention of the uterus can be considered for a patient who might desire to avail herself of advanced reproductive technologies that can allow her to carry a donated ovum.

ECTOPIC PREGNANCY

Ectopic pregnancies are defined as **gestations implanted in areas other than the lining of the endometrial cavity**. Implantation sites include the fallopian tube (interstitial, isthmic, ampullary, or fimbrial ectopics), the cervix, the ovary, and the abdominal cavity (Figure 45–3). The ectopic pregnancy rate, usually quoted as the number of ectopics per reported pregnancies, has been steadily increasing in recent decades in the United States and throughout the world. The rate of ectopic pregnancies per 1000 reported pregnancies in the United States tripled from 4.5 per 1000 in 1970 to 14 per 1000 in 1983 and has roughly paralleled the increasing incidence of sexually transmitted infections reported during the same period. In the United States, greater than one out of every 100 reported pregnancies will be ectopic, and roughly 40 women die annually as the result of ectopic pregnancy.

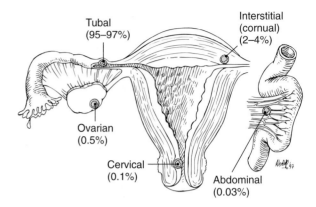

Figure 45–3. Location and incidence of ectopic pregnancy.

Fortunately, medical advances have lead to a steady decline in the mortality rate for ectopic pregnancy, from 3.5 deaths per 1000 ectopic cases in 1970 to 0.5 per 1000 in 1987. Despite these advances, physician misdiagnosis and treatment delays occur in roughly 50% of fatal ectopic cases. The ectopic mortality rate per case is three times higher in black than in white women, and 1.7 times higher in unmarried than in married women of any race.

ETIOLOGY

Previous tubal damage secondary to salpingitis is the leading cause of ectopic pregnancy. Tubal occlusion has been estimated to occur in 13%, 35%, and 75% of patients with one, two, or three or more past pelvic infections. Patients able to conceive after an episode of PID have roughly a 5% chance that the conception will be ectopic.

Various contraceptive methods also increase the risk of ectopic pregnancy, should contraceptive failure occur. Accidental conception with an IUD is associated with a 5% chance of ectopic, presumably because of the device's ability to lower the success of intrauterine implantation, while leaving the chances of extrauterine implantation unaffected. Former users of an IUD do not appear to have an increased future risk of ectopic gestation, with the exception of past users of the Dalkon Shield (an IUD associated with a very high rate of PID). Patients conceiving while using progesterone-only hormonal contraceptive methods appear to have an increased ectopic risk, presumably the result of the alteration of tubal motility by progesterone. Hormonal imbalance might also explain the increased risk of ectopic gestation of patients undergoing ovulation induction for infertility or other assisted reproductive techniques.

Patients who conceive after tubal sterilization have an increased ectopic risk. If the tubal sterilization was via laparoscopic electrocoagulation, then a future conception would have as high as a 50% chance of being ectopic. Nonlaparoscopic methods, if they fail, are associated with roughly a 15% ectopic rate. Multiple induced abortions might increase subsequent ectopic risk, as would an illegally performed abortion, presumably because of the cumulative or acute risk of salpingitis.

Anatomic alteration of the fallopian tubes, such as is seen in patients exposed to diethylstilbestrol (DES) in utero, is associated with increased ectopic rates, as is prior tubal surgery. Depending on the tubal surgery performed (eg, lysis of adhesions, fimbrioplasty, salpingostomy, tubal reanastamosis), ectopic rates will vary from 2–7%. A previous tubal gestation, whether treated medically or surgically, is associated with a 10–20% chance of recurrent ectopic in a future conception. If the first conception is a tubal gestation, the chance of a repeat ectopic is 30%, and only 30% will ever carry an intrauterine pregnancy to term.

DIAGNOSIS

Prior to the advent of transvaginal ultrasonography and sensitive β-hCG assays, roughly 90% of patients with ectopic pregnancies presented acutely with tubal rupture. In some recent series, over 85% of patients with an ectopic pregnancy were diagnosed prior to rupture. The classic triad of a tubal ectopic pregnancy is pelvic pain, abnormal bleeding, and an adnexal mass. A history of all medications currently being used and all risk factors for ectopic gestation should be obtained from the patient. Menstrual history, reproductive history, contraceptive history, sexual history, surgical history, and medical history should all be noted.

There is no distinct menstrual history that is characteristic for ectopic pregnancy. From 50%–80% of patients with ectopic gestations report some type of recent abnormal menstrual bleeding. Roughly 15% report 12 weeks or more of amenorrhea, while a similar number report a normal last menses within the preceding 4 weeks. Abdominal pain is the most consistent symptom, reported in over 90% of patients with an ectopic pregnancy. Other symptoms and physical signs of ectopic pregnancy are listed in Tables 45–9 and 45–10. As with PID, abdominal tenderness and adnexal tenderness on bimanual examination are present in the majority of patients with an ectopic pregnancy. The bimanual examination is reported as normal in 10% of patients, and a slightly enlarged uterus (less than that of an 8-week gestation) is reported in another third. An adnexal mass representing the ectopic gestation is palpated only 30% of the time. Distinguishing an adnexal mass distinct from the uterus and ovaries can be difficult, especially when the examination is painful and the patient is guarding.

Patients presenting with a ruptured ectopic implant may have a profound anemia, although there is no particular hematocrit or white blood cell count that is characteristic

Table 45–9. Symptoms of ectopic pregnancy.

Symptoms	% Patients With Symptom
Abdominal pain	90–100
Amenorrhea	75–95
Vaginal bleeding	50–80
Dizziness, fainting	20–35
Urge to defecate	5–15
Pregnancy symptoms	10–25
Passage of tissue	5–10

Reprinted, with permission, from Weckstein LN: Current perspective on ectopic pregnancy. Obstet Gynecol Surv 1985;40:259.

of an ectopic pregnancy. Hypovolemic shock occurs in less than 5% of patients. Active intraperitoneal bleeding can be reflected by tachycardia or hypotension, but these are not consistently present with an ectopic pregnancy. Patients are rarely febrile.

Culdocentesis is a procedure than can be rapidly performed to assess whether there is free blood in the peritoneal cavity. Using a long 18- or 20-gauge needle, culdocentesis involves the transvaginal aspiration of fluid from the cul-de-sac. Aspiration of at least 0.5 cc of nonclotting blood with a hematocrit of 15% or more is deemed a positive tap, and this is the finding in 70–90% of cases of ectopic gestation. Failure to obtain fluid is nondiagnostic. A bleeding corpus luteum or abdominal abnormality other than an ectopic implant can result in nonclotting blood on culdocentesis, however, the hematocrit of the fluid in this case is usually lower than 15%.

With a clinical presentation suspicious for ectopic pregnancy, a positive pregnancy test, and a positive culdocentesis, an ectopic pregnancy is correctly identified over 95% of the time, and further diagnostic delay can be avoided. A positive culdocentesis in the presence of an ectopic gestation does not necessarily indicate tubal rupture, as 40–60% of unruptured ectopics have a positive culdocentesis. Conversely, the culdocentesis will be negative in up to 10% of patients with ectopic gestations, indicating only that tubal rupture has not occurred.

The single most useful laboratory test in the clinical

Table 45–10. Signs of ectopic pregnancy.

Sign	% Patients With Sign
Adnexal tenderness	75–90
Abdominal tenderness	80–95
Adnexal mass[1]	50
Uterine enlargement	20–30
Orthostatic changes	10–15
Fever	5–10

[1]20% present on the side opposite the ectopic pregnancy.
Reprinted, with permission, from Weckstein LN: Current perspective on ectopic pregnancy. Obstet Gynecol Surv 1985;40:259.

evaluation of ectopic pregnancy is the β-hCG assay. Assays sensitive to 5–10 mIU/mL of the First International Reference Preparation (IRP) for the beta subunit of human chorionic gonadotropin (β-hCG) will be positive in virtually every patient with an intrauterine or ectopic pregnancy. In cases in which immediate surgical exploration is not indicated by hemodynamic status, ultrasonography can help to discriminate between ectopic and intrauterine gestations. The principal use of ultrasonography is to rule out ectopic gestation by demonstrating an intrauterine gestation.

A discriminatory level for β-hCG of 6000–6500 mIU/mL (IRP) has been described, above which all normal intrauterine pregnancies should be visible on transabdominal ultrasonography in the form of an intrauterine gestational sac. A β-hCG level above this value and an inability with transabdominal ultrasonography to visualize a gestational sac within the endometrial cavity is presumptive of an ectopic gestation.

Unfortunately, the β-hCG levels in as many as 75% of ectopic gestations never reach the 6000–6500 mIU/mL (IRP) discriminatory threshold needed for transabdominal sonography. For this reason, transvaginal ultrasonography has become the preferred imaging modality for the diagnosis of ectopic pregnancies. The β-hCG discriminatory level for transvaginal imaging is 2000 mIU/mL (IRP). Inability to visualize an intrauterine sac on transvaginal ultrasonography at values of β-hCG above 2000 mIU/mL indicates an ectopic gestation. In patients with ectopic pregnancies, 60–90% will have a cystic or complex mass in the adnexae on ultrasonography, and 30% will have free fluid visible in the cul-de-sac. These findings are nonspecific, however, and are easily confused with a corpus luteum, hydrosalpinx, a paratubal cyst, and so forth. Direct ultrasonographic diagnosis of an ectopic within the adnexae is most accurate, of course, when a fetal pole and fetal cardiac activity are seen within the adnexal mass. This occurs, however, in a minority of cases (10–15%).

Patients without evidence of an intrauterine pregnancy on transvaginal ultrasonography, but with a β-hCG that is below the transvaginal discriminatory level of 2000 mIU/mL, may have either an intra- or extra-uterine gestation. These patients, if they are stable, can be followed with serial serum β-hCG levels taken every 2–3 days. In normal early intrauterine gestations (prior to 8–10 weeks of gestation), serum β-hCG levels in the mother double roughly every 3 days and rise by 66% every 2 days. Pregnancies in which the β-hCG levels plateau or rise by less than 50% every 2 days are abnormal, whether they are in the uterus or in an ectopic location.

Dilation and curettage at this time to remove intrauterine tissue for pathologic diagnosis will assist in locating the gestational tissue. Absence of villous tissue on endometrial sampling points to an ectopic gestation or to a complete spontaneous abortion. A continued rise or a plateau in β-hCG levels post-curettage indicates persistence of ectopic gestational tissue.

Patients with a normal or near normal rise in β-hCG levels can be followed until the discriminatory level is reached. Transvaginal ultrasonography can then be used to confirm the diagnosis.

Falling β-hCG levels in a patient that is stable can be closely followed down to normal without active intervention. Possible explanations for falling β-hCG levels include spontaneous abortion or spontaneous resolution of an ectopic pregnancy.

A single measurement of the patient's serum progesterone level can also be useful in the diagnosis of ectopic pregnancy. Levels greater than 25 ng/mL exclude the diagnosis of ectopic pregnancy, with a sensitivity of 97.5%. Levels of 5 ng/mL or less indicate nonviability of the pregnancy, whether the pregnancy is intrauterine or ectopic, and allow definitive diagnostic uterine curettage to proceed.

MANAGEMENT

Expectant management might be appropriate in select circumstances if the patient is compliant and has easy access to immediate medical care. Data suggest that up to 60% of tubal gestations will spontaneously resolve over 3 to 6 weeks. Unfortunately, clear criteria for distinguishing patients likely to have spontaneous resolution from those likely to experience tubal rupture with hemorrhage are not available. Patients with tubal gestations and falling β-hCG levels, although still at some risk for tubal rupture, can generally be safely followed expectantly until β-hCG levels normalize. Patients with ectopic tubal gestations of less than 2 cm diameter, with less than 50 ml of hematoperitoneum on ultrasonography, and with β-hCG levels less than 1000 mIU/mL on initial presentation, appear to be more likely to experience spontaneous resolution of their ectopic pregnancy.

Surgical Treatment

Laparoscopy is the standard method for confirming the diagnosis of ectopic pregnancy and for the surgical treatment of tubal gestations. Diagnostically, laparoscopy has both a false-negative and false-positive rate of 2–5%. Laparoscopy for the treatment of tubal gestations has been shown to achieve the same surgical result as is accomplished via a standard laparotomy incision, but with less morbidity and faster recovery. Laparoscopy is not recommended if the patient is unstable, if a laparoscopic approach is generally contraindicated, or if the surgeon lacks expertise in this modality.

Conservative or radical surgical therapy for tubal gestation may be performed either via laparoscopy or laparotomy. **Conservative surgery** involves preservation of the involved fallopian tube. Retention of the diseased tube appears to increase subsequent conception rate without significantly altering subsequent repeat ectopic rates. The repeat ectopic rate is approximately 15%, whether the affected tube is preserved via conservative methods or is completely removed by radical total salpingectomy.

The original conservative procedure for ectopic gestation was a linear salpingotomy performed via a laparotomy incision. With linear salpingotomy, an incision is made along the antimesenteric surface of the tube, and the trophoblastic tissue is gently expressed or irrigated out. The incision is then closed with fine nonreactive suture. The conservative procedure more commonly in use today is the **laparoscopic linear salpingostomy**: a procedure identical to linear salpingotomy except that suture closure of the tube is eliminated in favor of allowing the tube to heal spontaneously by secondary intention. No advantage of suture closure over spontaneous closure has been demonstrated, and elimination of laparoscopic suturing simplifies the procedure. Hemostasis in both procedures is facilitated by the injection of a weak vasopressor solution into the mesosalpinx beneath the intended site of incision.

Problems with the conservative approach to tubal gestation include the possibility of persistent trophoblastic tissue (3–5%) and continued bleeding from the tube. For these reasons, only women who desire preservation of their reproductive potential and who are hemodynamically stable should undergo conservative tubal surgery. Other contraindications to the conservative approach include ectopic implant greater than 5 cm and a ruptured tube with anything more than minimal tubal disruption.

Radical surgery for tubal pregnancy, called **salpingec-**

tomy, is indicated when the tube is severely diseased or distorted (including ruptured) or when the patient has no desire for future fertility, has an ectopic implant greater than 5 cm, or is hemodynamically unstable. Salpingectomy involves total removal of the affected tube (Figure 45–4).

Partial salpingectomy followed by either immediate or delayed tubal reanastamosis is a technique used by some for ectopic implants located in the narrow isthmic portion of the tube. Results have not shown this method to have any distinct advantage over the simpler linear salpingotomy, and it does require special microsurgical skills and increased time.

Ectopic pregnancies in the interstitial transmyometrial portion of the tube are handled differently. Although interstitial implantation occurs in only 2–4% of tubal pregnancies, it accounts for 10–20% of mortalities from ectopics. The increased mortality from this type of implantation is the result of the thick myometrial wall that surrounds the gestation at this location, which allows it to grow larger and to become more vascularized prior to rupture. Management involves removal of the tube and a wedge of the myometrium from the cornu of the uterus.

Cervical and abdominal implantations are fairly rare

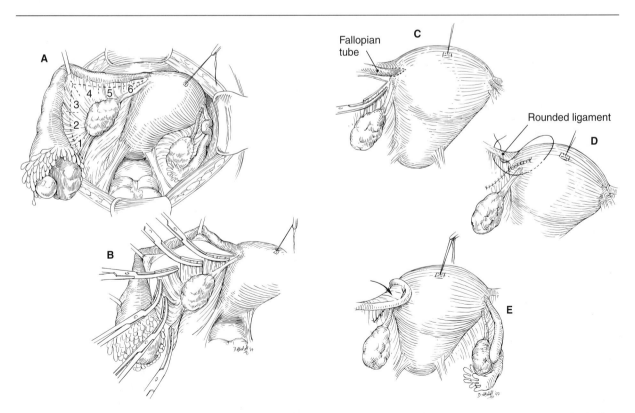

Figure 45–4. Total salpingectomy for tubal pregnancy. ***A, B:*** The mesosalpinx of the involved tube is cut in a sequential fashion. ***C:*** Each clamp is replaced by an absorbable suture. A wedge of intramural tube is excised from the uterine cornu, and the freed tube is removed. The site of the cornual wedge excision is oversewn. ***D, E:*** A stitch through the posterior uterus and peritoneum beneath the round ligament is taken as shown, thereby advancing round ligament over the site of the cornual excision.

and require special management strategies that are beyond the scope of this chapter. Ovarian pregnancies are exceedingly rare, but when present can usually be managed by wedge resection of a portion of the involved ovary. Oophorectomy is rarely necessary.

Medical Treatment

A variety of medicinal agents have been used to treat ectopic gestations, but none have approached the popularity of methotrexate for this purpose. Although methotrexate has produced success rates, complication rates, and subsequent pregnancy rates equivalent to those achieved with surgical therapy, its use has not become standard in many centers.

The great benefits of medical over surgical therapy are its lesser cost, morbidity, and convalescent time. Of course, if laparoscopy is required for diagnosis, then the benefits of medical therapy are obviated, and immediate surgical resolution of the tubal gestation is preferred. Simplified dosing of methotrexate (50 mg/m² of body surface area in one intramuscular dose, repeated weekly if needed) has been described. β-hCG levels are followed until undetectable. If levels plateau or rise, repeat dosing is necessary. Pelvic pain may increase a few days after injection of methotrexate, possibly reflecting involution of the ectopic tissue and/or abortion of the gestation out the fimbriated end of the tube. The increased pain may be difficult to differentiate from that of tubal rupture. Methotrexate therapy can also be used in cases of persistent ectopic tissue following linear salpingotomy.

Prognosis for future fertility following surgical or medical treatment of ectopic pregnancy depends upon a variety of factors, such as patient age, previous infertility, extent of pelvic adhesions, and so forth. In general, a 60–80% chance of future conception associated with a 15% chance of repeat ectopic pregnancy can be expected.

UTERINE LEIOMYOMATA

Uterine leiomyomata are whorl-like bundles of interlacing smooth muscle cells of the uterus that can range in size from microscopic to well over 20 cm in diameter (Figure 45–5). The most common tumors found in the pelvis, leiomyomas are present in roughly 25% of reproductive age women and in up to 50% of women at autopsy. They are three to nine times more common in black women than in white women.

Myoma growth is partly dependent upon estrogen stimulation, as is evidenced by the rarity of myomas prior to menarche, the degree of enlargement that usually occurs during the reproductive years, and the involution frequently seen in the hypoestrogenic conditions of menopause. These smooth muscle tumors, often inaccurately called "fibroids," are one of the leading indications for hysterectomy and can cause considerable reproductive

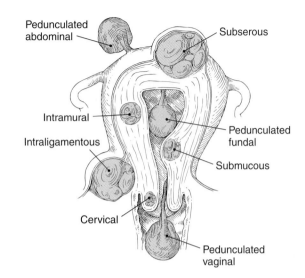

Figure 45–5. Leiomyomata of the uterus, with characteristic whorl-like appearance.

tract dysfunction, including prolonged and irregular menses (**menometrorrhagia**), painful menses (**dysmenorrhea**), pelvic pain, infertility, and spontaneous abortions.

Uterine myomas are nearly uniformly benign. Leiomyosarcoma is found in less than 0.1% of cases. A variety of benign degenerative changes (more frequent in the larger myomas) commonly occur within uterine leiomyomas. Some of the more common include hyaline, fatty (myxomatous), calcific, liquefactive (cystic), and carneous (red) degenerative changes. Carneous degeneration most commonly occurs during pregnancy. The congested and reddish appearance of the myoma is caused by venous thrombosis and interstitial hemorrhage. Such infarction-like degenerative changes can cause pain, but usually are self-limiting. Occasionally, superinfection of a degenerating myoma will occur.

DIAGNOSIS

The signs and symptoms of uterine myomas often relate to their position in the uterus. Myomas can be pedunculated, subserous, intramural, or submucosal. Myomas such as the submucosal type, which impinge on the endometrial cavity and the endometrial lining, are frequently associated with menstrual disturbances, such as menorrhagia or erratic bleeding patterns (**metrorrhagia**). Myomas within the muscular wall of the uterus (intramural type) can frequently cause painful or heavy periods. Myomas such as the subserous or pedunculated types, which principally grow away from the uterus, are less frequently associated with menstrual disturbance and dysmenorrhea.

Pedunculated myomas can occasionally torse on their pedicle and cause severe persistent pain. Submuous myomas can occasionally extend into the uterine cavity on a pedicle and prolapse through the cervical os. Such aborting myomas present as a cervical or endocervical mass and often are associated with irregular bleeding and secondary infection from colonization by the vaginal flora.

Most myomas grow slowly, and symptoms most often occur in an insidious fashion, with progressive dysmenorrhea, menometrorrhagia, and pelvic pressure. Except for necrosis or torsion, myomas do not usually present with acute onset of symptoms. Progressive growth can lead to pressure on the bladder, causing urinary frequency and sometimes stress incontinence. Urinary retention from obstruction of the bladder neck by fibroids is a rare occurrence. Ureteral obstruction from the uterine mass is occasionally seen.

Diagnosis is usually first suggested by pelvic examination in which an enlarged or irregularly shaped uterus is palpated or a large central pelvic mass is found. A uterus of normal size, but of unusual firmness on palpation, also suggests the diagnosis. When an enlarged mass is found, other diagnoses, such as pregnancy or ovarian neoplasm, need to be considered and excluded. Measuring the depth of the uterine cavity with a transcervical sound can confirm that the uterus is greatly enlarged (> 10 cm). An x-ray of the pelvis occasionally will reveal calcified myomas.

Ultrasonography can often give precise information regarding the number of fibroids, their size, and their relative positions within the uterus. Ovarian neoplasms can usually be ruled out by ultrasonography; however, excessive uterine enlargement can at times obscure visualization of the normal adnexae. A CT scan can also delineate the location and size of fibroids. A CT scan or intravenous pyelogram can determine whether hydronephrosis or hydroureter is present. Magnetic resonance imaging (MRI) can very clearly distinguish myomas from surrounding myometrium and can very accurately give information regarding their size, number, and location within the uterus.

MANAGEMENT

The mere presence of uterine myomas does not dictate therapeutic intervention. Treatment usually is considered in patients who request relief of symptoms attributable to the tumors. Some suggest surgical intervention when the uterus reaches the size of a 12- to 14-week gestation. Such size limits are arbitrary, however. Avoidance of surgical intervention in the perimenopausal years is frequently practiced, in hopes that menopause will bring regression of the tumors. Rapidly growing myomas or myomas that grow during the menopause are at higher risk for leiomyosarcoma and are best managed surgically. Women with unexplained infertility except for the presence of myomas and women who have a history of recurrent spontaneous abortions can potentially improve their reproductive

outcome by surgical removal of the myomas. Removal of myomas during pregnancy is not recommended.

Surgical therapy can be either conservative, with preservation of the uterus, or definitive, in the form of hysterectomy. With the advent of assisted reproductive technologies, more women are requesting conservation of the uterus when appropriate.

Myomectomy is the procedure of choice when preservation of the uterus is desired. Although most frequently performed via a laparotomy, hysteroscopic resection of submucosal fibroids is also an option. Laparoscopic myomectomy is occasionally performed in select cases (eg, pedunculated myoma, or single subserous myoma). However, generalized application of the laparoscopic myomectomy technique has not yet been sufficiently studied for it to be used routinely. Some preliminary success with electrical coagulation of myomas using bipolar cautery needles has also been described.

Hysterectomy is the definitive procedure for symptomatic uterine myomas in women not desiring to retain the uterus. Removal of the uterus eliminates the chance of myoma recurrence, assures resolution of disordered or painful menses, and decreases the potential for postsurgical pelvic adhesion formation. In the case of large or multiple myomas, blood loss is frequently less when hysterectomy, rather than myomectomy, is performed.

ENLARGED ADNEXAL STRUCTURES

Enlargements of the adnexae (ovaries and tubes) are often found incidentally at the time of laparotomy. Such enlargements may also present with acute symptomatology requiring immediate intervention, while at other times they are completely asymptomatic and are found on routine bimanual examination. Acute symptoms of adnexal enlargement can occur when torsion of the adnexa on its vascular base results in infarction and ischemia or when rupture of cyst contents results in peritoneal irritation.

Ovarian enlargements can be the result of normal physiologic processes, dysfunctional physiologic processes, or neoplastic and non-neoplastic processes (Table 45–11).

PHYSIOLOGIC OVARIAN ENLARGEMENTS

In reproductive-age women, formation of a preovulatory follicle and a corpus luteum occurs each cycle as a normal physiologic part of the menstrual cycle. Such cysts are usually no more than 2 cm in diameter, with the preovulatory cyst containing clear fluid, and the corpus luteum having a yellow and vascularized appearance. They are, for the most part, asymptomatic and can be seen routinely on ultrasonographic evaluations of the ovary. Rupture of the dominant follicle at the time of ovulation can be associated with transient unilateral discomfort (usually

Table 45–11. Common ovarian disorders.

Physiologic processes
    Preovulatory follicle
    Corpus luteum

Dysfunctional physiologic processes
    Persistent follicular cyst
    Corpus luteum cyst
    Polycystic ovaries
    Theca-lutein cysts

Nonphysiologic processes (non-neoplastic)
    Endometriosis
    Inflammatory cysts

Benign neoplastic processes
Epithelial
    Serous cystadenoma
    Mucinous cystadenoma
    Endometrioid cystadenoma
    Clear cell (mesonephroid) tumors
    Brenner tumors
Germ cell
    Mature cystic teratomas
    Struma ovarii
Stromal
    Fibroma
    Granulosa cell tumor

no more than 24–48 hours in duration), which is termed **mittelschmerz** (middle pain). The appearance, size, and location of these normal physiologic structures will vary with each menstrual cycle, and no intervention is necessary.

DYSFUNCTIONAL PHYSIOLOGIC OVARIAN ENLARGEMENTS

The most common ovarian enlargements occurring during the reproductive years are cysts that respond physiologically to sex steroid and gonadotropin stimulation. Persistent follicular cysts and corpus luteum cysts are the most common of these dysfunctional cysts. Representing temporary dysfunction of regular physiologic events, these cysts often present in association with transient menstrual dysfunction or irregularity.

Persistent follicular cysts, which most often result from a failure to ovulate, are usually unilateral and thin-walled, with clear or occasionally blood-stained fluid, and range from 2–8 cm in diameter. During the menstrual cycle, the corpus luteum routinely undergoes limited internal bleeding, filling its center with blood that ultimately is reabsorbed and replaced with a fluid-filled cystic cavity lined by yellow-orange luteinized cells. If bleeding is brisk or excessive, the final cystic space can range from 3–10 cm in diameter, with an average size of 4 cm. Persistent corpus luteum cysts are usually colored red-brown from internal hemorrhage, and can, if persistent, continue to secrete progesterone and cause menstrual irregularity.

Rupture can occasionally occur, spilling blood into the peritoneal cavity. Such bleeding can occasionally be massive and require immediate surgical intervention. Ectopic pregnancy should be considered in the differential diagnosis in such cases and can be ruled out by a sensitive pregnancy test that is negative for β-hCG.

Management of palpable adnexal masses can be aided by the use of transvaginal or transabdominal ultrasonography. A unilateral, unilocular cyst measuring 6 cm or less in diameter can usually be followed over one to two menstrual cycles for spontaneous resolution. Surgery is indicated if the cyst persists over two cycles, if excessive peritoneal fluid is present, if the cyst has significant solid elements or measures greater than 8 cm in diameter on ultrasonography, or if the signs or symptoms progress such that expectant managment can no longer be entertained.

Expectant management is predicated on the high frequency with which benign, self-limited, dysfunctional physiologic cysts are seen in reproductive-age women. Premenarchal girls or postmenopausal women are much less likely to develop such physiologic cysts, and expectant management is less often entertained in these age groups. In postmenopausal women, however, there has been a recent trend toward expectant managment in the case of cysts less than 3 cm in diameter, provided that the cyst is unilocular and unilateral, and without septations or ascites on ultrasonography. Measurement of serum levels of CA-125 (an epithelial ovarian cancer tumor marker) and followup ultrasonography have been used as part of the expectant management of such patients.

Surgery for dysfunctional physiologic cysts in the reproductive-age woman is rarely needed. When it does become necessary, cystectomy with ovarian conservation and closure of the dead space within the ovary usually is sufficient. Incidental cystectomy of a physiologic cyst found during abdominal surgery for another indication should be avoided, given the natural history of this self-limited process and the tendency for ovarian incisions to develop extensive postsurgical adhesions that can compromise fertility.

Polycystic ovarian disease is a syndrome associated with infertility and anovulation that occurs in reproductive-age women. Hirsutism and obesity are also frequent findings in these women. Polycystic ovaries are characterized by bilateral ovarian enlargements in which the ovarian capsule is pearl-white, smooth, and thickened. Multiple small cysts can be found beneath the cortex. Treatment of this condition is primarily hormonal, and surgical extirpation of such ovaries is not indicated.

Theca-lutein cysts of the ovary are fairly uncommon bilateral dysfunctional physiologic enlargements of the ovary. They are frequently associated with elevated levels of human chorionic gonadotropin (hCG) and are often found in conjunction with molar pregnancies, choriocarcinomas, twin gestations, diabetic pregnancies, or any pregnancy condition associated with an enlarged placenta. They are sometimes incidentally noted at the time of a caesarean section. Ovaries with theca-lutein cysts can be greatly enlarged (20 cm or greater), with multiple small, blue-grey cysts that form a "honeycomb" appearance. Incision or drainage of such cysts can result in severe hemorrhage and should be avoided. Spontaneous resolution occurs after the gestation or gestational tissues is removed.

OTHER OVARIAN ENLARGEMENTS

Endometriosis of the ovary with endometrioma formation is a relatively common nonphysiologic and non-neoplastic cause of ovarian enlargement. Most patients will have concurrent pelvic endometriosis. Ovarian endometriomas usually appear as dark, hemorrhagic cysts varying in size from a few millimeters to over 10 cm in diameter, and are oftentimes filled with old blood that resembles liquified milk chocolate (chocolate cysts). Spontaneous rupture of such cysts is often associated with acute peritoneal irritation of a magnitude that justifies surgical exploration. Such cysts usually have a distinct capsule that can be stripped from the cyst cavity. The dead space is usually closed with a fine purse string suture.

Dermoid cysts of the ovary (benign cystic teratoma) is one of the most common of the neoplastic disorders of the ovary. Dermoid cysts consist of elements from all three germ cell layers and often contain a combination of hair, sebaceous fluid, bone, teeth, cartilage, and so forth. Most are less than 10 cm in diameter, but larger sizes can be achieved. Dermoid cysts are bilateral in roughly 15% of cases, and only roughly 1% contain malignant elements. Rupture or leakage of such cysts is usually accompanied by severe chemical peritonitis. Functional thyroid tissue is present in roughly 10% of dermoids. When this is the principle tissue found, the dermoid is referred to as a **struma ovarii**. Thyrotoxicosis is a rare event with such tumors.

Dermoids can appear cystic or solid on ultrasonography or a combination of both. They are most often unilocular. A flat plate of the abdomen can often detect the calcified elements within such tumors. MRI can improve the diagnositic precision by identifying the increased fat density within the dermoid. Surgical treatment usually entails cystectomy when preservation of functional ovarian tissue is desired. A distinctly cystic capsule can often be dissected away from the surrounding ovarian tissue without rupturing the cyst, and any remaining ovarian capsule can be gathered together by a purse-string suture. Reconstitution of functioning ovarian tissue will usually occur, even in cases in which only a thin shell of ovary remains after cystectomy.

Fibromas, the most common of the benign solid neoplasms of the ovary, appears white and has a whorled appearance on cross-section. Fibromas are bilateral in 10% of cases. Fibromas can achieve diameters of 20 cm or more, but the great majority are smaller. Ascites can form from transudation of fluid from the surface of the fibroma, increasing in volume with increasing fibroma size. In cases with excessive ascites, hydrothorax can also occur. The triad of ovarian fibroma, ascites, and hydrothorax is

termed **Meigs' syndrome**. A solid tumor of the ovary in the presence of ascites should be assumed to be malignant until surgical pathology proves otherwise.

A **serous cystadenoma** is a fairly common benign epithelial neoplasm of the ovary that is bilateral in 15% of cases and is usually smaller than 10 cm in diameter. The cyst or cysts are rounded and thin-walled, usually containing clear-to-yellowish fluid. Oophorectomy of the involved ovary is indicated. Bilateral oophorectomy would be appropriate in the perimenopausal or postmenopausal woman. In the premenopausal age range, however, a contralateral ovary that looks grossly normal can be retained.

Mucinous cystadenomas have a tendency to achieve greater size than the serous tumors, at times reaching enormous proportions and weighing several pounds. They are bilateral in 10% of cases. Rupture of these tumors can establish mucin-producing epithelium on the peritoneal lining, a condition called **pseudomyxoma peritonei**. Mucinous cystadenomas are managed in the same manner as are their serous counterparts.

Ovarian tumors associated with ascites, peritoneal or omental growths, enlarged para-aortic nodes, or gross excrescences on the ovarian surface should all be suspected for malignancy and confirmed by frozen section at the time of surgery. Ovarian tumors suspicious for malignancy are generally approached through a midline incision in order to allow a thorough exploration of the entire abdominal cavity by which staging and subsequent treatment and prognosis can be based. The entire abdominal cavity, including the liver, diaphragm, and para-aortic lymph nodes, should be assessed for metastases. Any suspicious areas should be biopsied. In cases with no obvious intraperitoneal extension of the tumor, cytologic washing of all quadrants of the abdominal cavity becomes important for staging. Surgical treatment for ovarian cancer entails total abdominal hysterectomy, bilateral salpingo-oophorectomy, omentectomy, and debulking of as much intra-adominal tumor load as possible.

OVIDUCT ENLARGEMENTS

Enlargements of the fallopian tube can also be found, causing generalized adnexal enlargement that can be difficult to distinguish from ovarian enlargement on preoperative evaluation. The majority of these fallopian tube enlargements are benign. The two most common enlargements of the fallopian tube are the paratubal cyst and the hydrosalpinx.

Paratubal cysts are benign structures, usually arising from the remnants of mesonephric (müllerian) or paramesonephric (wolffian) structures within the mesosalpinx. They are thin-walled structures filled with clear fluid that can be seen in conjunction with other such cysts around the fallopian tube and ovary and can vary in size from a few millimeters to over 20 cm. The fallopian tube can, in some instances, be seen to be compressed and stretched over the capsule of a large paratubal cyst. Simple removal of the cyst, with care to avoid devascularizing the tube or ovary, is all that is required.

A **hydrosalpinx** is often the result of a previous pelvic infection in which the fimbriated ends of the fallopian tube become obstructed. Serous fluid can then accumulate within the tubal lumen, gradually enlarging the oviduct, and causing compression and eventual destruction of the endosalpinx. An adnexal enlargement due to a hydrosalpinx can at times be suspected on the basis of the tubular appearance of the cystic accumulation seen on ultrasonography. A hydrosalpinx can be managed by complete removal of the tube (**salpingectomy**) or by reopening the scarred fimbrial end (**salpingostomy**). Although salpingostomy can be accomplished in most cases, occlusion of the interstitial portion of the tube or destruction of the fimbria and endosalpinx can result in continued infertility, despite distal tubal patency.

SUGGESTED READING

Berger GS, Weström LV, Wolner-Hanssen P: Definition of pelvic inflammatory disease. In: Berger GS, Weström LV (editors): *Pelvic Inflammatory Disease*. Raven Press, 1992.

Centers for Disease Control and Prevention: 1993 Sexually Transmitted Diseases Treatment Guidelines. MMWR 1993;42 (No. RR-14):75.

Droegemueller W: Benign gynecologic lesions. In: Droegemueller W et al (editors): *Comprehensive Gynecology*. Mosby, 1987.

Droegemueller W: Upper genital tract infections. In: Droegemueller W et al (editors): *Comprehensive Gynecology*. Mosby, 1987.

Hadgu A, Weström L, Brooks CA et al: Predicting acute pelvic inflammatory disease: A multivarate analysis. Am J Obstet Gynecol 1986;155:956.

Jacobson LJ: Differential diagnosis of acute pelvic inflammatory disease. Am J Obstet Gynecol 1980;138:1007.

Kani J, Adler MW: Epidemiology of pelvic inflammatory disease. In: Berger GS, Weström LV (editors): *Pelvic Inflammatory Disease*. Raven Press, 1992.

Mishell DR: Ectopic pregnancy. In: Droegemueller W et al (editors): *Comprehensive Gynecology*. Mosby, 1987.

Paavonen J, Weström LV: Diagnosis of pelvic inflammatory disease. In: Berger GS, Weström LV (editors). *Pelvic Inflammatory Disease*. Raven Press, 1992.

Rock JA: Ectopic pregnancy. In: Thompson JD, Rock JA (editors). *Operative Gynecology*, 7th ed. Lippincott, 1992.

Rock JA: Surgery for benign disease of the ovary. In: Thompson JD, Rock JA (editors): *Operative Gynecology*, 7th ed. Lippincott, 1992.

Soper DE: Treatment of pelvic inflammatory disease. In: Berger GS, Weström LV (editors). *Pelvic Inflammatory Disease*. Raven Press, 1992.

Thompson JD, Spence MR: Pelvic inflammatory disease. In: Thompson JD, Rock JA (editors): *Operative Gynecology*, 7th ed. Lippincott, 1992.

Wallach EE: Myomectomy. In: Thompson JD, Rock JA (editors). *Operative Gynecology*, 7th ed. Lippincott, 1992.

Weckstein LN: Current perspective on ectopic pregnancy. Obstet Gynecol Surv 1985;40:259.

Weström LV, Wolner-Hanssen P: Differential diagnosis of pelvic inflammatory disease. In: Berger GS, Weström LV (editors). *Pelvic Inflammatory Disease*. Raven Press, 1992.

46

Pediatric Surgery

Jeffrey R. Lukish, MD, & Kurt D. Newman, MD

► Key Facts

- ► The spectrum of disease that affects infants and children is uniquely different from that which affects adults.

- ► At birth, the fetus must quickly adapt to life outside the uterus. This adaptation includes a rapid shift of circulation from the fetal pattern, in which blood bypasses the pulmonary circulation, to the neonatal/adult pattern, in which blood flow to the pulmonary circulation is maximized to achieve gas exchange.

- ► The newborn has a metabolic rate that is 2.5 times that of the adult. In the absence of disease, surgery, or trauma, newborns require 110–120 kcal/kg/d for growth.

- ► The combination of decreased renal function, unloading of excess fetal water, and increased in-

sensible water losses makes the neonate particularly susceptible to injudicious fluid and electrolyte management.

- ► Inguinal hernia is the most frequent condition requiring surgical intervention in children.

- ► Traumatic injuries surpass all major diseases as a risk for children. The three most common causes of death are airway obstruction, blood loss, and CNS injury.

- ► Pediatric cancer is the second most common cause of death in children under 14 years of age.

- ► The two most common solid tumors of childhood, after brain tumors, are neuroblastoma and Wilms' tumor, followed by soft tissue sarcomas, teratomas, and hepatic tumors.

The spectrum of diseases that affect infants and children is uniquely different from that which affect adults. This factor, coupled with certain anatomic and physiologic differences, has led to the evolution of pediatric surgery; a surgical discipline dedicated to the skills and knowledge required to optimize the care of children.

ANATOMY & PHYSIOLOGY

CARDIOVASCULAR

At birth, the fetus must quickly adapt to life outside the uterus. This transition occurs following a rapid shift from the fetal to the neonatal circulation pattern. Fetal circulation is characterized by a right-to-left shunt that diverts blood from the right heart pulmonary circulation to the left heart systemic circulation via the foramen ovale (intracardiac shunt) and the ductus arteriosus (pulmonary artery to aortic shunt). This circulatory pattern is maintained by the high pulmonary vascular resistance of the fetal lung and the relatively low systemic vascular resistance associated with the placental circulation. The transition to a normal circulatory pattern occurs as a result of decreased pulmonary vascular resistance due to ventilation of the infant's lungs at birth and subsequent oxygenation. Simultaneously, the systemic vascular resistance increases due to the loss of the low-resistance placenta circulation.

The ductus arteriosus usually closes within the first 24 hours of life and the foramen ovale closes during the first month. Persistent pulmonary hypertension of the newborn, intracardiac shunts, or immaturity may keep the ductus arteriosus open. Failure of the ductus arteriosus to close will lead to congestive heart failure. In cases where the ductus arteriosus remains patent, agents that block prostaglandin production, such as indomethacin, have been shown to facilitate closure. If the ductus fails to close following medical management, surgery is usually required to prevent cardiac failure.

The neonatal cardiac output is primarily rate-dependent, as opposed to the adult heart. Since the ability to increase stroke volume is limited, cardiac output may fall dramatically with bradycardia. The normal cardiovascular parameters for infants and children are shown in Figures 46–1 and 46–2.

PULMONARY

Although the lung does not reach full maturity until approximately 8 years of age, it undergoes rapid maturation in the last trimester of fetal development. A useful marker for fetal lung maturity is the ratio of lecithin to sphingomyelin in amniotic fluid (**L/S ratio**). Lecithin (phosphotidycholine) is the principal component of surfactant.

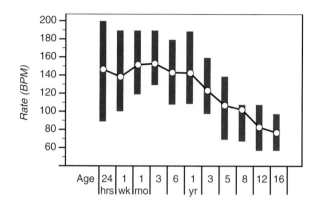

Figure 46–1. Heart rate by age. BPM = Beats per minute. (Reprinted, with permission, from Tepas JJ et al: Evaluation and management of the injured child. Bull Am Coll Surg 1995;80:36.)

Surfactant is produced by the type II alveolar cells and is extremely important in the prevention of alveolar collapse in the neonate. Lecithin is secreted into the fetal pulmonary airways, which communicate with the amniotic fluid; increasing levels in the amniotic fluid, therefore, correlate with increasing pulmonary development. Amniotic sphingomyelin levels remain essentially constant throughout gestation. An L/S ratio over 2 is considered compatible with relatively mature lung function.

Synthetic or animal surfactant is given routinely to premature infants with immature lungs. Glucocorticoids have been found to decrease problems associated with the premature newborn lungs and are often administered to mothers to induce lung maturation in the fetus if birth is imminent prior to 34 weeks gestation.

At birth, the "normal" respiratory rate can reach as high as 60 (Figure 46–3). The tidal volume is between 6 to 10 mL/kg. The infant airway is small and easily obstructed

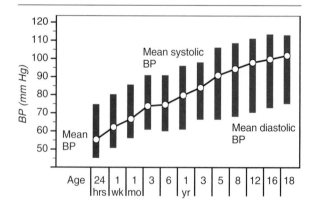

Figure 46–2. Blood pressure by age. (Reprinted, with permission, from Tepas JJ et al: Evaluation and management of the injured child. Bull Am Coll Surg 1995;80:36.)

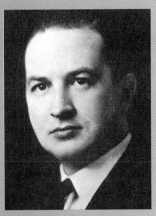

Robert E. Gross, MD.

Robert E. Gross became the first president of the American Pediatric Surgical Association in 1970 and was a pioneer in the development of the specialty. After training at the Peter Bent Brigham Hospital, he decided to devote his study to the problems of children with congenital malformations. Following his tenure as chief resident in surgery at Boston Children's Hospital, he developed a surgical approach to the closure of the patent ductus arteriosus and performed the first successful ligation in 1939. Dr Gross actively pursued the treatment of anomalies of the heart and great vessels in children, which led to his development of a practical method of preserving and using aortic homografts to repair vascular anomalies and injuries. He introduced modern cardiac and vascular surgery in children.

In 1947, Dr Gross was named Professor of Children's Surgery at Harvard Medical School and Surgeon-in-Chief of the Boston Children's Hospital. He trained and educated students, residents, and a number of renowned surgeons. He developed many innovative surgical techniques. Among the most noteworthy was the repair of congenital diaphragmatic hernias. Although he published numerous articles, many feel his most important contribution to the literature was his classic textbook, *Surgery of Infancy and Childhood.*

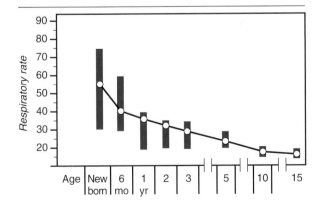

Figure 46–3. Respiratory rates by age. (Reprinted, with permission, from Tepas JJ et al: Evaluation and management of the injured child. Bull Am Coll Surg 1995;80:36.)

with secretions. The internal tracheal tube diameter for neonates is usually 2.5 to 3.5 mm. Infants are obligate nasal and diaphragmatic breathers and are usually unable to breathe by mouth effectively. Any condition that obstructs the nasal passages or reduces diaphragmatic function may cause respiratory embarrassment. Therefore, all gastric and tracheal tubes are best maintained through the oral route.

As a result of shunting and a more rapid respiratory rate, baseline arterial blood gases are slightly different from those in the adult. The PaO_2, $PaCO_2$, and pH for infants are approximately 75 mm Hg, 35 mm Hg, and 7.30–7.35, respectively.

GASTROINTESTINAL

The neonatal gastrointestinal tract is approximately 30% of the length of that found in an adult. However, the enhanced absorptive and digestive function allows the newborn to meet the caloric demands of a metabolic rate that is 2.5 times that of the adult. In the absence of disease, surgery, or trauma, newborns require 110 to 120 kcal/kg/d for growth. The calories should be provided as: 50% from carbohydrates, 35% from fats, and 15% from protein. The digestion and absorption physiology is similar to that found in adults with a few important exceptions. The newborn is deficient in pancreatic amylase and lipase, and the bile salt pool is 50% of that found in adults.

The lack of amylase has minimal effects on carbohydrate absorption because of the presence of amylase activity in human milk and the presence of a glycoamylase among the small bowel brush border enzymes. Most infant formulas use lactose as the principal carbohydrate, which requires lactase (not amylase) for absorption. This diet is usually well tolerated. However, since lactase is very sensitive to any illness that affects the gastrointestinal tract, including gastrointestinal surgery, the enzymatic activity may be diminished in these cases, resulting in diarrhea. It is for this reason that the postoperative infant is fed low-osmolar nonlactose formulas.

The deficiency in lipase and the reduced bile salt pool can lead to poor fat absorption. However, the newborn does have lingual lipase, which is secreted by the salivary glands, and does not depend on bile salts for its activity. In the neonate with conditions that result in fat malabsorption (eg, obstructive jaundice), medium-chain triglycerides (which do not require bile salts or lipase for absorption) can be used for supplementation. Cow milk fat (butter fat) is the least well tolerated by the infant. Human milk fat is usually well tolerated. Vegetable fats (corn, coconut, and soy) are the fats present in most formulas, along with medium-chain triglycerides.

In diseases such as short bowel syndrome, necrotizing enterocolitis, intestinal atresia, Crohn's disease, and cancer, it may not be possible to provide adequate nutrition via the gastrointestinal tract. In many of these children, normal growth is only possible by supplementation with parenteral nutrition. This approach provides calories via an intravenous (usually a central vein) route.

The optimal solution is made up of a 25% carbohydrate concentration, 2.5 gm/kg of protein, and approximately 4 gm/kg of lipids, to maintain a 150:1 ratio of nonprotein calories to a gram of nitrogen. Multivitamins and trace minerals are also added to the solution.

Technical complications, such as line sepsis, bleeding, pneumothorax, vein perforation, thrombosis, and pulmonary embolism, can produce significant problems. Metabolic complications include edema secondary to fluid overload, hypoglycemia and hyperglycemia, hypocalcemia, mineral and fatty acid deficiency, hepatic steatosis, and cholestatic jaundice. These complications can often be avoided by close monitoring and meticulous attention to subtle changes in the physical examination and laboratory tests.

RENAL

Neonatal renal function is not fully developed at birth. The infant can only concentrate urine to a maximum of 600 mOsm/kg, compared to 1200 mOsm/kg of the adult. This inability to concentrate urine appears to result from insensitivity of the collecting tubule to antidiuretic hormone. The glomerular filtration rate of a 2-week-old infant is approximately 50 mL/min/m^2 and does not reach the adult level of 100 mL/min/m^2 until 1.5 to 2 years of age. Despite decreased renal function, the newborn effectively reduces its total body water, which is 80% of its body weight at birth, to adult levels by 1.5 years of age.

The combination of decreased renal function, unloading of excess fetal water, and increased insensible water losses makes the neonate particularly susceptible to injudicious fluid and electrolyte management. Maintenance fluid requirements in the full-term infant are 100–120 mL/kg/d and increase up to 140 mL/kg/d in the premature infant in order to maintain a urine output of approximately 2 mL/kg/h. Potassium and sodium requirements are 2 to 3 meq/kg/d. Maintenance intravenous (IV) fluid is typically 5% dextrose in 25% or 30% normal saline with 10 meq of potassium chloride per liter. Fluid losses from vomiting, diarrhea, drainage tubes, and enterostomies must be accounted for to maintain appropriate fluid balance. The most precise method to accomplish this is to collect and analyze fluid losses and replace them appropriately.

Total blood volume in the infant is approximately 85 mL/kg, which makes up 8% of total body weight. A standard transfusion is 10 mL/kg of packed red blood cells, and a standard IV fluid bolus for hypotension is 20 mL/kg of lactated Ringer's solution.

CONGENITAL NECK LESIONS

FUNDAMENTAL CONSIDERATIONS

Neck masses in the pediatric population are a common occurrence and usually cause significant parental concern. The differential diagnosis is broadly classified into three categories: infectious, congenital, and neoplastic. Further subclassification is made in terms of whether these lesions are located in the midline or in a lateral position in the neck.

The most common lesion is **lymphadenitis**, often as a result of a local infection (eg, tonsillitis, otitis media). These are characteristically lateral neck masses, however, they can occur in the midline. They are often red, tender, and indurated. When they become fluctuant, incision and drainage is required. The infectious organism is most often *Staphylococcus* or *Streptococcus* species and is usually responsive to appropriate antibiotics.

Lymphadenitis that fails to resolve is concerning. Chronic indolent infectious agents, such as atypical mycobacteria (tuberculosis and mycobacteria other than tuberculosis), and neoplastic processes must be considered. In these cases, tissue biopsy (usually excisional biopsy) should be performed. The specimen should be sent for pathological and infectious evaluation, including fungal and mycobacterial cultures. If atypical mycobacterium is present with a draining skin sinus, the entire lesion, including the sinus tract, must be excised to achieve cure.

Tumors, both benign and malignant, can occur in the neck of the infant or child. Although these lesions are uncommon, they must be considered when neck masses persist or enlarge. Lymphoma, teratoma, neurofibroma, neuroblastoma, leukemia, thyroid tumors, and parathyroid tumors can occur primarily in the neck. Early biopsy is essential to direct therapy.

THYROGLOSSAL DUCT CYST & SINUS

Diagnosis

These lesions are generally midline and originate from the base of the tongue at the foramen caecum. They can pass either above, below, or through the hyoid bone. Infection is the most common presentation and results from failure of the duct to obliterate, creating a persistent, patent connection with the tongue. The differential diagnosis includes lymphadenopathy, ectopic thyroid, and dermoid cyst. Lymphadenopathy should resolve with appropriate therapy; an ectopic thyroid can be identified with ultrasonography; and dermoid cysts are usually small, nontender, palpable masses filled with keratin material. The thyroglossal duct cyst usually moves with swallowing because of its connection with the tongue and hyoid bone.

Management

The preferred treatments are (1) complete excision of the cyst; (2) resection of the central portion of the hyoid bone; and (3) high ligation of the duct at the foramen caecum. Complete excision is necessary to prevent recurrence.

BRANCHIAL CLEFT CYSTS & SINUSES

Diagnosis

These lesions present as lateral neck masses, usually occurring along the anterior border of the sternocleidomastoid muscle. The branchial cleft anomalies are remnants of the four paired embryonic branchial arches, clefts, and pouches; they present as sinuses, fistulae, and cysts. Second branchial cleft anomalies are the most common, presenting as draining sinuses in infants, or as cysts in young children.

Management

The treatment is surgical excision with complete removal of the cyst and the entire tract. If inadequate tract excision is performed, these children will commonly develop a recurrent cyst or sinus. Second branchial cleft sinus tracts usually pass under the digastric muscle be-

tween the internal and external carotid artery and under the hypoglossal nerve to end in the tonsillar fossa.

A fine lacrimal duct probe or methylene blue injection can be used to facilitate excision. Frequently, two incisions are required to gain adequate exposure of the inferior and superior elements of the sinus.

CYSTIC HYGROMA

Diagnosis

This lesion is a congenital lymphangioma, presumptively resulting from obstruction of the lymph vessels during development. It can occur in any location where lymph vessels exist, however, it most commonly arises in the neck, axilla, groin, or mediastinum.

When in the neck, congenital lymphangiomas are usually discrete lateral neck masses, however, they can become quite large, encompassing the entire cervical area. These lesions can be noted prenatally or at birth. Often, they come to attention following a respiratory infection in a young child.

Preoperative evaluation usually includes ultrasonography to define the anatomy and extent of the lesion. The most common finding is a multilocular cystic mass.

Management

The treatment is complete surgical excision, which in most cases prevents recurrence. However, the lesions can be intimately involved with vital structures, in which case conservative resection with unroofing of the remaining cyst tissue is appropriate. Closed suction drainage following excision is also advisable to prevent the persistent collection of lymph fluid. It is not unusual for these masses to recur, requiring repeated operations.

CONGENITAL DIAPHRAGMATIC HERNIA

Diagnosis

During the 10th week of fetal development, by an unknown mechanism, the abdominal viscera return to the fetal abdomen from the amniotic space. If a diaphragmatic defect is present, the viscera may enter the thoracic cavity. The abdominal organs then act as a space-occupying lesion, preventing normal lung development. There is usually pulmonary hypoplasia and pulmonary hypertension of the lung of the affected hemithorax. At birth, ventilation and perfusion of the affected lung is poor. As the infant swallows air, the bowel becomes distended, further compromising respiration. The resulting mediastinal shift compromises the ventilation in the contralateral lung, causing severe respiratory distress.

The infant's appearance is virtually diagnostic: a cyanotic, tachypneic baby with an increased chest diameter and a scaphoid abdomen. A chest film demonstrates air-filled viscera in the chest, confirming the diagnosis. The diagnosis is often made during prenatal ultrasonography, permitting antenatal consultation. The child is then delivered to a tertiary care medical center that offers the appropriate resources.

Management

Mortality is related to the degree of pulmonary hypoplasia. Physiologically, this correlates with the severity of pulmonary hypertension and the ability to oxygenate the infant. Therefore, the first principle of management is to correct the hypoxemia and the respiratory acidosis. This requires endotracheal intubation and ventilatory support.

Many types of ventilatory management have proven effective: pressure control, volume control, high-frequency ventilation, oscillation, and inverse-ratio ventilation. The concepts are similar: maintain a high respiratory rate to induce respiratory alkalosis, ensuring maximal pulmonary vasodilation that will facilitate oxygenation.

It is important to minimize ventilatory pressure to avoid barotrauma. Vasodilators (prostaglandins, tolazoline, amrinone lactate, etc) are given to reduce the persistent pulmonary hypertension. Some infants can be resuscitated and stabilized while maintaining a PaO_2 of greater than 100 mm Hg and an arterial-alveolar gradient of less than 600 mm Hg. These infants undergo diaphragmatic repair immediately.

If all conventional attempts to ventilate and oxygenate the infant fail, extracorporeal membrane oxygenation (ECMO) is instituted. Following stabilization and resolution of the pulmonary hypertension, the infant is weaned from the ECMO circuit, which may require days to weeks, and the operative diaphragmatic repair is performed. Some surgeons repair the defect while the infant is still on the ECMO circuit and begin to wean the infant postoperatively (Figure 46–4).

Operative repair is best accomplished by the transabdominal approach. The viscera are gently reduced into the abdomen, taking care to avoid injury to the spleen and liver. In some cases, there is enough diaphragmatic tissue to approximate the edges and close the defect. However, when the diaphragm is deficient or absent, the repair is accomplished with a synthetic patch. In some cases, the abdomen is too small after the repair to contain the viscera, and a Silastic silo can be constructed over the incision (see section on Abdominal Wall Defects), with reduction of the viscera into the abdomen over time.

Unfortunately, some infants have such severe pulmonary hypoplasia that it is impossible to reverse the persistent pulmonary hypertension. Despite successful repair and the use of ECMO, these children still have a high mortality rate. Future management may include fetal intervention to correct the defect in utero. There have been several anecdotal reports of success with open fetal surgery.

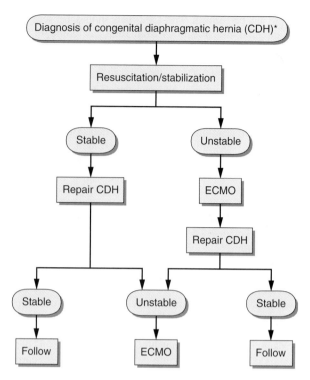

*In some cases of prenatal diagnosis, fetal intervention may be appropriate.

Figure 46–4. Algorithm depicting the management of congenital diaphragmatic hernia.

RESPIRATORY DISTRESS IN THE NEWBORN

The newborn that develops respiratory distress shortly after birth should be evaluated for other surgically correctable lesions in addition to congenital diaphragmatic hernia (CDH). The differential diagnosis includes lobar emphysema, pulmonary sequestrations, and cystic adenomatoid malformation.

Lobar emphysema represents hyperexpansion of one or more lobes of the lung. The infant usually presents in the first few months of life with severe tachypnea, dyspnea, and often cyanosis. The etiology is often an intrinsic bronchial obstruction or an extrinsic compression from a mass. These conditions allow air to enter the involved lobe but not exit. The hyperaerated lobe compresses the ipsilateral lung and causes a mediastinal shift to the other side, resulting in cardiopulmonary distress. A chest x-ray reveals a tracheal shift away from a hyperlucent area of lung. The treatment of choice is thoracotomy and resection of the affected lung.

Pulmonary sequestration refers to a condition in which there is nonfunctioning lung tissue that has no communication to the tracheobronchial tree. It is vascularized by an aberrant blood supply. There are two types, extralobar and intralobar. The **extralobar lesion** is far less common, has its own pleural investment, and is completely separate from the lung. It derives its arterial blood supply from a direct connection to the aorta, and its venous drainage is via the azygous system. The **intralobar lesion** occurs in association with the normal lung parenchyma. The arterial blood supply is similar to the extralobar lesion, however, the venous drainage is via the pulmonary veins.

The extralobar type is commonly asymptomatic, whereas the intralobar lesion presents with cough, hemoptysis, and recurrent pulmonary infections and abscess. The extralobar lesion can be cured with a local resection, however, the intralobar lesion usually requires lobectomy. Careful attention to the aberrant vascular supply is essential.

Congenital cystic adenomatoid malformation (CCAM) may present with similar findings to diaphragmatic hernia. Shortly after birth, the infant develops severe respiratory distress with persistent pulmonary hypertension. A chest x-ray reveals a characteristic "swiss cheese" appearance of the affected lung. This x-ray appearance of CCAM can be difficult to distinguish from the air-filled loops of bowel associated with CDH. The location of the distal end of a nasogastric tube in the thorax is consistent with a left-sided CDH as opposed to an abdominal position, which is found in normal infants and in those with CCAM. In recent years, many cases have been detected on prenatal ultrasound. The treatment of choice is lobectomy of the involved lung parenchyma.

TRACHEOESOPHAGEAL MALFORMATIONS

Diagnosis

The fetal development of the esophagus and trachea originates from a single ventral diverticulum of the foregut. Although the esophagus and trachea divide into separate tubes by the fifth week of gestation, this early common origination potentiates a number of malformations. These malformations occur in approximately one in 3000 live births.

The most common malformation is esophageal atresia, with a distal tracheoesophageal fistula (TE) occurring in 85% of cases. Pure esophageal atresia without a fistulous connection occurs in 8%, followed by a TE fistula without atresia in 4% ("H" type). Proximal esophageal atresia with a double TE fistula and proximal esophageal atresia with a proximal TE fistula are much less common, occurring in 1–2% of cases (Figure 46–5).

As many as 70% of these infants have associated anomalies. There is a clear association with Down's and trisomy 18 syndromes, and over 10% have the **VACTERL** association. VACTERL is an acronym for a series of associated but nonhereditary birth defects: *V*, vertebral or vas-

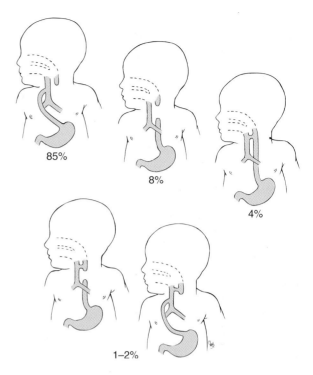

Figure 46–5. Tracheoesophageal (TE) fistulas. Esophageal atresia with distal TE fistula occurs in 85% of patients, followed by pure esophageal atresia without fistulous connection (8%), TE fistula without atresia (4%), proximal esophageal atresia with a double TE fistula (1–2%), and proximal esophageal atresia with a proximal TE fistula (1–2%).

cular defects; *A*, anorectal anomalies; *C*, cardiac anomalies; *T*, TE fistula; *E*, esophageal atresia; *R*, radial or renal anomalies; and *L*, limb defects.

The diagnosis of esophageal atresia and TE fistula is most commonly made shortly after birth, when the affected neonate exhibits respiratory distress following the first feeding. The infant may appear to hypersalivate or drool constantly. It may choke, cough, or even become cyanotic during the initial feeding. Attempts to pass a nasogastric tube will be unsuccessful, however, anterior-posterior (AP) and lateral chest x-rays with the tube in place will define the air-filled upper pouch. An abdominal x-ray is important, because if there is no air in the gastrointestinal tract then a distal fistula is unlikely, representing "pure" atresia. A cardiac echo is frequently part of the diagnostic work-up to define the location of the aortic arch or any anomalies.

Management

The most important aspect of management is decompression of the blind esophageal pouch and control of oral secretions. This is accomplished by means of a sump tube with constant suction. Following this maneuver, the infant is resuscitated, stabilized, and started on parenteral antibiotics. The infant is then evaluated for associated anomalies, primarily cardiac and renal defects. Infants with stable cardiac and respiratory status are immediately repaired.

Those infants for immediate repair undergo thoracotomy with an extrapleural dissection. The extrapleural dissection reduces the risk of empyema if an anastomotic leak occurs. The fistula is divided from the trachea, and the tracheal opening is oversewn and is covered with pleura to reduce the risk of a recurrent fistula. A primary esophagoesophagostomy is performed in an end-to-end fashion. In order to obtain adequate length to perform the anastomosis without tension, the proximal pouch is mobilized. Care must be taken during the dissection of the proximal and distal esophagus because the blood supply is often tenuous, particularly to the distal fistula. Myotomies may be useful to provide additional length of the proximal pouch (**Livaditis technique**). A drain is usually placed in the extrapleural space. A barium swallow is often obtained 1 week after the operation, and if there is no leak, feeding is initiated.

In those infants too unstable to undergo immediate repair or who have a wide defect (usually pure esophageal atresia), a gastrostomy is placed for enteral nutrition and gastric decompression. The repair then follows stabilization or, in the case of large defects, it is completed after a 6- to 8-week course of proximal pouch dilation and growth. In some patients, division of the fistula is required to prevent reflux and aspiration. The repair can be performed later when the ends have grown closer and anastomosis is possible. If reapproximation of the native esophagus is not possible, then esophageal replacement with a colon interposition or gastric tube may be required.

Long-term follow-up evaluation is important. These children are at risk for esophageal dysmotility, gastroesophageal reflux, anastomotic strictures, tracheomalacia, and recurrent TE fistulas, all of which may require surgery for resolution.

ABDOMINAL WALL DEFECTS

FUNDAMENTAL CONSIDERATIONS

There are two types of defects: gastroschisis and omphalocele. These defects share a similar presentation in that a portion of the abdominal contents are extra-abdominal. However, because they are developmentally different and require uniquely different therapy, these lesions should be considered separately.

GASTROSCHISIS

Diagnosis
Although the embryogenesis of gastroschisis is uncertain, the defect is believed to be the result of a defect that occurs at the site where the second umbilical vein invo-

lutes, allowing a hernia of the umbilical cord. These infants have a large amount of viscera protruding through an opening in the surface of a completely developed abdominal wall. There is usually a small defect at the right edge of the umbilicus. The viscera lie freely outside the abdomen with no apparent covering. The viscera often appear thickened, edematous, and discolored. They are frequently covered with an exudate as a result of the irritating effects of amniotic fluid. The bowel is usually foreshortened and nonrotated and can be associated with intestinal atresia in as many as 15% of cases (see section on Intestinal Obstruction). However, in contrast to omphalocele, other associated anomalies are rare.

Gastroschisis is often detected during prenatal ultrasonography. The mother should be delivered to a tertiary care medical center with the appropriate resources. There is no evidence that cesarean section improves outcome, therefore, vaginal delivery is reasonable, in most cases. A majority of these infants are premature or small for gestational age.

Management
The infant with gastroschisis has enormous insensible fluid losses secondary to the eviscerated organs. Hypothermia, hypovolemia, and sepsis are common complications in the perinatal period. At delivery, the lower half of the infant, including the viscera, should be placed into a sterile plastic bowel bag. If this is unavailable, sterile gauze soaked in normal saline should be applied, covered with plastic wrap. This reduces volume requirements, however, these infants characteristically require much more fluid than the normal newborn.

Fluid resuscitation continues until urine output is established. Acid/base levels and electrolytes are closely monitored. An orogastric tube is placed and the infant is started on parenteral antibiotics.

At operation, the defect is increased longitudinally in both the cephalad and caudad directions to facilitate replacement of the viscera into the abdominal cavity. The abdominal wall is stretched, the gastrointestinal tract is decompressed, and an attempt is made to reduce the viscera into the abdomen. Reduction followed by primary repair is often successful. However, some infants, because of respiratory distress associated with reduction, require a staged repair.

A Silastic silo is created, which acts as a temporary extra-abdominal housing. The viscera can be reduced over time with gentle pressure on the silo. This reduction is usually completed within a week. Since these infants usually have a prolonged ileus requiring parenteral nutrition, a central venous catheter placed at the time of operation is helpful. The current survival for all infants with gastroschisis is greater than 90%.

OMPHALOCELE

Diagnosis
Omphalocele results from incomplete closure of the somatic folds of the anterior abdominal wall in the fetus.

The incomplete closure leads to a defect of the entire umbilical ring, into which the abdominal contents herniate. The herniated mass is covered by a sac composed of an outer layer of amnion and an inner layer of peritoneum. The liver and small bowel are the most common organs present in the hernia sac.

Unlike gastroschisis, serious anomalies are associated with this defect. Beckwith-Wiedemann syndrome (gigantism, macroglossia, and an umbilical defect), chromosomal abnormalities (trisomy 13, 18), exstrophy of the bladder or cloaca, and the pentalogy of Cantrell (omphalocele, diaphragmatic hernia, cleft sternum, absent pericardium, and intracardiac defects) can occur in as many as 50% of infants with omphalocele. The size of the defect varies from 1 to 10 cm, however, the smaller the defect the better the prognosis.

Management

The essentials of management are similar to those used in the care of the infant with gastroschisis. Protection of the abdominal contents, control of insensible and thermal losses, and fluid resuscitation are of utmost importance. Associated anomalies should be evaluated prior to operative repair.

Many therapeutic options exist, and the choice of appropriate management depends on the condition of the infant. Small defects can be closed primarily; larger defects may require a staged repair using a Silastic silo with reduction of the viscera over time. Since the viscera are covered with a physiologic sac, conservative nonoperative management is an option. Infants with serious anomalies or poor cardiopulmonary function may be candidates for this conservative topical therapy. Escharotic agents can be directly applied to the sac, allowing it to thicken and even epithelialize. Definitive repair can be delayed until the infant is stable. The overall survival is related to the size and location of the defect and to the presence of associated anomalies. The overall mortality rate is approximately 40%.

PYLORIC STENOSIS

Diagnosis

Pyloric stenosis is caused by hypertrophy of the muscular layer of the pylorus, causing a gastric outlet obstruction. It is relatively common, occurring in one in 750 births, and is predominant in males (male-to-female ratio 4:1), often seen in the first-born male. The children of a woman with pyloric stenosis have a 10 times greater chance of developing pyloric stenosis than those with unaffected mothers.

These infants present during the first month of life with a history of progressive, nonbilious, projectile vomiting, which usually starts during the second week of life. They are profoundly dehydrated with a concomitant hypokalemic,

hypochloremic metabolic alkalosis secondary to vomiting. On physical examination, a midepigastric mass in the right upper quadrant can often be palpated (midepigastric "olive"). Ultrasonography confirms the diagnosis by demonstrating an elongated pyloric channel (> 15 mm) and a thickened muscular wall (> 3.5 mm). The radiographic gastrointestinal series can also be used, demonstrating an elongated pyloric channel with an antral shoulder (the "string" sign).

Management

Correction of the fluid deficits and gastrointestinal decompression are fundamental in the preoperative management of these infants. The electrolyte abnormalities and alkalosis will resolve with proper resuscitation. These children often require significant fluid resuscitation to correct the dehydration and establish an adequate urine output of 1–2 mL/kg/h. The infant is appropriately resuscitated and ready for operative repair when the serum bicarbonate is less than 28 meq/dL, the serum chloride is greater than 92 meq/dL, and adequate urine output has been established.

The surgical procedure, **pyloromyotomy**, is curative. This operation is performed by an incision of the serosa over the pylorus followed by division of its hypertrophic muscular fibers, taking care to avoid entering the duodenum or stomach. Gentle spreading of the muscular fibers with a hemostat or Ramstedt forceps allows the submucosa and mucosa to protrude and relieve the obstruction. Independent motion of the two sides of the pylorus indicates an adequate pyloromyotomy.

Postoperatively, the infant can be started on electrolyte infant formula or a glucose and water solution within 4–6 hours of surgery. Feeding should be initiated with small volumes and can usually be advanced quickly to full feedings.

BILIARY ATRESIA

Diagnosis

Biliary atresia is a disease that leads to fibrosis of both the intrahepatic and extrahepatic biliary ductal system, occurring in approximately one in 15,000 infants. Although the initiating events are unknown, it is thought to be the result of an acquired inflammatory process, possibly viral in etiology, that preferentially targets the neonatal biliary ducts.

Clinically, the infant presents with progressive neonatal jaundice with an onset in the first few weeks of life. Infants with biliary atresia usually have a normal physical examination except for icterus and, occasionally, hepatomegaly. Laboratory studies reveal a conjugated hyperbilirubinemia. Liver function tests, however, may or may not be abnormal, depending on the degree of liver damage from cholestasis (duration of disease). Although neonatal physiologic jaundice is common, persistent jaundice beyond the first month of life must be thoroughly evaluated.

The success of therapy for this disease is primarily a function of timeliness of diagnosis and age at repair; that is, the more expeditious the diagnosis and the younger the patient the less time the liver is subjected to cholestatic injury. Since there are many causes of neonatal cholestatic syndromes, the work-up is intended to differentiate anatomic obstruction of the biliary tree from other causes of cholestasis.

Radioisotope scanning is virtually 100% sensitive for biliary atresia, with a specificity of approximately 90%. The radioisotope is promptly taken up by the liver, however, there is no excretion into the gut in children with biliary atresia. Alternatively, patients with hepatocellular disease take up the isotope slowly and have delayed excretion. The diagnostic yield can be increased with the use of phenobarbital, which acts to stimulate the hepatocyte and hepatic microsomal enzymes. Abdominal ultrasonography to evaluate the liver, gallbladder, and biliary tree is also important. In biliary atresia, this study usually reveals an absent gallbladder and common bile duct, and a liver without intrahepatic ductal dilation. Percutaneous liver biopsy is often helpful in establishing an early diagnosis.

Management

The principle that governs the diagnosis of biliary atresia is that prompt laparotomy, liver biopsy, and operative cholangiography should be performed in any suspicious case. It is now clear that the success of surgical correction of biliary atresia is much improved when done in the first 2 months of life, and that after 3 months success is unlikely.

The extent of repair is mitigated by the type of atresia present. Five percent of infants present with a **"correctable"** type (a blind-ending cystic dilation of the common hepatic duct), which is repaired by direct anastomosis with a Roux-en-Y loop of jejunum. The remaining infants have a **"noncorrectable"** type: either fibrous obliteration of the gallbladder with a fibrous duct up to the porta hepatis (80% of infants), or a patent gallbladder and distal common duct with no evidence of proximal ducts (15% of infants). These infants will require the **Kasai procedure**, which is a hepatoportoenterostomy. Briefly, the porta hepatis is dissected out, biopsied, and a loop of jejunum is anastomosed to the liver hilus, incorporating the area where the hepatic ducts should ordinarily be.

Two factors primarily influence the prognosis for these patients: age at the time of repair and the microscopic evaluation of the porta hepatis biopsy. As stated previously, some infants repaired prior to 2 months of age do well, and approximately 30% will never require liver transplantation. The porta hepatis biopsy allows histologic evaluation of the biliary ductules. If the ductules are greater than 150 μm in diameter, then the prognosis is good for bile flow. Those infants with ductules less than

110 μm have a poor prognosis for bile flow and may be candidates for early transplantation.

Postoperatively, these infants are placed on prophylactic antibiotics to reduce the incidence of cholangitis. They are often given phenobarbital to stimulate bile flow. Despite the apparent success of surgery and decompression of the biliary tree, biliary fibrosis frequently fails to resolve and cirrhosis and liver failure result. For children who fail to improve after the Kasai procedure and for those children referred at a late age, orthotopic liver transplantation is now an option, with a 70–90% 2-year survival following successful transplantation.

INTESTINAL OBSTRUCTION

FUNDAMENTAL CONSIDERATIONS

The differential diagnosis of neonatal intestinal obstruction includes not only intestinal malrotation and atresia but entities such as meconium ileus, intussusception, necrotizing enterocolitis, intestinal webs, and many others. Fundamental to the diagnosis of these disorders is the ability to recognize and understand the essential signs and symptoms: bilious vomiting; failure to pass meconium; maternal polyhydramnios; and abdominal distension.

Bilious vomiting is always a pathological finding that must be promptly evaluated. Although it may be due to ileus, correctable surgical conditions must be ruled out first. Characteristically, bilious vomiting indicates an obstruction distal to the ampulla of Vater. These infants have dark green bilious emesis; in many cases this is the first sign of malrotation, a surgical emergency.

Failure to pass meconium in the first 24 hours of life can be associated with intestinal obstruction. **Meconium** is the intestinal debris that accumulates during fetal life. It is typically black and viscous, and up to 200 g may be passed per rectum. Failure to pass this material in the first day of life may be indicative of a pathologic obstruction.

Polyhydramnios is characterized by the presence of greater than 2000 mL of fluid in the amniotic sac. This is often secondary to a bowel obstruction because the fetus normally swallows and absorbs approximately 50% of the amniotic fluid by the fifth month of gestation. Excess fluid represents either a failure to swallow or absorb the fluid, sometimes due to a proximal obstruction. Distal obstructions may not cause polyhydramnios, since the fetal gastrointestinal tract absorbs this amniotic fluid via the proximal and middle jejunum.

In the normal neonate, air swallowing begins at birth, and air should reach the proximal small intestine in 15 minutes and the large intestine by 2 hours. This rate of air transport is relatively constant. Therefore, abdominal distension characterized by a number of air-filled loops of bowel usually indicates a distal obstruction.

MALROTATION & MIDGUT VOLVULUS

Diagnosis

The **midgut** (duodenum to mid-transverse colon) develops extra-abdominally, migrating intraperitoneally by the 12th week of gestation. During this migration the midgut undergoes a 270-degree counterclockwise rotation around the axis of the superior mesenteric artery and vein. The C-loop of the duodenum, the right colon, and transverse colon trace this rotational path, resulting in the cecum becoming fixed in the right lower quadrant, the right colon becoming attached to the right paracolic gutter, and the duodenum becoming fixed to the retroperitoneum. The small bowel becomes tethered from its mesentery, extending from the left upper quadrant (ligament of Treitz) to the right lower quadrant (cecum). Failure of intestinal rotation leads to a right upper quadrant cecum, lack of appropriate fixation of the small bowel, and the duodenum remaining to the right of the superior mesenteric artery. The clinical consequences of this orientation creates the potential for a partial duodenal obstruction from adhesions (Ladd's bands). Secondly, the small bowel hangs from a short, narrow mesenteric pedicle that can easily twist, causing volvulus.

Infants with malrotation usually present with the acute onset of bilious vomiting. The infant may have abdominal distension and mild diffuse tenderness, however, many children present with minimal physical findings. The passage of bloody stool occurs late and is a sign of bowel ischemia and necrosis often associated with midgut volvulus. These infants quickly become seriously ill. The abdominal x-ray often shows a paucity of bowel gas or the "double bubble" sign, representing air in the stomach and proximal duodenum. A more reliable study is the upper gastrointestinal series, in which the duodenal C-loop does not extend to the left of the vertebral bodies, a finding pathognomonic for malrotation. A majority of infants with malrotation present with midgut volvulus in the first year of life; therefore, bilious vomiting in infants less than 1 year of age should be aggressively evaluated.

Management

Midgut volvulus is a surgical emergency. Following diagnosis the infant is promptly taken to the operating room, where the volvulus is reduced by counterclockwise rotation of the bowel. The Ladd procedure involves reduction of the volvulus, lysis of the adhesions between the cecum and the duodenum, and appendectomy. Appendectomy is performed because the cecum remains in the left upper quadrant, therefore, signs of future appendicitis would be misleading. The duodenum is placed to the right; fixation sutures are not required. When significant bowel ischemia has occurred, all compromised bowel is returned to the abdomen and a "second look" operation is planned 24 hours later at which time bowel resection may occur.

These infants have a 10% chance of recurrent volvulus, usually occurring in the early postoperative period. These infants suffer significant morbidity, primarily from short bowel syndrome as a result of the extensive intestinal resection. The mortality of midgut volvulus is as high as 25%.

Simple malrotation without volvulus does occur. Typically these children or young adults have a history of chronic abdominal pain and obstructive-like symptoms that seem to resolve with nasogastric suction. Upper gastrointestinal (UGI) series reveals an abnormal duodenal C-loop. This is treated by the Ladd procedure.

INTESTINAL ATRESIA

Diagnosis

Atresia, which is a congenital obstruction of the intestinal lumen, can occur throughout the gastrointestinal tract. Duodenal atresia probably occurs because of failure of the duodenum to recanalize during early fetal life; jejunal, ileal, and colonic atresias, however, occur as a result of in utero fetal vascular accidents causing ischemia to a segment of bowel. Duodenal atresia is associated with other anomalies (trisomy 21, VACTERL complex, and annular pancreas). Since small bowel and colonic intestinal atresia are not usually due to an embryologic maldevelopment, associated anomalies are rare.

The diagnosis of duodenal atresia is easily made since the infants are totally obstructed. Diagnosis is often by ultrasonography. Maternal polyhydramnios is present in as many as 50% of cases. The atresia is usually distal to the ampulla of Vater. These infants develop bilious vomiting with a scaphoid abdomen shortly after birth. Abdominal x-rays reveal the characteristic **"double bubble"** sign, signifying air in the stomach and duodenum. As mentioned above (see section on diagnosis of malrotation), this sign can occur with malrotation and volvulus. Therefore, if treatment is going to be delayed, an UGI must be performed to rule out malrotation.

The clinical presentation of distal intestinal atresia varies with the level of obstruction. Jejunal atresia is slightly more common than ileal atresia. These infants typically present with bilious vomiting after the first 24 hours of life. The passage of meconium does not rule out atresia, because the distal gastrointestinal tract may have developed prior to the vascular accident. Abdominal x-rays show different degrees of obstruction but are nonspecific as to the level of blockage. A clue to the diagnosis is calcification in the abdomen on a plain x-ray. These signify **meconium peritonitis**, which occurs following fetal perforation of the bowel. The intraperitoneal meconium causes an intense inflammatory reaction that later becomes calcified. A UGI is helpful and may be the most appropriate first study to rule out malrotation. If nondiagnostic, a contrast enema is then ordered, which will reveal colonic and potentially low ileal atresia.

Management

Although these lesions do not constitute absolute emergencies, they should be repaired as expeditiously as possible to prevent complications. Preoperative management includes gastrointestinal decompression, fluid resuscitation, and initiation of broad-spectrum antibiotics. In duodenal atresia, the preoperative management should include a thorough genetic, cardiac, pulmonary, and renal evaluation. All infants with intestinal atresia should be evaluated for cystic fibrosis.

The goal of operative management is to reestablish gastrointestinal continuity. In duodenal atresia, usually a duodenoduodenostomy can be performed. If a web is present, a duodenotomy is performed, the web excised, and the duodenotomy closed. If an annular pancreas is present, it is bypassed, taking care to avoid injuring the pancreas. The duodenal stenosis that occurs as a result of the annular pancreas is the obstructing lesion, not the annular pancreas itself. Any attempt to resect the pancreatic lesion will significantly increase morbidity and mortality.

In small bowel and colonic atresia, the procedure of choice is an end-to-end anastomosis. This may be difficult when the proximal end is significantly dilated and the distal end atrophied. In some cases, the bowel length is marginal, and the need to preserve all of the remaining intestine exists. However, the proximal dilated segment is often atonic and should be resected, if possible. Prior to closure, the gastrointestinal tract should be thoroughly examined to ensure that multiple atresias do not exist.

Postoperatively, these infants have a significant ileus and may require parenteral nutrition. Survival after duodenal atresia is a function of the associated anomalies. Prognosis is usually good. Survival following small bowel and colonic atresias is essentially 100%, if bowel length is adequate.

INGUINAL HERNIA

Diagnosis

The inguinal hernia is the most frequent condition requiring surgical intervention in children. The incidence varies with age, from approximately 10% in preterm infants to 5% in full-term infants. It is more common in males. There is an increased incidence of hernias in those children whose peritoneal cavities are used for absorptive purposes (ventriculoperitoneal shunt, peritoneal dialysis) or in any state that increases abdominal pressure (ascites). The etiology of the inguinal hernia is a failure of obliteration of the processus vaginalis (a projection of peritoneum that follows the testis into the scrotum). Different degrees of patency of the processus vaginalis can lead to a variety of anomalies: scrotal hernia, proximal hernia with fusion of the distal projection, communicating hydrocele (where the processus or hernia sac continues to communicate with the peritoneum), hydrocele of the cord, and hydrocele of the tunica vaginalis.

The major risks of inguinal hernias are incarceration of a loop of bowel, or in females, incarceration of the ovary,

fallopian tube, or both. The incidence of incarceration is as high as 30% in the first year of life compared to 15% in the general pediatric age group. Those children who are repaired following incarceration have a much greater postoperative complication rate than those children who are repaired electively (20% versus 1%). This is the rationale behind the current recommendations to repair a hernia as soon as possible after making the diagnosis. However, in premature infants, the risks from anesthesia must be balanced against the need for repair.

The classic presentation is that of a bulge in the groin, scrotum, or labia, usually occurring at times of increased intra-abdominal pressure (crying or coughing). The mass usually disappears with resolution of the crying or coughing. On physical examination, if no mass is present, one may feel a thickening over the external ring or spermatic cord, which represents the hernia sac. This is referred to as the **"silk glove sign."** If a herniated mass is present, it is usually easily reducible. Parents may also report a change in size of the scrotum; this is due to the fluid exchange between the hernia sac and the peritoneum that is characteristic of a communicating hydrocele.

An undescended testicle can present as a hernia. It must be differentiated from a retractile testicle. A **retractile testicle** is one that typically resides above the scrotum or in the inguinal canal and can be brought into the scrotum with gentle retraction; this is managed nonoperatively because these testicles usually descend over the first year of life. A testicle that cannot be brought into the scrotum is an **undescended testicle** and should be repaired. In those children who do appear to have an undescended testicle, current recommendations are for early orchiopexy at 1 year of age. In evaluating a child with a potential hernia, care should be taken during the initial examination to palpate and capture the testicle in the scrotum prior to palpating for the hernia or the silk glove sign; this will prevent misdiagnosis.

Management

Inguinal hernias should be repaired shortly after diagnosis except in premature infants. Infants and children who present with an incarcerated hernia (in which the hernia contents may be entrapped) may require admission. An attempt at reduction should be made after the patient is sedated. Reduction is usually successful with gentle downward motion on the hernia sac from above the inguinal ring, with simultaneous compression of the hernia contents and sac from below. If reduction is successful, these children should be hydrated and the defect repaired within 24 hours. If unsuccessful, patients should be taken to the operating room immediately following resuscitation, as they are at risk for intestinal strangulation and ischemia.

Most children and infants can be managed by high ligation of the indirect hernia sac at the internal ring. Rarely is a floor repair necessary. Care must be taken to avoid injury to the vas deferens and spermatic vessels. Controversy exists with respect to the need for contralateral groin exploration, however, most pediatric surgeons will explore the contralateral side in girls under 2 and boys under 1 year of age. Some surgeons are employing laparoscopy to assess the contralateral side. Hernia repair is routinely performed on an outpatient basis and is well tolerated with minimal morbidity, except for the occasional scrotal hematoma, and rare recurrence.

"IMPERFORATE ANUS"

Diagnosis

The rectum and anus develop from the urorectal septum in embryonic life. Abnormal termination of the descent of this septum leads to failure of normal separation and development of the urinary and hind gut systems. A variety of anorectal anomalies can occur, ranging from a fistulous opening in the perineal area, a rectovaginal fistula, a rectourethral fistula, or a completely blind ending of the rectum. These anomalies occur once in 20,000 live births, affecting males and females equally. Imperforate anus is broadly classified as high, intermediate, and low, depending on whether the rectum ends above, at the level of, or below the puborectalis sling, respectively (Figure 46–6). Males more commonly have high types and females commonly have low types. A majority of infants with this anomaly have a fistulous tract from the rectum. In males, low types usually have tracts to the perineum. Intermediate and high types have fistula tracts to the urethra near the prostate. In females, low types track to the perineum, and intermediate and high types track to the vagina. Ten percent of these anomalies have a blind-ending rectum or anus.

Anorectal anomalies are associated with other anomalies, commonly of the genitourinary tract. Renal agenesis, renal dysplasia, hypospadias, epispadias, and bladder exstrophy can occur in as many as 40% of patients with imperforate anus. Tracheoesophageal fistulas, cardiac anomalies, sacral agenesis, and spina bifida also occur with some frequency.

Although the diagnosis of imperforate anus is relatively straightforward, determination of the type and level of the lesion is critical for appropriate management. These infants should have an extensive perineal examination; in females, a thorough vaginal examination is crucial for a correct diagnosis. The urine should be evaluated for meconium (rectourethral fistula). These infants have a high incidence of urinary tract infections and hyperchloremic acidosis from colonic absorption of chloride. If no fistula is apparent, the use of transperitoneal injection of contrast media, pelvic computed tomography (CT), ultrasonography, or magnetic resonance imaging (MRI) can usually delineate the anatomy.

Management

The goal of operative repair is to recreate normal anorectal anatomy with preservation of continent function. Low-type lesions are repaired by a **V-Y** anoplasty. Essentially, the skin is divided over the anal atresia or anocutaneous fistula, and the anus is brought down and sewn to the skin. Intermediate-type lesions are usually treated by a **transplantation anoplasty**, where the rectal connection to the vagina or urethra is divided and the rectum is brought down posterior to the perineal body. High-type lesions are typically repaired by a **posterior sagittal anoplasty** developed by Pena and DeVries. This is a complex procedure that requires dividing the levator ani muscles and external sphincter complex in the midline posteriorly and bringing down the rectum after sufficient length is achieved. The muscles are then reconstructed around the rectum. A colostomy is utilized to divert the fecal stream until the reconstruction has healed.

The prognosis for normal continent function is related to the type of lesion and whether there is associated neurologic dysfunction associated with spina bifida or sacral

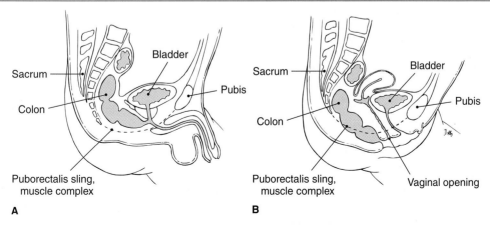

Figure 46–6. Imperforate anus anomaly. **A:** High lesion in male. **B:** Low lesion in female.

agenesis. However, the higher the rectal atresia, typically, the poorer the likelihood of successful function. Long-term care and follow-up are required, sometimes employing anal dilation. Families must be counseled not to expect the normal progression of toilet training. These children may not achieve socially acceptable continence until 6 to 9 years of age, and then only with a bowel management program.

HIRSCHSPRUNG'S DISEASE

Diagnosis

Hirschsprung's disease is caused by the congenital absence of parasympathetic ganglion cells in the wall of the colon. These ganglion cells are derived from neural crest cells that migrate, from proximal to distal, in the gastrointestinal tract. This process is usually complete by the 12th week of fetal life. Premature termination of migration leads to **aganglionosis**, which presents as a failure of the affected bowel segment to relax and allow normal peristalsis. In children with this disease the rectum is always involved; aganglionosis may extend to the proximal bowel. In 80% of children, the rectosigmoid area is affected; 10% have extension to the ascending colon, and 10% have the entire colon and distal ileum afflicted. The male-to-female ratio is 4:1, except when the entire colon is involved, in which case this ratio is reversed. There is a clear familial predisposition, with an approximately 10% risk to siblings.

More than 95% of these children fail to pass meconium in the first 24 hours of life. Newborns present with abdominal distension and bilious vomiting consistent with obstruction. Although unusual, it should be suspected in any child who presents with abnormal bowel habits dating back to infancy. Older children present with a history of constipation and failure to thrive. A small percentage of patients (10%) present with enterocolitis, which carries a high mortality rate.

The diagnosis is suspected by history and physical examination, specifically the rectal examination. Characteristically, these children have increased sphincter tone and an empty rectum. If only a narrow distal segment is involved, rectal examination is followed by explosive diarrhea. The diagnosis is confirmed by barium enema and tissue biopsy. The barium enema reveals spasm and a narrowed lumen in the affected bowel. Children exhibit a transition zone, showing dilated proximal gut and narrowed distal gut, however, newborns may not have this dramatic "cut off" point. The **transition zone** indicates the most distal area where ganglion cells are present. Tissue biopsy of the wall of the colon is then performed and the tissue examined for the presence of ganglion cells. This is done by either full-thickness transrectal biopsy or seromuscular biopsy at the time of laparotomy. Many surgeons perform a suction rectal biopsy, which can be done in the office, however, this requires an experienced pathologist for interpretation.

Management

The goal of repair is generally to remove the involved bowel and to restore gastrointestinal continuity with continent anal function. Most children have a colostomy performed first, which allows the dilated bowel to return to normal size. Some surgeons are performing primary repair in the newborn period. The colostomy is positioned proximal to the transition zone, and the presence of ganglion cells at the stoma site is verified by frozen section biopsy at the time of operation. Multiple biopsies are often taken, starting distally and moving proximally, looking for the presence of ganglion cells, in order to verify the proximal extent of disease.

Following a 3- to 6-month period, to allow the colon to return to normal size, a definitive pull-through procedure is performed. The three operations most commonly performed are named the Swenson, Duhamel, and Soave operations. The **Swenson** procedure is a rectosigmoidectomy with coloanal anastomosis. The involved colon is excised to within 1 cm of the anal mucocutaneous margin. Most pediatric surgeons use the Duhamel or Soave procedure. The **Duhamel** is a retrorectal coloanal anastomosis. The involved colon is excised at the peritoneal reflection and the normal colon is tunnelled between the sacrum and rectum and is anastomosed end-to-side to the remaining anorectum. The **Soave** procedure is an endorectal coloanal anastomosis. The involved colon is excised at the level of the pelvic peritoneal reflection. The mucosa in the remaining rectum is removed and the proximal normal bowel is pulled through the stripped anorectal segment and anastomosed to the anus.

Prognosis overall is excellent. However, those infants and children who initially presented with enterocolitis are more likely to have this complication postoperatively and must be monitored closely. Problems with constipation or fecal soiling occasionally occur, however, most infants are continent, with only a small percentage having severe fecal soilage.

NECROTIZING ENTEROCOLITIS

Diagnosis

Necrotizing enterocolitis (NEC) is a disease that occurs almost exclusively in premature and low-birth-weight infants. Its incidence is approximately 10% in infants weighing less than 800 grams. Among those infants with classic NEC, the overall mortality is 29%. Although the etiology is unknown, it is suspected to result from gut ischemia, which leads to bacterial invasion and intestinal gangrene.

A number of conditions predispose the infant to NEC. These include respiratory distress syndrome, sepsis, congenital cardiac anomalies, shock, hypoxia, apneic episodes, and umbilical artery catheters. The disease usually occurs in the first month of life. Early symptoms and signs are formula intolerance, abdominal distension, vomiting (usually bilious), and either occult or gross bloody stools. Late findings include fever or hypothermia, abdominal wall erythema, abdominal mass, and apnea and bradycardia. Thrombocytopenia, leukopenia or leukocytosis, acidosis, and coagulation defects are common. Abdominal x-rays are used to aid in diagnosis and to follow the infant's clinical course. Findings include fixed dilated loops of bowel, pneumatosis intestinalis, pylephlebitis, and pneumoperitoneum. The key to reducing morbidity is early suspicion on the part of the physician, followed by prompt evaluation and management.

Management

The primary treatment is medical support. This includes cessation of feedings, gastrointestinal decompression with a large oral gastric tube, intravenous fluid support, ventilator support as needed, parenteral antibiotics, and blood or platelet transfusions as necessary. Some infants respond dramatically. The abdomen becomes less distended and the pneumatosis intestinalis and the distended loops of bowel slowly resolve. Operative therapy may be indicated in as many as 30% of these patients. Indications for surgery include pneumoperitoneum, peritonitis, a fixed abdominal mass, and deterioration despite optimal medical therapy.

At surgery, the treatment is individualized depending on findings. Some infants are too ill to undergo laparotomy, in which case peritoneal drains are inserted under local anesthesia. Patients with necrosis and perforation require bowel resection. Reanastomosis is rarely advisable and a diverting proximal ostomy and distal mucous fistula are constructed. For infants with extensive involvement of the entire midgut, resection is not performed. These severely ill infants are closed and drained, and a second-look laparotomy is performed 24 hours later, in the hope that viable bowel is present.

Postoperative complications are common, including persistent sepsis, bowel necrosis, disseminated intravascular coagulation, wound infection, and dehiscence. Management includes continued nasogastric decompression, antibiotics, and fluid support. Parenteral nutrition is usually initiated early, and oral feedings are not started until 10–14 days following resolution of the acute disease. These infants require long-term follow-up care, because as many as 20% develop intestinal strictures or short gut syndrome. Recent reviews have shown an increase in survival, up to 80%.

PEDIATRIC TRAUMA

Fundamental Considerations

The incidence of pediatric traumatic injuries surpasses that of all major diseases of children and young adults, making it a very important health care issue. The order and priority of evaluation and treatment is the same as in the adult, however, the anatomic and physiologic differences of this population require special consideration.

Since children are small, the energy resulting from a fall, collision, or projectile is associated with greater force applied per unit area. When applied to a body with less fat and connective tissue, a close proximity of vital organs, and an incompletely calcified, pliable skeleton, multisystem injuries result. Children with multiple injuries require specialized care and can deteriorate rapidly. Therefore, trauma-related injuries are optimally evaluated at a facility capable of handling serious injuries in the pediatric population. The three most common causes of death are airway obstruction, blood loss, and central nervous system (CNS) injury. Therefore, the evaluation and management focuses on these critical issues.

Evaluation & Management

Rapid assessment and stabilization of the airway, breathing, circulation, and disability (CNS/head evaluation) are fundamental in reducing trauma-related morbidity.

A child's airway is very different from that of an adult. The tonsils and tongue are large, the larynx is anterior and high in the neck, and the trachea is short. These anatomic factors result in an easily occluded airway that is difficult to visualize during intubation. The "sniffing" position is used to maintain the airway in a conscious child. If obstruction by the tongue or foreign material occurs, the chin lift or jaw thrust maneuver can be used. For an unconscious child, an oral airway can be gently inserted and the child ventilated with bag and mask. If intubation is required to protect the airway, the orotracheal route is preferred. Should orotracheal intubation prove to be unsuccessful, needle cricothyroidotomy is preferred over tracheostomy. Children should be ventilated at a rate of approximately 20 breaths per minute and infants at 40 breaths per minute, with a tidal volume of 7–10 mL/kg (see Figure 46–3).

The injured child with significant blood loss can present without evidence of hypotension and only mild tachycardia. In fact, hypovolemia in children causes tachycardia and peripheral vasoconstriction before hypotension. Hypotension does not usually occur until approximately one quarter of the blood volume is lost. The care provider must be alert for early shock, which may have subtle signs. Any evidence of tachycardia or hypotension should be evaluated by a surgeon as soon as possible (see Figures 46–1 and 46–2, for appropriate vital signs). Adequate urine output must be maintained; infant 2 mL/kg/h, child 1.5 mL/kg/h, adolescent 1 mL/kg/h (see Figure 46–7 for proper guidelines for resuscitation from hypovolemia).

Head and CNS injuries are common. Survival is related more to the presence of associated injuries than to the head injury itself. Children are particularly susceptible to secondary brain injury as a result of hypotension, hypoxia,

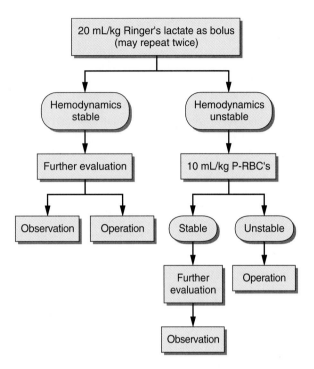

Figure 46–7. Algorithm depicting resuscitation procedure for hypovolemia due to traumatic injury. (Reprinted and modified, with permission, from Tepas JJ et al: Evaluation and management of the injured child. Bull Am Coll Surg 1995;80:36.)

seizures, and hypothermia. In order to optimize cerebral perfusion, adequate restoration of an appropriate circulating blood volume is mandatory, and hypoxia must be avoided. A young child may not develop signs of increasing intracranial pressure, because the cranium can expand via open fontanelles or mobile cranial sutures. Any child with bulging fontanelles or suture diastasis should be considered to have a severe head injury; early neurosurgical evaluation is essential. Children with CNS injuries should be hyperventilated to maintain a Pco_2 of 30 torr.

All children should have a complete neurologic evaluation, with completion of a Glasgow Coma Scale. Children with a decreased level of consciousness or suspected loss of consciousness should undergo a CT of the head, unless other injuries require more urgent care.

The physician must be aware of the battered, abused child syndrome. Children who die within the first year of life from injury frequently do so as the result of child abuse. A thorough history and physical examination is critical to avoid unnecessary injury and death.

Suspect child abuse if: history and degree of physical injury do not correlate; there is a delay between injury and treatment; repeated injury is present; a changing history and inappropriate parental responses are evident. The following physical findings suggest child abuse: perioral injuries; retinal hemorrhages; multiple subdural hematomas; ruptured viscera without history of trauma; old fractures; genitalia injuries; long bone fractures in children under the age of three; and bizarre injuries. It is the responsibility of all health care providers to report child abuse, if suspected, to the appropriate personnel.

Although survival following trauma has improved, it is far from 100%. The key to improvement is prevention. Preventive programs and laws to mandate safety are essential. Mortality is zero if the injury is prevented.

NEOPLASTIC DISEASE

Although significant advances have been made with regard to pediatric cancer, it still remains the second most common cause of death in children under 14 years of age. Survival, however, continues to improve, which is a direct result of the multidisciplinary approach currently used to diagnose and manage childhood tumors. The two most common solid tumors of childhood, after brain tumors, are neuroblastoma and Wilms' tumor, followed by soft tissue sarcomas, teratomas, and hepatic tumors.

WILMS' TUMOR

Diagnosis

Wilms' tumor or nephroblastoma originates in the kidney. These children are usually between 1 and 3 years of age and typically present when parents report palpating an asymptomatic flank mass. Children often complain of abdominal pain and anorexia. Hematuria and hypertension can occur in as many as 15%.

This neoplasm is associated with other congenital anomalies, such as aniridia, hemihypertrophy, cryptorchidism, urinary tract anomalies, abnormal karyotypes, neurofibromatosis, and the Beckwith-Wiedemann syndrome. Preliminary diagnostic studies include ultrasonography followed by CT scan. This neoplasm is located intrarenally (bilateral 5%) and can have intravascular extension. Ultrasonography can confirm the location and determine whether there is intravascular extension. The CT scan allows assessment of the size of the mass, evaluation of the contralateral kidney, and assessment of all pertinent anatomic relationships as well as the presence of direct extension. The lung is the most common site of metastasis.

Management

Surgery is the mainstay of treatment, however, the multidisciplinary approach is crucial for optimizing survival. The initial postoperative treatment is based on the surgical stage. Current staging is as follows:

I. Tumor is limited to kidney, completely resected.
II. Tumor extends beyond the kidney but is completely resected.

III. Residual intra-abdominal tumor remains, including tumor rupture or biopsy, or lymph node involvement.
IV. There is hematogenous metastasis.
V. There is bilateral renal involvement.

The standard operation includes en bloc resection of the tumor, exploration of the abdomen, periortic lymph node sampling, and assessment of the contralateral kidney. Any organs involved with direct extension should be partially resected (liver, adrenal, diaphragm), if possible. If safe en bloc resection is not possible, biopsy only is performed. A reexploration for resection follows several courses of chemotherapy to shrink the tumor.

Postoperative treatment is based on stage and histologic cell type and incorporates chemotherapy and radiation therapy. Overall survival for patients with favorable histology is 90% for all stages. Those children with unfavorable histology and stages II–V have a much poorer prognosis.

NEUROBLASTOMA

Diagnosis

Neuroblastoma is a neoplasm that originates from neural crest cells. It can derive from the adrenal gland(s) or anywhere in the sympathetic nervous system. It is the most common extracranial solid tumor of childhood, occurring once in every 7000–10,000 live births. A majority of these tumors (65%) occur in the adrenal gland or the retroperitoneum. Most children are less than 8 years of age, with half being younger than 2 years. Neuroblastoma can be associated with other conditions, such as Hirschsprung's disease, fetal alcohol syndrome, Beckwith syndrome; children whose mothers took phenylhydantoin for seizures may also be affected. The tumor itself can secrete several vasoactive substances and hormones, leading to unusual presentations.

Symptoms vary according to tumor location and the presence of metastasis. Metastatic spread can involve the liver, lung, skin, bone, and bone marrow. Most children present with complaints of abdominal pain and a mass. Neurologic symptoms can occur from nerve compression, such as Horner's syndrome. Bone metastasis can present with intractable leg pain and periorbital ecchymosis secondary to orbital metastasis. Skin lesions are firm, nontender, and bluish. These patients can also have any number of paraneoplastic syndromes as a result of the secreted hormones and peptides, such as hypertension (secondary to catecholamine secretion), which occurs in 25% of patients.

Diagnosis can be confirmed by various laboratory and radiologic studies. Urine should be sent for various byproducts of catecholamines. A skeletal survey and chest x-ray are helpful in revealing bone and pulmonary metastasis. An abdominal x-ray may show calcifications within the lesion. A CT or MRI scan allows full visualization of the tumor and its possible invasion or metastasis into adja-

cent organs. Biopsy of the bone marrow may reveal neuroblastoma cells.

Management

Unlike other solid tumors, the survival of children with neuroblastoma has not changed over the last few decades. Many children present with evidence of metastatic disease at diagnosis, and complete surgical excision is impossible. Therapy is based on preoperative clinical and operative staging. Although there are many staging classifications, the classic Evans staging is as follows:

I. Tumor is confined to organ of origin.
II. Tumor is not confined and does not cross the midline; regional lymph nodes can be involved.
III. Tumor extends beyond the midline.
IV. There is distant metastasis.
IV-S. The child is less than 1 year of age and the tumor does not cross the midline; remote disease is confined to the liver, bone marrow without bone involvement, or the subcutaneous tissues.

Stage I disease is rare, however, when present, resection alone is often curative. Stage II disease can usually be completely resected, especially if the tumor has favorable histology. Stages III and IV require aggressive chemotherapy and radiotherapy; some protocols use bone marrow transplantation. Operative therapy in these later stages permits tumor debulking and lymph node evaluation. Treatment for stage IV-S disease is controversial, because in some children the tumor resolves without treatment.

The prognosis has remained poor despite advances in antineoplastic therapy. The key elements that influence survival are age at diagnosis and stage of disease. Those children diagnosed at less than 1 year of age have a markedly improved prognosis. The overall survival is dismal at 44%.

FETAL INTERVENTIONS

Advances in prenatal ultrasonography have permitted the early diagnosis of many congenital fetal abnormalities. Many of these anomalies are theoretically amenable to surgical repair, however, until recently, repair could not occur until the infant was delivered. Research on animal models has led to the realization that fetal surgical intervention is not only possible, but, in certain anomalies, is the most logical alternative. During the last decade in utero surgery for a number of fetal anomalies, including congenital hydronephrosis, saccrococcygeal teratoma, cystic adenomatoid malformation, congenital diaphragmatic hernia, chylothorax, and simple types of congenital heart disease has become a reality (Figure 46–8).

Continued research and success in the treatment of the unborn surgical patient will certainly increase the survival for certain infants with previously lethal anomalies.

A

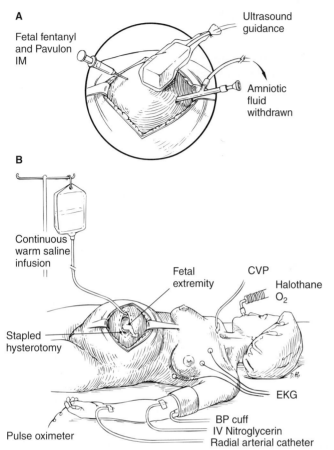

Fetal fentanyl and Pavulon IM

Ultrasound guidance

Amniotic fluid withdrawn

B

Continuous warm saline infusion

Stapled hysterotomy

Fetal extremity

CVP

Halothane O₂

Pulse oximeter

BP cuff

IV Nitroglycerin

Radial arterial catheter

EKG

Figure 46–8. Diagram depicting positioning and monitoring of mother during fetal surgery. **A:** The uterus is exposed via a laparotomy, and the placenta is localized using ultrasonography. A portion of blood and amniotic fluid is withdrawn in order to make the uterus softer. **B:** Careful positioning is important in order to avoid compression of the vena cava by the gravid uterus. Hysterotomy is made away from the placenta, so only the pertinent fetal anatomy is exposed. Monitoring may include a radial arterial line and a subclavian venous catheter. (Reprinted and modified, with permission, from Adzick NS, Harrison MR: The unborn surgical patient. Curr Probl Surg 1994;31:1.)

SUGGESTED READING

Adzick NS, Harrison MR: The unborn surgical patient. Curr Probl Surg 1994;31:1.

Peña A: *Surgical Management of Anorectal Anomalies.* Springer-Verlag, 1990.

Grosfeld JL: Pediatric surgery. In: Sabiston D (editor): *Textbook of Surgery*, 14th ed. Saunders, 1991.

Guzzetta PC et al: Pediatric surgery. In: Schwartz S et al (editors): *Principles of Surgery*, 6th ed. McGraw Hill, 1994.

Hays DM (editor): *Pediatric Surgical Oncology.* Grune & Stratton, 1986.

Smith S: Physiology of the pediatric patient. In: Simmons RL, Steed DL (editors): *Basic Science Review for Surgeons.* Saunders, 1992.

Welch KW et al (editors): *Pediatric Surgery*, 5th ed. Year-Book Medical Publishers, 1991.

Index

NOTE: Page numbers in bold face type indicate a major discussion. A *t* following a page number indicates tabular material and an *i* following a page number indicates an illustration. Drugs are listed under their generic names. When a drug trade name is listed, the reader is referred to the generic name.